Practical Guidelines on Fluid Therapy

THIRD EDITION

Dr. Sanjay Pandya

M.D. (Medicine), D.N.B. (Nephrology)
Consulting Nephrologist
Rajkot, Gujarat, INDIA

First Edition 2002

Second Edition 2005

Third Edition 2024

Author and Publisher:
Dr. Sanjay Pandya
Rajkot - 360002 (Gujarat, INDIA)
E-mail: fluidtherapy2024@gmail.com

ISBN: 978-93-6128-363-5

ISBN (eBook): 978-93-6128-860-9

NOTICE

Medicine is an ever-changing science. Every effort has been made to ensure that the information provided in this book is accurate and in accord with the standards accepted at the time of publication. However, in view of the possibility of human error or changes in medical sciences, neither the author nor the publisher will be held responsible for any inadvertent errors.

The information in this book is meant to supplement, not replace, proper training and education in the field of medicine. The author and publisher expressly disclaim responsibility for any adverse effects arising from the use or application of the information contained in this book.

Practical Guidelines on Fluid Therapy and its cover design are trademarks of Dr. Sanjay Pandya.

Dedicated to

To my beloved parents,

Who gifted me the art of learning, teaching, and writing.

and my family,

Whose constant encouragement and support made this task possible.

With all my love and gratitude!

Table of Contents

Table of Contents

Table of Contents

Preface

To the Third Edition

I am delighted to introduce the third edition of "Practical Guidelines in Fluid Therapy," a comprehensive compendium on fluid, electrolyte, and acid-base disorders.

The journey from the first edition to the third has been incredible, marked by unwavering support and appreciation from clinicians and postgraduate students alike. This overwhelming response has not only fueled my passion for this subject but also motivated me to bring you the third edition of this unique and comprehensive book on fluid, electrolyte, and acid-base disorders.

As we embark on this latest edition, our commitment to providing up-to-date, practice-oriented information remains steadfast. The core theme of this book, to offer practical insights into these crucial clinical aspects, remains unchanged.

OUTSTANDING FEATURES

This monogram provides complex concepts in simple, digestible language, addressing the common clinical challenges clinicians face in prescribing fluid therapy in their day-to-day practice. It provides quick and efficient guidelines tailored to meet the needs of clinicians in emergency patient care. Each chapter begins with an outline to offer a quick overview and enhanced clarity.

Separate chapters dedicated to commercially available IV fluids and managing fluid, electrolyte, and acid-base disorders in medical, surgical, and pediatric patients offer valuable insights to meet diverse clinical requirements. Our commitment to reader-friendliness continues, with evidence-based information presented through tables, charts, and figures. Recognizing the critical role of Parenteral Nutrition (PN) in life-saving therapy, practical guidance on its indications, requirements, and monitoring in significant clinical disorders is included.

NEW TO THIS EDITION

To provide comprehensive information in a single source, this new edition includes sections on parenteral additives, fluid replacement strategies (including planning and prescribing fluid therapy, maintenance fluid therapy, resuscitation fluids, fluid therapy in elderly patients), fluid therapy in obstetrics, and hemodynamic monitoring. Our emphasis remains on providing clear, practical, and practice-based information on management strategies.

This book is an indispensable companion for clinicians managing acutely ill patients. This book caters to the needs of clinicians across various specialties, including intensivists, physicians, emergency physicians, anesthesiologists, internists, surgeons, pediatricians, obstetricians, and other specialists who deal with critical as well as hospitalized patients.

I trust this edition will meet your expectations, and we welcome any suggestions you may have to make this resource even more useful; please feel free to email us with your feedback, and we are thankful for your input.

Dr. Sanjay Pandya

Acknowledgments

I would like to thank all without whose support this book would not have been possible.

- I take this opportunity to express my heartfelt gratitude to all my teachers, colleagues, and postgraduate students, who have been a constant source of inspiration, encouragement, and unwavering support.

- My most profound appreciation goes to my esteemed teachers, Prof. V. H. Yagnik, Prof. P. S. Kulkarni, Prof. Y. K. Oza, and Prof. B. K. Shah, whose inspiration and encouragement led me to embark on this project, which initially was not my idea to write a book.

- I am immensely grateful to Prof. Dr. Kumud Mehta, the late Prof. Sugandha Doshi, Prof. Dr. Bakul Javadekar, Dr. Sadanand Kulkarni, Dr. Abhay Gaglani, and Dr. Sishir Gang for their invaluable assistance, feedback, suggestions, and support during the preparation of the previous editions of this book.

- I extend my heartfelt thanks to my doctor friends from various specialties for their valuable contributions, reviews, and suggestions in their respective fields during the preparation of this edition, including Intensivist Dr. Rajesh Mishra, Dr. Naman Shastri, and Dr. Navubha Sodha; Pediatrician Dr. Yagnesh Popat; Gynecologists Dr. Jigna Ganatra and Dr. Dipal Solanki; Nephrologist Dr. Rajen Mathur; Anesthetist Dr. Dipti Mehta; Plastic Surgeon Dr. Hitesh Dhruv; and Physicians Dr. Vijay Maniyar and Dr. Miren Patel.

- I would like to express my gratitude to my hospital doctor and staff team for their continuous support in efficiently managing my clinical responsibilities, allowing me more time for book preparation. I would also like to extend my appreciation to my PA, Mr. Vishal Aadthakkar, who played an invaluable role in assisting me throughout this journey, providing various forms of logistic academic support, including book formatting.

- I take this opportunity to express my gratitude to Hemant Bhalani and Himanshu Bhalani of Bhalani Medical Book House for their unwavering guidance and suggestions and, most importantly, for their widespread distribution of this book.

- Finally, I am deeply grateful to my wife, Priti, for her unwavering support and selfless sacrifices, which allowed me to dedicate years to completing this monumental work. Her contributions were absolutely crucial to the successful culmination of this project. I also want to thank my children, Isha and Rohan, for their encouragement and understanding, which allowed me to devote the necessary time to this book. Additionally, my loyal companion, Leo, my Golden Retriever, who has been by my side during countless work hours, consistently boosted my enthusiasm and morale.

About the Author

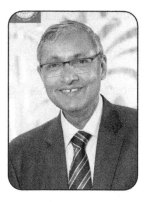

Dr. Sanjay Pandya
M.D. (Medicine), D.N.B. (Nephrology)

- Dr. Sanjay Pandya is a senior nephrologist based in Rajkot, Gujarat, India. He earned his Doctor of Medicine (Internal Medicine) degree from M. P. Shah Medical College, Jamnagar, Gujarat 1986. He subsequently completed his DNB in Nephrology at the Institute of Kidney Diseases and Research Center, Ahmedabad, in 1989. Since 1990, Dr. Pandya has been dedicated to practicing as a nephrologist in Rajkot, Gujarat.

- Driven by his passion for education, Dr. Pandya authored and published the pioneering book titled "Practical Guidelines on Fluid Therapy," which marked the first Indian publication on fluid, electrolytes, and acid-base disorders. Dr. Pandya is widely recognized as a proficient educator on this subject.

- Over the course of two decades, Dr. Pandya's book has garnered remarkable acclaim and tremendous success. His unwavering commitment continues to provide comprehensive, up-to-date, and evidence-based practical information on fluid therapy and related topics. To fulfill this dream, the latest fully revised and rewritten third edition (2024) has been prepared to benefit medical professionals and students alike.

- Beyond his significant contributions to educating medical professionals, he has made an outstanding global impact by educating laypeople about kidney diseases.

- Dr. Pandya is the visionary founder and Chief Mentor of the Kidney Education Foundation, leading a global team of over 100 nephrologists in disseminating crucial information on kidney disease prevention and care. His pioneering initiative, the Kidney Education website (www.KidneyEducation.com), available in 40 languages, provides easily understandable guidance on preventing and managing common kidney diseases through free access to a 200-page book titled 'Save Your Kidneys.' With over 100 million hits and over 1 million PDF downloads, this platform, free of external funding, has made valuable information accessible worldwide.

- Recognized and endorsed by over 20 prominent global kidney organizations and renowned nephrologists, the work of the global team has earned accolades from prestigious institutions such as the American Society of Nephrology, the International Society of Nephrology, and the European Renal Association. Notably, the Kidney Education Website holds the world record for the 'eBook in the highest number of languages'.

- Dr. Pandya's remarkable educational contributions to medical professionals and his philanthropic endeavors in preventing and caring for kidney diseases, alongside his global team, serve as an exemplary and inspiring model for young medical professionals worldwide.

Foreword

To the First Edition

Even though Indian doctors are good clinicians they need sound knowledge of fluid, electrolyte and acid-base disorders for optimal management of critical patients. It thus gives me great pleasure to introduce the book "Practical Guidelines on Fluid Therapy" - the only book of its kind from an Indian author.

Understanding and managing fluid, electrolyte and acid-base disorders has been difficult for most doctors. It is true even for Indian doctors because it is poorly emphasized in medical schools and partly due to lack of good laboratory support in many hospitals including teaching institutions.

Most books on this subject discuss basic physiology and principles of managing different disorders. This book, in addition, provides practical guidelines for each clinical situation. This is made simpler by providing guidelines in the form of questions and answers. Every clinical situation that one can conceive has been taken into consideration, including disorders commonly seen in children and adults with medical and surgical problems. It can thus be of use to pediatricians, physicians and surgeons. Most important is the fact that it provides detailed information about intravenous fluid preparations available in our country.

This book by Dr. Sanjay Pandya will undoubtedly be a very useful text for all residents and practising doctors in day-to-day management of patients.

Dr. Bharat V. Shah
M.D. (Medicine), D.N.B. (Nephrology)
Consultant Nephrologist
Global Hospital,
Mumbai, India

Foreword

To the Second Edition

There have been many developments at the sub-cellular level on the mechanisms operating in maintaining the normal homeostasis. Our commitment to learn by understanding the various compartments of the body constituted by fluid, electrolytes, acids and bases is reinforced by old and new information. A teaching based on sound physiology, biochemistry, anatomy and molecular biology pose numerous challenges.

The second edition of "Practical Guidelines on Fluid Therapy" is written with emphasis on understanding basic pathophysiologic approach to the fluid and the electrolyte balance we encounter in our day-to-day practice. The presentation of the contents is aimed at medical students, doctors in postgraduate training in medicine, surgery, obstetrics, gynecology, anesthesia, pediatrics and neurosciences. The chapters in the book are compiled for a quick reference for general practitioners as well as practicing consultants. The emphasis on instructive case discussions dealing with "Acid-Base Disorders" has been problem based to reinforce the clinical message. The concepts of fluid and electrolyte balance are a simplified set of guidelines which can be easily practiced in the day-to-day management of the patients. Additional information is also provided in tables so as not to distract the reader and disrupt the flow of thought.

The second edition of the practical guidelines on fluid therapy by Dr. Sanjay Pandya will be a very useful hand book for the medical profession.

Dr. Georgi Abraham
MBBS, MD, FRCP (UK)
MGM Healthcare, Indian Institute of Technology Madras, Tanker Foundation, Kerala Kidney Research Foundation, Chennai, India

Part 1

Physiology

1 | Basic Physiology

INTRODUCTION

Water is the most abundant component of the body. Body fluid is essential for the life as it helps in transport of nutrients, electrolytes, gases, and wastes and also helps to maintain body temperature and cell shape. An understanding of the physiology of body fluids is essential to plan appropriate management of patients' fluid and electrolyte disorders. In this chapter, we will discuss the body's fluid compartments (i.e., their location, size, and composition), normal water balance, electrolytes, and their distribution, and finally, the units of measurement.

TOTAL BODY WATER

The total body water (TBW) content of a person varies mainly with body weight, but it also varies with age, sex,

and fat content [1]. Total body water content is about 60% of body weight in a young adult male and about 50% in a young adult female [2]. Because the water content of adipose tissue is relatively low, an obese person will have proportionately less body water as compared to a lean person. The highest percentage of TBW is found in newborns (as high as 80%), which declines with age. The average total body water in different groups is shown in Table 1.1. The measurement of TBW can be performed via indicator dilution techniques using Deuterium oxide ($2H_2O$), tritium oxide ($3H_2O$), oxygen-18 labelled water, or more recently via bioelectrical impedance analysis [3].

Distribution of body fluid

Total body water is commonly divided into two volumes: the intracellular fluid

Age	Adult male	Adult female	Elderly	Adult obese	Infant	Neonate
Total body water (% of body weight)	60%	50%	50%	50%	70%	80%

Table 1.1 Average total body water as a percentage of body weight

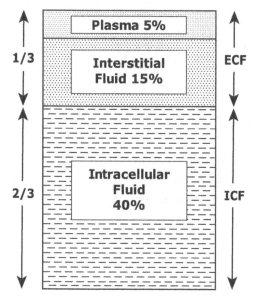

Figure 1.1 Body fluid compartments.

(ICF) volume and the extracellular fluid (ECF) volume (Figure 1.1) [4].

Intracellular fluid

ICF is defined as all the body water within cells. The ICF is normally two third of total body water and 40% of total body weight. Water balance regulates the ICF volume.

Extracellular fluid

ECF is defined as all body water outside the cells - within the tissue spaces (interstitial fluid), the blood vessels (intravascular fluid or plasma), and the lymphatic vessels (lymph). The ECF is normally one third of total body water and 20% of total body weight. As shown in Figure 1.1, ECF is subdivided into extravascular (interstitial) fluid (3/4th of

ECF or 15% of total body weight) and plasma or intravascular volume (1/4th of ECF, 1/12 total body water or 5% of total body weight). There is another small compartment of ECF that is referred to as transcellular fluid. This compartment includes cerebrospinal fluid and fluid in the synovial, peritoneal, pericardial, and intraocular spaces. Sodium balance regulates the ECF volume.

For better understanding, the distribution of fluid volume in a 70 kg man is summarized in Table 1.2.

BODY FLUID AND ELECTROLYTES MOVEMENT

The movement of water and electrolytes between ICF and ECF compartments is regulated to stabilize their distribution and the composition of body fluids. The cell membranes that separate fluid compartments are selectively permeable. Water passes freely and readily through cell membranes in response to changes in solute concentration; therefore, the osmolalities in all compartments are equal. Two major determinants of water and electrolyte movements from one compartment to another are hydrostatic pressure and oncotic pressure [5]. Major water retaining solutes in ECF, ICF, and intravascular compartments are sodium, potassium, and plasma protein, respectively.

Unlike water, solutes cannot pass freely through cell membranes even though there is a significant difference in solute concentration between ICF and ECF. The movement of solutes occurs

Table 1.2 Distribution of fluid volume in body compartments					
Fluid type	**Total**	**ICF**	**ECF**	**Interstitial**	**Plasma**
% of body weight	60%	40%	20%	15%	5%
Volume for 70 kg weight	42.0 L	28.0 L	14.0 L	10.5 L	3.5 L

through active and passive transport mechanisms. Active transport by sodium-potassium pumps (Na$^+$-K$^+$-ATPase) is the major force maintaining the difference in cation concentration between the ICF and ECF [2]. Sodium and potassium are compartmentalized into extracellular and intracellular spaces, respectively, by sodium-potassium pumps present in all cell membranes.

NORMAL WATER BALANCE

A healthy adult person consumes an average of 2000 ml of water per day. Fluid intake and output are balanced during steady-state conditions as summarized in Figure 1.2.

Daily water intake

Major sources of water intake are oral intake in the form of liquids (drinking water or beverages), water in food, and water synthesized in the body by oxidation. Thirst primarily regulates water intake. The loss of water increases osmotic pressure in the extracellular fluid, stimulating osmoreceptors in the brain's hypothalamus thirst center, which, in turn, triggers a sensation of thirst, prompting individuals to drink. Conversely, drinking and the resulting stomach distension inhibit the thirst mechanism.

Daily water loss

Routes of water loss are kidneys, feces, sweat (sensible perspiration), evaporation of water from the skin (insensible perspiration), and lungs during breathing. The kidney plays a major role in water balance. By regulating volume of urine, kidneys adjust water output from the body.

Oral or intravenous (IV) fluid intake and urine output are important measurable parameters of body fluid

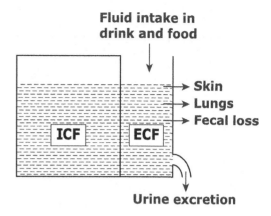

Figure 1.2 Daily water intake and loss in the body.

balance. While calculating the daily fluid requirement of the body, it is important to know and consider insensible fluid input and loss.

Insensible fluid input = 300 ml water due to oxidation.

Insensible fluid loss = 1000 ml (500 ml through the skin, 400 ml through the lung, and 100 ml through stool)

Normal daily insensible fluid loss = fluid loss − fluid input = 1000 − 300 ml = 700 ml

Water loss is increased during exercise, excessive sweating, fever, burns, and surgery. This basic information is necessary to determine daily fluid requirements for patients receiving IV fluids. The daily fluid requirement for a normal person is calculated by adding together the amount of fluid lost in urine and insensible losses. In a normal person, the insensible daily loss is about 700 ml. So, daily fluid requirement = urine output + 700 ml.

DISTRIBUTION OF ELECTROLYTES

The normal electrolyte compositions of each fluid compartment differ markedly, as summarized in Tables 1.3 and 1.4.

Table 1.3 The electrolyte concentration of body fluids		
Electrolytes	**ECF (mEq/L)**	**ICF (mEq/L)**
Sodium	142.00	10.00
Potassium	4.30	150.00
Chloride	104.00	2.00
Bicarbonate	24.00	6.00
Calcium	5.00	0.01
Magnesium	3.00	40.00
Phosphate and sulphate	8.00	15.00

Table 1.4 Major ions in ECF and ICF		
	ECF	**ICF**
Major cation	Sodium	Potassium and magnesium
Major anion	Chloride and bicarbonate	Phosphate, sulphate and protein

For example, the ECF compartment contains a high concentration of sodium, chloride, and bicarbonate but only a small quantity of potassium. In contrast, the ICF compartment contains a high concentration of potassium, magnesium, phosphate, sulfate, and proteins. Furthermore, as sodium is confined chiefly to the ECF compartment, sodium-containing fluids are distributed throughout the ECF. As a result, sodium-containing fluids expand the volume of both the interstitial and intravascular spaces (the interstitial space expansion is approximately three times as much as the plasma).

UNITS OF MEASUREMENTS

It is important to understand the basic terminology used to measure the concentration and composition of body fluids and their interrelationship.

Ions: An ion is an atom or group of atoms with an electric charge. Ions are divided into anions and cations as shown in Figure 1.3.

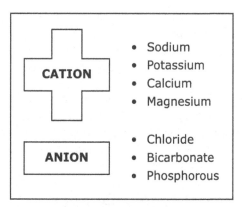

- Sodium
- Potassium
- Calcium
- Magnesium

- Chloride
- Bicarbonate
- Phosphorous

Figure 1.3 Major Cations and Anions.

Anion: When an ion has a negative electric charge, it is called an anion (i.e., Cl^-, HCO_3^-, phosphate).

Cation: When an ion has a positive electric charge, it is called a cation (i.e., Na^+, K^+, Mg^{2+}).

If cation and anion are confusing, here is a simple method to remember.

Anion: **"n"** - negative charge

Cation: **"t"** - + positive charge

Different ways by which solute concentrations can be measured are milligram per decilitre (mg/dL), milliequivalent per liter (mEq/L), or milliosmoles per liter or kg (mOsmol/L or mOsmol/kg).

Moles and millimoles

The unit millimole (mmol) is used in practice instead of mole (mol) for convenience as it is smaller and more practical to handle in medical and scientific settings.

$$6.022 \times 10^{23}$$

A mole represents a specific number of particles. One mole of any non-dissociable substance contains approximately 6.022×10^{23} particles. To clarify with an example, consider salt (NaCl). It contains an equal number of atoms: one sodium (Na^+) atom for

Table 1.5 Atomic and molecular weights of important substances		
Substances	**Symbol or formula**	**Atomic or molecular weight**
Calcium	Ca^{2+}	40.1
Carbon	C	12.0
Chloride ion	Cl^-	35.5
Hydrogen ion	H^+	1.0
Magnesium ion	Mg^{2+}	24.3
Oxygen	O	16.0
Phosphorus	P	31.0
Potassium ion	K^+	39.1
Sodium ion	Na^+	23.0
Ammonium	NH_4^+	18.0
Bicarbonate ion	HCO_3^-	61.0
Phosphate ion	PO_4^{3-}	95.0
Water	H_2O	18.0

every chloride (Cl^-) atom, even though they have different atomic weights, with 23 mg for Na^+ and 35.5 mg for Cl^-. If we compare one dozen mangoes to one dozen bananas, they represent the same quantity of fruit, but their weights differ.

Mole: One mole (mol) of any substance is defined as the atomic or molecular weight of that substance in gm.

Similarly, one millimole (mmol) is equals to one-thousandth of a mole or the molecular (or atomic) weight in milligrams.

So to determine the amount of any substance in one mole, we need to know the atomic (molecular) weight of that substance (Table 1.5).

The atomic weight of Na^+ is 23. Thus, 23 mg of Na^+ represents 1 mmol. Therefore, 23 mg of Na^+ in 1 liter of water results in a Na^+ concentration of one mmol/L.

Equivalent and milliequivalent

The equivalent is a relative term; it refers to a mole of ionic charges.

Equivalent: The equivalent weight of an element is its atomic weight in gm multiplied by its valence.

For ions that carry a single charged mole equals an equivalent (i.e., Na^+, K^+, Cl^-, H^+). But if the ion carries a charge that is greater than one, numbers are no longer equal. So, for example, one mole of calcium ion (Ca^{2+}) equals two equivalents.

So, Equivalents = Moles × Valence

A comparison of the normal value of serum electrolytes concentration in mmol/L and mEq/L is shown in Table 1.6.

Molecules must be quantified in moles (e.g., a mole of glucose) because they carry no charge. However, in practice, they are usually measured in mg or gm because of their simplicity and convenience. The following formula can be used to convert mg/dL to mmol/L.

Ions can be quantified as either moles or equivalents.

$$mmol/L = \frac{mg/dL \times 10}{Atomic\ Weight}$$

Table 1.6 Normal plasma electrolyte concentrations		
Electrolyte	**mmol/L**	**mEq/L**
Cations		
Sodium	136 to 145	136 to 145
Potassium	3.5 to 5.0	3.5 to 5.0
Calcium total*	2.2 to 2.6	4.5 to 5.6
Ionized*	1.05 to 1.3	2.2 to 2.6
Magnesium*	0.70 to 0.85	1.4 to 1.7
Anions		
Chloride	96 to 106	96 to 106
Bicarbonate	22 to 26	22 to 26
*Value in mg/dL: The normal values for total calcium and ionized calcium are 8.5-10.5 mg/dL and 4.3-5.3 mg/dL, respectively. The normal value of magnesium is 1.7–2.1 mg/dL.		

Why are the terms "mmol" or "mEq" used instead of "moles" or "equivalents"?

In routine practice, we prefer using "mmol" (millimoles) or "mEq" (milli-equivalents) to express concentrations rather than "moles" or "equivalents." This preference arises from the extremely low concentrations of most molecules and ions in serum.

In day-to-day practice, we use a millimeter, which is 1/1000 of the meter. Similarly, "mmol" or "mEq" represents 1/1000 of a mole or equivalent. For example, consider the serum potassium value, which might be expressed as 0.004 moles or equivalents per liter. However, converting it to 4 mmol/L or mEq/L provides a more practical, straightforward, and convenient value for everyday use in clinical practice.

The relationship between mEq and mg

Formula to convert mg/dL to mEq/L: To convert from milligrams per deciliter (mg/dL) to milliequivalents per liter (mEq/L), you can use the following formula:

$$mEq/L = \frac{mg/dL \times 10 \times Valence}{Mol.\ Weight}$$

Example: If 1 gm of salt (NaCl) is added to 1 liter of water, what will be its concentration in mEq/L?

NaCl 1 gm/L = 1,000 mg/L = 100 mg/dL valence of NaCl = 1 molecular weight = 58.5 (Na$^+$ mol. wt. 23 and Cl$^-$ mol. wt. 35.5).

$$mEq/L = \frac{100 \times 10 \times 1}{58.5} = 17.1$$

1 gm NaCl/L = 17.1 mEq/L 1 gm of NaCl contains 17.1 mEq sodium and 17.1 mEq chloride, or the Na$^+$ concentration of NaCl = 17.1 mEq/gm.

Formula to convert mEq/L to mg/dL: To convert mEq/L to mg/dL, you can use the following formula:

$$mg/dL = \frac{mEq/L \times Mol.\ Weight}{10 \times Valence}$$

Example: If 1 liter of NaCl solution contains 154 mEq of NaCl, what is the amount of NaCl in mg/dL?

NaCl mEq/L = 154

Molecular Weight = 58.5 (Na$^+$ mol. wt. 23 and Cl$^-$ mol. wt. 35.5)

Valence = 1

$$So,\ mg/dL = \frac{154 \times 58.5}{10 \times 1} = 900.9$$

So, in a 1-liter solution of NaCl with 154 mEq of NaCl, there is 9009 mg/L of NaCl salt.

When 9009 is divided by 154, the result is 58.5.

Therefore, 100 ml of NaCl solution containing 1 mEq of NaCl has 58.5 mg of salt.

These values, derived from both equations (Na$^+$ concentration is 17.1 mEq/gm of NaCl, and 1 mEq contains 58.5 mg NaCl), are useful for the calculation and interchangeability of routinely used substances.

Conversion factors helpful in day-to-day practice are summarized in Table 1.7.

Examples of conversion

Find out K$^+$ concentration in mEq in 10 ml ampoule of 15% potassium chloride (KCl)

10 ml of 15% KCl = 1.5 gm KCl/ampoule

1 gm of KCl contains 13 mEq of K$^+$ (as per Table 1.7).

So, 1.5 gm KCl = 1.5 × 13 = 19.5 mEq of K$^+$.

Answer: 10 ml amp. of 15% KCl contains 19.5 mEq of potassium.

Find out Na$^+$ concentration in mEq in a 25 ml ampoule of 7.5% sodium bicarbonate (NaHCO$_3$)

25 ml of 7.5% NaHCO$_3$ = 1.86 gm of NaHCO$_3$ per ampoule

Table 1.7 Conversion between mEq and mg		
Salt	mEq cation or anion/ gm of salt	mg of salt/ mEq
Sodium chloride	17	58
Potassium chloride	13	75
Sodium bicarbonate	12	84
Calcium gluconate	4	224
Calcium chloride	14	73
Magnesium sulfate	8	123

1 gm of $NaHCO_3$ contains 12 mEq of Na^+ (as per Table 1.7).

So, 1.86 gm of $NaHCO_3$ = 1.86 × 12 = 22.3 mEq of Na^+.

Answer: A 25 ml ampoule of 7.5% $NaHCO_3$ contains 22.3 mEq of Na^+.

Osmotic pressure and osmolality

Osmotic pressure

Osmotic pressure determines the distribution of water among the different fluid compartments, particularly between the ECF and ICF.

The osmotic pressure generated by a solution is proportional to the number of particles per unit volume of solvent, not to the type, valence, or weight of the particles. To generate osmotic pressure, the solute must be unable to cross the cell membrane.

Osmole (Osm)

It is the unit of measurement of osmotic pressure. One osmole is defined as 1 gm molecular weight (1 mol) of any nondissociable substance (such as glucose) and contains 6.022×10^{23} particles.

Milliosmoles (mOsm)

mOsm is 1/1000 of an osmole. So in relatively diluted fluids in the body,

the osmotic pressure is measured in milliosmole per kg of water (mOsm/kg).

An osmole (or mOsm) of a substance, such as glucose which does not dissociate into ions, is the same as a mole (or mmol). However, a mole of salts such as sodium chloride, which dissociates almost completely into sodium and chloride ions, equals 2 osmoles.

Osmolality and osmolarity

These laboratory values reflect the relationship between solute and solvent.

Osmolality

The osmolality of a solution is determined by the amount of solute dissolved in a solvent (i.e., water) measured in weight (kg).

If a solute is dissolved in 1 kg of water (solvent), the concentration of the solution is called osmolality and is expressed as mOsm/kg of the water solvent.

When osmolality is high, the solution is more concentrated, and when osmolality is low solution is diluted.

Osmolarity

The osmolarity of a solution is determined by the amount of solute dissolved in a solvent (i.e., water) measured in volume (liter).

If a solute is dissolved in 1 litre of water (solvent), the concentration of solution is called osmolarity and is expressed as mOsm/L.

Remember

When the solvent is measured in lite**r - "r"** - Osmolarity

and when the solvent is measured in Kilogram - **"l"** - Osmolality

As the temperature can affect the volume of solvent and solute in the solution, it can affect the value of the solution's osmolarity.

So osmolality (mOsm/kg), determined by the solvent's weight, is more accurate than osmolarity. However, the difference between these two values is negligible, and osmolarity is easier to measure, so it is used more commonly.

The osmolality of any solution is measured by measurement of its freezing point.

Plasma osmolality

Plasma osmolality is primarily determined largely by sodium salts, with a lesser contribution from ions, glucose, and urea. Normal plasma osmolality is 285 (275–295) mOsm/kg.

Plasma Osmolality

$$= 2 \times Na^+ + \frac{Glucose\ (mg/dL)}{18} + \frac{BUN\ (mg/dL)}{2.8}$$

Effective osmolality

Those solutes determine the effective osmolality of the extracellular fluid (ECF), which does not freely permeate the cell membrane and act to hold water within the ECF.

Lipid-soluble solutes like urea, which can pass through cell membranes, do not affect the difference in osmotic pressure between the ECF and ICF. So, urea which contributes to the calculation of plasma osmolality does not contribute to effective osmolality. Therefore, total osmolality and effective osmolality are different.

Effective Osmolality (mOsm / kg)

$$= 2 \times Na^+\ (mEq/L) + \frac{Glucose\ (mg/dL)}{18}$$

Under normal circumstances, glucose accounts for only 5 mOsm/kg in effective osmolality. So normally, plasma sodium concentration is the determinant and reflector of the plasma osmolality.

REFERENCES

1. Bradbury MW. Physiology of body fluids and electrolytes. British Journal of Anaesthesia. 1973;45(9):937–944.

2. Bhave G, Neilson EG. Body fluid dynamics: back to the future. J Am Soc Nephrol. 2011;22(12):2166–81.

3. Armstrong LE. Hydration assessment techniques. Nutr Rev. 2005;63(6 Pt 2):S40–54.

4. Hall JE. Guyton and Hall Textbook of Medical Physiology. 2016; 13th edition, Chapter 25.

5. Shier D, Jackie BJ, Lewis R. Hole's Human Anatomy & Physiology. 2017; 11th edition, Chapter 21.

Part 2

Basics of Intravenous Fluids and Solutions

2 | Overview of Intravenous Fluids

INTRODUCTION

A significant number of hospitalized patients across various medical specialties require intravenous (IV) fluid therapy. Understanding the fundamental principles is crucial for the safe and effective administration of IV fluids [1]. Inadequate fluid management can exacerbate patient outcomes and prolong hospital stays [2].

To prescribe appropriate fluid therapy, it is essential to consider the following:

- The underlying cause of fluid deficit and the type of electrolyte imbalance present.
- Coexisting medical conditions (e.g., diabetes, hypertension, ischemic heart disease, renal or hepatic disorders.).
- Clinical status, including factors like age, hydration level, vital signs, urine output, etc.

To ensure rational and adequate fluid therapy, it is imperative to address the following questions:

- When is IV fluid administration appropriate, and when should it be avoided?
- Which type of fluid should be infused, and why?
- How much fluid should be administered, and what is the calculation method?
- At what rate should IV fluid be infused, and how is the drop rate calculated?
- What are the contraindications for various types of IV fluids, and what are the reasons behind them?
- How do you select IV fluids to correct electrolyte imbalances?
- When and how should specific fluids be used?

Following a comprehensive evaluation, the necessary fluid therapy is planned and prescribed.

BASIC PRINCIPLES OF FLUID THERAPY

As a principle, the oral route is always preferred over the IV route. But IV fluid

Table 2.1 Composition of common IV solutions

	Dext.*	Calories	Na+	K+	Cl-	Acet.	Lact.	NH4	Ca2+	Mg2+	HPO4	Gluc.	Citr.	Osm.	SID
	gm/L	kcals/L	mEq/L	mEq/L	mEq/L	mEq/L	mEq/L	mEq/L	mEq/L	mEq/L	mEq/L	mEq/L	mEq/L	mOsm/L	mEq/L
5% dextrose	50	170	-	-	-	-	-	-	-	-	-	-	-	252	0
10% dextrose	100	340	-	-	-	-	-	-	-	-	-	-	-	505	0
0.45% saline	-	-	77	-	77	-	-	-	-	-	-	-	-	154	0
D5W, 0.45% saline	50	170	77	-	77	-	-	-	-	-	-	-	-	406	0
Normal (0.9%) saline	-	-	154	-	154	-	-	-	-	-	-	-	-	308	0
Dextrose saline	50	170	154	-	154	-	-	-	-	-	-	-	-	560	0
Ringer's lactate	-	-	130	4.0	109	-	28	-	3.0	-	-	-	-	273	28
Ringer's acetate	-	-	130	5.0	112	27	-	-	3.0	2.0	-	-	-	276	27
PlasmaLyte	-	-	140	5.0	98	27	-	-	-	3.0	-	23	-	295	50
Sterofundin	-	-	145	4.0	127	24	-	-	5.0	2.0	-	-	-	309	29
Isolyte-G	50	170	63	17	150	-	-	70	-	-	-	-	-	578	NA
Isolyte-M	50	170	37	35	37	20	-	-	-	-	15	-	-	415	NA
Isolyte-P	50	170	25	20	24	23	-	-	-	3.0	3.0	-	-	348	NA
Isolyte-E	50	170	140	10	103	47	-	-	5.0	3.0	-	-	8.0	595	57
Isolyte-S	-	-	141	5.0	98	27	-	-	5.0	3.0	1.0	23	-	295	NA

Dext.: Dextrose

Na+: Sodium

K+: Potassium

Cl-: Chloride

Acet.: Acetate

Lact.: Lactate

NH4: Ammonium

Ca2+: Calcium

Mg2+: Magnesium

HPO4: Phosphate

Citr.: Citrate

Osm.: Osmolality

SID: Strong ion difference

Gluc.: Gluconate

*Dextrose concentration is in gms/L

therapy has great importance and is life-saving in various clinical problems.

The basic principles of IV fluid therapy are summarized.

Indications

Fluid therapy is widely used for resuscitation, for proving the maintenance need of fluids, replacing and restoring fluids and electrolytes deficits, as a drug carrier, and for nutrition [3]. The most common and important indications for fluid administration includes:

1. For resuscitation in moderate to severe dehydration and shock, where urgent and rapid fluid replacement is needed.

2. To provide maintenance need in conditions when oral intake is not possible or is insufficient (i.e., coma, anesthesia, surgery).

3. To restore or replace fluid losses (e.g., severe vomiting, diarrhea, fever, burns, etc.), third space fluid loss (e.g., sepsis, burns, ascites, pancreatitis, or ileus), or blood losses (e.g., trauma or surgery).

4. To correct electrolytes and acid-base disorders.

5. To correct severe hypoglycemia, where IV 25% dextrose is life-saving.

6. As a vehicle for various IV medications (e.g., antibiotics, chemotherapeutic agents, insulin, vasopressor agents, etc.).

7. To provide parenteral nutrition.

8. Treatment of critical problems: Shock, anaphylaxis, severe asthma, cardiac arrest, forced diuresis in drug overdose, poisoning, etc.

9. To monitor hemodynamic functions and administer diagnostic reagents.

Contraindications

1. IV fluid should be avoided if the patient can take oral fluid.

2. Preferable to avoid IV fluid in a patient with congestive heart failure or volume overload.

Advantages

1. A perfect, controlled, and predictable way of fluid administration.

2. Immediate response is achieved through direct infusion into the intravascular compartment.

3. Rapid correction of life-threatening fluid and electrolyte disturbances.

Disadvantages

1. More expensive and needs strict asepsis.

2. Feasible only in hospitalized patients under supervision.

3. Improper selection of the type of fluid used can lead to serious problems.

4. The inappropriate volume and rate of infusion of fluid can be life-threatening.

5. The incorrect administration technique can lead to complications.

Complications

1. **Local:** Haematoma, infiltration, and infusion phlebitis.

2. **Systemic:** Circulation overload with rapid or large volume infusion, especially in patients with cardiac problems. Rigors, air embolism, and septicemia.

3. **Others:** Fluid contamination, fungus in IV fluids, mixing of incompatible drugs, an incorrect infusion technique, IV set or IV catheter-related problems, and human error-related problems.

OVERVIEW OF COMPOSITION OF IV FLUIDS

It is important to know the compositions of different commercially available IV fluids (Table 2.1) when making an appropriate choice for specific situations.

Bird's eye view of IV fluid characteristics

Before discussing the detailed composition and pharmacology of IV fluids, let's first assess and clarify the fundamental concept of IV fluids.

The physiological IV fluids

Balanced crystalloids such as Ringer's lactate (RL), PlasmaLyte, and Sterofundin are physiological IV fluids. Among these, RL is the most commonly used balanced crystalloid, with its electrolyte contents similar to the composition of the extracellular fluid (ECF) (Na^+-130 mEq/L, K^+-4 mEq/L, Cl^-109 mEq/L, lactate (bicarbonate) 28 mEq/L, and Ca^{2+}-3 mEq/L).

Daily normal maintenance requirement and preventing starvation ketosis in adults

Understanding the daily normal maintenance requirements for water, sodium, potassium, and the amount of

dextrose needed to prevent starvation ketosis in adults is essential. These details are summarized in Table 2.2 [4].

Sodium content in various IV fluids

Understanding the sodium content in commonly used IV fluids is crucial. Among these fluids, normal saline (NS) and dextrose saline (D5NS) contain the maximum amount of sodium, with 154 mEq/L or 9 gm of NaCl per liter. (Note: 1 gm of NaCl contains 17.1 mEq Na^+). For detailed information on the sodium content of various IV fluids, refer to Table 2.3.

Chloride content in various IV fluids

Determining the chloride content in commonly used IV fluids is important. Among these fluids, normal saline, D5NS, and Isolyte-G all contain the maximum chloride concentration at 154 mEq/L.

Potassium content in various IV fluids

Understanding the potassium content in different IV fluids is essential. The potassium content of various IV fluids is summarized in Table 2.4.

It's crucial to note that Isolyte-M has the highest potassium content, with 35 mEq/L. In contrast, balanced crystalloids such as RL, PlasmaLyte, and Sterofundin contain only 4–5 mEq/L of potassium.

Table 2.2 Maintenance requirement of water, sodium, potassium and dextrose

	Water	Sodium	Potassium	Dextrose
Normal requirement	25–30 mL/kg/day	1 mEq/kg/day	1 mEq/kg/day	100 gm/day to prevent starvation ketosis

Table 2.3 Sodium concentration of IV fluids

IV Solutions	NS D5NS	Sterofundin	Plasma-Lyte	RL	0.45% NaCl	Isolyte-G	Isolyte-M	Isolyte-P	3% NaCl
Sodium mEq/L	154.0	145.0	140.0	130.0	77.0	63.0	37.0	25.0	513.0

Table 2.4 Potassium concentration of IV fluids						
IV solutions	Isolyte-M	Isolyte-P	Isolyte-G	PlasmaLyte	RL and sterofundin	Inj. potassium chloride 15%
Potassium (mEq/L)	35.0	20.0	17.0	5.0	4.0	20 mEq/10 ml

Magnesium content in various IV fluids

IV fluids that contain magnesium include Ringer's acetate and Sterofundin, which contain 2 mEq/L, and solutions like PlasmaLyte, Isolyte-P, Isolyte-E, and Isolyte-S, which contain 3 mEq/L.

Calcium content in various IV fluids

IV fluids that contain calcium include Ringer's lactate and Ringer's acetate, which contain 2 mEq/L, while Sterofundin, Isolyte-E, and Isolyte-S contain 5 mEq/L.

Phosphate content in various IV fluids

Phosphate-containing IV fluids include Isolyte-M, which contains 15 mEq/L, and Isolyte-P, which contains 3 mEq/L.

Correction of acidosis with IV fluids

Understanding which IV fluids can directly correct acidosis and its mechanism is essential. Some IV fluids contain bicarbonate precursors, such as lactate and acetate [5]. Ringer's lactate, for example, contains 28 mEq/L of lactate, which is converted into bicarbonate in the liver, effectively correcting metabolic acidosis. Additionally, fluids like PlasmaLyte, Sterofundin, Isolyte-P, and Isolyte-M contain acetate (PlasmaLyte = 27 mEq/L, Sterofundin = 24, Isolyte-P = 23, and Isolyte-M = 20 mEq/L). Acetate also undergoes conversion into bicarbonate, both in the liver and peripheral tissues, aiding in the correction of metabolic acidosis.

Correction of metabolic alkalosis with IV fluids

Understanding which IV fluids can directly correct metabolic alkalosis is important. Isolyte-G stands out as the only IV fluid capable of directly addressing metabolic alkalosis. This effect is achieved through the presence of ammonium chloride (NH_4Cl = 70 mEq/L) in Isolyte-G, which undergoes conversion into H^+ ions and urea in the liver. The addition of H^+ ions effectively corrects the alkalosis.

Cautious use of IV fluids in renal failure

It is essential to exercise caution when using certain IV fluids in patients with renal failure. IV fluids with high sodium content, such as normal saline, dextrose saline (154 mEq/L sodium or 9 gm of salt per liter), and Ringer's lactate (130 mEq/L or approximately 7 gm of salt per liter), are administered with care due to their potential risk of fluid overload.

Furthermore, IV fluids containing a high potassium content, such as Isolyte-M, Isolyte-P, and Isolyte-G, should also be used cautiously in renal failure patients because of the potential risk of hyperkalemia.

Additionally, it's important to note that ammonium chloride in Isolyte-G undergoes conversion into hydrogen ions and urea, which can potentially exacerbate uremic acidosis, further emphasizing the need for caution when administering this fluid to individuals with renal issues.

Glucose-free IV fluids

It's important to note that normal saline, Ringer's lactate, PlasmaLyte, and Sterofundin do not contain glucose. Therefore, they can be administered without the risk of worsening hyperglycemia.

Sodium and chloride free IV fluids

Among commonly used IV fluids, 5%, 10%, and 20%-dextrose are the only fluids that do not contain sodium and chloride. On the other hand, fluids like Isolyte-M and Isolyte-P have relatively low sodium and chloride content.

Potassium-free IV fluids

IV fluids such as normal saline, dextrose saline (D5NS), and 5%, 10%, and 20%-dextrose do not contain potassium.

CLASSIFICATION OF FLUIDS

The solutions used in intravenous fluid therapy are classified into the following based on the composition of fluids, osmolality, presence of buffers (in balanced solutions), and electrolytes.

Classification based on composition

The solutions used in intravenous fluid therapy are classified into three groups based on composition:

A. Crystalloids

B. Colloids

C. Whole blood and blood products

A. Crystalloids

Crystalloids are solutions in sterile water which contain varying concentrations of electrolytes and dextrose.

B. Colloids

Colloids are a solution containing water, electrolytes, and plasma-derived protein or semi-synthetic starch molecules that remain uniformly distributed and do not readily cross semi-permeable membranes. Colloids are frequently called volume expanders or plasma expanders. Commonly used Colloids include albumin, hydroxyethyl starch, gelatine, and dextran.

Classification of crystalloids based on osmolality

Crystalloids are classified into three categories according to their osmolality (Table 2.5).

A. Isotonic crystalloids

A crystalloid solution that has the same concentration of electrolytes as the body plasma. Isotonic fluids have an osmolality of 270–310 mOsm/L. When an isotonic crystalloid is administered, the infused isotonic solution remains within the extracellular fluid compartment (distributed between the intravascular and interstitial spaces), and therefore, isotonic IV fluids expand the intravascular compartment more effectively than hypotonic IV fluids [3]. Isotonic fluids don't move into cells, and thus cells neither swell nor shrink with the isotonic fluid infusion.

Examples of isotonic solutions with their respective osmolarity values include 0.9% sodium chloride (308 mOsm/L), Ringer's lactate (273 mOsm/L), Ringer's acetate (276 mOsm/L), PlasmaLyte (295 mOsm/L), and Sterofundin (309 mOsm/L).

B. Hypotonic crystalloids

Crystalloid solutions with a lower concentration of electrolytes than body plasma are hypotonic fluids. Hypotonic fluids have an osmolality of less than 270 mOsm/L (lower than serum osmolarity). When hypotonic crystalloid is administered, the fluid will quickly move from the intravascular space into the cells and interstitial spaces. These solutions will hydrate cells causing them to swell. Examples of hypotonic solutions are 0.45% sodium chloride, 0.33% sodium chloride, 5% dextrose, 10% dextrose and D5W + 0.45% NaCl.

Table 2.5 Classification of crystalloid solutions according to osmolality						
Characteristics	Isotonic solutions		Hypotonic solutions		Hypertonic solutions	
Osmolality (mOsm/L)	270–310		Lesser than 270		Greater than 310	
Distribution and effect on fluid compartment	Remains within ECF and expands ECF compartment		Fluid quickly moves from the intravascular space into the cells		Pull water from the cells into the intravascular space	
Effect on cell size	No effect		Swollen		Shrink	
Examples	Solutions	Osmolality mOsm/L	Solutions	Osmolality mOsm/L	Solutions	Osmolality mOsm/L
Normal serum osmolality is 275–295 mOsm/kg	0.9% NaCl	308	0.45% NaCl	154	3% NaCl	1026
	Ringer's lactate	273	0.33% NaCl	103	D5W + 0.9% NaCl	560
	PlasmaLyte	290	-	-	-	-

The 5% dextrose solution, with an osmolality of 252 mOsm/L, is often considered near isotonic in the bag. However, once it enters the body, dextrose is rapidly metabolized, leaving behind pure water, which becomes hypotonic. Similarly, the 10% dextrose solution has an osmolality of 505 mOsm/L in vitro, but it becomes pure hypotonic water in vivo with zero osmolality.

Additionally, D5W + 0.45% NaCl is hypertonic in the bag, with an osmolality of 406 mOsm/L. Nevertheless, once administered in the body, dextrose is rapidly metabolized, leaving behind a solution containing only 0.45% NaCl, which offers an osmolality of just 154 mOsm/L, making it hypotonic. Therefore, when using the above-mentioned IV fluids, selection should be based on the expected in vivo osmolality rather than what is mentioned on the package label [6].

Use hypotonic fluid with caution. As hypotonic fluid quickly moves from the intravascular space into the cells, vascular bed volume decrease. Depletion of intravascular fluid volume can exacerbate preexisting hypovolemia and hypotension and carries the risk of cardiovascular collapse. As hypotonic fluid can cause or exacerbate cerebral edema, avoid it in patients who are at risk for increased intracranial pressure (stroke, head injury, or neurosurgery) [7].

C. Hypertonic crystalloids

Crystalloid solutions with a higher concentration of electrolytes than body plasma are considered hypertonic fluids, which have an osmolarity of more than 310 mOsm/L or higher. Among the most widely used hypertonic solutions are 3% sodium chloride and 5% dextrose in 0.9% saline.

When hypertonic crystalloid solutions are administered, they draw water from the cells into the intravascular space, causing the cells to shrink and increasing extracellular fluid volume. This characteristic makes 3% sodium chloride a mainstay of treatment for cerebral edema since it can shrink brain cell size without the risk of hypotension, due to its ability to expand the extracellular fluid volume.

5% dextrose in 0.9% saline is not used for the treatment of cerebral edema because, in vivo, after the metabolism of glucose, it becomes similar to normal saline, which is an isotonic fluid.

As hypertonic fluid increases extracellular fluid volume, it carries the risk of volume overload and pulmonary edema and, therefore, should be avoided in cardiac or renal patients with circulatory overload. As hypertonic fluid causes cell shrinkage, it should be avoided in conditions causing cellular dehydration.

Classification of crystalloids based on buffers and electrolytes

For proper selection of crystalloids, we need to know the composition, pharmacological basis, important indications, and contraindications of commonly used IV fluids. The following crystalloids are discussed here.

A. Dextrose and sodium chloride solutions

5% dextrose, normal saline, dextrose saline, half normal saline, and half normal saline with dextrose.

B. Balanced crystalloids

Ringer's lactate, ringer's acetate, PlasmaLyte, and sterofundin.

C. Multiple electrolyte solutions

Isolyte-G, isolyte-M, isolyte-P, isolyte-E and isolyte-S.

METHODS FOR CALCULATING DROP RATES PER MINUTE FOR FLUID INFUSION

In most non-ICU setups, electronic pump systems are unavailable, and fluids are administered via either macrodrip tubing (conventional, routine IV sets) or microdrip tubings. In such scenarios, manual calculation is necessary to determine the volume of fluid administered within a given time frame at required rates of drops per minute. It's essential to verify the drop factor of the administration set, which is used to ensure accurate fluid delivery during infusion therapy. Calculations differ based on either macrodrip tubing, which delivers larger-sized drops, or microdrip tubing, which provides smaller-sized drops.

A. Calculation for macro drip tubing

Commercially available macro drip tubing delivers larger drops, with the specific drop factor varying depending on the manufacturer's location and practices worldwide. Each milliliter of fluid administered through macro drip tubing typically delivers 10, 15, or 20 drops of fluid, known as the administration set drop factor (drops/mL).

- A drop factor of 10 drops/mL means that 10 drops of fluid will equal one milliliter.
- A drop factor of 15 drops/mL means that 15 drops of fluid will equal one milliliter.
- A drop factor of 20 drops/mL means that 20 drops of fluid will equal one milliliter.

The method used to calculate macro drop rates per minute for fluid infusion:

Step 1: First, convert the total volume of fluid to be delivered over a given time period into volume in an hour.

Volume/hour = Total Volume of Fluid (ml) / Duration of Time (hour)

Step 2: Convert the volume of fluid to be delivered in an hour into the volume given in a minute.

Volume/min =Total Volume of Fluid (ml) / 60

Step 3: Convert the volume of fluid to be delivered in a minute into the number of macro drops to be delivered in a minute.

Macro Drops/min = Total Volume of Fluid (ml) × Drop Factor of Macro Drip Tubing

Example: A patient needs 600 mL of intravenous fluids over 5 hours using macrodrip tubing with a drop factor of 15 drops/mL. Calculate the macro drop rates per minute.

- Volume/hour = 600 ml/5 hours = 120 ml/hour
- Volume/min = 120 ml/60 min = 2 ml/min
- Macro drops/min = 2 ml × 15 = 30 macro drop rates per min

Simple formulas for macro drip tubing with a drop factor of 15 drops/mL: A simple, practical, and user-friendly method for roughly calculating drop rates when macro drip tubing with a drop factor of 15 drops/mL is used to infuse IV fluids is summarized below.

Rule of ten: Multiply the volume of IV fluid to be delivered in liters over 24 hours by ten to obtain the drop rate per minute.

IV Fluid in liters/24 hours × 10 = Macro Drop Rate/min

- 2.0 liters in 24 hours = 2.0 × 10 = 20 macro drops/min
- 3.5 liters in 24 hours = 3.5 × 10 = 35 macro drops/min
- Calculation for 1 liter in 8 hours = 3.0 liters in 24 hours = 3.0 × 10 = 30 macro drops/min
- Calculation for 1 liter in 6 hours = 4.0 liters in 24 hours = 4.0 × 10 = 40 macro drops/min

Rule of four: Divide the volume of fluid (in ml) to be infused in one hour by four to obtain the macro drop rate per minute.

Volume in ml/hour ÷ 4 = Macro drop rate/min

- 60 ml/hour = 60 ÷ 4 = 15 drops/min
- 200 ml/hour = 200 ÷ 4 = 50 drops/min

B. Calculation for micro drip tubing

Commercially available micro drip tubing delivers small-sized drops, with typically 1 mL providing 60 micro drops.

The formula to calculate micro drop rates per minute is simple.

Volume in ml/hour = Number of Micro drops/min

- 30 ml/hour = 30 Micro drops/min
- 45 ml/hour = 45 Micro drops/min

REFERENCES

1. Floss K, Borthwick M, Clark C. Intravenous fluid therapy – Background and principles. Pharmaceutical Journal Sept, 1 2008.
2. Hilton AK, Pellegrino VA, Scheinkestel CD. Avoiding common problems associated with intravenous therapy. Med J Aust. 2008;189(9):509–13.
3. Hoorn EJ. Intravenous fluids: balancing solutions. J Nephrol. 2017;30(4):485–492.
4. Intravenous fluid therapy in adults in hospital. London: National Institute for Health and Care Excellence, 2013 (https://www.nice.org.uk/guidance/cg174).
5. Ergin B, Kapucu A, Guerci P, et al. The role of bicarbonate precursors in balanced fluids during haemorrhagic shock with and without compromised liver function. Br J Anaesth. 2016;117:521–528.
6. Mertzlufft F, Brettner F, Crystal GJ, et al. Intravenous fluids: issues warranting concern. Eur J Anaesthesiol. 2022;39(4):394–396.
7. van der Jagt M. Fluid management of the neurological patient: a concise review. Crit Care. 2016;20(1):126.

3 | Dextrose and Sodium Chloride Solutions

Crystalloids are solutions in sterile water which contain varying concentrations of electrolytes and dextrose. Dextrose and sodium chloride containing crystalloid solutions are discussed (Summarized in Table 3.1).

5% DEXTROSE (D5W)

Composition

One liter of fluid contains:
  Hydrous Dextrose USP 50 gm
  Osmolality 252 mOsm/L
  Caloric value 170 kcal/L
  pH 4.3 (3.2 to 6.5)
Each 100 ml of 5% Dextrose contains Hydrous Dextrose USP 5 gm

Pharmacological basis

5% dextrose (usually abbreviated as D5W) provides free water with glucose without electrolytes. D5W is selected when there is a need for water but not electrolytes.

When a patient requires pure water, we administer intravenous 5% dextrose. Intravenous administration of free water is avoided due to its potential to cause hemolysis of red blood cells. However, the addition of dextrose renders the fluid near isotonic (252 mOsm/L) and does not result in hemolysis within the body.

5% dextrose packed in the bag is an isotonic solution, but once infused becomes a hypotonic solution in the

Table 3.1 Composition of dextrose and sodium chloride solutions					
	5% Dextrose (D5W)	**Normal saline (0.9% NaCl)**	**Dextrose saline/ (D5NS)**	**Half normal saline (0.45% NaCl)**	**Half normal saline with dextrose (D5-1/2NS)**
Tonicity	Isotonic*	Isotonic	Hypertonic	Hypotonic	Hypertonic
Osmolality (mOsm/L)	252	308	560	154	406
Sodium (mEq/L)	-	154	154	77	77
Chloride (mEq/L)	-	154	154	77	77
NaCl (gm/L)	-	9.0	9.0	4.5	4.5
Dextrose (gm/L)	50	-	50	-	50
Caloric value (kcals/L)	170	-	170	-	170
*5% Dextrose isotonic in the bag but hypotonic effect after administration in body					

body as dextrose is consumed rapidly, and the remaining plain water is hypotonic [1].

When D5W is infused, dextrose is metabolized, and the remaining water is distributed uniformly in all body compartments. As about 67% of the volume of infused D5W will be distributed in the intracellular compartment, D5W is the best agent to correct intracellular dehydration [2].

Because the infusion of D5W expands the intravascular compartment by 83 ml, just 8% of its infused volume, D5W is not a suitable agent for intravascular plasma volume expansion and therefore is avoided for the fluid resuscitation in hypovolemia and hypotension [3].

5% dextrose solution (50 gm dextrose per liter) provides 170 kcal/L (3.4 kcal/gm of dextrose). The calories provided by D5W help to prevent starvation ketosis but are inadequate to meet normal nutritional requirements.

Indications

1. A commonly used fluid in conditions like preoperative fluid replacement for preventing and treating dehydration caused by prolonged fasting.

2. As a diluent and vehicle for administrating intravenous drugs.

3. For the treatment or prevention of ketosis during starvation and in cases of high-grade fever.

4. Correction of hypernatremia due to pure water loss (e.g., diabetes insipidus). Hypernatremia due to salt poisoning or excessive use of electrolyte solution needs an infusion of 5% dextrose with furosemide to promote sodium excretion and correction of hypernatremia.

Caution: In severe hypernatremia, a fast infusion of 5% dextrose will rapidly correct hypernatremia. Rapid lowering of plasma sodium concentration causes osmotic water movement into the brain leading to an increase in brain size and resulting in cerebral edema. The cerebral edema can then lead to headache, nausea or vomiting, dizziness, seizures, permanent neurologic damage, or even death. So the rate of infusion of 5% dextrose should be adjusted in such a way that the correction of hypernatremia will occur slowly.

5. Infusing small volume of fluid for a prolong period to keep a vein.

6. To treat hypoglycemia.

Contraindications

1. Cerebral edema: Because of its hypotonic nature, 5% dextrose aggravates cerebral edema [4].

2. Neurosurgical procedures: As 5% dextrose increases intracranial pressure, it can cause damage during neurosurgery and so must be avoided [5].

3. Acute ischaemic stroke: Glucose containing fluid should not be used after acute ischaemic stroke in non-hypoglycemic patients, as hyperglycemia aggravates cerebral ischaemic brain damage [6].

4. Hypovolemic shock: Avoid 5% dextrose for fluid resuscitation because of its minimal and transient effects on blood volume expansion [7]. Moreover, fast replacement by a large volume of D5W can lead to hyperglycemia and osmotic diuresis, leading to increased urine output. So the correction of dehydration will be delayed.

5. Hyponatremia and water intoxication: By providing electrolyte free water, 5% dextrose worsens both conditions [7].

6. Blood transfusion: 5% dextrose and whole blood should not be administered through the same intravenous (IV) line as hemolysis can occur [8].

7. Uncontrolled diabetes and severe hyperglycemia.

8. Maintenance IV fluid: 5% dextrose is routinely used to provide free water with calories. But 5% dextrose as a sole IV solution is not a suitable maintenance IV fluid for two reasons. Dextrose concentration is just 5% in D5W, so calories provided by D5W are inadequate to meet normal nutritional requirements, and 5% dextrose is an electrolyte-free solution, so it cannot fulfill the daily electrolyte need of the body.

9. Severe hypokalemia: Rapid administration of 5% dextrose will cause hyperglycemia and stimulate insulin release, which will push potassium into the intracellular compartment. Shifting extracellular potassium into the cells in severe hypokalemia will further aggravate the existing severe hypokalemia, which can be dangerous. Therefore, avoid the rapid administration of 5% dextrose in a patient with severe hypokalemia.

Precautions

1. IV administration of dextrose solution (especially hypertonic) may cause local pain, vein irritation, and thrombophlebitis.

2. Prolonged IV administration of 5% dextrose can cause hypokalemia, hypomagnesemia, and hypophosphatemia.

3. Respiratory compromised patients: High glucose intake leads to increased CO_2 production (high respiratory quotient as compared to lipids). The elevated production of CO_2 increases the workload of respiratory muscles and may precipitate respiratory decompensation, prolong the need for mechanical ventilator assistance, or delay weaning from the ventilator. Therefore, carbohydrate is not preferred as the only source of calorie in respiratory compromised patients and patients weaning from ventilator support.

Rate of administration

Dextrose in water can be given intravenously safely at a rate of 0.5

gm/kg/hour without causing glycosuria [9]. This is equivalent to 10 mL/kg/hour of 5% dextrose, 5 mL/kg/hour of 10% dextrose, 2 mL/kg/hour of 25% dextrose, and 1 mL/kg/hour of 50% dextrose respectively, which will not cause glycosuria. It is useful to test the urine for sugar at regular intervals during dextrose infusion to rule out glycosuria and the associated fluid loss due to osmotic diuresis.

NORMAL SALINE
(0.9% NaCl - Isotonic Saline)

Composition

One liter of fluid contains:
   Sodium 154.0 mEq
   Chloride 154.0 mEq
   Osmolality 308 mOsm/L
   pH around 5.5

Each 100 ml contains 0.9 gm of Sodium Chloride

Pharmacological basis

It is the most widely used crystalloid solution prescribed for fluid resuscitation [10]. The commonly used terms for a solution of 0.9% of sodium chloride are normal saline (because its osmolarity is nearly the same as that of blood) and isotonic saline (because it closely approximates isotonic solution).

As sodium and chloride are present chiefly in the extracellular fluid compartment, infused normal saline is distributed primarily in extracellular fluid. So normal saline is an extracellular fluid (ECF) replacement fluid. If one liter of normal saline is infused, about 25% (250 ml) of it stays in the intravascular compartment, and 75% (750 ml) enters the interstitial fluid [11].

Normal saline can be infused safely with packed red blood cells because it is isotonic with blood, so there is no risk of hemolysis. Additionally, it is devoid of calcium, so there is no risk of binding with citrate anticoagulants used in blood products.

The term 'normal' saline is a misnomer because:

- The chloride in normal saline is 154 mEq/L which is supraphysiological (50% higher compared to the normal plasma chloride value of 102 mEq/L) [12].

- Normal saline is not isotonic (osmolality 308 mOsm/L, which is higher than plasma osmolality 275–295 mOsm/L).

- The sodium in normal saline is 154 mEq/L, which is about 10% higher compared to the normal plasma value of 140 mEq/L.

- The pH of normal saline is 5.0, which is lower than the normal plasma pH of 7.4.

Because of the higher chloride concentration of normal saline:

- It is the preferred IV fluid for patients with hypochloremic metabolic alkalosis and volume depletion caused by the upper gastrointestinal tract (vomiting or nasogastric suction) [13].

- Avoid a large volume of normal saline infusion, as it can lead to hyperchloremic metabolic acidosis [14]. Hyperchloremia carries a high risk of acute kidney injury due to increased renal vasoconstriction leading to decreased renal blood flow and glomerular filtration [15, 16]. To avoid hyperchloremic acidosis and other potential complications of normal saline, limit its use to less than 2 liter (or 20–30 mL/kg) for resuscitation [17].

Indications

1. For fluid resuscitation and treatment of hypovolemic shock. In septic shock, at least 30 mL/kg of normal saline should be given within the first 3 hours for initial resuscitation [18].

2. Treatment of hypochloremic metabolic alkalosis (e.g., vomiting) with dehydration [13].

3. Treatment of severe salt depletion or hypovolemic hyponatremia [19].

4. Water and salt depletion, as in vomiting, nasogastric suction, excessive diuresis, or excessive perspiration.

5. In traumatic brain injury for initial resuscitation for volume expansion [20–22].

6. The use of normal saline as a maintenance IV fluid is the current standard of care in acutely ill hospitalized children [23].

7. Perioperative fluid therapy in children [24]. The risk of postoperative hyponatremia is higher in children than in adults [25].

8. Diabetic ketoacidosis (DKA): DKA leads to high plasma osmolarity, and a rapid reduction in plasma osmolarity carries the risk for cerebral edema. So normal saline is preferred for the initial fluid therapy in DKA rather than hypo-osmolar and hypotonic fluids [26].

9. Miscellaneous uses:
   - Treatment of hypercalcemia.
   - The fluid challenge in prerenal AKI (acute kidney injury).
   - Treatment of hypernatremia with hypotension.
   - Sterile irrigation medium for washing of wounds, parts of the body, or medical equipment.
   - Gut irrigation for bowel preparation.
   - As a vehicle for certain drugs.
   - Most common fluid for co-administration with blood because saline does not contain calcium. Administration of calcium-containing solutions like Ringer's lactate should be avoided with the infusion of blood because citrate, used as an anticoagulant in the blood, can mix with calcium and result in clot formation.
   - As a priming fluid in the hemodialysis procedure.

Contraindications and precautions

Use normal saline cautiously or avoid in:

1. Volume overload due to congestive heart failure, renal disease, and cirrhosis.

2. Severe uncontrolled hypertension. Cautious use in preeclamptic patients.

3. Hypoproteinemia, hypernatremia, as well as patients who are very young, elderly, or debilitated.

4. Hyponatremia due to the syndrome of inappropriate antidiuresis hormone (SIADH) and cerebral salt wasting syndrome (CSWS) in whom the urine osmolality is high (>500 mOsm/kg).

5. Hyperkalemia: When a large volume (>2L) of saline is administered rapidly, it can lead to hyperchloremic acidosis [27]. Hyperchloremic acidosis shifts potassium out of cells. As 98% of total body potassium is intracellular, and just 2% is extracellular, even the slightest shift of intracellular potassium out of cells can lead to clinically significant hyperkalemia. So in patients with hyperkalemia, the rapid infusion of a large volume of saline can be harmful [28–30].

6. Dehydration with severe hypokalemia: In cases of severe hypokalemia, where there is a deficit of intracellular potassium, infusing normal saline without additional potassium supplementation will worsen the intracellular electrolyte imbalance.

DEXTROSE SALINE

(5% Dextrose with 0.9% NaCl Solution, D5NS)

Composition

One liter of fluid contains:
   Hydrous Dextrose USP 50 gm
   Sodium 154 mEq
   Chloride 154 mEq
   Osmolality 560 mOsm/L
   Caloric value 170 kcal/L

Each 100 ml contains: Hydrous Dextrose USP 5.0 gm and Sodium Chloride 0.90 gm

Pharmacological basis

5% dextrose-0.9% saline (dextrose saline, D5NS) solution has the advantage of both normal saline (to provide salt) and 5%-dextrose (to provide minimal carbohydrate calories). So D5NS solution is useful to supply major extracellular electrolytes (sodium and chloride), provides calories (50 gm dextrose/liter, which provides 170 kcal/L), prevents ketone formation, and provides fluid to correct dehydration.

As the D5NS solution is distributed chiefly in the ECF compartment, unlike D5W, it does not correct intracellular dehydration. Instead, this solution provides sodium and chloride and effectively expands ECF, like normal saline.

While theoretically, the D5NS solution could be considered for resuscitation in hypovolemic shock, the rapid infusion of a large volume of this solution (at a rate of 16 mL/kg/hour of 5% dextrose) results in a substantial glucose load (>0.8 gm/kg/hour), leading to hyperglycemia and subsequent osmotic diuresis [9]. Increased urine output in the presence of incompletely or partially corrected hypovolemic shock is undesirable and can mislead the clinician when determining the appropriate rate of fluid infusion.

Indications

1. Correction of vomiting or nasogastric aspiration induced alkalosis and hypochloremia along with a supply of calories.

2. Fasting ketosis and alcoholic ketoacidosis: Infusion of both components, saline and 5% dextrose, are essential and beneficial. Saline replenishes circulating volume and increases the elimination of ketoacids. Dextrose increases insulin secretion and decreases glucagon secretion leading to decreased ketone production and correction of metabolic acidosis [31]. Caution: Correct hypokalemia before glucose administration because insulin stimulated by dextrose will worsen hypokalemia.

3. Adrenal crisis and acute adrenal insufficiency: Hyponatremia, hypoglycemia, and hypotension are common in adrenal insufficiency. As D5NS corrects all these abnormalities, D5NS is a preferred fluid for uniform infusion over 24 hours to correct volume deficit and as a maintenance IV fluid [32].

4. Maintenance fluid in pediatric patients: Hyponatremia due to the use of hypotonic maintenance IV fluids has become increasingly

recognized as a cause of morbidity and mortality in hospitalized children. Recent literature suggests the use of isotonic D5NS as a standard maintenance IV solution in children to avoid the development of hyponatremia [23].

Precautions

1. Anasarca: Cautious use in anasarca of cardiac, hepatic, and renal disease.

2. Hypovolemic shock: In severe hypovolemic shock, when rapid replacement with a larger volume of fluid is required, D5NS is not a preferred solution. Rapid infusion of D5NS can cause hyperglycemia, which causes osmotic diuresis and urinary fluid loss (even in the presence of fluid deficit). So the simple logic to use D5NS for supplying a salt solution to correct shock and simultaneously providing energy is not correct.

3. Hypokalemia: Excessive administration of potassium-free D5NS may cause significant hypokalemia. Dextrose in this fluid stimulates the release of insulin, which shifts potassium into cells with a possible worsening of hypokalemia.

HALF NORMAL SALINE

(0.45% NaCl Solution)

Composition

One liter of fluid contains:
Sodium 77 mEq
Chloride 77 mEq
Osmolality 154 mOsm/L (hypotonic saline)
pH 4.0 (3.2 to 6.5)

Each 100 ml contains: Sodium Chloride 0.45 gm

Pharmacological basis

Half normal saline (0.45% NaCl) is often written as half isotonic saline (0.45% is half of 0.9%). Half normal saline contains 50% salt as compared to normal saline and therefore is used when there is a need for more water and lesser sodium and chloride replacement. Because of the low concentration of sodium (77 mEq/L), this fluid carries the risk for hyponatremia, especially in sick children, women, elderly patients, postoperatively patients, and persons with psychogenic polydipsia.

Indications

1. Maintenance fluid therapy in adults: 2 liters per day of half normal saline with 5% Dextrose and potassium (20 mEq/L) added is a suitable combination for maintenance requirements in adults [33].

2. Treatment of severe or chronic hypernatremia: As half normal saline corrects hypernatremia gently, it avoids cerebral edema and is therefore safe in treatment of severe or chronic hypernatremia [34]. But avoid excess use or too rapid infusion of half normal saline, as it may cause a rapid reduction in serum sodium and carries the risk of cerebral edema in severe or chronic hypernatremia.

3. Gastric fluid loss from nasogastric suction or vomiting. Half normal saline with potassium of 10 mmol/L is the preferable repletion fluid for loss of gastric fluid [35].

4. Diabetic ketoacidosis and hyperosmolar hyperglycemic state (HHS): In these patients, rapid infusion of normal saline is initially recommended to correct hypovolemia or hypovolemic

shock. But after the correction of hypotension, the IV fluid is generally switched to half normal saline in patients who are hypernatremic or eunatremic. However, in patients with hyponatremia, normal saline should be continued [36–38].

In DKA and HHS, urinary losses of electrolytes due to osmotic diuresis are usually hypotonic, similar to half normal saline [39]. Therefore, switching to half normal saline is beneficial after volume re-expansion because it matches the osmolality of the lost fluid. Additionally, low chloride (77 mEq/L) containing half normal saline avoids hyperchloremia, which is likely to occur with the infusion of a large volume of chloride-rich (154 mEq/L) normal saline.

5. Potassium replacement in DKA or HHS: Hypokalemia is common in DKA or HHS, and potassium chloride (KCl) is added to IV fluids for potassium replacement [40]. When potassium chloride is added to half-normal saline, the osmolality of the infused fluid becomes more physiological. However, adding potassium to normal saline results in a hypertonic solution, which can exacerbate serum osmolarity.

For example, when 40 mEq of potassium chloride is added to 1 liter of half-normal saline, the solution's osmolality becomes 234 mOsm/L (154 mOsm/L of 0.45% NaCl and 80 mOsm/L of 40 mEq potassium chloride). Conversely, when 40 mEq of potassium chloride is added to 1 liter of normal saline, the solution's osmolality becomes 388 mOsm/L (308 mOsm/L of 0.9% NaCl and 80 mOsm/L of 40 mEq potassium chloride) [41].

Contraindications

1. Maintenance fluid therapy in children: Currently, isotonic solutions (normal saline or Ringer's lactate) are recommended as maintenance fluid because the risk of hyponatremia was greater in children who received hypotonic solutions such as 0.45% NaCl [23].

2. Hyponatremia, hypervolemia, and severe renal insufficiency (with oliguria/anuria).

3. Replacement fluid in severe dehydration due to diarrhea and vomiting where there is a need for fluid with high sodium.

4. As this fluid is hypotonic, avoid it in patients with cerebral edema, liver disease, trauma, or burns.

HALF NORMAL SALINE WITH DEXTROSE

(0.45% NaCl with 5% Dextrose Solution, D5-1/2NS)

Composition

One liter of fluid contains:
   Sodium 77 mEq
   Chloride 77 mEq
   Hydrous Dextrose USP 50 gm
   Osmolality 405 mOsm/L (hypertonic)
   Caloric value is 170 kcal/L
   pH 4.4 (3.5 to 6.5)

Each 100 ml contains: Hydrous Dextrose USP 5.0 gm and Sodium Chloride 0.45 gm

Pharmacological basis

In this solution, dextrose is added to half normal saline, and therefore its pharmacological basis is almost the same. Half normal saline with dextrose is often written as D5-1/2NS. The benefit of this fluid is that it provides minimal carbohydrate calories (170 kcal/L) and therefore is more appropriate as a maintenance fluid. An added benefit of dextrose addition is the prevention of the lysis of red blood cells that may occur with the rapid infusion of hypotonic fluids.

Indications

1. Maintenance fluid therapy in adults: Half normal saline with dextrose solution with the addition of potassium (20 mEq/L), is a suitable combination for maintenance requirements in adults [33].

2. The recovery phase of diabetic ketoacidosis. In the treatment of DKA, when the blood glucose concentration is approximately 250 mg per dL or less, half normal saline with dextrose is preferred as a hydration fluid [42]. Dextrose content in this solution allows the continued administration of insulin until ketonemia is controlled and avoids hypoglycemia. Additionally, this solution also prevents hyperchloremia due to the infusion of a large volume of normal saline.

3. Postoperative surgical patient: In the absence of shock and hyponatremia, this fluid is used as a postoperative intravenous maintenance fluid therapy in adults. The dextrose content in this solution stimulates basal insulin secretion and prevents muscle breakdown when the patient cannot to eat or drink [43].

4. Vomiting: As this solution provides dextrose and sodium chloride, it is used for hydration in vomiting without hyponatremia, hypotension, and shock.

Contraindication

Caution and contraindications are similar to Half normal saline, as discussed previously.

REFERENCES

1. Sweeney RM, McKendry RA, Bedi A. Perioperative intravenous fluid therapy for adults. Ulster Med J 2013;82(3):171–178.

2. Asim M, M Alkadi MM, Asim H, et al. Dehydration and volume depletion: how to handle the misconceptions. World J Nephrol. 2019;8(1):23–32.

3. Popescu M. Albumin therapy in critically ill patients. Cleveland clinic pharmacotherapy Update 2009; Volume XII, No. V.

4. Zornow MH, Prough DS. Fluid management in patients with traumatic brain injury. New Horiz. 1995;3(3):488–98.

5. Ali Z, Prabhakar H. Fluid management during neurosurgical procedures. J NeuroanaesthesiolCrit Care 2016;3:S35–S40.

6. Jauch EC, Saver JL, Adams Jr HP, et al. Guidelines for the early management of patients with acute ischemicstroke: a guideline for healthcare professionals from the American HeartAssociation/ American Stroke Association. Stroke. 2013;44(3):870–947.

7. National Clinical Guideline Centre (UK). Intravenous fluid therapy: Intravenous fluid therapy in adults in hospital [Internet]. London: Royal College of Physicians (UK); 2013 Dec. (NICE Clinical Guidelines, No. 174.) 7, Intravenous Fluid Therapy for Fluid Resuscitation. Available from: https://www.ncbi.nlm.nih.gov/books/NBK333097/.

8. Ryden SE, Oberman HA. Compatibility of common intravenous solutions with CPD blood. Transfusion. 1975;15(3):250–5.

9. Gahart BL, Nazareno AR, Ortega M. Gahart's 2019 Intravenous Medications: A handbook for nurses and health professionals. 2019 35thEdition.

10. Myburgh JA, Mythen MG. Resuscitation Fluids. N Engl J Med. 2013;369:1243–51.

11. Yartsev A. Response to 1L of Hartmann's compound sodium lactate. Deranged physiology June 25, 2015 (https://derangedphysiology.com/main/core-topics-intensive-care/manipulation-fluids-and-electrolytes/Chapter%202.3.4/response-1l-hartmanns-compound-sodium-lactate).

12. Semler MW, Rice TW. Saline is not the first choice for crystalloid resuscitation fluids. Crit Care Med. 2016;44(8):1541–4.

13. Hoorn EJ. Intravenous fluids: balancing solutions. J Nephrol 2017;30:485–492.

14. Lobo DN, Awad S. Should chloride-rich crystalloids remain the mainstay of fluid resuscitation to prevent "pre-renal" acute kidney injury? con. Kidney International. 2014;86(6):1096–1105.

15. Li H, Sun SR, Yap JQ, et al. 0.9% saline is neither normal nor physiological. J Zhejiang Univ Sci B. 2016;17(3):181–187.

16. Yunos NM, Bellomo R, Glassford N, et al. Chloride-liberal vs. Chloride-restrictive intravenous fluid administration and acute kidney injury: an extended analysis. Intensive Care Med 2015;41:257–64

17. Nickson C. Chloride in critical illness. LITFL. reviewed and revised 21 March 2017 https://litfl.com/chloride-in-critical-illness/ Accessed on 12 May 2019.

18. Rhodes A, Evans LE, Alhazzani W, et al. Surviving sepsis campaign: international guidelines for management of sepsis and septic shock: 2016. Crit Care Med 2017;45(3):486–552.

19. Sahay M, Sahay R. Hyponatremia: A practical approach. Indian J Endocrinol Metab. 2014;18(6):760–771.

20. Finfer S, Bellomo R, Boyce N, et al. A comparison of albumin and saline for fluid resuscitation in the intensive care unit. (SAFE Study) N Engl J Med 2004;350:2247–56.

21. Haddad SH, Arabi YM. Critical care management of severe traumatic brain injury in adults. scandinavian journal of trauma, resuscitation and emergency medicine. 2012;20:12.

22. Ertmer C, Van Aken H. Fluid therapy in patients with brain injury: what does physiology tell us? Crit Care. 2014;18(2):119.

23. Feld LG, Neuspiel DR, Foster BA, et al. Clinical practice guideline: maintenance intravenous fluids in children. Pediatrics 2018;142(6):e20183083.

24. Wright C. Perioperative Intravenous Fluids prescription and monitoring in children 3 months to 16 years. NHSClinical Guideline. 2017.

25. Andersen C, Afshari A. Impact of perioperative hyponatremia in children: a narrative review. World J Crit Care Med. 2014;3(4):95–101.

26. Gosmanov AR, Gosmanova EO, Dillard-Cannon E. Management of adult diabetic ketoacidosis. diabetes, metabolic syndrome and obesity: targets and therapy. 2014;7:255–64.

27. Ding X, Cheng Z, Qian Q. Intravenous fluids and acute kidney injury. Blood Purif 2017;43:163–172.

28. Khajavi MR, Etezadi F, Moharari RS, et al. Effects of normal saline vs. lactated ringer's during renal transplantation. Ren Fail. 2008;30(5):535–9.

29. Farkas, J. Myth-busting: lactated ringers is safe in hyperkalemia, and is superior to NS. PulmCrit.org (EMCrit) 2014 (https://emcrit.org/pulmcrit/myth-busting-lactated-ringers-is-safe-in-hyperkalemia-and-is-superior-to-ns/).

30. Weinberg L, Harris L, Bellomo R, et al. Effects of intraoperative and early postoperative normal saline or PlasmaLyte148® on hyperkalaemia in deceased donor renal transplantation: a double-blind randomized trial. Br J Anaesth. 2017;119(4):606–615.

31. McGuire LC, Cruickshank AM, Munro PT. Alcoholic ketoacidosis. Emerg Med J. 2006;23(6):417–20.

32. Bowden SA, Henry R. Pediatricadrenal insufficiency: diagnosis, management, and new therapies. International Journal of Pediatrics Volume 2018;110(20):1504–1516.

33. Sterns RH, Emmett M, Forman JP. Maintenance and replacement fluid therapy in adults. UptoDate (accessed 19.05.2019).

34. Reynolds RM, Padfield PL, Seckl JR. Disorders of sodium balance. BMJ. 2006;332:702.

35. Anigilaje EA. Management of diarrhoeal dehydration in childhood: a review for clinicians in developing countries. Frontiers in Pediatrics 2018;6:28.

36. Kitabchi AE, Umpierrez GE, Miles JM, et al. Hyperglycemic crises in patients with diabetes. Diabetes Care. 2009;32(7):1335–43.

37. Basnet S, Venepalli PK, Andoh J, et al. Effect of normal saline and half normal saline on serum electrolytes during recovery phase of diabetic ketoacidosis. J Intensive Care Med. 2014;29(1):38–42.

38. Goguen J, Gilbert J. Hyperglycemicemergencies in adults. 2018 clinical practice guidelines. Diabetes Canada clinical practice guidelines expert committee. Can J Diabetes 2018;42:S109–S114.

39. Jivan D. Management of diabetic ketoacidosis, Journal of Endocrinology, Metabolism and Diabetes of South Africa 2011;16(1):10–14.

40. Perilli G, Saraceni C, Daniels MN, et al. Diabetic ketoacidosis: a review and update. CurrEmerg Hosp Med Rep 2013;1:10–17.

41. Hirsh I, Emmett M, Nathan DM, et al. Diabetic ketoacidosis and hyperosmolar hyperglycaemic state in adults: treatment. UptoDate (accessed 19.05.2019).

42. Kitabchi A, Wall BM. Management of diabetic ketoacidosis. Am Fam Physician. 1999;60(2):455–464.

43. Siparsky N, Cochran A, Sterns RH. Overview of postoperative fluid therapy in adults. UptoDate (accessed 19.05.2019).

4 | Balanced and Multi-electrolyte Solutions

Balanced and a few multi-electrolyte solutions are discussed in this chapter. Crystalloids with a composition closely resembling extracellular fluid have been termed 'balanced' or 'physiological' solutions [1, 2]. Balanced crystalloids are also distributed throughout the extracellular fluid (ECF) and are, therefore, of similar efficacy to normal saline (0.9% NaCl) in terms of plasma volume expansion.

Balanced crystalloids contain somewhat less sodium and significantly less chloride and therefore have advantages over normal saline solution when used for resuscitation or routine maintenance. Due to the instability of bicarbonate-containing solutions in plastic containers, alternative buffers such as lactate, acetate, gluconate, and malate are used to provide bicarbonate in balanced crystalloids [3]. Ringer's lactate is the most widely used balanced crystalloid.

RINGER'S LACTATE (RL)

Ringer's lactate solution is also known as Hartmann's solution, sodium

32

lactate solution, or lactated Ringer's solution (LR).

Composition

One liter of fluid contains:
Sodium 130 mEq
Chloride 109 mEq
Potassium 4 mEq
Calcium 3 mEq
Lactate 28 mEq
Osmolality is 273 mOsm/L
pH 6.5 (6.0 to 7.5)

Each 100 ml contains: Sodium Lactate 320 mg, Sodium Chloride 600 mg, Potassium Chloride 40 mg and Calcium Chloride 27 mg

Pharmacological basis

1. Effectively expand ECF: Because of its high sodium concentration (130 mEq/L), RL is primarily distributed within the extracellular fluid (approximately 25% of the fluid will increase plasma volume, while the remaining 75% will expand interstitial fluid) [4]. The effective expansion of plasma volume by RL renders it a valuable option in the treatment of severe hypovolemia and shock.

2. Physiological fluid: Ringer's lactate is a balanced physiological fluid with electrolyte contents (sodium, chloride, potassium, calcium, and bicarbonate from lactate conversion) closely resembling those in plasma. Due to its balanced composition, large volumes of RL can be rapidly infused without the risk of causing electrolyte imbalances. However, it's important to note that RL does not provide calories, magnesium, or phosphorus.

3. Provides HCO_3: Lactate in RL is metabolized and converted into bicarbonate by the liver [5] after infusion, even in the presence of hemorrhagic shock. This property makes RL valuable in the treatment of metabolic acidosis. Ringer's lactate not only supplies all necessary electrolytes but also provides bicarbonate, it is advantageous in various surgical conditions.

For its buffering effect, which corrects metabolic acidosis, RL contains lactate instead of bicarbonate, as sodium lactate is more stable in intravenous (IV) fluids during storage. However, it's essential to note that in conditions like lactic acidosis, sepsis, or liver failure, the conversion of sodium lactate to bicarbonate may be impaired [6].

4. Understanding Ringer's lactate and lactic acidosis: The belief that Ringer's lactate causes lactic acidosis is a common misconception [7, 8]. To address this misunderstanding, it's essential to differentiate between the terms "lactate" and "lactic acid." Understanding the distinction between lactic acid and the sodium lactate content in Ringer's lactate solution is both crucial and fascinating.

Lactate is an anion, a negatively charged ion, present in both lactic acid and sodium lactate. Lactic acid contains a positively charged cation, hydrogen (H^+ ion), which binds with lactate, making it acidic, with a pH ranging from approximately 2.44 to 3.51. In contrast, sodium lactate has a positively charged cation, sodium (Na^+ ion), binding with lactate, resulting in an alkaline pH range of 6.0 to 7.3. Therefore, the pH of both substances is the complete opposite.

It's important to note that lactic acid is indeed an "acid" and can be harmful due to the presence of hydrogen ions, leading to acidosis.

On the other hand, sodium lactate in Ringer's lactate is benign. Ringer's lactate will never induce lactic acidosis because it contains sodium lactate, which is a "conjugate base." Interestingly, sodium lactate absorbs hydrogen ions during its metabolism, leading to metabolic alkalosis [4, 6].

5. Effect on lactate level: The administration of RL does not increase serum lactate concentrations in hemodynamically stable adults [9]. However, when RL is administered to patients with frank hepatic failure, it can result in lactate accumulation, leading to elevated lactate concentrations in the bloodstream. As the serum lactate level serves as a valuable tool for assessing the severity of lactic acidosis, an increase in serum lactate levels due to RL can lead to confusion in interpretation [7].

   However, it's important to note that any increase in serum lactate levels due to RL is generally minimal and lacks clinical significance [10].

6. Effect on chloride level: The chloride concentration of RL is 109 mEq/L, which closely matches the normal plasma chloride level and therefore avoids the risk of hyperchloremic acidosis (unlike normal saline).

7. Effect on potassium level: The potassium concentration of RL is 4 mEq/L, which is similar to that of plasma but is insufficient to correct severe potassium deficiency.

   In hyperkalemia, potassium containing RL should be avoided, and potassium free normal saline is safe is a myth [11, 12]. Ringer's lactate is preferable to normal saline in hyperkalemia [13, 14].

Here are three reasons for the low risk of aggravation of hyperkalemia with RL:

1. Potassium is a predominantly intracellular ion. 98% of potassium is distributed in the intracellular compartment, and the alkalinizing effect of RL prevents potassium from shifting from intracellular fluid (ICF) to ECF compartments. On the contrary, large-volume normal saline-induced hyperchloremic acidosis can significantly shift the potassium out of the cells and aggravate hyperkalemia.

2. In hyperkalemic patients (serum potassium >5.5 mEq/L), administration of lower potassium containing Ringer's lactate (4 mEq/L) will actually lower the serum potassium level.

3. With the addition of just 4 mEq of potassium in large ECF volume (20% of body weight in adults, 12 liters in 60 kg person), the rise in serum potassium is negligible.

Indications

Balanced crystalloids are increasingly recommended as first line resuscitation fluids in surgical patients, trauma, and burns:

1. Resuscitation fluid: Currently, RL is increasingly advocated as a first-line resuscitation fluid [15–18]. RL is commonly used for correcting severe hypovolemia with a rapid fluid infusion. When a large volume of fluid administration is required for resuscitation, compared to normal saline, RL is preferred because it does not cause hyperchloremia and acidosis [19]. RL's chloride content is more physiological compared to normal saline (109 vs. 154 mEq/L) [20], and RL additionally

provides 28 mEq/L bicarbonate to correct acidosis.

2. For replacing the fluid in trauma and surgical patients:

   • Preoperative patients: To correct hypotension due to blood loss and to replace losses due to diarrhea or bowel preparation [21].

   • Induction of anesthesia: About 500 ml or 20 mL/kg of RL is administered rapidly (within the first 5–10 min) as a bolus, simultaneously with spinal anesthesia (co-load), to prevent spinal anesthesia induced hypotension [22, 23].

   • Intraoperative and postoperative patients: To replace the loss of a small volume of blood and to maintain normal ECF fluid and electrolyte balance during and after surgery [24].

3. Aggressive fluid replacement: RL is a preferred fluid for aggressive fluid replacement in sepsis [25], burns [26], fractures, and acute pancreatitis [27, 28]. In acute pancreatitis, Ringer's lactate is the preferred choice for fluid resuscitation due to its lower risk of systemic and local complications, as well as its association with improved outcomes including reduced need for intensive care, shorter hospitalization, and decreased severity and mortality [27, 28].

4. Diarrhea induced hypovolemia with hypokalemic metabolic acidosis is effectively treated with RL. RL is the fluid of choice for the initial treatment of diarrhea induced dehydration, even in pediatric practice.

5. **Diabetic ketoacidosis:** The use of RL is increasingly considered in treating patients with diabetic ketoacidosis (DKA) because it lacks dextrose, has a chloride concentration of 109 mEq/L (thereby reducing the risk of hyperchloremic metabolic acidosis), and effectively addresses acidosis by providing bicarbonate. Various trials have demonstrated the benefits of balanced crystalloids, such as lower total cost, lower rates of cerebral edema [29], and earlier and faster resolution of acidosis [30, 31]. Therefore, its use is included in recent guidelines for treating DKA [32, 33].

6. Used to wash the eyes after a chemical burn because it neutralizes and flushes out irritants and reduces the risk of further damage to the eyes.

7. Sterile irrigation of body cavity, wounds, burns, etc.

Contraindications and precautions

1. In severe liver failure and severe hemorrhagic shock, Ringer's lactate is usually avoided due to the impaired capacity of the liver to regenerate bicarbonate from lactate [12, 34]. When RL is used for the resuscitation of moderate hypovolemic shock, generally, it does not increase lactate levels substantially or adversely affect the outcome.

2. Avoid RL in head injury and brain edema. As the osmolality of RL is low compared to plasma (273 vs. 290 mOsm/L), RL may exacerbate cerebral edema [35].

3. In renal failure, congestive heart failure and anasarca use RL cautiously because of the risk of volume overload due to sodium overload.

4. In vomiting, continuous nasogastric aspiration, and metabolic alkalosis:

Loss of hydrochloric acid containing gastric juice can lead to metabolic alkalosis. As RL provides 28 mEq/L bicarbonate, it can cause worsening of metabolic alkalosis and therefore is not preferred in such patients.

5. Metformin-associated lactic acidosis: As hepatic metabolism of the lactate is impaired in metformin-associated lactic acidosis, avoid RL in such diabetic patients [10].

6. Along with blood transfusion: Calcium in RL binds with the citrate anticoagulant in the transfused blood, which can inactivate the anticoagulant effect of citrate and promote the formation of clots in donor blood. Because of the potential risk of clotting, simultaneous infusion of RL and blood products in one IV line is usually avoided [36]. However, few studies have reported that Ringer's lactate can be administered safely in patients requiring rapid blood transfusions [37, 38].

7. Avoid RL with an injection ceftriaxone. Do not mix, reconstitute, or simultaneously infuse ceftriaxone with Ringer's lactate. Mixing of calcium containing RL solution with ceftriaxone causes the formation of the insoluble ceftriaxone calcium salt.

8. The calcium in RL binds with certain drugs (i.e., amphotericin, thiopental, ampicillin, doxycycline, etc.), and reduces their bioavailability and efficiency.

WHAT IS RINGER'S SOLUTION?

Ringer's solution was invented in 1880 by British physician Sydney Ringer. Ringer's solution is an isotonic fluid with 147 mEq/L of sodium, 4 mEq/L of potassium, 4 mEq/L of calcium, and 156 mEq/L of chloride. As compared to RL, sodium and chloride concentration are high in Ringer's solution, and it doesn't contain lactate (Table 4.1).

With its balanced composition offering more advantages, RL received greater acceptance and, over time, replaced the standard Ringer's solution as the preferred choice for routine use.

WHAT IS HARTMANN'S SOLUTION?

Hartmann's solution is routinely known as "Ringer's lactate solution". In 1930, American pediatrician Alexis Hartmann added lactate to correct acidosis in Ringer's solution and, therefore, named "Hartmann's solution".

NEWER BALANCED CRYSTALLOID SOLUTIONS

Newer balanced crystalloids are designed in such a way that its composition (sodium, potassium, osmolality) is similar to plasma and has better buffering agents (metabolizable anions). In preparing newer balanced crystalloids, lactate is replaced with metabolizable anions such as acetate, gluconate, and maleate as a precursor of bicarbonate (Table 4.1) [1, 39]. Balanced crystalloids containing acetate as a buffer show better buffering effects than lactate-buffered balanced crystalloids like RL [40]. The advantages of acetate over lactate are as follows:

• Acetate is metabolized in whole body cells and not only in the liver and therefore is safe and effective in patients with liver dysfunction [40, 41].

• Better buffering action because acetate makes bicarbonate faster than lactate (just 15 minutes after infusion) [41, 42].

• In shock, the ability to metabolize acetate is preserved, while lactate

Table 4.1 Composition of plasma, saline, and balanced crystalloids

Electrolyte mEq/L	Plasma	Normal saline	Ringer's lactate	Hartman's solution	Ringer's acetate	PlasmaLyte	Braun's sterofundin
Sodium	135–140	154	130	131	130	140	140
Potassium	3.5–5.5	0	4.0	5.0	5.0	5.0	4.0
Chloride	98–106	154	109	111	112	98	127
Calcium	4.5–5.5	0	3.0	4.0	3.0	0	5.0
Magnesium	1.5–3.0	0	0	0	2.0	3.0	2.0
Buffers	HCO_3 22–26	0	Lactate 28	Lactate 29	Acetate 27	Acetate 27 Gluconate 23	Acetate 24 Maleate 5.0
SID	40	0	28	27	27	50	29
pH	7.35–7.45	3.5–6.5	6.0–7.5	5.0–7.0	6.0–8.0	7.4	4.6–5.4
Osmolality mOsm/L	290	308	273	278	276	295	309

SID: Strong ion difference; Calcium 2 mEq/L: 1 mmol; Magnesium 2 mEq/L: 1 mmol; PlasmaLyte® from Baxter; Sterofundin® from B Braun

metabolism may be significantly impaired [43].

- Acetate is more efficiently metabolized than lactate, consuming less oxygen and producing less CO_2. Acetate has a lower respiratory quotient (0.5) than lactate; and for every 2 moles of acetate, only 1 mole of carbon dioxide is produced [44]. Lactate requires higher oxygen to produce bicarbonate [45].

- It does not affect serum lactate levels, so it will not misguide serial serum lactate measurements in shock states.

The newer generation of "balanced" solutions (such as the crystalloid solutions PlasmaLyte or Sterofundin ISO) also contains magnesium. As hypomagnesemia is associated with increased cardiac arrhythmia, longer ICU stays, higher mortality, and worse prognosis; magnesium in newer balanced crystalloid is beneficial.

The composition of different IV fluids is summarized in Table 4.1.

WHAT IS RINGER'S ACETATE SOLUTION?

The composition of Ringer's acetate solution is similar to RL, but the lactate buffer is replaced by acetate. The metabolism of both lactate and acetate results in the formation of bicarbonate in the body. Acetate is metabolized effectively, regardless of liver failure or severe shock [40]. Acetate is metabolized faster and in most tissues [46], so Ringer's acetate solution is a reasonable alternative to RL in patients with liver dysfunction. Ringer's acetate is the better solution, also in the presence of a compromised circulation in shock [43].

PLASMALYTE SOLUTION

PlasmaLyte, a newer balanced crystalloid solution, and Ringer's lactate are two commonly used balanced crystalloids [47]. PlasmaLyte 148 (Multiple Electrolytes Injection, Type 1, USP) is a newer balanced crystalloid solution closely mimics human plasma in terms of electrolyte content, osmolality, and pH [44, 48, 49].

Composition

One liter of fluid contains:
    Sodium 140 mEq
    Potassium 5 mEq
    Magnesium 3 mEq
    Chloride 98 mEq
    Acetate 27 mEq
    Gluconate 23 mEq
    Osmolality 294 mOsm/L
    pH 7.4 (6.5 to 8.0)

Each 100 ml contains: Sodium Chloride 526 mg, Sodium Gluconate 502 mg, Sodium Acetate Trihydrate 368 mg, Potassium Chloride 37 mg, and Magnesium Chloride 30 mg

Pharmacological basis

1. PlasmaLyte is a further refined form of balanced crystalloid with the concentration of sodium, chloride, and potassium, as well as pH and osmolality, similar to that of plasma [50].

2. The composition of balanced solution PlasmaLyte is similar to Ringer's lactate with the following difference:

    • PlasmaLyte is isotonic compared to the mildly hypotonic Ringer's lactate (osmolality 295 and 273 mOsm/L, respectively). PlasmaLyte has 140 mEq/L sodium as compared to 130 mEq/L sodium in RL.

    • As a bicarbonate precursor, PlasmaLyte has acetate and gluconate as compared to lactate in RL [44]. Acetate has better buffering action compared to lactate. As Gluconate is excreted in the urine after its partial metabolism by the liver, it does not contribute to the buffering effect of PlasmaLyte [40].

    • PlasmaLyte contains magnesium instead of calcium in RL.

3. As PlasmaLyte contains magnesium instead of calcium and has normal pH (pH 7.4), it is compatible with blood or blood components (unlike RL) [42]. PlasmaLyte can be infused concurrently with blood components or can be used as a diluent for red blood cells (RBC) transfusions.

Indications

Literature for recommendation to use the PlasmaLyte is growing. As PlasmaLyte is a better designed balanced solution, it is used for similar indications as balanced crystalloid RL.

1. Resuscitation of the critical patient: PlasmaLyte, is presumably the best choice for most critically ill patients who need fluid resuscitation [51], particularly in cases of septic shock [52] or hemorrhagic shock [53].

2. Diabetic ketoacidosis: Normal saline is the preferred fluid for resuscitation in the initial phase of diabetic ketoacidosis [54]. But the administration of large volume normal saline in DKA can cause harmful effects like hyperchloremia and hyperchloremic metabolic acidosis, and therefore is not the ideal fluid to use [55]. PlasmaLyte is dextrose free and may have a beneficial role instead of saline because of higher bicarbonate levels with faster initial resolution of metabolic acidosis, less hyperchloremia, and transiently improved blood pressure profile and urine output [56–58].

3. Liver dysfunction, liver resection, and liver transplantation: During hepatic

resection, the use of balanced crystalloids is recommended [59]. Amongst balanced crystalloids, PlasmaLyte has the advantage compared to RL in the presence of liver dysfunction, hepatic resection, and liver transplantation. During liver transplantation, major liver surgery, or in patients with acute or chronic liver insufficiency, hepatic metabolism of lactate in RL may be impaired, leading to hyperlactatemia [42]. The plasma lactate level is an important prognostic marker after liver resection [60], and a rise in lactate due to RL can create confusion in the interpretation of lactate levels [12]. Metabolism of acetate into bicarbonate is not entirely dependent on liver metabolism, and therefore acetate based resuscitation fluids (PlasmaLyte) would have a superior buffering effect than non-acetate-based fluids (RL) in the presence of liver dysfunction [40, 43, 61].

4. Kidney transplantation: Infusion of PlasmaLyte maintains better acid-base and electrolyte balance than normal saline and RL in kidney transplantation patients [62, 63].

5. Along with blood transfusions: As PlasmaLyte is calcium free, it is compatible with blood and blood products, unlike RL [42].

6. Intraoperative: PlasmaLyte is used for Intraoperative fluid replacement because of its better metabolic profile. However, there is currently insufficient evidence for routine clinical use of PlasmaLyte over other commercially available buffered or nonbuffered crystalloids [42, 50].

7. Head injury: For resuscitation, balanced crystalloids are preferred over normal saline [17]. But in traumatic brain injury, the large volume of balanced crystalloid RL is avoided because it is hypo-osmolar (osmolality 254 mOsm/L) and, therefore, may worsen cerebral edema leading to increased intracranial pressure causing increased mortality in neurosurgical patients [64, 65]. Recent systematic reviews have revealed that the use of balanced crystalloids, including isotonic solutions like PlasmaLyte (osmolality 295 mOsm/L), resulted in adverse outcomes in patients with aSAH and traumatic brain injury (TBI) [66, 67]. Therefore, it emphasizes the importance of avoiding the use of balanced crystalloids, including PlasmaLyte, in these patients.

8. Fluid therapy in children: According to NICE guidance, PlasmaLyte meets the requirements for use in children and young people and can be used for maintenance, replacement, and resuscitation fluid [49].

9. Diabetic ketoacidosis: The use of dextrose-free PlasmaLyte, with its balanced composition, is gaining popularity in the treatment of patients with diabetic ketoacidosis as it reduces the risk of hyperchloremic metabolic acidosis, corrects acidosis by providing bicarbonate and offers benefits like early and faster acidosis resolution, and reduced ICU and hospital stays leading to decreased total cost [30, 68, 69].

Contraindications and precautions

1. Use with caution or avoid PlasmaLyte in patients with metabolic or respiratory alkalosis, hypermagnesemia, hypocalcemia, fluid overload, or renal failure with oliguria or anuria.

2. In patients with hypermagnesemia, PlasmaLyte, which contains 1.5 mmol/L of magnesium, should be used with caution. Magnesium can induce bradycardia and increase peripheral vascular resistance leading to a decrease in microcirculation and worsening of organ ischemia [44].

3. Like most other crystalloid fluids, administration of a large volume of PlasmaLyte can lead to volume overload, weight gain due to swelling, and pulmonary edema [44].

STEROFUNDIN

Isotonic electrolyte solution Sterofundin/ Ringerfundin are lactate free, newer balanced crystalloid solutions with electrolyte composition similar to that of plasma [70].

Composition

One liter of fluid contains:
Sodium 145 mEq
Potassium 4 mEq
Calcium 5 mEq
Magnesium 2 mEq
Chloride 127 mEq
Acetate 24 mEq
Malate 5.0 mEq
Osmolality 309 mOsm/L
pH 5.5 (5.1 to 5.9)

Each 100 ml contains: Sodium Chloride 680 mg, Sodium Acetate Trihydrate 327 mg, Potassium Chloride 30 mg, Magnesium Chloride Hexahydrate 20 mg, Calcium Chloride Dihydrate 37 mg, and L-Malic acid 67 mg

Pharmacological basis

The composition of this newer balanced solution is similar to plasma with the following difference with Ringer's lactate:

• As compared to RL, Sterofundin has higher sodium (130 vs. 145 mEq/L), chloride (100 vs. 127 mEq/L) and osmolality (273 vs. 309 mOsm/L) [70].

• Both fluids contain potassium and calcium, but Sterofundin also contains magnesium, unlike RL.

• As a bicarbonate precursor, Sterofundin has two metabolizable ions, acetate, and malate, compared to only one metabolizable ion, lactate, in RL. Metabolism of acetate occurs early, while malate is metabolized slowly.

Indications

Lactate free balanced crystalloid Sterofundin is used for intraoperative fluid management [71, 72] and replacement of extracellular fluid losses where acidosis is present or imminent.

Contraindications and precautions

Use with caution or avoid in patients with fluid overload, severe congestive heart failure, or renal failure with oliguria or anuria, hyperkalemia, hypercalcemia, and metabolic alkalosis.

ISOLYTE-G

Isolyte-G (Electrolyte-G) is a multi-electrolyte solution used to replace the loss of gastric juice.

Composition

One liter of fluid supplies:
Hydrous Dextrose USP 50 gm
Sodium 65 mEq
Chloride 150 mEq
Potassium 17 mEq
Ammonium 69 mEq
Caloric value 170 kcal/L

Each 100 ml of fluid contains: Hydrous Dextrose USP 5.0 gm, Sodium Chloride

0.370 gm, Potassium Chloride 0.130 gm, Ammonium Chloride 0.370 gm

Pharmacological basis

During vomiting or continuous nasogastric aspiration, gastric juice is lost. Gastric juice contains 60 mEq/L sodium, 10 mEq/L potassium, 130 mEq/L chloride, and acidic content. So vomiting or continuous nasogastric aspiration will lead to hypochloremic, hypokalemic metabolic alkalosis. Isolyte-G is a gastric replacement solution. It provides all electrolytes lost by gastric juice, corrects alkalosis, and provides calories. Ammonium ions in Isolyte-G are converted into urea and hydrogen ions by the liver. Hydrogen ions produced will replace the deficit of hydrogen ions caused by the loss of gastric juice. Isolyte-G is the only available IV fluid which directly corrects metabolic alkalosis of any nature.

Indications

1. In vomiting and continuous gastric aspiration to replace the loss of gastric juice.
2. In the treatment of metabolic alkalosis, Isolyte-G provides hydrogen ions.

Contraindications

1. Hepatic failure: In severe liver disease, ammonium ions in Isolyte-G will not be converted into hydrogen ions. Accumulation of such unchanged ammonium ions may precipitate hepatic precoma in severe liver disease. Moreover, this process of conversion of ammonium ions into hydrogen ions will be an additional load to the already sick liver cells.

2. Renal failure: Isolyte-G may aggravate uremic acidosis (due to the addition of H^+ ions) and may lead to hyperkalemia in renal failure (due to 17 mEq/L potassium). So, Isolyte-G should be used judiciously or avoided in patients with renal failure.

3. Metabolic acidosis: By providing hydrogen ions, Isolyte-G will aggravate metabolic acidosis.

4. Severe vomiting with shock: Isolyte-G is contraindicated for the initial therapy of shock due to vomiting because it carries the risk of hyperkalemia due to its high potassium concentration and its poor ability to raise blood pressure due to low sodium concentration.

ISOLYTE-M

(Maintenance solution with 5% Dextrose)

Isolyte-M (Electrolyte-M) is a multi-electrolyte solution with dextrose, which is used to correct hypokalemia and to provide various electrolytes, calories, and water.

Composition

One liter of fluid supplies:
 Hydrous Dextrose USP 50 gm
 Sodium 37 mEq
 Chloride 49 mEq
 Potassium 35 mEq
 Phosphate 15 mEq
 Acetate 20 mEq
 Osmolality 390 mOsm/L
 pH 5.0 (4.0 to 6.0)
 Caloric value 170 kcal/L

Each 100 ml Contains: Hydrous Dextrose USP 5.0 gm, Sodium Chloride 0.091 gm, Sodium Acetate 0.280 gm, Potassium Chloride 0.150 gm, Dibasic Potassium Phosphate 0.130 gm

Pharmacological basis

Amongst different commercially available multi-electrolyte IV solutions, Isolyte-M is the richest source of potassium (35 mEq/L) and therefore is useful in the treatment of hypokalemia. Always ensure good urine output or normal renal status before its infusion.

The proportion of electrolytes in Isolyte-M is almost similar to the maintenance requirements of the body. As per NICE clinical guidelines for IV fluid therapy in adults in hospital (2013, updated 2017), the requirement of water is 25–30 mL/kg/day, and the requirement of sodium, potassium, and chloride is approximately 1 mEq/kg/day [73]. Based on this recommendation, for a person with 35 kg weight, the daily maintenance requirement of water is about 1,000 ml with 35 mEq of sodium and potassium. As Isolyte-M contains 37 mEq/L of sodium and 35 mEq/L of potassium, its composition closely matches with NICE recommendations for routine maintenance IV fluids in adults.

Furthermore, Isolyte-M corrects acidosis, provides energy, and supplies phosphate. So, this fluid fulfills the needs of body electrolytes, pH maintenance, caloric supply, and water requirements and, therefore, is a suitable fluid for maintenance fluid therapy and is named Isolyte-M. As the sodium concentration of Isolyte-M is low (37 mEq/L), avoid it in patients with hyponatremia.

It is not the preferred IV fluid in patients with significant salt and water depletion.

Avoid rapid infusion of Isolyte-M because it is rich in potassium (35 mEq/L) and phosphate (15 mEq/L); therefore, rapid infusion carries the risk of hyperkalemia; and hypocalcemia or tetany.

Indications

1. Suitable as a maintenance fluid for adults. But carefully observe and monitor patients for the development of hyponatremia as the sodium concentration of Isolyte-M is low (37 mEq/L).
2. To correct hypokalemia secondary to diarrhea, bilious vomiting, prolonged infusion of potassium free IV fluids, ulcerative colitis, etc.

Contraindications

1. Hyperkalemia and renal failure: As the potassium content of Isolyte-M is high (35 mEq/L), it should be avoided in patients with hyperkalemia and should be used cautiously or avoided in oliguric patients and the presence of significant renal failure due to potential risk of hyperkalemia.
2. Hyponatremia and water intoxication: As the sodium concentration of Isolyte-M is low (37 mEq/L), it should be avoided in such patients.
3. Adrenocortical insufficiency: As hyponatremia and hyperkalemia are common in adrenal insufficiency, Isolyte-M with high potassium and low sodium should be avoided in these patients.
4. Burns: In patients with severe burns, potassium concentration may be abnormally high due to tissue destruction and acidosis. Moreover, such patients require fluid with high sodium concentration, such as Ringer's lactate, rather than hypotonic fluid, such as Isolyte-M.
5. Hyperphosphatemia: As the phosphate content of Isolyte-M is very high (15 mEq/L), avoid it in patients with hyperphosphatemia.
6. Metabolic or respiratory alkalosis: Isolyte-M contains acetate (20

mEq/L), which gets converted into bicarbonate and aggravates alkalosis and, therefore, should be avoided.

ISOLYTE-P

(Electrolyte-P in Dextrose 5% parenteral solution)

Composition

One liter of fluid supplies:
  Hydrous Dextrose USP 50 gm
  Sodium 25 mEq
  Potassium 20 mEq
  Magnesium 3 mEq
  Chloride 22 mEq
  Acetate 23 mEq
  Phosphate (HPO4) 3 mEq
  Caloric value 170 kcal/L

Each 100 ml contains: Glucose 5.0 gm, Sodium Acetate 0.260 gm, Potassium Chloride 0.130 gm, Magnesium Chloride 0.031 gm, Dibasic Potassium Phosphate 0.026 gm

Pharmacological basis

Isolyte-P is a hypotonic multi-electrolyte fluid composition of which is based on the fluid and electrolyte requirement in healthy children at rest [74]. For over six decades, this hypotonic solution was used as a standard maintenance IV fluid for hospitalized children worldwide [75]. This solution provides electrolytes (Sodium, potassium, phosphate, magnesium, and chloride), maintains pH (acetate gets converted into bicarbonate), supplies calories, and replaces water deficit.

A prevailing to use hypotonic maintenance fluid, Isolyte-P, may be appropriate for a healthy child. Still, it may not apply to hospitalized children who are more likely to have a nonosmotic stimulus for antidiuretic hormone (ADH) production, such

as anxiety, stress, pain, etc. The administration of hypotonic maintenance fluid in hospitalized children with high ADH leads to water retention, causing iatrogenic hyponatremia and neurologic complications [76]. A patient-safety alert issued by the National Health Service recommended removing 0.18% saline from general-use areas for children, such as the emergency department and pediatric ward [77]. The unanimous current global recommendation is to avoid the use of hypotonic maintenance (Isolyte-P) as a maintenance IV fluid for hospitalized children [78–81].

Indications

Used in selected adult patients as a source of low sodium containing, potassium rich solution with multiple electrolytes, calories, and water for hydration. Additionally, it is an alkalinizing agent:

1. Excessive water loss or inability to concentrate urine (i.e., diabetes insipidus).

2. Hypernatremia. Because of low sodium, Isolyte-P may be used in adult patients with hypernatremia.

Contraindications

1. Hyponatremia and as a maintenance IV fluid: Isolyte-P has a low concentration of sodium (25 mEq/L), so it will aggravate pre-existing hyponatremia. Previously used as a maintenance fluid in infants and children, but currently abandoned because of the increased risk of hyponatremia.

2. Renal failure: Cautiously used in renal failure due to the high concentration of potassium (20 mEq/L).

3. Resuscitation fluid: Avoid Isolyte-P as a resuscitation fluid to correct

hypovolemic shock due to the following reasons:

- Because of low Na$^+$ concentration, the ability of Isolyte-P to correct intravascular volume and hypotension is poor.

- In an oliguric child, the rapid infusion of fluid with high potassium concentration (20 mEq/L) is not safe.

- Rapid infusion of a large volume of Isolyte-P can cause hyperglycemia and osmotic diuresis even in a child with a fluid deficit, which is not desirable.

REFERENCES

1. Guidet B, Soni N, Della Rocca G, et al. A balanced view of balanced solutions. Crit Care 2010;14:325.
2. Hoorn JE. Intravenous fluids: balancing solutions. J Nephrol 2017;30:485–492.
3. Myburgh JA, Mythen MG. Resuscitation fluids. N Engl J Med. 2013;369(13):1243–51.
4. Alex Yartsev. Response to 1L of Hartmann's compound sodium lactate. Deranged Physiology June 25, 2015. https://derangedphysiology.com/main/core-topics-intensive-care/manipulation-fluids-and-electrolytes/Chapter%202.3.4/response-1l-hartmanns-compound-sodium-lactate.
5. Gladden LB. Lactate metabolism: A new paradigm for the third millennium. J. Physiol. 2004;558:5–30.
6. Palevsky PM. Intravenous fluids. CJASN 2018;13(12):1912–1914.
7. Farkas J. Three myths about plasmalyte, normosol and LR. PulmCrit January 26, 2015. https://emcrit.org/pulmcrit/three-myths-about-plasmalyte-normosol-and-lr/.
8. Paul Marik. iSepsis – The lactate myths - EMCrit January 7, 2018 https://emcrit.org/isepsis/isepsis-lactate-myths/.
9. Didwania A, Miller J, Kassel D, et al. Effect of intravenous lactated Ringer's solution infusion on the circulating lactate concentration: Part 3. Results of a prospective randomized, double-blind, placebo-controlled trial. Crit Care Med 1997;25:1851–4.
10. Farkas J. Fluid selection & pH-guided fluid resuscitation. Pulmcrit (EMCrit) June 2019 https://emcrit.org/ibcc/fluid/.
11. Farkas, J. Myth-Busting: Lactated Ringers is safe in hyperkalemia and is superior to NS. Retrieved from PulmCrit.org (EMCrit) 2014, September 29. https://emcrit.org/pulmcrit/myth-busting-lactated-ringers-is-safe-in-hyperkalemia-and-is-superior-to-ns/.
12. Singh S, Davis D. Ringer's lactate. In: StatPearls [Internet]. Treasure Island (FL): StatPearls Publishing; 2019 Jan. Available from: https://www.ncbi.nlm.nih.gov/books/NBK500033/.
13. Weinberg L, Harris L, Bellomo R, et al. Effects of Intraoperative and early postoperative normal saline or Plasmalyte 148® On Hyperkalaemia in deceased donor renal transplantation: A double-blind randomized trial. Br J Anaesth. 2017;119(4):606–615.
14. Modi MP, Vora KS, Parikh GP, et al. A comparative study of impact of infusion of Ringer's lactate solution versus normal saline on acid–base balance and serum electrolytes. Saudi J Kidney Dis Transplant. 2012;23(1):135–7.
15. Miller TE, Bunke M, Nisbet P, et al. Fluid resuscitation practice patterns in intensive care units of the USA: a cross-sectional survey of critical care physicians. Perioper Med (Lond) 2016;5:15.
16. Jonsson, AB, Perner A. Changes from 2012 to 2015 in intravenous fluid solutions issued to hospital departments. Acta Anaesthesiol Scand. 2017;61(5):532–538.
17. Semler MW, Self WH, Wanderer JP, et al. Balanced crystalloids versus saline in critically ill adults. New Engl J Med 2018;378:829–839.
18. Semler MW, Kellum JA. Balanced crystalloid solutions. Am J Respir Crit Care Med. 2019;199(8):952–960.
19. Lehr AR, Rached-d'Astous S, Parker M, et al. Impact of balanced versus unbalanced fluid resuscitation on clinical outcomes in critically ill children: protocol for a systematic review and meta-analysis.Syst Rev. 2019;8(1):195.
20. Martini WZ, Cortez DS, Dubick MA. Comparisons of normal saline and lactated ringer's resuscitation on hemodynamics, metabolic responses, and coagulation in pigs after severe hemorrhagic shock. Scand J Trauma ResuscEmerg Med. 2013;21:86.
21. Spahn DR, Bouillon B, Cerny V, et al. The European guideline on management of major bleeding and coagulopathy following trauma: Fifth edition Critical Care 2019;23:98.
22. Loubert C. Fluid and vasopressor management for Cesarean delivery under spinal anesthesia: continuing professional development. Can J Anaesth 2012;59:604–19.
23. Kinsella SM, Carvalho B, Dyer RA, et al. International Consensus Statement on the Management of Hypotension with Vasopressors during Caesarean Section under Spinal Anaesthesia. Anaesthesia 2018;73:71–92.
24. Miller TE, Myles PS. Perioperative fluid therapy for major surgery. Anesthesiology 2019;130(5):825–832.
25. Crosignani A, Spina S, Marrazzo F, et al. Intravenous fluid therapy in patients with severe acute pancreatitis admitted to the intensive care unit: a narrative review. Ann Intensive Care. 2022;12(1):98.
26. Mehta M, Tudor GJ. Parkland Formula. [Updated 2023 Jun 19]. In: StatPearls [Internet]. Treasure Island (FL): StatPearls Publishing; 2023 Jan-. Available from: https://www.ncbi.nlm.nih.gov/books/NBK537190/
27. Aziz M, Ahmed Z, Weissman S, et al. Lactated Ringer's vs normal saline for acute pancreatitis: An updated

systematic review and meta-analysis. Pancreatology. 2021;21(7):1217–1223.

28. Ocskay K, Mátrai P, Hegyi P, et al. Lactated Ringer's Solution Reduces Severity, Mortality, Systemic and Local Complications in Acute Pancreatitis: A Systematic Review and Meta-Analysis. Biomedicines. 2023;11(2):321.

29. Bergmann KR, Abuzzahab MJ, Nowak J, et al. Resuscitation with Ringer's lactate compared with normal saline for pediatric diabetic ketoacidosis. Pediatr Emerg Care 2021;37(5):e236–e242.

30. Jahangir A, Jahangir A, Siddiqui FS, et al. Normal Saline Versus Low Chloride Solutions in Treatment of Diabetic Ketoacidosis: A Systematic Review of Clinical Trials. Cureus. 2022;14(1):e21324.

31. Catahay JA, Polintan ET, Casimiro M, et al. Balanced electrolyte solutions versus isotonic saline in adult patients with diabetic ketoacidosis: A systematic review and meta-analysis. Heart Lung. 2022;54:74–79.

32. JBDS. JBDS-IP Joint British Diabetes Societies Inpatient Care Group. The Management of Diabetic Ketoacidosis in Adults, March 2023 Update: JBDS Guidelines [Internet]. London: ABCD; 2023 Mar. Available from: https://abcd.care/sites/abcd.care/files/site_uploads/JBDS_Guidelines_Current/JBDS_02_DKA_Guideline_with_QR_code_March_2023.pdf.

33. Gripp K, Trottier ED, Thakore S, et al. Current recommendations for management of paediatric diabetic ketoacidosis. Paediatr Child Health. 2023;28(2):128–138.

34. Hussmann B, Lendemans S, de Groot H, et al. Volume replacement with ringer-lactate is detrimental in severe hemorrhagic shock but protective in moderate hemorrhagic shock: studies in arat model. Crit Care. 2014;18(1):R5.

35. Diringer MN. New trends in hyperosmolar therapy? Curr Opin Crit Care. 2013;19(2):77–82.

36. Ryden SE, Oberman HA. Compatibility of common intravenous solutions with CPD blood. Transfusion. 1975;15(3):250–5.

37. Lorenzo M, Davis JW, Negin S, et al. Can Ringer's lactate be used safely with blood transfusions? Am J Surg 1998;175(4):308–10.

38. Albert K, van Vlymen J, James P, et al. Ringer's lactate is compatible with the rapid infusion of AS-3 preserved packed red blood cells. Can J Anaesth. 2009;56(5):352–6.

39. Langer T, Santini A, Scotti E, et al. Intravenous balanced solutions: from physiology to clinical evidence. Anaesthesiology Intensive Therapy. 2015;47(1):s78–88.

40. Ergin B, Kapucu A, Guerci P, et al. The role of bicarbonate precursors in balanced fluids during haemorrhagic shock with and without compromised liver function. British Journal of Anaesthesia 2016;117(4):521–528.

41. Hamada T, Yamamoto M, Nakamaru K, et al. The pharmacokinetics of D-lactate, L-lactate and acetate in humans. Masui 1997;46(2):229–236.

42. Weinberg L, Collins N, Van Mourik K, et al. Plasmalyte 148: a clinical review. World J Crit Care Med 2016;5(4):235–250.

43. Kveim M, Nesbakken R. Utilization of exogenous acetate during canine haemorrhagic shock. Scand J Clin Lab Invest 1979;39(7):653–658.

44. Rizoli S. PlasmaLyte. J Trauma 2011;70:S17–8.

45. Hofmann-Kiefer KF, Chappell D, Kammerer T, et al. Influence of acetate and a lactate-based balanced infusion solution on acid base physiology and hemodynamics: an observational pilot study. Eur J Med Res. 2012;17(1):21.

46. Reddy S, Weinberg L, Young P. Crystalloid fluid therapy. Crit Care. 2016;20:59.

47. Kwong YD, Liu KD. Selection of intravenous fluids. Am J Kidney Dis. 2018;72(6):900–902.

48. Pfortmueller CA, Fleischmann E. Acetate-buffered crystalloid fluids: current knowledge, a systematic review. J Crit Care 2016;35:96–104.

49. Edwards ED, Mason BW. Plasmalyte for intravenous fluid maintenance, replacement or resuscitation as an alternative to other intravenous fluids in paediatric patients: a systematic review. J Pedia Health Care Med 2018;1(1):23–26.

50. Chatrath V, Ranjana, Kaur J, et al. A comparison of Plasmalyte a vs 0.9% saline for intraoperative fluid replacement in abdominal surgeries. International Journal of Contemporary Medical Research 2016;3(12):3579–3583.

51. Liu C, Mao Z, Hu P, et al. Fluid resuscitation in critically ill patients: a systematic review and network meta-analysis. Ther Clin Risk Manag. 2018;14:1701–1709.

52. Garnacho-Montero J, Fernández-Mondéjar E, Ferrer-Roca R, et al. Crystalloids and colloids in critical patient resuscitation. Med Intensiva. 2015;39(5):303–315.

53. Noritomi DT, Pereira AJ, Bugano DDG, et al. Impact of Plasmalyteph 7.4 on acid-base status and hemodynamics in a model of controlled hemorrhagic shock. Clinics. 2011;66(11):1969–1974.

54. Type1 diabetes in adults: diagnosis and management. NICE, 2015. Available at: www.nice.org.uk/ng17.

55. Farkas J. Four DKA Pearls. PulmCrit blog. May 2014 Available at https://emcrit.org/pulmcrit/four-dka-pearls/ Accessed June 9, 2019.

56. Chua HR, Venkatesh B, Stachowski E, et al. Plasmalyte 148 vs 0.9% saline for fluid resuscitation in diabetic ketoacidosis. J Crit Care. 2012;27(2):138–45.

57. Mahler SA, Conrad SA, Wang H, et al. Resuscitation with balanced electrolyte solution prevents hyperchloremic metabolic acidosis in patients with diabetic ketoacidosis. Am J Emerg Med. 2011;29(6):670–674.

58. Oliver WD, Willis GC, Hines MC, et al. Comparison of Plasmalyte A and sodium chloride 0.9% for fluid resuscitation of patients with diabetic ketoacidosis. Hosp Pharm. 2018;53(5):326–330.

59. Melloul E, HübnerM, ScottM, et al. Guidelines for perioperative care for liver surgery: Enhanced Recovery after Surgery (ERAS) Society recommendations. World J Surg 2016;40(10):2425–40.

60. Watanabe I, Mayumi T, Arishima T, et al. Hyperlactemia can Predict the prognosis of liver resection. Shock. 2007;28(1):35–8.

61. Shin WJ, Kim YK, Bang JY, et al. Lactate and liver function tests after living donor right hepatectomy: a comparison of solutions with and without lactate. Acta Anaesthesiol Scand. 2011;55(5):558–64.

62. Collins MG, Fahim MA, Pascoe EM, et al. Balanced crystalloid solution versus saline in deceased donor kidney transplantation (BEST-Fluids): a pragmatic, double-blind, randomised, controlled trial. Lancet. 2023;402(10396):105–117.

63. Venkataraman K, McTaggart SJ, Collins MG. Choosing fluids to reduce the risks of acute electrolyte disturbances in children after a kidney transplant. Kidney Int. 2024;105(2):247–250.

64. Alvis-Miranda HR, Castellar-Leones SM, Moscote-Salazar LR. Intravenous fluid therapy in traumatic brain injury and decompressive craniectomy. Bull Emerg Trauma. 2014;2(1):3–14.

65. Rowell SE, Fair KA, Barbosa RR, et al. The impact of pre-hospital administration of lactated ringer's solution versus normal saline in patients with traumatic brain injury. J Neurotrauma. 2016;33(11):1054–9.

66. Mistry AM, Magarik JA, Feldman MJ, et al. Saline versus Balanced Crystalloids for Adults with Aneurysmal Subarachnoid Hemorrhage: A Subgroup Analysis of the SMART Trial. Stroke Vasc Interv Neurol. 2022;2(4):e000128.

67. Zampieri FG, Damiani LP, Biondi RS, et al. Effects of balanced solution on short-term outcomes in traumatic brain injury patients: a secondary analysis of the BaSICS randomized trial. Rev Bras Ter Intensiva. 2022;34(4):410–417.

68. Ramanan M, Attokaran A, Murray L, et al. Sodium chloride or Plasmalyte-148 evaluation in severe diabetic ketoacidosis (SCOPE-DKA): a cluster, crossover, randomized, controlled trial. Intensive Care Med. 2021;47(11):1248–1257.

69. Othman MI, Nashwan AJ, Alfayoumi M, et al. Plasmalyte-148 Versus Normal Saline 0.9% in Diabetic Ketoacidosis Management: A Review. Cureus. 2023;15(6):e41079.

70. Hassan HM, Hasbullah AN, Ali S, et al. Ringer's lactate versus sterofundin ® ISOinpaediatric surgical patients: the acid base and electrolytes assessment. Journal of Anesthesiology. 2018;6(1):33–39.

71. Shariffuddin, Bathumana APP, Adeline C, et al. A comparison of Sterofundin and Ringer's lactate on intraoperative acid base and electrolytes status in children: a randomized controlled trial. Anaesth Critic Care Med J 2018;3(1):000128.

72. Hafizah M, Liu CY, Ooi JS. Normal saline versus balanced-salt solution as intravenous fluid therapy during neurosurgery: effects on acid-base balance and electrolytes. Journal of Neurosurgical Sciences2017;61(3):263–270.

73. Clinical guideline for intravenous fluid therapy in adults in hospital (2013, updated 2017). National Institute for Health and Care Excellence 2017.

74. Holliday MA, Segar WE. The maintenance need for water in parenteral fluid therapy. Pediatrics 1957;19(5):823–32.

75. Saba TG, Fairbairn J, Houghton F, et al. A randomized controlled trial of isotonic versus hypotonic maintenance intravenous fluids in hospitalized children. BMC Pediatrics. 2011;11:82.

76. Skippen P, Adderley R, Bennett M, et al. Iatrogenic hyponatremia in hospitalized children: can it be avoided? Paediatr Child Health. 2008;13(6):502–506.

77. National Patient Safety Agency. Patient Safety Alert 22. Reducing the risk of hyponatraemia when administering intravenous infusions to children. 2007. https://www.sps.nhs.uk/wp-content/uploads/2018/02/2007-NRLS-0409-Hyponatraemia-cen-PSA-2007-03-28-v1.pdf.

78. Moritz ML, Ayus JC. Maintenance intravenous fluids in acutely ill patients. N Engl J Med 2015;373(14):1350–60.

79. Duke T. Maintenance intravenous fluids for children: enough evidence, now for translation and action. Paediatr Int Child Health 2016;36(3):165–7.

80. Padua AP, Macaraya JR, Dans LF, et al. Isotonic versus hypotonic saline solution for maintenance intravenous fluid therapy in children: a systematic review. Pediatr Nephrol 2015;30(7):1163–72.

81. Feld LG, Neuspiel DR, Foster BA, et al. Clinical practice guideline: maintenance intravenous fluids in children. Pediatrics 2018;142(6):e20183083.

5 | Colloid Solutions

INTRODUCTION

Colloids are volume expanders commonly used in clinical practice for fluid resuscitation in hypovolaemic patients. Colloids are electrolyte solutions fortified with large molecular weight molecules that do not pass through semipermeable membranes and therefore are retained within the vascular system. Theoretically, colloids are more effective as plasma volume expanders and improve blood pressure more rapidly than crystalloids because of their intravascular distribution, the property of drawing fluid from extravascular spaces (due to their higher oncotic pressure), and prolonged effect [1, 2].

Compared to crystalloid fluids, colloids are three times more effective in expanding blood volume and increasing cardiac output [3]. So, when plasma or blood is not available immediately, the infusion of colloids to correct circulatory fluid volume is vital and often life-saving in patients with hemorrhagic shock. However, a blood transfusion is subsequently required to maintain the adequate capacity to carry oxygen. The potency of colloid fluids as plasma volume expanders differs with different commercially available colloid fluids, as shown in Table 5.1.

The major advantages and disadvantages of colloids are summarized in Table 5.2 [4]. Colloids vs. crystalloids in resuscitation is a long-standing debate. The colloids were an attractive and preferred choice for resuscitation before a decade [5]. The potential benefits of colloids are greater, rapid, and

Table 5.1 Plasma volume expansion with 100 ml of different colloid solutions

Type of fluid	Effective plasma volume expansion	Duration of plasma volume expansion
5% Albumin	90–100 ml	12–24 hrs
25% Albumin	300–500 ml	12–24 hrs
6% Hydroxyethyl starch	100 ml	6–24 hrs
10% Pentastarch	150 ml	12–24 hrs
10% Dextran-40	100–150 ml	1–2 6 hrs
6% Dextran-70	100 ml	8–12 hrs

more prolonged intravascular volume expansion with smaller volume [3, 6–9] and lesser salt and water overload and edema. The benefit of speedier achievement of hemodynamic goals with colloids is less organ damage and a decreased incidence of organ failure [3].

But various recent studies and meta-analyses of reviews on colloids vs. crystalloids in fluid resuscitation failed to show an improvement in the long-term outcomes with colloids [10]. Therefore, because of higher cost, greater adverse effects (e.g., worsening of acute kidney injury (AKI), coagulopathy, and anaphylaxis), and lack of proven better outcome benefits, the trend to use colloids as compared to crystalloids is decreasing [11–14].

Table 5.2 Advantages and disadvantages of colloids

Advantages	Disadvantages
• More rapid plasma volume expansion	• Greater cost
• Smaller volume than crystalloids needed for rapid resuscitation	• Risk of allergy/anaphylactic reaction
	• Renal dysfunction
• Prolonged increase in plasma volume	• Coagulopathy
	• Pruritus
• Lesser risks of edema than with crystalloids	• May interfere with crossmatch

There are currently no indications to use colloids instead of crystalloids routinely [9, 15], and colloids are recommended as adjunctive therapy as second-line resuscitation fluids [16, 17].

When the requirement of the crystalloid volume is large, it carries the risk of adverse effects. So colloids are used selectively along with balanced solutions to limit the amount of total fluid administered in such patients [3, 13, 18, 19]. In surgical and trauma patients with severe blood loss, colloids may be administered (usually in a 1:1 ratio) to achieve hemodynamic stability [20]. Currently, colloids are used sparingly in surgical and trauma patients; but avoided in sepsis, critically ill patients, and in patients with impaired renal function [21].

There are two types of colloids: Natural and semisynthetic. Natural colloids are derived from plasma protein, and human albumin is a commonly used solution. Three commonly used semisynthetic colloids are hydroxyethyl starches (HES), gelatin solutions, and dextran.

HUMAN ALBUMIN SOLUTION

Albumin is the most abundant, negatively charged natural plasma protein (3.5–5 gm/dL). Albumin represents approximately 50% of the total body protein content. Human albumin solution used in therapy is prepared from donated human blood and is commercially available as iso-oncotic 4–5% solutions and hyperoncotic 20–25% solutions. Albumin solutions do not require compatibility. Iso-oncotic 4–5% albumin solutions are used chiefly as a plasma volume expander in hypovolemic patients and for therapeutic plasmapheresis [22]. Hyperoncotic 20–25% albumin solutions (also referred to as "salt-poor" albumin) are appropriate in hypoproteinemic patients with edema where fluid and sodium intake is restricted. Human albumin solution is the costliest type of colloid. 20 to 100 times higher cost of albumin solution compared to crystalloid fluids is the major limitation of using albumin in practice [23].

The functions of albumin are:

- Maintains intravascular colloid oncotic pressure (responsible for 75–80% of the total colloid oncotic pressure of the plasma).

- Plays a significant role in the regulation of fluid body distribution.

- Maintains microvascular integrity.

- Binds and transports low molecular substances like bilirubin, hormones, vitamins, drugs, fatty acids, as well as minerals throughout the body.

- Major and predominant antioxidant in plasma, and functions as a free-radical scavenger.

Pharmacological basis

The physiological Properties of albumin solutions are summarized in Table 5.3. 5% albumin solution (50 gm/L) has a colloid osmotic pressure of 20 mm of Hg (which is similar to that of plasma) and expands the plasma volume to roughly the same as the infused volume. The oncotic effects of albumin last for about 12 to 24 hrs. Therefore, in hypovolemic patients, 5% albumin is a preferred solution.

The 25% human albumin solution has high osmotic pressure (70 mm Hg), while the 5% solution has osmotic pressure similar to plasma (20 mm Hg). Thus, the 25% solution is a potent plasma volume expander, increasing plasma volume by 4 to 5 times the amount infused (100 ml of 25% albumin can increase the plasma volume by 400–500 ml). 25% albumin is reserved for hypoalbuminemic patients with intravascular volume depletion but total body volume overload. In such patients with anasarca and oliguria, albumin infusion will shift fluid from the interstitial space to the intravascular space, and plasma volume expansion helps the kidney to excrete fluid from the body and reduce anasarca.

Infusion of 25% albumin solution causes 4 to 5 times greater volume expansion due to fluid shifts from the extravascular to the intravascular compartment. Because of this reason, avoid 25% albumin for volume resuscitation in hypovolemic patients or

Table 5.3 Physiological properties of albumin solutions						
Albumin solutions	Tonicity	Osmolality mOsmol/kg	Oncotic pressure (mm of Hg)	Plasma volume expansion	Duration of effect hrs	Sodium content mEq/L
5% albumin	Hypotonic	260	20–30	Same volume	12–24	130–160
25% albumin	Hypertonic	312	70–100	4 to 5 times	12–24	130–160

Table 5.4 Use of albumin solutions	
Recommended	Large volume paracentesis, Spontaneous bacterial peritonitis, Hepatorenal syndrome, Therapeutic plasma exchange
Selective use	Plasma volume expansion, Sepsis and septic shock, Nephrotic syndrome with massive refractory edema, Adult respiratory distress syndrome
Inappropriate use	Hypoalbuminemia with stable hemodynamics, Nutritional support as a source of protein

should be infused after adequate hydration with intravenous (IV) crystalloid solutions.

Indications

Major indications for using albumin infusion are summarized in Table 5.4 [24]:

1. **Plasma volume expansion:** When rapid volume expansion is required, as in acute hypovolemia with or without shock, burns, and severe acute albumin loss, albumin is an effective solution for replacement [25]. In hypovolemia, albumin solution is considered as an adjunct to crystalloids when a patient is unresponsive to crystalloids, requires substantial amounts of crystalloids to achieve hemodynamic endpoints, cannot tolerate large-volume crystalloid resuscitation [6, 26], or non-protein colloids are contraindicated [27]. As albumin is more expensive than crystalloids [28], its short supply is frequent [9], and is not superior to crystalloids (little or no difference in mortality, need for blood transfusion or need for renal replacement therapy); it is used selectively as the second line of treatment in resuscitation [10, 26]. Besides effectiveness, efficiency, and safety, do not use albumin when other therapeutic options are available [20].

2. **Sepsis and septic shock:** In patients with sepsis and septic shock who require substantial amounts of crystalloids, the use of 5% albumin along with crystalloids is beneficial for early resuscitation and intravascular volume replacement [19, 26, 29]. Albumin administration stabilizes hemodynamics, but it is not associated with mortality improvement compared with crystalloids [24, 25].

3. **Paracentesis:** Large volume paracentesis (removal of more than 5 L of ascitic fluid in a single session) is the first line of treatment for patients with tense and refractory ascites. It exerts lesser side effects than diuretics [30, 31]. Intravenous albumin replacement is the best available therapy after large volume paracentesis, which reduces paracentesis associated complications [32, 33]. After large volume paracentesis (>5 L) in cirrhotic ascites, replace 6–8 gm of albumin for every 1L of drained ascites [34]. The risk of development of post-paracentesis circulatory dysfunction (PPCD) is about 70% without albumin replacement [35]. Infusion of 25% albumin reduces the risk of PPCD, hyponatremia, and mortality among patients with cirrhosis and tense ascites [36, 37]. When ≤4 to 5 L of ascitic fluid is removed, albumin is not necessary because paracentesis induced circulatory dysfunction can be managed with electrolyte replacement [38].

4. **Spontaneous bacterial peritonitis:** Bacterial infection of the ascitic fluid in patients with cirrhosis is known as spontaneous bacterial peritonitis. In spontaneous bacterial peritonitis, correction of hypoalbuminemia and hypovolemia with 25% albumin prevents hemodynamic complications and reduces the incidence of renal impairment and mortality [39, 40]. The recommended dose of IV 25% albumin in spontaneous bacterial peritonitis is 1.5g/kg at the time of diagnosis (within six hours), followed by an additional 1g/kg infusion given on day 3 [31, 37].

5. **Hepatorenal syndrome:** Hepatorenal syndrome (HRS) is a life-threatening complication that occurs in patients with severe liver damage, most commonly caused by cirrhosis. It is characterized by progressive kidney failure due to a decrease in effective arterial blood volume [41]. HRS carries high morbidity and mortality and poor prognosis. A combination of 20 or 25% albumin with terlipressin (arteriolar vasoconstrictor in the splanchnic region) in hepatorenal syndrome helps to reduce the release of vasoconstrictors such as angiotensin and expands the effective arterial blood volume, which leads to improvement in renal function. A combination of 25% albumin infusion with terlipressin is an effective strategy for improving renal function. It carries a higher chance of recovery and increases the survival of patients with HRS [37, 42, 43]. The recommended dose of IV 25% albumin with terlipressin in HRS is 1g/kg/d (up to 100g/d) for at least two consecutive days with diuretic withdrawal, followed by a reduction of the dose to 20–40 gm daily days [31, 42–44].

6. **Therapeutic plasma exchange:** In therapeutic plasma exchange (TPE), 5% albumin is used as an exchange fluid to replace removed large volume plasma. As a human albumin solution is expensive, the cost of plasma exchange significantly increases when albumin is used as a replacement fluid. However, the benefit is that albumin is safer [45].

7. **Nephrotic syndrome:** 25% albumin infusion with furosemide is safe and effective in the treatment of hypoalbuminemia in diuretic resistant nephrotic syndrome with severe symptomatic edema (e.g., tense ascites limiting movement of the diaphragm, massive pleural effusions causing respiratory distress, oliguria with incipient acute kidney injury, etc.) or marked hypovolemia or [46–48]. But definitive recommendations about these treatment modalities are not established [49, 50].

8. **Correction of hypoalbuminemia:** 25% albumin is beneficial in treating hypoalbuminemia in liver cirrhosis with severe refractory ascites [51, 52]. Avoid using albumin to treat hypoalbuminemia in the absence of severe edema or acute hypotension.

9. **Ovarian hyperstimulation syndrome:** It is a severe iatrogenic complication of ovulation induction that results from the administration of human menopausal gonadotropin. In the severe form of OHSS, vascular permeability increases, which leads to massive fluid shifts from the intravascular compartment to the abdominal and pleural space. The resultant clinical presentation is rapid weight gain, oliguria, abdominal pain, vomiting, tense ascites, dyspnea, and hemodynamic instability.

Administration of 25% albumin is suggested as a plasma volume expander in severe OHSS [53], but its role is controversial [54, 55].

10. **Adult respiratory distress syndrome (ARDS):** A combination of 25% albumin with furosemide may improve oxygenation and hemodynamics without survival benefits in ARDS patients [56, 57].

Adverse effects

Adverse effects are rare such as nausea, vomiting, febrile reaction, and allergic reaction, including anaphylactic shock. Furthermore, as commercially available albumin solution is heat-treated preparation of human serum albumin (pasteurized for 10–11 hours at 60 °C), the risk of viral transmission is very low.

Precautions and contraindications

1. Volume overload: Rapid infusion of albumin expands circulatory volume rapidly with the potential risk of vascular overload and pulmonary edema.

2. Infuse albumin solution with caution in patients with severe anemia, congestive heart failure, kidney failure, or a history of hypersensitivity.

3. Traumatic brain injury: Avoid albumin infusion as a resuscitation fluid in patients with traumatic brain injury because albumin had worse outcomes than saline treated patients [58, 59].

4. Avoid 25% albumin for volume resuscitation in hypovolemic patients. 25% albumin can be used to treat hypovolemia after achieving adequate hydration or in the presence of edema is present.

5. The most common inappropriate use of albumin solution in clinical practice is its administration to correct hypoalbuminemia per se in hemodynamically stable patients or for parenteral nutrition [60, 61]. During the perioperative period, the use of albumin solution is not recommended to treat hypoalbuminemia if the patient is hemodynamically stable [24]. Albumin solution as a source of parenteral nutrition is unsuitable, insufficient, and expensive [62]. A decision to use albumin infusion should be made after consideration of underlying disease and patient conditions.

6. Albumin solution should not be added to parenteral nutrition solutions because of the potential for complications such as infections and physical as well as chemical incompatibility and instability.

Administration

Albumin infusion is compatible with IV fluids such as normal saline, Ringer's lactate, PlasmaLyte, and 5% Dextrose.

Rate of infusion

The infusion rate of albumin solutions is determined based on the patient's condition. High rates of albumin infusion can cause circulatory overload and pulmonary edema. Therefore, the recommended infusion rate for safe administration is 1 to 2 mL/min for 5% albumin solutions and less than 1 mL/min for 25% albumin solutions.

How much to give?

The amount of albumin solution to be administered will depend upon the patient's clinical condition and response to treatment.

For adults, it is suggested to administer an initial infusion of 25 gm, which can be achieved with 500 mL of a 5% albumin solution or 100 mL of a 25% solution. A suggested rate is 1 to 2 ml per minute for 5% albumin or less than 1 ml per minute for 25% albumin, although high rates may be required for the treatment of shock.

HYDROXYETHYL STARCH

Hydroxyethyl starch (HES) solutions are synthetic colloids used as a volume expander to prevent and treat hypovolemic shock following severe blood loss. HES solutions are low cost and are highly effective for increasing the intravascular volume for sustained periods [63, 64]. HES solutions for decades were most widely used for fluid resuscitation [65], but as recent data suggested a high risk of renal injury and death [66], its use is restricted and discouraged [30, 67, 68].

Hydroxyethyl starch solutions are composed of modified polysaccharides derived from natural starch. They contain more than 90% esterified amylopectin. Starch solutions are unstable because they are rapidly hydrolyzed by α-amylase. Hydroxyethylation of amylopectin retards its degradation,

which leads to longer plasma volume expansion. Corn (Maize), wheat, and potato are common sources of amylopectin.

Pharmacological basis

Hydroxyethyl starch solution expands circulatory plasma volume like serum albumin and dextran. Hydroxyethyl starch solutions are classified according to concentration, average molecular weight, molar substitution, and C2/C6 ratio (Summarized in Table 5.5) [1, 69].

1. **Concentration:** HES solutions are available as 6% and 10%. The concentration of the HES solution determines the initial volume expansion. For example, initial volume expansion with isooncotic 6% HES will close to 100% of infused volume, whereas, with hyperoncotic 10% solution, it will be considerably exceeding the infused volume (about 145%).

2. **Average molecular weight (MW):** Based on molecular weight, HES is classified into low (<70 kDa), medium (130–270 kDa), or high (>450 kDa) molecular weight solutions. The molecular weight of

Table 5.5 Classification of HES according to physiochemical properties				
Criteria	**Available options**			**Clinical effect**
Concentration	Hypooncotic	Iso-oncotic	Hyperoncotic	Determines the oncotic value and, therefore, the degree of volume expansion.
	3%	6%	10%	
Molecular weight (MW) kDa	Low	Medium	High	Determines the duration of persistence in intravascular space. Higher MW HES stays longer in circulation.
	70	130–270	>450	
Molar substitution (MS)	Low	Medium	High	MS and C2/C6 ratios determine the rates of HES degradation by serum α-amylase. A higher value of both suggests slower degradation and longer intravascular persistence.
	0.4	0.5	0.7	
C2/C6 ratio	Low		High	
	<8		>8	

initially marketed older HES solutions (i.e., hetastarch) was large (450 kDa). HES with higher MW takes a longer time to metabolize, stays longer in circulation, and, therefore, can expand intravascular volume for a longer duration. But to reduce complications, lower molecular sized (130 kDa) newer HES solutions (i.e., tetrastarch) are currently used.

3. **Molar substitution (MS):** HES solutions are prepared by hydroxyethylation of starch solutions. Hydroxyethylation retards starches' degradation, leading to their longer intravascular persistence. Molar substitution is defined as the average number of hydroxyethyl groups per unit of glucose. Based on the degree of molar substitution, HES are classified into high (0.7), medium (0.5), and low substituted (0.4) preparations. Commercially available HES solutions are divided into hetastarch (0.7), pentastarch ($\approx$0.5), and tetrastarch ($\approx$0.4) based on molar substitution (Table 5.5).

4. **C2/C6 ratio:** The C2/C6 ratio refers to the preferential hydroxyethylation site of the carbon atoms in the glucose ring. HES solutions are classified into low (<8) or high (>8) C2/C6 ratios. When the C2/C6 ratio of HES solutions is high, the half-life is longer, and the persistence in the blood is prolonged.

5. **Carrier solutions:** The two types of carrier solutions currently used as a base of HES solutions are normal (0.9%) saline and "balanced" solutions. Voluven is 6% hydroxyethyl starch 130/0.4 in 0.9% sodium chloride, and Volvulyte is 6% hydroxyethyl starch 130/0.4 in a balanced electrolyte solution.

How to interpret the formulation of hydroxyethyl starch solutions?

Three numbers identify the structural properties of hydroxyethyl starch preparations. In HES solutions, the first number indicates the concentration of the solution; the second number indicates the mean molecular weight, and the third number indicates the molar substitution ratio [1].

Interpretation of structural properties of 6% HES 130/0.4 solution

The first number 6% is the concentration of HES solution; the second number 130 is molecular weight, and the third number 0.4 is the molar substitution ratio. This HES solution is iso-oncotic (6% concentration) with medium molecular weight (130 kDa MW); and low molar substitution ratio (0.4 MS).

How do older and newer preparations of hydroxyethyl starch solutions differ?

HES introduced in the market in 1970 was improvised continuously, and currently, several preparations are available in the market (Summarized in Table 5.6). Older HES preparations such as 10% HES 200/0.5 are hyperoncotic (10% highly concentrated), have a high molecular weight (>200 kDa), and have a high degree of molar substitution (>0.6). Older, hyperoncotic HES preparations are associated with an increased risk of acute kidney injury, increased need for renal replacement therapy (RRT), pruritus, and prolongation of clotting times [70, 71].

To solve these problems, manufacturers produced and marketed new HES solutions. Newer HES Tetrastarch preparations such as 6% HES 130/0.4 are isooncotic (6% concentration), have a lower molecular weight (130 kDa),

Table 5.6 Preparations of hydroxyethyl starch solutions			
Generation	First	Second	Third
Preparation	Hetastarch	Pentastarch	Tetrastarch
Formulation	6% Hydroxyethyl starch 450/0.7	10% Hydroxyethyl starch 200/0.5	6% Hydroxyethyl starch 130/0.4
Molecular weight	450 kDa	200 kDa	130 kDa
Molar substitution	0.7	0.5	0.4
Duration of action	24–36 hours	6–12 hours	4–8 hours
Product name	Hespan	Pentaspan	Voluven

and have less degree of molar substitution (0.4).

Newer preparation Hydroxyethyl starch 130/0.4 does not accumulate in plasma compared to pentastarch and hetastarch solutions. Plasma clearance of hydroxyethyl starch 130/0.4 is about 20 times higher than hetastarch and considerably higher than for pentastarch.

IV infusions of hydroxyethyl starch solutions with a lower molecular weight (i.e., tetrastarch) are readily excreted in the urine. In comparison, a solution with a larger molecular weight (i.e., hetastarch) is metabolized and eliminated slowly. Data from recent literature demonstrate that third-generation HES has a much-improved safety profile [72].

Advantage

1. Nonantigenic, with fewer antigenic properties as compared to dextran.
2. HES does not interfere with blood grouping or crossmatching.
3. HES solutions are less expensive than albumin.
4. Expands plasma volume greater and for a longer period than crystalloids.
5. In trauma volume of HES required is equal to the volume of blood loss and has a greater and quicker effect in preventing hypotension over crystalloids [3].

Disadvantage

1. Serum amylase concentration increases during and for 3–5 days after discontinuing high molecular weight HES (hetastarch). Since high serum amylase concentration is an important tool for assessing acute pancreatitis, HES infusion-induced elevated serum amylase levels can be misleading and may result in diagnostic inaccuracies.
2. Like other colloids, it has no oxygen carrying capacity, so one should not allow hematocrit to fall below 25 to 30% after an infusion.

Adverse effects

1. **Allergic reactions:** HES can cause allergic or sensitive reactions such as vomiting, feverishness, urticaria, and wheezing. Pruritus is the most common, and anaphylactic reactions are extremely rare adverse effects of HES.
2. **Acute kidney injury:** The use of HES in severe sepsis and critically ill patients is associated with an increased incidence of acute kidney injury and a higher requirement for renal replacement therapy [10,

73–76]. Therefore, HES should be discontinued at the first indication of renal injury. As an increased need for renal replacement therapy is reported till 90 days, monitor kidney functions closely for a longer period following the administration of HES [77]. Administration of HES increases mortality compared to crystalloids [66], and among all colloids, HES is the only solution that increases mortality [6].

3. **Coagulopathy:** The use of HES is associated with a risk of coagulopathy due to the dilution of coagulation factors and its binding and inactivation of factor VIII and von Willebrand's factor. HES causes larger intraoperative blood loss compared to crystalloid therapy and an increased need for blood products [10, 78, 79]. The risk of dilutional coagulopathy associated with colloids varies in a dose-dependent manner among different colloids. Risk is greatest in dextran, moderate in HES and gelatins, and least in albumin [80–82].

Indications

HES was widely used because of its low cost and ability to expand intravascular volume for a prolonged period effectively [63].

Because of safety concerns, the use of HES solution as a volume expander is currently restricted to prevent and treat hypovolemic shock following a severe loss of blood that cannot be corrected by crystalloids alone [77, 83]. However, in surgical patients, meticulously administered HES is found to be safe in some studies and literature [9, 14, 84–88].

Currently, HES is recommended to be used at the lowest effective dose for the shortest period (dose less than 30 mL/kg and maximum duration <24 hours) for the initial phase of volume resuscitation [83].

Contraindications

1. Due to the risk of kidney injury and increased mortality, hydroxyethyl starch should not be used in patients with sepsis, burn injuries, or critical illness (Recommendation by both EMA - European Medicines Agency and USA FDA) [89, 90].

2. HES is contraindicated in patients with severe coagulopathy, congestive heart failure, dehydration, severe liver disease, intracranial or cerebral hemorrhage, impaired renal function, or in patients receiving renal replacement therapy and organ transplant patients. [83, 90].

3. Do not use HES as a maintenance IV fluid [83].

Administration

The rate of administration is variable depending on the blood loss and hemodynamic status of the patient but is usually less than 20 mL/kg. Because of possible anaphylactoid reactions, an initial 10 to 20 ml of HES should be infused slowly, under close observation.

The total daily dose of 6% HES 130/0.4 (Voluven) should not exceed 50 mL/kg, and the total daily dose of hetastarch (Hepspan, Hextnd) should not exceed 20 mL/kg.

In patients treated with HES, monitor renal function, liver function, and coagulation status closely.

GELATIN POLYMERS

Gelatin solutions are a type of intravenous colloid used for plasma volume expansion. In the last decade, the use of gelatin-based colloids has increased. It is commonly used as a potential alternative to HES due to the growing incidence of harmful effects and regulations to avoid HES [91]. However, the practice of using gelatines varies between countries. For example, gelatines are not available in the USA [19], while in the UK, it is the most frequently used colloid [65, 92].

Gelatines are sterile, pyrogen-free solutions prepared by hydrolysis of bovine collagen [93]. As gelatin is a degradation product of animal collagen, it is readily available and is the most cost effective choice of synthetic colloid [94].

Gelatin solutions contain a relatively low molecular weight (30–35 kD) polymer of the degraded gelatin with electrolytes [95]. The immediate plasma expansion effect of gelatin solutions is 80–100% of the administered volume. So compared to crystalloids, smaller volumes of gelatin solutions are required to produce the same expansion of intravascular volume. Gelatins are metabolized and excreted chiefly by the kidney. As Gelatins are excreted rapidly, their plasma volume expanding effect is short (just 1–2 hours), and therefore repeated infusions are necessary to maintain intravascular volume [96].

Commercially available three common preparations of gelatin solutions are urea-linked gelatines-polygeline (e.g., Haemaccel), succinylated gelatins (e.g., Gelofusine), and Oxypolygelatins (e.g., Gelifundol).

Composition

Hemaccel (urea-linked gelatin–polygeline)

Mean molecular weight 30,000 Dalton

Osmolality 301 mOsm/L

3.5% w/v solution contains: 35 gm polygeline polypeptides of degraded gelatin, 8.5 gm sodium chloride, 0.38 gm potassium chloride and 0.70 gm calcium chloride per 1000 ml (1L)

Sodium 145 mEq/L
Calcium 12.5 mEq (6.25 mmol)/L
Chloride 145 mEq/L
Potassium 5.1 mEq/L

Gelofusine (succinylated gelatin)

Mean molecular weight 26,500 Dalton.
Osmolality 274 mOsm/L

4% w/v solution contains: 40 gm succinylated gelatine and 7.0 gm sodium chloride per 1000 ml (1L)

Sodium 154 mEq/L
Chloride 120 mEq/L

Difference: Compared to Hemaccel, Gelofusine has low chloride content and no calcium and potassium.

Indications

1. For the rapid expansion of intravascular volume and correction of hypotension in shock, trauma, burns, and intraoperative or postoperative blood loss [97]. If acute hypovolaemia cannot be adequately treated using crystalloids alone, gelatin solutions may be considered [98]. But because of harmful effects and few trials supporting their use, gelatins cannot be recommended as a routine plasma expander and should be used cautiously [26, 91, 94, 99–101].

2. For priming Extra-corporeal circulation (e.g. heart-lung machine) [102].

3. Volume pre-loading prior to regional anesthesia [98].

Advantage

1. It is readily available and cheaper than albumin and other synthetic colloids.

2. Stable, long shelf lives, and can be stored at room temperature.

3. It does not affect coagulation, blood grouping, or cross matching.

4. No infusion ceiling, so large volume can be infused as compared to starches and dextrans [1].

5. Compared to starches and dextrans, the risk of acute kidney injury is lower with gelatins [103]. Gelatins are small sized molecules and, therefore, readily excreted by the kidney.

Adverse effects and precautions

1. Allergic reactions like flushing, urticaria, and rigor can occur.

2. Anaphylaxis: Gelatins carry the highest, three times higher risk of an anaphylactic reaction than other synthetic colloids [20, 100, 104]. In previous literature, anaphylactic reactions were reported to be fairly common (0.35%) but rarely severe [105]. However, in recent literature, the incidence is found to be low (6.2 per 100,000 exposures) [92] but usually severe or even life-threatening [106]. "Reaction presents with Latency" is a noteworthy and surprising feature of gelatin induced anaphylaxis. In the recent largest reported case series, latency (a median delay of 15 min) was observed between the administration of gelatin solutions and the development of the anaphylactic reaction [106]. The delayed presentation carries the risk of a missing diagnosis of a severe, life-threatening anaphylactic reaction.

The most frequent presenting sign of gelatin induced perioperative anaphylaxis is hypotension, which occurs even before the cutaneous manifestations develop [106], and therefore can lead to diagnostic confusion. So closely monitor all patients who receive gelatin solutions; and watch for unexplained hypotension or symptoms of anaphylaxis for early diagnosis and timely management. The surgeon and anesthetists should be aware that the reaction to gelatin infusions is one of the causes of acute worsening of hypotension intraoperatively.

3. In previous studies, the increased risk of acute kidney injury [107] and impairment of coagulation [108] were documented with gelatins. But in recent literature, gelatins have not shown increased acute kidney injury, clinically relevant bleeding, or mortality [26, 29].

4. It contains no preservatives, so ensure a clear solution before infusion.

5. Gelatin is a plasma expander like dextran, so it needs almost similar precautions.

6. As Hemaccel contains calcium, it should not be administered with citrated blood because it carries a risk of clotting. On the other hand, Gelofusine is calcium free and, therefore, can be given concomitantly with blood.

DEXTRAN

Dextran, a synthetic colloid, is a highly branched polysaccharide synthesized by the fermentation of natural sources of sugar, such as sucrose, by the bacterium Leuconostoc [109]. Dextran is commercially available in two forms, with a molecular weight of 70,000 (high-molecular weight dextran, Dextran 70) and with a molecular weight of 40,000 (low molecular weight dextran, Dextran 40) [110]. Dextrans are used primarily as antithrombotic agents and to lower blood viscosity rather than for volume expansion [111].

Pharmacological basis

1. Plasma volume expansion: Both forms effectively expand the intravascular volume, but dextran is not a substitute for whole blood because it has no oxygen carrying property. It is not a substitute for plasma proteins because it has many limitations, including a lack of clotting factors.

   - Dextran-40, as a 10% solution, produces a greater expansion of plasma volume (twice the infused volume) than dextran 70 as a 6% solution. But the duration of volume expansion of Dextran-40 is shorter (2–4 hours) due to its rapid renal excretion [112].

   - A solution of 6% dextran 70 expands the plasma volume slightly larger than the infused volume, and it remains in the intravascular space for a longer period (expand plasma volume for 6–8 hours), and therefore, is preferred over Dextran-40 for fluid resuscitation [1].

2. Improvement of microcirculation and prevention of thromboembolism: Low molecular dextran decreases blood viscosity and improves microcirculation independently of just volume expansion. It minimizes the sludging of blood that may accompany shock, prevents intravascular aggregation of red blood cells (RBC), and improves microcirculation in conditions or procedures associated with impaired circulation.

Indications

1. Correction of hypovolemia: For short term rapid expansion of plasma volume in conditions such as shock or impending shock from burns, surgery, hemorrhage, or trauma. Currently, the use of dextrans for resuscitation is not favored, and its use is declining because of adverse effects [99], lack of benefits over crystalloids [10], and lack of supporting safety evidence [6, 29].

2. Prophylaxis of deep vein thrombosis and postoperative and post traumatic thromboembolism. Current literature suggests limited clinical utility for its routine use because of its side effect and recommends safer and more effective agents for venous thromboembolism [113, 114].

3. To improve blood flow and microcirculation in threatened vascular gangrene [115].

4. Use as a priming fluid in pump oxygenators during extracorporeal circulation.

Adverse effects

1. Hypersensitivity reaction: As dextran is a potent antigen, sensitivity reactions are known to occur, but with better manufacturing techniques, incidences have decreased (less than 10%). Untoward reactions include itching, urticaria, joint pain, and rarely anaphylactic reactions [116]. An anaphylactic reaction induced by dextran is a rare but serious complication that can occur even with small doses [117, 118]. If the patient develops a hypersensitivity reaction, discontinue the drug immediately and treat it with epinephrine (Adrenalin) and/or antihistamines. Pretreatment with 20 ml of dextran 1 reduces the risk of anaphylactic reactions [119].

2. Acute kidney injury: In patients with reduced urine flow, rapid renal excretion of dextran-40 can result in high urinary concentration,

increasing urinary viscosity and potentially causing oliguria or acute kidney injury [120, 121].

3. Antithrombotic effects: Dextran-70 prolongs clot amplification time [122, 123] and may reduce the coagulability of the blood, and may increase blood loss [124].

4. Dextran may interfere with blood grouping and cross matching.

Contraindications

1. Bleeding disorders such as thrombocytopenia, hypofibrinogenemia, etc.

2. Known hypersensitivity to dextran.

3. Severe oligo-anuria and renal failure.

4. Severe CHF, pulmonary edema, or circulatory overload.

5. Severe dehydration.

Precautions

1. Dextran should be cautiously administered in a patient with:
   - Impaired renal function or oliguria.
   - Active hemorrhage.
   - Chronic liver disease and diabetes mellitus.
   - Patients at risk of developing pulmonary edema or CHF.

2. The hematocrit should not be allowed to fall below 30.

3. Correct dehydration before or at least during dextran infusion to maintain adequate urine flow and prevent AKI.

4. The anticoagulant effect of heparin is enhanced by dextran.

5. Dextran may interfere with blood grouping and cross matching, so collect and preserve blood samples prior to the infusion of dextran.

6. Along with dextran infusion, the patient may require blood, coagulation factors, or electrolytes.

Administration

Dextran-40

It is given by IV infusion as a 10% solution in 0.9% NaCl or 5% glucose. The dosage depends on the patient's need:

- In shock: An adult person with shock usually requires 500 ml of rapid IV infusion. In the first 24 hours, the total dose should not exceed 20 mL/kg. Dextran-40 can be given subsequently in dose of 10 mL/kg/day up to 5 days [125].

- Regimen for surgical prophylaxis: 500 ml of dextran 40 given preoperatively and daily postoperatively for 3 days.

- Extracorporeal circulation: In pump oxygenators, 10 to 20 mL/kg of a 10% dextran-40 solution is used as a priming fluid (alone or as an additive to other fluids).

Dextran-70

- Dextran-70, as a 6% solution, is given IV in emergencies for plasma volume expansion. The total dose should not exceed 1.2 gm/kg (20 mL/kg) in the first 24 hrs.

REFERENCES

1. Mitra S, Khandelwal P. Are all colloids same? How to select the right colloid? Indian J Anaesth 2009;53(3):592–607.

2. Severs D, Hoorn EJ, Rookmaaker MB. A Critical appraisal of intravenous fluids: from the physiological basis to clinical evidence. Nephrol Dial Transplant. 2015;30(2):178–87.

3. László I, Demeter G, Öveges N, et al. Volume-replacement ratio for crystalloids and colloids during bleeding and resuscitation: An Animal Experiment. Intensive Care Med Exp. 2017;5(1):52.

4. Colloids vs. crystalloids as resuscitation fluids. Deranged Physiology 2016 (https://derangedphysiology.com/main/required-reading/electrolytes-and-fluids/Chapter%202.2.5/colloids-vs.-crystalloids-resuscitation-fluids-0).

5. Sara J. Allen. Fluid therapy and outcome: balance is best. JECT. 2014;46(1):28–32.

6. Martin GS, Bassett P. Crystalloids vs. colloids for fluid resuscitation in the intensive care unit: a systematic

review and meta-analysis. Journal of Critical Care 2019;50:144–154.

7. Cortés DO, Barros TG, Njimi H, et al. Crystalloids versus colloids: exploring differences in fluid requirements by systematic review and meta-regression. Anesthesia Analgesia. 2015;120(2):389–402.

8. Hahn RG, Lyons G. The half-life of infusion fluids: An educational review. Eur J Anaesthesiol. 2016;33(7):475–482.

9. Kabon B, Sessler DI, Kurz A, et al. Effect of intraoperative goal-directed balanced crystalloid versus colloid administration on major postoperative morbidity: a randomized trial. Anesthesiology 2019;130(5):728–744.

10. Lewis SR, Pritchard MW, Evans DJ, et al. Colloids versus crystalloids for fluid resuscitation in critically ill people. Cochrane Database Systematic Reviews 2018;8(8):CD000567.

11. Miller TE, Bunke M, Nisbet P, et al. Fluid resuscitation practice patterns in intensive care units of the USA: a cross-sectional survey of critical care physicians. Perioper Med (Lond) 2016;5:15.

12. Jonsson AB, Perner A. Changes from 2012 to 2015 in intravenous fluid solutions issued to hospital departments. Acta Anaesthesiol Scand. 2017;61(5):532–538.

13. Heming N, Lamothe L, Jaber S, et al. Morbidity and mortality of crystalloids compared to colloids in critically ill surgical patients: a subgroup analysis of a randomized trial. Anesthesiology 2018;129(6):1149–1158.

14. Joosten A, Delaporte A, Mortier J, et al. Long-term impact of crystalloid versus colloid solutions on renal function and disability-free survival after major abdominal surgery. Anesthesiology 2019;130(2):227–236.

15. Spahn DR, Bouillon B, Cerny V, et al. The European guideline on management of major bleeding and coagulopathy following trauma: Fifth edition Critical Care 2019;23(1):98.

16. Perner A, Junttila E, Haney M, et al. Scandinavian clinical practice guideline on choice of fluid in resuscitation of critically ill patients with acute circulatory failure. Acta Anaesthesiol Scand. 2015;59(3):274–85.

17. Myburgh JA. Fluid resuscitation in acute medicine: what is the current situation? J Intern Med 2015;277(1):58–68.

18. Guidet B, Soni N, Rocca GD, et al. A balanced view of balanced solutions. Crit Care. 2010;14(5):325.

19. Vincent JL. Fluid management in the critically ill. Kidney International 2019;96(1):52–57.

20. Rehm M, Hulde N, Kammerer T, et al. State of the art in fluid and volume therapy: A user-friendly staged concept Anaesthesist 2019;68(Suppl 1):1–14.

21. Qureshi SH, Rizvi SI, Patel NN, et al. Meta-analysis of colloids versus crystalloids in critically ill, trauma and surgical patients. Br J Surg. 2016;103(1):14–26.

22. Clarke G, Yan M. Clinical Guide to Transfusion - Professional Education – Canadian Blood Services 2018. Chapter 3: Albumin. https://professionaleducation.blood.ca/en/transfusion/clinical-guide/albumin.

23. Jiang L, Jiang S, Zhang M, et al. Albumin versus other fluids for fluid resuscitation in patients with sepsis: a meta-analysis. PLoS One. 2014;9(12):e114666.

24. Yasumura S, Makino S, Matsumoto M, et al. Evidence-based guidelines for the use of albumin products. Japan Society of Transfusion Medicine and Cell Therapy. 2017;63(5):641–663.

25. Caironi P, Tognoni G, Masson S, et al. ALBIOS study investigators. Albumin replacement in patients with severe sepsis or septic shock. N Engl J Med. 2014;370:1412–1421.

26. Rhodes A, Evans LE, Alhazzani W, et al. Surviving sepsis campaign: International guidelines for management of sepsis and septic shock: 2016. Crit Care Med 2017;45(3):486–552.

27. Liumbruno GM, Bennardello F, Lattanzio A, et al. Recommendations for the use of albumin and immunoglobulins. Blood Transfus 2009;7(3):216–234.

28. Vincent JL, Russell JA, Jacob M, et al. Albumin administration in the acutely ill: what is new and where next? Crit Care 2014;18(4):231.

29. Martin C, Cortegiani A, Gregoretti C, et al. Choice of fluids in critically ill patients. BMC Anesthesiology 2018;18(1):200.

30. Annamalai A, Wisdom L, Herada M, et al. Management of refractory ascites in cirrhosis: are we out of date? World J Hepatol 2016;8(28):1182–1193.

31. European Association for the Study of the Liver. EASL Clinical Practice Guidelines for the management of patients with decompensated cirrhosis. J Hepatol. 2018;69(2):406–460.

32. Runken MC, Caraceni P, Fernandez J, et al. The cost-effectiveness of albumin in the treatment of decompensated cirrhosis in Germany, Italy, and Spain. Health Econ Rev. 2019;9(1):22.

33. Bernardi M, Caraceni P, Navickis RJ. Does the evidence support a survival benefit of albumin infusion in patients with cirrhosis undergoing large-volume paracentesis? Expert Rev Gastroenterol Hepatol. 2017;11(3):191–192.

34. Valerio C, Theocharidou E, Davenport A, et al. Human albumin solution for patients with cirrhosis and acute on chronic liver failure: beyond simple volume expansion. World J Hepatol 2016;8(7):345–354.

35. Kwok CS, Krupa L, Mahtani A, et al. Albumin reduces paracentesis-induced circulatory dysfunction and reduces death and renal impairment among patients with cirrhosis and infection: a systematic review and meta-analysis. Biomed Res Int. 2013;2013:295153.

36. Bernardi M, Caraceni P, Navickis RJ, et al. Albumin infusion in patients undergoing large-volume paracentesis: a meta-analysis of randomized trials. Hepatology 2012;55(4):1172–81.

37. AISF-SIMTI Position Paper: The appropriate use of albumin in patients with liver cirrhosis. Dig Liver Dis. 2016;48(1):4–15.

38. Runyon BA, AASLD. Introduction to the revised American association for the study of liver diseases practice guideline management of adult patients

with ascites due to cirrhosis 2012. Hepatology 2013;57(4):1651–1653.

39. Salerno F, Navickis RJ, Wilkes MM. Albumin infusion improves outcomes of patients with spontaneous bacterial peritonitis: a meta-analysis of randomized trials. Clin Gastroenterol Hepatol 2013;11(2):123–30.e1.

40. Nottingham antibiotic guidelines committee. Guidelines for the management of adult patients with spontaneous bacterial peritonitis or liver cirrhosis with upper gastrointestinal bleed. 2018 (https://www.nuh.nhs.uk/download.cfm?doc=docm93jijm4n627.pdf&ver=4771).

41. Dundar HZ, Yılmazlar T. Management of hepatorenal syndrome. World J Nephrol 2015;4(2):277–286.

42. Loftus M, Brown RS Jr, El-Farra NS, et al. Improving the Management of Hepatorenal Syndrome-Acute Kidney Injury Using an Updated Guidance and a New Treatment Paradigm. Gastroenterol Hepatol (N Y). 2023;19(9):527–536.

43. Bai Z, Méndez-Sánchez N, Romeiro FG, et al. Use of albumin infusion for cirrhosis-related complications: An international position statement. JHEP Rep. 2023;5(8):100785.

44. Wong F, Pappas SC, Curry MP, et al. Terlipressin plus Albumin for the Treatment of Type 1 Hepatorenal Syndrome. N Engl J Med 2021;384(9):818–828.

45. Winters JL, Brown D, Hazard E, et al. Cost-minimization analysis of the direct costs of TPE and IVIg in the treatment of guillain-barre syndrome. BMC Health Serv Res 2011;11:101.

46. Cyriac J, Balasubramanian R. Management of childhood nephrotic syndrome: Nottingham university hospitals NHS trust clinical guideline 2018.

47. Dharmaraj R, Hari P, Bagga A. Randomized cross-over trial comparing albumin and frusemide infusions in nephrotic syndrome. Pediatr. Nephrol. 2009;24(4):775–82.

48. Ellis D. Pathophysiology, evaluation, and management of edema in childhood nephrotic syndrome. Front. Pediatr. 2016;3:111.

49. Duffy M, Jain S, Harrell N, et al. Albumin and furosemide combination for management of edema in Nephrotic Syndrome: a review of clinical studies. Cells 2015;4(4):622–630.

50. Ho JJ, Adnan AS, Kueh YC, et al. Human albumin infusion for treating oedema in people with nephrotic syndrome. Cochrane Database of Systematic Reviews 2019;7(7):CD009692.

51. Di Pascoli M, Fasolato S, Piano S, et al. Long-term administration of human albumin improves survival in patients with cirrhosis and refractory ascites. Liver Int 2019;39(1):98–105.

52. Tajiri K, Futsukaichi Y, Yasuda I. Albumin administration for refractory ascites in cirrhotic patients. AME Med J 2019;4:10.

53. Royal College of Obstetricians and Gynaecologists. The Management of Ovarian Hyperstimulation Syndrome. Green-top Guideline 5. London: RCOG, 2016.

54. Prevention and treatment of moderate and severe ovarian hyperstimulation syndrome: a guideline.

Practice Committee of the American Society for Reproductive Medicine. Fertility and sterility. 2016;106(7):1634–1647.

55. Darii N, Pavlovic M, Doroftei B, et al. Unsuspected adverse effect of albumin in severe ovarian hyperstimulation syndrome: a case report. JBRA Assist Reprod. 2019;23(4):430–433.

56. Uhlig C, Silva PL, Deckert S, et al. Albumin versus crystalloid solutions in patients with the acute respiratory distress syndrome: a systematic review and meta-analysis. Critical Care 2014;18(1):R10.

57. Itagaki Y, Yoshida N, Banno M, et al. Efficacy of albumin with diuretics in mechanically ventilated patients with hypoalbuminemia: A systematic review and meta-analysis. Medicine (Baltimore). 2022;101(37):e30276.

58. SAFE Study Investigators; Australian and New Zealand Intensive Care Society Clinical Trials Group; Australian Red Cross Blood Service; et al. Saline or albumin for fluid resuscitation in patients with traumatic brain injury. N Engl J Med. 2007;357(9):874–84.

59. Rossi S, Picetti E, Zoerle T, et al. Fluid management in acute brain injury. Curr Neurol Neurosci Rep 2018;18(11):74.

60. Mirici-Cappa F, Caraceni P, Domenicali M, et al. How albumin administration for cirrhosis impacts on hospital albumin consumption and expenditure. World J Gastroenterol. 2011;17(30):3479–86.

61. Caraceni P, Domenicali M, Tovoli A, et al. Clinical indications for the albumin use: still a controversial issue. Eur J Intern Med. 2013;24(8):721–8.

62. Executive committee of the German medical association on the recommendation of the scientific advisory board. Cross-sectional guidelines for therapy with blood components and plasma derivatives: Chapter 5 Human albumin – revised. Transfus Med Hemother 2016;43(3):223–232.

63. Bunn F, Trivedi D. Colloid solutions for fluid resuscitation. Cochrane Database Syst Rev. 2012;2012(7):CD001319.

64. Jungheinrich C, Neff TA. Pharmacokinetics of hydroxyethyl starch. Clin Pharmacokinet. 2005;44(7):681–699.

65. Finfer S, Liu B, Taylor C, et al. Resuscitation fluid use in critically ill adults: an international cross-sectional study in 391 intensive care units. Crit. Care 2010;14:R185.

66. Zarychanski R, Abou-Setta AM, Turgeon AF, et al. Association of hydroxyethyl starch administration with mortality and acute kidney injury in critically ill patients requiring volume resuscitation: a systematic review and meta-analysis. JAMA 2013;309(7):678–688.

67. European Medicines Agency. Hydroxyethyl-starch solutions for infusion to be suspended – CMDh endorses PRAC recommendation: suspension due to serious risks of kidney injury and death in certain patient populations. EMA http://www.ema.europa.eu/ema/index.jsp?curl=pages/news_and_events/news/2018/01/news_detail_002892.jsp&mid=WC0b01ac058004d5c1 (2018).

68. Ünal MN, Reinhart K. Understanding the harms of HES: a review of the evidence to date. Turk J Anaesthesiol Reanim 2019;47(2):81–91.

69. Westphal M, James MF, Kozek-Langenecker S, et al. Hydroxyethyl starches: different products - different effects. Anesthesiology 2009;111(1):187–202.

70. Brunkhorst FM, Engel C, Bloos F, et al. Intensive insulin therapy and pentastarch resuscitation in severe sepsis. N. Engl.J. Med. 2008;358(2):125–139.

71. Myburgh JA, Mythen MG. Resuscitation fluids. N Engl J Med 2013;369:1243–1251.

72. McConnell M, Baisden J, Duncan E. Pro: third-generation hydroxyethyl starch solution is safe and effective for plasma volume expansion during cardiac surgery. Journal of Cardiothoracic and Vascular Anesthesia. 2018;32(1):570–575.

73. Myburgh JA, Finfer S, Bellomo R, et al. Hydroxyethyl starch or saline for fluid resuscitation in intensive care. N Engl J Med 2012;367:1901–1911.

74. Perner A, Haase N, Guttormsen AB. Hydroxyethyl starch 130/0.42 versus Ringer's acetate in severe sepsis. N Engl J Med. 2012;367(2):124–34.

75. Muller RB, Haase N, Lange T, et al. Acute kidney injury with hydroxyethyl starch 130/0.42 in severe sepsis. Acta Anaesthesiologica Scandinavica 2015;59(3):329–36.

76. Liu C, Zhi Mao Z, Hu1 P, et al. Fluid resuscitation in critically ill patients: a systematic review and network meta-analysis. Therapeutics and Clinical Risk Management 2018;14:1701–1709.

77. European Medicines Agency. Hydroxyethyl-starch Solutions (HES) no longer to be used in patients with sepsis or burn injuries or in critically ill patients EMA/809470/2013.

78. Haase N, Perner A, Hennings LI, et al. Hydroxyethyl starch 130/0.38–0.45 versus crystalloid or albumin in patients with sepsis: systematic review with meta-analysis and trial sequential analysis. BMJ 2013;346:f839.

79. Rasmussen KC, Secher NH, Pedersen T. Effect of perioperative crystalloid or colloid fluid therapy on hemorrhage, coagulation competence, and outcome: a systematic review and stratified meta-analysis. Medicine (Baltimore) 2016;95(31):e4498.

80. Kozek-Langenecker SA. Fluids and coagulation. Curr Opin Crit Care 2015;21(4):285–291.

81. Toyoda D, Shinoda S, Kotake Y. Pros and cons of tetra starch solution for critically ill patients. Journal of Intensive Care 2014;2:23.

82. Fenger-Eriksen C, Tonnesen E, Ingerslev J, et al. Mechanisms of hydroxyethyl starch-induced dilutional coagulopathy. J Thromb Haemost 2009;7(7):1099–1105.

83. European Medicines Agency. Hydroxyethyl starch solutions: CMDh introduces new measures to protect patients. Internet Document: 29 Jun 2018.

84. Martin C, Jacob M, Vicaut E, et al. Effect of waxy maize-derived hydroxyethyl starch 130/0.4 on renal function in surgical patients. Anesthesiology. 2013;118(2):387–94.

85. Van der Linden P, James M, Mythen M, et al. Safety of modern starches used during surgery. Anesth Analg. 2013;116(1):35–48.

86. Gillies MA, Habicher M, Jhanji S, et al. Incidence of postoperative death and acute kidney injury associated with IV 6% hydroxyethyl starch use: systematic review and meta-analysis. Br J Anaesth 2014;112(1):25–34.

87. Schetz M, Shaw AD, Vincent JL. Is the literature inconclusive about the harm of HES? We are not sure. Intensive Care Med. 2017;43(10):1526–1528.

88. Ertmer C, Zwißler B, Van Aken H, et al. Fluid therapy and outcome: a prospective observational study in 65 German intensive care units between 2010 and 2011. Ann Intensive Care. 2018;8(1):27.

89. Wiedermann C, Eisendle K. Comparison of hydroxyethyl starch regulatory summaries from the food and drug administration and the european medicines agency. Journal of Pharmaceutical Policy and Practice. 2017;10:12.

90. Food and drug administration FDA safety communication: boxed warning on increased mortality and severe renal injury, and additional warning on risk of bleeding, for use of hydroxyethyl starch solutions in some settings (2013). Available online at: http://wayback.archive-it.org/7993/20170112095648/http://www.fda.gov/BiologicsBloodVaccines/SafetyAvailability/ucm358271.htm.

91. Boer C, Bossers SM, Koning NJ. Choice of fluid type: physiological concepts and perioperative indications. Br J Anaesth. 2018;120(2):384–396.

92. Cook TM, Harper NJN, Farmer L, et al. Anaesthesia, surgery, and life-threatening allergic reactions: protocol and methods of the 6th National Audit Project (NAP6) of the Royal College of Anaesthetists. Br J Anaesth. 2018;121(1):124–133.

93. Davies MJ. Polygeline. Dev Biol Stand 1987;67:129–31.

94. Riley TT, Sanchez CK, Gauthier-Lewis M, et al. A concise review of colloids for fluid resuscitation in severe sepsis and septic shock. Austin J Pharmacol Ther 2014;2(3):1019.

95. Niemi TT, Miyashita R, Yamakage M. Colloid solutions: a clinical update. J Anesth. 2010;24(6):913–925.

96. Finfer S, Myburgh J, Bellomo R. Intravenous fluid therapy in critically ill adults. Nat Rev Nephrol 2018;14(9):541–557.

97. Shah S, Singh A, Kala S, et al. Polygeline in patients with hypovolemia caused by accidental trauma: a prospective, multicentric, safety study. Int Surg J 2018;5(4):1432–1437.

98. Marx G, Schindler AW, Mosch C, et al. Intravascular volume therapy in adults: guidelines from the association of the scientific medical societies in Germany. Eur J Anaesthesiol 2016;33(7):488–521.

99. Saw MM, Chandler B, Ho KM. Benefits and risks of using gelatin solution as a plasma expander for perioperative and critically ill patients: a meta-analysis. Anaesth Intensive Care 2012;40(1):17–32.

100. Moeller C, Fleischmann C, Thomas-Rueddel D, et al. How safe is gelatin? A systematic review and meta-analysis of Gelatin-containing plasma expanders vs crystalloids and albumin. Journal of Critical Care 35 2016;75–83.

101. Thomas-Rueddel DO, Vlasakov V, Reinhart K, et al. Safety of Gelatin for volume resuscitation – a systematic review and meta-analysis. Intensive Care Medicine 2012;38(7):1134–42.

102. Ghijselings I, Himpe D, Rex S. Safety of Gelatin solutions for the priming of cardiopulmonary bypass in cardiac surgery: a systematic review and meta-analysis. Perfusion. 2017;32(5):350–362.

103. Bayer O, Reinhart K, Sakr Y, et al. Renal effects of synthetic colloids and crystalloids in patients with severe sepsis: a prospective sequential comparison. Crit Care Med. 2011;39(6):1335–1342.

104. Laxenaire MC, Charpentier C, Feldman L. Anaphylactoid reactions to colloid plasma substitutes: incidence risk factors mechanisms. A French multicenter prospective study. Ann Fr Anest Reanim. 1994;13(3):301–10.

105. Hahn RG. Clinical pharmacology of infusion fluids. Acta medica lituanica. 2012;19(3):210–212.

106. Farooque S, Kenny M, Marshall SD. Anaphylaxis to intravenous Gelatin-based solutions: a case series examining clinical features and severity. Anaesthesia 2019;74(2):174–179.

107. Bayer O, Reinhart K, Kohl M, et al. Effects of fluid resuscitation with synthetic colloids or crystalloids alone on shock reversal, fluid balance, and patient outcomes in patients with severe sepsis: a prospective sequential analysis. Crit. Care Med. 2012;40(9):2543–2551.

108. Schramko A, Suojaranta-Ylinen R, Kuitunen A. et al. Hydroxyethylstarch and Gelatin solutions impair blood coagulation after cardiac surgery: a prospective randomized trial. British Journal of Anaesthesia 2010;104(6):691–7.

109. Naessens M, Cerdobbel A, Soetaert W, et al. Leuconostoc dextransucrase and dextran: production, properties and applications. J. Chem. Technol. Biotechnol. 2005;80:845–860.

110. Atik M. Dextran-40 and dextran-70. A review. Arch Surg 1967;94(5):664–67.

111. Perner A, Aneman A, Guttormsen AB, et al. Preferences for colloid use in scandinavian intensive care units. Acta Anaesthesiol Scand. 2008;52(6):750–8.

112. Dextran 1 - GLOWM (Internet) https://www.glowm.com/resources/glowm/cd/pages/drugs/d023.html.

113. Farber A, Tan TW, Rybin D, et al. Intraoperative use of dextran is associated with cardiac complications after carotid endarterectomy. J Vasc Surg. 2013;57(3):635–641.

114. Kozek-Langenecker S, Fenger-Eriksen C, Thienpont E, et al. European guidelines on perioperative venous thromboembolism prophylaxis: surgery in the elderly. Eur J Anaesthesiol. 2018;35(2):116–122.

115. Bag S, Behera A, Khandelwal N, et al. Improvement in blood supply after "Heparin-Dextran" therapy in patients of buerger's disease with critical limb ischemia. Indian J Surg. 2013;75(6):462–468.

116. Michelson E. Anaphylactic reaction to Dextrans. New Engl J Med 1968;278:552.

117. Ljungström KG, Renck H, Strandberg K, et al. Adverse reactions to dextran in Sweden 1970–1979. Acta Chirurgica Scandinavica, 1983;149(3):253–262.

118. Shiratori T, Sato A, Fukuzawa M, et al. Severe dextran-induced anaphylactic shock during induction of hypertension-hypervolemia-hemodilution therapy following subarachnoid hemorrhage hindawi publishing corporation case reports in critical care Volume 2015, Article ID 967560, 5 pages.

119. Zinderman CE, Landow L, Wise RP. Anaphylactoid reactions to dextran 40 and 70: reports to the United States food and drug administration, 1969 to 2004. J Vasc Surg 2006;43(5):1004–9.

120. Ferraboli R, Malheiro PS, Abdulkader RC, et al. Anuric acute renal failure caused by dextran 40 administration. Renal Failure 1997;19(2):303–306.

121. Dickenmann M, Oettl T, Mihatsch MJ. Osmotic nephrosis: acute kidney injury with accumulation of proximal tubular lysosomes due to administration of exogenous solutes Am J Kidney Dis 2008;51(3):491–503.

122. Sigurjonsson J, Hedman D, Bansch P, et al. Comparison of dextran and albumin on blood coagulation in patients undergoing major gynaecological surgery Perioperative Medicine 2018;7:21.

123. Schott U, Kander T, Bentzer P. Effects of dextran-70 and albumin on coagulation in experimental hemorrhage in the guinea pig. SHOCK 2018;50(3):366–372.

124. Rasmussen KC, Hoejskov M, Johansson PI, et al. Coagulation competence for predicting perioperative hemorrhage in patients treated with lactated Ringer's vs. Dextran - randomized controlled trial. BMC Anesth 2015;15:178.

125. 10% LMD in 5% Dextrose, 10% LMD in 0.9% Sodium Chloride (Dextran 40) [prescribing information]. Hospira, Inc. Revised: 8/2018.

Part 3

Fluid Replacement Strategies

6 | Principles, Planning, and Prescribing Fluid Therapy

INTRODUCTION AND IMPORTANCE

Fluid administration is commonly needed in hospitalized patients, especially in an emergency, ICU, and surgical units.

Why is it important to plan and prescribe fluid therapy meticulously?

- Fluid administration is an essential and most commonly required intravenous treatment in acutely ill hospitalized patients [1, 2].

- Timely, appropriate, and properly designed intravenous fluid administration is lifesaving [2, 3].

- The prescription plans of fluid therapy vary markedly in different dynamic phases, demanding frequent attention, evaluation, and necessary changes.

- Prescribing intravenous fluids is complex. Unfortunately, doctors' basic knowledge and understanding of prescribing intravenous (IV) fluids are poor, and errors in planning appropriate fluid type, rate, or volume lead to morbidity and mortality, which is preventable [4-7].

- IV fluids are not just an innocent bag of water; their under or over-administration may be potentially harmful [8-11].

- Fluid overload is one of the most common complications of overzealous IV fluid administration, which is often overlooked but is harmful [10, 12-18].

Because of the possibilities of multifactorial errors and harmful effects, it is recommended to use the right type of fluid, in the right volume at the right time, by the right route (in a similar way as using any other pharmacological prescription antibiotics or drugs), and tailor the fluid therapy to meet the patient's individualized needs which reduces the risks and improves the outcome [2, 10, 19, 20].

GOALS OF FLUID THERAPY

- To correct life-threatening imbalances (shock and hyperkalemia) urgently with a top priority.

- To provide daily maintenance needs of water, electrolytes, and nutrients.

- To replace preexisting water and electrolyte deficits.

- To replace ongoing fluid and electrolyte losses.

- To avoid complications or new disturbances as a result of improper therapy.

- To prescribe IV fluid in a proper order which can be easily understood and followed.

- To select proper IV fluid with the correct composition and determine the appropriate infusion rate.

PRINCIPLES OF FLUID THERAPY

For appropriate administration of IV fluids, it is essential to consider all aspects of given patients, such as indications, contraindications, potential benefits, and harms, in addition to clinical status and laboratory tests. To provide a basic understanding for planning and prescribing safe, effective, and personalized fluid therapy in individual patients, standard guidelines and protocols suggested are [20]:

1. 5 Rs (Resuscitation, Routine maintenance, Replacement, Redistribution, and Reassessment) recommended in NICE guidelines for fluid therapy in adults (summarized in Figure 6.1) [8].

2. The concept of four dynamic phases (SOS-D: Salvage/Rescue, Optimization, Stabilization, and De-escalation) of fluid therapy in treating shock is recommended by the ADQI (Acute Dialysis Quality Initiative) group is summarized in Figure 6.2 [2, 21].

3. The ROSE concept (Resuscitation, Optimization, Stabilization, Evacuation) of fluid therapy recommended by Malbrain et al. is summarized in Figure 6.3 [22].

4. The concept "Four D's" of fluid therapy: drug, dosing, duration, and de-escalation as summarized in Figure 6.4 [20, 23, 24].

PLANNING AND PRESCRIBING OF FLUID THERAPY

When a patient needs IV fluids, important considerations in planning fluid therapy are:

- The first and most important steps are detailed history and meticulous clinical examination (See, Chapter 15 "Fluid Assessment and Monitoring").

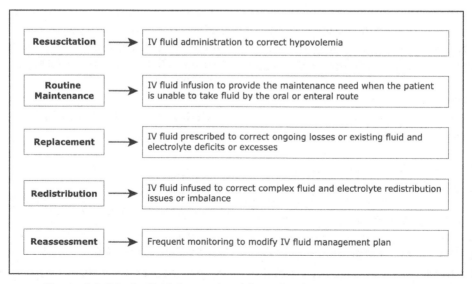

Resuscitation	→	IV fluid administration to correct hypovolemia
Routine Maintenance	→	IV fluid infusion to provide the maintenance need when the patient is unable to take fluid by the oral or enteral route
Replacement	→	IV fluid prescribed to correct ongoing losses or existing fluid and electrolyte deficits or excesses
Redistribution	→	IV fluid infused to correct complex fluid and electrolyte redistribution issues or imbalance
Reassessment	→	Frequent monitoring to modify IV fluid management plan

Figure 6.1 5 Rs for fluid therapy in adults NICE clinical guideline 174 [8].

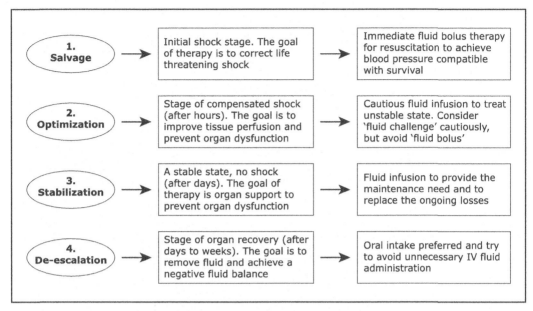

Figure 6.2 SOS-D concept of 4 phases in the treatment of shock [2, 21].

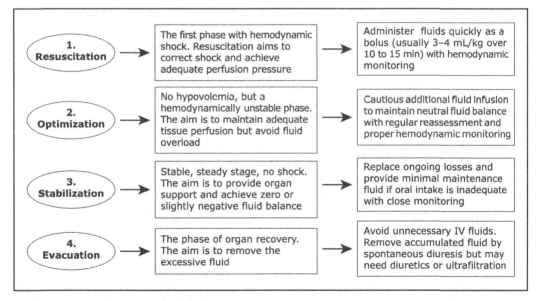

Figure 6.3 ROSE concept of 4 phases in the treatment of shock [22].

- Determine the treatment priorities based on the clinical status and laboratory parameters (emergency measures for the resuscitation first, followed by fluid administration to provide the maintenance needs, replace ongoing losses, and correct existing fluid and electrolyte deficits).

- What imbalances (deficit/excess) are present, their magnitude, and which underlying causative disorders are responsible?

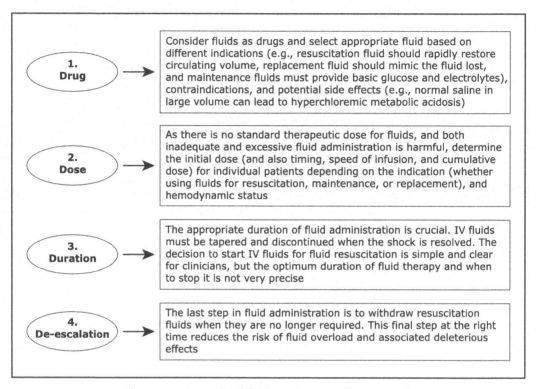

Figure 6.4 Four D's of fluid management [20, 23, 24].

- Consider renal, cardiac, and hepatic status and its severity while determining the requirements of individuals.

- Select appropriate IV fluid considering all the above factors (See, Chapters 2, 3, and 4). Plan volume, route, rate and administration duration judiciously to provide the optimum benefits but to avoid harmful effects.

- Reassessment and close monitoring to modify the management plan.

INDICATIONS

In clinical practice, the major indications of fluid administration are resuscitation, maintenance, replacing ongoing losses [20], and as a vehicle for administering medications. For example, in a study by Van Regenmortel et al., the need to administer fluids in about 15,000 hospitalized patients on the first day was 19.6% for resuscitation, 41.3% for maintenance and replacement, 6.2% for nutrition, and 26.3% for the administration of medications [14].

RESUSCITATION FLUIDS

Fluid resuscitation is the mainstay of therapy in hypovolemic shock or intravascular volume depletion due to significant and sudden fluid or blood losses. Details of timing, rate of fluid administration, and selection of fluids for resuscitation are discussed in Chapter 8 "Resuscitation Fluids".

MAINTENANCE FLUIDS

Haemodynamically stable patients who are unable or not allowed to drink water to meet their daily requirements of water and electrolytes need maintenance IV fluids. However, maintenance IV fluids should be administered cautiously because they may be a greater source of iatrogenic harm than resuscitation fluids due to excessive sodium, chloride, and water loading. The volume, composition, rate of fluid administration, and selection of fluids for maintenance are discussed in the Chapter 7 "Maintenance Fluid Therapy".

REPLACEMENT FLUIDS

In hemodynamically stable patients, in addition to routine maintenance IV fluids, replacement fluids are administered to correct deficits that cannot be compensated by oral intake alone.

Goals

The replacement fluid therapy aims to correct ongoing and existing fluid and electrolyte losses.

The volume of IV fluids

The volume of fluid lost is variable, and its accurate estimate is difficult. However, close clinical evaluation and frequent monitoring of laboratory tests provide a rough guide in determining the volume of fluid to be administered. In addition, the recent weight change (difference in pre-and post-deficit body weight) is a reliable parameter for accurately predicting the volume of fluid lost.

Rate of administration

The severity of volume depletion determines the fluid replacement rate. Hemodynamic monitoring helps in the effective and optimum speed of fluid administration. Cautious administration of fluid replacement is essential to avoid iatrogenic complications such as volume overload, osmotic demyelination

syndrome (when the hyponatremia is corrected too rapidly), and hyperkalemia (with generous potassium replacement).

Selection of replacement IV fluids

Replacement fluids are chosen in such a way that their composition mimics the fluid that is lost. Normal saline (0.9% sodium chloride), balanced crystalloid solutions, and dextrose 5% (with or without additional potassium as appropriate) are the most widely used replacement solutions [25]. Approximate electrolyte contents lost in common disorders (based upon the NICE guideline-2013) and empirically selected replacement fluids for initial administration are summarized in Table 6.1.

- Broad guidelines in selecting replacement fluids are administering saline to correct upper gastrointestinal (GI) losses, balanced crystalloids to correct lower GI losses, and providing additional potassium and bicarbonate supplementing based on individuals' needs.

- Upper GI losses (vomiting/nasogastric (NG) tube loss) contain higher concentrations of chloride and hydrogen and cause hypovolemic, hypochloremic metabolic alkalosis with hypokalemia. Preferred fluids for the administration are normal saline or dextrose saline with potassium supplementation.

- Losses during diarrhea are rich in potassium and bicarbonate and cause hypovolemic, hyperchloremic, metabolic acidosis with hypokalemia. Preferred IV fluids for the administration are balanced crystalloids (e.g., Ringer's lactate) when oral rehydration solution consumption is not possible or is inadequate.

Table 6.1 Composition of different body fluids lost and selection of IV fluids for their replacement								
Type of fluid loss	**Major electro-lytes lost**	**Approximate electrolyte content (mEq)**					**Initial re-placement fluid**	**Additional supplemen-tation**
		Na⁺	**K⁺**	**Cl⁻**	**H⁺**	**HCO₃**		
Vomiting/NG tube loss	Cl^-, H^+, Na^+	20–40	14	140	60–80	-	Saline	K^+
Diarrhea/excess colostomy loss	HCO_3, K^+	30–140	30–70	-	-	20–80	Balanced crystalloids	HCO_3, K^+
Jejunal loss (stoma/fistula)	Na^+, Cl^-	140	5.0	135	-	8.0	Saline	K^+
High volume ileal loss via a new stoma	Na^+, Cl^-	100–140	4.0–5.0	75–125	-	0–30	Balanced crystalloids	K^+, HCO_3
Lower volume ileal loss via established stoma or low fistula	Na^+, Cl^-, HCO_3	50–100	4.0–5.0	25–75	-	0–30	Balanced crystalloids	K^+, HCO_3
Pancreatic drain or fistula loss	Na^+, HCO_3	125–138	8.0	56	-	85	Balanced crystalloids	HCO_3, K^+
Biliary drainage loss	Na^+, Cl^-	145	5.0	105	-	30	Balanced crystalloids	HCO_3, K^+
Inappropriate urinary loss	Highly variable, monitor serum electrolytes closely						Selected as per electrolytes status	
"Pure" water loss (e.g., fever, dehydration, hyperventilation)	Fluid loss is poor in electrolytes and carries the risk of hypernatremia						Supplement hypotonic fluids based on the electrolyte status	

HCO_3: Bicarbonate; Cl^-: Chloride; H^+: Hydrogen; K^+: Potassium; Na^+: Sodium

Specific treatment is provided considering underlying disorders (e.g., diarrhea, vomiting, burns, diuretic therapy, diabetic ketoacidosis, diabetes insipidus, SIADH, etc.) and coexisting electrolyte disorders (e.g., hypernatremia, hyponatremia, hyperkalemia, hypokalemia, hypomagnesemia, and hypochloremia, etc.) and acid-base disorders (e.g., metabolic acidosis or metabolic alkalosis) which are discussed in different chapters.

REFERENCES

1. Finfer S, Myburgh J, Bellomo R. Intravenous fluid therapy in critically ill adults. Nat Rev Nephrol. 2018;14(9):541–557.

2. Martin C, Cortegiani A, Gregoretti C, et al. Choice of fluids in critically ill patients. BMC Anesthesiology 2018;181):200.

3. Hoste EA, Maitland K, Brudney CS, et al. Four phases of intravenous fluid therapy: a conceptual model. Br J Anaesth. 2014;113(5):740–747.

4. Ramsay G, Baggaley A, Vaughan Shaw PG et al. Variability in the prescribing of intravenous fluids: A cross sectional multicentre analysis of clinical practice. Int J Surg 2018;51:199–204.

5. Mathur A, Johnston G, Clark L. Improving intravenous fl¬uid prescribing. J R Coll Physicians Edinb 2020;50(2):181–187.

6. Drummond GB. Why is knowledge about fluid prescribing so poor? J R Coll Physicians Edinb 2020;50(3):343–350.

7. Leach R, Crichton S, Morton N, et al. Fluid management knowledge in hospital physicians: 'Greenshoots' of improvement but still a cause for concern. Clin Med (Lond). 2020;20(3):e26–e31.

8. National Clinical Guideline Centre (UK). Intravenous Fluid Therapy: Intravenous Fluid Therapy in Adults

in Hospital [Internet]. London: Royal College of Physicians (UK); 2013 Dec.

9. Benes J, Kirov M, Kuzkov V, et al. Fluid Therapy: Double-Edged Sword during Critical Care? Biomed Res Int. 2015;2015:729075.

10. Hawkins WA, Smith SE, Newsome AS, et al. Fluid Stewardship during Critical Illness: A Call to Action. J Pharm Pract. 2020;33(6):863–873.

11. Malbrain M. Optimising Fluid Therapy in the Critically Ill: Introduction to the 7D conceptual framework. iFAD 2021 Visit: https://www.fluidacademy.org/blog-foam/item/optimising-fluid-therapy-in-the-critically-ill.html.

12. Boyd JH, Forbes J, Nakada TA, et al. Fluid resuscitation in septic shock: a positive fluid balance and elevated central venous pressure are associated with increased mortality. Crit Care Med. 2011;39(2):259–265.

13. Mitchell KH, Carlbom D, Caldwell E, et al. Volume overload: prevalence, risk factors, and functional outcome in survivors of septic shock. Ann Am Thorac Soc. 2015;12(12):1837–1844.

14. Van Regenmortel N, Verbrugghe W, Roelant E, et al. Maintenance fluid therapy and fluid creep impose more significant fluid, sodium, and chloride burdens than resuscitation fluids in critically ill patients: a retrospective study in a tertiary mixed ICU population. Intensive Care Med. 2018;44(4):409–417.

15. Claure-Del Granado R, Mehta RL. Fluid overload in the ICU: evaluation and management. BMC Nephrol. 2016;17(1):109.

16. Neyra JA, Li X, Canepa-Escaro F, et al. Cumulative fluid balance and mortality in septic patients with or without acute kidney injury and chronic kidney disease. Crit Care Med. 2016;44(10):1891–1900.

17. Perez Nieto OR, Wong A, Lopez Fermin J, et al. Aiming for zero fluid accumulation: First, do no harm. Anaesthesiol Intensive Ther. 2021;53(2):162–178.

18. Barhight MF, Nelson D, Chong G, et al. Non-resuscitation fluid in excess of hydration requirements is associated with higher mortality in critically ill children. Pediatr Res. 2022;91(1):235–240.

19. Chappell D, Jacob M, Hofmann-Kiefer K, et al. A rational approach to perioperative fluid management. Anesthesiology. 2008;109(4):723–40.

20. Malbrain MLNG, Langer T, Annane D, et al. Intravenous fluid therapy in the perioperative and critical care setting: Executive summary of the International Fluid Academy (IFA). Ann Intensive Care. 2020;10(1):64.

21. Vincent JL, De Backer D. Circulatory shock. N Engl J Med 2013;369(18):1726–34.

22. Malbrain ML, Marik PE, Witters I, et al. Fluid overload, de-resuscitation, and outcomes in critically ill or injured patients: a systematic review with suggestions for clinical practice. Anaesthesiol Intensive Ther. 2014;46(5):361–380.

23. Malbrain ML, Van Regenmortel N, Owczuk R. It is time to consider the four D's of fluid management. Anaesthesiol Intensive Ther. 2015;47(Spec No):s1–s5.

24. Malbrain MLNG, Van Regenmortel N, Saugel B, et al. Principles of fluid management and stewardship in septic shock: it is time to consider the four D's and the four phases of fluid therapy. Ann Intensive Care. 2018;8(1):66.

25. National Institute for Health and Care Excellence Guideline for Intravenous fluid therapy in adults in hospital (CG174), 2013-Updated May 2017 (https://www.nice.org.uk/guidance/cg174).

7 | Maintenance Fluid Therapy

MAINTENANCE FLUIDS

Patients who are euvolemic, hemodynamically stable but unable to take adequate fluid by oral or enteral route need maintenance intravenous (IV) fluids to replace anticipated insensible (such as respiration, perspiration, and stools) and sensible (such as urine) losses [1].

PHYSIOLOGICAL BASIS

The goal of maintenance IV fluid is to replace the ongoing daily physiologic losses such as urine, feces, and sweat, maintain normal water and electrolyte balance and provide adequate calories to avoid starvation ketosis [1, 2].

Ideal maintenance IV fluid should provide adequate water and electrolytes to preserve the extracellular volume and ensure proper tissue perfusion without causing volume depletion, fluid overload, or electrolyte disturbances, along with supplementation for optimal calories [1].

Sodium concentration of maintenance fluids

Sodium concentration of maintenance IV fluids is a crucial but debatable issue discussed in many studies, which needs special consideration because of its two common and potentially harmful effects, hyponatremia [3, 4] and volume overload [5, 6].

How much sodium concentration is appropriate for the maintenance IV fluids in adult patients?

The concepts of appropriate sodium concentration of maintenance IV fluids in adults are changing like a pendulum shift.

A. Initially, the use of hypotonic fluids as a maintenance IV fluid was recommended in children

Administering hypotonic fluids (0.18–0.3% sodium chloride) as a maintenance fluid was a routine practice for about half a century, based on the Holliday–Segar formula published in 1957 [7].

B. The use of isotonic fluids as maintenance IV fluids recommended to avoid hyponatremia

Since the 1990s, multiple studies have shown strong evidence of increased risk of hyponatremia with hypotonic fluids, especially in children, and therefore the use of hypotonic fluids as a maintenance fluid is strongly discouraged [3, 8–12].

Current guidelines (2015 NICE guideline, 2015 North American publication, and 2018 American Academy of Pediatrics) have strongly recommended isotonic fluids for maintenance fluid therapy and abandoned hypotonic fluids as a maintenance fluid in children [1, 13, 14].

Even in adults, hospital-acquired hyponatremia is 'reported' with hypotonic fluid [15–17], and therefore, North American publication (Mortiz and Ayus 2015) disapprove the use of hypotonic maintenance fluid and recommends the use of isotonic fluid (glucose 5% sodium chloride 0.9%) as the first choice for routine maintenance fluids in acutely ill and major surgical patients [1].

C. Recent trend is to restrict the use of isotonic fluids to avoid iatrogenic fluid accumulation in adults

The trend is changing to use hypotonic maintenance fluid and use isotonic maintenance fluid judiciously in adults because:

- Compared to resuscitation fluids, maintenance fluids may be the largest source of iatrogenic harm [6, 18, 19], so the right selection of fluid is critical.

- The kidney can absorb sodium efficiently under the influence of aldosterone but lacks the dedicated mechanism for sodium excretion. So, the administration of sodium-rich maintenance fluids, even in patients with normal kidney function, can result in a positive cumulative fluid balance due to reduced urine output and inefficient renal sodium excretion [20–22].

- Fluid overload can cause harmful effects (e.g., heart failure, pulmonary edema, impaired bowel function, delayed wound healing, wound infections, and pressure ulcers, and is associated with increased incidence of acute kidney injury and longer mechanical ventilation), prolonged hospital stay, and high morbidity and mortality [5, 6, 23–28]. So, prevent isotonic maintenance fluid-induced avoidable sodium burdens, volume overload, and complications by special patient-specific approach and proper monitoring [21].

- The amount of sodium in maintenance fluid is an important determinant of iatrogenic fluid overload [20]. In a recent TOPMAST trial (2019), sodium-rich isotonic maintenance solutions (Na+ 154 mEq/L) compared to low sodium (Na+ 54 mEq/L) containing hypotonic fluids demonstrated a more positive cumulative fluid balance [29]. In contrast, this TOPMAST trial also demonstrated that despite lower sodium concentration, hypotonic fluids were associated with mild and asymptomatic hyponatremia, supporting the safety of using hypotonic maintenance fluids in adults [29].

Efforts of the current literature are to trade-off between the harmful effect of isotonic (e.g., sodium accumulation and volume overload) [21] and hypotonic (e.g., dangers of hyponatremia) [4] maintenance IV fluids.

Unphysiological sodium administration through maintenance IV fluids therapy and fluid creep needs increased attention because it is potentially harmful but avoidable [21].

Avoid iatrogenic fluid overload

The combined volume of maintenance fluids and the volume used as a vehicle to administer medications amounts to almost 60% of the total fluid administered and is a major cause of fluid overload [6]. Measures to avoid iatrogenic sodium and fluid overload in patients receiving such maintenance IV fluids and fluid creep are [21, 30, 31]:

- Use of hypotonic maintenance fluids instead of sodium-rich (Na$^+$ 154 mEq/L) isotonic maintenance fluids.

- Use a lesser volume of dilution fluids for administering medications (fluid creep) to reduce sodium burden.

- Use the lowest possible volume of diluent for preparing continuous infusion.

- Use 5% dextrose instead of normal saline as a diluent for medications.

- If the oral bioavailability of drugs is good, use oral or enteral instead of the parenteral route.

What is fluid creep, and why is it important to know about it?

Fluid creep is the sum of the volumes of fluids administered as a vehicle to dissolve medications or keep intravenous lines open (hidden fluids).

It is the largest (up to 40% of total fluid intake), hidden, unintentional, and often overlooked source of sodium in daily fluid administered, which is a common cause of harmful sodium load and positive fluid balance in hospitalized patients [6, 21, 32–35].

PRESCRIBING MAINTENANCE IV FLUIDS

For prescribing maintenance fluids, it is essential to consider indications, select the appropriate type, determine the volume of fluids required, and determine the optimal rate of administration.

Indications of maintenance IV fluids

Maintenance fluid is commonly prescribed for patients as follows:

- Poor oral intake: Patients unable to consume fluids orally due to issues like severe nausea and vomiting.

- Kept nil by mouth: Patients in specific medical situations, such as severe acute pancreatitis, bowel obstruction, ileus, acute abdomen, prolonged preoperative or postoperative fasting, critically ill patients with neurological injuries and dysphagia (without enteral feeding tubes), or those at risk of airway compromise and requiring ventilator support.

However, avoid the administration of maintenance fluids if the patient can eat and drink sufficiently to prevent fluid overload and fluid creep [27].

Selection of maintenance IV fluids

No single IV fluid is the most appropriate as a maintenance IV fluid in adults because a controversy exists regarding its optimum volume, composition, and rate of administration [1]. Available guidelines provide rough estimates about the initial water, sodium, and potassium

Table 7.1 NICE recommendation for IV maintenance fluids [2]	
Volume	25–30 mL/kg/day of water
Electrolytes	1 mEq/kg/day of sodium, potassium, and chloride
Calories	100 gm/day (1–1.5 gm/kg/day) of glucose to provide adequate calories to prevent hypoglycemia, starvation ketosis and restrict tissue catabolism, but it is not sufficient to provide complete nutritional support

requirements, but further prescriptions need modifications based on the vital signs, physical examination, strict measurements of intake and output, daily weight, and serum electrolytes.

The most widely used NICE guidelines for the initial prescription of maintenance IV fluids for euvolemic adult patients are summarized in Table 7.1 [2, 36].

Type of maintenance IV fluids

Based on the clinical and biochemical status of the patients, the type of maintenance IV fluids is selected.

A. Hypotonic fluids

Considering all the above evidence of the role of the sodium concentration of maintenance IV fluids into account, currently, hypotonic fluids are recommended for the initial prescription of maintenance IV fluids for euvolemic adult patients [21].

Hypotonic maintenance IV fluids should contain a low sodium concentration (30–77 mEq/L) to provide 1 mEq/kg/day of sodium.

Different options to administer hypotonic maintenance IV fluids suggested are:

- Administer solution containing sodium chloride 0.18% (fluids containing 31 mEq/L Na⁺) in 4%

glucose with added potassium [2].

- Administer a mixture of Dextrose 5% and normal saline (0.9% NaCl) bags in a ratio of 2:1 (two bags of Dextrose 5% with one bag of normal saline) with added potassium [2].

- If a solution containing 40 mEq/L sodium is administered at a rate of 25 mL/kg/day, it will provide 1 mEq/kg/day of sodium [21].

- In recent literature, the use of half-normal saline (0.45% NaCl = 77 mEq/L NaCl) in 5% dextrose with the addition of 20 mEq/L of potassium chloride as a maintenance IV fluid is suggested [37]. Sodium concentration of half-normal saline is greater than 0.18% Saline (NICE recommendation) [2] but lesser than isotonic fluid (North American publication) [1]. For patients who are not at risk for increased antidiuretic hormone secretion, this approach will reduce the hypotonic fluid-related risk of hyponatremia and will avoid the potential risk of salt and fluid overload due to an isotonic fluid.

B. Monitoring and modification

Serum sodium should be monitored daily in the patient receiving hypotonic maintenance IV fluids:

- If the serum sodium falls, discontinue using hypotonic fluids and start more concentrated isotonic maintenance IV fluids such as normal saline (154 mEq/L sodium) or balanced crystalloid solutions (Ringer's lactate-RL 130 mEq/L sodium and PlasmaLyte 140 mEq/L sodium).

- Use hypotonic fluids with a lower sodium concentration in patients with hypernatremia or clinically significant renal concentrating defect with ongoing free-water losses.

- The amount of potassium to be added in maintenance IV fluid needs modifications considering the change in serum potassium concentration.

The volume of maintenance IV fluids

As per the NICE recommendation (2013) [2], the requirements for the maintenance IV fluids for adult patients are 25–30 mL/kg/day.

Factors affecting the volume of maintenance IV fluid:

- The maintenance fluid requirement is higher in children than in adults [38].

- However, in obese patients (for those weighing more than 75kg.), the fluid requirement is in the lower range of volumes per kg (usually do not need more than 2.5 liters of fluid per day) [2].

- The fluid requirement is less (about 20–25 mL/kg/day or less) in older, edematous patients, those with renal impairment, cardiac failure, SIADH, and malnourished patients at risk of refeeding syndrome [2].

- Do not forget to calculate the amount of fluid provided by other sources (e.g., medication and nutrition) and subtract it from the estimated volume of maintenance fluids to determine the total volume of maintenance fluids.

- The fluid requirement increases if the patient has a fever, excessive sweating, increased respiratory rate, hypermetabolic states, burns, drains, polyuria, or ongoing significant gastrointestinal losses.

The rate of administration of maintenance IV fluids

There is no recommendation regarding the most appropriate rate of administration, but administration of maintenance IV fluid during daytime hours to promote sleep and well-being [2, 36].

Cautions while using maintenance fluid

- The NICE recommendation is to avoid prescribing >2.5 L/day for patients weighing more than 75 kg due to the potential risk of hyponatremia [2]. In addition, avoid giving maintenance fluids at a rate of more than 100 ml/hour.

- Allow oral fluid intake whenever possible and deduct this volume from the total amount of maintenance IV fluid.

- Do not use maintenance fluids for volume resuscitation, to replace abnormal ongoing losses (e.g., diarrhea, vomiting, blood loss, etc.), or provide nutritional support.

- Reassess patients receiving maintenance IV fluids closely. Monitor intake and output strictly, measure weight daily, watch for signs and symptoms of fluid retention and monitor serum electrolytes, and modify the composition and rate of IV fluid according to an individual's need.

- Discontinue maintenance fluids when no longer needed. Consider nasogastric fluid or enteral feeding when maintenance needs are more than 3 days [2].

REFERENCES

1. Moritz ML, Ayus JC. Maintenance intravenous fluids in acutely ill patients. N Engl J Med. 2015;373(14):1350–1360.

2. National Institute for Health and Care Excellence Guideline for Intravenous fluid therapy in adults in hospital (CG174), 2013-Updated May 2017 (https://www.nice.org.uk/guidance/cg174).

3. Foster BA, Tom D, Hill V. Hypotonic versus isotonic fluids in hospitalized children: A systematic review and meta-analysis. J Pediatr. 2014;165(1):163–169.

4. McNab S, Duke T, South M, et al. 140 mmol/L of sodium versus 77 mmol/L of sodium in maintenance intravenous fluid therapy for children in hospital (PIMS): a randomised controlled double-blind trial. Lancet. 2015;385(9974):1190–7.

5. Mitchell KH, Carlbom D, Caldwell E, et al. Volume overload: prevalence, risk factors, and functional outcome in survivors of septic shock. Ann Am Thorac Soc. 2015;12(12):1837–1844.

6. Van Regenmortel N, Verbrugghe W, Roelant E, et al. Maintenance fluid therapy and fluid creep impose more significant fluid, sodium, and chloride burdens than resuscitation fluids in critically ill patients: a retrospective study in a tertiary mixed ICU population. Intensive Care Med. 2018;44(4):409–417.

7. Holliday Ma, Segar We. The maintenance need for water in parenteral fluid therapy. Pediatrics 1957;19(5):823–32.

8. Shafiee MA, Bohn D, Hoorn EJ, et al. How to select optimal maintenance intravenous fluid therapy. QJM 2003;96(8):601–10.

9. Koczmara C, Wade AW, Skippen P, et al. Hospital-acquired acute hyponatremia and reports of pediatric deaths. Dynamics 2010;21(1):21–6.

10. Padua AP, Macaraya JR, Dans LF, et al. Isotonic versus Hypotonic saline solution for maintenance intravenous fluid therapy in children: a systematic review. Pediatr Nephrol 2015;30(7):1163–72.

11. Robles CMF, García CAC. A prospective trial comparing isotonic with hypotonic maintenance fluids for prevention of hospital-acquired hyponatraemia. Paediatr Int Child Health. 2016;36(3):168–174.

12. Hall AM, Ayus JC, Moritz ML. Things we do for no Reason: the default use of hypotonic maintenance intravenous fluids in pediatrics. J. Hosp. Med 2018;13(9):637–640.

13. National Institute for Health and Care Excellence. Intravenous fluid therapy in children and young people in hospital. NICE guideline [NG29]. December 2015. Available from: https://www.nice.org.uk/guidance/ng29.

14. Feld LG, Neuspiel DR, Foster BA, et al. Clinical practice guideline: maintenance intravenous fluids in children. Pediatrics 2018;142:e20183083.

15. Aronson D, Dragu RE, Nakhoul F, et al. Hyponatremia as a complication of cardiac catheterization: a prospective study. Am J Kidney Dis 2002;40(5):940–6.

16. Moritz ML, Ayus JC. Hospital-Acquired Hyponatremia – Why are hypotonic parenteral fluids still being used? Nat Clin Pract Nephrol 2007;3(7):374–82.

17. Nair V, Niederman MS, Masani N, et al. Hyponatremia in community acquired pneumonia. Am J Nephrol 2007;27(2):184–90.

18. Bihari S, Peake SL, Seppelt I, et al. George Institute for Global Health; Australian and New Zealand Intensive Care Society Clinical Trials Group. Sodium administration in critically ill patients in Australia and New Zealand: a multicentre point prevalence study. Crit Care Resusc. 2013;15(4):294–300.

19. Bihari S, Watts NR, Seppelt I, et al. George Institute for Global Health and the Australian and New Zealand Intensive Care Society Clinical Trials Group. Maintenance fluid practices in intensive care units in Australia and New Zealand. Crit Care Resusc. 2016;18(2):89–94.

20. Van Regenmortel N, De Weerdt T, Van Craenenbroeck AH, et al. Effect of isotonic versus hypotonic maintenance fluid therapy on urine output, fluid balance, and electrolyte homeostasis: a crossover study in fasting adult volunteers. Br J Anaesth. 2017;118(6):892–900.

21. Van Regenmortel N, Moers L, Langer T, et al. Fluid-induced harm in the hospital: look beyond volume and start considering sodium. From physiology towards recommendations for daily practice in hospitalized adults. Ann Intensive Care. 2021;11(1):79.

22. Van Regenmortel N, Langer T, De Weerdt T, et al. Effect of sodium administration on fluid balance and sodium balance in health and the perioperative setting. Extended summary with additional insights from the MIHMoSA and TOPMAST studies. J Crit Care. 2022;67:157–165.

23. Hawkins WA, Smith SE, Newsome AS, et al. Fluid Stewardship during Critical Illness: A Call to Action. J Pharm Pract. 2020;33(6):863–873.

24. Boyd JH, Forbes J, Nakada TA, et al. Fluid resuscitation in septic shock: a positive fluid balance and elevated central venous pressure are associated with increased mortality. Crit Care Med. 2011;39(2):259–265.

25. Claure-Del Granado R, Mehta RL. Fluid overload in the ICU: evaluation and management. BMC Nephrol. 2016;17(1):109.

26. Neyra JA, Li X, Canepa-Escaro F, et al. Cumulative fluid balance and mortality in septic patients with or without acute kidney injury and chronic kidney disease. Crit Care Med. 2016;44(10):1891–1900.

27. Perez Nieto OR, Wong A, Lopez Fermin J, et al. Aiming for zero fluid accumulation: First, do no harm. Anaesthesiol Intensive Ther. 2021;53(2):162–178.

28. Barhight MF, Nelson D, Chong G, et al. Non-resuscitation fluid in excess of hydration requirements is associated with higher mortality in critically ill children. Pediatr Res. 2022;91(1):235–240.

29. Van Regenmortel N, Hendrickx S, Roelant E et al. 154 compared to 54 mmol per liter of sodium in intravenous maintenance fluid therapy for adult patients undergoing major thoracic surgery (TOPMAST): a single-center randomized controlled double-blind trial. Intensive Care Med 2019;45(10):1422–1432.

30. Giordano M, Ciarambino T, Castellino P, et al. Diseases associated with electrolyte imbalance in the ED: age-related differences. Am J Emerg Med 2016;34(10):1923–1926.

31. Bihari S, Prakash S, Potts S, et al. Addressing the inadvertent sodium and chloride burden in critically ill patients: a prospective before-and-after study in a tertiary mixed intensive care unit population. Crit Care Resusc. 2018;20(4):285–93.

32. Choo WP, Groeneveld AB, Driessen RH, et al. Normal saline to dilute parenteral drugs and to keep catheters open is a major and preventable source of hypernatremia acquired in the intensive care unit. J Crit Care. 2014;29(3):390–4.

33. Bihari S, Peake SL, Prakash S, et al. Sodium balance, not fluid balance, is associated with respiratory dysfunction in mechanically ventilated patients: a prospective, multicentre study. Crit Care Resusc. 2015;17(1):23–8.

34. Langer T, D'Oria V, Spolidoro G, et al. Fluid therapy in mechanically ventilated critically ill children: the sodium, chloride and water burden of fluid creep. BMC Pediatr 2020;20(1):424.

35. Gamble KC, Smith SE, Bland CM, et al. Hidden Fluids in Plain Sight: Identifying Intravenous Medication Classes as Contributors to Intensive Care Unit Fluid Intake. Hospital Pharmacy 2021.

36. Padhi S, Bullock I, Li L, et al. Intravenous fluid therapy for adults in hospital: summary of NICE guidance. BMJ 2013;347:f7073.

37. Sterns RH, Emmett M, Forman JP. Maintenance and replacement fluid therapy in adults. UptoDate 2019.

38. Meyers RS. Pediatric fluid and electrolyte therapy. J Pediatr Pharmacol Ther 2009;14(4):204–211.

8 | Resuscitation Fluids

INTRODUCTION

Fluid resuscitation is defined as a rapid administration of intravenous fluids used to restore or maintain a patient's circulatory volume during severe hypovolemia or shock due to significant and sudden fluid or blood losses. The most common indications of fluid resuscitation in critically ill patients are severe hypovolaemia, sepsis, trauma, burn, and perioperative volume loss [1]. The objective of fluid resuscitation is to quickly administer a large fluid volume to restore circulating volume, stabilize hemodynamics, and thereby restore tissue perfusion and oxygen delivery without causing harm due to fluid overload [2]. Identifying the cause of shock and treating it simultaneously is vital.

TIMING AND RATE OF FLUID ADMINISTRATION

Hypovolemic shock is a medical emergency, and fluid resuscitation should begin immediately. Delay in therapy can lead to ischemic injury and possibly to irreversible shock and multiorgan system failure. For initial fluid resuscitation, crystalloid fluids containing 130–154 mEq/L sodium are infused as a bolus of 500 mL within 15 minutes [1, 3]. Usually, one to two liters of fluid is administered rapidly to establish hemodynamic stability, maintain adequate blood flow to organs, and improve tissue perfusion. Fluid resuscitation should be done under close monitoring in high-risk patients who have kidney impairment or congestive heart failure to avoid fluid overload.

As per Surviving Sepsis Campaign recommendations (2021), in the resuscitation from sepsis-induced hypoperfusion, at least 30 mL/kg of intravenous (IV) crystalloid fluid should be given within the first 3 hours [4]. The use of an average fluid volume of around 30 mL/kg was supported by the PROCESS [5], ARISE [6], and PROMISE trials [7], where patients, on average, received this volume of fluid before randomization.

As early aggressive fluid resuscitation with large-bore IV cannulas is crucial in severe sepsis and septic shock, fluid resuscitation should be initiated earliest (after obtaining blood for measuring lactate and blood cultures) and should be completed within the first 3 hours. Earlier fluid resuscitation (within the first 3 hours) improves survival in patients with severe sepsis and septic shock [4]. Delayed administration of fluid (>2 hours after diagnosis) is the most crucial predictor of the fluid refractory state, which is associated with longer hospital stays and higher mortality [8].

If the patient does not respond to adequate fluid resuscitation, consider using vasopressors and inotropes and rule out other causes of shock besides hypovolemia (e.g., cardiogenic shock, sepsis) [9]. Consider earlier use of vasopressors in patients at risk of volume overload and to achieve the initial mean arterial pressure (MAP) target more rapidly.

An initial target of fluid resuscitation is to achieve a mean arterial pressure of 65 mmHg [4]. Following initial fluid resuscitation, additional fluid infusion is planned based on a frequent assessment of clinical parameters, hemodynamic status, and laboratory tests.

The requirement for IV fluids changes over time. During the early salvage phase of shock (0–24 h), rapid fluid replacement in an adequate volume is essential. Fluid requirements decrease subsequently during optimization and stabilization phases (24–96 h), so the volume of fluids infusion should be reduced. Restrictive strategy during the last de-escalation phase (>96 h) is associated with better outcomes [10, 11].

TYPE OF FLUIDS FOR RESUSCITATION

The choice of resuscitation fluid depends on the severity and etiology of hypovolemic shock. Three major categories of fluids used for resuscitation are crystalloid fluids (normal saline, Ringer's lactate (RL), and other chloride-restrictive balanced crystalloids such as PlasmaLyte); colloids (albumin, hydroxyethyl starch (HES), dextran, and gelatine), and blood products (packed red blood cells).

THE PHYSIOLOGY OF FLUID SELECTION

Understating the basic physiology of the distribution of infused fluids helps in the selection of appropriate fluid for a given patient. When different IV fluids are infused, their distribution in various compartments of body fluids differs depending upon their composition (Table 8.1 and Figure 8.1). The ability of infused IV fluids to expand intravascular volume determines its effectiveness in raising blood pressure.

Avoiding 5% dextrose in the treatment of hypovolemic shock: 5% dextrose is typically avoided in the treatment of hypovolemic shock for several reasons:

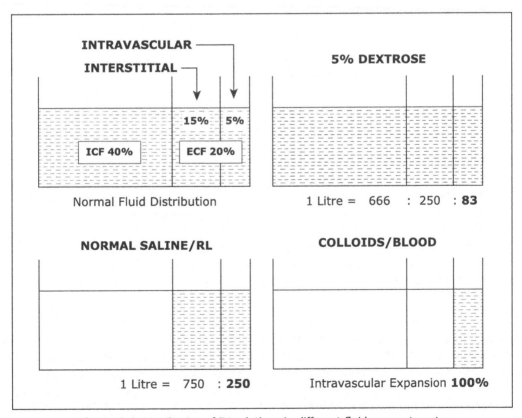

Figure 8.1 Distribution of IV solutions in different fluid compartments.

Table 8.1 Distribution of IV solutions in body fluid compartments				
Fluid distribution (1000 ml)	5% Dextrose	0.45% Saline	RL and 0.9% saline	Colloids/Blood products
Intracellular fluid (ml)	667	333	0	0
Extracellular fluid (ml)	333	667	1000	1000
Interstitial fluid (ml)	250	500	750	0
Intravascular fluid (ml)	83	167	250	1000

1. **Poor expansion of intravascular volume:** 1000 ml of 5% dextrose increases the extracellular fluid (ECF) volume by only 330 ml, with just 83 ml (or 1/4 of the ECF) remaining in the intravascular space [12]. As 1 liter of 5% dextrose will increase the intravascular volume only by about 83 ml (8%), the rise in blood pressure will be poor in the patient with shock.

2. **Increased urine output due to osmotic diuresis:** Administering a large volume of 5% dextrose at a faster rate results in a glucose load of more than 25 gm/hour, inducing osmotic diuresis. So, even in the presence of hypovolemia, there will be increased urine output, which delays the correction of dehydration.

   Increased urine output will also create a false impression that the fluid deficit has been resolved. In such a setting, the rate of fluid replacement may be slowed down despite hypovolemia; therefore, hypotension may not improve. So, 5% dextrose should be avoided in the treatment of shock.

Selecting normal saline and Ringer's lactate as initial fluids for treating Hypovolemic shock: Crystalloid fluids such as normal saline and Ringer's lactate are sodium-rich electrolyte solutions and therefore are distributed only in the ECF compartment (25% in intravascular and 75% in interstitium). Infusion of 1 liter of these fluids will expand intravascular volume by about 250 ml, so the blood pressure rise will be much more rapid compared to 5%-dextrose [13].

As normal saline, Ringer's lactate and other chloride-restrictive balanced crystalloids are dextrose-free in an emergency when the patient's glycemic status is unknown; these fluids are safe for initial resuscitation. Moreover, compared to colloids, these fluids are inexpensive, readily available, noninfectious, reaction-free, and easy to store, so they are preferred for the initial treatment of shock.

The use of dextrose saline infusion for fluid resuscitation: Avoid using dextrose saline infusion for fluid resuscitation. 1000 ml of Dextrose saline contains 50 gm of dextrose (5% dextrose) and 154 mEq of sodium and chloride (0.9% NaCl). Faster infusion of fluid with 5% dextrose will cause hyperglycemia and resultant osmotic diuresis and increased urine output. Increased urine output in the presence of hypovolemia delays the correction of dehydration, which is not desirable. Therefore, all dextrose-containing fluids are not appropriate for fluid resuscitation [14].

Colloids and blood products: the most potent options for rapidly raising blood pressure during shock: For the prompt rise of blood pressure in shock, natural colloids (such as albumin), synthetic colloids (such as hydroxyethyl starches, gelatin solutions, and dextran), and blood products are more potent agents.

Large molecules of these agents do not readily cross the capillary membrane and, therefore, are primarily restricted to the intravascular compartment. In contrast to normal saline, where 3/4 of it enters the interstitium, the total volume of infused colloids and blood products remains in the vascular space. As 100% of the infused volume stays in the vascular space and selectively expands the plasma volume, they will raise blood pressure rapidly.

Colloids carry a lesser risk of pulmonary edema since the increase in plasma oncotic pressure favors fluid movements out of the interstitium into the vascular space.

Despite the physiological potency and benefits of colloids, they are not the preferred or superior solution over crystalloids in clinical practice, as discussed later.

SELECTING IV FLUID FOR RESUSCITATION

From a variety of available choices, to choose the appropriate fluid for resuscitation, consider the composition, effectiveness, benefits, and disadvantages of different solutions. Three common IV replacement fluids used to manage hypovolemic shock are crystalloids, colloids, and blood products:

- Crystalloids: The most widely used first-line therapy in managing hypovolemic shock comprises crystalloids such as normal saline, Ringer's lactate, and PlasmaLyte.

- Colloids: Colloids are second-line resuscitation therapy used in selected patients with hypotension. Among colloids, the use of natural colloids

like albumin, which is safe but highly expensive, is recommended in specific clinical settings. However, the use of synthetic colloids such as hydroxyethyl starch, dextran, and gelatin is not recommended, and they are avoided or discouraged due to their harmful effects and lack of benefits.

- Blood Products: Packed red blood cells or blood substitutes are essential for effective resuscitation for patients with significant blood loss or anemia associated with hypotension.

Each type of fluid comes with its characteristics and is chosen based on the specific needs and conditions of the patient.

CRYSTALLOID RESUSCITATION: FIRSTLINE THERAPY

Crystalloids like Normal saline and balanced crystalloids like Ringer's lactate and PlasmaLyte are the most frequently prescribed crystalloid solutions for resuscitation.

The selection between normal saline and balanced crystalloids depends on their respective clinical benefits and safety profiles, not solely on physiological characteristics. This choice remains a subject of ongoing controversy. To provide a clear and comprehensive understanding of the appropriate use of crystalloids, key studies, and guidelines that provide comparative insights are summarized below:

- Composition of commonly used IV crystalloids.

- Physiological basis, advantages, disadvantages, and preferred indications for using normal saline and balanced crystalloids.

- A literature review to address the ongoing controversy between saline and balanced crystalloids.

- Conclusions and current recommendations for appropriate use of crystalloids.

The composition of commonly used IV crystalloids

Understanding the composition of commonly used IV crystalloids is crucial for their appropriate use in resuscitation; a comparison of these compositions with human plasma is summarized in Table 8.2.

A. Normal saline

Normal saline, or 0.9% saline (0.9% NaCl), often referred to as "Isotonic saline," is among the most commonly used crystalloids for resuscitation worldwide. Below are the advantages and disadvantages of using normal saline.

Advantages

Major advantages of normal saline for resuscitation include:

- **Availability and compatibility:** It is readily available, cost-effective, and compatible with the co-infusion of blood products and medications like ceftriaxone [15].

- **Volume expansion:** With 154 mEq/L of sodium, it effectively expands intravascular volume and corrects hypotension.

- **Safe for specific conditions:** It is the preferred option for patients with brain injury, hypochloremia, hypovolemic hyponatremia, and metabolic alkalosis. As the osmolarity of normal saline is 308 mOsm/L (compared to normal plasma osmolality of about 285 mOsm/kg), its use for resuscitation in neurological patients is without the risk of cerebral edema.

- **Glucose-free:** Ideal for scenarios with unknown glycemic statuses due to its lack of glucose content.

Disadvantages

The use of normal saline can be harmful, as it is neither "normal" nor "physiological" [16]. Major disadvantages of normal saline for resuscitation include:

Nonphysiological composition: Normal saline differs from the balanced crystalloid Ringer's lactate in three key aspects:

1. It has a significantly higher chloride concentration (154 versus 109 mEq/L).

2. It lacks a buffer, essential for maintaining pH.

3. It does not contain several electrolytes, like potassium and calcium, that are present in plasma.

Table 8.2 Composition of plasma and IV crystalloid resuscitation fluids										
	Na⁺ mEq/L	K⁺ mEq/L	Cl⁻ mEq/L	Acet. mEq/L	Lact. mEq/L	Ca²⁺ mEq/L	Mg²⁺ mEq/L	Gluc. mEq/L	Osm. mOsm/L	SID mEq/L
Plasma	136–145	3.5–5.0	98–106	-	-	2.2–2.6	0.8–1.0	-	285–295	40
0.9% NaCl	154	-	154	-	-	-	-	-	308	0
RL	130	4.0	109	-	28	3.0	-	-	273	28
PlasmaLyte	140	5.0	98	27	-	-	3.0	23	295	50
Sterofundin	145	4.0	127	24	-	5.0	2.0	-	309	29

Acet.: Acetate; Ca²⁺: Calcium; Cl⁻: Chloride; Gluc.: Gluconate; Lact.: Lactate; Mg²⁺: Magnesium; Osm.: Osmolality; K⁺: Potassium; Na⁺: Sodium; SID: Strong ion difference

Harmful effects: Normal saline contains supraphysiologic chloride concentrations (154 mEq/L) -50% higher than human serum chloride concentration [17]. The infusion of large volumes of this high chloride-containing fluid can lead to hyperchloremic acidosis [18, 19], an increased risk of acute kidney injury [18, 20], a greater need for renal replacement therapy, higher hospital mortality [21–23], coagulopathy [24], hyperkalemia, and more pronounced interstitial fluid retention [25].

Hyperchloremic metabolic acidosis

Infusing a large volume of normal saline often results in a normal anion gap hyperchloremic metabolic acidosis [26, 27]. This effect can be attributed to factors such as the strong ion difference (SID), reduced bicarbonate (HCO_3) reabsorption, and dilution of bicarbonate [28]:

- The SID of normal saline is zero; therefore, its infusion decreases plasma SID, leading to metabolic acidosis (SID: Normal value = 40; Normal saline = 0; RL = 28, PlasmaLyte = 50) [16, 29].

- Administering a large volume of normal saline reduces renal bicarbonate reabsorption, decreasing bicarbonate levels [30].

- Using large volumes of bicarbonate-free fluids like normal saline dilutes the bicarbonate concentration in the body, inducing dilutional acidosis [2, 31].

Risk of acute kidney injury (AKI)

Administering a large volume of normal saline can lead to hyperchloremia and an increase in chloride concentration in the distal tubular fluid. This elevated chloride level is sensed by macula densa cells located in the distal convoluted tubule. These tubular cells then transmit signals to the afferent arterioles, triggering vasoconstriction (known as "Tubuloglomerular Feedback"). This vasoconstriction, in turn, diminishes renal perfusion and reduces the glomerular filtration rate (GFR), potentially leading to acute kidney injury [16, 20, 27, 32, 33].

Use in hyperkalemia

Infusing a large volume of normal saline can induce hyperchloremic metabolic acidosis, promoting the shift of potassium out of cells and potentially causing or worsening hyperkalemia. So, the simple logic that normal saline, because it does not contain potassium, is safe to use in hyperkalemia is a myth. On the contrary, Ringer's lactate does not cause any acidosis, and in a patient with hyperkalemia, it will actually lower his serum potassium level and, therefore, is safe. Thus, Ringer's lactate is often preferred over normal saline in cases of hyperkalemia [34–36].

B. Balanced crystalloids

Emerging evidence suggests that using normal saline as a resuscitation fluid leads to complications like hyperchloremic metabolic acidosis, AKI, etc. Balanced crystalloids (buffered or chloride-restrictive solutions or balanced salt solutions) are the result of a search for safer fluid for resuscitation. Balanced crystalloids are more physiological than normal saline and are increasingly advocated as a first-line resuscitation fluid [15].

To provide a comprehensive overview of RL's optimal use, the sections below outline its basic physiology, benefits, applications in various electrolyte and clinical disorders, and potential disadvantages.

Balanced electrolyte composition

Balanced crystalloid solutions are formulated to closely mirror the electrolyte composition, osmolality, and pH of human plasma, enabling the administration of large volumes without the risk of electrolyte disturbances.

Provides buffer to prevent or correct metabolic acidosis

Balanced crystalloids contain precursors of bicarbonate (e.g., lactate and acetate) that are metabolized into bicarbonate, helping to correct metabolic acidosis [37–39]. This buffering effect is a significant advantage over normal saline, which lacks this buffering capacity. Since bicarbonate-containing solutions are unstable in plastic containers, alternative metabolizable anions like lactate, acetate, gluconate, and malate are used to formulate balanced crystalloids to ensure stability and efficacy.

Reduces the risks of hyperchloremia

Balanced crystalloid solutions containing significantly less chloride than normal saline, effectively reduce the incidence of an increase in plasma chloride levels [40]. The potential benefit of balanced crystalloid solutions comes from their lower chloride content (<112 mEq/L) and a strong ion difference that closely matches that of human plasma. The chloride concentrations in Ringer's lactate (109 mEq/L) and PlasmaLyte A (98 mEq/L) are similar to that of human plasma (102 mEq/L), contrasting with the high chloride concentration in normal saline (154 mEq/L) [41, 42].

Effect of RL on serum lactate levels

Despite each liter of Ringer's lactate containing 28 mmol of sodium lactate, its infusion in hemodynamically stable adults only transiently elevates lactate levels or does not significantly increase them compared to normal saline solution [43–46]. As the rise in serum lactate levels is very minimal (<1.00 mmol/L) following the infusion of RL, it may not significantly interfere with the interpretation of serial lactate measurements as an index of the severity of acidosis [44, 47].

Use in lactic acidosis misconceptions and facts

Contrary to a common misconception, the infusion of Ringer's lactate does not induce lactic acidosis. The avoidance of this solution due to fears of exacerbating lactic acidosis is based on a misunderstanding.

Clarification is needed regarding the difference between lactic acid and the sodium lactate contained in Ringer's lactate. Remember that lactic acid, consisting of anion lactate plus cation hydrogen and with a pH of 2.44 to 3.51, is an "acid," and it's harmful.

However, the sodium lactate in Ringer's lactate, a "conjugate base" consisting of anion lactate and cation sodium with a pH of 6.0 to 7.3, is benign, contrasting the harmful nature of lactic acid. So, in conclusion, interestingly, RL not only has the capacity to absorb hydrogen ions, potentially correcting acidosis or leading to metabolic alkalosis, but also, importantly, it does not cause lactic acidosis [48, 49].

Safety in hyperkalemia

Ringer's lactate contains 4 mEq/L potassium, whereas the potassium content of normal saline is zero. The common apprehension that potassium-containing Ringer's lactate is unsafe and should be avoided in patients with hyperkalemia is a myth [35, 50]. As the potassium concentration of Ringer's lactate is just 4 mEq/L, its administration cannot raise the value of serum potassium higher than its potassium concentration (i.e., 4 mEq/L) and, therefore, cannot lead to hyperkalemia. In contrast, the low potassium content in Ringer's lactate may cause the potassium level of a hyperkalemic patient to trend toward 4 mEq/L [51, 52].

98% of potassium is distributed within the intracellular compartment, and serum potassium levels are significantly influenced by a change in pH that shifts potassium. Acidosis triggers a shift of potassium from the intracellular fluid (ICF) to the extracellular fluid. Since Ringer's lactate rectifies acidosis, it not only prevents hyperkalemia but can actually reduce serum potassium levels, supporting its safety for patients with hyperkalemia. So, we can conclude that Ringer's lactate is safer than normal saline in hyperkalemia [34, 36, 52].

Safety in neurological disorders

RL is a hypotonic fluid with a plasma osmolarity of 273 mOsm/L, lower than the normal plasma osmolality of about 285 mOsm/kg. Because of its hypotonicity, RL can cause or exacerbate cerebral edema and should, therefore, be avoided in cases with a risk of raised intracranial pressure, such as aneurysmal subarachnoid hemorrhage (aSAH), traumatic brain injury (TBI), and in patients undergoing neurosurgery [53–55].

Use in liver disorders

The lactate in RL is primarily metabolized into bicarbonate in the liver. The administration of RL is not an absolute contraindication for patients with liver dysfunction or cirrhosis, and its clinical impact remains unknown [56–58]. However, for those with severe or frank liver failure or post-liver transplantation, where a significant reduction in lactate metabolism is observed, bicarbonate-buffered solutions are often preferred over lactate-buffered ones [47, 59]. Balanced crystalloids, like PlasmaLyte, contain acetate instead of lactate, and acetate metabolism occurs in all body tissues and is not limited to liver tissues. So, PlasmaLyte can be used instead of RL in severe liver diseases.

Use in diabetic ketoacidosis

RL may be considered over normal saline for treating patients with diabetic ketoacidosis (DKA) because it is dextrose-free and reduces the risk of hyperchloremic metabolic acidosis. Additionally, it provides bicarbonate to correct acidosis and offers other benefits such as lower total cost, shorter hospital stays, and quicker, more efficient resolution of acidosis [60–63].

Precautions

Large volumes of balanced crystalloids may result in hyperlactatemia, metabolic alkalosis, and hypotonicity. As the osmolality of RL is low compared to plasma (273 vs. 290 mOsm/L), RL may exacerbate cerebral edema and therefore avoided in head injury and brain edema. As the capacity of the liver to metabolize lactate and generate bicarbonate is impaired in severe liver failure, the use of RL is avoided in such patients. Since Ringer's lactate contains calcium, it may not be suitable for co-infusion with blood products through the same IV line [15].

C. Saline vs. balanced crystalloids: A review of literature

To resolve the dilemma of choosing between normal saline and balanced crystalloids, establish the superiority of one fluid over the other, and provide evidence-based insights, we conducted an extensive review and analysis of various clinical trials, meta-analyses, and society guidelines. In this comprehensive review, evidence is categorized based on the superiority of each fluid, findings indicating no significant difference between the two, and insights from meta-analyses and society guidelines; a summary of conclusions and current recommendations is provided below.

1. Trials suggestive of the superiority of balanced crystalloids

- **Shaw et al. (Ann Surg 2012)** compared adult patients undergoing major open abdominal surgery who received either normal saline (30,994 patients) or a PlasmaLyte (926 patients) on the day of surgery. This study concluded that PlasmaLyte was associated with less postoperative morbidity than normal saline [64].

- **Yunus et al. (JAMA 2012)** compared the association of a chloride-restrictive vs. chloride-liberal IV fluid strategy with AKI in 760 critically ill patients. This study concluded that the chloride-restrictive strategy in a tertiary ICU was associated with a significant decrease in the incidence of AKI and the use of renal replacement therapy (RRT) [20].

- **McCluskey et al. (Anesth Analg 2013)** compared the impact of postoperative hyperchloremia in 22,851 patients undergoing noncardiac surgery. This study concluded that postoperative hyperchloremia was associated with increased mortality, renal dysfunction, and length of hospital stay [65].

- **Raghunathan et al. (Crit Care Med 2014)** compared the outcome

after resuscitation with balanced versus non-balanced fluids in 53,448 patients with sepsis in an ICU. This study concluded that among critically ill adults with sepsis, resuscitation with balanced crystalloids was associated with a lower risk of in-hospital mortality [66].

- **SMART Trial (Semler et al. NEJM 2018)** is a very large study that compared normal saline with balanced crystalloids among 15,802 critically ill adults. This study concluded that using balanced crystalloids resulted in a lower rate of death from any cause, RRT, or persistent renal dysfunction than using saline [67].

- **SALT-ED Trial (Self et al. NEJM 2018)** compared normal saline with balanced crystalloids among 13,347 noncritically ill adults. This study concluded that there was no difference in hospital-free days between both groups, but the use of balanced IV fluid resulted in a lower rate of death from any cause, RRT, or persistent renal dysfunction than the use of saline [68].

2. Trials and analysis suggestive of no difference between both groups

- **The SPLIT Trial (Young et al. JAMA 2015)** compared normal saline with PlasmaLyte in 2278 ICU patients and concluded that using a buffered crystalloid compared with saline did not reduce the risk of AKI [69]. A major limitation of this study was the median administration of a small volume of saline (<2 liters) and, therefore, a lesser risk of developing hyperchloremia.

- **The SALT Trial (Semler et al. Am J Respir Crit Care Med 2017)** compared normal saline with balanced crystalloids in 974 ICU patients and concluded no difference in the overall incidence of AKI or major adverse kidney events [70].

- **The BaSICS Trial (Zampieri et al. JAMA 2021)**, a multicenter, double-blind RCT involving 11,000 patients, compared normal saline with balanced crystalloids and concluded that there were no significant differences in mortality rates or AKI incidence [71].

- **The PLUS Study (Finfer et al. NEJM 2022)**, a multicenter, double-blind RCT involving 5,000 patients, compared normal saline to balanced crystalloids and concluded that the balanced crystalloid group did not demonstrate reduced mortality or kidney injury [72].

3. Meta-analysis and society guidelines

- **Krajewski et al. (Br J Surg 2015)** reported in a meta-analysis of 21 studies involving 6,253 patients that the use of high-chloride fluids in perioperative or intensive care settings was associated with an increased risk of acute kidney injury, with no observed benefits on mortality [32].

- **Cochrane Database Syst Rev. (2017)** reported that perioperative administration of buffered versus non-buffered crystalloid fluids showed insufficient evidence of impacting mortality and organ system function but noted a significant reduction in postoperative hyperchloremia and metabolic acidosis with the use of buffered fluids [73].

- **Surviving Sepsis Campaign Guidelines (Evans et al. Crit Care Med 2021):** The guidelines advise using crystalloids for both initial resuscitation and ongoing intravascular volume replenishment in adult patients with sepsis and septic shock [4]. The previous Surviving Sepsis Guidelines (2017) [74] suggested using either balanced crystalloids or saline, but in 2021, guidelines suggested using balanced crystalloids instead of normal saline for resuscitation [4].

- **Hammond NE et al. (NEJM Evid 2022)** conducted a Systematic Review with Meta-Analysis comparing balanced crystalloids to saline in critically ill adults and demonstrated reduced mortality in patients who received balanced crystalloids [75].

- **Beran A et al. (J Clin Med 2022)** demonstrated in their systematic review and meta-analysis that adults with sepsis treated with balanced crystalloids showed reduced mortality and AKI compared to those who received normal saline [76].

- **Isha et al. (Front Med 2023)** conducted a retrospective analysis that compared normal saline with balanced crystalloids in 2022 patients and found no significant difference in mortality rates, hospital stay, ICU admission rates, mechanical ventilation needs, oxygen therapy, and renal replacement therapy [77].

- Zampieri et al. (Lancet Respir Med. 2024) conducted a systematic review and meta-analysis, demonstrating lower in-hospital mortality associated with the use of balanced solutions compared to saline in the ICU [78].

Various systematic reviews with meta-analyses and guidelines [4, 32, 73, 75, 76, 78], except the recent one performed by Isha et al. on a small number of patients [77], suggesting that using balanced crystalloids offers some benefits compared to normal saline.

4. Trials suggestive of the superiority of normal saline

- To date, not a single study has demonstrated the superiority of saline over balanced crystalloids in the selection of appropriate resuscitation fluids. The absence of evidence establishing the superiority of saline indirectly reinforces the preference for using balanced crystalloids. This is consistent with the existing body of evidence highlighting the efficacy of balanced crystalloids in fluid resuscitation, even in the absence of high-quality reference evidence.

D. Crystalloids: conclusions and current recommendations

There is no clear consensus on recommending one crystalloid over others [79, 80]. However, suggestions are made based on the literature, as mentioned earlier, and various recent studies. However, it's crucial to acknowledge that the preference for using balanced crystalloids is without high-quality evidence [74, 81]. Given the low risk of harm and the real possibility of benefit, the use of balanced crystalloids could be a prudent choice in clinical practice [82]. Selecting resuscitation fluids considering history, cause, acid-base, and electrolyte disorders will be wise.

1. Balanced crystalloids preferred firstline modality

- The current trend in literature favors the use of isotonic, balanced crystalloids as preferred resuscitation fluids [67, 83–95]. The benefits of using balanced crystalloids are more evident in patients with metabolic acidosis, hyperchloremia, increased creatinine, or those at risk of kidney injury [96].

- Ringer's lactate is suggested as the preferred resuscitation fluid in sepsis [37, 42, 82], acutely ill critical patients [97–99], surgical patients [64, 100], trauma [101, 102], high risk for acute kidney injury [103], acute pancreatitis [104–106], diarrhea, burns [107]. Benefits of balanced solutions are more evident when administering fluid in large volumes, particularly for septic patients [108, 109].

- Patients with acidosis should receive balanced crystalloids with an "alkalinizing" effect, while patients with alkalosis and hypochloremia should be treated with normal saline [110].

- Ringer's lactate should be avoided or used with caution in patients with severe metabolic alkalosis and hypochloremia (e.g., due to profound vomiting) [18], those with frank hepatic failure [111], and individuals with traumatic brain injury or at risk of increased intracranial pressure [18, 53].

- Although lactate metabolism may be impaired in patients with severe lactic acidosis, sepsis, or liver failure, Ringer's lactate does not cause or aggravate lactic acidosis [49, 50].

- Besides the fact that balanced crystalloids contain a small amount of potassium, the risk of hyperkalemia is significantly lower compared to normal saline [18, 35, 50].

2. Normal saline: selective use preferred

- Infusion of large quantities (>2 L) of supraphysiologic chloride containing normal saline can cause hyperchloremic metabolic acidosis, acute kidney injury [112], coagulopathy, increased hemodynamic instability, and potential mortality and therefore is harmful [113].

- Avoid administering large volumes of chloride-rich normal saline to all patients, especially those at high risk for AKI or incipient AKI, due to the potential risk of acute kidney injury [103, 114].

- Small to moderate amounts of normal saline do not increase the incidence of acute kidney injury [69]. Thus, modest volumes of normal saline can be administered to patients with normal kidney function in the absence of hyperchloremia and sepsis [115–117].

- Normal saline is the fluid of choice for patients with metabolic alkalosis, hypovolemia due to vomiting or upper gastrointestinal suction, traumatic brain injury, and those receiving blood products [18, 39, 88, 118–120].

SELECTION OF BALANCED CRYSTALLOID

The evidence supporting the use of balanced crystalloid solutions as preferred resuscitation fluids over saline is growing [1]. In addition to Ringer's lactate, other newer balanced crystalloids like PlasmaLyte, Sterofundin, and Ringer's acetate are commercially available. Table 8.2 provides a detailed comparison of the composition of these balanced crystalloids with the body's natural serum concentrations. However, selecting the appropriate one for practical use presents a dilemma. To choose the most suitable balanced crystalloid, considerations include:

- Understanding the difference between lactate and Acetate buffer.

- Physiological basis for limitations of Ringer's lactate.

- Understanding the composition of PlasmaLyte and its advantages.

- Evidence comparison of Ringer's lactate vs. PlasmaLyte.

- Summary and clinical indications of newer balanced crystalloids.

A. Understanding the difference between lactate and acetate buffer

Balanced crystalloids contain lactate and acetate as buffers and provide bicarbonate. Lactate is primarily metabolized in the liver, a process that can be impaired in patients with substantial liver dysfunction, extreme hypoxia, severe sepsis and septic shock, or tissue hypoperfusion due to any form of pronounced hypotension [121, 122]. In contrast, acetate is metabolized in tissues throughout the body, not just the liver, making it a more adaptable choice for patients with severe liver dysfunction [42, 123]. Importantly, metabolizing capacity of acetate is preserved in shock [39, 124]. Additionally, acetate is rapidly converted into bicarbonate and doesn't require significant oxygen, enhancing its suitability for diverse patient populations [42, 123].

B. Physiological basis for limitations of Ringer's lactate

Ringer's lactate remains the default choice among balanced crystalloids and is widely used as an effective resuscitation fluid in various clinical scenarios. However, certain compositional characteristics can make it a less suitable choice for specific patient populations. These limitations are associated with its:

- **Use of lactate as a buffer:** In cases of severe liver impairment, hypoxia, acidaemia, or shock, the body's ability to convert lactate into bicarbonate is compromised [121, 122]. This impairment leads to not only a lack of buffering benefits but also lactate accumulation and a rise in serum lactate levels [44]. Consequently, using lactate levels as markers for resuscitation effectiveness becomes challenging.

- **Lower osmolality:** As RL is a hypotonic fluid (osmolality of RL 278 mOsmol/L vs. plasma osmolality 290 mOsmol/L), use it with caution in neurological patients with cerebral edema [39].

- **Lower sodium content:** Since RL contains less sodium than plasma (130 mEq/L vs. 140 mEq/L serum sodium), administering it in large volumes can lead to hyponatremia.

- **Calcium content:** The presence of calcium in RL can lead to precipitation when mixed with citrate in blood transfusions [15].

C. Understanding the composition of PlasmaLyte and its advantages

The growing preference for PlasmaLyte is attributed to its unique composition, which closely mimics human plasma in terms of electrolyte content, osmolality, and pH [125]. The advantages of PlasmaLyte include not only the correction of volume and electrolyte deficits but also the improvement of acidosis. Here are the key compositional features that determine its benefits, as discussed below:

- **Use of acetate as a buffer in PlasmaLyte:** PlasmaLyte replaces the lactate in RL with anions like acetate, gluconate, and maleate as bicarbonate precursors. Acetate's ability to be metabolized both in the liver and other tissues of the body allows it to ensure the conversion to bicarbonate even in severe liver failure and shock [42, 123]. PlasmaLyte has better buffering agents and effects. Furthermore, PlasmaLyte doesn't affect serum lactate levels, ensuring accurate readings during shock.

- **Osmolality equal to plasma:** PlasmaLyte, having an osmolality equal to plasma (290 mOsmol/L), does not carry the risk of causing cerebral edema, unlike hypotonic fluids.

- **Sodium concentration similar to plasma:** The sodium concentration in PlasmaLyte is identical to that of plasma (140 mEq/L), reducing the risk of hyponatremia or hypernatremia during large-volume fluid infusion [42].

- **Free of calcium content:** Being free of calcium, PlasmaLyte mitigates the risk of calcium overload and avoids complications associated with the co-administration of blood products containing citrate, which can lead to calcium precipitation.

- **Magnesium content:** Hypomagnesemia is common in critically ill patients, and PlasmaLyte, containing 1.5 mmol/L of magnesium, can be beneficial in these cases. However, it should be used cautiously in patients at risk for hypermagnesemia.

D. A comparative review of literature on Ringer's lactate vs. acetate buffered solutions

While acetate-buffered solutions like PlasmaLyte have distinct compositional benefits, a thorough review of the existing literature is needed to determine their edge over Ringer's lactate. Recent literature offering insights into this ongoing debate is summarized below.

Evidence suggesting Acetate buffered solutions/PlasmaLyte is superior

- **Curran et al. (2021):** This systematic review with a meta-analysis of 24 trials noted that PlasmaLyte led to lower serum chloride and lactate levels and a higher base excess compared to Ringer's lactate, although the evidence is of low certainty [126].

- **Ellekjaer et al. (2022):** Another systematic review with a meta-analysis of five RCTs involving 390 patients found very limited, low-quality evidence supporting the use of acetate over lactate-buffered solutions in hospitalized patients for all-cause mortality [127].

- **Priyanka et al. (2023):** A study involving 80 children indicated a preference for PlasmaLyte over RL during perioperative fluid therapy for abdominal surgeries due to enhanced acid-base, serum electrolytes, and blood lactate profiles [128].

- **Abdellatif et al. (2023):** In a study with 80 children undergoing cardiac surgery, PlasmaLyte showed better lactate and calcium levels than Ringer's lactate when used as a priming solution [129].

- The inclusion of PlasmaLyte as a balanced crystalloid in recent major saline vs. balanced crystalloid trials such as SPLIT (2015), SALT (2017), SMART (2018), SALT-ED (2018), BaSICS (2021), and PLUS (2022) emphasizes its recognition and utility as a valuable option among balanced crystalloids [67–72].

Evidence suggesting equal effectiveness of Ringer's lactate and Acetate buffered solutions

- **Weinberg et al. (2018):** In a trial with 50 adults, PlasmaLyte and Hartmann's solution showed no significant differences in plasma bicarbonate levels, complications, or length of ICU and hospital stays during elective cardiac surgery with CPB [130].

- **Pfortmueller et al. (2019):** In a study of seventy-five patients undergoing cardiac surgery, the use of RL and Ringer's acetate showed similar effects on hemodynamic stability and the progression of acid-base parameters [131].

- **Rawat et al. (2020):** A study of fifty adult ICU patients with metabolic acidosis revealed no significant advantage of acetate solution over RL in either the speed or extent of acidosis correction [132].

- **Chaussard et al. (2020):** A comparison involving twenty-eight burn patients showed similar alkalinizing effects between PlasmaLyte and Ringer's lactate during fluid resuscitation. However, using PlasmaLyte resulted in significantly lower ionized calcium levels [133].

E. Summary and clinical indications of newer balanced crystalloids

The studies comparing different lactate vs. acetate-based balanced crystalloids are limited and often involve small patient cohorts, leading to no consensus on the preference for a single balanced solution [88, 134, 135]. Amongst balanced solutions, Ringer's lactate is the most preferred fluid as it is inexpensive, readily available, and its composition is favorable and more physiological. In contrast, an acetate-buffered crystalloid solution like PlasmaLyte is known for its distinct compositional advantages and is an excellent choice in specific scenarios where RL is relatively contraindicated [47]. However, it is essential to note that this preference has not yet escalated to the level of a strong recommendation. The trend to use newer balanced solutions like PlasmaLyte is growing, especially among critically ill patients with multiple organ failure and shock; however, their higher cost can be a limiting factor. The common conditions where the use of PlasmaLyte is suggested are outlined below:

- **Diabetic ketoacidosis:** The use of dextrose-free PlasmaLyte reduces the risk of hyperchloremic metabolic acidosis, corrects acidosis by providing bicarbonate, and offers benefits like early and faster acidosis resolution, and reduces ICU and hospital stays leading to decreased total cost [61, 136, 137].

- **Perioperative fluid therapy:** The use of PlasmaLyte may result in improved acid-base status, serum electrolytes, and blood lactate profiles [128]. It may be useful in major open gastrointestinal (GI) and liver surgeries, including liver transplantation and complex cardiac surgeries [42, 138].In postoperative patients, using PlasmaLyte for fluid replacement on the day of major surgery has been linked to lower mortality than normal saline [64].

- **Critically ill patients:** PlasmaLyte is likely the optimal choice for fluid resuscitation in most critically ill, trauma patients, except those with traumatic brain injury [139–141].

- **Priming the CPB circuit:** Using PlasmaLyte for priming in cardiopulmonary bypass can be associated with reduced metabolic acidosis and improved calcium levels [129, 142].

- **Deceased donor kidney transplantation:** Using PlasmaLyte may reduce the incidence of delayed graft function in deceased donor kidney transplantation in adults [143] and decrease the risk of acute electrolyte disturbances in children [144]. Based on the findings of the 'BEST-Fluids' trial , PlasmaLyte should be preferred over normal saline as the fluid of choice in deceased donor kidney transplantation [143].

COLLOIDS: SECOND-LINE THERAPY FOR SELECTIVE USE

Colloids are potent resuscitation agents that rapidly improve hemodynamics with small volumes for longer periods. However, they are recommended for fluid resuscitation in only a select few patients and not as a routine practice. Commercially available colloids include natural colloids, such as albumin, and synthetic colloids, such as hydroxyethyl starch, dextran, and gelatin. Among these colloids, judicious use of albumin in selected patients is recommended, but synthetic colloids like hydroxyethyl starch, dextran, and gelatin are usually avoided or discouraged. The rationale for limited use or recommendation against the use of various colloids is summarized below, considering the literature on their benefits, disadvantages, and adverse effects.

A. The rationale for using colloids in resuscitation

- Greater volume expansion: As colloid solutions remain in the vascular space, plasma volume expansion is greater with colloids as compared to crystalloids [145, 146]. As the volume of colloids required to correct hypovolemic shock is less [147, 148], colloids prevent complications associated with the large volume of crystalloids, such as hyperchloremic acidosis, dilutional coagulopathy, and tissue edema. Accumulation of crystalloids in tissues, including lungs and incision sites, can cause weight gain, anasarca, and delayed tissue healing [149, 150].

- Faster volume expansion: Colloids are statistically more effective than crystalloids in reaching resuscitative hemodynamic endpoints [151]. The benefit of speedier achievement of hemodynamic goals with colloids compared to crystalloids is less organ damage and a decreased incidence of organ failure [146].

- More prolonged volume expansion: Because of longer intravascular half-life, colloids remain in circulation for a longer period, resulting in lesser volume requirement and better hemodynamic stability compared to crystalloids [152–154].

Review of literature

Theoretical advantages of larger and rapid intravascular volume expansion with colloids are not translated to improvement in safety and long-term outcomes in several large studies and randomized controlled trials. Summaries of significant trials, systematic reviews, meta-analyses, and guidelines comparing crystalloids with colloids are provided below.

Albumin trials

- **Cochrane Injuries Group Albumin Reviewers (BMJ 1998):** Administration of albumin for fluid resuscitation in critically ill patients may increase mortality [155].
- **SAFE Study (Finfer et al. NEJM 2004):** In ICU, using 4% albumin

or saline for fluid resuscitation results in similar outcomes at 28 days [156].

- **Cochrane Database Syst Rev (Roberts et al 2011):** The review of 38 trials involving patients with hypovolemia concluded that there is no evidence suggesting that albumin decreases mortality among critically ill patients with burns and hypoalbuminemia [157].

- **Meta-analysis of five RCTs (Xu et al 2014):** In this meta-analysis involving 3,658 patients with severe sepsis, those resuscitated with albumin, compared to crystalloid and saline, demonstrated a trend toward reduced 90-day mortality [158].

- **Systematic review and meta-analysis (Patel et al 2014):** In a study of 16 primary clinical trials including 4190 critically ill adults with sepsis, compared to crystalloids, albumin did not reduce all-cause mortality [159].

- **ALBIOS Trial (Caironi et al. NEJM 2014):** Comparing 20% albumin to crystalloid in 1800 septic patient resuscitation. No differences in mortality at 28 or 90 days [160].

Hydroxyethyl starch trials

- **6S Trial (Perner et al. NEJM 2012):** Increased incidence of renal replacement therapy after HES and significantly higher 90-day mortality [161].

- **CHEST Trial (Myburgh et al. NEJM 2012):** Increased incidence of renal replacement therapy after HES [162].

- **Cochrane Database Syst Rev 2013:** The review highlighted an overall increased risk of AKI and RRT in individuals treated with HES, indicating the detrimental effects of

HES on kidney function compared to alternative fluids [163].

- **Recommendation of European Medicines Agency (PRCA 2013):** HES should be used at the lowest effective dose for the shortest period. HES should not be used for more than 24 hours and monitor patients' kidney function for 90 days. HES should no longer be used in patients with sepsis, burns, or critically ill patients. HES should only be used to treat hypovolaemia caused by acute blood loss when crystalloids alone are insufficient [164].

- **Recommendation of European Medicines Agency (PRCA July 2018):** Because of potential adverse effects, HES should be used with additional measures of protection in selected patients with acute blood loss, where for resuscitation, 'crystalloids' alone are not sufficient. HES should be used at the lowest effective dose for the shortest duration (dose less than 30 mL/kg and maximum duration <24 hours) for the initial phase of volume resuscitation [165].

- **Recommendation of European Medicines Agency (July 2022):** The PRAC noted the persistent use of HES solutions in contraindicated populations, increasing the risk of severe harm and mortality. Given that the associated risks outweigh the benefits, they suspended the marketing of HES and recommended opting for safer therapeutic alternatives in line with clinical guidelines [166].

Colloids vs. crystalloids: Trials and reviews

- **CRISTAL Trial (Annane et al. JAMA 2013):** No significant difference in 28-day mortality but lower 90-day mortality in patients receiving colloids [148].

- **Cochrane Database Review of 78 RCTs (2013):** Colloids are not associated with an improvement in survival and are much more expensive than crystalloids. Because of the lack of survival benefits and higher costs, the routine use of colloids in clinical practice cannot be justified [167].

- **Cochrane Database Review (2018):** Using colloids versus crystalloids probably makes little or no difference to mortality. Starches probably slightly increase the need for blood transfusion and RRT. With the use of albumin or fresh frozen plasma (FFP), there is little or no difference in the need for renal replacement therapy [168].

- **A systematic review and meta-analysis (Martin et al. 2019):** A recent meta-analysis of 55 randomized clinical trials by Martin and Bassett concluded that crystalloids were less effective than colloids in stabilizing resuscitation endpoints in patients with a critical illness (e.g., shock, trauma, and sepsis) [151].

- **Surviving Sepsis Campaign Guidelines (Evans et al. Crit Care Med 2021):** The guidelines advise using crystalloids for both initial resuscitation and ongoing intravascular volume replenishment in adult patients with sepsis and septic shock [4].

B. Colloids: Current recommendations

Based on the physiological basis, literature discussed above, and other recent reviews, various colloids' current roles, advantages, and disadvantages in fluid resuscitation are summarized below.

Colloids are potent but not safe or preferred over crystalloids

- Crystalloids and colloids are both effective, but evidence of comparative superiority and significant benefits of colloids are lacking; therefore, current trends and recommendations favor crystalloids over colloids for the resuscitation of nonseptic and septic patients [83, 84, 95, 101, 168–170], and no indications currently exist for the routine use of colloids over crystalloids [154].

- The potential benefit of colloids to provide better hemodynamic stability is due to their effectiveness in achieving greater, rapid, and prolonged intravascular volume expansion [171].

- During resuscitation, colloids are usually used along with crystalloids when patients are likely to require a large volume of crystalloids to expand the intravascular volume [172]. Adding colloids can achieve hemodynamic stability with a smaller fluid volume, thereby reducing the risk of positive fluid balance and the associated complications, such as fatal pulmonary edema and systemic organ dysfunction, that can arise from administering larger volumes of crystalloids [151].

- Colloid solutions other than albumin (e.g., Hydroxyethyl starch dextran, gelatin) are not used routinely because of lack of benefits, safety, and potential adverse effects. Several studies have demonstrated increased risks, including tubular necrosis and acute kidney injury, associated with synthetic colloid treatment [173].

Albumin: Safe, potent but costly option, use selectively

- Albumin is not recommended as the first-line fluid for resuscitation in both nonseptic and septic patients; instead, it should be considered a second-line option for fluid resuscitation, along with crystalloids [4, 174]. Albumin is indicated as an adjunct to crystalloids when a patient is unresponsive to crystalloids, requires substantial amounts of crystalloids to achieve hemodynamic endpoints, or cannot tolerate large-volume crystalloid resuscitation [4, 88, 151, 175]. Albumin helps to reduce the total infused volume of crystalloids for hemodynamic stability [4, 134, 176]. IV human albumin solution is more effective for resuscitation when patients have hypoalbuminemia [176]. In septic patients, early administration of the combination of albumin (particularly 20% albumin) with balanced crystalloids within the first 24 hours of treatment decreases mortality [93, 177–179]. The use of albumin is recommended in treatment of spontaneous bacterial peritonitis, hepatorenal syndrome, and large-volume paracentesis (>5 L) [174].

- The 30 to 100 times higher cost of albumin compared to crystalloids, along with occasional supply shortages, serves as a significant limiting factor for its use [154, 180–183].

- Avoid albumin for resuscitation in patients with severe TBI [54, 55, 93, 184–186]. The most likely mechanism of increased mortality in patients with severe TBI is the increased intracranial pressure associated with using albumin for resuscitation. 4% albumin is hypotonic (260 mOsmol/kg) and therefore increases brain edema [118].

Hydroxyethyl starch is harmful; avoid it

- Hydroxyethyl starch (HES) was once the most commonly used colloid, but due to its adverse effects, current recommendations are against its use [187]. HES is currently indicated as an adjuvant therapy for treating hypovolemia induced by acute blood loss when crystalloids alone are insufficient [188].

- HES is associated with several adverse effects including an increased risk of acute kidney injury, a higher need for renal replacement therapy, excessive postoperative bleeding, an increased need for blood transfusions, and a higher mortality rate [161].

- **Strict limitations and cautious use of HES:** Both the US Food and Drug Administration (FDA) [189] and the European Medicines Agency (EMA) have raised concerns about the safety of HES due to its significant harmful effects. Responding to these concerns, the EMA issued guidelines in 2013 restricting the use of HES, and these guidelines were further tightened in July 2018 [165]. According to the revised guidelines, HES should only be administered during the initial phase of fluid resuscitation, and its dosage should not exceed 30 mL/kg. Additionally, the treatment duration should be as short as possible, not extending beyond 24 hours, and it is mandatory to monitor the patient's kidney function for at least 90 days following the administration of HES [165].

- **Advise against using HES:** Despite implementing risk minimization measures in 2018, the use of HES persisted in populations where

it posed significant health risks, including an increased mortality rate. Owing to non-compliance with product guidelines and its misuse beyond approved recommendations, the EMA suspended the use of HES on 24 June 2022 [190].

Dextrans and gelatins are not recommended

- Gelatin use is associated with an increased risk of anaphylaxis, AKI, bleeding, and mortality [171, 191–193]. Given that the side effects outweigh the potential benefits [80], the Surviving Sepsis Campaign Guidelines (2021) advise against using gelatin for acute resuscitation in adults with sepsis and septic shock [4].

- Dextrans are frequently utilized in vascular surgery due to their beneficial effects, such as reducing blood viscosity and potentially enhancing microvascular circulation, particularly following grafting procedures [88]. However, their use is restricted due to associated adverse effects like antithrombotic actions [194], renal dysfunction [195], hypersensitivity reactions [196], and interference with blood grouping and cross-matching. Notably, dextrans present a higher risk of severe anaphylactic reactions compared to gelatines or starches [145].

GUIDELINES FOR BLOOD TRANSFUSION IN HYPOVOLEMIC SHOCK

In the management of hypovolemic shock resulting from massive blood loss or active bleeding, administering blood transfusions in addition to fluid replacement and hemorrhage control is essential for restoring hemodynamic stability.

Transfusion decisions should always be based on the patient's clinical state:

1. In hospitalized, hemodynamically stable adult patients, blood transfusion is necessary if the hemoglobin level drops to ≤7 gm/dL (hematocrit ≤21%) [197].

2. In patients at high risk of adverse effects, including those undergoing cardiac surgery or exhibiting evidence of myocardial or other organ ischemia, a blood transfusion is required if hemoglobin drops to ≤8 gm/dL, aiming to maintain the hemoglobin level at ≥8 gm/dL.

3. In patients with ongoing significant bleeding and hypovolemia, the need for transfusion is determined based on pulse and blood pressure, the rate of bleeding, and estimated blood loss rather than solely relying on serial hemoglobin measurements. When a large volume of blood is needed, infuse one unit of plasma, one unit of platelets, and one unit of red blood cells (1:1:1 ratio), as suggested by the massive transfusion protocol [198].

4. Avoid liberal blood transfusion; hemoglobin and hematocrit should not be raised over 10 gm/dL and 30%, respectively [199]. A higher hematocrit level is unnecessary for oxygen transport and may increase blood viscosity, leading to stasis in the already impaired capillary circulation.

REFERENCES

1. Hoste EA, Maitland K, Brudney CS, et al. Four phases of intravenous fluid therapy: a conceptual model. Br J Anaesth 2014;113(5):740–7.

2. Hoorn EJ. Intravenous fluids: balancing solutions. J Nephrol. 2017;30(4):485–492.

3. Padhi S, Bullock I, Li L, et al. Intravenous fluid therapy for adults in hospital: summary of NICE guidance. BMJ 2013;347:f7073.

4. Evans L, Rhodes A, Alhazzani W, et al. Surviving sepsis campaign: international guidelines for management of sepsis and septic shock 2021. Crit Care Med 2021;49:e1063–143.

5. Yealy DM, Kellum JA, Huang DT, et al. ProCESS Investigators: A randomized trial of protocol-based care for early septic shock. N Engl J Med 2014;370(18):1683–1693.

6. Peake SL, Delaney A, Bellomo R, et al. ARISE Investigators: Goal-directed resuscitation in septic shock. N Engl J Med 2015;372(2):190–191.

7. Mouncey PR, Osborn TM, Power GS, et al. ProMISe Trial Investigators: Trial of early, goal-directed resuscitation for septic shock. N Engl J Med 2015;372(14):1301–1311.

8. Leisman DE, Doerfler ME, Schneider SM, et al. Predictors, Prevalence, and Outcomes of Early Crystalloid Responsiveness Among Initially Hypotensive Patients With Sepsis and Septic Shock. Crit Care Med. 2018;46(2):189–198.

9. Pollard S, Edwin SB, Alaniz C. Vasopressor and inotropic management of patients with septic shock ſ pharmacy and therapeutics. 2015;40(7):438–50.

10. Rewa O, Bagshaw SM. Principles of fluid management. Crit Care Clin 2015;31(4):785–801.

11. Myburgh JA. Fluid resuscitation in acute medicine: what is the current situation? Journal of Internal Medicine 2015;277(1):58–68.

12. Popescu M. Albumin therapy in critically ill patients. Cleveland clinic pharmacotherapy Update 2009; Volume XII, No. V.

13. Yartsev A. Response to 1L of normal saline. Deranged physiology 2015 (https://derangedphysiology.com/main/core-topics-intensive-care/manipulation-fluids-and-electrolytes/Chapter%202.3.3/response-1l-normal-saline).

14. Chin KJ, Macachor J, Ong KC, et al. A comparison of 5% dextrose in 0.9% normal saline versus non-dextrose-containing crystalloids as the initial intravenous replacement fluid in elective surgery. Anaesth Intensive Care 2006;34(5):613–7.

15. Myburgh JA, Mythen MG. Resuscitation fluids. N Engl J Med. 2013;369(13):1243–51.

16. Li H, Sun SR, Yap JQ, et al. 0.9% saline is neither normal nor physiological. J Zhejiang Univ Sci B. 2016;17(3):181–187.

17. Awad S, Allison SP, Lobo DN. The history of 0.9% saline. Clin Nutr. 2008;27(2):179–188.

18. Lobo DN, Awad S. Should chloride-rich crystalloids remain the mainstay of fluid resuscitation to prevent "pre-renal" acute kidney injury?: con. Kidney International. 2014;86(6):1096–1105.

19. Besen BA, Gobatto AL, Melro LM, et al. Fluid and electrolyte overload in critically ill patients: An overview. World J Crit Care Med 2015;4(2):116–129.

20. Yunos NM, Bellomo R, Hegarty C, et al. Association between a chloride-liberal vs chloride-restrictive

intravenous fluid administration strategy and kidney injury in critically ill adults. JAMA 2012;308(15):1566–72.

21. Neyra JA, Canepa-Escaro F, Li X, et al. Acute kidney injury in critical illness study G. Association of hyperchloremia with hospital mortality in critically ill septic patients. Crit Care Med. 2015;43(9):1938–44.

22. Sen A, Keener CM, Sileanu FE, et al. Chloride content of fluids used for large-volume resuscitation is associated with reduced survival. Crit Care Med. 2017;45(2):e146–e153.

23. Kim HJ, Oh TK, Song IA, et al. Association between fluctuations in serum chloride levels and 30-day mortality among critically ill patients: a retrospective analysis BMC Anesthesiol 2019;19(1):79.

24. Fisher AD, Carius BM. Three reasons not to use normal saline or crystalloids in trauma. JEMS March 2018; https://www.jems.com/2018/03/14/three-reasons-not-to-use-saline-or-crystalloids-in-trauma/.

25. Farkas J. Nine reasons to quit using normal saline for resuscitation. EMCrit Project. https://emcrit.org/pulmcrit/smart/. Published 2018. Accessed 2018.

26. Scheingraber S, Rehm M, Schmisch C, et al. Rapid saline infusion produces hyperchloremic acidosis in patients undergoing gynecologic surgery. Anesthesiology. 1999;90(5):1265–1270.

27. Yunos NM, Bellomo R, Story D, et al. Bench-to-bedside review: chloride in critical illness. Critical Care; 2010;14(4):226.

28. Reddi BAJ. Why is saline so acidic (and does it really matter?) Int J Med Sci 2013;10(6):747–750.

29. Morgan TJ. The meaning of acid-base abnormalities in the intensive care unit–effects of fluid administration. Crit Care. 2005;9(2):204–11.

30. Nagami GT. Hyperchloremia - Why and how. Nefrologia 2016;36(4):347–353.

31. Adrogué HJ, Madias NE. Management of life-threatening acid-base disorders. First of two parts. N Engl J Med. 1998;338(1):26–34.

32. Krajewski ML, Raghunathan K, Paluszkiewicz SM, et al. Meta-analysis of high- versus low-chloride content in perioperative and critical care fluid resuscitation. Br J Surg 2015;102(1):24–26.

33. Ginter D, Gilfoyle E, Wade A, et al. Hyperchloremia and association with acute kidney injury in critically ill children. Pediatr Nephrol. 2023;38(7):2233–2242.

34. Khajavi MR, Etezadi F, Moharari RS, et al. Effects of normal saline vs. Lactated ringer's during renal transplantation. Ren Fail. 2008;30(5):535–9.

35. Farkas J. Myth-busting: lactated Ringers is safe in hyperkalemia, and is superior to ns. PulmCrit.org (EMCrit) 2014 (https://emcrit.org/pulmcrit/myth-busting-lactated-ringers-is-safe-in-hyperkalemia-and-is-superior-to-ns/).

36. Weinberg L, Harris L, Bellomo R, et al. Effects of intraoperative and early postoperative normal saline or Plasmalyte 148® on hyperkalaemia in deceased donor renal transplantation: a double-blind randomized trial. Br J Anaesth. 2017;119(4):606–615.

37. White SA, Goldhill DR. Is Hartmann's the solution? Anaesthesia 1997;52(5):422–427.

38. Metabolic fate of lactate, acetate, citrate and gluconate. June, 2015. http://www.derangedphysiology.com/main/core-topics-intensive-care/manipulation-fluids-and-electrolytes/Chapter%204.1.4/metabolic-fate-lactate-acetate-citrate-and-gluconate.

39. Reddy S, Weinberg L, Young P. Crystalloid fluid therapy. Critical Care; 2016;20:59.

40. Raman S, Gibbons KS, Mattke A, et al. Effect of Saline vs Gluconate/Acetate-Buffered Solution vs Lactate-Buffered Solution on Serum Chloride Among Children in the Pediatric Intensive Care Unit: The SPLYT-P Randomized Clinical Trial. JAMA Pediatr. 2023;177(2):122–131.

41. Semler MW, Rice TW. Saline is not the first choice for crystalloid resuscitation fluids. Crit Care Med. 2016;44(8):1541–1544.

42. Weinberg L, Collins N, Mourik KV, et al. Plasma-lyte 148: a clinical review. World Journal of Critical Care Medicine. 2016;5(4):235–250.

43. Didwania A, Miller J, Kassel D, et al. Effect of intravenous lactated Ringer's solution infusion on the circulating lactate concentration: Part 3. Results of a prospective, randomized, double-blind, placebo-controlled trial. Crit Care Med. 1997;25(11):1851–4.

44. Zitek T, Skaggs ZD, Rahbar A, et al. Does Intravenous Lactated Ringer's Solution Raise Serum Lactate? J Emerg Med. 2018;55(3):313–318.

45. Hernandez G, Bellomo R, Bakker J. The ten pitfalls of lactate clearance in sepsis. Intensive Care Med. 2019;45(1):82–85.

46. Limapichat T, Pattanapong K. Normal Saline Solution or Lactated Ringer's Solution to Enhance Lactate Clearance in Septic Patients After Initial Resuscitation in the ED: A Retrospective Cohort Trial. Open Access Emerg Med. 2021;13:511–519.

47. Farkas J. Fluid selection & pH-guided fluid resuscitation. Pulmcrit (EMCrit) June 2019 https://emcrit.org/ibcc/fluid/.

48. Yartsev A. Response to 1L of Hartmann's compound sodium lactate. Deranged Physiology June 25, 2015 https://derangedphysiology.com/main/core-topics-intensive-care/manipulation-fluids-and-electrolytes/Chapter%202.3.4/response-1l-hartmanns-compound-sodium-lactate.

49. Farkas J. Three myths about Plasmalyte, Normosol, and LR. PulmCrit January 26, 2015 https://emcrit.org/pulmcrit/three-myths-about-plasmalyte-normosol-and-lr/.

50. Singh S, Davis D. Ringer's Lactate. [Updated 2019 Mar 22]. In: StatPearls [Internet]. Treasure Island (FL): StatPearls Publishing; 2019 Jan. Available from: https://www.ncbi.nlm.nih.gov/books/NBK500033/.

51. O'Malley CMN, Frumento RJ, Hardy MA, et al. A randomized, double-blind comparison of lactated Ringer's solution and 0.9% NaCl during renal transplantation. Anesth Analg. 2005;100(5):1518–1524.

52. Modi MP, Vora KS, Parikh GP, et al. A Comparative study of impact of infusion of Ringer's lactate solution versus normal saline on acid–base balance and serum electrolytes. Saudi J Kidney Dis Transplant. 2012;23(1):135–137.

53. Tommasino C, Picozzi V. Volume and electrolyte management. Best Pract Res Clin Anaesthesiol. 2007;21(4):497–516.

54. Ryu T. Fluid management in patients undergoing neurosurgery. Anesth Pain Med (Seoul). 2021;16(3):215–224.

55. Rossaint R, Afshari A, Bouillon B, et al. The European guideline on management of major bleeding and coagulopathy following trauma: sixth edition. Crit Care. 2023;27(1):80.

56. Yoo HK, Cheong MA, Jong Won Lee JW, et al. Effects of Lactated Ringer's Solution on Acid-Base and Serum Electrolyte Levels during Liver Surgery in Cirrhosis Patients. Korean J Anesthesiol. 2004;47(3):361–367.

57. Singh S, Kerndt CC, Davis D. Ringer's Lactate. [Updated 2023 Aug 14]. In: StatPearls [Internet]. Treasure Island (FL): StatPearls Publishing; 2023 Jan-. Available from: https://www.ncbi.nlm.nih.gov/books/NBK500033/.

58. Jimenez JV, Garcia-Tsao G, Saffo S. Emerging concepts in the care of patients with cirrhosis and septic shock. World J Hepatol 2023;15(4):497–514.

59. Ellekjaer KL, Perner A, Jensen MM, et al. Lactate versus acetate buffered intravenous crystalloid solutions: a scoping review. Br J Anaesth. 2020;125(5):693–703.

60. Bergmann KR, Abuzzahab MJ, Nowak J, et al. Resuscitation with Ringer's lactate compared with normal saline for pediatric diabetic ketoacidosis. Pediatr Emerg Care 2021;37(5):e236–e242.

61. Jahangir A, Jahangir A, Siddiqui FS, et al. Normal Saline Versus Low Chloride Solutions in Treatment of Diabetic Ketoacidosis: A Systematic Review of Clinical Trials. Cureus. 2022;14(1):e21324.

62. Catahay JA, Polintan ET, Casimiro M, et al. Balanced electrolyte solutions versus isotonic saline in adult patients with diabetic ketoacidosis: A systematic review and meta-analysis. Heart Lung. 2022;54:74–79.

63. Alghamdi NA, Major P, Chaudhuri D, et al. Saline Compared to Balanced Crystalloid in Patients With Diabetic Ketoacidosis: A Systematic Review and Meta-Analysis of Randomized Controlled Trials. Critical Care Explorations. 2022;4(1):e0613.

64. Shaw AD, Bagshaw SM, Goldstein SL, et al. Major complications, mortality, and resource utilization after open abdominal surgery: 0.9% saline compared to plasma-lyte. Ann Surg 2012;255(5):821–829.

65. McCluskey SA, Karkouti K, Wijeysundera D, et al. Hyperchloremia after noncardiac surgery is independently associated with increased morbidity and mortality: a propensity-matched cohort study. Anesth Analg 2013;117(2):412–21.

66. Raghunathan K, Shaw A, Nathanson B, et al. Association between the choice of IV crystalloid and in-hospital mortality among critically ill with sepsis. Crit Care Med 2014;42(7):1585–91.

67. Semler MW, Self WH, Wanderer JP, et al. Balanced crystalloids versus saline in critically ill adults. (SMART Trial) N Engl J Med 2018;378(9):829–39.

68. Self WH, Semler MW, Wanderer JP, et al. Balanced crystalloids versus saline in noncritically ill adults. (SALT-ED Trial) N Engl J Med 2018;378(9):819–28.

69. Young P, Bailey M, Beasley R, et al. Effect of a buffered crystalloid solution vs saline on acute kidney injury among patients in the intensive care unit: the SPLIT randomized clinical trial. JAMA 2015;314(16):1701–1710.

70. Semler MW, Wanderer JP, Ehrenfeld JM, et al. Balanced crystalloids versus saline in the intensive care unit. The SALT randomized trial. Am J Respir Crit Care Med 2017;195(10):1362–1372.

71. Zampieri FG, Machado FR, Biondi RS, et al. Effect of Intravenous Fluid Treatment With a Balanced Solution vs 0.9% Saline Solution on Mortality in Critically Ill Patients: The BaSICS Randomized Clinical Trial. JAMA. 2021;326(9):1–12.

72. Finfer S, Micallef S, Hammond N, et al. PLUS Study Investigators and the Australian New Zealand Intensive Care Society Clinical Trials Group. Balanced Multielectrolyte Solution versus Saline in Critically Ill Adults. N Engl J Med. 2022;386(9):815–826.

73. Bampoe S, Odor PM, Dushianthan A, et al. Perioperative administration of buffered versus non-buffered crystalloid intravenous fluid to improve outcomes following adult surgical procedures. Cochrane Database Syst Rev 2017;9(9):CD004089.

74. Rhodes A, Evans LE, Alhazzani W, et al. Surviving sepsis campaign: international guidelines for management of sepsis and septic shock: 2016. Crit Care Med. 2017;45(3):486–552.

75. Hammond NE, Zampieri FG, Di Tanna GL, et al. Balanced Crystalloids versus Saline in Critically Ill Adults — A Systematic Review with Meta-Analysis. NEJM Evid 2022;1(2).

76. Beran A, Altorok N, Srour O, et al. Balanced Crystalloids versus Normal Saline in Adults with Sepsis: A Comprehensive Systematic Review and Meta-Analysis. J Clin Med. 2022;11(7):1971.

77. Isha S, Satashia PH, Yarrarapu SNS, et al. A retrospective analysis of normal saline and lactated ringers as resuscitation fluid in sepsis. Front Med (Lausanne). 2023;10:1071741.

78. Zampieri FG, Cavalcanti AB, Di Tanna GL, et al. Balanced crystalloids versus saline for critically ill patients (BEST-Living): a systematic review and individual patient data meta-analysis. Lancet Respir Med. 2024;12(3):237–246.

79. Shankar M, Trinidad C, Tannor EK, et al. Balanced Solutions Versus Saline to Reduce AKI: A #NephJC Editorial on the BaSICS Trial. Kidney Med. 2022;4(6):100472.

80. Moschopoulos CD, Dimopoulou D, Dimopoulou A, et al. New Insights into the Fluid Management in Patients with Septic Shock. Medicina (Kaunas). 2023;59(6):1047.

81. Antequera Martín AM, Barea Mendoza JA, Muriel A, et al. Buffered solutions versus 0.9% saline for resuscitation in critically ill adults and children. Cochrane Database Syst Rev 2019;7(7):CD012247.

82. Drew D, Hendin A, Eagles D. Which crystalloid should we be using for the resuscitation of septic patients? CJEM. 2023;25(1):20–21.

83. Miller TE, Bunke M, Nisbet P, et al. Fluid resuscitation practice patterns in intensive care units of the USA:

a cross-sectional survey of critical care physicians. Perioper Med (Lond) 2016;5:15.

84. Jonsson AB, Perner A. Changes from 2012 to 2015 in intravenous fluid solutions issued to hospital departments. Acta Anaesthesiol Scand. 2017;61(5):532–538.

85. Severs D, Hoorn EJ, Rookmaaker MB. A critical appraisal of intravenous fluids: from the physiological basis to clinical evidence. Nephrol Dial Transplant 2015;30(2):178–87.

86. Glassford NJ, French CJ, Bailey M, et al. Changes in intravenous fluid use patterns in Australia and New Zealand: evidence of research translating into practice. Crit Care Resusc. 2016;18(2):78–88.

87. Semler MW, Kellum JA. Balanced Crystalloid Solutions. Am J Respir Crit Care Med. 2019;199(8):952–960.

88. Mayerhöfer T, Shaw AD, Wiedermann CJ, et al. Fluids in the ICU: which is the right one? Nephrol Dial Transplant. 2023;38(7):1603–1612.

89. Zampieri FG, Bagshaw SM. Making (numerical) sense of recent trials comparing balanced and normal saline intravenous solutions in the critically ill. Br J Anaesth. 2023;131(1):e10–e13.

90. Nam JH, Kwack HJ, Ha WS, et al. Resuscitation Fluids for Patients at High Risk of Multiple Organ Dysfunction Syndromes: A Systematic Review and Meta-analysis. Korean J Clin Pharm 2022;32(3):251–259.

91. Kherallah M. Balanced fluid or saline for critically-ill patients? ICU Reach. Updated 2022 Oct 7. Available from: https://www.icureach.com/post/balanced-fluid-or-saline-for-critically-ill-patients.

92. Qayyum S, Shahid K. Fluid Resuscitation in Septic Patients. Cureus. 2023;15(8):e44317.

93. Tseng CH, Chen TT, Wu MY, et al. Resuscitation fluid types in sepsis, surgical, and trauma patients: a systematic review and sequential network meta-analyses. Crit Care. 2020;24(1):693.

94. Guarino M, Perna B, Cesaro AE, et al. 2023 Update on Sepsis and Septic Shock in Adult Patients: Management in the Emergency Department. Journal of Clinical Medicine. 2023;12(9):3188.

95. Yealy DM, Mohr NM, Shapiro NI, et al. Early Care of Adults With Suspected Sepsis in the Emergency Department and Out-of-Hospital Environment: A Consensus-Based Task Force Report. Ann Emerg Med. 2021;78(1):1–19.

96. Prabhakar A, Bhargava V. Balanced Salt Solutions: Are We Crystal Clear or Still Murky? ASN Kidney News 2022;14(12):25–26.

97. Raghunathan K, Murray PT, Beattie WS, et al. Choice of fluid in acute illness: what should be given? An international consensus. Br J Surg 2014;113(5):772–83.

98. Martin C, Cortegiani A, Gregoretti C, et al. Choice of fluids in critically ill patients. BMC Anesthesiology 2018;18(1):200.

99. Hammond DA, Lam SW, Rech MA, et al. Balanced Crystalloids Versus Saline in Critically Ill Adults: A Systematic Review and Meta-analysis. Ann Pharmacother. 2020;54(1):5–13.

100. Miller TE, Myles PS. Perioperative fluid therapy for major surgery. Anesthesiology 2019;130(5):825–832.

101. Spahn DR, Bouillon B, Cerny V, et al. The European guideline on management of major bleeding and coagulopathy following trauma: Fifth edition Critical Care 2019;23(1):98.

102. Cantle PM, Cotton BA. Balanced resuscitation in trauma management. Surg Clin North Am. 2017;97(5):999–1014.

103. Ostermann M, Liu K, Kashani K. Fluid management in acute kidney injury. Chest 2019;156(3):594–603.

104. Iqbal U, Anwar H, Scribani M. Ringer's lactate versus normal saline in acute pancreatitis: A systematic review and meta-analysis. J Dig Dis. 2018;19(6):335–341.

105. Guzmán-Calderón E, Diaz-Arocutipa C, Monge E. Lactate Ringer's Versus Normal Saline in the Management of Acute Pancreatitis: A Systematic Review and Meta-Analysis of Randomized Controlled Trials. Dig Dis Sci. 2022;67(8):4131–4139.

106. Yaowmaneerat T, Sirinawasatien A. Update on the strategy for intravenous fluid treatment in acute pancreatitis. World J Gastrointest Pharmacol Ther. 2023;14(3):22–32.

107. ISBI Practice Guidelines Committee; Steering Subcommittee; Advisory Subcommittee. ISBI Practice Guidelines for Burn Care. Burns. 2016;42(5):953–1021.

108. Zampieri FG, Machado FR, Veiga VC, et al. Determinants of fluid use and the association between volume of fluid used and effect of balanced solutions on mortality in critically ill patients: a secondary analysis of the BaSICS trial. Intensive Care Med. 2024;50(1):79–89.

109. Klouche K, Monnet X, Zarbock A. Balanced solution versus saline in critically ill patients: a new piece to the puzzle! Intensive Care Med. 2024;50(1):134–135.

110. Yartsev A. Normal saline vs balanced crystalloids as resuscitation fluid. Deranged Physiology. June 10, 2016 https://derangedphysiology.com/main/required-reading/electrolytes-and-fluids/Chapter%202.2.6/normal-saline-vs-balanced-crystalloids-resuscitation-fluid.

111. Lactated Ringers FDA prescribing information. Mar 1, 2019 - Accessed on 24 Sept 2019. https://www.drugs.com/pro/lactated-ringers.html.

112. Yunos NM, Bellomo R, Glassford N, et al. Chloride-liberal vs. Chloride-restrictive intravenous fluid administration and acute kidney injury: an extended analysis. Intensive Care Med 2015;41(2):257–64.

113. Pfortmueller CA, Kabon B, Schefold JC, et al. Crystalloid fluid choice in the critically ill: current knowledge and critical appraisal. Wien Klin Wochenschr 2018;130(7–8):273–82.

114. Rein J, Coca S. I don't get no respect": the role of chloride in acute kidney injury. Am J Physiol Renal Physiol. 2019;316(3):F587–F605.

115. Palevsky PM. Intravenous Fluids Finding the right balance. Clin J Am Soc Nephrol 2018;13(12):1912–1914.

116. Lim JY, Kang PJ, Jung SH, et al. Effect of high-versus low-volume saline administration on acute kidney injury after cardiac surgery. J Thorac Dis 2018;10(12):6753–62.

117. Romagnoli S, Ricci Z. Intravenous sodium and chloride: not too much, not too quick, and only to healthy kidneys! J Thorac Dis. 2019;11(9):S1180–S1183.

118. Ertmer C, Van Aken H. Fluid therapy in patients with brain injury: what does physiology tell us? Crit Care. 2014;18(2):119.

119. Berend K, de Vries AP, Gans RO. Physiological approach to assessment of acid-base disturbances. N Engl J Med 2014;371(15):1434–1445.

120. Haddad SH, Arabi YM. Critical care management of severe traumatic brain injury in adults. Scandinavian Journal of Trauma, Resuscitation and Emergency Medicine. 2012;20:12.

121. Sterling SA, Puskarich MA, Jones AE. The effect of liver disease on lactate normalization in severe sepsis and septic shock: a cohort study. Clin Exp Emerg Med. 2015;2(4):197–202.

122. Andersen LW, Mackenhauer J, Roberts JC, et al. Etiology and therapeutic approach to elevated lactate levels. Mayo Clin Proc. 2013;88(10):1127–40.

123. Ergin B, Kapucu A, Guerci P, et al. The role of bicarbonate precursors in balanced fluids during haemorrhagic shock with and without compromised liver function. Br J Anaesth 2016;117(4):521–528.

124. Kveim M, Nesbakken R. Utilization of exogenous acetate during canine haemorrhagic shock. Scand J Clin Lab Invest 1979;39(7):653–658.

125. Rizoli S. PlasmaLyte. J Trauma. 2011;70(5):S17–8.

126. Curran JD, Major P, Tang K, et al. Comparison of Balanced Crystalloid Solutions: A Systematic Review and Meta-Analysis of Randomized Controlled Trials. Crit Care Explor. 2021;3(5):e0398.

127. Ellekjaer KL, Perner A, Sivapalan P, et al. Acetate-versus lactate-buffered crystalloid solutions: A systematic review with meta-analysis and trial sequential analysis. Acta Anaesthesiol Scand. 2022;66(7):782–794.

128. Priyanka A, Ganapathy U, Choudhary R, et al. A Comparative Study of Peri-Operative Fluid Therapy With Ringer Lactate and PlasmaLyte in Children Undergoing Intra-Abdominal Surgery: A Randomized Control Trial. Cureus. 2023;15(5):e39124.

129. Abdellatif AE, Alassal MA, Ul-Haq R, et al. Plasmalyte and Ringer Lactate as Priming Solutions in Pediatric Cardiopulmonary Bypass: A Comparative Study. Cardiometry 2023;28:34–42.

130. Weinberg L, Chiam E, Hooper J, et al. Plasma-Lyte 148 vs. Hartmann's solution for cardiopulmonary bypass pump prime: a prospective double-blind randomized trial. Perfusion. 2018;33(4):310–319.

131. Pfortmueller CA, Faeh L, Müller M, et al. Fluid management in patients undergoing cardiac surgery: effects of an acetate- versus lactate-buffered balanced infusion solution on hemodynamic stability (HEMACETAT). Crit Care. 2019;23(1):159.

132. Rawat N, Sahni N, Yaddanapudi L. Comparison of Commercially Available Balanced Salt Solution and Ringer's Lactate on Extent of Correction of Metabolic Acidosis in Critically Ill Patients. Indian J Crit Care Med. 2020;24(7):539–543.

133. Chaussard M, Dépret F, Saint-Aubin O, et al. Physiological response to fluid resuscitation with Ringer lactate versus Plasmalyte in critically ill burn patients. J Appl Physiol (1985). 2020;128(3):709–714.

134. Lira A, Pinsky MR. Choices in fluid type and volume during resuscitation: impact on patient outcomes. Annals of Intensive Care. 2014;4:38.

135. Pfortmueller CA, Fleischmann E. Acetate-buffered crystalloid fluids: current knowledge, a systematic review. J Crit Care. 2016;35:96–104.

136. Ramanan M, Attokaran A, Murray L. SCOPE-DKA Collaborators and Queensland Critical Care Research Network (QCCRN). Sodium chloride or Plasmalyte-148 evaluation in severe diabetic ketoacidosis (SCOPE-DKA): a cluster, crossover, randomized, controlled trial. Intensive Care Med. 2021;47(11):1248–1257.

137. Othman MI, Nashwan AJ, Alfayoumi M, et al. Plasma-Lyte-148 Versus Normal Saline 0.9% in Diabetic Ketoacidosis Management: A Review. Cureus. 2023;15(6):e41079.

138. Raghunathan K, Khangulov VS, Peyerl FW, et al. The association between choice of balanced intravenous crystalloid and subsequent major in-hospital outcomes among adult patients undergoing cardiac surgery. Value in Health 2015;18(3):A133.

139. Liu C, Zhi Mao Z, Hu P, et al. Fluid resuscitation in critically ill patients: a systematic review and network meta-analysis. Therapeutics and Clinical Risk Management 2018;14:1701–1709.

140. McCague A, Dermendjieva M, Hutchinson R, et al. Sodium acetate infusion in critically ill trauma patients for hyperchloremic acidosis. Scand J Trauma Resusc Emerg Med. 2011;19:24.

141. Young JB, Utter GH, Schermer CR, et al. Saline versus Plasma-Lyte A in initial resuscitation of trauma patients: a randomized trial. Ann Surg. 2014;259(2):255–62.

142. Surabhi S, Kumar M. Comparison of ringer's lactate and plasmalyte-A as cardiopulmonary bypass prime for bypass associated acidosis in valve replacement surgeries. Ann Card Anaesth. 2021;24(1):36–41.

143. Collins MG, Fahim MA, Pascoe EM, et al. Balanced crystalloid solution versus saline in deceased donor kidney transplantation (BEST-Fluids): a pragmatic, double-blind, randomised, controlled trial. Lancet. 2023;402(10396):105–117.

144. Venkataraman K, McTaggart SJ, Collins MG. Choosing fluids to reduce the risks of acute electrolyte disturbances in children after a kidney transplant. Kidney Int. 2024;105(2):247–250.

145. Mitra S, Khandelwal P. Are all colloids same? How to select the right colloid? Indian J Anaesth 2009;53(5):592–607.

146. László I, Demeter G, Öveges N, et al. Volume-replacement ratio for crystalloids and colloids during bleeding and resuscitation: an animal experiment. Intensive Care Med Exp. 2017;5(1):52.

147. Cortés DO, Barros TG, Njimi H, et al. Crystalloids versus colloids: exploring differences in fluid requirements by systematic review and meta-regression. Anesthesia Analgesia. 2015;120(2):389–402.

148. Annane D, Siami S, Jaber S, et al. Effects of fluid resuscitation with colloids vs crystalloids on mortality in critically ill patients presenting with hypovolemic shock: The CRISTAL Randomized Trial. JAMA 2013;310(17):1809–17.

149. Doherty M, Buggy DJ. Intraoperative fluids: how much is too much? Br J Anaesth. 2012;109(1):69–79.

150. Voldby AW, Brandstrup B. Fluid therapy in the perioperative setting-a clinical review. J Intensive Care 2016;4:27.

151. Martin GS, Bassett P. Crystalloids vs. colloids for fluid resuscitation in the intensive care unit: a systematic review and meta-analysis. Journal of Critical Care 2019;50:144–154.

152. Kwan I, Bunn F, Chinnock P, et al. Timing and volume of fluid administration for patients with bleeding. Cochrane Database of Systematic Reviews 2014;2014(3):CD002245.

153. Hahn RG, Lyons G. The half-life of infusion fluids: An educational review. Eur J Anaesthesiol. 2016;33(7):475–482.

154. Kabon B, Sessler DI, Kurz A, et al. Effect of intraoperative goal-directed balanced crystalloid versus colloid administration on major postoperative morbidity: a randomized trial. Anesthesiology 2019;130(5):728–744.

155. Cochrane injuries group albumin reviewers. Human albumin administration in critically ill patients: systematic review of randomised controlled trials. BMJ. 1998;317(7153):235–40.

156. Finfer S, Bellomo R, Boyce N, et al. A comparison of albumin and saline for fluid resuscitation in the intensive care unit. (SAFE study) N Engl J Med 2004;350(22):2247–56.

157. Roberts I, Blackhall K, Alderson P, Bunn F, Schierhout G. Human albumin solution for resuscitation and volume expansion in critically ill patients. Cochrane Database Syst Rev. 2011;11:CD001208.

158. Xu JY, Chen QH, Xie JF, et al. Comparison of the effects of albumin and crystalloid on mortality in adult patients with severe sepsis and septic shock: a meta-analysis of randomized clinical trials. Crit Care. 2014;18(6):702.

159. Patel A, Laffan MA, Waheed U, et al. Randomised trials of human albumin for adults with sepsis: systematic review and meta-analysis with trial sequential analysis of all-cause mortality. BMJ. 2014;349:g4561.

160. Caironi P, Tognoni G, Masson S, et al. Albumin replacement in patients with severe sepsis or septic shock (ALBIOS Trial). N Engl J Med. 2014;370(15):1412–1421.

161. Perner A, Haase N, Guttormsen AB, et al. Hydroxyethyl starch 130/0.42 versus Ringer's acetate in severe sepsis. (6S Trial) N Engl J Med 2012;367(2):124–34.

162. Myburgh JA, Finfer S, Bellomo R, et al. Hydroxyethyl starch or saline for fluid resuscitation in intensive care. (Chest Trial) N Engl J Med 2012;367(20):1901–1911.

163. Mutter TC, Ruth CA, Dart AB. Hydroxyethyl starch (HES) versus other fluid therapies: effects on kidney function. Cochrane Database Syst Rev 2013;(7):CD007594.

164. European Medicines Agency. Hydroxyethyl starch solutions (HES) should no longer be used in patients with sepsis or burn injuries or in critically ill patients. EMA http://www.ema.europa.eu/docs/en_GB/document_library/Referrals_document/Solutions_for_infusion_containing_hydroxyethyl_starch/European_Commission_final_decision/WC500162361.pdf (2014).

165. European Medicines Agency. Hydroxyethyl starch solutions: CMDh introduces new measures to protect patients. Internet Document: 17 July 2018. https://www.ema.europa.eu/en/documents/referral/hydroxyethyl-starch-article-107i-referral-hydroxyethyl-starch-solutions-cmdh-introduces-new-measures_en.pdf.

166. European Medicines Agency. Hydroxyethyl starch (HES) solutions for infusion: suspension of marketing authorisations due to continued use in contraindicated patient populations with increased risk of serious harm. Update as of 26 July 2022 [Internet]. Available from: https://www.ema.europa.eu/en/documents/dhpc/direct-healthcare-professional-communication-dhpc-hydroxyethyl-starch-hes-solutions-infusion_en.pdf.

167. Perel P, Roberts I, Ker K. Colloids versus crystalloids for fluid resuscitation in critically ill patients. Cochrane Database Syst Rev 2013;(2):CD000567.

168. Lewis SR, Pritchard MW, Evans DJ, et al. Colloids versus crystalloids for fluid resuscitation in critically ill people. Cochrane Database of Systematic Reviews 2018;(8):CD000567.

169. Hammond NE, Taylor C, Finfer S, et al. Patterns of intravenous fluid resuscitation use in adult intensive care patients between 2007 and 2014: an international cross-sectional study. PLoS One. 2017;12(5):e0176292.

170. Heming N, Lamothe L, Jaber S, et al. Morbidity and mortality of crystalloids compared to colloids in critically ill surgical patients: a subgroup analysis of a randomized trial. Anesthesiology 2018;129(6):1149–1158.

171. Boer C, Bossers SM, Koning NJ. Choice of fluid type: physiological concepts and perioperative indications. Br J Anaesth. 2018;120(2):384–396.

172. Vincent JL. Fluid management in the critically ill. Kidney International 2019;96(1):52–57.

173. Mårtensson J, Bellomo R. Are all fluids bad for the kidney? Curr Opin Crit Care. 2015;21(4):292–301.

174. Callum J, Skubas NJ, Bathla A, et al. Use of Intravenous Albumin: A Guideline from the International Collaboration for Transfusion Medicine Guidelines. Chest. 2024:S0012-3692(24)00285-X.

175. Wiedermann CJ. Human Albumin Infusion in Critically Ill and Perioperative Patients: Narrative Rapid Review of Meta-Analyses from the Last Five Years. Journal of Clinical Medicine. 2023;12(18):5919.

176. Wiedermann CJ. Moderator Effect of Hypoalbuminemia in Volume Resuscitation and Plasma Expansion with Intravenous Albumin Solution. Int. J. Mol. Sci. 2022;23(22):14175.

177. Zhou S, Zeng Z, Wei H, et al. Early combination of albumin with crystalloids administration might be beneficial for the survival of septic patients: a retrospective analysis from MIMIC-IV database. Ann Intensive Care. 2021;11(1):42.

178. Geng L, Tian X, Gao Z, et al. Different Concentrations of Albumin Versus Crystalloid in Patients with Sepsis and Septic Shock: A Meta-Analysis of Randomized Clinical Trials. J Intensive Care Med. 2023;38(8):679–689.

179. Raynor B, Huang A, Udrea D, et al. The Role of Albumin in the Resuscitation of Hypotensive Patients. Curr Emerg Hosp Med Rep 2023:11:89–94.

180. Caironi P, Gattinoni L. The clinical use of albumin: the point of view of a specialist in intensive care. Blood Transfus. 2009;7(4):259–267.

181. Vincent JL, Russell JA, Jacob M, et al. Albumin administration in the acutely ill: what is new and where next? Crit Care 2014;18(4):231.

182. Jiang L, Jiang S, Zhang M, et al. Albumin versus other fluids for fluid resuscitation in patients with sepsis: a meta-analysis. PLoS One. 2014;9(12):e114666.

183. Altawalbeh SM, Almestarihi EM, Khasawneh RA, et al. Cost-effectiveness of intravenous resuscitation fluids in sepsis patients: a patient-level data analysis in Jordan. J Med Econ. 2024;27(1):126–133.

184. Rossi S, Picetti E, Zoerle T, et al. Fluid management in acute brain injury. Curr Neurol Neurosci Rep 2018;18(11):74.

185. Oddo M, Poole D, Helbok R, et al. Fluid therapy in neurointensive care patients: ESICM consensus and clinical practice recommendations. Intensive Care Med. 2018;44(4):449–463.

186. Ma HK, Bebawy JF. Albumin Use in Brain-injured and Neurosurgical Patients: Concepts, Indications, and Controversies. J Neurosurg Anesthesiol. 2021;33(4):293–299.

187. Schmidt AP, Bilotta F. Hydroxyethyl starch for perioperative fluid management: a critical appraisal. Braz J Anesthesiol. 2023;73(5):529–531.

188. Joosten A, Coeckelenbergh S, Alexander B, et al. Hydroxyethyl starch for perioperative goal-directed fluid therapy in 2020: a narrative review. BMC Anesthesiol. 2020;20(1):209.

189. Landow L, Wei S, Song L, et al. Recent U.S. Food and Drug Administration Labeling Changes for Hydroxyethyl Starch Products Due to Concerns about Mortality, Kidney Injury, and Excess Bleeding. Anesthesiology. 2022;136(5):868–870.

190. Hydroxyethyl starch: CMDh Scientific Conclusion and Condition for Lifting suspension of the marketing authorisations. 24 June 2022 Available at: https://www.ema.europa.eu/en/documents/psusa/hydroxyethyl-starch-cmdh-scientific-conclusions-conditions-lifting-suspension-marketing/h/n/psr/j/0031_en.pdf.

191. Thomas-Rueddel DO, Vlasakov V, Reinhart K, et al. Safety of gelatin for volume resuscitation–a systematic review and meta-analysis. Intensive Care Med. 2012;38(7):1134–42.

192. Moeller C, Fleischmann C, Thomas-Rueddel D, et al. How safe is gelatin? A systematic review and meta-analysis of gelatin-containing plasma expanders vs crystalloids and albumin. J Crit Care 2016;35:75–83.

193. Farooque S, Kenny M, Marshall SD. Anaphylaxis to intravenous gelatin-based solutions: a case series examining clinical features and severity. Anaesthesia. 2019;74(2):174–179.

194. Sigurjonsson J, Hedman D, Bansch P, et al. Comparison of dextran and albumin on blood coagulation in patients undergoing major gynaecological surgery Perioperative Medicine 2018;7:21.

195. Dickenmann M, Oettl T, Mihatsch MJ. Osmotic nephrosis: acute kidney injury with accumulation of proximal tubular lysosomes due to administration of exogenous solutes Am J Kidney Dis 2008;51(3):491–503.

196. Shiratori T, Sato A, Fukuzawa M, et al. Case reports: severe dextran-induced anaphylactic shock during induction of hypertension-hypervolemia-hemodilution therapy following subarachnoid hemorrhage. Critical Care 2015:967560.

197. Carson JL, Guyatt G, Heddle NM, et al. Clinical practice guidelines from the AABB. JAMA. 2016;316(19):2025–2035.

198. Holcomb JB, Tilley BC, Baraniuk S, et al. Transfusion of Plasma, Platelets, and Red Blood Cells in a 1:1:1 Vs a 1:1:2 Ratio and Mortality in Patients with Severe Trauma:The Proppr Randomized Clinical Trial. JAMA 2015;313(5):471–82.

199. Yaddanapudi S, Yaddanapudi LN. Indications for blood and blood product transfusion. Indian J Anaesth 2014;58(5):538–42.

9 | Fluid Therapy in the Elderly

Globally, Life expectancy is increasing steadily [1], so there is a need to understand the medical problems of the larger elderly population.

PHYSIOLOGICAL BASIS

To understand fluid and electrolyte disorders in the elderly, it is essential to understand physiological changes related to fluid balance in older adults. Significant relevant physiological changes are [2–5]:

- Decrease in total body water by about 10–15% due to reduced lean body mass.
- A reduction in thirst perception due to central nervous system dysfunction controlling thirst.
- Progressive reduction in renal blood flow, glomerular filtration rate and loss of renal mass.
- Impaired renal ability to concentrate urine and conserve water makes older adults prone to dehydration.
- Significant increase in atrial natriuretic peptide (ANP) activity and reduction in renin and aldosterone serum concentrations. These hormonal changes lead to an impaired ability

to retain sodium, causing a greater risk of developing hyponatremia and hypovolemia.

Why understanding dehydration in the elderly is important?

It is essential to understand about dehydration in the elderly because:

- Hypovolemia is a common fluid and electrolyte disorder in the elderly [6, 7], which affects about 20% to 30% of older adults [8].
- Dehydration is the most common cause requiring hospitalization in the elderly [9, 10].
- Dehydration in the elderly is associated with a longer stay in the hospital, increased health care costs, morbidity and mortality [11–13].
- Dehydration in the elderly can cause problems like acute confusion, constipation, urinary tract infections, kidney stones, exhaustion, and pressure ulcers [14–16]. Elderly patients with dehydration can have orthostatic hypotension leading to impaired brain perfusion and dizziness, causing an increased risk of falls and bone fractures [17].

- Timely aggressive fluid administration can improve clinical outcomes in dehydration [18].

Why are elderly patients being more prone to develop dehydration?

Reasons for the higher risk of dehydration in the elderly are:

- Reduced total body water (TBW) as a portion of body weight, so the risk of dehydration even with a loss of less volume of fluids.
- Inability to access water due to physical limitations and lack of help.
- Inadequate water intake due to decreased thirst sensation and altered awareness or mental status [5].
- With aging, renal function and ability to concentrate urine and retain fluid decline [16].
- Among older people, the habit is drinking less water than younger people [19], and the daily fluid intake of older people is below the recommended daily requirement [16].
- Common medications for the elderly such as diuretics for hypertension, increase the risk of dehydration.

DIAGNOSIS OF DEHYDRATION

In the elderly, commonly used signs and tests such as skin turgor, mouth dryness, weight change, urine color, specific gravity, or bioelectrical impedance are not useful in assessing hydration status [20, 21]. However, clinical clues like mental confusion, non-fluent speech, extremity weakness, dry mucous membranes, dry tongue, furrowed tongue, and sunken eyes provide important clues in diagnosing volume depletion in the elderly (the presence of ≥4 criteria out of 7 indicates volume depletion) [21].

Directly measured serum osmolality >300 mOsm/kg is a reliable test to diagnose dehydration in the elderly [11, 21].

NORMAL FLUID REQUIREMENT

The total fluid intake recommended for all ages by ESPEN (2022) and European Food Safety Authority (EFSA) 2010 guidelines is 2.5 L/day for men and 2.0 L/day for women [21, 22]. Out of total fluid consumed, drinking water or beverages account for 70–80%, and 20% come from consumed food [23].

Daily fluid intake is a minimum of 2.0 L/day for elderly males, and 1.6 L/day for elderly females is recommended by ESPEN and EFSA guidelines [21, 22].

PREVENTION OF DEHYDRATION

Dehydration is highly costly in older people as it causes multiple complications and is associated with morbidity and mortality. On the other hand, optimum fluid intake and prevention of dehydration offer mental, physical, and general health benefits, provides a better quality of life for older people, and save money for healthcare systems [24].

Simple steps to prevent dehydration in older persons are to ensure access to oral fluids, frequent offering of drinks, and encourage the older adult to increase their fluid intake according to their preferences throughout the day [21, 25, 26].

As dehydration is expected in the elderly, all hospitalized old adult patients should be screened carefully for early detection, preventive measures, and treatment if required, followed by frequent assessment of urine outputs and fluid balance during the hospital stay.

If diuretics are prescribed to the elderly, adjust their dose appropriately.

MANAGEMENT

The basic principles of fluid management are:

- To provide the maintenance need for fluids and to correct volume depletion, elderly patients should be given fluids, preferably orally or nasogastrically.

- Euvolemic patients who may be nothing by mouth (NPO) may need intravenous maintenance fluids. The maintenance intravenous fluid requirement is lesser in the elderly. Maintenance of intravenous fluids recommended by NICE guidelines is about 20–25 mL/kg/day in the elderly, while intravenous (IV) fluid requirement in an adult person is approximately 25–30 mL/kg/day [27].

- Elderly patients have low body weight and lesser total body water (about 45–50% of body weight in the elderly compared to 50–60% of body weight in adults), so prescribe the total volume of fluids carefully.

- Cardiac or renal impairment is common in these patients, so avoid prescribing large volumes without assessing the patient's fluid status.

The choice of IV fluids: Hypovolemic older adults who cannot drink isotonic fluids should be administered intravenously [21]. The selection of IV fluids should be individualized based on the type of fluid lost and its composition and the electrolyte and acid-base status of the patient:

- Ringer's lactate and normal saline are the most widely used IV fluids for resuscitation in hypovolemia and hypotension.

- Hypovolemia with hypernatremia due to water losses or poor intake needs supplementation of hypotonic fluid.

- In patients with diarrhea or metabolic acidosis, preferred IV fluids are balanced crystalloids like Ringer's lactate.

- Normal saline is preferred in patients with vomiting, hypovolemic hyponatremia, and metabolic alkalosis.

The volume of IV fluids administered needs careful attention and is determined based on appropriate clinical assessment, an accurate daily body weight, maintaining strict fluid intake and output chart, and measuring serum electrolyte, renal function, and serum osmolarity. Improvement in blood pressure and urine output usually suggests a response to fluid administration.

REFERENCES

1. Vaupel JW, Villavicencio F, Bergeron-Boucher. Demographic perspectives on the rise of longevity. PNAS 202;118(9):e201953611.

2. Weinstein JR, Anderson S. The aging kidney: physiological changes. Adv Chronic Kidney Dis. 2010;17(4):302–7.

3. Sands JM. Urine concentrating and diluting ability during aging. J Gerontol A Biol Sci Med Sci. 2012;67(12):1352–7.

4. El-Sharkawy AM, Sahota O, Maughan RJ, et al. The pathophysiology of fluid and electrolyte balance in the older adult surgical patient. Clin Nutr. 2014;33(1):6–13.

5. Begg DP. Disturbances of thirst and fluid balance associated with aging. Physiol Behav. 2017;178:28–34.

6. Begum MN, Johnson CS.A review of the literature on dehydration in the institutionalized elderly. e-SPEN Eur. E-J. Clin. Nutr. Metab. 2010;5:e47–e53.

7. Wotton K, Crannitch K, Munt R. Prevalence, risk factors and strategies to prevent dehydration in older adults. Contemp Nurse. 2008;31(1):44–56.

8. Miller HJ. Dehydration in the Older Adult. J Gerontol Nurs. 2015;41(9):8–13.

9. Wakefield BJ, Mentes J, Holman JE, et al. Risk factors and outcomes associated with hospital admission for dehydration. Rehab Nurs. 2008;33(6):233–41.

10. Marshall KA, Burson R, Gall K, et al. Hospital admission for malnutrition and dehydration in patients with dementia. Home Healthc Now. 2016;34(1):32–7.

11. Lacey J, Corbett J, Forni L, et al. A multidisciplinary consensus on dehydration: definitions, diagnostic methods and clinical implications. Ann Med. 2019;51(3–4):232–251.

12. Ko SY, Esteve Cuevas LM, Willeboer M, et al. The association between intravenous fluid resuscitation and mortality in older emergency department patients with suspected infection. Int J Emerg Med. 2019;12(1):1.

13. Edmonds CJ, Foglia E, Booth P, et al. Dehydration in older people: A systematic review of the effects of dehydration on health outcomes, healthcare costs and cognitive performance. Arch Gerontol Geriatr. 2021;95:104380.

14. Botigué T, Masot O, Miranda J, et al. Prevalence and Risk Factors Associated With Low Fluid Intake in Institutionalized Older Residents. J Am Med Dir Assoc. 2019;20(3):317–322.

15. Anjo I, Amaral TF, Afonso C, et al. Are hypohydrated older adults at increased risk of exhaustion? J Hum Nutr Diet. 2020;33(1):23–30.

16. Masot O, Miranda J, Santamaría AL, et al. Fluid Intake Recommendation Considering the Physiological Adaptations of Adults Over 65 Years: A Critical Review. Nutrients. 2020;12(11):3383.

17. Hamrick I, Norton D, Birstler J, et al. Association Between Dehydration and Falls. Mayo Clin Proc Innov Qual Outcomes. 2020;4(3):259–265.

18. Thomas DR, Tariq SH, Makhdomm S, et al. Physician misdiagnosis of dehydration in older adults. J Am Med Dir Assoc. 2004;5(2 Suppl):S30–4.

19. Rosinger A, Herrick K. Daily Water Intake among U.S. Men and Women, 2009–2012. NCHS Data Brief No. 242, April 2016. Available online: https://www.cdc.gov/nchs/products/databriefs/db242.htm (accessed on 2 October 2022).

20. Hooper L, Abdelhamid A, Attreed NJ, et al. Clinical symptoms, signs and tests for identification of impending and current water-loss dehydration in older people. Cochrane Database Syst Rev. 2015;2015(4):CD009647.

21. Volkert D, Beck AM, Cederholm T, et al. ESPEN guideline on clinical nutrition and hydration in geriatrics. Clin Nutr. 2022;41(4):958–989.

22. European Food Safety Authority (EFSA). Scientific opinion on dietary reference values for water. EFSA J. 2010;8:1459.

23. Kant AK, Graubard BI, Atchison EA. Intakes of plain water, moisture in foods and beverages, and total water in the adult US population--nutritional, meal pattern, and body weight correlates: National Health and Nutrition Examination Surveys 1999–2006. Am J Clin Nutr. 2009;90(3):655–63.

24. Nakamura Y, Watanabe H, Tanaka A, et al. Effect of Increased Daily Water Intake and Hydration on Health in Japanese Adults. Nutrients. 2020;12(4):1191.

25. Schols JM, De Groot CP, van der Cammen TJ, et al. Preventing and treating dehydration in the elderly during periods of illness and warm weather. J Nutr Health Aging. 2009;13(2):150–157.

26. Crogan NL. Nutritional Problems Affecting Older Adults. Nurs Clin North Am. 2017;52(3):433–445.

27. National Institute for Health and Care Excellence Guideline for Intravenous fluid therapy in adults in hospital (CG174), 2013-Updated May 2017 (https://www.nice.org.uk/guidance/cg174).

Part 4

Parenteral Additives

10 | Calcium Gluconate, Calcium Chloride, and Hypertonic Dextrose Solutions

Commonly used special solutions are calcium chloride, calcium gluconate, dextrose 25% and 50%, hypertonic saline, magnesium sulfate, potassium chloride, potassium phosphate, and sodium bicarbonate (Table 10.1).

Table 10.1 Composition of commonly used special solutions				
Injection	Content in mEq/ml	Volume of amp (mL)	Content in mEq/amp	gm/10 ml amp
Calcium gluconate 10%	$Ca^{2+} = 0.45$	10	$Ca^{2+} = 4.5/10$ ml	1.0
Calcium chloride 10%	$Ca^{2+} = 1.36$	10	$Ca^{2+} = 13.6/10$ ml	1.0
Hypertonic (3%) saline	$Na^+ = 0.5$	100	$Na^+ = 51/100$ ml	3.0
Magnesium sulphate 50%	$Mg^{2+} = 4$	2.0	$Mg^{2+} = 8/2$ ml	1.0
Potassium chloride 15%	$K^+ = 2.0$	10	$K^+ = 20/10$ ml	1.5
Potassium phosphates	$K^+ = 4.4$ $PH_4 = 3.0$	15	$K^+ = 66/15$ ml $PH_4 = 45/15$ ml	-
7.5% $NaHCO_3$	$HCO_3 = 0.9$	10	$HCO_3 = 9/10$ ml	0.75
8.4% $NaHCO_3$	$HCO_3 = 1.0$	20	$HCO_3 = 10/10$ ml	0.84

HCO_3: Bicarbonate; Ca^{2+}: Calcium; Mg^{2+}: Magnesium; PH_4: Phosphate; K^+: Potassium; Na^+: Sodium; $NaHCO_3$: Sodium bicarbonate

CALCIUM GLUCONATE AND CALCIUM CHLORIDE

Calcium gluconate and calcium chloride are two different salt forms commonly used in various emergency conditions.

Composition

Injection 10% Calcium Gluconate

Each ml contains:
    9.3 mg of Calcium ion/mL
    0.22 mmol of Calcium ion/mL
    0.465 mEq of Calcium ion/mL
    Osmolarity 680 mOsm/L

Available as 10 ml ampules:
    10 ml contains 1 gm of Calcium Gluconate

Injection 10% Calcium Chloride

Each ml contains:
    27.3 mg of Calcium ion/mL
    0.68 mmol of Calcium ion/mL
    0.136 mEq of Calcium ion/mL
    Osmolarity 2000 mOsm/L

Available as 10 ml ampules:
    10 ml contains 1 gm of Calcium Chloride

Pharmacological basis

Injection calcium gluconate and calcium chloride are available as a 10% solution in 10 ml ampoule (Table 10.2). Each 10 ml or 1 gm of calcium gluconate solution contains 2.2 mmol or 4.5 mEq of elemental calcium. Conversely, 10 ml or 1 gm of calcium chloride solution contains 6.8 mmol or 13.6 mEq of elemental calcium [1]. While calcium chloride solution provides three times more elemental calcium than calcium gluconate (i.e., 10 ml or one ampule of calcium chloride is equivalent to 30 ml or three ampules of calcium gluconate), current literature suggests that both solutions have similar onset of action and efficacy [2].

Calcium chloride is more potent than calcium gluconate but is highly irritant with a greater risk of tissue necrosis, extravasation, and risk of venous thrombophlebitis, and requires a central line for administration. On the contrary, calcium gluconate is less irritant and better tolerated through a peripheral intravenous (IV), with a less significant risk of venous thrombophlebitis and tissue necrosis if it extravasates. Because of these benefits, calcium gluconate is preferred in emergencies, where a central line is unavailable [3].

Both solutions should be administered intravenously slowly, preferably after dilution, with an equal amount of sterile water for injection, 5% dextrose, or normal saline.

Rapid infusion carries the risk of hypotension, bradycardia, cardiac arrhythmias, syncope, and cardiac arrest.

The maximum rate of administration recommended is 1.5 ml/minute for calcium gluconate and 1.0 ml/minute for calcium chloride.

Table 10.2 Composition of injection calcium gluconate and calcium chloride				
Calcium salt	Elemental calcium per gm			Osmolarity mOsm/L
	mg	mmol	mEq	
10% Calcium gluconate (monohydrate) 10 ml	93	2.2	4.5	680
10% Calcium chloride (dihydrate) 10 ml	273	6.8	13.6	2000

Indications and usage

A. Hyperkalemia

Intravenous calcium administration is the first step in the emergency management of hyperkalemia and is lifesaving in severe hyperkalemia.

The role of calcium is to antagonize the depolarizing effects of hyperkalemia, stabilize cardiac cell membranes, and thereby protect the heart against the risk of arrhythmias. In addition, calcium rapidly decreases the effect of hyperkalemia without lowering serum potassium levels, and this benefit persists even in normocalcemic patients [4].

Indications: Calcium should be administered promptly in [1] severe hyperkalemia, [2] in patients where hyperkalemia is strongly suspected based on the electrocardiogram (ECG) changes (i.e., presence of conduction abnormalities such as absent P waves, prolonged PR interval, a wide QRS complex, or sine-wave pattern), without waiting for the laboratory reports, and [3] in cardiac arrest [5–8].

Dose and effect: One ampule or 10 ml of 10% calcium gluconate is infused IV slowly over 2 to 3 minutes under continuous ECG monitoring [9]. The effect of calcium infusion starts fastest among all measures (just in 1 to 3 minutes) and it lasts for about 30 to 60 minutes. IV calcium provides protection against the life-threatening cardiac side effect of hyperkalemia till other measures act.

One ampule of calcium gluconate is usually not enough to achieve a desirable effect, and the dose is adjusted based on ECG improvement (three ampules are often needed to see the improvement in the ECG changes of hyperkalemia) [10]. It is very important to reassess ECG after 5 minutes, and the dose of calcium should be repeated if ECG changes persist, worsen, or recur after initial improvement [2, 4].

Calcium chloride is preferred in hyperkalemic patients if a central venous line is available or the patient is in circulatory shock or cardiac arrest [2, 5]. The recommended rate of the administration of Inj. calcium chloride is slower, i.e., 0.5 to 1 mL of solution over 1 minute.

In digitalized patients with severe hyperkalemia, administer IV calcium very cautiously at a slower rate than usual (10 ml of 10% calcium gluconate diluted in 100 ml of D5W and infused over 20 to 30 minutes, rather than 5 minutes) to avoid acute hypercalcemia and resultant digitalis toxicity [10, 11].

B. Severe, acute, and/or symptomatic hypocalcemia

For the emergency management of severe acute hypocalcemia (ionized calcium <0.8 mmol/L), or hypocalcemic tetany, 10 to 20 ml of calcium gluconate diluted in 50–100 ml of 5% dextrose is infused intravenously slowly over 10 to 20 minutes under ECG monitoring [12, 13]. Calcium boluses can be repeated until the recovery of acute symptoms.

As boluses of calcium gluconate increase the serum calcium levels for a short duration (about 2–3 hours), subsequent continuous calcium infusion is necessary to prevent the recurrence of hypocalcemia. Calcium infusion is prepared by adding 100 ml or 10 Amp of calcium gluconate (22.5 mmol of calcium) in 1,000 ml of 5% dextrose or 0.9% saline and is administered at the rate of 50 ml/hour initially [12, 13].

Ionized calcium is monitored every 4 to 6 hours, and the dose is adjusted to maintain serum calcium at the lower end of the normal range. Once symptoms recover, and improved calcium levels remain stable, calcium infusion is gradually tapered over 24–48 hours.

C. Severe hypermagnesemia

Calcium is the antidote for cardiac and respiratory depression in magnesium overdose. Calcium antagonizes the effects of magnesium at the neuromuscular junction and effectively reverses cardiac arrhythmias, hypotension, and respiratory depression in patients with hypermagnesemia. Slow intravenous administration of 10 to 20 mL of 10% calcium gluconate is recommended for the initial emergency treatment. The patient is closely monitored, and the calcium dose is repeated until neuromuscular and cardiac disturbances improve. Magnesium toxicity is frequently encountered in obstetric patients receiving magnesium sulfate to prevent eclampsia.

D. Calcium-channel blocker overdose

IV calcium is recommended as first-line therapy for the initial temporary support in symptomatic patients of calcium channel blocker (CCB) overdose [14–17]. Calcium therapy aims to increase extracellular calcium concentrations, antagonize the CCB competitively, and overcome the cardiovascular toxicities of CCBs [18].

Recommended Initial dose is an IV bolus of 30–60 ml of 10% calcium gluconate or 10–20 ml of 10% calcium chloride to be administered slowly [14]. As the effect of calcium is transient, patient of CCB overdose may subsequently require an additional IV bolus or a continuous infusion of 0.6 to 1.2 mL/kg/h of 10% calcium gluconate or 0.2 to 0.4 mL/kg/h of 10% calcium

chloride. The infusion rate is titrated based on hemodynamic response and maintaining ionized calcium less than two times the normal [18].

E. ß-blocker overdose

IV calcium salts have an inotropic effect and reverse hypotension, but it does not improve bradycardia.

F. Prevent citrate toxicity

Citrate binds with ionized calcium causing a fall in ionized calcium concentration in citrate toxicity which can cause potentially fatal neurologic and cardiovascular dysfunction. It is important to remember that in citrate toxicity induced hypocalcemia, the value of total calcium is near normal, but the ionized fraction is reduced. As citrate metabolism is severely impaired in patients with major liver dysfunction, the risk of hypocalcemia is substantially greater.

Intravenous calcium is routinely used to treat citrate induced ionized hypocalcemia in patients receiving multiple blood transfusions, plasmapheresis, and continuous renal replacement therapy (CRRT) to avoid citrate induced hypocalcemia.

Multiple blood transfusions: Each unit of stored packed red cells contains approximately 3 gm citrate as an anticoagulant, which is metabolized in the liver within 5 minutes in healthy adults. Following multiple blood transfusions, citrate-induced ionized hypocalcemia occurs only when the transfusion rate exceeds one unit every five minutes or the patient has liver dysfunction [19].

Following multiple blood transfusions, 10 to 20 mL of 10% calcium gluconate is administered intravenously via a different vein for each 500 mL of blood transfused to prevent ionized hypocalcemia if indicated. However, in patients with abnormal liver function and severe symptomatic hypocalcemia, 10% calcium chloride is preferable to calcium gluconate, and just 2 to 5 mL is administered intravenously, preferably via central vein access, for each 500 mL of blood transfused [20].

Plasmapheresis: Hypocalcemia occurs in plasmapheresis because of the use of citrate as an anticoagulant, citrate content of fresh frozen plasma (FFP), and 5% albumin as a replacement fluid which is calcium free:

1. Citrate used as a regional anticoagulant. When blood enters the apheresis circuit, to prevent clotting, most apheresis machines use citrate as a regional anticoagulation which will chelate calcium and causes hypocalcemia.

2. Citrate content of FFP. When FFP is used as a replacement fluid in plasmapheresis, it carries the risk of hypocalcemia because FFP contains a high proportion of citrate (approximately 15% of citrate by volume) which binds with calcium [21, 22].

   Prophylactic administration of calcium reduces the incidence of citrate induced hypocalcemic symptoms [23]. Administration of 2–3 mL of 10% calcium gluconate (IV slow bolus over 10 minutes/continuous infusion to the return line) with each 100 mL FFP can prevent citrate toxicity [24].

3. Use of 5% albumin. The most preferred replacement fluid in plasmapheresis is 5% albumin, and its administration in large quantity during plasmapheresis can lead to hypocalcemia because:

   • Calcium depleted 5% albumin will bind with the physiologically

active ionized calcium leading to a drop in ionized calcium and resultant hypocalcemia [25].

• Dilutional effect of administration of large volume of calcium-free 5% albumin.

The addition of calcium gluconate as a concurrent continuous infusion (at the rate of 10 ml/liter to the return line) along with 5% albumin-based return fluid effectively reduces the incidence of citrate toxicity compared with IV bolus or oral calcium supplementation during plasmapheresis [26–28].

Citrate anticoagulant in CRRT: Regional citrate anticoagulation (RCA) is a safe and effective method recommended for anticoagulation in CRRT [29–32] because of advantages such as longer filter lifespan, reduced risk of bleeding complications, and lesser need for blood transfusion [33–37].

During RCA, citrate is infused in the arterial limb of the CRRT circuit, which chelates ionized Ca^{2+} forming calcium-citrate complexes and preventing blood coagulation. Calcium is administered post filter into the venous return line to replace calcium lost in the effluent, maintain the systemic ionized calcium concentration in the normal range and prevent hypocalcemia.

G. Hydrofluoric (HF) acid burns

Hydrofluoric acid (HF) is a potent and highly corrosive acid used in chrome or rust cleaners and multiple industries. Even in small amounts, it can cause severe local injury (i.e., severe pain and local necrosis) and significant systemic toxicity. It is standard practice to treat HF burns with calcium gluconate local gel, and If pain persists, intradermal 5% calcium gluconate into and around the affected areas [38].

H. Cardiac resuscitation

IV calcium may be beneficial during cardiac arrest in selected patients with hyperkalemia, hypocalcemia, or calcium channel blocker overdose [39, 40]. But IV calcium administration in cardiac arrest is not routinely recommended because the elevation in serum calcium concentrations can cause detrimental effects on the heart and vascular smooth muscle [41]. The usual adult bolus dose in these settings is 10 mL of 10% calcium gluconate or 5–10 mL of 10% calcium chloride.

Contraindications and precautions

Intramuscular or subcutaneous administration of these calcium solutions is avoided as it causes tissue necrosis and sloughing. As hypercalcemia potentiates the toxic effect of digitalis, calcium should be avoided or used cautiously in patients taking digitalis. Intravenous calcium administration is contraindicated in patients with hypercalcemia and ventricular fibrillation. Avoid coadministration of calcium and bicarbonate containing solutions because of the risk of precipitation of calcium carbonate. Also, avoid mixing calcium-containing solutions with ceftriaxone because of the risk of particulate formation [42].

HYPERTONIC DEXTROSE SOLUTIONS

Hypertonic or concentrated dextrose solutions commonly used in clinical practice are 25% and 50% dextrose.

Composition

25% Dextrose

Each 100 ml contains:
  Dextrose 25 gm
  Osmolality 1262 mOsm/L
  Caloric value 850 kcal/L

50% Dextrose

Each 100 ml contains:
  Dextrose 50 gm
  Osmolality 2525 mOsm/L
  Caloric value 1700 kcal/L
  Dextrose delivers 3.4 kcal/gm

Pharmacological basis

Dextrose is a nutrient replenisher which supplies calories, exerts a protein-sparing effect, and prevents catabolism. Hypertonic dextrose injections are a concentrated form of dextrose solution, so it is useful when a faster replacement of dextrose is needed (like in a hypoglycemic coma). In addition, when a patient requires fluid restriction (i.e., congestive heart failure, volume overload, cirrhosis, oliguric renal failure), hypertonic dextrose solutions in a minimal fluid volume are a rich source of calories.

Indications

1. Hypoglycemia: Rapid correction of insulin-induced hypoglycemia or hypoglycemic coma. Usually100 mL of 25% dextrose is infused, and the dose is repeated if needed.

2. Nutrition: Calorie dense 25% and 50% dextrose solutions are used to provide calorie and fluid replacement to the patient on maintenance fluid therapy or mixed with the amino acid solution as a part of the parenteral nutrition.

3. Hyperkalemia: When regular insulin is used to treat hyperkalemia, 25%-dextrose is co-administered to prevent hypoglycemia.

Contraindications

1. Patients with delirium tremens with dehydration, intracranial hemorrhage, and severe dehydration.

2. To be avoided in a diabetic patient unless there is severe hypoglycemia.

Adverse effects and caution

Rapid infusion of concentrated dextrose solutions can cause hyperglycemia leading to glycosuria, producing diuresis, and may result in dehydration.

So, in the absence of hypoglycemia, hypertonic dextrose solutions should be infused slowly, and serum glucose should be monitored closely to avoid hyperglycemia. While administering the dextrose solution in malnourished and chronic alcoholic patients, thiamine is routinely supplemented simultaneously to prevent the risk of Wernicke encephalopathy. Concentrated dextrose solutions should be tapered gradually because an abrupt withdrawal of the concentrated dextrose solutions may cause rebound hypoglycemia. Hypertonic dextrose solutions may cause local pain, vein irritation, and thrombophlebitis.

REFERENCES

1. Davey M, Caldicott D. Calcium salts in management of hyperkalaemia. Emerg Med J. 2002;19(1):92–3.
2. Long B, Warix JR, Koyfman A. Controversies in Management of Hyperkalemia. J Emerg Med. 2018;55(2):192–205.
3. Semple P, Booth C. Calcium chloride; a reminder. Anaesthesia 1996;51(1):93.
4. Weisberg LS. Management of severe hyperkalemia. Crit Care Med 2008;36(12):3246–51.
5. Truhlar A, Deakin CD, Soar J, et al., European resuscitation council guidelines for resuscitation 2015: Section 4. Cardiac arrest in special circumstances. Resuscitation, 2015;95:148–201.
6. Batterink J, Cessford TA, Taylor RAI. Pharmacological interventions for the acute management of hyperkalaemia in adults. Cochrane Database of Systematic Reviews 2015;10:CD010344.
7. Robert T, Joseph A, Mesnard L. Calcium salt during hyperkalemia. Kidney Int. 2016;90(2):451–452.
8. Wang CH, Huang CH, Chang WT, et al. The effects of calcium and sodium bicarbonate on severe hyperkalaemia during cardiopulmonary resuscitation: A retrospective cohort study of adult in-hospital cardiac arrest. Resuscitation,2016;98:105–11.
9. Vanden Hoek TL, Morrison LJ, Shuster M, et al. Part 12: cardiac arrest in special situations: 2010 American heart association guidelines for cardiopulmonary resuscitation and emergency cardiovascular care. Circulation. 2010;122:S829–S861.
10. Helman A, Baimel M, Etchells E. Emergency management of hyperkalemia. Emergency Medicine Cases. 2016 https://emergencymedicinecases.com/emergency-management-hyperkalemia/ Accessed 11 June 2020.
11. Ahee P, Crowe AV. The management of hyperkalaemia in the emergency department. J Accid Emerg Med. 2000;17(3):188–191.
12. Cooper MS, Gittoes NJL. Diagnosis and management of hypocalcaemia. BMJ 2008;336(7656):1298–1302.
13. Walsh J, Gittoes N, Selby P. Society for Endocrinology Endocrine Emergency Guidance: Emergency management of acute hypocalcemia in adult patients. Endocr Connect. 2016;5(5):G9–G11.
14. Rietjens SJ, de Lange DW, Donker DW, et al. Practical recommendations for calcium channel antagonist poisoning. Neth J Med 2016;74(2):60–67.
15. Graudins A, Lee H, Druda D. Calcium channel antagonist and beta-blocker overdose: Antidotes and adjunct therapies. Br J Clin Pharmacol 2016;81(3):453–461.
16. St-Onge M, Anseeuw K, Cantrell FL, et al. Experts consensus recommendations for the management of calcium channel blockerpoisoning in adults. Crit Care Med. 2017;45(3):e306–e315.
17. Kumar K, Biyyam M, Bajantri B, et al. Critical management of severe hypotension caused by amlodipine toxicity managed with hyperinsulinemia/euglycemia therapy supplemented with calcium gluconate, intravenous glucagon and other vasopressor support: Review of literature. Cardiol Res 2018;9(1):46–49.
18. Shah SK, Goswami SK, Babu RV, et al. Management of calcium channel antagonist overdose with hyperinsulinemia-euglycemia therapy: case series and review of the literature. Case Rep Crit Care. 2012;2012:927040.
19. Lima SK, Begum M, Gupta AK, et al. Management of Massive Blood Transfusion-a case study. Pulse 2014;5(1):39–43.
20. Hess JR, Silvergleid AJ. Massive blood transfusion. In: Post TW, editor. UpToDate. Waltham, MA: Wolters Kluwer Health. http://www.uptodate.com. Accessed 12 Sept 2020.
21. Basic-Jukic N, Kes P, Glavas-Boras S, et al. Complications of therapeutic plasma exchange: experience with 4857 treatments. Ther Apher Dial. 2005;9(5):391–5.
22. Lee G, Arepally GM. Anticoagulation techniques in apheresis: from heparin to citrate and beyond. J Clin Apher. 2012;27(3):117–125.
23. Sigler K, Lee J, Srivaths P. Regional citrate anticoagulation with calcium replacement in pediatric apheresis. J Clin Apher. 2018;33(3):274–7.
24. Szczepiorkowski ZM, Winters JL, Bandarenko N, et al. Guidelines on the use of therapeutic apheresis in clinical practice--evidence-based approach from the Apheresis Applications Committee of the American Society for Apheresis. J Clin Apher. 2010;25(3):83–177

25. Patterson ER, Winters JL. Hemapheresis. In: McPherson RA, Pincus MR, eds. Henry's Clinical Diagnosis and Management by Laboratory Methods E-Book. (23rd ed., pp. 779) St Louis, MO: Elsevier;2017.

26. Weinstein R. Prevention of citrate reactions during therapeutic plasma exchange by constant infusion of calcium gluconate with the return fluid. J Clin Apher. 1996;11(4):204–210.

27. Kankirawatana S, Huang ST, Marques MB. Continuous infusion of calcium gluconate in 5% albumin is safe and prevents most hypocalcemic reactions during therapeutic plasma exchange. J Clin Apher. 2007;22(5):265–269.

28. Krishnan RG, Coulthard MG. Minimising changes in plasma calcium and magnesium concentrations during plasmapheresis. Pediatr Nephroly 2007;22(10):1763–1766.

29. Section 5: Dialysis Interventions for Treatment of AKI. Kidney Int Suppl (2011). 2012;2(1):89–115.

30. Oudemans-van Straaten HM, Ostermann M. Bench-to-bedside review: Citrate for continuous renal replacement therapy, from science to practice. Crit Care 2012;16(6):249.

31. Kindgen-Milles D, Brandenburger T, Dimski T. Regional citrate anticoagulation for continuous renal replacement therapy. Curr Opin Crit Care. 2018;24(6):450–4.

32. Karkar A, Ronco C. Prescription of CRRT: a pathway to optimize therapy. Ann. Intensive Care 2020;10(1):32.

33. Wu MY, Hsu YH, Bai CH, et al. Regional citrate versus heparin anticoagulation for continuous renal replacement therapy: A metaanalysis of randomized controlled trials. Am J Kidney Dis 2012;59(6):810–818.

34. Stucker F, Ponte B, Tataw J, et al. Efficacy and safety of citrate-based anticoagulation compared to heparin in patients with acute kidney injury requiring continuous renal replacement therapy: a randomized controlled trial. Crit Care 2015;19(1):91.

35. Liu C, Mao Z, Kang H, et al. Regional citrate versus heparin anticoagulation for continuous renal replacement therapy in critically ill patients: a meta-analysis with trial sequential analysis of randomized controlled trials. Crit Care. 2016;20(1):144.

36. Davenport A, Tolwani A. Citrate anticoagulation for continuous renal replacement therapy (CRRT) in patients with acute kidney injury admitted to the intensive care unit. NDT Plus. 2009;2(6):439–447.

37. Morabito S, Pistolesi V, Tritapepe L, et al. Regional citrate anticoagulation in cardiac surgery patients at high risk of bleeding: a continuous veno-venous hemofiltration protocol with a low concentration citrate solution. Crit Care. 2012;16(3):R111.

38. McKee D, Thoma A, Bailey K, et al. A review of hydrofluoric acid burn management. Plast Surg (Oakv). 2014;22(2):95–98.

39. Guidelines 2000 for Cardiopulmonary Resuscitation and Emergency Cardiovascular Care. Part 6: advanced cardiovascular life support: section 6: pharmacology II: agents to optimize cardiac output and blood pressure. The American Heart Association in collaboration with the International Liaison Committee on Resuscitation. Circulation. 2000;102(8 Suppl):I129–135.

40. Australian Resuscitation Council. Section 11 – Adult advanced life support. ANZCOR Guideline 11.5 – Medications in Adult Cardiac Arrest August 2016 Available: https://resus.org.au/guidelines/.

41. Morrison LJ, Deakin CD, Morley PT, et al. Part 8: Advanced life support: 2010 International Consensus on Cardiopulmonary Resuscitation and Emergency Cardiovascular Care Science With Treatment Recommendations. Circulation. 2010;122(16 Suppl 2):S345–421.

42. Gin A, Walker S. Notice to Hospitals regarding Ceftriaxone-calcium incompatibility: What's a clinician to do? Can J Hosp Pharm. 2009;62(2):157–8.

11 | Hypertonic Saline

Hypertonic saline (HS) is a concentrated form of sodium chloride dissolved in water, and 3% and 5% hypertonic saline are commonly used solutions in clinical practice.

COMPOSITION

3% Hypertonic Saline

Each 100 ml of contains:
  Sodium 51.3 mEq
  Chloride 51.3 mEq
  Osmolality 1027 mOsm/L

100 ml of 3% NaCl contains 3 gm of Sodium Chloride

5% Hypertonic Saline

Each 100 ml of contains:
  Sodium 85.6 mEq
  Chloride 85.0 mEq
  Osmolality 1711 mOsm/L

100 ml of 5% NaCl contains 5 gm of Sodium Chloride

PHARMACOLOGICAL BASIS

Hypertonic saline solutions have higher sodium chloride concentration and serum osmolality as compared to normal serum values.

A. High sodium concentration promptly corrects hyponatremia

Sodium concentration of 3% and 5% hypertonic saline is 513 mEq/L and 856 mEq/L respectively compared to normal plasma concentration of 140 mEq/L. As a high sodium concentration of hypertonic saline can rapidly raise sodium and reduce cerebral edema, it is recommended in the treatment of life-threatening hyponatremia. Because of substantially higher concentrations of salt, this solution is selected to provide a large amount of sodium in a small amount of fluid (i.e., in a patient with euvolemic or hypervolemic hyponatremia who needs salt supplementation, but fluid restriction).

B. High osmolality decreases cerebral edema and intracranial pressure (ICP)

Osmolality of sodium-rich 3% and 5% hypertonic saline solutions is high (i.e., 1027 mOsm/L and 1711 mOsm/L respectively), compared to the osmolality of normal plasma (285 mOsm/L). Because of higher osmolality, hypertonic saline solutions have a stronger osmotic action which creates an osmotic gradient and pulls water out of the intracellular and extravascular water into the intravascular compartment [1]. Rapid mobilization of free water from the cranial vault reduces the cerebral water content leading to a decrease in brain edema and a reduction in ICP [2].

C. Greater plasma volume expansion with smaller infused volume

Hypertonic saline solutions with high sodium mobilize water from interstitial and intracellular compartments to the intravascular compartment and rapidly expand intravascular volume. Resultant benefits are several times plasma volume expansion with smaller infused volume without the interstitial fluid expansion and occurrence of edema [3–5]. As hypertonic saline stimulates the release of vasopressin from the pituitary gland [6], it leads to a decrease in the loss of water through the kidneys. Plasma volume expansion increases blood pressure and improves the microcirculation of the brain [7, 8].

INDICATIONS

Hypertonic saline is frequently used in the following indications:

A. Severe symptomatic hyponatremia

Hypertonic saline is the first-line therapy and only rapidly effective modality in the emergency management of acute symptomatic hyponatremia [9–14]. Hypertonic saline is a lifesaving

treatment as it rapidly corrects hyponatremia causing a reduction in cerebral edema and the prevention of fatal brain herniation [15].

Various formulas to guide administration of hypertonic saline are proposed but are not perfect because none of these formulas can consider the effect of ongoing renal loss of water or sodium on the concentration of sodium [14]. So, to determine the desirable rate of hypertonic saline infusion, serial measurement of sodium is mandatory.

Simple and easy to use the formula for the immediate initial therapy is to administer 1 mL/kg/h of 3% hypertonic saline which increases serum sodium roughly by 1 mEq/L/h [14].

Additional two common approaches for the management of patients with severe symptomatic hyponatremia are:

- As per United States guidelines, a 100 mL bolus of 3% hypertonic saline is infused over 10 minutes. If symptoms persist, up to two additional boluses of 100 mL of 3% hypertonic saline is repeated (total infused volume 300 mL) [10].

- As per European recommendations, 150 mL of 3% hypertonic saline is infused over 20 minutes. After the initial dose, if the serum sodium does not increase by 4 to 6 mEq/L, the second bolus of 150 mL of 3% hypertonic saline is infused [11].

As a 4–6 mEq/L increase in serum sodium is adequate to reverse the manifestations of acute or severely symptomatic hyponatremia [9], discontinue 3% hypertonic saline once the correction goal of 4 to 6 mEq/L is achieved.

To prevent the rapid correction of hyponatremiaand resultant risk of osmotic demyelination syndrome, gentle correction of hyponatremia (increase in serum sodium less than 10 mEq/L in the first 24 hours and less than 18 mEq/L in the first 48 hours) is desired.

In patients with anasarca, furosemide is added with hypertonic saline to prevent the worsening of hypervolemia [16].

B. Osmotherapy for cerebral edema and raised intracranial pressure

Hypertonic saline effectively reduces brain swelling due to osmotic gradient driven strong fluid shift [17]. Previously mannitol was considered as a gold standard medical treatment for cerebral edema, but now the trend is changing [18, 19].

During the last two decades, data supporting the use of hypertonic saline over mannitol are emerging and hypertonic saline is found to be a safe, effective, and superior modality for the initial treatment of intracranial hypertension [20–25].

Benefits of hypertonic saline over mannitol are:

- **Better hemodynamic stability:** Hypertonic saline causes volume expansion (because of the fluid shift from extravascular to an intravascular compartment) [26], while mannitol leads to volume depletion due to diuresis. So, hypertonic saline is beneficial and preferred in patients with blood loss, or hypotension due to trauma.

- **More effective reduction of intracranial pressure:** When administering in an equimolar dose, reduction of intracranial pressure with hypertonic saline is rapid, more pronounced, and more sustained than mannitol [21, 22, 25, 27–33].

Even in patients with refractory intracranial hypertension or in whom mannitol had failed, hypertonic saline is found to be effective [34–39]. In a few studies, hypertonic saline and mannitol are found to be equally effective [37, 40, 41].

- **Better cerebral perfusion:** As compared to mannitol, hypertonic saline has an additional and stronger effect on cerebral perfusion [25, 41, 42].

- **Better oxygenation of brain tissue:** As compared to mannitol, hypertonic saline is associated with a significant increase in brain oxygenation [42].

- **Greater reflection coefficient:** The reflection coefficient determines how well a particular substance crosses the blood-brain barrier. As the reflection coefficient of hypertonic saline is higher than that of mannitol (1.0 vs 0.9, respectively), the risk of leak of hypertonic saline into brain tissue is less [43, 44]. Because of low blood-brain barrier permeability, hypertonic saline generates a greater osmotic gradient compared to mannitol in equimolar dosage [45].

Besides all physiological benefits seen with hypertonic saline over mannitol, mortality and outcome benefits compared with mannitol are not documented, and therefore hypertonic saline cannot be recommended as a first-line treatment in the management of cerebral edema and severe traumatic brain injury [23, 46–50].

Administration: 3% hypertonic saline is commonly used for the management of cerebral edema, which is administered at the rate of 1 mL/kg/hr as a continuous infusion with the initial sodium goal of approximately 145 to 155 mEq/L [51].

For the emergency management of severe cerebral edema with signs of herniation, infusion of 30 ml bolus of 23.4% hypertonic saline intravenous (IV) slowly over 10 minutes through a central line, is life-saving (i.e., reduces intracranial pressure rapidly and helps in the reversal of transtentorial herniation) [52]. Currently, symptom-based bolus administration of hypertonic saline is preferred over sodium target based continuous infusion for the management of cerebral edema [25].

C. Plasma volume expansion

Hypertonic saline rapidly expands intravascular volume considerably more than the volume infused, by drawing water from interstitial and intracellular space [3–5, 53]. As hemodynamic goals are achieved with lower volumes of hypertonic saline, the total fluid requirement for resuscitation is lesser with a resultant reduction in total fluid accumulation [4, 5, 54–57]. So, protection from fluid overload is the advantage of hypertonic saline in edematous patients with volume depletion [4]. But there are no mortality benefits with hypertonic saline compared to isotonic fluids, so routine use of hypertonic saline cannot be recommended for "small-volume" resuscitation [3, 5, 58–61].

D. Acute decompensated heart failure

Several studies described the potential use of combined administration of intravenous hypertonic saline plus intravenous furosemide in the management of diuretic-resistant, refractory acute decompensated heart failure (ADHF) [16, 62–66]. Rapidly administration of 3% hypertonic saline along with high dose loop diuretics

is reported to increase diuretic efficiency, greater fluid and weight loss, improvement of serum sodium, chloride, and creatinine concentrations, reduced length of hospitalization, reduced risk of ADHF-related re-hospitalization, and decreases all-cause mortality [65, 67–73]. For hyperdiuresis, there are no fixed guidelines. The protocol used in the large - SMAC-HF study was the administration of 150 ml of 3% hypertonic saline along with 250 mg IV furosemide infused over 30 minutes [65].

Traditionally salt is restricted in heart failure, so the recommendation to administer hypertonic saline in acute decompensated heart failure is a paradox and challenges our understanding. Proposed mechanisms by which hypertonic saline effectively augments the effect of loop diuretics are [74]:

1. Because of the osmotic gradient, hypertonic saline pulls fluid into the intravascular space. The resultant expansion of intravascular fluid volume promotes the diuretic effect of furosemide.

2. As hypochloremia is responsible for sodium retention and diuretic resistance, by raising chloride levels hypertonic saline reverses the sodium retaining effects of hypochloremia and facilitates diuresis [75, 76].

3. Hypertonic saline induced intravascular fluid volume expansion by temporarily suppressing renin/angiotensin/aldosterone system permits diuresis.

Although the effectiveness of this therapy is supported by a moderate amount of clinical evidence, currently data supporting its administration routinely in diuretic-resistant acute decompensated heart failure is insufficient [73, 74, 77].

E. Cystic fibrosis

Hypertonic saline inhalation is an effective, safe, and inexpensive adjunctive therapy for all children with cystic fibrosis older than six years of age [78–80]. The recommended timing of hypertonic saline inhalation for cystic fibrosis is twice a daily [79, 81].

Hypertonic saline inhalation improves mucociliary clearance and lung health by generating an osmotic gradient that draws water into the airway lumen which hydrates the mucus and makes it easier to cough out [82–85]. Nebulized hypertonic saline can also cause airway irritation and promotes cough, which helps in the breaking up and clearance of mucus [86].

CONTRAINDICATIONS AND ADVERSE EFFECTS

There are no absolute contraindications. But because of high sodium content, hypertonic saline is avoided or used cautiously in patients with hypernatremia or congestive heart failure, or renal insufficiency with volume overload.

Common adverse effects of 3% hypertonic saline are infection at the injection site, thrombophlebitis, hypernatremia, and hypervolemia. Overly rapid sodium correction of hyponatremia may develop osmotic demyelination syndrome especially in higher-risk patients with serum sodium 105 mEq/L or less at presentation, female gender, hypokalemia, alcoholism, malnutrition, and advanced liver disease [10, 87].

REFERENCES

1. Hinson HE, Stein D, Sheth KN. Hypertonic saline and mannitol therapy in critical care neurology. J Intensive Care Med 2013;28(1):3–11.

2. Busey K, Samai K. Hypertonic Saline for ICP Reduction in Traumatic Brain Injury Patients: An Evolving Practice. J Trauma Nurs. 2017;24(4):222–223.

3. Bunn F, Roberts I, Tasker R, et al. Hypertonic versus near isotonic crystalloid for fluid resuscitation in critically ill patients. Cochrane Database Syst Rev. 2004;2004(3):CD002045.

4. Pfortmueller CA, Schefold JC. Hypertonic saline in critical illness - A systematic review. J Crit Care. 2017;42:168–177.

5. Orbegozo D, Vincent JL, Creteur J, et al. Hypertonic Saline in Human Sepsis: A Systematic Review of Randomized Controlled Trials. Anesth Analg. 2019;128(6):1175–1184.

6. Hashimoto K, Suemaru S, Hirasawa R, et al. Effect of hypertonic saline on the corticotropin-releasing hormone and arginine vasopressin content of the rat pituitary neurointermediate lobe. Endocrinol Jpn. 1990;37(5):599–606.

7. Mazzoni MC, Borgstrom P, Arfors KE, et al. Dynamic fluid redistribution in hyperosmotic resuscitation of hypovolemic hemorrhage. Am J Physiol. 1988;255(3 Pt 2):H629–37.

8. Strandvik GF. Hypertonic saline in critical care: a review of the literature and guidelines for use in hypotensive states and raised intracranial pressure. Anaesthesia. 2009;64(9):990–1003.

9. Sterns RH, Nigwekar SU, Hix JK. The treatment of hyponatremia. Semin Nephrol 2009;29(3):282–299.

10. Verbalis JG, Goldsmith SR, Greenberg A, et al. Diagnosis, evaluation, and treatment of hyponatremia: expert panel recommendations. Am J Med 2013;126(10 Suppl 1):S1–42.

11. Spasovski G, Vanholder R, Allolio B, et al. Clinical practice guideline on diagnosis and treatment of hyponatraemia. Eur J Endocrinol 2014;170(3):G1–47.

12. Ayus JC, Caputo D, Bazerque F, et al. Treatment of hyponatremic encephalopathy with a 3% sodium chloride protocol: a case series. Am J Kidney Dis 2015;65(3):435–42.

13. Weismann D, Schneider A, Höybye C. Clinical aspects of symptomatic hyponatremia. Endocr Connect. 2016;5(5):R35–R43.

14. Seay NW, Lehrich RW, Greenberg A. Diagnosis and Management of Disorders of Body Tonicity—Hyponatremia and Hypernatremia: Core Curriculum 2020. Am J Kidney Dis. 2020;75(2):272–286.

15. Sterns RH. Treatment of Severe Hyponatremia. Clin J Am Soc Nephrol 2018;13(4):641–649.

16. Okuhara Y, Hirotani S, Naito Y, et al. Intravenous salt supplementation with low-dose furosemide for treatment of acute decompensated heart failure. J Card Fail. 2014;20(5):295–301.

17. Shah S, Kimberly WT. Today's Approach to Treating Brain Swelling in the Neuro Intensive Care Unit. Semin Neurol. 2016;36(6):502–507.

18. Hays AN, Lazaridis C, Neyens R, et al. Osmotherapy: use among neurointensivists. Neurocritical Care. 2011;14(2):222–228.

19. Marko NF. Hypertonic saline, not mannitol, should be considered gold-standard medical therapy for intracranial hypertension. Crit Care. 2012;16(1):113.

20. Ogden AT, Mayer SA, Connolly ES. Hyperosmolar agents in neurosurgical practice: the evolving role of hypertonic saline. Neurosurgery. 2005;57(2):207–215.

21. Ware ML, Nemani VM, Meeker M, et al. Effects of 23.4% sodium chloride solution in reducing intracranial pressure in patients with traumatic brain injury: a preliminary study. Neurosurgery 2005;57(4):727–36.

22. Kamel H, Navi BB, Nakagawa K, et al. Hypertonic saline versus mannitol for the treatment of elevated intracranial pressure: A meta-analysis of randomized clinical trials. Crit Care Med. 2011;39(3):554–9.

23. Mortazavi MM, Romeo AK, Deep A, et al. Hypertonic saline for treating raised intracranial pressure: literature review with meta-analysis. J Neurosurg. 2012;116(1):210–221.

24. Rickard AC, Smith JE, Newell P, et al. Salt or sugar for your injured brain? A meta-analysis of randomised controlled trials of mannitol versus hypertonic sodium solutions to manage raised intracranial pressure in traumatic brain injury. Emerg Med J. 2014;31(8):679–683.

25. Cook AM, Morgan JG, Hawryluk GWJ, et al. Guidelines for the Acute Treatment of Cerebral Edema in Neurocritical Care Patients. Neurocrit Care. 2020;32(3):647–666.

26. Riou B, Carli P. Hypertonic sodium chloride and hemorrhagic shock. Ann Fr Anesth Reanim. 1990;9:536–46.

27. Vialet R, Albanèse J, Thomachot L, et al. Isovolume hypertonic solutes (sodium chloride or mannitol) in the treatment of refractory posttraumatic intracranial hypertension: 2 mL/kg 7.5% saline is more effective than 2 mL/kg 20% mannitol. Crit Care Med 2003;31(6):1683–7.

28. Battison C, Andrews PJ, Graham C, et al. Randomized, controlled trial on the effect of a 20% mannitol solution and a 7.5% saline/6% dextran solution on increased intracranial pressure after brain injury. Crit Care Med 2005;33(1):196–202.

29. Mangat HS, Chiu Y-L, Gerber LM, et al. Hypertonic saline reduces cumulative and daily intracranial pressure burdens after severe traumatic brain injury. J Neurosurg. 2015;122(1):202–10.

30. Li M, Chen T, Chen SD, et al. Comparison of equimolar doses of mannitol and hypertonic saline for the treatment of elevated intracranial pressure after traumatic brain injury: a systematic review and meta-analysis. Medicine (Baltimore) 2015;94(17):e668.

31. Burgess S, Abu-Laban RB, Slavik RS, et al. A systematic review of randomized controlled trials comparing hypertonic sodium solutions and mannitol for traumatic brain injury: implications for emergency department management. Ann Pharmacother. 2016;50(4):291–300.

32. Alnemari AM, Krafcik BM, Mansour TR, et al. A comparison of pharmacologic therapeutic agents used for the reduction of intracranial pressure after traumatic brain injury. World Neurosurg 2017;106:509–528.

33. Mangat HS, Wu X, Gerber LM, et al. Hypertonic saline is superior to mannitol for the combined effect on intracranial pressure and cerebral perfusion pressure

34. Horn P, Munch E, Vajkoczy P, et al. Hypertonic saline solution for control of elevated intracranial pressure in patients with exhausted response to mannitol and barbiturates. Neurol Res. 1999;21:758–764.

35. Schwarz S, Georgiadis D, Aschoff A, et al. Effects of hypertonic (10%) saline in patients with raised intracranial pressure after stroke. Stroke. 2002;33(1):136–40.

36. Harutjunyan L, Holz C, Rieger A, et al. Efficiency of 7.2% hypertonic saline hydroxyethyl starch 200/0.5 versus mannitol 15% in the treatment of increased intracranial pressure in neurosurgical patients—a randomized clinical trial. Crit Care. 2005;9(5):R530–40.

37. Sakellaridis N, Pavlou E, Karatzas S, et al. Comparison of mannitol and hypertonic saline in the treatment of severe brain injuries. J Neurosurg. 2011;114(2):545–548.

38. Lewandowski-Belfer JJ, Patel AV, Darracott RM, et al. Safety and efficacy of repeated doses of 14.6 or 23.4% hypertonic saline for refractory intracranial hypertension. Neurocrit Care 2014;20(3):436–42.

39. Gu J, Huang H, Huang Y, et al. Hypertonic saline or mannitol for treating elevated intracranial pressure in traumatic brain injury: a meta-analysis of randomized controlled trials. Neurosurg Rev 2019;42(2):499–509.

40. Francony G, Fauvage B, Falcon D, et al. Equimolar doses of mannitol and hypertonic saline in the treatment of increased intracranial pressure. Crit Care Med. 2008;36(3):795–800.

41. Cottenceau V, Masson F, Mahamid E, et al. Comparison of effects of equiosmolar doses of mannitol and hypertonic saline on cerebral blood flow and metabolism in traumatic brain injury. J Neurotrauma 2011;28(10):2003–12.

42. Oddo M, Levine JM, Frangos S, et al. Effect of mannitol and hypertonic saline on cerebral oxygenation in patients with severe traumatic brain injury and refractory intracranial hypertension. J Neurol Neurosurg Psychiatry 2009;80(8):916–20.

43. Rozet I, Tontisirin N, Muangman S, et al. Effect of equiosmolar solutions of mannitol versus hypertonic saline on intraoperative brain relaxation and electrolyte balance. Anesthesiology 2007;107(5):697–704.

44. Boone MD, Oren-Grinberg A, Robinson TM, et al. Mannitol or hypertonic saline in the setting of traumatic brain injury: What have we learned? Surg Neurol Int 2015;6:177.

45. Singla A, Mathew PJ, Jangra K, et al. A comparison of hypertonic saline and mannitol on intraoperative brain relaxation in patients with raised intracranial pressure during supratentorial tumors resection: A randomized control trial. Neurol India 2020;68(1):141–5.

46. Chen H, Song Z, Dennis JA. Hypertonic saline versus other intracranial pressure-lowering agents for people with acute traumatic brain injury. Cochrane Database Syst Rev. 2019;12(12):CD010904.

47. Roquilly A, Moyer JD, Huet O, et al. Effect of Continuous Infusion of Hypertonic Saline vs Standard Care on 6-Month Neurological Outcomes in Patients

With Traumatic Brain Injury: The COBI Randomized Clinical Trial. JAMA. 2021;325(20):2056–2066.

48. Han C, Yang F, Guo S, et al. Hypertonic Saline Compared to Mannitol for the Management of Elevated Intracranial Pressure in Traumatic Brain Injury: A Meta-Analysis. Front Surg. 2022;8:765784.

49. Bernhardt K, McClune W, Rowland MJ, et al. Hypertonic Saline Versus Other Intracranial-Pressure-Lowering Agents for Patients with Acute Traumatic Brain Injury: A Systematic Review and Meta-analysis. Neurocrit Care. 2023.

50. Iqbal U, Kumar A, Arsal SA, et al. Efficacy of hypertonic saline and mannitol in patients with traumatic brain injury and cerebral edema: a systematic review and meta-analysis. Egypt J Neurosurg. 2023;38:54.

51. Hauer EM, Stark D, Staykov D, et al. Early continuous hypertonic saline infusion in patients with severe cerebrovascular disease. Crit Care Med. 2011;39(7):1766–1772.

52. Koenig MA, Bryan M, Lewin IJL, et al. Reversal of transtentorial herniation with hypertonic saline. Neurology. 2008;70(13):1023–1029.

53. Cooper DJ. Hypertonic saline resuscitation for head injured patients. Critical Care and Resusctiation 1999;1(2):161.

54. Joseph B, Aziz H, Snell M, et al. The physiological effects of hyperosmolar resuscitation: 5% vs 3% hypertonic saline. Am. J. Surg. 2014;208(5):697–702.

55. Shrum B, Church B, McArthur E, et al. Hypertonic salt solution for peri-operative fluid management. Cochrane Database Syst Rev. 2016;(6):CD005576.

56. Jarvela K, Rantanen M, Koobi T, et al. Hypertonic saline-hydroxyethyl starch solution attenuates fluid accumulation in cardiac surgery patients: a randomized controlled double-blind trial. Anaesthesiol Intensive Ther 2018;50(2):122–127.

57. Loftus TJ, Efron PA, Bala TM, et al. Hypertonic saline resuscitation following emergent laparotomy and temporary abdominal closure. J Trauma Acute Care Surg. 2018;84(2):350–357.

58. Bulger EM, May S, Kerby JD, et al. Out-of-hospital hypertonic resuscitation after traumatic hypovolemic shock. Ann Surg. 2011;253(3):431–441.

59. Vahidi E, Naderpour Z, Saeedi M. Hypertonic Saline in the Treatment of Hemorrhagic Shock. Adv J Emerg Med. 2017;1(1):e8.

60. Wu MC, Liao TY, Lee EM, et al. Administration of Hypertonic Solutions for Hemorrhagic Shock: A Systematic Review and Meta-analysis of Clinical Trials. Anesth Analg. 2017;125(5):1549–1557.

61. Blanchard IE, Ahmad A, Tang KL, et al. The effectiveness of prehospital hypertonic saline for hypotensive trauma patients: a systematic review and meta-analysis. BMC Emerg Med. 2017;17(1):35.

62. Paterna S, Parrinello G, Amato P, et al. Tolerability and efficacy of high-dose furosemide and small-volume hypertonic saline solution in refractory congestive heart failure. Adv Ther. 1999;16(5):219–228.

63. Paterna S, Di Pasquale P, Parrinello G, et al. Effects of high-dose furosemide and small-volume hypertonic saline solution infusion in comparison with a high dose of furosemide as a bolus, in refractory congestive heart failure. Eur J Heart Fail. 2000;2(3):305–313.

64. Licata G, Di Pasquale P, Parrinello G, et al. Effects of high-dose furosemide and small-volume hypertonic saline solution infusion in comparison with a high dose of furosemide as bolus in refractory congestive heart failure: long-term effects. Am Heart J 2003;145(3):459–66.

65. Paterna S, Fasullo S, Parrinello G, et al. Short-term effects of hypertonic saline solution in acute heart failure and long-term effects of a moderate sodium restriction in patients with compensated heart failure with New York Heart Association class III (Class C) (SMAC-HF Study). Am J Med Sci. 2011;342(1):27–37.

66. Engelmeier RS, Le TT, Kamalay SE, et al. Randomized trial of high dose furosemide-hypertonic saline in acute decompensated heart failure with advanced renal disease. Journal of the American College of Cardiology. 2012;59:e958.

67. Gandhi S, Mosleh W, Myers RB. Hypertonic saline with furosemide for the treatment of acute congestive heart failure: a systematic review and meta-analysis. Int J Cardiol 2014;173(2):139–145.

68. Yayla Ç, Akyel A, Canpolat U, et al. Comparison of three diuretic treatment strategies for patients with acute decompensated heart failure. Herz. 2015;40(8):1115–1120.

69. De Vecchis R, Esposito C, Ariano C, et al. Hypertonic saline plus i.v. furosemide improve renal safety profile and clinical outcomes in acute decompensated heart failure: A meta-analysis of the literature. Herz 2015;40(3):423–35.

70. Lafrenière G, Béliveau P, Bégin J, et al. Effects of hypertonic saline solution on body weight and serum creatinine in patients with acute decompensated heart failure. World J Cardiol. 2017;9(8):685–692.

71. Wan Y, Li L, Niu H, et al. Impact of Compound Hypertonic Saline Solution on Decompensated Heart Failure. Int Heart J. 2017;58(4):601–607.

72. Crane A, Hertel C, Hobza, et al. Does hypertonic saline infusion with furosemide improve outcomes for patients with acute CHF exacerbation? Evidence-Based Practice 2018;21(2):5–6.

73. Griffin M, Soufer A, Goljo E, et al. Real world use of hypertonic saline in refractory acute decompensated heart failure: a U.S. center's experience. JACC: Heart Failure 2020;8(3):199–208.

74. Farkas J. Hyperdiuresis: Using hypertonic saline to facilitate diuresis. PulmCrit December 9, 2019. https://emcrit.org/pulmcrit/pulmcrit-hyperdiuresis-using-hypertonic-saline-to-facilitate-diuresis/.

75. Hanberg J, Rao V, Ter M, et al. Hypochloremia and diuretic resistance in heart failure: mechanistic insights. Circ Heart Fail. 2016;9(8):10.

76. Masella C, Viggiano D, Molfino I, et al. Diuretic resistance in cardio-nephrology: role of pharmacokinetics, hypochloremia, and kidney remodeling. Kidney Blood Press Res 2019;44(5):915–927.

77. Regolisti G, Antoniotti R, Pastorini G, et al. Management of congestion and diuretic resistance in heart failure. Nephrology @ Point of Care. 2016;2(1):73–87.

78. Elkins MR, Robinson M, Rose BR, et al. A controlled trial of long-term inhaled hypertonic saline in patients with cystic fibrosis. N Engl J Med 2006;354(3):229–40.

79. Flume PA, O'Sullivan BP, Robinson KA, et al. Cystic fibrosis pulmonary guidelines: chronic medications for maintenance of lung health. Am J Respir Crit Care Med 2007;176(10):957–69.

80. Wark P, McDonald VM. Nebulised hypertonic saline for cystic fibrosis. Cochrane Database Syst Rev 2018;9(9):CD001506.

81. Elkins M, Dentice R. Timing of hypertonic saline inhalation for cystic fibrosis. Cochrane Database of Systematic Reviews 2020;2(2):CD008816.

82. Donaldson SH, Bennett WD, Zeman KL, et al. Mucus clearance and lung function in cystic fibrosis with hypertonic saline. N. Engl. J. Med. 2006;354(3):241–250.

83. Elkins MR, Bye PT. Mechanisms and applications of hypertonic saline. R Soc Med 2011;104(Suppl 1):S2–5.

84. Reeves EP, McCarthy C, McElvaney OJ, et al. Inhaled hypertonic saline for cystic fibrosis: reviewing the potential evidence for modulation of neutrophil signalling and function. World J Crit Care Med. 2015;4(3):179–191.

85. Tildy BE, Rogers DF. Therapeutic options for hydrating airway mucus in cystic fibrosis. Pharmacology 2015;95(3–4):117–132.

86. Rubin BK. Aerosol medications for treatment of mucus clearance disorders respiratory care 2015;60(6):825–832.

87. George JC, Zafar W, Bucaloiu ID, et al. Risk Factors and Outcomes of Rapid Correction of Severe Hyponatremia. Clin J Am Soc Nephrol 2018;13(7):984–992.

12 | Magnesium Sulfate

Injection Magnesium sulfate (MgSO$_4$) is the most common parenterally used magnesium salt in clinical practice.

COMPOSITION

Injection Magnesium sulfate is available in different concentrations.

Injection 50% Magnesium Sulfate
Each ml contains:
  Magnesium Sulfate USP 500 mg
  4.06 mEq or 2.03 mmol Magnesium ions
  Osmolarity 4,060 mOsm/L

50% Magnesium Sulfate per ampoule: 1 gm/2 ml and 5 gm/10 ml

Injection 20% Magnesium Sulfate
  Magnesium Sulfate USP 2 gm/10 ml

Injection 10% Magnesium Sulfate
  Magnesium Sulfate USP 1 gm/10 ml

Conversion relationships: Magnesium Sulfate 1 gm = 4 mmol mg = 8 mEq mg

PHARMACOLOGICAL BASIS

Magnesium is the second most common intracellular cation. It is an essential co-factor in many biochemical reactions and plays a vital role in nerve transmission, neurochemical transmission, cardiac excitability, muscular excitability, and vasomotor tone. It also affects the regulation of calcium and potassium.

A. Preeclampsia and eclampsia

Magnesium sulfate is an effective

treatment for eclampsia, but the exact mechanism of action remains unclear and is suggested to be multi-factorial (works through both vascular and neurological mechanisms) [1]. Different proposed mechanisms are:

1. Vasodilation: The calcium antagonist effect of magnesium on cerebrovasculature and peripheral vascular smooth muscle leads to vasodilation. Arterial relaxation due to magnesium lowers cerebral vascular resistance and relieves vasospasm during eclampsia, resulting in reduced cerebral ischemia [1]. Magnesium induced vasodilatation reduces total peripheral (predominantly arteriolar) vascular resistance, and therefore have a role in lowering the blood pressure [2]. A low to moderate dose of magnesium can cause flushing and sweating, while a high dose may lead to hypotension.

2. Protection of the blood-brain barrier and reduction of cerebral edema formation [3, 4].

3. Central anticonvulsant action: Magnesium, by inhibiting calcium entry into the nerve terminal, reduces the amount of calcium-mediated acetylcholine release and thus blocks the transmission between nerves and muscles [5, 6]. As a result, impaired neuromuscular transmission leads to the slowing of muscle contraction and prevents or controls seizures.

B. Preterm labor

The mechanism of action of magnesium sulfate in preterm labor is not well understood, but it probably blocks intracellular calcium channels, decreases the availability of calcium within the muscle, inhibits contractility, and promotes relaxation of the uterine muscle [7, 8].

C. Asthma

The proposed mechanism of action of magnesium in asthma is the inhibition of calcium influx by blocking the voltage-dependent calcium channels causing relaxation of bronchial smooth muscle, which reverses bronchospasm and leads to bronchodilation [9, 10].

D. Cardiac arrhythmias

Although magnesium is effective and frequently used for arrhythmias, it is not an antiarrhythmic drug and should be used as adjuvant therapy. Magnesium is an essential cofactor that regulates the Na^+-K^+-ATPase pump, controls the outward K^+ movement across cell membranes, and influences myocardial excitability [11, 12]. Hypomagnesemia by inhibiting the Na^+-K^+-ATPase pump reduces the amount of intracellular potassium resulting in shortened action potential and increased susceptibility to arrhythmias [13].

Administration of magnesium causes an increase in intracellular potassium, delays atrioventricular node conduction time, prolongs the atrial refractory period, and decreases the frequency of arrhythmias [14]. As arrhythmias are resistant to both antiarrhythmic drugs and cardioversion in the presence of magnesium deficiency, its correction is essential [15].

E. Hypokalemia

Mechanism of renal potassium wasting in hypomagnesemia: Normal or high intracellular magnesium concentration blocks the renal outer medullary potassium (ROMK) channel pores and prevents potassium secretion [16]. Because of the decrease in intracellular magnesium in hypomagnesemia, there is a lack of inhibitory effect on ROMK channels, which will promote potassium secretion from the cell into the lumen leading to an increase in urinary potassium excretion with resultant hypokalemia.

F. Tetanus

Central actions of tetanus toxins cause autonomic dysfunction (leading to increased release of catecholamines, predominantly epinephrine), which is a major cause of mortality from tetanus [17]. Magnesium sulfate is useful as a first-line treatment to reduce the effect of autonomic dysfunction and also helps to control spasms of muscle in tetanus [18–20].

Magnesium is a pre-synaptic neuromuscular blocker. Magnesium, by blocking pre-synaptic neuromuscular excitation, inhibits the release of catecholamines from nerves and reduces the responsiveness of receptors to already released neurotransmitters [21, 22]. With this action, magnesium controls spasms and protects against the ill effects of autonomic dysfunction.

Magnesium helps in the prevention or control of seizures also by blocking peripheral neuromuscular transmission and inhibiting the calcium-dependent acetylcholine release.

INDICATIONS

Because of its multifactorial actions, parenteral magnesium sulfate is frequently used to manage different critical and non-critical patients. The major benefits of using intravenous magnesium are low cost, easy availability, and high therapeutic-to-toxic ratio.

A. Hypomagnesemia

In hospitalized patients, hypomagnesemia is common (in ICU, the prevalence ranges from 20 to 61%) [23–25]

and harmful (increases the duration of mechanical ventilation days, morbidity, and mortality) [26–28].

Intravenous magnesium sulfate is a safe, effective, and low cost which is indicated in patients with severe (serum magnesium concentration 1 mg/dL [0.4 mmol/L or 0.8 mEq/L] or less), and symptomatic (seizures, tetany, or life-threatening arrhythmias, or severe neuromuscular irritability) hypomagnesemia [29, 30].

The dose and rate of magnesium replacement are determined on the basis of the degree of hypomagnesemia, severity of symptoms, and clinical indications (summarized in Table 12.1):

- **Severe hypomagnesemia in hemodynamically unstable symptomatic patients:** In life-threatening conditions (e.g., with torsade de pointes associated with a long QT interval), initially 1 to 2 gm (8 to 16 mEq) magnesium sulfate bolus (diluted in 10 mL D5W) is infused over 2 to 15 minutes followed by a continuous infusion [31, 32].

- **Severe hypomagnesemia in hemodynamically stable patients:** In symptomatic patients with severe magnesium depletion (plasma magnesium <1 mg/dL), initially 1 to 2 gm of magnesium sulfate diluted in 50 to 100 mL of D5W can be infused over one hour. Subsequently, 4 to 8 gm (32 to 64 mEq) of magnesium sulfate infusion is administered slowly over 12 to 24 hours [33]. Patients with severe hypomagnesemia may require repeat doses for 3–7 days to replenish total body stores and to return the plasma magnesium concentration to 1.5 mEq/kg or higher [30].

- **Moderate hypomagnesemia (plasma magnesium 1 to 1.5 mg/dL):** In patients with moderate

Table 12.1 Administration of IV magnesium in clinical practice		
Clinical settings	**Suggested doses of magnesium**	**Ref.**
Severe symptomatic hypomagnesemia	A. Hemodynamically unstable patients 2 gm MgSO$_4$ as a bolus over 2–15 min followed by a continuous infusion	[31, 32]

	B. Hemodynamically stable patients
	   Initial dose: 1 to 2 gm of magnesium infused over one hour.
	   Subsequent dose: 4 to 8 gm of magnesium as a continuous infusion over 12 to 24 hours
		[33]

Moderate hypomagnesemia	2 to 4 gm of magnesium infused over 4 to 12 hours.	[33]
Mild hypomagnesemia	1 to 2 gm of magnesium given over 1 to 2 hours (If the patient is unable to tolerate oral magnesium and mid symptoms present.)	
Preeclampsia	4–6 gm IV over 20 to 30 min followed by a maintenance dose of 1–2 gm/hr as a continuous infusion	[34]
Fetal neuroprotection	4 gm IV over 30 min followed by a 1 gm/hr infusion for 24 hours or until birth, whichever occurs earlier	[35]
Asthma (severe exacerbations)	A single dose of 2 gm of magnesium infused over 20 min	[36]
Tetanus	5 gm magnesium infused over 20 min followed by a 2–3 gm/hr infusion until spasm control is achieved	[37]
50% magnesium sulfate 2 ml = 1 gm = 4 mmol Mg^{2+} = 8 mEq Mg^{2+}		

magnesium depletion, 2 to 4 gm (16 to 32 mEq) of magnesium sulfate is infused slowly over 4 to 12 hours (at a maximum rate of 1 gm/hr) [33].

- **Mild hypomagnesemia (plasma magnesium 1.6 to 1.9 mg/dL):** If the patient is unable to take or tolerate oral magnesium supplementation, 1 to 2 gm (8 to 16 mEq) magnesium sulfate is infused slowly over one to two hours in patients with mild magnesium depletion and mild symptoms.

- **Rules of thumb:** In critically ill mild to moderate hypomagnesemia patients, 1 gm of intravenous (IV) Mg^{2+} will roughly increase the serum Mg^{2+} concentration by 0.15 mEq/L within 18 to 30 h [38].

- **In renal failure:** Assess renal function before initiating of magnesium supplementation because by regulating the excretion of administered magnesium, kidneys maintain the plasma magnesium concentration within the normal range [39]. In patients with renal insufficiency, administer 50% or less of the suggested empirical magnesium dose to reduce the risk of hypermagnesemia [33].

- **Duration of therapy:** When magnesium is administered intravenously, uptake by the cells is slow, but renal elimination is rapid (acute rise in serum magnesium inhibits its renal reabsorption, and up to 50% of administered magnesium is excreted in the urine) [40]. Administration of magnesium at a slow rate (over 8 to 24 hours) and for a longer period (at least for 1 to 2 days after achieving the normal serum magnesium concentration) is important because sustained supplementation allows a longer time for magnesium uptake by cells, reduces renal wasting and thereby correct hypomagnesemia effectively.

B. Obstetric practice

Magnesium sulfate is used for preventing and treating seizures in severe preeclampsia or eclampsia before early preterm delivery for neuroprotection to reduce the risk of cerebral palsy and for the short-term prolongation of pregnancy (as a tocolytic agent) in women who are at risk of preterm labor within 7 days.

1. Preeclampsia and eclampsia

Magnesium sulfate therapy is the first line, most preferred, time-tested, and superior therapy for the preventing and treating of seizures in preeclampsia with severe features and eclampsia [34, 41–45]. However, it is essential to remember that magnesium sulfate therapy is not used to treat hypertension.

The large multicentre Magpie trial demonstrated a more than 50% reduction in the seizure rate in preeclampsia with this treatment [46].

Although magnesium sulfate is routinely administered for the prevention of seizures in gestational hypertension or mild preeclampsia, there is no consensus regarding the same [34, 47, 48]. In preeclampsia without severe features, the clinician or institution decides to administer magnesium sulfate for seizure prophylaxis considering the preferences of the patient and the risk-benefit trade-off of each strategy [34].

The benefits of magnesium sulfate therapy are low-cost, avoids producing central nervous system depression, and this modality is safer and more effective than phenytoin, diazepam, nimodipine,

or lithic cocktail (chlorpromazine, promethazine, and pethidine) for the prevention of recurrent seizures in eclampsia [49–53].

Administration

- Timing: As labor and delivery is a more likely time to develop convulsions, seizure prophylaxis with magnesium sulfate in women with preeclampsia-eclampsia is usually initiated before onset or induction of labor, and for women requiring cesarean delivery, magnesium infusion should be started before surgery [34, 54, 55].

- Route of administration: Magnesium sulfate is typically administered intravenously, preferably using an infusion pump if available. But in patients with a lack of facility to establish venous access, the intramuscular route is used, which is as effective as intravenous administration [56].

- Intravenous regimen: A loading dose of 4–6 gm of magnesium sulfate diluted in 100 mL of IV fluid administered intravenously over 20 to 30 minutes, followed by a maintenance dose of 1–2 gm/hour as a continuous infusion (ACOG recommended dosing) [34].

- Intramuscularly regimen: A loading dose of 5 gm of 50% magnesium sulfate is injected deeply intramuscularly into each buttock (total of 10 gm), followed by a maintenance dose of 5 gm intramuscularly every four hours (maybe mixed with 1 mL of 2% xylocaine in the same syringe to reduce pain [34].

- Recurrent seizures: Treated with an additional 2–4 gm bolus infused over 5 to 15 minutes [42].

- Duration of therapy: Magnesium sulfate is continued throughout delivery, whether vaginal or caesarean, and continued for at least 24 hours after delivery or the last convulsion, whichever occurs later [34, 57].

- Monitor for magnesium toxicity: To detect the signs of early magnesium toxicity, monitor urine output hourly (magnesium sulfate is excreted almost exclusively in the urine), assess deep tendon reflexes every 10 minutes for the first 2 hours and then every 30 minutes, and closely monitor respiratory rate and O_2 saturation. Loss of patellar reflex is the earliest and foremost sign of magnesium toxicity.

- Stop or delay magnesium infusion if patellar reflexes are absent, respiratory rate <16 breaths/minute, oxygen saturation <90%, or urine output <30 ml per hour in the preceding four hours.

- Antidote: Administer 10% Calcium gluconate 10 ml IV slowly over 3 minutes if respiratory depression.

- Caution: In myasthenia gravis, magnesium sulfate is contraindicated because it can exacerbate symptoms of myasthenia and may precipitate a severe myasthenic crisis. As magnesium sulfate is excreted by the kidneys, in women with renal dysfunction, adjust the maintenance dose (but not the loading dose) and monitor serum magnesium levels closely.

2. Fetal neuroprotection

Antenatal administration of magnesium sulfate plays an important role in fetal neuroprotection in women of less than 32 weeks of gestation at risk of preterm delivery within the next 24 hours [58–60]. Maternal administration of magnesium sulfate has strongly demonstrated a decreased risk of cerebral palsy in different trials [61, 62] and meta-analyses [63–66] and therefore is recommended for fetal neuroprotection [35, 57]. Loading dose of 4 gm intravenously slowly over 20 minutes, followed by a 1 gm/hr infusion, is administered for 24 hours or until birth, whichever occurs earlier [35].

3. Preterm labor

The use of magnesium sulfate is recommended for short-term (up to 48 hours only) prolongation of pregnancy (as a tocolytic agent), as it can alter myometrial contractility and may inhibit labor [67]. Magnesium sulfate is also recommended in women between 24 and 34 weeks of gestation who are at risk of preterm delivery within 7 days so that it permits time for the maternal administration of antenatal corticosteroids [68]. In neonates with preterm birth, maternal administration of corticosteroids in the antenatal period helps to improve fetal lung maturity and increases the chances of neonatal survival. FDA issues the safety alert warning against continuous maternal use of IV magnesium sulfate beyond 5 to 7 days, as it may cause fetal hypocalcemia, bone abnormalities, and predispose to risk of fractures in the neonate [69].

C. Severe exacerbations of acute asthma

IV magnesium sulfate is not used routinely in acute asthma. Still, administration of a single dose of magnesium sulfate (2 gm infused over 20 min) is recommended in severe exacerbations of acute asthma with inadequate response to standard intensive initial treatment [36, 70–72].

IV magnesium sulfate as an adjunct to standard therapy in moderate to severe exacerbations of acute asthma improves respiratory function, decreases the need for hospitalization [36, 71, 73–75], shortens the length of stay [76], and reduces the requirement of mechanical ventilation support [77].

But on administering nebulized magnesium sulfate in acute asthma, no significant benefits were demonstrated on respiratory function or hospital admission [71, 78, 79].

D. Cardiac arrhythmia

Magnesium deficiency is associated with an increased risk of atrial fibrillation (even in individuals without cardiovascular disease) [80, 81], ventricular arrhythmias [82], and sudden death [83].

Administration of IV magnesium helps in the prevention of atrial fibrillation following coronary artery bypass or cardiac surgery [84–87]. In addition, as adjuvant therapy, IV magnesium helps to control the ventricular rate in acute onset rapid atrial fibrillation [88–90].

IV magnesium also reduced ventricular and supraventricular arrhythmias effectively and significantly [91].

ESC (2015) and ACLS (2018) Guidelines recommend IV magnesium as the treatment of choice in the management of patients with torsades de pointes (i.e., polymorphic VT associated with long-QT interval); however, its routine use during resuscitation of cardiac arrest is not recommended [92, 93].

E. Refractory hypokalemia

The rationales for using IV magnesium in the treatment of refractory hypokalemia are:

- Magnesium deficiency is common in hypokalemia (in about 40% of hypokalemic patients) [94].

- Serum magnesium levels do not necessarily correlate with body magnesium stores. Therefore, even with normal serum magnesium levels, magnesium deficiency can exist [95, 96]. So, consider magnesium depletion even with a normal serum magnesium level in refractory hypokalemia (when suspected on clinical background, i.e., the presence of severe diarrhea or obvious malnutrition) [97].

- Hypomagnesemia by increasing urinary potassium excretion aggravates hypokalemia and can cause treatment-resistant hypokalemia [16].

So, in refractory hypokalemia, suspected and treat hypomagnesemia adequately. Symptomatic patients usually need about 3 to 6 gm of magnesium/day for 3–5 days [95].

F. Refractory hypocalcemia

Magnesium deficiency is a common cause of hypocalcemia, and it occurs due to decreased parathyroid hormone (PTH) secretion and end-organ resistance to the PTH effect. In hypomagnesemia, hypocalcemia will be refractory to calcium and vitamin D treatment unless magnesium is administered.

G. Tetanus

Inj. magnesium sulfate is helpful as first-line therapy in controlling spasms and autonomic dysfunction (as an adjunct to sedation) in patients with tetanus [18, 20, 98]. A loading dose of 5 gm (or 75 mg/kg) of magnesium is given over 20 minutes to control spasms in tetanus, followed by a 2–3 gm per hour infusion until spasm control is achieved [37].

H. Migraine

Intravenous magnesium sulfate is found to be beneficial in the treatment of an acute attack of migraine [99–101], but the evidence is inadequate, and therefore, such use is not recommended in recent guidelines [102–104]. However, literature and guidelines support its use in migraine to control pain beyond 1 hour, reduce the duration of aura [102–105], and reduce the need for rescue analgesia compared to other medications [106–108]. Usually, 1–2 gm of magnesium is infused IV slowly over 10 to 20 minutes in the treatment of migraine [102].

I. Aneurysmal subarachnoid hemorrhage

Magnesium sulfate is proposed to have a neuroprotective effect as it antagonizes calcium and reduces cerebral vasospasm. The beneficial effect of magnesium in aneurysmal subarachnoid hemorrhage by preventing cerebral vasospasm and the resultant reduction of cerebral ischemia and the risk of developing infarction is shown in several studies [109–114]. However, multiple studies, systematic reviews, and meta-analyses failed to demonstrate improvement in neurological outcomes in aneurysmal subarachnoid hemorrhage with intravenous magnesium, and therefore its routine use is not recommended [115–121].

J. Chronic obstructive pulmonary disease (COPD)

Hypomagnesemia is common in COPD patients, and administration of IV magnesium sulfate (2 gm infused over 20 minutes as a single dose) may be useful as an adjunctive therapy in the treatment of acute exacerbations of COPD who are not improving with inhaled bronchodilator therapy because of its potential benefits like decrease in hospital admissions, reduced length of hospital stay and symptoms of dyspnea [122–124].

CONTRAINDICATIONS AND PRECAUTIONS

Magnesium is avoided or used with caution in severe renal failure, myasthenia gravis, cardiac ischemia, and heart block.

A. **Renal failure:** As magnesium is excreted by the kidney, in patients with renal failure (e.g., GFR <30 ml/min), there is a risk of accumulation of magnesium and resultant toxicity [125]. So, in patients with renal failure, magnesium should be used cautiously with a reduction of dose by 25% to 50%, and its serum level should be monitored closely [126, 127].

B. **Myasthenia gravis:** As magnesium interferes with neuromuscular transmission and inhibits the release of acetylcholine, it potentiates neuromuscular weakness and can precipitate a severe myasthenic crisis [128, 129].

C. **Heart block:** As hypermagnesemia (>4 mEq/L) may cause conduction defects and bradycardia, the administration of magnesium is contraindicated in patients with heart block.

ADVERSE EFFECTS

At a different magnesium level, the usual adverse effects are summarized below in Table 12.2.

ADMINISTRATION

Intramuscular: Inj. magnesium sulfate 50% is used for deep intramuscular (IM)

Table 12.2 Plasma concentration of magnesium and clinical effects				
Plasma concentration of magnesium				**Clinical effects**
Level	**mg/dL**	**mEq/L**	**mmol/L**	
Low	<1.2	<1.0	<0.5	Arrhythmias, tetany, or seizures
	1.2–1.8	1.0–1.5	0.5–0.75	Hypokalemia, hypocalcemia, neuromuscular irritability
Normal	1.8–2.5	1.5–2.1	0.75–1.05	No clinical effect
High	2.5–5.0	2.1–4.2	1.05–2.1	Clinically asymptomatic
	5.0–7.0	4.2–5.8	2.1–2.9	Nausea, lethargy, drowsiness, impaired patellar reflexes
	7.0–12	5.8–10	2.9–5.0	Loss of deep tendon reflexes, bradycardia, hypotension, hypoventilation, and ECG changes (P-Q interval prolongation, widen QRS complex)
	>12	>10	>5.0	Complete heart block, respiratory failure, cardiac arrest

administration and may be mixed with 1 mL of 2% xylocaine to reduce pain.

Intravenous: Never use undiluted 50% magnesium sulfate for IV administration. For IV infusion, dilute magnesium sulfate to a concentration of at least 20% or less before administration.

As each mL of 50% magnesium sulfate contains 500 mg of magnesium, to prepare 10 or 20% solution, add 20 ml (10 gm) of 50% magnesium to 80 ml or 40 ml of diluent, respectively. Use 5% dextrose and 0.9% sodium chloride as a diluent. The advantages of using a smaller volume of the bag (e.g., 250 to 500 mL) for dilution are delivery of a limited amount of magnesium in case of accidental rapid infusion and ease of differentiating from one-liter bags of hydrating solutions and medications [130].

MONITORING

While administering IV magnesium, closely monitor heart rate, blood pressure, respiratory rate, patellar reflex, urine output, and oxygen saturation

(SpO_2) to avoid its serious adverse effects. Discontinue IV administration of magnesium if:

- Respiratory rate of less than 12 breaths/minute.

- Absent of knee jerks.

- Urine output of less than 25 mL/hour or less than 100 mL over 4 hours.

- Diastolic blood pressure decreases more than 15 mmHg below the baseline.

Monitor serum magnesium at least once daily during the administration of IV magnesium. The administration is usually discontinued once serum magnesium levels are 1.5 mg/dL (1.25 mEq/L or 0.625 mmol/L) or higher. A high level of magnesium concentration may benefit patients with eclampsia or preeclampsia, recent cardiac surgery, or the presence of arrhythmias and digitalis toxicity.

ANTIDOTE

In hypermagnesemia, IV calcium chloride or gluconate is used as an antidote along with the discontinuation of magnesium infusion.

REFERENCES

1. Euser AG, Cipolla MJ. Magnesium sulfate for the treatment of eclampsia: A brief review. Stroke. 2009;40(4):1169–75.

2. Vigorito C, Giordano A, Ferraro P, et al. Hemodynamic effects of magnesium sulfate on the normal human heart. Am J cardiol 1991;67(16):1435–7.

3. Kaya M, Ahishali B. The role of magnesium in edema and blood brain barrier disruption. In: Vink R, Nechifor M, editors. Magnesium in the Central Nervous System [Internet]. Adelaide (AU): University of Adelaide Press; 2011. Available from: https://www.ncbi.nlm.nih.gov/books/NBK507252/.

4. Li X, Han X, Yang J, et al. Magnesium sulfate provides neuroprotection in eclampsia-like seizure model by ameliorating neuroinflammation and brain edema. Mol Neurobiol 2017;54:7938–7948.

5. Swaminathan R. Magnesium metabolism and its disorders. Clin Biochem Rev. 2003;24(2):47–66.

6. Zwer F. Factors affect neuromuscular transmission and block. J Anesth Crit Care Open Access 2016;6(1):00216.

7. Dube L, Granry JC. The therapeutic use of magnesium in anesthesiology, intensive care and emergency medicine: a review. Can J Anaesth 2003;50(7):732–746.

8. Abramovici A, Cantu J, Jenkins SM. Tocolytic therapy for acute preterm labor. ObstetGynecol Clin North Am. 2012;39(1):77–87.

9. Gourgoulianis KI, Chatziparasidis G, Chatziefthimiou A, et al. Magnesium as a relaxing factor of airway smooth muscles. J Aerosol Med 2001;14(3):301–307.

10. Kelly HW. Magnesium sulfate for severe acute asthma in children. J PediatrPharmacolTher. 2003;8(1):40–45.

11. Skou JC, Butler KW, Hansen O. The effect of magnesium, ATP, P i, and sodium on the inhibition of the (Na++ K+)-activated enzyme system by g-strophanthin. BiochimBiophys Acta. 1971;241(2):443–61.

12. Agus MS, Agus ZS. Cardiovascular actions of magnesium. Crit Care Clin. 2001;17(1):175–86.

13. Millane TA, Ward DE, Camm AJ. Is hypomagnesemia arrhythmogenic? Clin Cardiol 1992;15(2):103–8.

14. DiCarlo LA Jr, Morady F, de Buitleir M, et al. Effects of magnesium sulfate on cardiac conduction and refractoriness in humans. J Am Coll Cardiol. 1986;7(6):1356–62.

15. Kasaoka S, Tsuruta R, Nakashima K, et al. Effect of intravenous magnesium sulfate on cardiac arrhythmias in critically ill patients with low serum ionized magnesium. JpnCirc J. 1996;60(11):871–5.

16. Huang CL, Kuo E. Mechanism of hypokalemia in magnesium deficiency. J Am Soc Nephrol. 2007;18(10):2649–2652.

17. Thwaites CL, Yen LM, Cordon SM, et al. Urinary catecholamine excretion in tetanus. Anaesthesia 2006;61(4):355–359.

18. Attygalle D, Rodrigo N. Magnesium as first line therapy in the management of tetanus: A prospective study of 40 patients. Anaesthesia 2002;57(8):778–817.

19. Kole AK, Roy R, Kar SS, et al. Experience of use of magnesium sulfate in the treatment of tetanus in a tertiary referral infectious disease hospital, Kolkata, India. Ann Trop Med Health 2013;6:456–9.

20. Rodrigo C, Fernando D, Rajapakse S. Pharmacological management of tetanus: an evidence-based review. Crit Care 2014;18(2):217.

21. Cook TM, Protheroe RT, Handel JM. Tetanus: a review of the literature, Br J Anaesth, 2001;87(3):477–87.

22. Thwaites CL, Yen LM, Cordon SM, et al. Effect of magnesium sulphate on urinary catecholamine excretion in severe tetanus. Anaesthesia 2008;63(7):719–725.

23. Soliman HM, Mercan D, Lobo SS, et al. Development of ionized hypomagnesemia is associated with higher mortality rates. Crit Care Med 2003;31(4):1082–7.

24. Chernow B, Bamberger BSS, Stoiko M, et al. Hypomagnesemia in patients in postoperative intensive care. Chest 1989;95(2):391–397.

25. Deheinzelin D, Negri EM, Tucci MR, et al. Hypomagnesemia in critically ill cancer patients: A prospective study of predictive factors. Braz J Med Biol Res 2000;33(12):1443–8.

26. Rubeiz GJ, Thill-Baharozian M, Hardie D, et al. Association of hypomagnesemia and mortality in acutely ill medical patients. Crit Care Med. 1993;21(2):203–9.

27. Limaye CS, Londhey VA, Nadkar MY, et al. Hypomagnesemia in critically ill medical patients. J Assoc Physicians India. 2011;59:19–22.

28. Fairley J, Glassford NJ, Zhang L, et al. Magnesium status and magnesium therapy in critically ill patients: A systematic review. J Crit Care. 2015;30(6):1349–1358.

29. Martin KJ, Gonzalez EA, Slatopolsky E. Clinical consequences and management of hypomagnesemia. J. Am. Soc. Nephrol. 2009;20(11):2291–2295.

30. Velissaris D, Karamouzos V, Pierrakos C, et al. Hypomagnesemia in critically ill sepsis patients. J Clin Med Res. 2015;7(12):911–8.

31. Neumar RW, Otto CW, Link MS, et al. Part 8: adult advanced cardiovascular life support: 2010 American Heart Association guidelines for cardiopulmonary resuscitation and emergency cardiovascular care. Circulation. 2010;122(18 Suppl 3):729–67.

32. Tzivoni D, Banai S, Schuger C, et al. Treatment of torsade de pointes with magnesium sulfate. Circulation. 1988;77(2):392–7.

33. Kraft MD, Btaiche IF, Sacks GS, et al. Treatment of electrolyte disorders in adult patients in the intensive care unit. Am J Health Syst Pharm. 2005;62(16):1663–82.

34. Gestational Hypertension and Preeclampsia: ACOG Practice Bulletin, Number 222. Obstet Gynecol. 2020;135(6):e237–e260.

35. Magee LA, De Silva DA, Sawchuck D, et al. 376-Magnesium Sulphate for Fetal Neuroprotection. SOGC Clinical practice guideline 2019;41(4):505–522.

36. Kew KM, Kirtchuk L, Michell CI. Intravenous magnesium sulfate for treating adults with acute asthma in the emergency department. Cochrane Database of Systematic Reviews 2014;28(5):CD010909.

37. Current recommendations for treatment of tetanus during humanitarian emergencies. WHO Technical Note. World Health Organization January 2010.

38. Hammond DA, Stojakovic J, Kathe N, et al. Effectiveness and safety of magnesium replacement in critically ill patients admitted to the medical intensive care unit in an academic medical center: a retrospective, cohort study. J Intensive Care Med. 2019;34(11–12):967–972.

39. Van de Wal-Visscher ER, Kooman JP, van der Sande FM. Magnesium in chronic kidney disease: should we care?. Blood Purif. 2018;45(1–3):173–178.

40. Agus ZS. Hypomagnesemia. J Am Soc Nephrol 1999;10(7):1616–22.

41. Pritchard JA. The use of the magnesium ion in the management of eclamptogenictoxemias. SurgGynecolObstet 1955;100(2):131–40.

42. Which anticonvulsant for women with eclampsia? Evidence from the Collaborative Eclampsia Trial. Lancet. 1995;345(8963):1455–63.

43. WHO recommendations for Prevention and treatment of pre-eclampsia and eclampsia. World Health Organization 2011.

44. Magee LA, Pels A, Helewa M, et al. Diagnosis, evaluation, and management of the hypertensive disorders of pregnancy: executive summary. J ObstetGynaecol Can 2014;36(5):416–41.

45. Hypertension in pregnancy: diagnosis and management. NICE guideline [NG133] Published: 25 June 2019. Visit: www.nice.org.uk/guidance/ng133.

46. Altman D, Carroli G, Duley L, et al. Do women with preeclampsia, and their babies, benefit from magnesium sulphate? The Magpie Trial: a randomised placebo-controlled trial. Magpie Trial Collaboration Group. Lancet 2002;359(9321):1877–90.

47. Livingston JC, Livingston LW, Ramsey R, et al. Magnesium sulfate in women with mild preeclampsia: a randomized controlled trial. Obstet Gynecol 2003;101(2):217–20.

48. Cahill AG, Macones GA, Odibo AO, et al. Magnesium for seizure prophylaxis in patients with mild preeclampsia. ObstetGynecol 2007;110(3):601–7.

49. Duley L, Henderson-Smart DJ, Chou D. Magnesium sulphate versus phenytoin for eclampsia. Cochrane Database of Systematic Reviews 2010;(10):CD000128.

50. Duley L, Gülmezoglu AM, Henderson-Smart DJ, et al. Magnesium sulphate and other anticonvulsants for women with pre-eclampsia. Cochrane Database of Systematic Reviews. 2010;2010(11):CD000025.

51. Duley L, Henderson-Smart DJ, Walker GJA, et al. Magnesium sulphate versus diazepam for eclampsia. Cochrane Database of Systematic Reviews 2010;2010(12):CD000127.

52. Belfort MA, Anthony J, Saade GR, et al. A comparison of magnesium sulfate and nimodipine for the prevention of eclampsia. Nimodipine Study Group. N Engl J Med 2003;348(4):304–11.

53. Duley L, Gülmezoglu AM, Chou D. Magnesium sulphate versus lytic cocktail for eclampsia. Cochrane Database of Systematic Reviews 2010;2010(9):CD002960.

54. Cunningham FG, Leveno KJ, Bloom SL, et al. Hypertensive Disorders. In: Williams Obstetrics, 25th edition McGraw-Hill Education, 2018.p.710.

55. Hall DR, Odendaal HJ, Smith M. Is the prophylactic administration of magnesium sulphate in women with pre-eclampsia indicated prior to labour? BJOG 2000;107(7):903–8.

56. Salinger DH, Mundle S, Regi A, et al. Magnesium sulphate for prevention of eclampsia: are intramuscular and intravenous regimens equivalent? A population pharmacokinetic study. BJOG 2013;120(7):894–900.

57. Managing complications in pregnancy and childbirth: a guide for midwives and doctors – 2nd ed. Geneva: World Health Organization;2017.

58. Chollat C, Marret S. Magnesium sulfate and fetal neuroprotection: overview of clinical evidence. Neural Regen Res 2018;13(12):2044–2049.

59. Jayaram PM, Mohan MK, Farid I, et al. Antenatal magnesium sulfate for fetal neuroprotection: a critical appraisal and systematic review of clinical practice guidelines. J Perinat Med 2019;47(3):262–269.

60. Society for Maternal-Fetal Medicine (SMFM), Martins JG, Biggio JR, et al. Society for Maternal-Fetal Medicine Consult Series #52: Diagnosis and management of fetal growth restriction: (Replaces Clinical Guideline Number 3, April 2012). Am J Obstet Gynecol. 2020;223(4):B2–B17.

61. Crowther CA, Hiller JE, Doyle LW, et al. Effect of magnesium sulfate given for neuroprotection before preterm birth: a randomized controlled trial. JAMA 2003;290(20):2669–76.

62. Rouse DJ, Hirtz DG, Thom E, et al. A randomized, controlled trial of magnesium sulfate for the prevention of cerebral palsy. N Engl J Med 2008;359(9):895–905.

63. Doyle LW, Crowther CA, Middleton P, et al. Magnesium sulphate for women at risk of preterm birth for neuroprotection of the fetus. Cochrane Database Syst Rev 2009;(1):CD004661.

64. Nguyen TMN, Crowther CA, Wilkinson D, et al. Magnesium sulphate for women at term for neuroprotection of the fetus. Cochrane Database Syst Rev 2013;(2):CD009395.

65. Zeng X, Xue Y, Tian Q, et al. Effects and safety of magnesium sulfate on neuroprotection: a meta-analysis based on PRISMA guidelines. Medicine (Baltimore) 2016;95(1):e2451.

66. Crowther CA, Middleton PF, Voysey M, et al. Assessing the neuroprotective benefits for babies of antenatal magnesium sulphate: An individual participant data meta-analysis. PLoS Med. 2017;14(10):e1002398.

67. Committee Opinion No 652: Magnesium Sulfate Use in Obstetrics. Obstet Gynecol. 2016;127(1):e52–e53.

68. American College of Obstetricians and Gynecologists Committee on Obstetric Practice Society for Maternal-Fetal Medicine. Committee Opinion No. 573: Magnesium sulfate use in obstetrics. Obstet Gynecol. 2013;122(3):727–8.

69. FDA recommends against prolonged use of magnesium sulfate to stop pre-term labor due to bone changes in exposed babies. https://www.fda.gov/media/85971/download (Accessed on July 25, 2020).

70. Cheuk DKL, Chau TC, Lee SL. A meta-analysis on intravenous magnesium sulphate for treating acute asthma. Arch Dis Child. 2005;90(1):74–7.

71. Su Z, Li R, Gai Z. Intravenous and nebulized magnesium sulfate for treating acute asthma in children: a systematic review and meta-analysis. PediatrEmerg Care. 2018;34(6):390–395.

72. 2020 GINA Pocket Guide - Global Initiative for Asthma. Pocket guide for asthma management and prevention (for adult and children older than 5 years). A Pocket Guide for Health Professionals Updated 2020.

73. Silverman RA, Osborn H, Runge J, et al. Acute Asthma/Magnesium Study Group. IV magnesium sulfate in the treatment of acute severe asthma: a multicenter randomized controlled trial. Chest. 2002;122(2):489–97.

74. Griffiths B, Kew KM. Intravenous magnesium sulfate for treating children with acute asthma in the emergency department. Cochrane Database Syst Rev. 2016;29(4):CD011050.

75. Özdemir A, Doğruel D. Efficacy of magnesium sulfate treatment in children with acute asthma. Med PrincPract. 2020;29(3):292–298.

76. Irazuzta JE, Paredes F, Pavlicich V, et al. High-dose magnesium sulfate infusion for severe asthma in the emergency department: efficacy study. Pediatr Crit Care Med. 2016;17(2):e29–33.

77. Torres S, Sticco N, Bosch JJ, et al. Effectiveness of magnesium sulfate as initial treatment of acute severe asthma in children, conducted in a tertiary- level university hospital: a randomized, controlled trial. Arch Argent Pediatr. 2012;110(4):291–6.

78. Mathew JL, Walia M. Systematic review on efficacy of magnesium (intravenous or nebulized) for acute asthma episodes in children. Indian Pediatr 2017;54(2):133–137.

79. Knightly R, Milan SJ, Hughes R, et al. Inhaled magnesium sulfate in the treatment of acute asthma. Cochrane Database Syst Rev 2017;11(11):CD003898.

80. Khan AM, Lubitz SA, Sullivan LM, et al. Low serum magnesium and the development of atrial fibrillation in the community. Circulation 2013;127(1):33–38.

81. Markovits N, Kurnik D, Halkin H, et al. Database evaluation of the association between serum magnesium levels and the risk of atrial fibrillation in the community. Int J Cardiol 2016;205:142–146.

82. Ceremuzynski L, Gebalska J, Wolk R, et al. Hypomagnesemia in heart failure with ventricular arrhythmias. Beneficial effects of magnesium supplementation. J Intern Med. 2000;247(1):78–86.

83. Eisenberg MJ. Magnesium deficiency and sudden death. Am Heart J. 1992;124(2):544–549.

84. Alghamdi AA, Al-Radi OO, Latter DA. Intravenous magnesium for prevention of atrial fibrillation after coronary artery bypass surgery: a systematic review and meta-analysis. Journal of Cardiac Surgery 2005;20(3):293–299.

85. Gu WJ, Wu ZJ, Wang PF, et al. Intravenous magnesium prevents atrial fibrillation after coronary artery bypass grafting: a meta-analysis of 7 double-blind, placebo-controlled, randomized clinical trials. Trials. 2012;13:41.

86. Burgess DC, Kilborn MJ, Keech AC. Interventions for prevention of post-operative atrial fibrillation and its complications after cardiac surgery: a meta-analysis. European Heart Journal 2006;27(23):2846–57.

87. Miller S, Crystal E, Garfinkle M, et al. Effects of magnesium on atrial fibrillation after cardiac surgery: a meta-analysis. Heart. 2005;91(5):618–623.

88. Ho KM, Sheridan DJ, Paterson T. Use of intravenous magnesium to treat acute onset atrial fibrillation: a meta-analysis. Heart. 2007;93(11):1433–40.

89. Onalan O, Crystal E, Daoulah A, et al. Meta-analysis of magnesium therapy for the acute management of rapid atrial fibrillation. Am J Cardiol 2007;99(12):1726–32.

90. Bouida W, Beltaief K, Msolli MA, et al. Low-dose magnesium sulfate versus high dose in the early management of rapid atrial fibrillation: randomized controlled double-blind study (LOMAGHI study). AcadEmerg Med. 2019;26(2):183–191.

91. Salaminia S, Sayehmiri F, Angha P, et al. Evaluating the effect of magnesium supplementation and cardiac arrhythmias after acute coronary syndrome: a systematic review and meta-analysis. BMC Cardiovasc Disord 2018;18(1):129.

92. Priori SG, Blomstrom-Lundqvist C, Mazzanti A, et al. 2015 ESC Guidelines for the management of patients with ventricular arrhythmias and the prevention of sudden cardiac death. Europace 2015;17(11):1601–87.

93. Panchal AR, Berg KM, Kudenchuk PJ, et al. 2018 American heart association focused update on advanced cardiovascular life support use of antiarrhythmic drugs during and immediately after cardiac arrest: an update to the American heart association guidelines for cardiopulmonary resuscitation and emergency cardiovascular care. Circulation 2018;138:e740–e749.

94. Whang R, Whang DD, Ryan MP. Refractory potassium repletion. A consequence of magnesium deficiency. Arch Intern Med. 1992;152(1):40–5.

95. Abbott LG, Rude RK. Clinical manifestations of magnesium deficiency. Miner Electrolyte Metab 1993;19(4–5):314–22.

96. Baker WL. Treating arrhythmias with adjunctive magnesium: identifying future research directions. Eur Heart J Cardiovasc Pharmacother. 2017;3(2):108–117.

97. Hansen BA, Bruserud Ø. Hypomagnesemia in critically ill patients. J Intensive Care 2018;6:21.

98. Rodrigo C, Samarakoon L, Fernando SD, et al. A meta-analysis of magnesium for tetanus. Anaesthesia 2012;67(12):1370–4.

99. Corbo J, Esses D, Bijur PE, et al. Randomized clinical trial of intravenous magnesium sulfate as an adjunctive medication for emergency department treatment of migraine headache. Ann Emerg Med. 2001;38(6):621–7.

100. Demirkaya S, Vural O, Dora B, et al. Efficacy of intravenous magnesium sulfate in the treatment of acute migraine attacks. Headache. 2001;41(2):171–7.

101. Chiu HY, Yeh TH, Huang YC, et al. Effects of intravenous and oral magnesium on reducing migraine: a meta-analysis of randomized controlled trials. Pain Physician 2016;19(1):E97–112.

102. Orr SL, Friedman BW, Christie S, et al. Management of adults with acute migraine in the emergency department: the american headache society evidence

assessment of parenteral pharmacotherapies. Headache. 2016;56(6):911–40.

103. Miller AC, K Pfeffer B, Lawson MR, et al. Intravenous magnesium sulfate to treat acute headaches in the emergency department: a systematic review. Headache. 2019;59(10):1674–1686.

104. The State of the Migraine Nation, Migraine care rapid research review. Migraine nation - The Migraine Trust 2020.

105. Bigal ME, Bordini CA, Tepper SJ, et al. Intravenous magnesium sulphate in the acute treatment of migraine without aura and migraine with aura. A randomized, double-blind, placebo-controlled study. Cephalalgia. 2002;22(5):345–353.

106. Shahrami A, Assarzadegan F, Hatamabadi HR, et al. Comparison of therapeutic effects of magnesium sulfate vs. dexamethasone/metoclopramide on alleviating acute migraine headache. J Emerg Med. 2015;48(1):69–76.

107. Baratloo A, Mirbaha S, Delavar KH, et al. Intravenous caffeine citrate vs. magnesium sulfate for reducing pain in patients with acute migraine headache; a prospective quasi-experimental study. The Korean Journal of Pain. 2017;30(3):176–182.

108. Delavar KH, Amiri M, Negida A, et al. Ketorolac versus magnesium sulfate in migraine headache pain management; a preliminary study. Emergency (Tehran, Iran). 2017;5(1):e2.

109. Chia RY, Hughes RS, Morgan MK. Magnesium: a useful adjunct in the prevention of cerebral vasospasm following aneurysmal following aneurysmal subarachnoid haemorrhage. J Clin Neurosci. 2002;9(3):279–81.

110. Dorhout MSM, van den Bergh WM, Algra A, et al. Achieved serum magnesium concentrations and occurrence of delayed cerebral ischaemia and poor outcome in aneurysmal subarachnoid haemorrhage. J Neurol Neurosurg Psychiatry. 2007;78(7):729–731.

111. Zhao XD, Zhou YT, Zhang X, et al. A meta-analysis of treating subarachnoid haemorrhage with magnesium sulfate. J ClinNeurosci. 2009;16(11):1394–7.

112. Westermaier T, Stetter C, Vince GH, et al. Prophylactic intravenous magnesium sulfate for treatment of aneurysmal subarachnoid hemorrhage: a randomized, placebo-controlled, clinical study. Crit Care Med. 2010;38(5):1284–1290.

113. Kunze E, Lilla N, Stetter C, et al. Magnesium protects in episodes of critical perfusion after aneurysmal SAH, Translational Neuroscience 2018;9(1):99–105.

114. Soliman R, Zohry G. Effect of magnesium sulphate and milrinone on cerebral vasospasm after aneurysmal subarachnoid hemorrhage: a randomized study. Rev Bras Anestesiol. 2019;69(1):64–71.

115. Muir KW, Lees KR, Ford I, et al. Magnesium for acute stroke (Intravenous Magnesium Efficacy in Stroke trial): randomised controlled trial. Lancet. 2004;363(9407):439–45.

116. Dorhout MSM, Algra A, Vandertop WP, et al. Magnesium for aneurysmal subarachnoid haemorrhage (MASH-2): a randomized placebo-controlled trial. Lancet. 2012;380(9836):44–49.

117. Steiner T, Juvela S, Unterberg A, et al. European Stroke Organization guidelines for the management of intracranial aneurysms and subarachnoid haemorrhage. Cerebrovasc Dis. 2013;35:93–112.

118. Golan E, Vasquez D, Ferguson N, et al. Prophylactic magnesium for improving neurologic outcome after aneurysmal subarachnoid haemorrhage: systematic review and meta-analysis. J CritCare. 2013;28(2):173–81.

119. Reddy D, Fallah A, Petropoulos JA, et al. Prophylactic magnesium sulfate for aneurysmal subarachnoid haemorrhage: a systematic review and meta-analysis. Neurocrit Care. 2014;21(2):356–64.

120. Saver JL, Starkman S, Eckstein M, et al. Prehospital use of magnesium sulfate as neuroprotection in acute stroke. N Engl J Med. 2015;372(6):528–536.

121. Avgerinos KI, Chatzisotiriou A, Haidich AB, et al. Intravenous magnesium sulfate in acute stroke: a systematic review and meta-analysis of randomized controlled trials. Stroke. 2019;50(4):931–938.

122. Ni H, Aye SZ, Naing C. Magnesium sulfate for acute exacerbations of chronic obstructive pulmonary disease. Cochrane Database Syst Rev. 2022;5(5):CD013506.

123. Jahangir A, Zia Z, Niazi MRK, et al. Efficacy of magnesium sulfate in the chronic obstructive pulmonary disease population: a systematic review and meta-analysis. Adv Respir Med. 2022;90(2):125–133.

124. Makwana S, Patel A, Sonagara M. Correlation Between Serum Magnesium Level and Acute Exacerbation in Patients With Chronic Obstructive Pulmonary Disease (COPD). Cureus. 2022;14(6):e26229.

125. Guerrera MP, Volpe SL, Mao JJ. Therapeutic uses of magnesium. Am Fam Physician. 2009;80(2):157–162.

126. Efstratiadis G, Sarigianni M, Gougourelas I. Hypomagnesemia and cardiovascular system. Hippokratia. 2006;10(4):147–152.

127. Xiong J, He T, Wang M, et al. Serum magnesium, mortality, and cardiovascular disease in chronic kidney disease and end-stage renal disease patients: a systematic review and meta-analysis. J. Nephrol. 2019;32(5):791–802.

128. Mehrizi M, Fontem RF, Gearhart TR, et al. Medications and Myasthenia Gravis (A Reference for Health Care Professionals). Department of Neurology, Indiana University School of Medicine, USA. 2012.

129. Singh P, Idowu O, Malik I, et al. Acute respiratory failure induced by magnesium replacement in a 62-year-old woman with myasthenia gravis. Tex Heart Inst J. 2015;42(5):495–7.

130. Grissinger M. Avoiding patient harm from a magnesium bolus dose. P T. 2014;39(2):81–129.

13 | Potassium Chloride and Potassium Phosphate

Potassium chloride and potassium phosphate are essential potassium salts used in clinical practice, with potassium chloride being the more common choice and is widely used for correcting hypokalemia. In contrast, potassium phosphate is less frequently administered and primarily used to manage or prevent hypophosphatemia.

INJECTION POTASSIUM CHLORIDE

Composition

Injection 15% Potassium Chloride
Each ml contains:
   2.0 mEq Potassium
   150 mg Potassium Chloride
   Osmolarity 4024 mOsmol/L (calc)
   pH 6.0 (4.0 to 8.0)
Available as 10 ml ampules which provides:
   20.0 mEq Potassium
   1.5 gm Potassium Chloride

Pharmacological basis

Potassium is distributed chiefly intracellularly with concentrations of 140 to 150 mEq/L and is the most abundant intracellular cation. The normal range for serum potassium is 3.5–5.0 mEq/L, and its presence in extracellular fluid (ECF) is very important for the regulation of nerve conduction and contraction of muscles, particularly in the heart.

The ability of kidneys to retain potassium is incomplete (unlike sodium). Therefore, potassium loss from the body continues in patients on a potassium-free diet and even in hypokalemia. So, potassium supplementation is required in the patient on maintenance fluid therapy to avoid hypokalemia.

Moreover, in many conditions where sodium and potassium both are lost (i.e., diarrhea, vomiting, diuretic therapy, etc.), under the influence of increased aldosterone, sodium is retained, and the potassium is lost by the kidney, which causes or aggravates hypokalemia. So adequate potassium supplementation is necessary along with the administration of sodium.

Indications

A. **Prevention of hypokalemia:** Potassium chloride is added to various intravenous (IV) fluids to prevent potassium deficiency in the patient on maintenance fluid therapy. The normal requirement of potassium in an adult is 1 mEq/kg/day (about 60 mEq/day) [1].

B. **Correction of hypokalemia:** Potassium chloride is useful in treatment of hypokalemia caused by abnormal potassium losses or deficit, such as diuretic therapy, vomiting, diarrhea, diabetic ketoacidosis, corticosteroid therapy, or in the treatment of digoxin toxicity, is necessary when oral potassium replacement is inadequate or not feasible.

C. **Addition to peritoneal dialysis fluid:** Potassium chloride is added to peritoneal dialysis fluid to customize or modify its potassium concentration.

D. **To induce cardioplegia:** During cardiac bypass surgery, concentrated potassium chloride is used to achieve cardiac standstill after the heart-lung bypass is prepared.

Adverse effects

Infusion of higher concentrations of potassium chloride solutions into a peripheral vein can cause local pain, phlebitis, or venous thrombosis. In addition, improper use of injection potassium chloride can cause hyperkalemia, which if severe can cause serious cardiac arrhythmia and can be life-threatening.

Contraindications

A. **Unknown potassium status:** Do not use injection potassium chloride without knowing potassium status.

B. **Kidney failure:** Cautious use of potassium chloride in renal failure because hyperkalemia is a potential risk.

C. **High risk for hyperkalemia:** Cautious use of potassium chloride is advised in conditions associated with a high risk of hyperkalemia, such as oliguria, severe adrenal insufficiency, crush syndrome, severe burns, severe hemolytic reactions, and concomitant use of ACEI, ARB, or potassium-sparing diuretic therapy.

Administration

General guidelines for replacement:

- Never administer an undiluted injection of potassium chloride as a direct intravenous push, as it may cause instant death. Always use it after dilution in the infusion [2].

- To prepare potassium infusion, add potassium chloride to saline rather than a dextrose solution because dextrose administration stimulates insulin release, leading to a transient reduction in the plasma potassium concentration and aggravating hypokalemia.

- Usually, the maximum concentration of injection potassium chloride is 40 mEq in 1L of solution.

- Every 10 mEq of IV potassium chloride replacement will roughly increase serum levels by about 0.1 mEq/L [3].

- When the peripheral vein is used to administer IV potassium infusion, the recommended maximum rate is 10 mEq/hour, and the maximum concentration is 40 mEq/L. The central line is essential for administering potassium at a faster rate or greater concentration.

- In patients with serum potassium >2.5 mEq/L, the maximum infusion rate should not normally exceed 10 mEq/hour, and the total dose should not exceed 200 mEq/day [4].

- In patients with symptomatic and severe (serum potassium <2.5 mEq/L) hypokalemia, the maximum rate of potassium infusion of up to 20 mEq/hour with continuous electrocardiogram (ECG) monitoring is safe [5].

- In critically ill patients with life-threatening severe hypokalemia (serum potassium <2.0 mEq/L), potassium can be infused very cautiously at a rate of up to 40 mEq/hour for the initial urgent correction (via the central line under close, continuous ECG monitoring and frequent lab assessment) [6–8].

- Ensure thorough mixing (by fully inverting the bag at least 10 times) while adding potassium chloride to intravenous solutions [2]. Potassium chloride solution is 'heavier', so it may settle in the bottom of the infusion bag if mixed improperly. Resultant inadvertent administration of potassium bolus can cause life-threatening cardiac arrhythmia. To avoid errors, prefer ready to use glucose-free, potassium-containing premixed diluted solutions, if available [1].

- In patients with impaired renal function, the dose of potassium should be ≤50% of the initial empirical dose [9].

- As hypokalemia is usually associated with hypomagnesemia, co-administrating of magnesium with potassium infusion is beneficial [10]. Hypomagnesemia, by promoting urinary potassium losses, can lead to refractory hypokalemia.

- Always label the potassium-containing solution carefully and clearly to avoid errors in administration.

INJECTION POTASSIUM PHOSPHATE

Potassium phosphates injection is commonly used as a rich source of phosphorus to treat hypophosphatemia, especially when it is associated with hypokalemia.

Composition

Injection Potassium Phosphates
Each ml contains:
    3 mmol Phosphate
    4.4 mEq Potassium
    224 mg of Monobasic Potassium Phosphate (KH_2PO_4)
    236 mg of Dibasic Potassium Phosphate (K_2HPO_4)
    Osmolarity 7400 mOsm/L

Available as 5 ml ampules which provides:
    15.0 mmol Phosphate
    22.0 mEq Potassium

Available as 15 ml ampules which provides:
    45.0 mmol Phosphate
    66.0 mEq Potassium

Available as 50 ml pharmacy bulk package vial which provides:
    150.0 mmol Phosphate
    220.0 mEq Potassium

Pharmacological basis

Phosphorus plays an important role in nearly all metabolic reactions as a constituent of nucleic acids, proteins, and some vitamins. Symptoms in hypophosphatemia are due to intracellular phosphate deficiency and resultant impaired energy production, protein synthesis, cell signaling, pH regulation, and a variety of other biological functions.

As severe hypophosphatemia frequently occurs in critically ill patients and is associated with increased risk of arrhythmia, skeletal muscle weakness, respiratory muscle dysfunction with resultant failure to wean from ventilation, longer ICU stay, and significant morbidity as well as mortality [11, 12], phosphate replacement is essential.

When hypophosphatemia is associated with hypokalemia, potassium phosphates are preferred due to their high potassium concentration, providing 4.4 mEq of potassium in each ml along with 3 mmol of phosphate.

Potassium phosphates solution should be diluted before use because it is extremely hypertonic, with an osmolality of 7400 mOsm/L. The osmolality of commonly used fluids, like 5% dextrose, Ringer's lactate, and normal saline, is much lower, with values of 252 mOsm/L, 273 mOsm/L, and 308 mOsm/L, respectively, which highlights the high hypertonicity of potassium phosphates solution.

Indications

A. **Hypophosphatemia:** Intravenous potassium phosphates injection supplementation is necessary for patients with severe hypophosphatemia (serum phosphate <1 mg/dL or 0.32 mmol/L), symptomatic patients with moderate hypophosphatemia, and other degrees of hypophosphatemia when oral or enteral intake is not possible, restricted, or contraindicated.

B. **Hypokalemia with hypophosphatemia:** Due to its high potassium content, potassium phosphates solution offers an advantage in hypophosphatemic patients with hypokalemia, such as those with diabetic ketoacidosis, refeeding syndrome, or chronic alcoholism. The potassium concentration in potassium phosphates solution (4.4 mEq/mL) is more than twice that of 15% potassium chloride solution (2.0 mEq/mL).

C. **Hypernatremia with hypophosphatemia:** In hypernatremic patients with hypophosphatemia, administration of sodium-free potassium phosphates is preferred over sodium phosphates solution.

D. **Parenteral nutrition (PN):** Intravenous potassium phosphates injection is used in the prevention of hypophosphatemia in patients receiving parenteral nutrition. In adult patients on PN, the approximate dose of phosphorus required is 20–40 mmol/day [13] or 10–15 mmol/L of PN solution to maintain normal serum phosphorus levels [14].

Adverse effects

IV phosphate administration has many potential side effects:

- Cardiovascular: Hypotension, cardiac arrhythmia, heart block, and cardiac arrest.

- Endocrine and metabolic: Hypocalcemia, hypomagnesemia, hyperkalemia, hyperphosphatemia.

- Neurological: Tingling, numbness, tremor, tetany, and seizures.

- Pulmonary: Embolism due to pulmonary vascular precipitates containing calcium phosphate complexes.

- Renal: Nephrocalcinosis due to calcium phosphate precipitates causing acute kidney injury.

- Local: Infusion into a peripheral vein can cause local pain, phlebitis, or venous thrombosis.

- Aluminum toxicity: As concentrated potassium phosphate contains aluminum, its prolonged use in patients with renal failure may cause aluminum toxicity.

Precautions and contraindications

As IV phosphate replacement may carry different side effects, it should be used cautiously:

- Avoid bolus: Do not infuse undiluted or rapid infusion of intravenous phosphate, as it can cause hyperkalemia, hypocalcemia, hypotension, arrhythmias, and cardiac arrest.

- Check serum potassium: Avoid or use IV phosphate cautiously if serum potassium is 4 mEq/dL or more because it is a potassium-rich solution (1 ml provides 4.4 mEq potassium). Use it cautiously in conditions carrying the risk of hyperkalemia (oliguria, severe adrenal insufficiency, extensive tissue breakdown {e.g., severe burns}, and concomitant use of ACEI, ARB, or potassium-sparing diuretic therapy).

- Attention to concomitant potassium content: It is important to remember that the administration of each 1 mmol of phosphate concomitantly provides 1.5 mEq of potassium, which needs to be calculated and considered in the total electrolytes infused.

- Renal insufficiency: Because of the risk of developing hyperphosphatemia and hyperkalemia, avoid it, or use it cautiously by reducing the dose of phosphate by 50%.

- Hypercalcemia: The binding of high phosphorous with high calcium may precipitate calcium-phosphate products in tissues (calciphylaxis).

- Significant hypocalcemia: Rapid infusion of phosphate may worsen pre-existing hypocalcemia causing acute severe life-threatening hypocalcemia with tetany and seizures [15]. So, check serum calcium concentration, and if low, normalize it before phosphate administration.

- Do not co-administer parenteral nutrition or IV fluids containing magnesium or calcium.

- Avoid venous damage and thrombosis: Use phosphate infusion after proper dilution or use the central line for administering concentrated or hypertonic solutions.

Administration

General guidelines for replacement:

Watch before you start: Check serum potassium, calcium, phosphate magnesium, and creatinine before administration of injection potassium phosphate to exclude hyperkalemia, hypocalcemia, hypomagnesemia, and renal failure. Calculate Ca × PO$_4$ product and If the product is greater than 60 mg/dL, avoid infusing phosphate as it carries the risk of precipitation of calcium phosphate in tissues.

Write a one-time order: Such planning for IV phosphate replacement helps to avoid potential side effects. After re-evaluation, subsequent orders are determined. Severely hypophosphatemic patients may need several doses. The prescription should clearly specify the dose of phosphate, type, and volume of diluent solution, route of infusion, and rate of administration.

Dilution: Potassium phosphates solution is hypertonic (osmolality 7400 mOsm/L) and potassium-rich (potassium concentration is 4.4 mEq/mL, which is double as compared to 2 mEq/mL in potassium chloride solution). So, this "high-alert" medication must be diluted in a sufficient volume of diluent (i.e., 100 to 500 mL of 5% dextrose or 0.9% sodium chloride), mixed thoroughly,

Table 13.1 Guidelines for IV phosphate therapy for hypophosphatemia				
Dose	**Serum phosphate concentration**		**Initial infusion**	
	mg/dL	**mmol/L**	**Clark et al [18]**	**Brown et al [19]**
Low	2.3 to 3.0	0.73 to 0.96	0.16 mmol/kg	0.32 mmol/kg
Intermediate	1.6 to 2.2	0.51 to 0.72	0.32 mmol/kg	0.64 mmol/kg
High	<1.6	<0.50	0.64 mmol/kg	1.0 mmol/kg

- Infuse potassium phosphate if serum potassium is <4 mEq/L. If serum potassium is >4 mEq/L, replace potassium phosphate by sodium phosphate.
- Administration of IV potassium phosphorus slowly at 7.5 mmol/hour is definitely safe. 1 ml contains 3.0 mmol phosphorus and 4.4 mEq potassium.
- As a part of parenteral nutrition, the dose of phosphate should not exceed 15 mmol/L.
- Discontinue phosphate replacement when the patient is asymptomatic and serum phosphate >2 mg/dL unless there is persistent loss or intake failure.

and should be administered IV slowly to avoid serious adverse effects. Do not use calcium-containing Ringer's lactate solution to dilute potassium phosphates because it causes calcium-phosphate precipitation.

Peripheral vs. central venous access: As the osmolarity of potassium phosphates is extremely high (7400 mOsm/L), the appropriate route of infusion is essential to avoid local irritation and damage.

For peripheral infusion, the maximum rate of administration is about 6.4 mmol phosphate per hour (10 mEq potassium/hour). The addition of 10 ml of potassium phosphates in 500 mL of diluent will provide 6 mmol phosphates and 8.8 mEq potassium per 100 mL of solution and this diluted solution is safe for peripheral administration.

Use central venous access when the required concentration and rate of administration are higher (i.e., 15 mmol per hour phosphate, which contains 22 mEq potassium). The addition of 30 ml of potassium phosphates in 500 mL of diluent (or 6 ml in 100 mL of diluent) will provide 18 mmol phosphates and 26.4 mEq potassium per 100 mL. The

resultant concentrated solution is suitable for central administration.

Dose and rate of administration: To avoid confusion and errors in prescribing the requirements of phosphate, the standard recommendation is to specify the dose of phosphate in millimoles (mmol) and the amount of potassium will be in mEq (i.e., administer 1 ml potassium phosphate to provide 3 mmol phosphates and 4.4 mEq potassium).

Currently, no agreement or guidelines exist, and different dosage regimens of phosphate are proposed in the literature based on the severity of the hypophosphatemia and the patient's weight (Table 13.1) [11, 16, 17].

Simple recommendations for phosphate administration in hypophosphatemia are:

- Serum phosphate 1.25 mg/dL (0.40 mmol/L) or more: Administer phosphate at the rate 0.08 to 0.24 mmol/kg over six hours (up to 30 mmol maximum total dose) [20].
- Serum phosphate 1.25 mg/dL (0.40 mmol/L) or less: Administer phosphate at the rate 0.25 to 0.50 mmol/kg over 8 to 12 hours (up to 80 mmol maximum total dose) [20].

- In symptomatic patients with severe hypophosphatemia (i.e., serum phosphate <1.5 mg/dL/0.48 mmol/kg), administer phosphate at a rate of up to 15 mmol/hour [21].

Monitoring: Serum phosphate and calcium concentration should be monitored every 6 to 12 hours, and serum sodium, potassium, magnesium, and creatinine should be monitored every 12 to 24 hours during therapy. ECG monitoring is recommended for infusions of >6.4 mmol phosphates (potassium >10 mEq) per hour.

REFERENCES

1. Intravenous fluid therapy in adults in hospital. London: National Institute for Health and Care Excellence, 2013 (https://www.nice.org.uk/guidance/cg174).

2. Gray A, Wright J, Goodey V, et al. Injectable drugs guide. London. Pharmaceutical Press; 2011:699–702.

3. Aboujamous H, Walton t, Doran JJ. Evaluation of the change in serum potassium levels after potassium administration. J Clin Nephrol Ren Care 2016;2:013.

4. Potassium Chloride Dosage by Drugs.com. Last updated on Aug 9, 2023. Available at: https://www.drugs.com/dosage/potassium-chloride.html Accessed on 12 January 2024.

5. Clase CM, Carrero JJ, Ellison DH, et al. Potassium homeostasis and management of dyskalemia in kidney diseases: conclusions from a Kidney Disease: Improving Global Outcomes (KDIGO) Controversies Conference. Kidney Int. 2020;97(1):42–61.

6. Hamill RJ, Robinson LM, Wexler HR, et al. Efficacy and safety of potassium infusion therapy in hypokalemic critically ill patients. Crit Care Med. 1991;19(5):694–699.

7. Du Y, Mou Y, Liu J. Efficiency evaluation and safety monitoring of tailored rapid potassium supplementation strategy for fatal severe hypokalemia. Exp Ther Med. 2019;17(4):3222–323.

8. Mount DB, Sterns RH, Emmett M. Clinical manifestations and treatment of hypokalaemia in adults. In: Post TW, editor. UpToDate. Waltham, MA: Wolters Kluwer Health. http://www.uptodate.com. Accessed 31 Aug 2020.

9. Kraft MD, Btaiche IF, Sacks GS, et al. Treatment of electrolyte disorders in adult patients in the intensive care unit. Am J Health Syst Pharm. 2005;62(16):1663–1682.

10. Huang CL, Kuo E. Mechanism of hypokalemia in magnesium deficiency. J Am Soc Nephrol. 2007;18(10):2649–2652.

11. Geerse DA, Bindels AJ, Kuiper MA, et al. Treatment of hypophosphatemia in the intensive care unit: a review. Crit Care 2010;14(4):R147.

12. Zhao Y, Zhihai LI, Shi Y, et al. Effect of hypophosphatemia on the withdrawal of mechanical ventilation in patients with acute exacerbations of chronic obstructive pulmonary disease. Biomedical Reports. 2016;4(4):413–6.

13. Mirtallo J, Canada T, Johnson D, et al, "Safe Practices for Parenteral Nutrition," JPEN J Parenter Enteral Nutr, 2004;28(6):S39–70.

14. Hicks W, Hardy G. Phosphate supplementation for hypophosphatemia and parenteral nutrition. CurrOpin Clin NutrMetab Care 2001;4(3):227–33.

15. Imel EA, Econs MJ. Approach to the hypophosphatemic patient. J Clin Endocrinol Metab. 2012;97(3):696–706.

16. Basri MN, Janattul AJ, Azrina MR, et al. Hypophosphatemia in the intensive care unit: incidence, predictors and management. IMJM 2012;11(1):31–36.

17. Geerse DA, Bindels AJ, Kuiper MA, et al. Approach to hypophosphataemia in intensive care units - a nationwide survey. Neth J Med. 2012;70(9):425–430.

18. Clark CL, Sacks GS, Dickerson RN, et al. Treatment of hypophosphatemia in patients receiving specialized nutrition support using a graduated dosing scheme: results from a prospective clinical trial. Crit Care Med. 1995;23(9):1504–10.

19. Brown KA, Dickerson RN, Morgan LM, et al. A new graduated dosing regimen for phosphorus replacement in patients receiving nutrition support. JPEN J Parenter Enteral Nutr 2006;30(3):209–14.

20. Yu ASL, Stubbs JR, Goldfarb S. Hypophosphatemia: Evaluation and treatment. In: Post TW, editor. UpToDate. Waltham, MA: Wolters Kluwer Health. http://www.uptodate.com. Accessed 12 Sept 2020.

21. Charron T, Bernard F, Skrobik Y, et al, Intravenous phosphate in the intensive care unit: more aggressive repletion regimens for moderate and severe hypophosphatemia. Intensive Care Med, 2003;29(8):1273–8.

14 | Sodium Bicarbonate

COMPOSITION

Injection 8.4% Sodium Bicarbonate

Each ml contains:
   1 mEq or 1 mmol of Sodium
   1 mEq or 1 mmol of Bicarbonate
   23.0 mg of Sodium and 61.0 mg of Bicarbonate
   84 mg Sodium Bicarbonate
   Osmolarity 2000 mOsmol/L

Injection 7.5% Sodium Bicarbonate

Each ml contains:
   0.89 mEq or 0.89 mmol of Sodium
   75 mg Sodium Bicarbonate
   Osmolarity 1786 mOsmol/L

Injection 4.2% Sodium Bicarbonate

Each ml contains:
   0.5 mEq or 0.5 mmol of Sodium
   0.5 mEq or 0.5 mmol of Bicarbonate
   42 mg Sodium Bicarbonate
   Osmolarity 1000 mOsmol/L

Electrolyte contents and osmolality of different strengths and volumes of solutions are summarized in Table 14.1. Every 10 ml of 4.2%, 7.5%, and 8.4% of sodium bicarbonate ($NaHCO_3$) solutions contain about 5 mEq, 9 mEq, and 10 mEq of bicarbonate as well as sodium, respectively.

Table 14.1 Sodium bicarbonate solutions: different strengths and composition									
Strength	4.2% NaHCO$_3$		7.5% NaHCO$_3$				8.4% NaHCO$_3$		
Volume (mL)	1.0	500	1.0	10	25	50	1.0	10	25	50
Sodium (mEq)	0.5	250	0.89	8.9	22.5	44.5	1.0	10	25	50
Bicarbonate (mEq)	0.5	250	0.89	8.9	22.5	44.5	1.0	10	25	50
Osmolality	1000 mOsm/L		1786 mOsm/L				2000 mOsm/L		

PHARMACOLOGICAL BASIS

The administration of sodium bicarbonate intravenously dissociates in the body to form sodium and bicarbonate. Bicarbonate anions act as a buffer and correct metabolic acidosis by combining with hydrogen ions ($HCO_3 + H^+ = H_2CO_3^-$ carbonic acid). In addition, by increasing pH and shifting potassium intracellularly, bicarbonate corrects hyperkalemia.

Bicarbonate is excreted readily in the urine in patients with normal renal function. An increase in plasma bicarbonate leads to greater urinary loss of bicarbonate and the resultant increase in urinary pH.

Because of the beneficial alkalinizing effect of intravenous (IV) sodium bicarbonate, this solution is useful in treating salicylate toxicity, phenobarbitone toxicity, tumor lysis syndrome, and rhabdomyolysis.

INDICATIONS

A. Metabolic acidosis

Sodium bicarbonate is used routinely in clinical practice to manage metabolic acidosis. However, the role of sodium bicarbonate in acute metabolic acidosis is controversial [1, 2], and bicarbonate therapy should be used selectively and not routinely in such patients [2].

Common indications of bicarbonate therapy in metabolic acidosis are:

- Normal anion gap (hyperchloremic) metabolic acidosis having pH <7.2 [1] or serum HCO_3 below 16–18 mEq/L [3]. As the loss of large quantities of bicarbonate is the most common cause of hyperchloremic metabolic acidosis, the replacement of bicarbonate is beneficial and hastens recovery [4, 5].

- Lactic acidosis: In lactic acidosis, the role of bicarbonate therapy is

controversial and is generally used only in life-threatening severe metabolic acidosis (pH<7.1) [6–9]. The 2021 Surviving Sepsis Campaign Guidelines discourage the use of sodium bicarbonate therapy to improve hemodynamics or reduce vasopressor requirements in adults with septic shock and hypoperfusion-induced lactic acidemia [9].

- In lactic acidosis, bicarbonate therapy is selectively administered with the goal of partial correction and is not recommended as a routine treatment due to the following reasons:

    1. Bicarbonate therapy can be harmful: Potential complications associated with bicarbonate therapy in lactic acidosis patients include the development of hypernatremia, extracellular fluid volume expansion, increased lactate production, elevation of $PaCO_2$ leading to paradoxical intracellular acidosis, central nervous system (CNS) acidosis, hypokalemia, hypocalcemia, and the potential for overshoot or rebound alkalosis [10].

    2. Mild to moderate lactic acidosis may have advantages and may not be harmful: A growing body of evidence suggests that avoiding bicarbonate therapy is a prudent approach for cases of mild to moderate acidosis [1, 2, 11, 12].

    3. Lack of evidence supporting its benefits: Currently, there is insufficient evidence to demonstrate the advantages of using bicarbonate in the treatment of metabolic lactic acidosis [13–17].

- Lactic acidosis with acute kidney injury (AKI): In lactic acidosis, even with less severe metabolic acidosis (pH≤7.2), bicarbonate therapy is recommended in patients with severe acute kidney injury [18–21]. Bicarbonate therapy is beneficial in this subgroup of patients with lactic acidosis and severe acute kidney injury and reduces 28-day mortality and the need for dialysis [18, 19, 22].

- Diabetic ketoacidosis (DKA): In DKA, bicarbonate's role is controversial and is rarely indicated. Bicarbonate therapy is used very selectively in patients with extremely severe acidosis with arterial pH less than 6.9 (recommendation by the American Diabetes Association) [23]. In recent literature, the role of bicarbonate in DKA has been discouraged [20, 24, 25].

B. Hyperkalemia

For the acute management of hyperkalemia, sodium bicarbonate is not recommended routinely, as a first-line therapy, or as a single agent [26–28].

In metabolic acidosis, bicarbonate therapy by increasing the pH shifts potassium into cells and thereby corrects hyperkalemia [29]. The administration of sodium bicarbonate is recommended selectively in severely hyperkalemic patients (serum potassium >6 mEq/L) having metabolic acidosis (pH<7.35, bicarbonate levels <17 mEq/L) [30], with intact renal function [31, 32], and either intravascular volume depletion or normal intravascular volume. Bicarbonate therapy is ineffective in patients without significant metabolic acidosis and in advanced chronic kidney disease (CKD) or stable hemodialysis patients [30, 31, 33–35].

Bicarbonate infusion vs. bolus: In hyperkalemia with metabolic acidosis, administration of bicarbonate is recommended as an isotonic infusion (e.g., 150 mEq in 1 L of 5% dextrose IV slowly over two to four hours), rather than a bolus form [33].

The assessment of volume status and sodium concentration is essential before administering sodium-rich bicarbonate infusion, as every 100 ml of 7.5% and 8.4% sodium bicarbonate solutions contains approximately 90 mEq and 100 mEq of sodium, respectively [36]. Isotonic bicarbonate infusion is an effective treatment modality in hyperkalemia with metabolic acidosis who can tolerate or require sodium fluid loading (i.e., having contracted intravascular volume), but not suitable or recommended in patients with the risk of volume overload (i.e., having heart failure or CKD) as it requires administration of a large volume of sodium-rich fluid [37].

Bicarbonate bolus: When 7.5% or 8.4% bicarbonate is administered as a bolus, it has a neutral effect on the potassium level due to its two opposite effects on the concentration of potassium [38]:

- By increasing the pH, bicarbonate shifts potassium intracellularly and reduces the serum potassium level.

- Hypertonic bicarbonate pulls water out of cells which also pulls out potassium along with it, causing an increase in the serum potassium level.

C. Cardiac arrest

Administration of bicarbonate is not recommended routinely for resuscitation in cardiac arrest [39] because of a lack of benefit evidence and potentially detrimental effects [17, 40–42]. However, bicarbonate may be reserved for resuscitation in patients with cardiac arrest having hyperkalemia, tricyclic antidepressant toxicity, preexisting severe metabolic acidosis (pH <7.1), or patients with prolonged (>10–20 min) cardiac arrest [39, 43].

The recommended initial dose of bicarbonate is 1 mEq/kg, with repeat administration based on arterial blood gas measurements. Bicarbonate should be administered in cardiac arrest only after cardiac compression, intubation, and adequate ventilation.

D. Tricyclic antidepressant (TCA) overdose

Sodium bicarbonate is an effective antidote and the cornerstone of treating tricyclic antidepressant poisoning [44–46]. Patients with tricyclic antidepressant poisoning are treated with sodium bicarbonate in the presence of hemodynamic instability, seizures, QRS prolongation (>100 msec), or ventricular arrhythmia.

Proposed mechanisms of benefit of sodium bicarbonate are [46–49]:

1. The increase in serum pH increases the protein binding of TCAs, which may reduce the concentration of biologically active free TCA, which may cause TCA toxicity.

2. Sodium rich bicarbonate increases the extracellular sodium concentration and thereby counteracts the TCA-induced blockade of rapid sodium channels. In TCA poisoning, QRS prolongation occurs due to TCA induced inhibition of the fast sodium channels and the resultant decrease in conduction velocity.

Initially, 1–2 mEq/kg bicarbonate is administered as a bolus, followed by an intravenous infusion containing 100–150 mEq sodium bicarbonate in 1000 ml of D5W.

The dose of bicarbonate is adjusted by monitoring improvement in hypotension and narrowing of widened QRS complexes on electrocardiogram (ECG). Also, monitor pH, serum sodium, potassium, and bicarbonate level during therapy [50].

The goal of this therapy is to achieve narrowing of the QRS complex (<100ms) and to maintain the serum pH between 7.5 and 7.55 and serum sodium 150–155 mEq/L [51].

E. Prevention of contrast-induced acute kidney injury

To prevent contrast-induced AKI (CI-AKI), the use of volume expansion with sodium bicarbonate solutions was recommended by the 2012 KDIGO guideline [52], various studies [53–55], and meta-analysis [56–58].

An isotonic sodium bicarbonate infusion consisting of 154 mL of 8.4% $NaHCO_3$ in 1000 mL of 5% Dextrose is administered at a rate of 3 mL/kg/h for 1 hour before the procedure and at a rate of 1 mL/kg/h for 6 hours after the procedure [53]. By making urine alkaline, sodium bicarbonate reduces the formation of contrast-induced injurious free radical formation and peroxide injury [59].

However, in a recent large trial (PRESERVE group 2018) and literature, for the volume expansion to prevent CI-AKI, the use of bicarbonate and saline demonstrated similar outcomes, and bicarbonate provides no additional benefit to saline [60–62]. So, the current literature recommends using both isotonic sodium bicarbonate and 0.9% sodium chloride for intravenous volume expansion in high-risk patients [63, 64]. But normal saline is preferred over bicarbonate solution because bicarbonate solution need pharmacist compounding, is more expensive, and does not have an additional benefit over saline [65, 66].

F. Urinary alkalinization

Administration of intravenous sodium bicarbonate to produce alkaline urine (pH≥7.5) is useful to increases the elimination of certain drug overdoses and toxic substances. The use of the term urine alkalinization emphasizes that in this therapy, manipulation of urine pH is important rather than a diuresis, and therefore has replaced the previously used terms like forced alkaline diuresis and alkaline dieresis [67].

1. Barbiturates poisoning

Urine alkalinization is used in barbiturate poisoning but is not a first-line treatment because of its low efficiency, and this therapy is effective only in long-acting barbiturates such as Phenobarbital [67–70].

2. Salicylate poisoning

Administration of bicarbonate is the mainstay and the first-line therapy in salicylate (aspirin) poisoning [49, 71, 72]. Bicarbonate by alkalinization of urine increases the renal excretion of salicylate substantially, and alkalinizing the plasma reduces the amount of circulating lipid-soluble salicylate [67, 73]. As lipid-soluble salicylate easily penetrates the blood-brain barrier, its reduction decreases the diffusion of salicylate anions into the central nervous system and the resultant neurotoxicity [49].

Indications: Administration of bicarbonate is indicated for alkalinization in all symptomatic patients of salicylate poisoning and salicylate level >40 mg/dL (>2.9 mM). Bicarbonate may be beneficial even in respiratory alkalosis (pH up to 7.55) to achieve urinary alkalinization.

Administration: An initial bolus of 1 mEq/kg of hypertonic sodium bicarbonate (8.4% $NaHCO_3$ provides 1 mEq/ml bicarbonate), followed by a 2 to 3 mL/kg per hour continuous infusion of isotonic bicarbonate solution (150 ml of 7.5% or 8.4% sodium bicarbonate added to 1 liter of D5W) is recommended for alkalinizing the urine [73]. The infusion rate is titrated to maintain a serum pH of 7.5–7.55 and urine pH of ≥7.5.

Risk of hypokalemia: As alkaline diuresis can cause hypokalemia, replace potassium aggressively by adding 40 mEq of potassium chloride (KCl)/L of IV infusion to prevent hypokalemia and to maintain serum potassium around 4.0–4.5 mEq/L (after ensuring adequate urine output and normal kidney function).

Discontinue bicarbonate therapy when salicylate levels fall below toxic levels (<40 mg/dL or <2.9 mM) and the patient is asymptomatic with a normal respiratory rate.

3. Tumor lysis syndrome

In the past, alkalinization of urine was recommended in tumor lysis syndrome due to the possibility that it makes uric acid more soluble and less likely to precipitate in the renal tubules.

But urinary alkalinization is currently NOT recommended in the prevention or treatment of tumor lysis syndrome [74–76] because:

- Urinary alkalinization decreases calcium–phosphate solubility and therefore promotes the precipitation of calcium phosphate in the renal tubules [77]. In patients who develop severe hyperphosphatemia due to rapid lysis of tumor cells, marked precipitation and deposition of calcium phosphate can occur in the renal tubules, heart, and other organs, which can be harmful.

- In patients treated with rasburicase, urinary alkalinization carries the risk of heavy calcium phosphate precipitation [78].

- Animal studies demonstrated that in minimizing uric acid precipitation, the administration of normal saline is as effective as alkalinization [79].

If alkalinization is needed, initiate it when hyperuricemia develops, but it should be discontinued when hyperphosphatemia develops [77].

4. Rhabdomyolysis

In patients with rhabdomyolysis, isotonic bicarbonate infusion is infused to prevent acute kidney injury when the serum creatine phosphokinase (CPK) level is above 5000 units/L, and there is severe muscle injury (e.g., crush injury) [80]. Avoid bicarbonate infusion in the presence of hypocalcemia and serum bicarbonate >30 mEq/L.

The rationale for using alkalinization is the prevention of heme-protein precipitation, which decreases the direct pigment injury, reduces myoglobin cast formation, and reduces the crystallization of uric acid [81, 82].

Besides theoretical benefits, clinical evidence that an alkaline diuresis is more effective than standard saline resuscitation in preventing AKI is lacking [83–86] and therefore is not recommended [87]. So, using alkaline diuresis in rhabdomyolysis as a single standard measure is discouraged [82]. However, it may be useful if diuresis occurs after volume repletion and in the presence of metabolic acidosis or hyperkalemia [85, 86].

ADVERSE EFFECTS AND CONTRAINDICATIONS

- **Metabolic alkalosis:** Due to the rapid alkalotic effect of sodium bicarbonate, it has the potential for worsening symptoms of alkalosis in patients with excessive Cl⁻ loss from vomiting or gastrointestinal (GI) suctioning or diuretic-induced hypochloremic alkalosis.

- **Hypernatremia:** As sodium bicarbonate is rich in sodium (89 and 100 mEq/dL in 7.5% and 8.4% of $NaHCO_3$, respectively), prolonged therapy or large volume infusion can precipitate or exacerbate hypernatremia.

- **Edematous or sodium retaining states:** As sodium bicarbonate is rich in sodium, it should be used cautiously in patients with congestive heart failure, cirrhosis, renal impairment with anasarca, oliguria, or anuria to avoid volume overload.

- **Hypocalcemia:** Bicarbonate administration carries the risk of developing alkalosis-induced tetany.

- **Respiratory acidosis:** Metabolism of bicarbonate produces carbon dioxide (CO_2) and water, so hypercapnia can worsen due to bicarbonate administration. Impaired removal of CO_2 due to hypoventilation carries the risk of respiratory acidosis.

- **Hypokalemia:** Risk of worsening of hypokalemia because administration of bicarbonate leads to alkalosis and resultant intracellular shift of potassium.

- **Avoid extravasation:** Hypertonic bicarbonate solutions carry a risk of vascular irritation, ulceration, and sloughing.

ADMINISTRATION

Precautions required during sodium bicarbonate administration are:

- Before administration of bicarbonate, exclude volume overload, hypocalce-mia, hypokalemia, alkalosis, respiratory acidosis, and ensure adequate ventilation and perfusion.

- To minimize venous irritation due to $NaHCO_3$, it is crucial to establish a large intravenous line for infusion.

- Avoid IV bolus of $NaHCO_3$, except in an emergency.

- Never treat just acidosis; treat its etiology simultaneously.

- Avoid $NaHCO_3$ administration if ventilation is inadequate, as it carries the risk of hypercapnia.

- Correct hypokalemia before correcting acidosis, as intracellular K^+ shifting can cause life-threatening hypokalemia.

- $NaHCO_3$ should be given with caution in circulatory overload.

- Avoid mixing calcium with $NaHCO_3$ to avoid precipitation.

- Avoid mixing $NaHCO_3$ with inotropes.

Isotonic bicarbonate infusion: When 150 mEq bicarbonate (150 ml of 8.4% sodium bicarbonate) is added to one liter of D5W, it becomes a 1.26% sodium bicarbonate solution. In the bag, it is hypertonic (552 mOsmol/L), but once infused, it becomes isotonic (300 mOsmol/L) in the body as dextrose is consumed rapidly [88].

Isotonic bicarbonate solution contains 150 mEq of sodium per liter and therefore does not cause hypernatremia. But the major limitation is the requirement of a large volume of fluid to raise bicarbonate. In a patient with severe hypovolemia and metabolic acidosis, the administration of isotonic bicarbonate will effectively provide both fluid volume and bicarbonate and can be administered at similar rates to other crystalloid solutions [88].

To prepare bicarbonate infusion, do not add 8.4% sodium bicarbonate

to normal saline because the resultant solution will be hypertonic (when 150 ml of 8.4% sodium bicarbonate is added to one liter of normal saline, the osmolarity of the resulting solution will be 608 mOsmol/L).

REFERENCES

1. Kraut JA, Madias NE. Treatment of acute metabolic acidosis: a pathophysiologic approach. Nat Rev Nephrol. 2012;8(10):589–601.

2. Forni LG, Hodgson LE, Se lby NM. The Janus faces of bicarbonate therapy in the ICU: not sure! Intensive Care Med. 2020;46(3):522–524.

3. Farkas J. Non-anion-gap metabolic acidosis (NAGMA) PulmCrit September 19, 2019 https://emcrit.org/ibcc/nagma/#treatment.

4. Sabatini S, Kurtzman NA. Bicarbonate therapy in severe metabolic acidosis. J. Am. Soc. Nephrol. 2009;20(4):692–695.

5. Adeva-Andany MM, Fernández-Fernández C, Mouriño-Bayolo D, et al. Sodium bicarbonate therapy in patients with metabolic acidosis. Scientific World Journal. 2014;2014:627673.

6. Boyd JH, Walley KR. Is there a role for sodium bicarbonate in treating lactic acidosis from shock? Curr Opin Crit Care. 2008;14(4):379–83.

7. Velissaris D, Karamouzos V, Ktenopoulos N, et al. The use of sodium bicarbonate in the treatment of acidosis in sepsis: a literature update on a long term debate. Crit Care Res Pract. 2015;2015:605830.

8. Ghauri S, Javaeed A, Mustafa K, et al. Bicarbonate therapy for critically ill patients with metabolic acidosis: a systematic review. Cureus 2019;11(3):e4297.

9. Achanti A, Szerlip HM. Acid-Base Disorders in the Critically Ill Patient. Clin J Am Soc Nephrol. 2023;18(1):102–112.

10. Rudnick MR, Blair GJ, Kuschner WG, et al. Lactic Acidosis and the Role of Sodium Bicarbonate: A Narrative Opinion. Shock. 2020;53(5):528–536.

11. Kimmoun A, Novy E, Auchet T, et al. Hemodynamic consequences of severe lactic acidosis in shock states: from bench to bedside. Crit Care. 2015;19(1):175.

12. Gehlbach BK, Schmidt GA. Bench-to-bedside review: treating acid-base abnormalities in the intensive care unit - the role of buffers. Crit Care. 2004;8(4):259–265.

13. Cooper DJ, Walley KR, Wiggs BR, et al. Bicarbonate does not improve hemodynamics in critically ill patients who have lactic acidosis: a prospective, controlled clinical study. Ann Intern Med 1990;112(7):492–498.

14. Mathieu D, Neviere R, Billard V, et al. Effects of bicarbonate therapy on hemodynamics and tissue oxygenation in patients with lactic acidosis: a prospective, controlled clinical study. Crit Care Med 1991;19(11):1352–1356.

15. Stacpoole PW, Wright EC, Baumgartner TG, et al. Natural history and course of acquired lactic acidosis in adults. Am J Med. 1994;97(1):47–54.

16. Kim HJ, Son YK, An WS. Effect of sodium bicarbonate administration on mortality in patients with lactic acidosis: a retrospective analysis. PLoS One 2013;8(6):e65283.

17. Ahn S, Kim YJ, Sohn CH, et al. Sodium bicarbonate on severe metabolic acidosis during prolonged cardiopulmonary resuscitation: a double-blind, randomized, placebo-controlled pilot study. J Thorac Dis. 2018;10(4):2295–2302.

18. Jaber S, Paugam C, Futier E, et al. Sodium bicarbonate therapy for patients with severe metabolic acidaemia in the intensive care unit (BICAR-ICU): a multicentre, open-label, randomised controlled, phase 3 trial. Lancet. 2018;392(10141):31–40.

19. Zhang Z, Zhu C, Mo L, et al. Effectiveness of sodium bicarbonate infusion on mortality in septic patients with metabolic acidosis. Intensive Care Med 2018;44(11):1888–1895.

20. Jung B, Martinez M, Claessens YE, et al. Diagnosis and management of metabolic acidosis: guidelines from a French expert panel. Ann Intensive Care. 2019;9(1):92.

21. Evans L, Rhodes A, Alhazzani W, et al. Surviving sepsis campaign: international guidelines for management of sepsis and septic shock 2021. Crit Care Med 2021;49(11):e1063–e1143.

22. Matyukhin I, Patschan S, Ritter O, et al. Etiology and management of acute metabolic acidosis: An Update. Kidney Blood Press Res. 2020;45(4):523–531.

23. Kitabchi AE, Umpierrez GE, Miles JM, et al. Hyperglycemic crises in adult patients with diabetes. Diabetes Care 2009;32(7):1335–43.

24. Duhon B, Attridge RL, Franco-Martinez AC, et al. Intravenous sodium bicarbonate therapy in severely acidotic diabetic ketoacidosis. Ann Pharmacother. 2013;47(7–8):970–5.

25. Patel MP, Ahmed A, Gunapalan T, et al. Use of sodium bicarbonate and blood gas monitoring in diabetic ketoacidosis: A review. World J Diabetes. 2018;9(11):199–205.

26. Alfonzo A, Soar J, MacTier R, et al. Clinical practice guidelines. Treatment of acute hyperkalaemia in adults. UK Renal Association 2014.

27. Batterink J, Cessford TA, Taylor RAI. Pharmacological interventions for the acute management of hyperkalaemia in adults. Cochrane Database of Systematic Reviews 2015;10:CD010344.

28. Bianchi S, Aucella F, De Nicola L, et al. Management of hyperkalemia in patients with kidney disease: a position paper endorsed by the Italian Society of Nephrology. J Nephrol. 2019;32(4):499–516.

29. Palmer BF. Regulation of potassium homeostasis. Clin J Am Soc Nephrol 2015;10(6):1050–1060.

30. Abuelo JG. Treatment of Severe Hyperkalemia: Confronting 4 Fallacies. Kidney Int Rep. 2017;3(1):47–55.

31. Sterns RH, Grieff M, Bernstein PL. Treatment of hyperkalemia: something old, something new. Kidney Int 2016;89(3):546–554.

32. Gibler WB, Racadio JM, Hirsch AL, et al. Hyperkalemia: Advancing care in the emergency department and intensive care unit. Proceedings monograph: EMCREG-International multidisciplinary Hyperkalemia Consensus Panel. 2018.

33. Blumberg A, Weidmann P, Shaw S, et al. Effect of various therapeutic approaches on plasma potassium and major regulating factors in terminal renal failure. Am J Med 1988;85(4):507–12.

34. Rafique Z, Chouihed T, Mebazaa A, et al. Current treatment and unmet needs of hyperkalaemia in the emergency department. Eur Heart J Suppl. 2019;21(Suppl A):A12–A19.

35. Dépret F, Peacock WF, Liu KD, et al. Management of hyperkalemia in the acutely ill patient. Ann. Intensive Care 2019;9(1):32.

36. Lindner G, Burdmann EA, Clase CM, et al. Acute hyperkalemia in the emergency department: a summary from a kidney disease: Improving Global Outcomes conference. Eur J Emerg Med. 2020;27(5):329–337.

37. Rossignol P, Legrand M, Kosiborod M, et al. Emergency management of severe hyperkalemia guidelines for best practice and opportunities for the future. Pharmacol Res. 2016;113(Pt A):585–591.

38. Farkas J. pH-guided fluid resuscitation & BICAR-ICU PulmCrit June 27, 2018. https://emcrit.org/pulmcrit/bicar-icu/.

39. Neumar RW, Otto CW, Link MS, et al. Part 8: adult advanced cardiovascular life support: 2010 American Heart Association Guidelines for Cardiopulmonary Resuscitation and Emergency Cardiovascular Care. Circulation. 2010;122(18 Suppl 3):S729–67.

40. Dybvik T, Strand T, Steen PA. Buffer therapy during out-of-hospital cardiopulmonary resuscitation. Resuscitation. 1995;29(2):89–95.

41. Vukmir RB, Katz L, Sodium Bicarbonate Study Group. Sodium bicarbonate improves outcome in prolonged prehospital cardiac arrest. Am J Emerg Med. 2006;24(2):156–61.

42. Kawano T, Grunau B, Scheuermeyer FX, et al. Prehospital sodium bicarbonate use could worsen long term survival with favorable neurological recovery among patients with out-of-hospital cardiac arrest. Resuscitation. 2017;119:63–69.

43. Velissaris D, Karamouzos V, Pierrakos C, et al. Use of sodium bicarbonate in cardiac arrest: Current Guidelines and Literature Review. J Clin Med Res. 2016;8(4):277–283.

44. Hoffman JR, Votey SR, Bayer M, et al. Effect of hypertonic sodium bicarbonate in the treatment of moderate-to-severe cyclic antidepressant overdose. Am J Emerg Med 1993;11(4):336–41.

45. Woolf AD, Erdman AR, Nelson LS, et al. Tricyclic antidepressant poisoning: an evidence-based consensus guideline for out-of-hospital management. Clin Toxicol (Phila). 2007;45(3):203–33.

46. Bruccoleri RE, Burns MM. A Literature Review of the Use of Sodium Bicarbonate for the Treatment of QRS Widening. J. Med. Toxicol. 2016;12(1):121–9.

47. Sasyniuk BI, Jhamandas V. Mechanism of reversal of toxic effects of amitriptyline on cardiac Purkinje fibers by sodium bicarbonate. J Pharmacol Exp Ther 1984;231(2):387–94.

48. Yartsev A. Tricyclic antidepressant overdose. Deranged

Physiology 12/07/2015. https://derangedphysiology. com/main/required-reading/pharmacology- and-toxicology/Chapter%2021/tricyclic- antidepressant-overdose.

49. Mirrakhimov AE, Ayach T, Barbaryan A, et al. The Role of Sodium Bicarbonate in the Management of Some Toxic Ingestions. Int J Nephrol. 2017;2017:7831358.

50. Sawhney R, McCullough PA. A commentary on treatment of tricyclic antidepressant overdose. J Clin Toxicol 2019;9(2):410.

51. Bradberry SM, Thanacoody HK, Watt BE et al. Management of the cardiovascular complications of tricyclic antidepressant poisoning: role of sodium bicarbonate. Toxicological Reviews 2005;24(3):195–204.

52. Kellum JA, Lameire N, Aspelin P, et al. Kidney Disease: Improving Global Outcomes (KDIGO) Acute Kidney Injury Work Group. KDIGO Clinical Practice Guideline for Acute Kidney Injury. Kidney Int Suppl. 2012;2(1):1–138.

53. Merten GJ, Burgess WP, Gray LV, et al. Prevention of contrast-induced nephropathy with sodium bicarbonate: a randomized controlled trial. JAMA 2004;291(19):2328–34.

54. Briguori C, Airoldi F, D'Andrea D, et al. Renal Insufficiency Following Contrast Media Administration Trial (REMEDIAL): a randomized comparison of 3 preventive strategies. Circulation 2007;115(110):1211–7.

55. Recio-Mayoral A, Chaparro M, Prado B, et al. The reno-protective effect of hydration with sodium bicarbonate plus N-acetylcysteine in patients undergoing emergency percutaneous coronary intervention: the RENO Study. J Am Coll Cardiol 2007;49(12):1283–8.

56. Navaneethan SD, Singh S, Appasamy S, et al. Sodium bicarbonate therapy for prevention of contrast-induced nephropathy: a systematic review and meta-analysis. Am J Kidney Dis. 2009;53(4):617–627.

57. Zhang B, Liang L, Chen W, et al. The efficacy of sodium bicarbonate in preventing contrast-induced nephropathy in patients with pre-existing renal insufficiency: a meta-analysis. BMJ Open. 2015;5(3):e006989.

58. Brown JR, Pearlman DM, Marshall EJ, et al. Metaanalysis of individual patient data of sodium bicarbonate and sodium chloride for all-cause mortality after coronary angiography. e Am J Cardiol. 2016;118(10):1473–1479.

59. Pisani A, Riccio E, Andreucci M, et al. Role of reactive oxygen species in pathogenesis of radiocontrast-induced nephropathy. Biomed Res Int. 2013;2013:868321.

60. Weisbord SD, Gallagher M, Jneid H, et al. Outcomes after angiography with sodium bicarbonate and acetylcysteine. N Engl J Med 2018;378:603–614.

61. Valette X, Desmeulles I, Savary B, et al. Sodium bicarbonate versus sodium chloride for preventing contrast-associated acute kidney injury in critically ill patients: a randomized controlled trial. Critical Care Medicine 2017;45(4):637–644.

62. Zapata-Chica CA, Bello Marquez D, Serna-Higuita LM, et al. Sodium bicarbonate versus isotonic saline solution to prevent contrast-induced nephropathy: a systematic review and meta-analysis. Colomb Med (Cali). 2015;46(3):90–103.

63. Acute kidney injury: prevention, detection and management. NICE guideline [NG148] 18 December 2019. https://www.nice.org.uk/guidance/ng148.

64. Patschan D, Buschmann I, Ritter O. Contrast-Induced Nephropathy: Update on the use of crystalloids and pharmacological measures. Int J Nephrol. 2018;2018:5727309.

65. Davenport MS, Perazella MA, Yee J, et al. Use of intravenous iodinated contrast media in patients with kidney disease: Consensus statements from the American College of Radiology and the National Kidney Foundation. Radiol. 2020;294(3):660–668.

66. Rudnick MR, Palevsky PM, Forman JP. Prevention of contrast-induced acute kidney injury associated with angiography. UpToDate 2020 https://www.uptodate. com/contents/prevention-of-contrast-induced-acute- kidney-injury-associated-with-angiography.

67. Proudfoot AT, Krenzelok EP, Vale JA. Position Paper on urine alkalinization. J Toxicol Clin Toxicol 2004;42(1):1–26.

68. Mawer GE, Lee HA. Value of forced diuresis in acute barbiturate poisoning. Br Med J. 1968;2(5608):790–793.

69. Roberts DM, Buckley NA. Enhanced elimination in acute barbiturate poisoning - a systematic review. Clin Toxicol (Phila). 2011;49(1):2–12.

70. Mactier R, Laliberté M, Mardini J, et al. Extracorporeal treatment for barbiturate poisoning: recommendations from the EXTRIP Workgroup. Am J Kidney Dis. 2014;64(3):347–58.

71. O'Malley GF. Emergency department management of the salicylate-poisoned patient. Emerg Med Clin North Am 2007;25(2):333–46.

72. Juurlink DN, Gosselin S, Kielstein JT, et al. Extracorporeal treatment for salicylate poisoning: systematic review and recommendations from the EXTRIP workgroup. Ann Emerg Med. 2015;66(2):165–81.

73. Palmer BF, Clegg DJ. Salicylate Toxicity N Engl J Med 2020;382(26):2544–55.

74. Coiffier B, Altman A, Pui CH, et al. Guidelines for the management of pediatric and adult tumor lysis syndrome: an evidence-based review. J Clin Oncol 2008;26(16):2767–78.

75. Wilson FP, Berns JS. Onco-nephrology: tumor lysis syndrome. Clin J Am Soc Nephrol. 2012;7(10):1730–1739.

76. Jones GL, Will A, Jackson GH, et al. British Committee for Standards in Haematology. Guidelines for the management of tumour lysis syndrome in adults and children with haematological malignancies on behalf of the British Committee for Standards in Haematology. Br J Haematol. 2015;169(5):661–71.

77. Howard SC, Jones DP, Pui C. The Tumor Lysis Syndrome. N Engl J Med 2011;364(19):1844–1854.

78. Matuszkiewicz-Rowinska J, Malyszko J. Prevention and treatment of tumor lysis syndrome in the era of onco-nephrology progress. Kidney Blood Press Res. 2020;45(5):645–660.

79. Conger JD, Falk SA. Intrarenal dynamics in the pathogenesis and prevention of acute urate nephropathy. J Clin Invest. 1977;59(5):786–93.

80. Ron D, Taitelman U, Michaelson M, et al. Prevention of acute renal failure in traumatic rhabdomyolysis. Arch Intern Med 1984;144(2):277–80.

81. Bosch X, Poch E, Grau JM. Rhabdomyolysis and acute kidney injury. N Engl J Med. 2009;361(1):62–72.

82. Somagutta MR, Pagad S, Sridharan S, et al. Role of bicarbonates and mannitol in rhabdomyolysis: a comprehensive review. Cureus 2020;12(8):e9742.

83. Homsi E, Barreiro MF, Orlando JM, et al. Prophylaxis of acute renal failure in patients with rhabdomyolysis. Ren Fail. 1997;19(2):283–8.

84. Huerta-Alardín AL, Varon J, Marik PE. Bench-to-bedside review: Rhabdomyolysis - an overview for clinicians. Crit Care 2005;9(2):158–69.

85. Scharman EJ, Troutman WG. Prevention of kidney injury following rhabdomyolysis: A systematic review. Ann Pharmacother 2013;47(1):90–105.

86. Chavez LO, Leon M, Einav S, et al. Beyond muscle destruction: a systematic review of rhabdomyolysis for clinical practice.Crit Care. 2016;20(1):135.

87. Michelsen J, Cordtz J, Liboriussen L, et al. Prevention of rhabdomyolysis-induced acute kidney injury - A DASAIM/DSIT clinical practice guideline. Acta Anaesthesiol Scand. 2019;63(5):576–586.

88. Farkas J. Fluid selection & pH-guided fluid resuscitation. PulmCrit (EMCrit) June 27, 2019 https://emcrit.org/pulmcrit/fluid/.

Part 5

Hemodynamic Monitoring

15 | Fluid Assessment and Monitoring

Both inadequate or excessive fluid replacement is detrimental [1, 2], and optimum fluid replacement is beneficial and, at times, lifesaving. So, meticulous evaluation and, on its basis, planning of proper administration of intravenous (IV) fluid is critical.

The accurate assessment of body fluid volume status requires proper history, clinical examination, hemodynamic monitoring, and laboratory investigations (Table 15.1). There is no single parameter that alone can precisely assess the hydration status [3]. Therefore, after initial resuscitation, frequent reassessment and monitoring are mandatory for the appropriate subsequent fluid administration.

HISTORY

Detailed history provides valuable information about body fluid volume status and associated illnesses. Important history to be elicited are:

Table 15.1 Assessment of volume status
• History
• Clinical examination and monitoring
• Hemodynamic monitoring
• Laboratory investigations

1. Fluid intake (volume and type of oral, nasogastric, or intravenous fluids).

2. Abnormal loss of fluid (diarrhea, vomiting, drains, high fever, and insensible losses).

3. Urine volume.

4. Symptoms of hypovolemia (increased thirst, oliguria, fatigue, weakness, or dizziness on standing).

5. Symptoms of hypervolemia (swelling, weight gain, shortness of breath with aggravation on exertion or lying down flat).

6. Coexisting illness and comorbidities (diabetes, hypertension, ischemic heart diseases, congestive heart failure, kidney failure, cirrhosis of the liver, hypoproteinemia, and malnutrition).

7. Medication (antihypertensive, diuretics, laxatives).

CLINICAL EXAMINATION

It is essential to assess the volume status of the patient by proper physical examination. Based on the clinical examination, the predictability of the severity of volume depletion is poor. However, in critical patients with severe volume depletion and shock, prompt clinical assessment and proper medical history are sufficient to initiate the right treatment [4]. It is essential to know the features of hypovolemia and hypervolemia to determine the volume status.

Signs of hypovolemia: Signs of volume depletion on clinical evaluation do not always correlate with the severity of hypovolemia. However, the features, based on the degree of extracellular fluid (ECF) volume depletion, are summarized below.

Mild volume depletion (<5% reduction of ECF)

- Diminished skin turgor
- Concentrated urine
- Loss of weight

Moderate volume depletion (5 to 10% reduction of ECF), as above plus

- Oliguria (<400 ml/day)
- Orthostatic tachycardia and hypotension (fall of ≥20 mm Hg systolic blood pressure or 10 mm Hg diastolic blood pressure)

Severe volume depletion (>10% reduction of ECF), as above plus

- Hypotension
- Low pulse volume, tachycardia, tachypnea
- Cold extremities, dry tongue, sunken eyeballs
- Prolonged capillary refill time (>2 seconds), and reduced skin turgor (doughy feel)
- Abnormal mental status and confusion

Difference between dehydration and hypovolemia: Terms dehydration and hypovolemia are often confusing and used interchangeably. But dehydration and hypovolemia are fundamentally different clinical disorders with different pathogenesis, clinical presentations, biochemical features, and management [5, 6]. The term dehydration refers to pure water loss producing hypertonicity and intracellular volume contraction. While hypovolemia refers to a combined loss of salt and water, causing extracellular fluid volume deficit and contraction of the blood volume. Characteristic features of dehydration are normal blood pressure, no orthostatic hypotension, and hypernatremia. Hypovolemia is characterized by orthostatic hypotension, tachycardia, decreased skin turgor, and normal or low serum sodium.

Signs of hypervolemia: Common signs of volume overload on clinical evaluation are:

- Peripheral edema, sacral edema in bedridden, and recent weight gain.
- Distended jugular vein.
- The third spacing of intravascular fluid causing ascites and pleural fluid.
- Tachycardia, tachypnea, and orthopnea.
- On auscultation, basal crepitation in the chest and third heart sounds.

MONITORING OF FLUID BALANCE

Important steps to monitor fluid balance are:

1. Intake and output chart: Maintain a proper chart of fluid administered (enterally or parenterally) and fluid losses (urine output, abnormal losses such as diarrhea, vomiting, or losses from gastrointestinal drainage tubes, and insensible losses) to assess the fluid balance.

2. Urine flow rate: Maintaining hourly urine output is a standard practice in all hemodynamically unstable patients. Urine output reflects

tissue perfusion and is an important indicator of hydration (in the absence of glycosuria, osmotic diuresis, or diuretic therapy). Fluid therapy aims to achieve a urine output of approximately 0.5 mL/kg/h or more.

3. Daily weight: The day-to-day weight chart is an accurate indicator for detecting the changes in the patient's volume status. Weight gain suggests fluid excess, while weight loss suggests fluid deficit. The inability to obtain weight is a limitation in sick patients.

HEMODYNAMIC MONITORING

Hemodynamic monitoring is a cornerstone in the management of hemodynamically unstable patients. The goal of hemodynamic monitoring is to ensure optimal tissue perfusion and to optimize the oxygenation of the tissues. Less than 50% of hemodynamically unstable

critical patients are 'fluid responders,' and in the rest 50% of patients, fluid administration may be harmful [7, 8], and therefore proper evaluation before administration of fluid is advisable.

Various hemodynamic monitoring techniques and parameters ranging from simple bedside examination to advanced complex methods are available (Table 15.2).

The selection of modality varies depending on the severity of the underlying disease, resources and local expertise available at each institution, predictability of the modality, and cost-effectiveness.

There is no single hemodynamic technique or parameter which is enough to provide sufficient information in all patients [9]. Less invasive systems are safer and therefore preferred for the initial evaluation. But invasive methods

Table 15.2 Techniques and parameters used for hemodynamic monitoring
A. Basic and non-invasive hemodynamic monitoring techniques
Non-invasive blood pressure measurement, pulse oximetry, continuous electrocardiography, ultra-sonogram, echocardiography, and X-ray chest
B. Static hemodynamic monitoring techniques
Inferior vena cava assessment, central venous pressure monitoring, arterial cannulation, and pulmonary artery catheter monitoring
C. Dynamic hemodynamic monitoring
1. Provocative techniques to detect fluid responsiveness The fluid challenge, passive leg raising, and end-expiratory occlusion test
2. Dynamic parameters to predict fluid responsiveness Pulse pressure variation, stroke volume variation, cardiac output, and plethysmographic variability index
3. Methods and monitors used for the assessment
a. Noninvasive cardiac output monitoring Transthoracic echocardiography, bioimpedance or bioreactance, radial applanation tonometry, volume clamp method, ultrasound cardiac output monitoring (USCOM), and plethysmographic variability index
b. Minimally invasive cardiac output monitoring Transesophageal echocardiography, transpulmonary thermodilution, lithium dilution, arterial pulse contour analysis, and partial CO_2 rebreathing
c. Invasive cardiac output monitoring Pulmonary thermodilution (Intermittent bolus or continuous)

provide more predictable information and therefore are preferred in critical, unstable patients or patients with shock who do not respond to initial therapy.

Non-critical patients who are hemodynamically stable require non-invasive monitoring techniques such as continuous ECG monitoring, frequent non-invasive blood pressure measurement, and peripheral pulse oximetry to assess their oxygen saturation.

The limitations of this primary monitoring modalities is a less precise or inaccurate data, but it avoids risks of harmful invasive approaches.

On the other hand, hemodynamically unstable critical patients need more precise or highly accurate data, so they require advanced hemodynamic monitoring approaches such as arterial pulse contour analysis, transesophageal echocardiography, and transpulmonary thermodilution for continuous hemodynamic monitoring [3, 10].

Noninvasive echocardiography and ultrasonogram are currently rapidly growing and preferred modalities for the initial hemodynamic assessment of shock and perioperative evaluation instead of more invasive technologies.

Dynamic parameters such as pulse pressure variation (PPV), stroke volume variation (SVV), and cardiac output (CO) are shown to be more accurate for the assessment of the volume status. Therefore, they are preferred in predicting fluid responsiveness over static invasive measures (e.g., central venous pressure and pulmonary artery catheters) [3].

However, monitoring these dynamic parameters is not routinely recommended for patients in shock who are responding well to initial treatment. Complex, high-risk patients who do not respond to initial fluid administration need measurements of dynamic parameters to evaluate the response to fluids or inotropes [3].

LABORATORY INVESTIGATIONS

Various laboratory investigations performed considering the clinical context for the monitoring of fluid therapy are:

- Routine investigations: CBC, BUN/creatinine, transaminases, and serum electrolytes.

- Additional investigations: Serum lactate level, arterial blood gas (ABG) analysis, cardiac biomarkers, coagulation profile, and urinary electrolytes.

Serum lactate

Serum lactate estimation is the most useful and valuable laboratory parameter for monitoring critically ill patients, and the high lactate level is strongly associated with the severity of sepsis [11, 12].

Elevated lactate is multifactorial: Increased serum lactate level reflects tissue hypoxia is a misconception [13]. Increased serum lactate level is a non-specific finding which can occur due to multiple causes such as impaired tissue oxygenation, stimulation of beta-2 adrenergic receptors due to increased aerobic glycolysis, medications (adrenaline, beta-2 agonists), liver failure, thiamine deficiency, or other causes [14]. So always interpret the value of serum lactate carefully in the clinical context.

Clinical application of lactate measurement

- A tool to diagnose severe sepsis or septic shock: The measurement of lactate is useful to establish the diagnosis of severe sepsis [15] and is included in the definition of recent major sepsis guidelines such as National Quality Forum Sepsis Update [16], and third international consensus definitions for sepsis and septic shock [17, 18].

- Prognostic marker on admission: Increased lactate level in the prehospital measurement or the emergency department is associated with increased mortality even in patients with initial normal vital signs [18–22]. So early elevated lactate is useful to detect occult shock, uncover subtle organ hypoperfusion, and help to detect patients who are at higher risk for deterioration and require aggressive management.

- As a component of resuscitative algorithms: Serum lactate is included as a component of resuscitative algorithms in different guidelines (e.g., Surviving Sepsis Campaign Bundle and Surviving Sepsis Campaign International Guidelines) [23, 24].

- Lactate monitoring for a shock: In addition to clinical assessment, trends in the blood lactate levels are useful to guide resuscitation [25]. Serial serum lactate measurements during resuscitation predict mortality among septic shock patients [26, 27]. So, serum lactate level is generally remeasured every 6 hours until it becomes normal [27, 28]. Lactate-guided therapy significantly reduces hospital mortality [29–31] and has a greater mortality benefit than even early goal-directed therapy [32].

- Lactate normalization predicts a favorable prognosis: Normalization of lactate within 6 hours of initial resuscitation is the strong predictor of survival [33–36]. In a recent study, even delayed normalization of lactate (i.e., within 24 hours),

independently predicts decreased mortality [37].

- Lactate clearance as a prognostic marker: Early lactate clearance reduces in-hospital mortality and strongly predicts the survivor [33, 38–41]. On the contrary, persistent hyperlactatemia increases morbidity and mortality and is a strong adverse prognostic factor [38, 42, 43].

REFERENCES

1. Mandal M. Ideal resuscitation fluid in hypovolemia: The quest is on and miles to go! Int J Crit Illn Inj Sci. 2016;6(2):54–55.

2. Claure-Del GR, Mehta RL. Fluid overload in the ICU: evaluation and management. BMC Nephrol 2016;17(1):109.

3. Cecconi M, De Backer D, Antonelli M, et al. Consensus on circulatory shock and hemodynamic monitoring. Task force of the European Society of Intensive Care Medicine. Intensive Care Med. 2014;40(12):1795–1815.

4. Marx G, Schindler AW, Mosch C, et al. Intravascular volume therapy in adults: Guidelines from the association of the scientific medical societies in Germany. Eur J Anaesthesiol 2016;33(7):488–522.

5. Bhave G, Neilson EG. Volume depletion versus dehydration: how understanding the difference can guide therapy. AJKD 2011;58(2):302–309.

6. Asim M, Alkadi MM, Asim H, et al. Dehydration and volume depletion: How to handle the misconceptions. World J Nephrol. 2019;8(1):23–32.

7. Marik PE, Monnet X, Teboul JL. Hemodynamic parameters to guide fluid therapy. Ann Intensive Care. 2011;1(1):1.

8. Bentzer P, Griesdale DE, Boyd J, et al. Will this hemodynamically unstable patient respond to a bolus of intravenous fluids? JAMA. 2016;316(12):1298–309.

9. Vincent JL, Rhodes A, Perel A, et al. Clinical review: Update on hemodynamic monitoring - a consensus of 16. Crit Care. 2011;15(4):229.

10. Aseni P, Orsenigo S, Storti E. et al. Current concepts of perioperative monitoring in high-risk surgical patients: a review. Patient Saf Surg 2019;13:32.

11. Gutiérrez HB, Concepción YA, Pérez JS1, et al. Prognostic value of serum lactate levels in critically ill patients in an intensive care unit. J Crit Care Med (Targu Mures). 2020;6(1):59–64.

12. Gattinoni L, Vasques F, Camporota L, et al. Understanding lactatemia in human sepsis: potential impact for early management. Am J Respir Crit Care Med 2019;200(5):582–589.

13. Levy B. Lactate and shock state: the metabolic view. Curr Opin Crit Care 2006;12(4):315–321.

14. Levy B, Desebbe O, Montemont C, et al. Increased aerobic glycolysis through beta2 stimulation is a common mechanism involved in lactate formation during shock states. Shock. 2008;30(4):417–21.

15. Fuller BM, Dellinger RP. Lactate as a hemodynamic marker in the crtically ill. Curr Opin Crit Care 2012;18(3):267–72.

16. National Quality Forum (NQF). #0500 Severe Sepsis and Septic Shock: Management Bundle, Last Updated: Jan 05, 2015 https://emcrit.org/wp-content/uploads/2015/06/0500.pdf Accessed May 23, 2020.

17. Shankar-Hari M, Phillips GS, Levy ML, et al. Developing a new definition and assessing new clinical criteria for septic shock: For the third international consensus definitions for sepsis and septic shock (Sepsis-3). JAMA 2016;315(8):775–87.

18. Singer M, Deutschman CS, Seymour CW, et al. The third international consensus definitions for sepsis and septic shock (Sepsis-3). JAMA 2016;315(8):801–10.

19. Jansen TC, van Bommel J, Mulder PG, et al. The prognostic value of blood lactate levels relative to that of vital signs in the pre-hospital setting: a pilot study. Crit Care. 2008;12(6):R160.

20. Mikkelsen ME, Miltiades AN, Gaieski DF, et al. Serum lactate is associated with mortality in severe sepsis independent of organ failure and shock. Crit Care Med. May 2009;37(5):1670–1677.

21. Soliman H, Vincent JL. Prognostic value of admission serum lactate concentrations in intensive care unit patients. Acta Clinica Belgica. 2010;65(3):176–81.

22. Casserly B, Phillips GS, Schorr C, et al. Lactate measurements in sepsis-induced tissue hypoperfusion: results from the Surviving Sepsis Campaign database. Crit Care Med. 2015;43(3):567–573.

23. Levy MM, Evans LE, Rhodes A. The surviving sepsis campaign bundle: 2018 update. Intensive Care Med 2018;44(6):925–928.

24. Rhodes A, Evans LE, Alhazzani W, et al. Surviving Sepsis Campaign: international guidelines for management of sepsis and septic shock: 2016. Intensive Care Med. 2017;43(3):304–77.

25. Weiss SL, Peters MJ, Alhazzani W, et al. Surviving sepsis campaign international guidelines for the management of septic shock and sepsis-associated organ dysfunction in children. Pediatr Crit Care Med. 2020;21(2):e52–e106.

26. Ryoo SM, Lee J, Lee YS, et al. Lactate level versus lactate clearance for predicting mortality in patients with septic shock defined by Sepsis-3. Crit Care Med 2018;46(6):e489–e495.

27. Ryoo SM, Ahn R, Lee J, et al. Timing of repeated lactate measurement in patients with septic shock at the emergency department. Am J Med Sci 2018;356(2):97–102.

28. Martin ND, Codner P, Greene W, et al. Trauma Surg Acute Care Open 2020;5(1):e000411.

29. Jansen TC, van Bommel J, Schoonderbeek FJ, et al. Early lactate-guided therapy in intensive care unit patients: a multicenter, open-label, randomized controlled trial. Am J Respir Crit Care Med. 2010;182(6):752–761.

30. Jones AE, Shapiro NI, Trzeciak S, et al. Lactate clearance vs central venous oxygen saturation as goals of early sepsis therapy: a randomized clinical trial. JAMA. 2010;303(8):739–746.

31. Lyu X, Xu Q, Cai G, et al. Efficacies of fluid resuscitation as guided by lactate clearance rate and central venous oxygen saturation in patients with septic shock. Zhonghua Yi Xue Za Zhi. 2015;95(7):496–500.

32. Ding XF, Yang ZY, Xu ZT, et al. Early goal-directed and lactate-guided therapy in adult patients with severe sepsis and septic shock: a meta-analysis of randomized controlled trials. J Transl Med. 2018;16(1):331.

33. Nguyen HB, Rivers EP, Knoblich BP, et al. Early lactate clearance is associated with improved outcome in severe sepsis and septic shock. Crit Care Med 2004;32(8):1637–42.

34. Puskarich MA, Trzeciak S, Shapiro NI, et al. Whole blood lactate kinetics in patients undergoing quantitative resuscitation for severe sepsis and septic shock. Chest. 2013;143(6):1548–1553.

35. Jones AE. Lactate clearance for assessing response to resuscitation in severe sepsis. Acad Emerg Med. 2013;20(8):844–847.

36. Chertoff J, Chisum M, Garcia B, et al. Lactate kinetics in sepsis and septic shock: a review of the literature and rationale for further research. J Intensive Care 2015;3:39.

37. Ryoo SM, Ahn R, Shin TG, et al. Lactate normalization within 6 hours of bundle therapy and 24 hours of delayed achievement were associated with 28-day mortality in septic shock patients. PLoS ONE 2019;14(6):e0217857.

38. Arnold RC, Shapiro NI, Jones AE, et al. Multicenter study of early lactate clearance as a determinant of survival in patients with presumed sepsis. Shock. 2009;32(1):35–9.

39. Zhang Z, Xu X. Lactate clearance is a useful biomarker for the prediction of all-cause mortality in critically ill patients: a systematic review and meta-analysis. Crit Care Med 2014;42(9):2118–25.

40. Gu WJ, Zhang Z, Bakker J. Early lactate clearance-guided therapy in patients with sepsis: a meta-analysis with trial sequential analysis of randomized controlled trials. Intensive Care Med 2015;41(10):1862–3.

41. Simpson SQ, Gaines M, Hussein Y, et al. Early goal-directed therapy for severe sepsis and septic shock: A living systematic review. J Crit Care 2016;36:43–48.

42. Zhang Z, Chen K, Ni H, et al. Predictive value of lactate in unselected critically ill patients: an analysis using fractional polynomials. J Thorac Dis. 2014;6(7):995–1003.

43. Dezman ZDW, Comer AC, Smith GS, et al. Failure to clear elevated lactate predicts 24-hour mortality in trauma patients. J Trauma Acute Care Surg. 2015;79(4):580–585.

16 | Basic and Non-Invasive Hemodynamic Monitoring Techniques

---

Various basic and non-invasive methods are routinely used in clinical practice, which help to plan, administer, and monitor fluid therapy in non-critical patients. The basic and non-invasive monitoring modalities are not the standard methods for hemodynamic monitoring and lack specificity and sensitivity, but it provides valuable help in the initial assessment and management of shock. Non-invasive cardiac output monitoring is discussed in detail separately in the subsequent chapter.

NON-INVASIVE BLOOD PRESSURE MEASUREMENT

Blood pressure monitoring is a basic and easy non-invasive parameter for hemodynamic monitoring in all patients.

Non-invasive blood pressure is measured either intermittently or continuously. Intermittently blood pressure is measured by an inflatable occluding cuff using a manual sphygmomanometer or automated oscillometric devices. Continuously blood pressure is measured by newer methods such as volume clamp method or arterial applanation tonometry. Details of these methods are included in the non-invasive cardiac output monitoring part of the Chapter 19 on "Cardiac Output Monitoring."

In mild hypovolemia, compensatory mechanisms prevent a fall in blood pressure. So, normal blood pressure does not exclude hypovolemia.

Postural hypotension is a fall of at least 20 mm Hg systolic blood pressure or 10 mm Hg diastolic blood pressure within 3 minutes of standing [1]. Postural hypotension is a strong indicator of hypovolemia in the absence of other causes such as medications, autonomic neuropathy, etc.

Mean arterial pressure is a better parameter for assessing tissue perfusion than systolic blood pressure (SBP) and diastolic blood pressure (DBP). Mean arterial pressure (MAP) is the average arterial pressure in one cardiac cycle.

Formula to calculate MAP is:

$$MAP = [SBP + (2 \times DBP)]/3$$

MAP of at least 60 mm Hg is necessary to maintain the adequate perfusion of vital organs. Recent Surviving Sepsis Campaign Guidelines recommended an initial MAP target of 65 mm Hg in patients with septic shock requiring vasopressors [2].

PULSE OXIMETRY

Pulse oximetry is used routinely worldwide for the rapid diagnosis of hypoxemia; It is referred to as "the fifth vital sign" [3].

Pulse oximetry is an inexpensive, non-invasive, compact, portable, and reliable technique that can continuously, rapidly, and accurately estimate arterial oxygen saturation (SpO_2) and thereby provide important information about tissue oxygenation.

Early diagnosis of hypoxemia is difficult clinically. Cyanosis is its late sign, so a pulse oximeter is used to monitor all types of patients at risk of developing hypoxemia [4]. In this easy-to-use method, the sensor probe is usually placed on fingers, toes, or ear lobes which measures two parameters, the oxygen saturation of hemoglobin in arterial blood and the pulse rate.

By using spectrophotometry, a pulse oximeter differentiates oxygenated versus non-oxygenated hemoglobin in the arterial blood and thereby measures the percentage of oxygenated hemoglobin in the blood (i.e., SpO_2). The accuracy of pulse oximeters is generally reliable when SpO_2 is in the range of 70% to 100%, but it is poor when SpO_2 values are <70% [5].

The normal value of SpO_2 in a healthy person is 96% to 100%, which correlates to the normal range of PaO_2 (i.e., 80 to 100 mm Hg). Less than 90% SpO_2 correlates to a PaO_2 of 60 mm Hg or less, which suggests significant hypoxemia, which can be dangerous [6]. When SpO_2 falls below 90%, the PaO_2 drops very rapidly. PaO_2 will be as low as 60–45 mm Hg when SpO_2 reduces from 90 to 80%, and when SpO_2 falls below 80%, it predicts life-threatening hypoxemia as the PaO_2 will be just 40 mm of Hg or even lesser [6].

Factors that can affect the accuracy of pulse oximetry are cold extremities, hypotension, poor circulation, patient movements, nail polish use, abnormal hemoglobins, and severe anemia [7].

Use of intravenous dyes like methylene blue (to treat methemoglobinemia, or to diagnose ureteral injury during surgical procedures) can result in low SpO_2 reading from a pulse oximeter but normal PaO_2 from a standard blood gas machine (known as "oxygen saturation gap") [8].

CONTINUOUS ELECTROCARDIOGRAPHY

Continuous electrocardiography monitoring is a standard practice in all unstable patients because it provides crucial information about rate, rhythm abnormality, cardiac ischemia, and abnormalities due to electrolyte abnormalities. Lead II and V1 are the most sensitive for detecting P waves and cardiac arrhythmias, while lead II, V2, and V5 are the most sensitive for detecting myocardial ischemia.

ECHOCARDIOGRAPHY

Echocardiography is a safe, simple, readily available, unique, and effective method for the initial assessment of hemodynamically unstable patients. Echocardiography is a widely used and preferred modality that helps to diagnose, monitor, manage, and follow up various clinical problems mentioned below [9–12].

- For the initial assessment of patients with hypovolemia, hemodynamic instability, and shock where it helps to differentiate various types of shock.
- To assess acute respiratory distress syndrome, right ventricular dysfunction, respiratory failure, or hypoxemia of unknown etiology.
- To diagnose pericardial effusion, cardiac tamponade, valvular obstructive or regurgitation lesions, cardiac thrombus, infective endocarditis, and pulmonary embolism.
- To assess the fluid status and by frequent evaluation guides in the tailored management of unstable patients.
- To determine the fluid responsiveness by measuring the size of the vena cava and assessing the effect of respiration, fluid challenge, and passive leg raising on it.

Respiratory variation in the vena cava, left ventricular function, right ventricular function size, and movement of the interventricular septum are the major parameters measured by echocardiography. These parameters are helpful in hemodynamic assessment and monitoring. In addition, echocardiography also provides information about cardiac output and pulmonary artery pressure, which helps to optimize patient management.

Two different echocardiography techniques used for hemodynamic monitoring are transthoracic echocardiography and transesophageal echocardiography.

Transthoracic echocardiography (TTE)

It is a simple tool in which an ultrasonic probe is placed on the chest or epigastrium of the subject to assess the heart and its blood vessels. For the hemodynamic assessment in patients with hypotension, TTE is performed first because it is a readily available, non-invasive, accurate, and precise technique that can be performed quickly at the bedside [13].

Transoesophageal echocardiography (TEE)

In TEE ultrasonic probe is placed into the esophagus and usually in a ventilated patient under sedation. As the probe is much closer to the heart in TEE, this method provides superior image quality of the heart and great vessels. Because TEE provides additional and more accurate information, it has higher diagnostic accuracy than TTE [14].

TEE is used selectively in the perioperative management of unstable surgical patients (e.g., cardiac surgical procedures, laparotomy, etc.) and in patients where TTE is not possible or provides insufficient information (i.e., chest wall injury, obese patients with poor echocardiographic window, etc.).

Although TEE provides accurate and more information than TTE, it is used in selected indications and not used routinely. Major limitations of this technique are higher cost, time-consuming method (compared to TTE), minimally invasive procedure (usually needs tracheal intubation), can be performed only on one patient at a time, and needs cleaning and disinfection after each use.

ULTRASONOGRAM

In hemodynamically unstable patients, ultrasonography may be useful in determining underlying causes for shock, such as hidden blood loss (intrathoracic intraabdominal, retroperitoneal, bladder, or extremity hematoma) or detecting the source of sepsis. Timely treatment of such potentially reversible causes of hemodynamic instability can be life-saving. Follow-up ultrasonography also helps to assess the treatment response (change in the volume of blood in pleural, pericardial or abdominal space, or improvement in the source of the infection).

LUNG ULTRASOUND

Lung ultrasound (LUS) is an increasingly used modality for assessing lung status and hemodynamic monitoring in critically unstable patients. Lung ultrasound is an easy-to-use, radiation-free, safe, less expensive, non-invasive, reliable, and reproducible bedside tool that helps in diagnosis as well as planning optimum fluid administration [15, 16].

Lung ultrasound is a powerful tool that helps to assess the fluid status and diagnose or exclude pleural effusion, pneumonia, and pneumothorax [17, 18]. In addition, bedside lung ultrasound is an effective and helpful tool for the initial evaluation of a patient with hypotension and shock, guiding fluid administration, monitoring treatment response, and detecting fluid overload early [19, 20].

Lung ultrasound is a more accurate, faster, and more convenient imaging technique than chest X-rays in emergency departments [20–22].

Pulmonary edema

Lung ultrasound is a useful tool that can reliably and sensitively detect pulmonary edema [16]. By assessing the volume of extravascular lung water, lung ultrasound can diagnose pulmonary edema before detecting it by any clinical signs [23]. Extravascular lung water is the amount of water in the

lungs outside the pulmonary circulation, i.e., accumulated in the interstitial and alveolar spaces [24]. Therefore, lung ultrasound is recommended as a first-line test to detect pulmonary congestion, which helps in the better management of fluid administration, monitoring the response of fluid therapy, and avoiding iatrogenic pulmonary edema [25–27].

On lung ultrasound, the presence and numbers of B-lines (also termed ultrasound lung comets) reflect the volume of extravascular lung water [28, 29]. The presence of B-lines is unanimously considered a pathological finding, and B-lines are generally absent in euvolemic patients (suggests "Dry" lungs) [30, 31].

B-lines score (BLS) is the sum of all B-lines used to quantify pulmonary congestion [32]. The normal value of BLS is <5, and >15 BLS reflects moderate/severe pulmonary congestion [33]. More than three B-lines in a particular view on lung ultrasound is also a reliable clue for pulmonary edema [34]. The new appearance of B-lines is an early sign of pulmonary congestion and guides clinicians to discontinue fluid administration [35].

Pleural effusion, consolidations and pneumothorax

In pleural effusion, lung ultrasonography is an essential tool in diagnosing, quantifying, following the course, decision-making to drain, deciding the best puncture site for tapping, guiding the drainage insertion procedure, and diagnosing co-existing lung diseases [36–39]. In pneumonia, bedside lung ultrasound is a first-line diagnostic tool with high accuracy (94% sensitivity and 96% specificity) [40–43]. In addition, lung ultrasound is a novel tool with high accuracy and reliability in diagnosing pneumothorax (91% sensitivity and 98% specificity) [44–46].

X-RAY CHEST

Chest X-ray (CXR) is routinely used in critical, unstable patients. The major advantage of chest X-rays is immediate panoramic imaging of the thoracic structures, which provides comprehensive information and helps clinicians to suspect or exclude many pulmonary disorders [47]. However, frequent exposure of X-rays carries the risk of radiation.

In hemodynamically unstable patients, chest X-ray helps to detect fluid overload, pleural effusion, pneumonia, pneumothorax, and complications of shock such as acute respiratory distress syndrome, pulmonary embolism, and aspiration pneumonia and provides information about cardiac size and shape. In addition, a chest X-ray is frequently taken after placement of the central line to check the position of the catheter tip and to rule out iatrogenic pneumothorax.

Common chest X-ray findings of fluid overload are cardiomegaly, septal Karley B-lines, congestive vascular hilum, bilateral diffuse perihilar alveolar infiltrates in a butterfly distribution suggestive of pulmonary edema, and signs of pleural effusion. A chest X-ray is not a very sensitive or specific diagnostic test for most of these disorders, but it may be a first step in providing some important clues.

REFERENCES

1. Bradley JG, Davis KA. Orthostatic hypotension. Am Fam Physician 2003;68(12):2393–2399.

2. Rhodes A, Evans LE, Alhazzani W, et al. Surviving Sepsis Campaign: international guidelines for management of sepsis and septic shock: 2016. Crit Care Med 2017;45(3):486–552.

3. Neff TA. Routine oximetry: a fifth vital sign? Chest 1988;94(4):227.

4. Pulse Oximetry Training Manual - World Health Organization 2011.

5. Chan ED, Chan MM, Chan MM. Pulse oximetry: Understanding its basic principles facilitates appreciation of its limitations. Respiratory Medicine 2013;107(6):789–799.

6. Madan A. Correlation between the levels of SpO2 and PaO2. Lung India. 2017;34(3):307–308.

7. Bowes WA, Corke BC, Hulka J. Pulse oximetry: a review of the theory, accuracy, and clinical applications. Obstet Gynecol. 1989;74(3 Pt 2):541–6.

8. Akhtar J, Johnston BD, Krenzelok EP. Mind the gap. J Emerg Med. 2007;33(2):131–2.

9. Hendy A, Bubenek-Turconi ŞI. The diagnosis and hemodynamic monitoring of circulatory shock: Current and Future Trends. J Crit Care Med (Targu Mures). 2016;2(3):115–123.

10. Casaroto E, Mohovic T, Pinto LM et al. Bedside echocardiography in critically ill patients. Einstein 2015;13(4):644–6.

11. Vignon P. What is new in critical care echocardiography? Critical Care 2018;22(1):40.

12. Longobardo L, Zito C, Carerj S, et al. Role of echocardiography in the intensive care unit: overview of the most common clinical scenarios. J Patient Cent Res Rev. 2018;5(3):239–43.

13. Mercado P, Maizel J, Beyls C, et al. Transthoracic echocardiography: an accurate and precise method for estimating cardiac output in the critically ill patient. Crit Care. 2017;21(1):136.

14. Hahn RT, Abraham T, Adams MS, et al. Guidelines for performing a comprehensive transesophageal echocardiographic examination: recommendations from the American Society of Echocardiography and the Society of Cardiovascular Anesthesiologists. J Am Soc Echocardiogr. 2013;26(9):921–64.

15. Demi L, Egan T, Muller M. Lung Ultrasound imaging, a technical review. Appl. Sci. 2020;10(2):462.

16. Grune J, Beyhoff N, Hegemann N, et al. From bedside to bench: lung ultrasound for the assessment of pulmonary edema in animal models. Cell and Tissue Research 2020.

17. Lichtenstein DA. BLUE-protocol and FALLS-protocol: Two applications of lung ultrasound in the critically ill. Chest 2015;147(6):1659–1670.

18. Lancellotti P, Price S, Edvardsen T, et al. The use of echocardiography in acute cardiovascular care: recommendations of the European Association of Cardiovascular Imaging and the Acute Cardiovascular Care Association. Eur Heart J Acute Cardiovasc Care. 2015;4(1):3–5.

19. Whitson MR, Mayo PH. Ultrasonography in the emergency department. Crit Care 2016;20(1):227.

20. Shrestha GS, Weeratunga D, Baker K. Point-of-care lung ultrasound in critically ill patients. Reviews recent Clinical trials. 2018;13(1):15–26.

21. Parlamento S, Copetti R, Di Bartolomeo S. Evaluation of lung ultrasound for the diagnosis of pneumonia in the ED. Am J Emerg Med. 2009;27(4):379–84.

22. Xirouchaki N, Magkanas E, Vaporidi K, et al. Lung ultrasound in critically ill patients: comparison with

bedside chest radiography. Intensive Care Med. 2011;37(9):1488–93.

23. Zieleskiewicz L, Contargyris C, Brun C, et al. Lung ultrasound predicts interstitial syndrome and hemodynamic profile in parturients with severe preeclampsia. Anesthesiology 2014;120(4):906–914.

24. Jozwiak M, Teboul J, Monnet X. Extravascular lung water in critical care: recent advances and clinical applications. Ann. Intensive Care 2015;5(1):38.

25. Mebazaa A, Yilmaz MB, Levy P, et al. Recommendations management on pre-hospital and hospital of acute heart failure: a consensus paper of the Heart Failure Association of the European Society of Cardiology, the European Society of Emergency Medicine and the Society of Academic Emergency Medicine. Eur Heart J 2015;17(6):544–558.

26. Lichtenstein D. Fluid administration limited by lung sonography: The place of lung ultrasound in assessment of acute circulatory failure (the FALLS-protocol). Expert Rev Respir Med. 2012;6(2):155–62.

27. Volpicelli G, Elbarbary M, Blaivas M, et al. International Liaison Committee on Lung Ultrasound (ILC-LUS) for International Consensus Conference on Lung Ultrasound (ICC-LUS). International evidence-based recommendations for point-of-care lung ultrasound. Intensive Care Med 2012;38(4):577–591.

28. Jambrik Z, Gargani L, Adamicza Á, et al. B-lines quantify the lung water content: A lung ultrasound versus lung gravimetry study in acute lung injury. Ultrasound Med Biol. 2010;36(12):2004–10.

29. Annamalai I, Balasubramaniam S, Fernando ME, et al. Volume assessment in hemodialysis: A comparison of present methods in clinical practice with sonographic lung comets. Indian J Nephrol. 2019;29(2):102–110.

30. Dietrich CF, Mathis G, Blaivas M, et al. Lung B-line artefacts and their use. J Thorac Dis 2016;8(6):1356–65.

31. Trezzi M, Torzillo D, Ceriani E, et al. Lung ultrasonography for the assessment of rapid extravascular water variation: evidence from hemodialysis patients. Intern Emerg Med 2013;8(5):409–15.

32. Picano E, Frassi F, Agricola E, et al. Ultrasound lung comets: a clinically useful sign of extravascular lung water. J Am Soc Echocardiogr 2006;19(3):356–363.

33. Picano E, Pellikka PA. Ultrasound of extravascular lung water: a new standard for pulmonary congestion. Eur Heart J. 2016;37(27):2097–2104.

34. Anile A, Russo J, Castiglione G, et al. A simplifed lung ultrasound approach to detect increased extravascular lung water in critically ill patients. Crit Ultrasound J 2017;9(1):13.

35. Caltabeloti FC, Monsel A, Arbelot C, et al. Early fluid loading in acute respiratory distress syndrome with septic shock deteriorates lung aeration without impairing arterial oxygenation: a lung ultrasound observational study. Crit Care 2014;18(3):R91.

36. Soni NJ, Franco R, Velez MI, et al. Ultrasound in the diagnosis and management of pleural effusions. J Hosp Med. 2015;10(12):811–816.

37. Ibitoye BO, Idowu BM, Ogunrombi AB, et al. Ultrasonographic quantification of pleural effusion: comparison of four formulae. Ultrasonography. 2018;37(3):254–260.

38. Brogi E, Gargani L, Bignami E, et al. Thoracic ultrasound for pleural effusion in the intensive care unit: a narrative review from diagnosis to treatment. Crit Care 2017;21(1):325.

39. Vetrugno L, Guadagnin GM, Orso D, et al. An easier and safe affair, pleural drainage with ultrasound in critical patient: a technical note. Crit Ultrasound J 2018;10:18.

40. Chavez MA, Shams N, Ellington LE, et al. Lung ultrasound for the diagnosis of pneumonia in adults: A systematic review and meta-analysis. Respir Res 2014;15(1):50.

41. Pagano A, Numis FG, Visone G, et al. Lung ultrasound for diagnosis of pneumonia in emergency department. Intern Emerg Med. 2015;10(7):851–4.

42. Ellington LE, Gilman RH, Chavez MA, et al. Lung ultrasound as a diagnostic tool for radiographically-confirmed pneumonia in low resource settings. Respir Med. 2017;128:57–64.

43. Najgrodzka P, Buda N, Zamojska A, et al. Lung ultrasonography in the diagnosis of pneumonia in children-a metaanalysis and a review of pediatric lung imaging. Ultrasound Q. 2019;35(2):157–163.

44. Alrajhi K, Woo MY, Vaillancourt C. Test characteristics of ultrasonography for the detection of pneumothorax: A systematic review and meta-analysis. Chest 2012;141(3):703–708.

45. Alrajab S, Youssef AM, Akkus NI, et al. Pleural ultrasonography versus chest radiography for the diagnosis of pneumothorax: review of the literature and meta-analysis. Crit Care 2013;17(5):R208.

46. Ebrahimi A, Yousefifard M, Mohammad KH, et al. Diagnostic accuracy of chest ultrasonography versus chest radiography for identification of Pneumothorax: A Systematic Review and Meta-Analysis. Tanaffos 2014;13(4):29–40.

47. Cardinale L, Priola AM, Moretti F, et al. Effectiveness of chest radiography, lung ultrasound and thoracic computed tomography in the diagnosis of congestive heart failure. World J Radiol. 2014;6(6):230–237.

17 | Static Hemodynamic Monitoring Techniques

Commonly used static hemodynamic monitoring methods are inferior vena cava assessment, central venous pressure (CVP) monitoring, arterial cannulation, and pulmonary artery catheter monitoring. Although these modalities are available more widely than compared to dynamic monitoring modalities, they lack precision and accuracy.

INFERIOR VENA CAVA ASSESSMENT

Echocardiography of the inferior vena cava (IVC) is a simple, routinely used, noninvasive tool that can rapidly measure maximal IVC diameter and respiratory variations in IVC diameter at the bedside for predicting the intravascular volume status and fluid responsiveness [1]. For the initial evaluation of shock, as compared to more invasive technologies, this modality is preferred to assess the hemodynamic status and fluid responsiveness [2, 3].

For the proper understanding clinical utility of this tool, it is discussed step by step as follows:

1. Physiological variations in IVC diameter during the respiratory cycle.

2. Measurement techniques.
3. Maximal IVC diameter in spontaneous breathing and patients on a ventilator.
4. Inferior vena cava diameter variation (IVC distensibility index (dIVC) in patients on mechanical ventilator and IVC collapsibility index (cIVC) during spontaneous breathing).

The diagnostic value of the variability of the superior vena cava is better than that of the IVC [4], but the limiting factor is a requirement of transoesophageal echocardiography for the measurement, which is minimally invasive and technically difficult [5].

Physiological principles

It is important to remember that amongst patients with spontaneous respiration, and in patients on positive pressure ventilation, physiological changes, values of variations of IVC parameters, and their interpretations differ markedly.

A. IVC in spontaneous respiration

In patients with spontaneous breathing, intrathoracic pressure decreases during inspiration, which increases the venous return of blood, resulting in the "collapse" of the vena cava. Inversely, intrathoracic pressure increases during expiration, which reduces the venous return of blood and thus causes the expansion of the vena cava.

IVC collapsibility index (cIVC): "Collapsibility index" is used to assess the respiratory variations in IVC diameter in patients with spontaneous respiration.

Calculation of the IVC collapsibility index: In spontaneous breathing patients, obtain the maximum IVC diameter (at the end of expiration) and minimum IVC diameter (at the end of inspiration) and calculate the index.

IVC Collapsibility Index
$$= \frac{\text{Maximum IVC} - \text{Minimum IVC}}{\text{Maximum IVC}} \times 100$$

B. IVC in patients on ventilator

In patients on positive pressure ventilation (on noninvasive ventilation or intubated and on the mechanical ventilator), IVC changes with respiration are just reversed compared with spontaneous breathing. During inspiration, intrathoracic pressure increases, which pushes blood back into the IVC from the right atrium causing "Distention" of IVC. While during expiration, intrathoracic pressure decreases, and venous return increases, which causes IVC collapse.

IVC distensibility index (dIVC): "Distensibility index" is used to assess the respiratory variations in IVC diameter in patients on a ventilator.

Calculation of the IVC distensibility index and IVC diameter variability: In patients on a ventilator, obtain the maximum IVC diameter (at the end of inspiration) and minimum IVC diameter (at the end of expiration) and calculate the mean of both (mean IVC), and calculate indexes [6].

IVC Distensibility Index
$$= \frac{\text{Maximum IVC} - \text{Minimum IVC}}{\text{Minimum IVC}} \times 100$$

IVC Diameter Variability
$$= \frac{\text{Maximum IVC} - \text{Minimum IVC}}{\text{Mean IVC}} \times 100$$

Why is the predictive value of variations in IVC diameter better in patients on a ventilator than in spontaneous breathing patients?

In spontaneous breathing patients, respiration is highly variable between different patients, and it varies from one to another respiratory cycle, even in the same patient. Additionally, in spontaneous breathing patients, changes in intrathoracic pressure are much smaller, and therefore variation in the size of the IVC is also smaller. So, during spontaneous breathing, respiratory variations in IVC diameter are nonuniform and smaller; therefore, its predictability for fluid responsiveness is inferior [7].

While in a patient on a ventilator, controlled large tidal volume and small positive end-expiratory pressure lead to uniform changes in intrathoracic pressure during the respiration cycle. As a result, changes in vena cava diameter are also uniform (without variability from one to another cycle of ventilation), and therefore, patients on ventilators predict fluid responsiveness better than spontaneous breathing patients.

Measurement techniques

Two types of techniques used for the IVC measurement are:

1. Transthoracic echocardiography (TTE): The diameter of the inferior vena cava can be quite easily and routinely measured by using transthoracic echocardiography using a subcostal view in a longitudinal section (measured approximately 1–2 cm caudal to the right atrium and IVC junction).

2. Transesophageal echocardiography (TEE): TEE provides an accurate view of the superior vena cava (SVC) and, therefore, provides more precise data for the calculation but is used infrequently and in selected patients as this method is minimally invasive (requires intubation) with many limitations.

Maximal IVC diameter

Assessment of maximal IVC diameter is a static parameter that may be

used to evaluate volume status and fluid responsiveness in spontaneously breathing patients [2]. In patients with shock, despite normalization of blood pressure after fluid resuscitation, inadequate dilatation of the IVC may be an important clue for insufficient circulating blood volume [8]. However, clinicians should use static IVC diameter cautiously because of its poor predictability [9]. Maximal IVC diameter is not useful in most patients, but very low or very high values may be helpful [10].

A. In spontaneous breathing

- Complete IVC collapse or end-expiratory IVC diameter less than 10 mm may suggest hypovolaemia and needs fluid administration in spontaneously breathing patients [11–14].

- IVC diameter of more than 25 mm may suggest hypervolemia in spontaneously breathing patients, and fluid administration is not appropriate [11, 15].

- In patients with marked volume overload, IVC is expanded and not collapsible [16]. However, noncollapsing large IVC diameter is not specific for volume overload, and it is essential to exclude multiple other causes [15].

B. In mechanically ventilated patients

A single static value of IVC diameter does not predict fluid status or fluid responsiveness in patients on a ventilator [6]. It is important to remember that IVC is often distended in patients on a mechanical ventilator due to increased intrathoracic pressure because of positive pressure ventilation. Therefore, a distended IVC in patients on a ventilator neither suggests volume overload nor excludes hypovolemia or fluid responsiveness.

However, an end-expiratory IVC diameter of less than 13 mm is a strong indicator of volume depletion, and an IVC diameter over 25 mm excludes fluid responsiveness in patients on a mechanical ventilator [10, 17].

Pitfalls: Between the vena cava and right atrium, there is no valve, and therefore, high right atrial pressure causes expansion of the vena cava and impairs the normal collapsibility of the vena cava. So, before diagnosing the volume status based on IVC parameters, consider other factors that can affect the IVC diameter and collapse, such as right atrial pressure, respiratory disorders affecting the degree of intrathoracic pressure change, and pressure within the abdominal cavity.

Remember that prerequisites to use IVC diameter and collapsibility to assess volume status effectively are controlled mode ventilator, tidal volume ≥8mL/kg with positive end-expiratory pressure (PEEP) ≤5 cm H_2O, intraabdominal pressure should be normal, and absence of acute cor pulmonale or severe right ventricular dysfunction [14, 15]. Fluid responsiveness is predicted poorly if tidal volumes <8 mL/kg or PEEP >5 cm H_2O [18].

Inferior vena cava diameter variation

In spontaneously breathing patients, the average diameter of IVC is about 18 mm, with approximately 50% collapse with inspiration [19].

Assessment of the change in diameter of the vena cava during respiration and calculation of the distensibility/collapsibility index on its basis is a widely

used tool for predicting intravascular volume status and fluid responsiveness. Variations in IVC diameter in response to fluid administration is a better indicator of adequate replacement of fluid than vital signs, and static maximal IVC diameter [9].

For the assessment of fluid responsiveness, the predictive value of variations in IVC diameter is better in patients on a ventilator compared to patients on spontaneous breathing [20, 21].

The measurement of inferior vena cava diameter is routinely performed in ICUs for both patients spontaneously breathing and on a ventilator. But it is important to remember that evidence about the predictive value of this modality in the assessment of volume status and fluid responsiveness in both groups is conflicting and the subject of debate [3, 17, 22–24].

A. In mechanically ventilated patients

There are controversies regarding the effectiveness of respiratory variation in IVC diameter and distensibility index to predict fluid responsiveness in mechanically ventilated patients. There are studies, systematic reviews, and meta-analyses supporting its predictive value and use [18, 20, 21, 25–32], and data not in favor of the same [4, 10, 33–35].

The distensibility index (dIVC) is a more accurate parameter in predicting the volume status as compared to the collapsibility index (CI-IVC) and variations in IVC (ΔIVC) in patients with positive pressure supports [36].

In patients on a ventilator:

- If the distensibility index is >18% or IVC diameter variability is >12%, it may predict fluid responsiveness [25–27].

- If the distensibility Index is <18%, the patient is not responsive to volume, and benefit from fluid administration is unlikely [37].

In patients on a ventilator, as compared to the measurement of IVC collapsibility, SVC collapsibility has better diagnostic accuracy in predicting fluid responsiveness [5]. The SVC collapsibility threshold of 36% can effectively differentiate between fluid responders and nonresponders patients (with a sensitivity of 90% and a specificity of 100%) [38]. But the measurement of SVC needs semi-invasive transesophageal echocardiography, which is the limiting factor.

B. In spontaneous breathing patients

Because of conflicting evidence, use IVC diameter variation and collapsibility index cautiously to predict fluid responsiveness in spontaneously breathing patients. Evidence supports its predictive value and uses [7, 9, 20, 39–44], and there is also literature not favoring the same [21, 45–48]. Remember that optimal thresholds of these parameters in spontaneous breathing are different from those described in patients on a ventilator [39].

In spontaneous breathing patients:

- Very collapsible IVC with higher amplitude respiratory variation, i.e., collapsibility index >40%, is a moderate predictor of fluid responsiveness [7, 40–42], but lower values (<40%) do not exclude volume responsiveness [9, 19].

- Very distended IVC with a collapsibility index <15% may suggest that the patient is not fluid responsive [49].

- The absence of respiratory variation is an important clue, which suggests that the patient is not fluid responsive [26].

Besides low sensitivity and less reliability in patients with spontaneous breathing, cautious use of this modality is preferred because it is readily available, easy to perform, noninvasive, and carries high specificity [40, 43, 44].

CENTRAL VENOUS PRESSURE MONITORING

Central venous pressure is the most frequently used method to assess the hemodynamic status and guide fluid resuscitation in ICU patients [50, 51].

What is CVP?

Central venous pressure is the pressure of blood measured in the vena cava at its junction with the right atrium. CVP is a simple method that can be easily measured in any patient with a central venous line, and the most frequently chosen access is the internal jugular vein.

CVP measures mean right atrial pressure and is an indicator of chiefly right ventricular preload and, to a lesser extent, left ventricular preload.

Factors determining CVP

CVP is influenced by multiple factors such as vascular volume status, right ventricular compliance, pulmonary vascular resistance, thoracic, pericardial, and abdominal pressures, peripheral vascular tone, and posture [11, 52]. In patients on a mechanical ventilator, the value of CVP increases proportionate to positive end-expiratory pressure (roughly 5 cmH_2O increase in PEEP will cause a 2.5 cmH_2O increase in CVP) [53].

CVP measurement is unreliable in the presence of pulmonary vascular disease and hypertension, right ventricular disease, congestive heart failure, valvular heart disease, tense ascites, and high intra-abdominal pressure.

Interpretation of the value of CVP

The value of CVP should always be interpreted with clinical status.

Normal value

The normal value of CVP is 2 to 6 mmHg (when measured continuously using electronic pressure transducers) or 3 to 10 cm H_2O (measured directly using water manometers).

Low CVP

1. True hypovolemia, as in blood loss, fluid loss, or fluid shift.
2. Relative hypovolemia caused by peripheral vasodilatation, as in spinal anesthesia, septicemia, and anaphylactic shock.

High CVP

1. Volume overload.
2. Cardiac causes like congestive heart failure, cardiac tamponade, constrictive pericarditis, and tricuspid regurgitation.
3. Pulmonary causes like embolism, pulmonary hypertension, tension pneumothorax, COPD, and cor pulmonale and positive pressure ventilation.

When and how to use CVP in clinical practice?

In the past, CVP monitoring was the most commonly used tool to assess volume status and to guide fluid resuscitation in critically ill patients [54]. However, in recent literature, the relationship between CVP and blood volume was poor, and CVP was unable to predict the hemodynamic response to a fluid challenge [2, 55, 56].

With recent evidence, the concept of using static marker CVP to assess intravascular volume or an indicator of fluid responsiveness is not recommended and is considered unreliable and potentially dangerous [57, 58].

However, CVP is still used in ICUs worldwide because other more accurate methods are not available easily [54].

In view of two contradictory facts (i.e., growing literature against the use and routine worldwide use in practice), different practical aspects related to indications and limitations of CVP monitoring are summarized.

Basic principles

- Normal CVP does not exclude volume depletion.
- A single value of CVP does not help in managing patients; it is always interpreted in the context of the clinical situation [57, 59].
- The "extreme" CVP values are important; it provides valuable guidance. The presence of "extreme" CVP values (CVP <6–8 mmHg and CVP >12–15 mmHg) can be of great help in predicting volume status and planning fluid administration [60–62].
- Using CVP to guide fluid administration is far from perfect, but when more accurate predictors of fluid responsiveness are not available, a reasonable CVP target is 8–12 mmHg [62, 63] during fluid administration. However, if the patient is stable, no attempt should be made to increase CVP to specific target values. Instead, the upper limit of CVP should be determined individually, considering

the potential benefit/risk of further fluid administration. The goal is to keep CVP as low as possible while maintaining adequate tissue perfusion [62].

Low CVP

- A low CVP can be normal but generally suggest hypovolemia. If CVP is normal, it does not exclude hypovolaemia [64].

- In patients with low CVP values (less than 6 mmHg), an initial moderate fluid bolus is unlikely to cause harm, and most patients will respond to fluids [59–62].

- Prognostic value: In patients with circulatory shock, lower CVP and increased cardiac output may improve the prognosis and renal function, so one should try to keep lower CVP with due caution to maintain adequate tissue perfusion [62, 65].

High CVP

- High CVP is always abnormal and has important therapeutic and prognostic values.

- An increase in CVP can occur due to increased total vascular volume, decreased cardiac function, or both.

- Patients with high CVP values (greater than 15 mmHg) do not respond to fluid administration, and therefore it is prudent to avoid the administration of fluids when the CVP is markedly elevated [61, 62].

- The upper threshold of CVP can alert the clinician to stop fluid therapy, and a positive trend reaching high values (CVP >8 mmHg) may warn the clinician that fluid replacement is no more needed [64]. So, the use of high CVP as a safety end-point and as a stopping rule for fluid

administration can minimize the risk of volume overload [66].

- Prognostic value: Elevated CVP (>10 mmHg) is associated with an increased risk of mortality, a higher incidence of acute kidney injury (AKI), and poor outcomes (i.e., death) in critical ICU patients [65, 67–71]. A high CVP causes an increase in renal venous pressure leading to increased renal venous congestion, and reduces renal perfusion pressure with AKI as a result [72]. Similarly, elevated venous pressure may impair the venous return and disturb microcirculatory blood flow, which may harm the functions of different organs, leading to poor outcomes and even high mortality [58, 68].

Conclusion: Except for the extreme values, CVP may provide inaccurate estimations of volume status and does not predict volume responsiveness. When more accurate methods to estimate a patient's fluid volume status are unavailable, clinicians should understand the limitations, dangers, and benefits of CVP and use it judicially and selectively rather than abandon it altogether.

ARTERIAL CANNULATION

Arterial cannulation is a frequently performed and preferred procedure for the hemodynamic monitoring of critically ill and high-risk surgical patients [64].

Use

Arterial catheterization is useful for:

1. **Continuous monitoring of arterial blood pressure:** Arterial catheterization is a low-risk method which provides reliable information about blood pressure in unstable patients. This beside technique continuously

and accurately measures beat-to-beat (as well as moment-to-moment) blood pressure and therefore recognizes the changes in blood pressure promptly and guides clinicians for quicker therapeutic interventions.

2. **Frequent blood sampling:** Arterial catheterization helps in repeated blood sampling for laboratory testing or arterial blood gas analysis.

3. **To predict fluid responsiveness:** An arterial catheter allows the analysis of arterial pressure waveforms. Analysis of respiration variations in the arterial waveform can determine fluid status and fluid responsiveness by calculating indices such as pulse pressure variation (PPV) and stroke volume variation (SVV). In addition, variations in the arterial waveform in response to fluid challenges or passive leg raising are reliable indices for assessing fluid responsiveness.

4. **Diagnostic or therapeutic interventions:** Arterial catheterization is used for various diagnostic and therapeutic coronary procedures such as vascular stenting or embolization and intra-aortic balloon pump (IABP).

Technique

Arterial cannulation is a relatively safe procedure in which a simple cannula is introduced by a Seldinger technique, usually in a radial or femoral artery, after local anesthesia. Hemorrhage or hematoma at the puncture site, arterial spasm or occlusion, embolization, distal ischemia, and local and catheter-related infection are common complications of arterial cannulation. Avoid using arterial lines to administer medication, as it can lead to serious tissue damage and cause considerable morbidity [73].

Indications

Common indications of arterial cannulation for hemodynamic monitoring are:

- In ICU for monitoring of critically ill patients with circulatory shock.
- Major surgery such as cardiothoracic surgery or major abdominal surgery.
- When noninvasive blood pressure measurements are unreliable or difficult such as with severe burns or trauma.

Contraindications

Common contraindications of arterial cannulation are:

- Severe peripheral vascular diseases, arterial atherosclerosis, insufficient collateral perfusion, or absent pulse.
- Anticoagulation therapy or the presence of coagulopathy.

Radial or femoral, which artery to select for the cannulation?

The radial artery is a common choice because of easy cannulation due to its superficial position, the adequate collateral blood supply to the hand via the ulnar artery (reduces the risk of hand ischemia due to catheter induced thrombosis of radial artery), low rates of complications, easy to compress for the control of bleeding during cannulation or following its removal, and early ambulation [74–77]. Perform the modified Allen test before cannulation of the radial artery to assess the collateral circulation to the hands.

The limitations of the radial arterial cannulation approach are:

- Significantly smaller average lumen diameter (less than 3 mm) makes the trans-radial approach difficult in small-sized patients.

- Higher risk of thrombosis and nerve injury.

- Locating the radial artery via palpation may be difficult in patients with severe hypotension, morbid obesity, and weak pulse due to atherosclerosis.

- In patients with severe peripheral vasoconstriction and sicker patients on higher vasopressor doses, the value of radial arterial blood pressure is lower and may underestimate the central blood pressure [78–80].

The femoral artery is the second most common cannulation site [81], but the trend to use the femoral artery first is increasing in many patients with critical illness [80] because:

- It is easiest to cannulate and therefore provides faster access during emergencies in patients with shock. In severely hypotensive patients with nonpalpable peripheral pulses, greater ease in locating and cannulating due to its large lumen.

- There may be discrepancies between radial and femoral arterial blood pressure measurements. However, patients with severe hypotension on higher vasopressor doses and hypothermia femoral approach provide accurate blood pressure measurement [82, 83]. So, the femoral approach of arterial cannulation is beneficial in high-risk patients undergoing longer surgical interventions and helps to avoid inappropriate administration of vasopressors and/or inotropic agents [84].

- More reliable functioning and less likely to fail because of inaccuracy, blockage, or accidental removal [85].

- The radial artery is thin, not palpable, or there may be contra-indication to intra-arterial catheter placement at the wrist in certain patients [86].

The limitations of the femoral arterial cannulation approach are:

- Higher risk of arterial catheter-related infection [87, 88].

- Limits mobility significantly, and in alert patients, delays ambulation.

- Difficult to control or prevent bleeding (unlike radial artery), carries a great risk of retroperitoneal hematoma, and its diagnosis is often delayed [86].

PULMONARY ARTERY CATHETER MONITORING

The pulmonary artery catheter (PAC) is an invasive diagnostic procedure in which a catheter is inserted through a central vein into a pulmonary artery. PAC was used widely and considered the gold standard for measuring cardiac output in the past. But currently, PAC is used sparingly for the management of critically ill or perioperative patients [89].

Description

A pulmonary artery or Swan-Ganz catheter is a pliable catheter made from polyvinyl chloride material with a four lumen and a thermodilution sensor.

Two ports, including the Red port used for balloon inflation and the Yellow port, along with the thermodilution sensor, open within the pulmonary artery lumen, while the remaining two ports, the Proximal (Blue) port, and the White port (Clear lumen), open within the right atrium, as summarized in Table 17.1.

Technique

For the measurement of pulmonary artery occlusion pressure (PAOP), the pulmonary artery or Swan-Ganz flexible balloon-tipped, flow-directed catheter is introduced through a large vein and is placed with the tip in a distal pulmonary artery. PAC is an invasive multi-lumen central line placed through a large vein such as an internal jugular, subclavian, or femoral vein.

By using a flow-directed balloon flotation technique and utilizing pressure waveform and or fluoroscopy/echocardiographic guidance, PAC traverses along with venous blood into the vena cava (superior or inferior), right atrium, tricuspid valve, right ventricle, pulmonic valve and finally placed in the pulmonary artery [90]. Continuous monitoring of catheter tip pressure provides clues about the position of the tip of the catheter that guides the clinician to traverse the catheter to the pulmonary artery. In addition, the X-ray chest and wedge pressure waveform helps to confirm the location of PAC [91].

What information does PAC provide?

PAC provides important information by directly measuring cardiac pressures (central venous pressure, right atrial and ventricular pressures, pulmonary arterial pressure, pulmonary artery occlusion pressure) and cardiac output [57, 92]. In addition, PAC also indirectly measures systemic and pulmonary vascular resistance, cardiac index, stroke volume, oxygen delivery, and mixed venous oxygen saturation (SvO_2).

Pulmonary artery occlusion pressure (PAOP)

Also known as pulmonary arterial wedge pressure (PAWP) or pulmonary capillary wedge pressure (PCWP), is a technique to measure pulmonary venous pressure and left atrial pressure indirectly by using PAC. In this method, the tip of a

	Location	Description	Function
Table 17.1 Sensor and lumens of pulmonary artery catheter			
Thermodilution sensor	Within the pulmonary artery lumen	Located 4 cm from the tip, proximal to the balloon	It measures the blood temperature in the pulmonary artery and assists in calculating cardiac output using the thermodilution technique
Lumen or ports			
Red port Balloon inflation port	Within the pulmonary artery lumen	It terminates in the balloon at the tip of the catheter, located approximately 2 cm from the distal end	The red port is used solely for inflating and deflating the balloon by using a custom syringe and air
Thermistor lumen Distal port Yellow port		The distal port terminates at the tip of the 110 cm long catheter, which should be positioned in the pulmonary artery	The yellow port useful for measuring pulmonary artery pressure, mixed venous samples, and allows continuous cardiac output monitoring
Proximal lumen Blue port CVP port	Within the right atrium	Located 30 cm from the tip of the catheter and rests within the right atrium	It is utilized for measuring and monitoring CVP, right atrial pressure as well as for fluid and drug administration
White port Clear lumen		Located 31 cm from the tip of the catheter and rests within the right atrium	The white port is used for infusing fluids and drugs

PAC is placed into a smaller, more distal pulmonary arterial branch. When the balloon at the distal tip of the PAC is inflated, it obstructs the forward blood flow in the distal branch of the pulmonary artery, and subsequently, measurements are obtained.

The pulmonary artery is in direct continuity with the left atrium and, therefore, with the left ventricle during diastole. So, PAOP, in addition to measurement of left atrial pressure, during diastole, reflects left ventricular end-diastolic pressure (LVEDP) and determines left ventricle (LV) function when mitral valve function is normal.

Cardiac output

PAC measures CO invasively using the thermodilution principle and was considered the gold standard method. Details about the same are covered in the invasive systems part of the Chapter 19 on "Cardiac Output Monitoring."

Mixed venous oxygen saturation (SvO$_2$)

It is a measurement of oxygen saturation from a blood sample from the pulmonary artery through a PAC. SvO$_2$ is the oxygen content of the blood that returns to the heart and is determined by cardiac output, hemoglobin concentration, oxygen supply (ventilatory settings, fraction of inspired oxygen, etc.), and tissue oxygen consumption [90].

Important causes of low SvO$_2$ are low or inadequate cardiac output, anemia, hypoxemia, or increased O$_2$ demand (sepsis, hyperthermia, burns, seizures, or shivering). The normal value of SvO$_2$ is 60–80%, and SvO$_2$ less than 65% is of poor prognostic value [93]. SvO$_2$ below 60% poses a serious risk of tissue hypoxia and needs urgent corrective measures.

Use of PAC in clinical practice. When and why?

The use of the PAC has decreased substantially and is not used routinely in most critically ill patients because:

1. PAC is a highly invasive technique with several complications. With the availability of less invasive hemodynamic monitoring techniques, the use of the PAC has declined in the last three decades [57, 94–96].

2. PAC failed to improve the outcome and survival [97–101].

3. Measurements of cardiac output by PAC are frequently inaccurate in critically ill patients [102, 103].

4. Static parameter like pulmonary artery occlusion pressure does not predict fluid volume [104, 105] or fluid responsiveness and therefore is not useful in fluid management in critically ill patients [106–108].

Indications

The unique feature of PAC monitoring is that it can directly measure the pressures in the right heart and pulmonary circulation [109]. PAC is the only device that efficiently assesses and continuously monitors the right ventricle function [110].

Currently, the use of PAC must be restricted to very few selected critically ill patients and complex clinical situations [92]. The most frequent indications are [2, 64, 111–113]:

- To differentiate the causes of various unexplained or multi-factorial shock states. PAC helps to differentiate cardiogenic and non-cardiogenic causes of severe shock.

- To evaluate right ventricular heart failure, pulmonary edema, pulmonary hypertension, or refractory shock, and helps in the planning of more precise fluid, inotropes, vasodilators, and diuretics treatment.

- Perioperatively in high-risk patients with severe pulmonary hypertension and acute right ventricular failure, PAC helps in the proper administration of fluids and vasopressors.

- To diagnose cardiac tamponade or constrictive pericarditis when clinical and echocardiographic findings are not conclusive.

- Preoperative assessment of intracardiac shunt, congenital heart disease, or right-sided valvular disease.

Complications

The common complications which may occur from the use of the PAC are cardiac arrhythmias, pulmonary artery rupture or thrombosis, pulmonary hemorrhage, balloon rupture, pneumothorax, catheter malposition or intra-cardiac knotting, tricuspid or pulmonary valve injury, right atrial thrombosis, internal jugular/subclavian vein stenosis, venous thromboembolism, electromechanical dissociation, and right-sided endocarditis and catheter-related bloodstream infection.

REFERENCES

1. Levitov A, Frankel HL, Blaivas M, et al. Guidelines for the appropriate use of bedside general and cardiac ultrasonography in the evaluation of critically ill patients - Part II: Cardiac ultrasonography. Crit Care Med. 2016;44(6):1206–27.

2. Cecconi M, De Backer D, Antonelli M, et al. Consensus on circulatory shock and hemodynamic monitoring. Task force of the European Society of Intensive Care Medicine. Intensive Care Med. 2014;40(12):1795–815.

3. Schmidt GA. POINT: Should acute fluid resuscitation be guided primarily by inferior vena cava ultrasound for patients in shock? Yes Chest. 2017;151(3):531–532.

4. Charbonneau H, Riu B, Faron M, et al. Predicting preload responsiveness using simultaneous recordings of inferior and superior vena cavae diameters. Crit Care. 2014;18(5):473.

5. Vignon P, Repesse X, Begot E, et al. Comparison of echocardiographic indices used to predict fluid responsiveness in ventilated patients. Am J Respir Crit Care Med. 2017;195(8):1022–1032.

6. Miller A, Mandeville J. Predicting and measuring fluid responsiveness with echocardiography. Echo Res Pract. 2016;3(2):G1–G12.

7. Muller L, Bobbia X, Toumi M, et al. Respiratory variations of inferior vena cava diameter to predict fluid responsiveness in spontaneously breathing patients with acute circulatory failure: need for a cautious use. Crit Care. 2012;16(5):R188.

8. Yanagawa Y, Sakamoto T, Okada Y. Hypovolemic shock evaluated by sonographic measurement of inferior vena cava during resuscitation in trauma patients. J Trauma. 2007;63(6):1245–8.

9. Airapetian N, Maizel J, Alyamani O, et al. Does inferior vena cava respiratory variability predict fluid responsiveness in spontaneously breathing patients? Crit Care. 2015;19:400.

10. Vieillard-Baron A, Evrard B, Repesse X, et al. Limited value of end-expiratory inferior vena cava diameter to predict fluid responsiveness impact of intra-abdominal pressure. Intensive Care Med 2018;44(2):197–203.

11. Marx G, Schindler AW, Mosch C, et al. Intravascular volume therapy in adults: guidelines from the Association of the Scientific Medical Societies in Germany. Eur J Anesthesiol. 2016;33(7):488–521.

12. Yanagawa Y, Nishi K, Sakamoto T, et al. Early diagnosis of hypovolemic shock by sonographic measurement of inferior vena cava in trauma patients. J Trauma. 2005;58(4):825–9.

13. Dipti A, Soucy Z, Surana A, et al. Role of inferior vena cava diameter in assessment of volume status: a meta-analysis. Am J Emerg Med. 2012;30(8):1414–1419.e1.

14. Furtado S, Reis L. Inferior vena cava evaluation in fluid therapy decision making in intensive care: practical implications. Rev. bras. ter. intensiva [online]. 2019;31(2):240–247.

15. Lee CW, Kory PD, Arntfield RT. Development of a fluid resuscitation protocol using inferior vena cava and lung ultrasound. J Crit Care. 2016;31(1):96–100.

16. Jardin F, Vieillard-Baron A. Ultrasonographic examination of the venae cavae. Intensive Care Med. 2006;32(2):203–206.

17. Millington SJ. Ultrasound assessment of the inferior vena cava for fluid responsiveness: easy, fun, but unlikely to be helpful Can J Anesth/J Can Anesth 2019;66(6):633–638.

18. Si X, Xu H, Liu Z, et al. Does respiratory variation in inferior vena cava diameter predict fluid responsiveness in mechanically ventilated patients? A systematic review and meta-analysis. Anesth Analg. 2018;127(5):1157–1164.

19. De Backer D, Fagnoul D. Intensive Care Ultrasound: VI. Fluid Responsiveness and Shock Assessment. Am Thorac Soc. 2014;11(1):129–36.

20. Zhang Z, Xu X, Ye S, et al. Ultrasonographic measurement of the respiratory variation in the inferior vena cava diameter is predictive of fluid responsiveness in critically ill patients: systematic review and meta-analysis. Ultrasound Med Biol. 2014;40(5):845–53.

21. Long E, Oakley E, Duke T, et al. Paediatric Research in Emergency Departments International Collaborative (PREDICT). Does respiratory variation in inferior vena cava diameter predict fluid responsiveness: A systematic review and meta-analysis. Shock 2017;47(5):550–559.

22. Kory P. COUNTERPOINT: should acute fluid resuscitation be guided primarily by inferior vena cava ultrasound for patients in shock? No. Chest. 2017;151(3):533–536.

23. Schmidt GA. Rebuttal from Dr Schmidt. Chest. 2017;151(3):536–537.

24. Kory P. Rebuttal from Dr Kory. Chest. 2017;151(3):537–538.

25. Barbier C, Loubieres Y, Schmit C, et al. Respiratory changes in inferior vena cava diameter are helpful in predicting fluid responsiveness in ventilated septic patients. Intensive Care Med 2004;30(9):1740–6.

26. Feissel M, Michard F, Faller JP, et al. The respiratory variation in inferior vena cava diameter as a guide to fluid therapy. Intensive Care Med 2004;30(9):1834–1837.

27. Moretti R, Pizzi B. Inferior vena cava distensibility as a predictor of fluid responsiveness in patients with subarachnoid hemorrhage. Neurocrit Care. 2010;13(1):3–9.

28. Machare-Delgado E, Decaro M, Marik PE. Inferior vena cava variation compared to pulse contour analysis as predictors of fluid responsiveness: a prospective cohort study. J Intensive Care Med 2011;26(2):116–24.

29. Mandeville JC, Colebourn CL. Can transthoracic echocardiography be used to predict fluid responsiveness in the critically ill patient? A systematic review. Crit Care Res Pract 2012;2012:513480.

30. Lu N, Xi X, Jiang L, et al. Exploring the best predictors of fluid responsiveness in patients with septic shock. Am J Emerg Med 2017;35(9):1258–1261.

31. Huang H, Shen Q, Liu Y, et al. Value of variation index of inferior vena cava diameter in predicting fluid responsiveness in patients with circulatory shock receiving mechanical ventilation: a systematic review and meta-analysis. Crit Care 2018;22(1):204.

32. Mohammad AWM, Saad-eldeen ES, Mohammad EK, et al. Distensibility index of inferior vena cava and pulse pressure variation as predictors of fluid responsiveness in mechanically ventilated shocked patients. Journal of Emergency Medicine, Trauma & Acute Care 2020;2020(1).

33. Sobczyk D, Nycz K, Andruszkiewicz P, et al. Ultrasonographic caval indices do not significantly contribute to predicting fluid responsiveness immediately after coronary artery bypass grafting when compared to passive leg raising. Cardiovasc Ultrasound 2016;14(1):23.

34. Zhang H, Zhang Q, Chen X, et al. Respiratory variations of inferior vena cava fail to predict fluid responsiveness in mechanically ventilated patients with isolated left ventricular dysfunction. Ann. Intensive Care 2019;9(1):113.

35. Orso D, Paoli I, Piani T, et al. Accuracy of ultrasonographic measurements of inferior vena cava to determine fluid responsiveness: a systematic review and meta-analysis. J Intensive Care Med. 2020;35(4):354–363.

36. Sarıtaş A, Zincircioğlu Ç, Uzun SP, et al. Comparison of inferior vena cava collapsibility, distensibility, and delta indices at different positive pressure supports and prediction values of indices for intravascular volume status. Turk J Med Sci. 2019;49(4):1170–1178.

37. Farcy DA, Jain A, Dalley M, et al. Pitfalls in using central venous pressure as a marker of fluid responsiveness. Emerg Med 2016;48(1):18–28.

38. Vieillard-Baron A, Chergui K, Rabiller A, et al. Superior vena caval collapsibility as a gauge of volume status in ventilated septic patients. Intensive Care Med 2004;30(9):1734–1739.

39. Lanspa MJ, Grissom CK, Hirshberg EL, et al. Applying dynamic parameters to predict hemodynamic response to volume expansion in spontaneously breathing patients with septic shock. Shock. 2013;39(2):155–60.

40. Preau S, Bortolotti P, Colling D, et al. Diagnostic accuracy of the inferior vena cava collapsibility to predict fluid responsiveness in spontaneously breathing patients with sepsis and acute circulatory failure. Crit Care Med. 2017;45(3):e290–e297.

41. Corl KA, George NR, Romanoff J, et al. Inferior vena cava collapsibility detects fluid responsiveness among spontaneously breathing critically-ill patients. J Crit Care. 2017;41:130–137.

42. Bortolotti P. Inferior vena cava respiratory variations. A useful tool at bedside to guide fluid therapy in spontaneously breathing patients. SHOCK 2018;49(2):235–236.

43. Bortolotti P, Colling D, Colas V, et al. Respiratory changes of the inferior vena cava diameter predict fluid responsiveness in spontaneously breathing patients with cardiac arrhythmias. Ann. Intensive Care 2018;8(1):79.

44. Szabó M, Bozó A, Darvas K, et al. Role of inferior vena cava collapsibility index in the prediction of hypotension associated with general anesthesia: an observational study. BMC Anesthesiol 2019;19:139.

45. Williams K, Ablordeppey E, Theodoro D, et al. The diagnostic accuracy of inferior vena cava collapsibility versus passive leg raise testing in determining volume responsiveness in emergency department patients with shock. Proceedings of the 40th Critical Care Congress, Society of Critical Care Congress. Crit Care Med 2011;39:8.

46. Corl K, Napoli AM, Gardiner F. Bedside sonographic measurement of the inferior vena cava caval index is a poor predictor of fluid responsiveness in emergency department patients. Emerg Med Australas. 2012;24(5):534–539.

47. Juhl-Olsen P, Vistisen ST, Christiansen LK, et al. Ultrasound of the inferior vena cava does not predict hemodynamic response to early hemorrhage. J Emerg Med 2013;45(4):592–597.

48. De Valk S, Olgers TJ, Holman M, et al. The caval index: an adequate non-invasive ultrasound parameter to predict fluid responsiveness in the emergency department? BMC Anesthesiology. 2014;14:114.

49. Block J, Mackenzie D. Fluid Responsiveness in a Hemodynamically Unstable Patient. EMresident15 Dec

2018 Visit: https://www.emra.org/emresident/article/fluid-responsiveness/.

50. McIntyre LA, Hébert PC, Fergusson D, et al. Canadian Critical Care Trials Group. A survey of Canadian intensivists' resuscitation practices in early septic shock. Crit Care. 2007;11(4):R74.

51. Cannesson M, Pestel G, Ricks C, et al. Hemodynamic monitoring and management in patients undergoing high risk surgery: a survey among North American and European anesthesiologists. Crit Care. 2011;15(4):R197.

52. Gelman S. Venous function and central venous pressure: a physiologic story. Anesthesiology. 2008;108(4):735–48.

53. Shojaee M, Sabzghabaei A, Alimohammadi H, et al. Effect of positive end-expiratory pressure on central venous pressure in patients under mechanical ventilation. Emerg (Tehran). 2017;5(1):e1.

54. Cecconi M, Hofer C, Teboul JL, et al. Fluid challenges in intensive care: the FENICE study: a global inception cohort study. Intensive Care Med 2015;41(9):1529–37.

55. Marik PE, Baram M, Vahid B. Does the central venous pressure predict fluid responsiveness? A systematic review of the literature and the tale of seven mares. Chest. 2008;134(1):172–8.

56. Marik PE, Cavallazzi R. Does the Central Venous Pressure (CVP) predict fluid responsiveness: An update meta-analysis and a plea for some common sense. Crit Care Med. 2013;41(7):1774–81.

57. Martin ND, Codner P, Greene W, et al. Contemporary hemodynamic monitoring, fluid responsiveness, volume optimization, and endpoints of resuscitation: an AAST critical care committee clinical consensus. Trauma Surg Acute Care Open 2020;5(1):e000411.

58. Chen C, Zhou Y, Wang P, et al. Elevated central venous pressure is associated with increased mortality and acute kidney injury in critically ill patients: a meta-analysis. Crit Care 2020;24(1):80.

59. Magder S. Value of CVP: an epidemiological or physiological question? Intensive Care Med 2016;42(3):458–459.

60. Eskesen TG, Wetterslev M, Perner A. Systematic review including re-analyses of 1148 individual data sets of central venous pressure as a predictor of fluid responsiveness. Intensive Care Med. 2016;42(3):324–332.

61. Biais M, Ehrmann S, Mari A, et al. Clinical relevance of pulse pressure variations for predicting fluid responsiveness in mechanically ventilated intensive care unit patients: the grey zone approach. Crit Care. 2014;18(6):587.

62. De Backer D, Vincent J. Should we measure the central venous pressure to guide fluid management? Ten answers to 10 questions. Crit Care 2018;22(1):43.

63. Rivers E, Nguyen B, Havstadt S, et al. Early goal-directed therapy in the treatment of severe sepsis and septic shock. N Engl J Med. 2001;345(19):1368–77.

64. Teboul JL, Saugel B, Cecconi M, et al. Less invasive hemodynamic monitoring in critically ill patients. Intensive Care Med. 2016;42(9):1350–1359.

65. Su L, Pan P, Li D, et al. Central Venous Pressure (CVP) reduction associated with higher Cardiac Output (CO) favors good prognosis of circulatory shock: a single-center, retrospective cohort study. Front Med (Lausanne). 2019;6:216.

66. Pinsky MR, Kellum JA, Bellomo R. Central venous pressure is a stopping rule, not a target of fluid resuscitation. Crit Care Resus 2014;16(4):245–246.

67. Boyd JH, Forbes J, Nakada TA, et al. Fluid resuscitation in septic shock: a positive fluid balance and elevated central venous pressure are associated with increased mortality. Crit Care Med. 2011;39(2):259–65.

68. Marik PE. Iatrogenic salt water drowning and the hazards of a high central venous pressure. Ann Intensive Care. 2014;4:21.

69. Lee J, De Louw E, Niemi M, et al. Association between fluid balance and survival in critically ill patients. J Intern Med. 2015;277(4):468–77.

70. Sondergaard S, Parkin G, Aneman A. Central venous pressure: soon an outcome-associated matter. Curr Opin Anaesthesiol. 2016;29(2):179–85.

71. Li D, Wang X, Liu D. Association between elevated central venous pressure and outcomes in critically ill patients. Ann. Intensive Care 2017;7(1):83.

72. Mullens W, Abrahams Z, Francis GS, et al. Importance of venous congestion for worsening of renal function in advanced decompensated heart failure. J Am Coll Cardiol. 2009;53(7):589–96.

73. Sen S, Chini EN, Michael J, et al. Complications after unintentional intra-arterial injection of drugs: risks, outcomes, and management strategies. Mayo Clin Proc. 2005;80(6):783–795.

74. Brzezinski M, Luisetti T, London MJ. Radial artery cannulation: a comprehensive review of recent anatomic and physiologic investigations. Anesth Analg. 2009;109(6):1763–81.

75. O'Grady NP, Alexander M, Burns LA, et al. Summary of recommendations: Guidelines for the Prevention of Intravascular Catheter-related Infections. Clin Infect Dis. 2011;52(9):1087–99.

76. Miller AG, Bardin AJ. Review of ultrasound-guided radial artery catheter placement. Respir Care. 2016;61(3):383–8.

77. Scheer B, Perel A, Pfeiffer UJ. Clinical review: complications and risk factors of peripheral arterial catheters used for hemodynamic monitoring in anaesthesia and intensive care medicine. Crit Care. 2002;6(3):199–204.

78. Camporota L, Beale R. Pitfalls in hemodynamic monitoring based on the arterial pressure waveform. Crit Care 2010;14(2):124.

79. Hatib F, Jansen JR, Pinsky MR. Peripheral vascular decoupling in porcine endotoxic shock. J Appl Physiol. 2011;111(3):853–60.

80. Farkas J. PulmCrit: A-lines in septic shock: the wrist versus the groin. Aug 2018 Visit: https://emcrit.org/pulmcrit/a-line/.

81. Koyuncu O, Leung S, Asha SA, et al. The present and future of indwelling arterial catheter: An anesthesiologist's perspective. Clin Res Trials, 2016;2(2):157–158.

82. Galluccio ST, Chapman MJ, Finnis ME. Femoral-radial arterial pressure gradients in critically ill patients. Crit Care Resusc. 2009;11(1):34–38.

83. Kim W, Jun J, Huh J, et al. Radial to femoral arterial blood pressure differences in septic shock patients receiving high-dose norepinephrine therapy. Shock. 2013;40(6):527–531.

84. Fuda G, Denault A, Deschamps A, et al. Risk factors involved in central-to-radial arterial pressure gradient during cardiac surgery. Anesth Analg. 2016;122(3):624–632.

85. Greer M, Carney S, McPheeters R, et al. Radial arterial lines have a higher failure rate than femoral. West J Emerg Med. 2018;19(2):364–371.

86. Lakhal K, Robert-Edan V. Invasive monitoring of blood pressure: a radiant future for brachial artery as an alternative to radial artery catheterisation? J Thorac Dis. 2017;9(12):4812–4816.

87. Lorente L, Santacreu R, Martín MM, et al. Arterial catheter-related infection of 2,949 catheters. Crit Care 2006;10(3):R83.

88. O'Horo JC, Maki DG, Krupp AE, et al. Arterial catheters as a source of bloodstream infection: a systematic review and meta-analysis. Crit Care Med 2014;42(6):1334–9.

89. Kalantari K, Chang JN, Ronco C, et al. Assessment of intravascular volume status and volume responsiveness in critically ill patients. Kidney Int. 2013;83(6):1017–28.

90. Lee CP, Bora V. Anesthesia monitoring of mixed venous saturation. StatPearls [Internet]. Feb 2020 Visit: https://www.ncbi.nlm.nih.gov/books/NBK539835/.

91. Nickson C. Pulmonary Artery Catheter. Life in the Fast Lane CCC. Sept 2019 Visit: https://litfl.com/pulmonary-artery-catheter/.

92. Demiselle J, Mercat A, Asfar P. Is there still a place for the Swan–Ganz catheter? Yes. Intensive Care Med 2018;44(6):954–956.

93. Hartog C, Bloos F. Venous oxygen saturation. Best Pract Res Clin Anaesthesiol. 2014;28(4):419–28.

94. Litton E, Morgan M. The PiCCO monitor: a review. Anaesthesia and intensive care. 2012;40(3):393–409.

95. Seifi A, Elliott RJ, Elshety MA. Usage of Swan-Ganz catheterization during the past 2 decades in United States. J Crit Care 2016;35:213–4.

96. De Backer D, Vincent JL. The pulmonary artery catheter: is it still alive? Current Opinion in Critical Care 2018;24(3):204–208.

97. Richard C, Warszawski J, Anguel N, et al. Early use of the pulmonary artery catheter and outcomes in patients with shock and acute respiratory distress syndrome: a randomized controlled trial. Journal of the American Medical Association 2003;290(20):2713–20.

98. Harvey S, Harrison DA, Singer M, et al. Assessment of the clinical effectiveness of pulmonary artery catheters in management of patients in intensive care (PAC-Man): a randomised controlled trial. Lancet. 2005;366(9484):472–7.

99. National Heart, Lung, and Blood Institute Acute Respiratory Distress Syndrome (ARDS) Clinical Trials Network, Wheeler AP, et al. Pulmonary-artery versus central venous catheter to guide treatment of acute lung injury. N Engl J Med. 2006;354(21):2213–24.

100. Harvey S, Young D, Brampton W, et al. Pulmonary artery catheters for adult patients in intensive care. Cochrane Database Syst Rev. 2006;(3):CD003408.

101. Rajaram SS, Desai NK, Kalra A, et al. Pulmonary artery catheters for adult patients in intensive care. Cochrane Database of Systematic Reviews 2013;2013(2):CD003408.

102. Phillips RA, Hood SG, Jacobson BM, et al. Pulmonary artery catheter (PAC) accuracy and efficacy compared with flow probe and transcutaneous Doppler (USCOM): an ovine cardiac output validation. Crit Care Res Pract 2012;2012:621494.

103. Marik PE. Obituary: pulmonary artery catheter 1970 to 2013. Ann Intensive Care. 2013;3(1):38.

104. Kumar A, Anel R, Bunnell E, et al. Pulmonary artery occlusion pressure and central venous pressure fail to predict ventricular filling volume, cardiac performance, or the response to volume infusion in normal subjects. Crit Care Med. 2004;32(3):691–9.

105. Oohashi S, Endoh H, Oohashi S, et al. Does central venous pressure or pulmonary capillary wedge pressure reflect the status of circulating blood volume in patients after extended transthoracic esophagectomy? J Anesth 2005;19(1):21–25.

106. Keller G, Sinavsky K, Desebbe O, et al. Combination of continuous pulse pressure variation monitoring and cardiac filling pressure to predict fluid responsiveness. J Clin Monit Comput. 2012;26(6):401–5.

107. Michard F, Teboul JL. Predicting fluid responsiveness in ICU patients: a critical analysis of the evidence. Chest. 2002;121(6):2000–2008.

108. Osman D, Ridel C, Ray P, et al. Cardiac filling pressures are not appropriate to predict hemodynamic response to volume challenge. Crit Care Med 2007;35(1):64–68.

109. Huygh J, Peeters Y, Bernards J, et al. Hemodynamic monitoring in the critically ill: an overview of current cardiac output monitoring methods. F1000Res. 2016;5:F1000.

110. Ventetuolo CE, Klinger JR. Management of acute right ventricular failure in the intensive care unit. Ann Am Thorac Soc 2014;11(5):811–822.

111. Chatterjee K. The Swan-Ganz catheters: past, present, and future. A viewpoint. Circulation. 2009;119(1):147–52.

112. Rhodes A, Evans LE, Alhazzani W, et al. Surviving Sepsis Campaign: International Guidelines for Management of Sepsis and Septic Shock: 2016. Intensive Care Med. 2017;43(3):304–377.

113. Ziccardi MR, Khalid N. Pulmonary Artery Catheterization. StatPearls [Internet]. Feb 2020 (Visit: https://www.ncbi.nlm.nih.gov/books/NBK482170/).

18 | Fluid Responsiveness: Provocative Techniques and Dynamic Parameters

Detection of fluid responsiveness is essential as it helps clinicians for the proper fluid management in critically ill patients. Various techniques are available to assess fluid responsiveness in hemodynamically unstable patients, including pulse pressure variation (PPV) and stroke volume variation (SVV), which are common dynamic measurements based on cardiopulmonary interaction derived from arterial waveform analysis.

Additionally, the plethysmographic variability index (PVI) is a simple, easily doable, noninvasive, and dynamic method that accurately predicts fluid responsiveness in mechanically ventilated patients by continuously and automatically estimating respiratory variations in the pulse oximeter waveform.

PROVOCATIVE TECHNIQUES TO DETECT FLUID RESPONSIVENESS

Why is it important to differentiate between fluid responsive from fluid nonresponsive patients by hemodynamic monitoring?

In hemodynamically unstable patients, prompt and adequate fluid administration is essential to increase blood volume, which increases venous return, cardiac output (CO), and organ perfusion. Assessment of volume responsiveness is vital in such patients because with fluid boluses, only 50% of patients with shock are benefited, and excess fluid may worsen patient outcomes [1, 2].

In which patients fluid responsiveness should be tested?

Patients do not require a test for fluid responsiveness if hypovolemia is evident on clinical examination. Avoid fluid challenge if volume overload is obvious clinically. Fluid responsiveness should be tested in hemodynamically unstable patients if fluid losses are not apparent.

Which dynamic methods are used to detect fluid responsiveness?

The use of dynamic variables is preferred over static variables to predict fluid responsiveness [3]. The fluid challenge, passive leg raising, and end-expiratory occlusion test are reliable provocative, dynamic methods used for the assessment of fluid status, which detects or unmasks the fluid responsive

Method	Fluid challenge	Passive leg raising	End-expiratory occlusion test
Nature	Non-invasive	Non-invasive	Invasive
Ventilation mode	Spontaneous	Spontaneous	Mechanical
Technique	Intravenous fluid loading	Internal volume challenge	Internal volume challenge
Effect of maneuver	Non-reversible	Reversible	Reversible
Parameters assessed	Cardiac output	Cardiac output	Cardiac output
Threshold	15% standard FC 6% mini FC	10%	5%
Methods to measure CO	Needs a very precise technique	Direct continuous measurement of CO	Direct continuous measurement of CO
	PCA, echocardiography	PCA, echocardiography, or bioreactance	PCA, echocardiography
Limitations/Exclusion criteria	Risk of volume overload	High intra-abdominal pressures, head trauma, and movement of the legs are not compatible	Non-intubated patients, 15 second respiration hold is not possible

Table 18.1 Summary of provocative dynamic methods to detect fluid responsiveness

ARDS: Acute respiratory distress syndrome; CO: Cardiac output; FC: Fluid challenge; PCA: Pulse contour analysis

state (Table 18.1). For the assessment of fluid responsiveness, parameters such as pulse pressure variation, stroke volume variation, Plethysmograph variability index, and cardiac output are measured with commercially available various devices and monitors.

Fluid challenge

In the fluid challenge, a small amount of fluid is administered quickly, and the left ventricle's ability to increase stroke volume (SV) is assessed precisely [4, 5].

Fluid challenge (FC) is an effective diagnostic intervention designed to identify the "fluid responsiveness" in hemodynamic compromise patients. The fluid challenge guides clinicians to administer the optimum volume of fluid to avoid over and under-fluid resuscitation [6]. The fluid challenge is usually performed in patients with hypotension and oliguria [7].

Balanced crystalloid solutions are usually preferred for the fluid challenge because the selection of the type of fluid does not affect the proportion of fluid responders [8]. Usually, 500 mL crystalloid is administered over 20–30 minutes (or 200–250 mL is administered over 5–10 minutes) [2, 7].

How to assess the response to the fluid challenge?

The "fluid responsiveness" cannot be predicted by heart rate, blood pressure measurements, clinical signs, or static hemodynamic parameters such as central venous pressure (CVP) or pulmonary artery occlusion pressure (PAOP) [9, 10].

The current recommendation is to monitor dynamic over static hemodynamic parameters after fluid challenge to predict the "fluid responsiveness" in mechanically ventilated patients [3, 10]. Even in spontaneously breathing patients, respiratory changes in dynamic parameters after fluid challenge predicts "fluid responsiveness" [11].

Cardiac output monitoring is used to assess pulse pressure variation, stroke volume, stroke volume variation, and cardiac index. Precise monitoring of these parameters is essential because the maximal effect on cardiac output occurs approximately one minute after the fluid challenge is over [12].

Which criteria define fluid responsiveness in the fluid challenge?

Usual parameters suggestive of fluid responsiveness are 10–15% increase in stroke volume [4] with a ≥15% increase in cardiac index [7]. Only fluid responsiveness patients should receive additional fluids [13].

Why is large volume fluid administration avoided for the fluid challenge?

The standard challenge with 300–500 mL of fluid is more a treatment than a test and, when repeated, carries the potential risk of volume overload. Volume overload is deleterious and probably more harmful than hypovolemia [14]. Potential harms of large volume fluid bolus are hypervolemia, pulmonary edema, bowel wall edema, endothelial glycocalyx damage, increased vascular permeability, tissue hypoxia, and organ dysfunctions [15, 16].

Positive fluid balance also increases the risk of acute kidney injury, slower recovery in acute respiratory distress syndrome, and higher mortality [17–21].

After large volume fluid bolus, clinical and physiological improvement occurs initially, but no long-term improvement, and on the contrary, causes higher mortality due to delayed cardiovascular collapse [22–24].

Why hemodynamics improvement following fluid bolus is short-lived?

Short-lived hemodynamics improvement following fluid bolus is because of rapid "Third" Spacing. In critical patients with leaky capillaries, 95% of the infused fluid shifts to interstitial space within 90 minutes, so transient benefit is lost rapidly [21, 25].

What is a mini-fluid challenge?

A mini-fluid challenge is an alternative approach that can reliably predict fluid responsiveness without a large amount of fluid infusion and the potential risk of fluid overload [26–29].

Protocols in the mini-fluid challenge includes:

- 100 ml of the crystalloid bolus is infused rapidly over one minute [26].
- A fluid bolus of 4 mL/kg of a balanced crystalloid solution is quickly infused over 5 minutes [30].

Fluid responsiveness in the mini-fluid challenge can be reliably predicted by velocity-time integral (VTI) measured by transthoracic echocardiography [29], pulse contour analysis derived from cardiac output [26], or changes in SVV [31]. As a small volume of fluid administration causes small and short-lived hemodynamic changes, response assessment should be monitored by very sensitive and precise techniques [26].

Passive leg raising test

The passive leg raising (PLR) test is a simple, safe, reliable non-invasive, and reproducible bedside test to evaluate fluid responsiveness in patients with spontaneous breathing, on a ventilator, low lung compliance, and even in the presence of cardiac arrhythmias [32–36]. Three metanalyses have confirmed the role of the PLR test in the assessment of fluid responsiveness [33, 37, 38].

In the PLR test, about 300 mL of blood from the lower extremities' veins is transferred into the thorax, which increases cardiac output [39]. The temporary gravitational shift of venous blood into the central circulation mimics a fluid challenge. Prediction of fluid responsiveness without administering a single drop of fluid avoids the risks of fluid overload. Rapidly reversible hemodynamic effects and no need for mechanical ventilation or sedation are the advantages of this test.

How to perform the passive leg raising test?

The basic method to perform the PLR test is [40]:

- Start the test by placing the patient 45 degrees head-up semi-recumbent (and not supine position) for 3 minutes and obtain the baseline hemodynamic values.

- The next step is to lower the patient's upper body and head to the horizontal position and passively raise legs at 45 degrees by changing the bed position (i.e., not manually) and holding in this position for one minute. Immediately assess the effects of PLR by obtaining the hemodynamic values again.

- As hemodynamic effects of the PLR test are short-term and transient, obtain the subsequent hemodynamic values fast within the first 90 seconds following leg elevation.

Assessment of the effect of the PLR test and its clinical utility

- To assess the hemodynamic effect of the PLR test, techniques which directly measure cardiac output should be used rather than methods that measure arterial pressure or pulse pressure [40]. Direct

measurement of cardiac output is the more reliable hemodynamic parameter to assess the effects of the PLR test [37].

- Positive PLR test is defined as a 10% or more increase in cardiac output/ stroke volume or pulse pressure, and it predicts fluid responsiveness [38, 41]. If, in response to the PLR test, an increase in cardiac output is less, it predicts a poor response to fluid administration.

- The most frequently used measurement/monitoring techniques for the direct measurement of cardiac output in the PLR test are arterial pulse contour analysis, transthoracic echocardiography, esophageal doppler, bioreactance, and contour analysis of the volume clamp-derived arterial pressure. In the PLR test, simple measurement and monitoring of systolic blood pressure by the oscillometric non-invasive method is not a sensitive or specific predictor of fluid responsiveness [42].

- During renal replacement therapy, a positive PLR test predicts subsequent hypotension even before fluid removal [43].

- As a positive PLR test predicts fluid responsiveness, a negative PLR test provides an important clinical clue to discontinue or stop fluid administration [40]. The negative PLR test helps the clinician to avoid fluid overload and guides them to select other measures like vasopressors rather than fluid administration in hemodynamically unstable patients.

- PLR test is not useful in patients with raised intra-abdominal pressure (may cause false-negative result), not feasible intraoperatively during anesthesia or in agitated patients, avoided in neurotrauma patients (may increase intracranial pressure), and in those requiring immobilization (traumatic hip or lower limb fractures) or using compression stocking [32, 44–46].

End-expiratory occlusion test

The end-expiratory occlusion (EEO) test is a simple test in patients undergoing mechanical ventilation, which predicts fluid responsiveness reliably in the operating room and ICU [27, 47, 48].

In this preload responsiveness test, a ventilator is interrupted for 15 seconds at the end of expiration, and cardiac output is measured. A more than 5% increase in cardiac output predicts fluid responsiveness with a high degree of accuracy [9, 49]. The standard method used to measure cardiac output in this test is pulse contour analysis, but recent evidence supports the use of even echocardiography [48, 50, 51].

Physiological basis [52, 53]:

- In patients on positive pressure ventilation, during inspiration, intrathoracic pressure increases, which pushes blood back from the right atrium and reduces the systemic venous return.

- In patients on a ventilator, during the expiratory phase, intrathoracic pressure reduces, which allows the return of systemic venous blood. When a ventilator is stopped for 15 seconds at the end-expiration, the reduced intrathoracic pressure will persist for additional 15 seconds, permit venous return for a more extended period, and allow a larger volume of venous blood return.

- The effect of increased venous return will be like a mini self-volume fluid challenge, a transient increase in the venous blood return with a resultant increase in the left ventricular stroke volume and cardiac output.

- With the EEO test, cardiac output will increase in fluid responsive patients while no significant increase in cardiac output in non-volume responders.

- When a 15-second end-inspiratory hold is added to hold in the end-expiratory phase, the combined effect induces more substantial cardiac output changes in fluid responders, increasing the diagnostic threshold of this test to 13% and the assessment possible by echocardiography examination [50].

Reliability, even in patients with cardiac arrhythmias, acute respiratory distress syndrome, low lung compliance, and low tidal volume, are the advantages of this easy-to-use test [9, 53–55]. But this test can be performed only in patients on a ventilator who can hold respiration for 15 seconds without interruption by a spontaneous breath.

EEO test is a preferred technique to measure CO in surgical patients in the operating theatre. It can be conveniently and safely performed in sedated patients on a ventilator and with the benefit of the assessment without fluid administration (i.e., risk of volume overload). In addition, it has no technical constraints like a passive leg raising test [27, 56].

DYNAMIC PARAMETERS TO PREDICT FLUID RESPONSIVENESS

Pulse pressure variation, stroke volume variation, and plethysmographic variability index are common dynamic measurements based on cardiopulmonary interaction derived from the arterial waveform analysis, which is used to predict fluid responsiveness.

Pulse pressure variation (PPV) and stroke volume variation (SVV)

Arterial waveform derived dynamic parameters such as pulse pressure variation and stroke volume variation are accurate and excellent predictors of fluid responsiveness in mechanically ventilated patients [57–60]. Dynamic parameters PPV and SVV are superior to traditionally used static indices to predict fluid responsiveness, such as central venous pressure and pulmonary artery occlusion pressure [57, 61–64].

PPV, SVV, and cardiac output can be easily recorded and automatically calculated by many modern commercially available bedside monitors.

Pulse pressure variation

Pulse pressure is the difference between systolic and diastolic blood pressure, which varies with respiration. Pulse pressure variation is calculated from the maximum pulse pressure (PPmax), minimum PP (PPmin), and mean PP (PPmean) during a respiratory cycle. These values can be obtained accurately by arterial catheters, and for the calculation, the values from three or more breaths are measured and averaged.

$$\text{Pulse Pressure Variation} = 100 \times \frac{\text{PPmax} - \text{PPmin}}{\text{PPmean}}$$

Interpretation of PPV for fluid administration:

1. PPV >13% is strongly associated with volume responsiveness [57, 58].

2. If PPV is low (<9), it suggests fluid unresponsiveness, and administration of fluids should be avoided [60].

3. PPV 9–13% is a grey zone value, and a definite strategy to administer intravenous (IV) fluid cannot be made on its basis [65, 66].

PPV has a higher predictive value for fluid responsiveness compared to SVV [67, 68]. Values of PPV are reliable, provided the patient is intubated and is on a volume cycled ventilator making no spontaneous respiratory efforts, tidal value >8 mL/kg body weight, and no arrhythmias [69, 70]. However, the accuracy of PPV in patients with increased intra-abdominal pressure is questionable as there is evidence supporting [71, 72] and against [73] its reliability.

Role of PPV to guide and monitor fluid administration in clinical practice [60]:

1. Surgical patients: Its applicability is higher during major surgery because PPV improves postoperative outcomes, and in patients on mechanical ventilator accuracy of PPV is greater.

2. ICU patients: Use of PPV is lesser in ICU because in the presence of commonly encountered conditions in ICU such as cardiac arrhythmias, spontaneous breathing, ventilatory support with low tidal volume, low lung compliance (e.g., acute respiratory distress syndrome), etc., the predictive value of PPV is unreliable.

3. Interpretation in low tidal volume ventilation: In patients on low tidal volume ventilation, PPV value can be misleading as it can be low even in fluid responsiveness patients. The 'tidal volume challenge' is a simple bedside test that helps to overcome the difficulty in interpretation in such patients. In this technique, tidal volume is increased from 6

to 8 mL/kg for 1 minute, and the resultant absolute changes in PPV are measured [69, 74]. If an increase in the absolute value of PPV is 3.5% or more, it predicts fluid responsiveness with excellent accuracy [74].

4. Interpretation in grey zone values of PPV: In patients with PPV 9% and 13% and tidal volume ≥8 mL/kg, PVV is inconclusive in predicting fluid responsiveness [65]. In such patients, augmented PPV (i.e., transient increase in tidal volume from 8 mL/kg to 12 mL/kg, known as a tidal volume challenge technique) can offer excellent predictability of fluid responsiveness [75].

Stroke volume variation

Left ventricular stroke volume variation, like PPV, is a dynamic parameter useful in diagnosing volume deficit and is a reliable predictor of fluid responsiveness in mechanically ventilated patients. Stroke volume variation is the percentage change between the maximal and minimal stroke volumes (SV) averaged over several respiratory cycles.

$$\frac{\text{Stroke Volume}}{\text{Variation}} = \frac{\text{SVmax} - \text{SVmin}}{\text{SVmean}}$$

SVV greater than 10% is associated with fluid responsiveness [76, 77]. The SVV is commonly measured by an arterial catheter but can also be measured by other methods such as esophageal doppler, bioimpedance, and bioreactance.

PPV and SVV are unreliable in patients with spontaneous breathing, on a mechanical ventilator with low tidal volume (<8 mL/kg), cardiac arrhythmias, right ventricular dysfunction, and low lung compliance [78–80].

Plethysmographic variability index

The plethysmographic variability index (PVI, Pleth variability index) is a simple, completely noninvasive, and dynamic method that accurately predicts fluid responsiveness in mechanically ventilated patients [81–83].

In this easy-to-use method, the pulse oximeter measures the light transmitted through the vascular bed of a finger and detects the dynamic change in the perfusion index during a complete respiratory cycle [84].

Continuous measurement derived from the plethysmographic waveform signals of the pulse oximetry is automatically calculated and displayed on the monitor's screen [85].

The PVI is calculated from the perfusion index (PI) variation between inspiration and expiration phases, as follows:

$$PVI = \frac{\text{PI Maximum} - \text{PI Minimumn}}{\text{PI Maximum}} \times 100\%$$

Generally, a PVI value >14% predicts preload dependence and is suggestive of fluid responsiveness [81, 86, 87].

PVI is a reasonably reliable predictor of fluid responsiveness in perioperative and critically ill patients with mechanical ventilation [88–92]. PVI guided goal-directed fluid management has been shown to improve outcomes in major surgery [93, 94]. However, in a recent meta-analysis, the reliability of PVI to predict fluid responsiveness was found to be limited, but it can play a role as a continuous bedside monitor in ICU [95].

Results of PVI are less reliable in pediatric patients with spontaneously breathing, with cardiac arrhythmias [88], probe malposition, patient motion, and in patients receiving norepinephrine (due to vasopressor induced dampened plethysmographic signals) [96, 97].

REFERENCES

1. Mackenzie DC, Noble VE. Assessing volume status and fluid responsiveness in the emergency department. Clin Exp Emerg Med. 2014;1(2):67–77.

2. Cecconi M, Hofer C, Teboul JL, et al. Fluid challenges in intensive care: the FENICE study: A global inception cohort study. Intensive Care Med 2015;41(9):1529–37.

3. Cecconi M, De Backer D, Antonelli M, et al. Consensus on circulatory shock and hemodynamic monitoring. Task force of the European Society of Intensive Care Medicine. Intensive Care Med. 2014;40(12):1795–1815.

4. Cecconi M, Parsons M, Rhodes A. What is a fluid challenge? Department of Intensive Care Medicine, St George's Healthcare NHS Trust, London, UK Current Opinion In Critical Care 2011;17(3):290–295.

5. Hasanin A. Fluid responsiveness in acute circulatory failure. J Intensive Care. 2015;3:50.

6. Vincent JL, Weil MH. Fluid challenge revisited. Crit Care Med 2006;34(5):1333–7.

7. Messina A, Longhini F, Coppo C, et al. Use of the fluid challenge in critically ill adult patients: A systematic review. Anesthesia and analgesia. 2017;125(5):1532–1543.

8. Toscani L, Aya HD, Antonakaki D, et al. What is the impact of the fluid challenge technique on diagnosis of fluid responsiveness? A systematic review and meta-analysis. Crit Care. 2017;21(1):207.

9. Marik PE, Monnet X, Teboul JL. Hemodynamic parameters to guide fluid therapy. Ann Intensive Care. 2011;1(1):1.

10. Rhodes A, Evans LE, Alhazzani W, et al. Surviving Sepsis Campaign: International Guidelines for Management of Sepsis and Septic Shock: 2016. Crit Care Med. 2017;45(3):486–552.

11. Lanspa MJ, Grissom CK, Hirshberg EL, et al. Applying dynamic parameters to predict hemodynamic response to volume expansion in spontaneously breathing patients with septic shock. Shock. 2013;39(2):155–160.

12. Aya HD, Ster IC, Fletcher N, et al. Pharmacodynamic analysis of a fluid challenge. Crit Care Med 2016;44(5):880–91.

13. Anand Swaminathan, "Fluid responsiveness and the six guiding principles of fluid resuscitation", REBEL EM blog, February 27, 2017. Available at: https://rebelem.com/fluid-responsiveness-and-the-six-guiding-principles-of-fluid-resuscitation/.

14. Farkas J. PulmCrit: Myth-busting the fluid bolus. June 3, 2019 Available at: https://emcrit.org/pulmcrit/bolus/.

15. Becker BF, Chappell D, Jacob M. Endothelial glycocalyx and coronary vascular permeability: The fringe benefit. Basic Res. Cardiol. 2010;105(6):687–701.

16. Malbrain MLNG, Van Regenmortel N, Saugel B, et al. Principles of fluid management and stewardship in septic shock: it is time to consider the four D's and the four phases of fluid therapy. Ann Intensive Care. 2018;8(1):66.

17. Vincent JL, Sakr Y, Sprung CL, et al. Sepsis in European intensive care units: results of the SOAP study. Crit Care Med. 2006;34(2):344–353.

18. Payen D, de Pont AC, Sakr Y, et al. Sepsis Occurrence in Acutely Ill Patients (SOAP) Investigators. A positive fluid balance is associated with a worse outcome in patients with acute renal failure. Crit Care. 2008;12(3):R74.

19. Prowle JR, Echeveri JE, Ligabo EV, et al. Fluid balance and acute kidney injury. Net Rev Nephrol. 2010;6(2):107–115.

20. Wiedemann HP, Wheeler AP, Bernard GR, et al. Comparison of two fluid-management strategies in acute lung injury. The New England Journal of Medicine. 2006;354(24):2564–75.

21. Malbrain ML, Marik PE, Witters I, et al. Fluid overload, de-resuscitation, and outcomes in critically ill or injured patients: a systematic review with suggestions for clinical practice. Anaesthesiol Intensive Ther. 2014;46(5):361–80.

22. Maitland K, Kiguli S, Opoka R, et al. Mortality after fluid bolus in African children with severe infection. N Engl J Med. 2011;364(26):2483–2495.

23. Andrews B, Semler M, Muchemwa L, et al. Effect of an early resuscitation protocol on in-hospital mortality among adults with sepsis and hypotension: a randomized clinical trial. JAMA. 2017;318(13):1233–1240.

24. Hjortrup PB, Haase N, Bundgaard H, et al. Restricting volumes of resuscitation fluid in adults with septic shock after initial management: the CLASSIC randomised, parallel-group, multicentre feasibility trial. Intensive Care Med. 2016;42(11):1695–1705.

25. Nunes TS, Ladeira RT, Bafi AT, et al. Duration of hemodynamic effects of crystalloids in patients with circulatory shock after initial resuscitation. Ann Intensive Care. 2014;4:25.

26. Biais M, de Courson H, Lanchon R, et al. Mini-fluid challenge of 100 ml of crystalloid predicts fluid responsiveness in the operating room. Anesthesiology 2017;127(3):450–456.

27. Messina A, Dell'Anna A, Baggiani M, et al. Functional hemodynamic tests: a systematic review and a metanalysis on the reliability of the end-expiratory occlusion test and of the mini-fluid challenge in predicting fluid responsiveness. Crit Care 2019;23(1):264.

28. Marik PE. Fluid therapy in 2015 and beyond: the mini-fluid challenge and mini-fluid bolus approach. Br J Anaesth. 2015;115(3):347–9.

29. Muller L, Toumi M, Bousquet PJ, et al. An increase in aortic blood flow after an infusion of 100 ml colloid over 1 minute can predict fluid responsiveness: the mini-fluid challenge study. Anesthesiology 2011;115(3):541–7.

30. Aya HD, Rhodes A, Ster IC, et al. Hemodynamic effect of different doses of fluids for a fluid challenge: a quasi-randomised controlled study. Crit Care Med. 2017;45(2):e161–e168.

31. Mallat J, Meddour M, Durville E, et al. Decrease in pulse pressure and stroke volume variations after mini-fluid challenge accurately predicts fluid responsiveness. Br J Anaesth. 2015;115(3):449–56.

32. Monnet X, Teboul JL. Passive leg raising. Intensive Care Med 2008;34(4):659–63.

33. Cavallaro F, Sandroni C, Marano C, et al. Diagnostic accuracy of passive leg raising for prediction of fluid responsiveness in adults: systematic review and meta-analysis of clinical studies. Intensive Care Med 2010;36(9):1475–83.

34. Duus N, Shogilev DJ, Skibsted S, et al. The reliability and validity of passive leg raise and fluid bolus to assess fluid responsiveness in spontaneously breathing emergency department patients. J Crit Care 2015;30(1):217.e1–5.

35. Monnet X, Marik PE, Teboul J. Prediction of fluid responsiveness: an update. Ann Intensive Care 2016;6(1):111.

36. Monnet X, Teboul JL. Assessment of fluid responsiveness: recent advances. Curr Opin Crit Care. 2018;24(3):190–195.

37. Cherpanath TG, Hirsch A, Geerts BF, et al. Predicting fluid responsiveness by passive leg raising: a systematic review and meta-analysis of 23 clinical trials. Crit Care Med. 2016;44(5):981–91.

38. Monnet X, Marik P, Teboul JL. Passive leg raising for predicting fluid responsiveness: a systematic review and meta-analysis. Intensive Care Med. 2016;42(12):1935–1947.

39. Jabot J, Teboul JL, Richard C, et al. Passive leg raising for predicting fluid responsiveness: importance of the postural change. Intensive Care Med. 2009;35(1):85–90.

40. Monnet X, Teboul JL. Passive leg raising: five rules, not a drop of fluid. Crit Care. 2015;19(1):18.

41. Monnet X, Rienzo M, Osman D, et al. Passive leg raising predicts fluid responsiveness in the critically ill. Crit Care Med 2006;34(5):1402–7.

42. Pickett JD, Bridges E, Kritek PA, et al. Noninvasive blood pressure monitoring and prediction of fluid responsiveness to passive leg raising. Am J Crit Care. 2018;27(3):228–237.

43. Monnet X, Flora CF, Laurent CL, et al. The passive leg raising test to guide fluid removal in critically ill patients. Ann. Intensive Care 2016;6(1):46.

44. Malbrain ML, Reuter DA. Assessing fluid responsiveness with the passive leg raising maneuver in patients with increased intra-abdominal pressure: be aware that not all blood returns. Crit Care Med. 2010;38(9):1912–1915.

45. Beurton A, Teboul JL, Girotto V, et al. Intra-Abdominal hypertension is responsible for false negatives to the passive leg raising test. Crit Care Med 2019;47(8):e639–e647.

46. Chacko CJ, Wise MP, Frost PJ. Passive leg raising and compression stockings: A note of caution. Crit. Care. 2015;19:237.

47. Monnet X, Osman D, Ridel C, et al. Predicting volume responsiveness by using the end-expiratory occlusion in mechanically ventilated intensive care unit patients. Crit Care Med. 2009;37(3):951–6.

48. Georges D, de Courson H, Lanchon R, et al. End-expiratory occlusion maneuver to predict fluid responsiveness in the intensive care unit: an echocardiographic study. Crit Care. 2018;22(1):32.

49. Monnet X, Teboul JL. End-expiratory occlusion test: please use the appropriate tools. Br J Anaesth. 2015;114(1):166–7.

50. Jozwiak M, Depret F, Teboul JL, et al. Predicting fluid responsiveness in critically ill patients by using combined end-expiratory and end-inspiratory occlusions with echocardiography. Crit Care Med. 2017;45(11):e1131–e1138.

51. Dépret F, Jozwiak M, Teboul JL, et al. Esophageal Doppler can predict fluid responsiveness through end-expiratory and end-inspiratory occlusion tests. Crit Care Med. 2019;47(2):e96–e102.

52. Biais M, Larghi M, Henriot J, et al. End-expiratory occlusion test predicts fluid responsiveness in patients with protective ventilation in the operating room. Anesth Analg 2017;125(6):1889–95.

53. Gavelli F, Teboul J, Monnet X. The end-expiratory occlusion test: please, let me hold your breath. Crit Care 2019;23:274.

54. Monnet X, Bleibtreu A, Ferré A, et al. Passive leg-raising and end-expiratory occlusion tests perform better than pulse pressure variation in patients with low respiratory system compliance. Crit Care Med 2012;40(1):152–157.

55. Shiva S, Jozwiak M, Teboul JL, et al. End-expiratory occlusion test predicts preload responsiveness independently of positive end-expiratory pressure during acute respiratory distress syndrome. Crit Care Med 2013;41(7):1692–701.

56. Xu LY, Tu GW, Cang J, et al. End-expiratory occlusion test predicts fluid responsiveness in cardiac surgical patients in the operating theatre. Ann Transl Med. 2019;7(14):315.

57. Marik PE, Cavallazzi R, Vasu T, et al. Dynamic changes in arterial waveform derived variables and fluid responsiveness in mechanically ventilated patients: a systematic review of the literature. Crit Care Med. 2009;37(9):2642–7.

58. Yang X, Du B. Does pulse pressure variation predict fluid responsiveness in critically ill patients? A systematic review and meta-analysis. Crit Care. 2014;18(6):650.

59. Hong JQ, He HF, Chen ZY, et al. Comparison of stroke volume variation with pulse pressure variation as a diagnostic indicator of fluid responsiveness in mechanically ventilated critically ill patients. Saudi Med J. 2014;35(3):261–8.

60. Teboul JL, Monnet X, Chemla D, et al. Arterial pulse pressure variation with mechanical ventilation. Am J Respir Crit Care Med. 2019;199(1):22–31.

61. Michard F, Teboul JL. Predicting fluid responsiveness in ICU patients: a critical analysis of the evidence. Chest 2002;121(6):2000–8.

62. Osman D, Ridel C, Ray P, et al. Cardiac filling pressures are not appropriate to predict hemodynamic response to volume challenge. Crit Care Med 2007;35(1):64–68.

63. Marik PE, Baram M, Vahid B. Does central venous pressure predict fluid responsiveness? A systematic review of the literature and the tale of seven mares. Chest 2008;134(1):172–8.

64. Perel A, Pizov R, Cotev S. Respiratory variations in the arterial pressure during mechanical ventilation reflect volume status and fluid responsiveness Intensive care med 2014;40(6):798–807.

65. Cannesson M, Le Manach Y, Hofer CK, et al. Assessing the diagnostic accuracy of pulse pressure variations for the prediction of fluid responsiveness: a "gray zone" approach. Anesthesiology 2011;115(2):231–241.

66. Biais M, Ehrmann S, Mari A, et al. Clinical relevance of pulse pressure variations for predicting fluid responsiveness in mechanically ventilated intensive care unit patients: the grey zone approach. Crit Care 2014;18(6):587.

67. Preisman S, Kogan S, Berkenstadt H, et al. Predicting fluid responsiveness in patients undergoing cardiac surgery: functional haemodynamic parameters including the Respiratory Systolic Variation Test and static preload indicators. British Journal of Anaesthesia. 2005;95(6):746–755.

68. Rathore A, Singh S, Lamsal R, et al. Validity of pulse pressure variation (PPV) compared with stroke volume variation (SVV) in predicting fluid responsiveness. Turk J Anaesthesiol Reanim 2017;45(4):210–217.

69. Myatra SN, Monnet X, Teboul JL. Use of 'tidal volume challenge' to improve the reliability of pulse pressure variation. Crit Care. 2017;21(1):60.

70. De Backer D, Heenen S, Piagnerelli M, et al. Pulse pressure variations to predict fluid responsiveness: influence of tidal volume. Intensive Care Med. 2005;31(4):517–523.

71. Renner J, Gruenewald M, Quaden R, et al. Influence of increased intra-abdominal pressure on fluid responsiveness predicted by pulse pressure variation and stroke volume variation in a porcine model. Crit Care Med 2009;37(2):650–8.

72. Jacques D, Bendjelid K, Duperret S, et al. Pulse pressure variation and stroke volume variation during increased intra-abdominal pressure: an experimental study. Crit Care 2011;15(1):R33.

73. Diaz F, Erranz B, Donoso A, et al. Influence of tidal volume on pulse pressure variation and stroke volume variation during experimental intra-abdominal hypertension. BMC Anesthesiol. 2015;15:127.

74. Myatra SN, Prabu NR, Divatia JV, et al. The changes in pulse pressure variation or stroke volume variation after a "tidal volume challenge" reliably predict fluid responsiveness during low tidal volume ventilation. Crit Care Med 2017;45(3):415–421.

75. Min JJ, Gil NS, Lee JH, et al. Predictor of fluid responsiveness in the 'grey zone': augmented pulse pressure variation through a temporary increase in tidal volume. Br J Anaesth. 2017;119(1):50–56.

76. Biais M, Nouette-Gaulain K, Cottenceau V, et al. Uncalibrated pulse contour-derived stroke volume variation predicts fluid responsiveness in mechanically ventilated patients undergoing liver transplantation. Br J Anaesth 2008;101(6):761–8.

77. Hofer CK, Müller SM, Furrer L, et al. Stroke volume and pulse pressure variation for prediction of fluid responsiveness in patients undergoing off-pump coronary artery bypass grafting. Chest 2005;128(2):848–54.

78. Lefrant JY, De Backer D. Can we use pulse pressure variations to predict fluid responsiveness in patients with ARDS? Intensive Care Med. 2009;35(6):966–8.

79. Lakhal K, Ehrmann S, Benzekri-Lefevre D, et al. Respiratory pulse pressure variation fails to predict fluid responsiveness in acute respiratory distress syndrome. Crit Care. 2011;15(2):R85.

80. Oliveira-Costa CD, Friedman G, Vieira SR, et al. Pulse pressure variation and prediction of fluid responsiveness in patients ventilated with low tidal volumes. Clinics (Sao Paulo). 2012;67(7):773–8.

81. Cannesson M, Attof Y, Rosamel P, et al. Respiratory variations in pulse oximetry plethysmographic waveform amplitude to predict fluid responsiveness in the operating room. Anesthesiology. 2007;106(6):1105–1111.

82. Cannesson M, Desebbe O, Rosamel P, et al. Pleth variability index to monitor the respiratory variations in the pulse oximeter plethysmographic waveform amplitude and predict fluid responsiveness in the operating theatre. Br J Anaesth 2008;101(2):200–6.

83. Desebbe O, Cannesson M. Using ventilation induced plethysmographic variations to optimize patient fluid status. Curr Opin Anaesthesiol 2008;21(6):772–8.

84. Keller G, Cassar E, Desebbe O, et al. Ability of pleth variability index to detect hemodynamic changes induced by passive leg raising in spontaneously breathing volunteers. Crit Care 2008;12(2):R37.

85. Cannesson M, Slieker J, Desebbe O, et al. The ability of a novel algorithm for automatic estimation of the respiratory variations in arterial pulse pressure to monitor fluid responsiveness in the operating room. Anesth Analg. 2008;106(4):1195–200.

86. Lu W, Dong J, Xu Z, et al. The pleth variability index as an indicator of the central extracellular fluid volume in mechanically ventilated patients after anesthesia induction: comparison with initial distribution volume of glucose. Med Sci Monit. 2014;20:386–392.

87. Feissel M, Teboul JL, Merlani P, et al. Plethysmographic dynamic indices predict fluid responsiveness in septic ventilated patients. Intensive Care Med 2007;33(6):993–9.

88. Yin JY, Ho KM. Use of plethysmographic variability index derived from the Massimo((R)) pulse oximeter to predict fluid or preload responsiveness: a systematic review and meta-analysis. Anaesthesia. 2012;67(7):777–783.

89. Chu H, Wang Y, Sun Y, et al. Accuracy of pleth variability index to predict fluid responsiveness in mechanically ventilated patients: a systematic review and meta-analysis. J Clin Monit Comput. 2015;30(3):265–74.

90. Bahlmann H, Hahn RG, Nilsson L. Pleth variability index or stroke volume optimization during open abdominal surgery: a randomized controlled trial BMC Anesthesiology 2018;18(1):115.

91. Kim DH, Shin S, Kim JY, et al. Pulse pressure variation and pleth variability index as predictors of fluid responsiveness in patients undergoing spinal surgery in the prone position. Therapeutics and Clinical Risk Management 2018;14:1175–1183.

92. Sandroni C, Cavallaro F, Marano C, et al. Accuracy of plethysmographic indices as predictors of fluid responsiveness in mechanically ventilated adults: a systematic review and meta-analysis. Intensive Care Med. 2012;38(9):1429–37.

93. Coeckelenbergh S, Delaporte A, Ghoundiwal D, et al. Pleth variability index versus pulse pressure variation for intraoperative goal-directed fluid therapy in patients undergoing low to-moderate risk abdominal surgery: a randomized controlled trial. BMC Anesthesiol. 2019;19(1):34.

94. Cesur S, Çardaközü T, Kuş A, et al. Comparison of conventional fluid management with PVI-based goal-directed fluid management in elective colorectal surgery. J Clin Monit Comput. 2019;33(2):249–57.

95. Liu T, Xu C, Wang M, et al. Reliability of pleth variability index in predicting preload responsiveness of mechanically ventilated patients under various conditions: a systematic review and meta-analysis. BMC Anesthesiol. 2019;19(1):67.

96. Biais M, Cottenceau V, Petit L, et al. Impact of norepinephrine on the relationship between pleth variability index and pulse pressure variations in ICU adult patients. Crit Care. 2011;15(4):R168.

97. Monnet X, Guerin L, Jozwiak M, et al. Pleth variability index is a weak predictor of fluid responsiveness in patients receiving norepinephrine. Br J Anaesth. 2013;110(2):207–13.

19 | Cardiac Output Monitoring

The accurate measurement of cardiac output (CO) is essential in all high-risk hemodynamically unstable patients.

Several devices for cardiac output measurement are available in the market, which is classified based on invasiveness (Non-invasive, minimally invasive, and invasive systems), the technology used (dilution technique, pulse contour analysis, doppler principle, applied Fick principle bioelectric properties, plethysmographic analysis, etc.), and calibration systems, as summarized (Table 19.1).

CALIBRATED VS. UNCALIBRATED DEVICES

Calibration is the process of comparing an instrument with the known standard. Subsequent adjustment of measured equipment achieves precision and accuracy and produces valid data. In calibrated monitoring devices, the bias in the continuous measurements is reduced or eliminated by calibration [1]. While in non-calibrated monitoring devices, bias is reduced by the pre-programmed correction factors in the monitoring device.

Table 19.1 Hemodynamic monitoring systems			
Methods	**Requirements**	**Calibration**	**Devices**
1. Non-invasive systems			
Transthoracic echocardiography	Thoracic echo probe	Calibrated	US, Echo
Bioimpedance or bioreactance	Specific cutaneous electrodes	Non-calibrated	BioZ Dx ECOM NICOM (Cheetah)
Radial applanation tonometry	Pressure sensor over the radial artery	Non-calibrated	T-line
Volume clamp method	Finger pressure cuff	Non-calibrated	CNAP Clearsight/Nexfin
Ultrasound cardiac output	Transthoracic doppler probe	Non-calibrated	USCOM
Plethysmographic variability index	Specific transcutaneous probe	Non-calibrated	MASSIMO
2. Minimally invasive systems			
Transesophageal echocardiography	Esophageal probe	Calibrated	Cardio Q WAKI TO
Transpulmonary thermodilution	Thermistor-tipped arterial catheter Central venous line	Calibrated	PiCCO VolumeView EV 1000
Lithium dilution	Arterial catheter Central venous line	Calibrated	LiDCO LiDCO Plus PulseCO
Arterial pulse contour analysis	Arterial catheter	Calibrated	PiCCO Plus LiDCO Plus
		Non-calibrated	Flotrac/Vigileo LiDCO rapid PRAM/MostCare ProAQT/PulsioFlex
Partial CO_2 rebreathing	Rebreathing circuit	Non-calibrated	NiCO
3. Invasive systems			
Pulmonary thermodilution	Pulmonary artery catheter Central venous line	Calibrated	Swan-Ganz pulmonary artery catheter

Cardiac output monitoring systems are divided into two groups, calibrated and uncalibrated devices, depending on the method of calibration [1, 2]. Cardiac output monitoring systems based on non-calibrated analysis have been emerging as the preferred modality in the last few years because of their minimally invasive nature and no need for calibration, usual independence from mechanical ventilation, and ease of use in practice [3]. Uncalibrated systems are used selectively in hemodynamically stable patients requiring cardiac output monitoring for a short period, e.g., during surgery [4]. Because of more accuracy and precision, calibrated techniques are preferred over uncalibrated methods in severely shocked hemodynamic unstable patients [2].

NON-INVASIVE SYSTEMS FOR CARDIAC OUTPUT MONITORING

Non-invasive techniques commonly used for measuring cardiac output are transthoracic echocardiography, thoracic electrical bioimpedance, thoracic bioreactance, applanation tonometry, and volume clamp method.

Transthoracic echocardiography

Measuring and monitoring cardiac output is valuable for diagnosing and managing critically ill patients. The trend to use transthoracic echocardiography (TTE) for the prompt measurement of cardiac output is increasing because it is a readily available, reproducible, and non-invasive, bedside method [5, 6].

In early literature, in stable patients, TTE was found to be accurate compared to the standard PA thermodilution technique [7–9], but in critically ill patients, predictability was found to be limited [10, 11].

With technological advancements, the ability of TTE to acquire high-quality images of critically ill patients improved [12, 13], and literature supporting the use of TTE to manage critical patients emerged [14–17].

Simultaneously, emerging literature supports the use of echocardiography for the measurement of cardiac output and its role in hemodynamic optimization [18–21].

In current literature, TTE is documented as a reliable, accurate, and highly valuable method to measure cardiac output, which provides rapid and vital diagnostic information and thereby guides clinicians for a wiser therapeutic strategy [6, 22–25].

Recent literature also documented that cardiac output measurement by transthoracic echocardiography was comparable to cardiac output measured by a pulmonary artery catheter thermodilution (TD) technique. Due to its wide availability, great potential to guide therapy, and noninvasive nature, TTE has become a routine and standard practice for bedside cardiac output measurement in the management of critical patients [26, 27].

How to measure and calculate cardiac output by TTE?

Parameters determined for the calculation of cardiac output by TTE are:

1. Left ventricular outflow tract velocity time integral (LVOT VTI): Velocity-time integral (VTI) is measured by pulsed wave doppler signal, most commonly at the level of the left outflow tract (LVOT) obtained in the apical 5 chamber view. LVOT-VTI reflects the column of blood that moves through the left ventricle (LV) outflow tract during each systole; therefore, it is a TTE parameter representing stroke volume.

2. Cross-sectional area (CSA): Measure the diameter of the LVOT in the parasternal long axis view in systole and calculate the area of the circle.

3. Heart rate (HR).

Calculation of cardiac output: After obtaining the above parameters by TTE, cardiac output is calculated with the formula below:

Cardiac Output = Stroke Volume × HR

Cardiac Output = [LVOT VTI × LVOT CSA] × HR

To measure cardiac output precisely, averaging three measurements within one TTE examination is recommended in patients with sinus rhythm, and averaging five measurements is necessary for patients with atrial fibrillation [28].

Limitations of TTE are:

- Accuracy is highly dependent on an operator, so the possibility of inter- and intra-observer variability. But even non-cardiologist ICU physicians, after brief training, can accurately estimate cardiac output by TTE [23].
- The probe's position needs to be very accurate, and errors in position can lead to misinterpretations.
- The accuracy of TTE to measure cardiac output is unreliable in patients with high cardiac output, low sedation, or with physiological structural changes.
- TTE provides only intermittent and not continuous cardiac output measurements.

TTE, in addition to calculating cardiac output, measures inferior vena cava diameter and left ventricular size, identifies wall motion abnormalities, and assesses left and right ventricular function. By providing this information, TTE improves diagnostic accuracy, narrows the possible differential diagnosis of shock, and achieves volume status optimization. Small LV size, hyperdynamic LV (left ventricular end-diastolic area in the parasternal short axis view <10 cm2), or papillary apposition (kissing ventricles) are strongly indicative of hypovolemia and predicts fluid responsiveness [29, 30]. Papillary apposition can be false positive in LVH, vasodilatation and high inotropes.

Thoracic electrical bioimpedance and bioreactance

Thoracic bioimpedance

Thoracic electrical bioimpedance (TEB) is a non-invasive method to continuously estimate cardiac output using pairs of high-frequency but low-voltage disposable electrodes placed on either side of the neck and the lateral aspect of the chest wall.

The fluid offers less resistance to electric flow. A greater volume of blood column during each systole will work as a larger electrical contrast medium, lowering the electrical impedance. This principle is used to calculate stroke volume [31].

A series of signals from sensing electrodes will travels through the thorax and will continuously and accurately measures the cyclic changes in thoracic electrical impedance, which occurs due to changes in intrathoracic blood volume with each heartbeat. Based on these changes in electrical impedance, cardiac output is calculated.

The reliability of TEB is poor in the exact measurement of cardiac output in surgical and critically ill patients [32, 33].

However, as TEB measures cardiac output continuously and non-invasively, its use is rapidly increasing as a bedside cardiac output trend analysis monitor [34, 35].

Thoracic bioimpedance is a simple, easy-to-use, totally safe, and low-cost method that provides rapid, real-time, continuous, and automated cardiac output monitoring. Various factors that can affect the measurement of cardiac output by this method are electrical interference, cardiac arrhythmias, pleural effusions, pulmonary edema, chest tubes, internal or external pacemakers, or patient movement.

Thoracic bioreactance

Thoracic bioreactance is a modified, improved bioimpedance technology which measures time delay called a phase shift in alternating current voltage across the thorax rather than changes in impedance.

Electrodes applied on either side of the chest detect phase shifts, which almost exclusively depend on pulsatile flow (e.g., blood flow) but are less affected by static fluids (e.g., intravascular and extravascular fluids), electrical noise, patient movement, electrode positioning, and respiratory effort. In addition, because of newer technology-related improvements in the signal-to-noise ratio, bioreactance is theoretically superior to bioimpedance [36].

Thoracic bioreactance is found to be a reliable technique to measure cardiac output in many studies (but not in all studies) [37–41]. In a recent meta-analysis of the accuracy and precision of non-invasive cardiac output monitoring devices, percentage errors were 42% for bioimpedance and bioreactance [42].

Applanation tonometry and volume clamp method

Radial artery applanation tonometry and volume clamp method are two non-invasive uncalibrated techniques that provide continuous blood pressure monitoring and real-time cardiac output from the pulse contour analysis.

Radial artery applanation tonometry

In this method, the transducer is strapped over the radial artery with a bone underneath. Optimal pressure is adjusted to flatten the artery, and using an electromechanically driven sensor; continuous arterial pressure waveform is recorded. Then, cardiac output is estimated with the help of autocalibrating pulse contour analysis.

As this novel method is extremely easy to use, and its initial clinical data are promising, it is an attractive alternative to measure cardiac output in practice [43, 44]. However, evidence suggests that this method is not suitable for measuring cardiac output in hemodynamically unstable critically ill patients [45–47].

Volume clamp method

In this technique, a non-invasive pulse oximeter using finger cuff devices continuously measures cardiac output and finger arterial blood pressure in addition to peripheral oxygen saturation [48].

This method is an extension of conventional photoplethysmography whereby using an inflatable cuff at the finger, the digital arterial waveform is obtained. With a photodiode device, the diameter of the artery in the finger is measured. By adjusting the pressure in the cuff, the diameter of the artery is kept constant during pressure waveform analysis. Arterial pressure waveform is continuously recorded from the pressure changes in the cuff, and cardiac output is calculated.

This simple and convenient method for cardiac monitoring is promising in surgical and non-critical cases [49–51], but its use is discouraged in obese, cardiac surgery, and ICU patients because of poor accuracy [52–57].

This method is not suitable for patients with gross peripheral edema or severe peripheral vasoconstriction.

MINIMALLY INVASIVE AND INVASIVE SYSTEMS FOR CARDIAC OUTPUT MONITORING

Minimally invasive and invasive methods for cardiac output monitoring are used in hemodynamically unstable patients in intensive care and perioperative medicine when initial resuscitation measures fail to improve the patient's hemodynamic and/or respiratory status. Accurate measurement of cardiac output with advanced hemodynamic monitoring will guide appropriate management with fluid resuscitation, vasopressors, or inotropic agents.

MINIMALLY INVASIVE SYSTEMS

Minimally invasive techniques commonly used for measuring cardiac output are transesophageal echocardiography, transpulmonary thermodilution, arterial pulse contour analysis, and partial CO_2 rebreathing [58].

Transesophageal echocardiographic

Transesophageal echocardiography (TEE) is a minimally invasive technique to measure cardiac output. This method is widely used for diagnosing and monitoring critical and perioperative patients.

Technique

In TEE ultrasonic probe is placed into the esophagus under sedation. Placement of the TEE probe is similar to the insertion of a nasogastric tube, and the depth of the tube inserted in the esophagus is to place the tip of the probe at descending thoracic aorta level (between the fifth and sixth intercostal space), which will be roughly 35–45 cm mark on the probe.

TEE probe obtains a doppler flow signal and measures the blood velocity in the descending thoracic aorta. From different data obtained, such as heart rate, peak velocity, flow time corrected (FTc), and others, hemodynamic monitor derives cardiac output, Stroke volume, and systemic vascular resistance.

The use of TEE is expanding with growing technology [59]. In addition to standard 2D technology, TEE probes are available with different modalities such as doppler, pulse wave doppler, continuous wave doppler, color flow doppler, and 3D echocardiography.

Use

TEE plays a vital role in the management of perioperative and critical patients by providing valuable diagnostic and therapeutic information such as:

- Assessment of the volume status (detects hypovolemia early or excludes volume overload).

- Serve as a dynamic parameter to assess fluid responsiveness and guides clinicians for fluid management (i.e., goal-directed fluid therapy).

- Measures cardiac output, detects ventricular dysfunction, and diagnose coexisting problems like valvular structural and functional abnormalities, pericardial effusion, and cardiac tamponade.

The results of studies about the reliability of TEE in predicting cardiac output were conflicting [60, 61]. However, in a recent systematic review and meta-analysis, cardiac output measurement by TEE was accurate [27].

Advantages

Different advantages of TEE are:

- Provides superior quality image, accurate assessment of heart and great vessels, and greater diagnostic accuracy than transthoracic echocardiography because the probe is much closer to the heart, and bone and lung tissue do not interfere with imaging [62].

- As the TEE probe is just adjacent to posterior cardiac structures, TEE provides its superior quality image. On the contrary, the point of examination of the TTE transducer is more distant from the posterior cardiac structures, i.e., at the anterior aspect of the chest. Therefore its visualization by TTE is poor.

- TEE monitoring does not disturb the surgical field and ensures continuous imaging in all stages of surgery [63].
- TEE is less dependent on the operator than TTE.

Indications

As TEE provides valuable information about several structural, functional, and hemodynamic parameters, its use is gaining popularity. But TEE is a semi-invasive method and therefore is used selectively when TTE cannot provide the required information, and the potential benefits of TEE outweigh the possible risks. Common indications of TEE are [62, 64–66]:

A. Intraoperative/Perioperative

TEE is indicated in high-risk surgical patients (e.g., significant coronary artery disease or poor cardiac status), patients with a risk of intraoperative hemodynamic instability (e.g., major vascular or abdominal surgery), major cardiac surgery like the repair of congenital heart lesions, repair of valvular lesions or thoracic aortic procedures, and as a rescue TEE in unexpected or unexplained hemodynamic unstable patients.

TEE monitoring and TEE-guided optimization of fluid administration improve outcomes, reduce postoperative complications, and shorten hospital stay in patients undergoing major or high-risk surgery [67–69].

B. Critically ill patients

TEE is useful in hemodynamically unstable critically ill patients because it calculates cardiac output, provides excellent visualization of cardiac structures, and is less dependent on the operator. TEE is used selectively in sedated ICU patients, usually on a mechanical ventilator [70]:

- For the assessment of unexplained persistent hypotension or hypoxemia when TTE or other modalities cannot obtain diagnostic information.
- For assessing volume status and cardiac output during fluid administration when no other hemodynamic monitoring systems are available.

C. Diagnostic modality

TEE is useful in diagnosing wall motion abnormalities, pericardial effusion, pulmonary hypertension, potential cardiac source of embolus, assessing valves for endocarditis, or excluding thrombi in patients with atrial fibrillation.

Contraindications

TEE's potential contraindications are previous esophagectomy, tracheo-esophageal fistula, postesophageal surgery, esophageal trauma, esophageal pathologies such as varices, diverticulum, stricture or tumor; coagulopathy, thrombocytopenia, upper gastrointestinal bleeding, and hiatus hernia [70, 71].

Limitations

Although TEE is more useful than TTE, it is used in selected indications and not used routinely. TEE is used more frequently in the operating theater than in the ICU [72]. Limitations of TEE are:

- The minimally invasive technique (usually needs tracheal intubation, under sedation).
- Do not calculate cardiac output continuously compared to other

hemodynamic monitoring devices, such as the pulmonary artery catheter (PAC) or transpulmonary thermodilution.

- Movement of the patient can change the position of the probe, and repositioning becomes necessary.

- Higher cost, time-consuming method (compared to TTE), can be performed only on one patient at a time and needs cleaning and disinfection after each use.

- Do not measure blood pressure, so critical patients need an additional device for continuous blood pressure measurement.

Transpulmonary thermodilution

Transpulmonary thermodilution (TPTD) is a minimally invasive technique (requires two catheters, a central venous catheter, and an arterial line), which is considered a new gold standard in measuring cardiac output [2, 73]. This advanced diagnostic modality using two distinct techniques, transpulmonary thermodilution and pulse contour analysis, provides continuous cardiac output measurements.

Technique

A bolus of a cold solution of known temperature is injected rapidly into the superior vena cava through an internal jugular or subclavian central venous catheter. The injected solution will mix with blood and traverse through the right heart chambers, pulmonary circulation, and finally, through the left heart chambers reaches the systemic artery.

An arterial cannula placed in a large peripheral artery (femoral, axillary, or brachial artery) with a thermistor tip will sense and measure the drop in blood temperature across the cardiopulmonary system [74]. Temperature fall between the injection site and measurement site is inversely proportional to cardiac output. Using a change in blood temperature over time, computer software plots a thermodilution curve and calculates cardiac output and other relevant hemodynamic parameters.

Calculation of cardiac output by transpulmonary thermodilution intermittently calibrates pulse contour analysis, and therefore TPTD provides precise, continuous, and real-time measurement of cardiac output by taking advantage of both techniques [74].

Use

Valuable information provided by TPTD is [74]:

1. Cardiac output: TPTD calculates cardiac output and stroke volume by analyzing an arterial pulse contour waveform. TPTD is a reliable method for the continuous and real-time monitoring of cardiac output [75]. This method also measures stroke volume variation (SVV)/PVV and predicts fluid responsiveness [76].

2. TPTD is also helpful in measuring various parameters such as, global end-diastolic volume, cardiac function index and global ejection fraction, extravascular lung water index, pulmonary vascular permeability index, which helps in assessment of volume status [74, 77–82].

Advantages

Transpulmonary thermodilution is used more frequently and has replaced the conventional intermittent thermodilution (TD) method through PAC to calculate cardiac output because:

- TPTD method is less invasive and avoids PAC-related serious complications [74].

- TPTD measures cardiac output with the same accuracy and is interchangeable with PAC thermodilution [83–86].

- It provides continuous and real-time monitoring of cardiac output in contrast to intermittent measurement by the conventional TD method.

- Provides robust support in the therapeutic management of hemodynamically unstable patients by providing several additional information such as measurement of SVV and pulse pressure variation (PPV) to predict fluid responsiveness, calculates extravascular lung water to quantify pulmonary edema, and estimates lung permeability to quantify the pulmonary leak [82].

Indications

This advanced but invasive hemodynamic monitoring is indicated over less invasive devices in selected most critically ill and/or complex patients such as:

- Perioperatively, during complex cardiac and prolonged major surgery.

- During major liver surgery, when less invasive techniques are unreliable [87].

- In ICU patients with severe shock, especially with acute respiratory distress syndrome, and high or increasing requirements of vasopressors [4, 72]. In ICU patients with severe shock, especially with acute respiratory distress syndrome, and high or increasing requirements of vasopressors [4, 72].

Limitations

- It is an invasive method that needs the placement of a central venous line and a large arterial line.

- This method does not provide information such as PA pressure and SvO_2 (unlike the PA thermodilution method).

- Needs manual calibration with cold water.

- It provides inaccurate measurements in patients with very low cardiac output (<2 L/min) [74].

- Unable to detect short-term hemodynamic changes induced by ventilation during passive leg raising or end-expiratory occlusion tests [74].

Lithium dilution

The lithium dilution technique is a minimally invasive method that measures cardiac output based on indicator dilution principles [88].

In this modality, a small dose of lithium is injected via any vein (peripheral vein or central), and a lithium-selective sensor connected to any peripheral arterial line (e.g., radial artery) measures the concentration of lithium ions in the arterial blood [89]. The lithium dilution curve (lithium concentration vs. time) is constructed, and cardiac output is derived from this data.

Lithium dilution is a less invasive method than transpulmonary thermodilution. It is performed using peripheral venous and arterial cannulation and, therefore, is without the risks of the pulmonary artery or central venous catheterization [90]. This method can measure cardiac output accurately [91].

Lithium is selected as an indicator for this dilution technique because this element is not found in the bloodstream; it is non-diffusible; a small dose is non-toxic but generates a plasma concentration that can be measured.

Lithium is not lost during the first pass in pulmonary circulation, so its assessment provides reliable value. Additionally, lithium is cleared rapidly from systemic circulation [92].

Avoid this technique during pregnancy and in patients weighing less than 40 kg, receiving lithium therapy, or high doses of nondepolarizing neuromuscular blockers [93].

Arterial pulse contour analysis

Arterial pulse contour analysis is a commonly used minimally invasive technique for continuous, beat-to-beat cardiac output measurement. Based on it, a computerized algorithm measures cardiac output.

In addition to cardiac output, arterial pulse contour analysis also calculates dynamic parameters such as pulse pressure variation and stroke volume variation, which is helpful for determining fluid responsiveness [4].

Several commercially available devices use pulse contour wave analysis for the continuous measurement of cardiac output and stroke volume. These devices are broadly divided into two groups, the calibrated (PiCCO Plus and LiDCO plus) and the uncalibrated systems (FloTrac/Vigileo and LiDCO rapid), as summarized in Table 19.1.

The advantages of the pulse contour analysis method are:

- Less invasive compared to cardiac output measurement by pulmonary artery catheter and transpulmonary thermodilution, as it requires only a peripheral arterial catheter (usually the radial artery).

- Easy method: An arterial line is frequently inserted in ICU so existing access can be utilized for pulse contour analysis.

- Continuously and real-time measurement of cardiac output.

- Effectively monitor volume responsiveness. In addition to the accurate measurement of stroke volume, cardiac output, and CI, pulse contour analysis also calculates dynamic indexes such as pulse pressure variation and stroke volume variation. These parameters help to determine response to a fluid challenge, passive leg raising, or end-expiratory occlusion in patients on a ventilator [4, 76].

- Operator independent and needs minimal training.

Limitations of arterial pulse contour wave analysis are:

- It is a less accurate technique in critically ill patients with low SVR (sepsis and chronic liver failure) [94], left ventricular dysfunction [95], norepinephrine infusion [96], in open aortic abdominal aneurysm repair [97], and off-pump coronary artery bypass surgery [98].

- An accuracy of PCA is low in patients with spontaneous breathing, cardiac arrhythmias, low tidal volume ventilation, positive-end expiratory pressure <5 mmHg, or abnormal abdominal pressure [99].

- Data suggesting that this device improve patient outcome are lacking [100, 101].

- This method is less reliable than the transpulmonary thermodilution technique in septic patients [102].

- The uncalibrated systems need frequent recalibration in patients with hemodynamic instability or requiring vasoactive drugs.

Partial CO_2 rebreathing

Partial CO_2 Rebreathing is a minimally invasive technique which uses indirect Fick's principle to calculate cardiac output [103]. This method can be used only in intubated, sedated patients on volume-controlled ventilation who are hemodynamically stable.

This technique is easy to use, safe, does not require a PAC, can be repeated every few minutes without substantial risk of CO_2 accumulation, and provides almost continuous cardiac output measurements.

This technique's accuracy and precision are similar to esophageal Doppler ultrasound, pulse contour analysis, and thoracic bioimpedance [33].

Currently, this technique is mainly focused on short-term intraoperative applications or mechanically ventilated postoperative patients [104].

This modality is not used routinely in ICU because its predictability is poor in common problems in critical patients like hemodynamic instability, anemia, or significant pulmonary disease (such as acute respiratory distress syndrome, pneumonia, atelectasis, shunting, etc.). Additionally, it does not provide information about the intravascular volume status or fluid responsiveness [105].

Avoid using this technique in patients with severe hypercapnia, raised intracranial pressure, or pulmonary hypertension because arterial CO_2 tension rises transiently in the rebreathing period, which may be harmful [106].

INVASIVE SYSTEMS

Pulmonary artery thermodilution is an invasive technique frequently used for hemodynamic monitoring.

Pulmonary artery thermodilution

Cardiac output measured invasively with the pulmonary artery using the thermodilution principle is traditionally considered as a gold standard method [107]. Modalities to measure cardiac output by pulmonary thermodilution (TD) are divided into two types: intermittent bolus and continuous cardiac output methods.

Intermittent thermodilution using the "bolus" technique

In the bolus technique of pulmonary thermodilution, about 10 ml of cold saline solution is injected via the proximal lumen of PAC in the right atrium. Cold saline mixes adequately with surrounding blood while traversing from the right atrium to the pulmonary artery (by passing through two valves and a right ventricle), which decreases blood temperature transiently. A thermistor on the tip of the PAC senses and measures changes in the blood temperature over time at a downstream side in the pulmonary artery [84].

The fall in the temperature is inversely proportional to the blood flow and cardiac output. Electronic monitors calculate cardiac output using a modified Stewart–Hamilton equation [108]. Usually, three measurements are performed and averaged to obtain a more reliable result [109].

Major advantages of the pulmonary artery thermodilution method are:

- Uses thermal energy (i.e., cold water) as an indicator which is non-toxic.

- Repeated measurement of cardiac output is safe, provided there is no constraint to administer the fluid.

- No requirement for manual calibration.

- The major advantage of this technique is that it provides an additional measurement of hemodynamic parameters such as pulmonary artery pressures, right-sided and left-sided filling pressures, and mixed venous oxyhemoglobin saturation (SvO_2).

Major limitations of the pulmonary artery thermodilution method are:

- The technique is invasive, so it carries the risk associated with placement and presence of a PAC, such as infection, pulmonary artery rupture, arrhythmias on insertion, thrombosis, and embolism [110].

- Fail to detect abrupt changes in cardiac output promptly because this technique measures cardiac output with some delay [107].

- Error in measuring cardiac output in the presence of low cardiac output, hypothermia, shunts, and cardiac valvular abnormalities.

- Error in measuring cardiac output in the presence of low cardiac output, hypothermia, shunts, and cardiac valvular abnormalities [111].

- Poor predictor of fluid responsiveness [112].

- Need to avoid magnetic resonance imaging as well as the use of electrocautery in patients with PAC.

Continuous thermodilution technique

Commercially available catheters with newer technologies now provide continuous cardiac output monitoring. This method uses the same thermodilution principles but uses a warmed bolus rather than a cold bolus [113].

This special catheter has a special blood-warming thermal filament or coil at the level of the right ventricle. Thermal filament heats the blood in a semi-random binary fashion. The thermistor at the tip of the PAC records changes in temperature and calculates the cardiac output by thermodilution.

This method's major benefits are a continuous display of cardiac output, avoidance of repeated boluses (which reduces the risk of infection), and avoids operator errors [114].

Details about pulmonary artery catheters, including description, insertion technique, use in clinical practice, indications, and complications, are covered in the pulmonary artery catheter monitoring part of the Chapter 17 on "Static Hemodynamic Monitoring Techniques."

REFERENCES

1. Peeters Y, Bernards J, Mekeirele M, et al. Hemodynamic monitoring: To calibrate or not to calibrate? Part 1 - Calibrated techniques. Anaesthesiol Intensive Ther. 2015;47(5):487–500.

2. Bernards J, Mekeirele M, Hoffmann B, et al. Hemodynamic monitoring: to calibrate or not to calibrate? Part 2 - Non-calibrated techniques. Anaesthesiology Intensive Ther. 2015;47(5):501–516.

3. Sakka SG. Hemodynamic monitoring in the critically ill patient – current status and perspective. Front Med (Lausanne). 2015;3;2:44.

4. Teboul JL, Saugel B, Cecconi M, et al. Less invasive hemodynamic monitoring in critically ill patients. Intensive Care Med. 2016;42(9):1350–9.

5. Ayuela Azcarate JM, Clau Terré F, Ochagavia A, et al. Role of echocardiography in the hemodynamic monitorization of critical patients. Med Intensiva. 2012;36(3):220–232.

6. Kiefer JJ, Raiten J, Gutsche J. Point-of-care transthoracic echocardiography: a growing body of evidence, an educational need J Cardiothorac Vasc Anesth. 2020;34(1):97–98.

7. Schuster AH, Nanda NC. Doppler echocardiographic measurement of cardiac output: comparison with a non-golden standard. Am J Cardiol 1984;53(1):257–259.

8. Evangelista A, Garcia-Dorado D, Del Castillo H. Cardiac index quantification by Doppler ultrasound in patients without left ventricular outflow tract abnormalities. J Am Coll Cardiol 1995;25(3):710–716.

9. Axler O, Megarbane B, Lentschener C. Comparison of cardiac output measured with echocardiographic

volumes and aortic Doppler methods during mechanical ventilation. Intensive Care Med 2003;29(2):208–217.

10. Vignon P, Mentec H, Terre S. Diagnostic accuracy and therapeutic impact of transthoracic and transesophageal echocardiography in mechanically ventilated patients in the ICU. Chest 1994;106(6):1829–1834.

11. Mayer SA, Sherman D, Fink ME. Noninvasive monitoring of cardiac output by Doppler echocardiography in patients treated with volume expansion after subarachnoid hemorrhage. Crit Care Med 1995;23(9):1470–1474.

12. Bergenzaun L, Gudmundsson P, Ohlin H, et al. Assessing left ventricular systolic function in shock: evaluation of echocardiographic parameters in intensive care. Crit Care. 2011;15(4):R200.

13. Dinh VA, Ko HS, Rao R, et al. Measuring cardiac index with a focused cardiac ultrasound examination in the ED. Am J Emerg Med. 2012;30(9):1845–51.

14. Mayo PH, Beaulieu Y, Doelken P. American College of Chest Physicians/La Société de Réanimation de Langue Française statement on competence in critical care ultrasonography. Chest 2009;135(4):1050–1060.

15. Expert Round Table on Ultrasound in ICU. International expert statement on standards for critical care ultrasonography. Intensive Care Med 2011;37(7):1077–1083.

16. Kanji HD, McCallum J, Sirounis D, et al. Limited echocardiography-guided therapy in subacute shock is associated with change in management and improved outcomes. J Crit Care 2014;29(5):700–5.

17. Orde S, Slama M, Hilton A, et al. Pearls and pitfalls in comprehensive critical care echocardiography. Crit Care 2017;21(1):279.

18. Marcelino P, Germano N, Marum S, et al. Hemodynamic parameters obtained by transthoracic echocardiography and Swan-Ganz catheter: a comparative study in liver transplant patients. Acta Med Port. 2006;19(3):197–205.

19. Tchorz KM, Chandra MS, Markert RJ, et al. Comparison of hemodynamic measurements from invasive and noninvasive monitoring during early resuscitation. J Trauma Acute Care Surg. 2012;72(4):852–60.

20. Gassner M, Killu K, Bauman Z, et al. Feasibility of common carotid artery point of care ultrasound in cardiac output measurements compared to invasive methods. J Ultrasound. 2014;18(2):127–33.

21. Olivieri PP, Patel R, Kolb S, et al. Echo is a good, not perfect, measure of cardiac output in critically ill surgical patients. J Trauma Acute Care Surg 2019;87(2):379–85.

22. Villavicencio C, Leache J, Marin J, et al. Basic critical care echocardiography training of intensivists allows reproducible and reliable measurements of cardiac output. Ultrasound J 2019;11:5.

23. Bergamaschi V, Vignazia GL, Messina A, et al. Transthoracic echocardiographic assessment of cardiac output in mechanically ventilated critically ill patients by intensive care unit physicians. Rev Bras Anestesiol. 2019;69(1):20–26.

24. Zarragoikoetxea I, Vicente R, Pajares A, et al. Quantitative transthoracic echocardiography of the

response to dobutamine in cardiac surgery patients with low cardiac surgery output syndrome. J Cardiothorac Vasc Anesth 2020;34(1):87–96.

25. Martin ND, Codner P, Greene W, et al. Contemporary hemodynamic monitoring, fluid responsiveness, volume optimization, and endpoints of resuscitation: an AAST critical care committee clinical consensus. Trauma Surg Acute Care Open 2020;5(1):e000411.

26. Gorrasi J, Pazos A, Florio L, et al. Cardiac output measured by transthoracic echocardiography and Swan-Ganz catheter. A comparative study in mechanically ventilated patients with high positive end-expiratory pressure. Rev Bras Ter Intensiva. 2019;31(4):474–482.

27. Zhang Y, Wang Y, Shi J, et al. Cardiac output measurements via echocardiography versus thermodilution: A systematic review and meta-analysis. PLoS ONE 2019;14(10):e0222105.

28. Jozwiak M, Mercado P, Teboul J, et al. What is the lowest change in cardiac output that transthoracic echocardiography can detect? Crit Care 2019;23(1):116.

29. Leung JM, Levine EH. Left ventricular end-systolic cavity obliteration as an estimate of intraoperative hypovolemia. Anesthesiology. 1994;81(5):1102–1109.

30. Mok KL. Make it SIMPLE: enhanced shock management by focused cardiac ultrasound. J Intensive Care. 2016;4:51.

31. Jakovljevic DG, Trenell MI, MacGowan GA. Bioimpedance and bioreactance methods for monitoring cardiac output. Best Practice & Research Clinical Anaesthesiology. 2014;28(4):381–394.

32. Nguyen LS, Squara P. Non-Invasive Monitoring of Cardiac Output in Critical Care Medicine. Front Med (Lausanne). 2017;4:200.

33. Peyton PJ, Chong SW. Minimally invasive measurement of cardiac output during surgery and critical care: a meta-analysis of accuracy and precision. Anesthesiology 2010;113(5):1220–1235.

34. Critchley LAH, Huang L, Zhang J. Continuous Cardiac Output Monitoring: What Do Validation Studies Tell Us? Curr Anesthesiol Rep 2014;4:242–250.

35. Harford M, Clark SH, Smythe JF, et al. Non-invasive stroke volume estimation by transthoracic electrical bioimpedance versus Doppler echocardiography in healthy volunteers, Journal of Medical Engineering & Technology 2019;43(1):33–37.

36. Saugel B, Cecconi M, Wagner JY, et al. Noninvasive continuous cardiac output monitoring in perioperative and intensive care medicine. Br J Anaesth 2015;114(4):562–575.

37. Squara P, Denjean D, Estagnasie P, et al. Noninvasive cardiac output monitoring (NICOM): a clinical validation. Intensive Care Med 2007;33(7):1191–1194.

38. Marik PE, Levitov A, Young A, et al. The use of bioreactance and carotid Doppler to determine volume responsiveness and blood flow redistribution following passive leg raising in hemodynamically unstable patients. Chest 2013;143(2):364–370.

39. Han S, Lee JH, Kim G, et al. Bioreactance Is Not Interchangeable with Thermodilution for Measuring Cardiac Output during Adult Liver Transplantation. PLoS One 2015;10(5):e0127981.

40. Jones TW, Houghton D, Cassidy S, et al. Bioreactance is a reliable method for estimating cardiac output at rest and during exercise. Br J Anaesth. 2015;115(3):386–91.

41. Galarza L, Mercado P, Teboul JL, et al. Estimating the rapid hemodynamic effects of passive leg raising in critically ill patients using bioreactance. Br J Anaesth 2018;121(3):567–573.

42. Joosten A, Desebbe O, Suehiro K, et al. Accuracy and precision of noninvasive cardiac output monitoring devices in perioperative medicine: A systematic review and meta-analysis. Br J Anaesth 2017;118(3):298–310.

43. Saugel B, Meidert AS, Langwieser N, et al. An autocalibrating algorithm for non-invasive cardiac output determination based on the analysis of an arterial pressure waveform recorded with radial artery applanation tonometry: a proof of concept pilot analysis. J Clin Monit Comput 2014;28(4):357–362.

44. Wagner JY, Sarwari H, Schön G, et al. Radial artery applanation tonometry for continuous noninvasive cardiac output measurement: A comparison with intermittent pulmonary artery thermodilution in patients after cardiothoracic surgery. Crit Care Med. 2015;43(7):1423–1428.

45. Compton F, Wittrock M, Schaefer JH, et al. Noninvasive cardiac output determination using applanation tonometry-derived radial artery pulse contour analysis in critically ill patients. Anesth Analg. 2008;106(1):171–4.

46. Wagner JY, Langemann M, Schön G, et al. Autocalibrating pulse contour analysis based on radial artery applanation tonometry for continuous non-invasive cardiac output monitoring in intensive care unit patients after major gastrointestinal surgery—A prospective method comparison study. Anaesthesia and intensive care 2016;44(3):340–345.

47. Gonzalez-Represas A, Mourot L. Stroke volume and cardiac output measurement in cardiac patients during a rehabilitation program: comparison between tonometry, impedancemetry and echocardiography. Int J Cardiovasc Imaging. 2020;36(3):447–455.

48. Bartels K, Thiele RH. Advances in photoplethysmography: beyond arterial oxygen saturation. Can J Anaesth. 2015;62(12):1313–28.

49. Broch O, Renner J, Gruenewald M, et al. A comparison of the Nexfin(R) and transcardiopulmonary thermodilution to estimate cardiac output during coronary artery surgery. Anaesthesia 2012;67(4):377–383.

50. Chen G, Meng L, Alexander B, et al. Comparison of noninvasive cardiac output measurements using the Nexfin monitoring device and the esophageal Doppler. J Clin Anesth 2012;24(4):275–283.

51. Pour-Ghaz I, Manolukas T, Foray N, et al. Accuracy of non-invasive and minimally invasive hemodynamic monitoring: where do we stand? Ann Transl Med. 2019;7(17):421.

52. Schraverus P, Kuijpers MM, Coumou J, et al. Level of agreement between cardiac output measurements using Nexfin® and thermodilution in morbidly obese patients undergoing laparoscopic surgery Anaesthesia 2016;71(12):1449–1455.

53. Fischer MO, Avram R, Cârjaliu I, et al. Non-invasive continuous arterial pressure and cardiac index monitoring with Nexfin after cardiac surgery. Br J Anaesth 2012;109(4):514–21.

54. Monnet X, Picard F, Lidzborski E, et al. The estimation of cardiac output by the Nexfin device is of poor reliability for tracking the effects of a fluid challenge. Crit Care 2012;16(5):R212.

55. Fischer MO, Coucoravas J, Truong J, et al. Assessment of changes in cardiac index and fluid responsiveness: a comparison of Nexfin and transpulmonary thermodilution Acta Anaesthesiol Scand 2013;57(6):704–712.

56. Taton O, Fagnoul D, De Backer D, et al. Evaluation of cardiac output in intensive care using a non-invasive arterial pulse contour technique (Nexfin((R))) compared with echocardiography. Anaesthesia 2013;68(9):917–923.

57. Fischera MO, Joosten A, Desebbe O, et al. Interchangeability of cardiac output measurements between non-invasive photoplethysmography and bolus thermodilution: A systematic review and individual patient data meta-analysis Anaesth Crit Care Pain Med. 2020;39(1):75–85.

58. Click RL, Abel MD, Schaff HV. Intraoperative transesophageal echocardiography: 5-year prospective review of impact on surgical management. Mayo Clinic Proceeding 2000;75(3):241–247.

59. Mahmood F, Shernan SK. Perioperative transoesophageal echocardiography: current status and future directions. Heart. 2016;102(15):1159–67.

60. Parra V, Fita G, Rovira I, et al. Transoesophageal echocardiography accurately detects cardiac output variation: a prospective comparison with thermodilution in cardiac surgery. Eur J Anaesthesiol 2008;25(2):135–43.

61. Møller-Sørensen H, Graeser K, Hansen KL, et al. Measurements of cardiac output obtained with transesophageal echocardiography and pulmonary artery thermodilution are not interchangeable. Acta Anaesthesiol Scand 2014;58(1):80–8.

62. Hahn RT, Abraham T, Adams MS, et al. Guidelines for performing a comprehensive transesophageal echocardiographic examination: recommendations from the American Society of Echocardiography and the Society of Cardiovascular Anesthesiologists. J Am Soc Echocardiogr. 2013;26(9):921–64.

63. Wally D, Velik-Salchner C. Perioperative transesophageal echocardiography in non-cardiac surgery. Update. Anaesthesist. 2015;64(9):669–682.

64. Rebel A, Klimkina O, Hassan ZU. Transesophageal echocardiography for the noncardiac surgical patient. Int Surg. 2012;97(1):43–55.

65. Fayad A, Shillcutt SK. Perioperative transesophageal echocardiography for non-cardiac surgery. Can J Anesth/J Can Anesth 2018;65(4):381–398.

66. Elsherbiny M, Abdelwahab Y, Nagy K, et al. Role of intraoperative transesophageal echocardiography in cardiac surgery: an observational study. Open Access Maced J Med Sci. 2019;7(15):2480–2483.

67. Abbas SM, Hill AG. Systematic review of the literature for the use of oesophageal Doppler monitor for fluid

replacement in major abdominal surgery. Anaesthesia 2008;63(1):44–51.

68. National Institute for Health and Clinical Excellence. Medical technologies guidance MTG3: CardioQ-ODM oesophageal doppler monitor. March 2011. http://www.nice.org.uk/MTG3 (accessed 19.4.20).

69. Dhawan R, Shahul S, Roberts JD, et al. Prospective, randomized clinical trial comparing use of intraoperative transesophageal echocardiography to standard care during radical cystectomy. Ann Card Anaesth. 2018;21(3):255–261.

70. Practice guidelines for perioperative transesophageal echocardiography. An updated report by the American Society of Anesthesiologists and the Society of Cardiovascular Anesthesiologists Task Force on transesophageal echocardiography. Anesthesiology. 2010;112(5):1084–96.

71. Hauser ND, Swanevelder J. Transoesophageal echocardiography (TOE): contra-indications, complications and safety of perioperative TOE. Echo Res Pract. 2018;5(4):R101–R113.

72. Cecconi M, De Backer D, Antonelli M, et al. Consensus on circulatory shock and hemodynamic monitoring. Task force of the European Society of Intensive Care Medicine. Intensive Care Med. 2014;40(12):1795–815.

73. Tibby S. Transpulmonary thermodilution: Finally, a gold standard for pediatric cardiac output measurement. Pediatr Crit Care Med. 2008;9(3):341–2.

74. Monnet X, Teboul JL. Transpulmonary thermodilution: advantages and limits. Critical Care. 2017;21(1):147.

75. Sakka SG, Reuter DA, Perel A. The transpulmonary thermodilution technique. J Clin Monit Comput. 2012;26(5):347–53.

76. Marik PE, Cavallazzi R, Vasu T, et al. Dynamic changes in arterial waveform derived variables and fluid responsiveness in mechanically ventilated patients: a systematic review of the literature. Crit Care Med 2009;37(9):2642–2647.

77. Perny J, Kimmoun A, Perez P, et al. Evaluation of cardiac function index as measured by transpulmonary thermodilution as an indicator of left ventricular ejection fraction in cardiogenic shock. BioMed Research International. 2014;2014:598029.

78. Michard F. Bedside assessment of extravascular lung water by dilution methods: temptations and pitfalls. Crit Care Med. 2007;35(4):1186–1192.

79. Jozwiak M, Teboul JL, Monnet X. Extravascular lung water in critical care: recent advances and clinical applications. Ann Intensive Care. 2015;5(1):38.

80. Sakka SG, Klein M, Reinhart K, et al. Prognostic value of extravascular lung water in critically ill patients. Chest 2002;122(6):2080–6.

81. Kushimoto S, Endo T, Yamanouchi S, et al. Relationship between extravascular lung water and severity categories of acute respiratory distress syndrome by the Berlin definition. Crit Care 2013;17(4):R132.

82. Beurton A, Teboul JL, Monnet X. Transpulmonary thermodilution techniques in the hemodynamically unstable patient. Curr Opin Crit Care. 2019;25(3):273–279.

83. Mielck F, Buhre W, Hanekop G, et al. Comparison of continuous cardiac output measurements in patients after cardiac surgery. J Cardiothorac Vasc Anesth. 2003;17(2):211–216.

84. Reuter DA, Huang C, Edrich T, et al. Cardiac output monitoring using indicator-dilution techniques: Basics, limits, and perspectives. Anesth Analg 2010;110(3):799–811.

85. Marik PE. Obituary: pulmonary artery catheter 1970 to 2013. Ann Intensive Care. 2013;3(1):38.

86. Vilchez Monge AL, Tranche Alvarez-Cagigas I, Perez-Peña J, et al. Cardiac output monitoring with pulmonary versus transpulmonary thermodilution during liver transplantation: interchangeable methods? Minerva Anestesiol. 2014;80(11):1178–87.

87. Benes J, Giglio M, Brienza N, et al. The effects of goal-directed fluid therapy based on dynamic parameters on post-surgical outcome: a meta-analysis of randomized controlled trials. Crit Care. 2014;18(5):584.

88. Linton RAF, Band DM, Haire KM. A new method of measuring cardiac output in man using lithium dilution. Brit J Anaesth.1993;71(2):262–266.

89. Jonas MM, Tanser SJ. Lithium dilution measurement of cardiac output and arterial pulse waveform analysis: an indicator dilution calibrated beat-by-beat system for continuous estimation of cardiac output. Curr Opin Crit Care. 2002;8(3):257–61.

90. Garcia-Rodriguez C, Pittman J, Cassell CH, et al. Lithium dilution cardiac output measurement: a clinical assessment of central venous and peripheral venous indicator injection. Crit Care Med. 2002;30(10):2199–2204.

91. Kurita T, Morita K, Kato S, et al. Comparison of the accuracy of the lithium dilution technique with the thermodilution technique for measurement of cardiac output. British Journal of Anaesthesia. 1997;79(6):770–775.

92. García X, Mateu L, Maynar J. Estimating cardiac output. Utility in the clinical practice. Available invasive and non-invasive monitoring. Med Intensiva. 2011;35(9):552–61.

93. Geerts BF, Aarts LP, Jansen JR. Methods in pharmacology: measurement of cardiac output. Br J Clin Pharmacol. 2011;71(3):316–330.

94. Grensemann J. Cardiac output monitoring by pulse contour analysis, the technical basics of less-invasive techniques. Front Med (Lausanne). 2018;5:64.

95. Wernly B, Lichtenauer M, Franz M, et al. Pulse contour cardiac output monitoring in acute heart failure patients: Assessment of hemodynamic measurements. Wien Klin Wochenschr. 2016;128(23-24):864–869.

96. Monnet X, Anguel N, Jozwiak M, et al. Third-generation floTrac/Vigileo does not reliably track changes in cardiac output induced by norepinephrine in critically ill patients. Br J Anaesth 2012;108(4):615–22.

97. Kusaka Y, Yoshitani K, Irie T, et al. Clinical comparison of an echocardiograph-derived versus pulse counter-derived cardiac output measurement in abdominal aortic aneurysm surgery. J Cardiothorac Vasc Anesth 2012;26(2):223–6.

98. Jeong YB, Kim TH, Roh YJ, et al. Comparison of uncalibrated arterial pressure waveform analysis

with continuous thermodilution cardiac output measurements in patients undergoing elective off-pump coronary artery bypass surgery. J Cardiothorac Vasc Anesth 2010;24(5):767–71.

99. Lansdorp B, Lemson J, van Putten MJ, et al. Dynamic indices do not predict volume responsiveness in routine clinical practice. Br J Anaesth 2012;108(3):395–401.

100. Marik PE. Non-invasive cardiac output monitors: a state-of-the-art review. J Cardiothorac Vasc Anesth. 2013;27(1):121–134.

101. Reisner A. Academic assessment of arterial pulse contour analysis: missing the forest for the trees? Br J Anaesth. 2016;116(6):733–736.

102. Sakka SG, Kozieras J, Thuemer O, et al. Measurement of cardiac output: a comparison between transpulmonary thermodilution and uncalibrated pulse contour analysis. Br J Anaesth 2007;99(3):337–342.

103. Jaffe MB. Partial CO2 rebreathing cardiac output - operating principles of the NICO system. J Clin Monit. 1999;15(6):387–401.

104. Miller RD, Cohen NH, Eriksson LI, et al. Miller's anesthesia. 8th ed. Philadelphia, PA: Saunders;2015.p.1391.

105. Chamos C, Vele L, Hamilton M, et al. Less invasive methods of advanced hemodynamic monitoring: principles, devices, and their role in the perioperative hemodynamic optimization. Perioper Med (Lond). 2013;2(1):19.

106. Kerstens MKM, Wijnberge M, Geerts BF. Non-invasive cardiac output monitoring techniques in the ICU. Neth J Crit Care 2018;26(3):104–110.

107. Lee AJ, Cohn JH, Ranasinghe JS. Cardiac output assessed by invasive and minimally invasive techniques. Anesthesiol Res Pract 2011;2011:475151.

108. Moise SF, Sinclair CJ, Scott DHT. Pulmonary artery blood temperature and the measurement of cardiac output by thermodilution Anaesthesia 2002;57(6):562–566.

109. Stetz CW, Miller RG, Kelly GE, et al. Reliability of the thermodilution method in the determination of cardiac output in clinical practice. The American Review of Respiratory Disease. 1982;126(6):1001–1004.

110. Drummond KE, Murphy E. Minimally invasive cardiac output monitors, Continuing Education in Anaesthesia Critical Care & Pain 2012;12(1):5–10.

111. Nishikawa T, Dohi S. Errors in the measurement of cardiac output by thermodilution. Can J Anaesth 1993;40(2):142–53.

112. Robin E, Costecalde M, Lebuffe G, et al. Clinical relevance of data from the pulmonary artery catheter. Critical Care 2006;10 Suppl 3(Suppl 3):S3.

113. Argueta EE, Paniagua D. Thermodilution cardiac output: A concept over 250 years in the making. Cardiol Rev. 2019;27(3):138–144.

114. Mehta Y, Arora D. Newer methods of cardiac output monitoring. World J Cardiol. 2014;6(9):1022–1029.

Part 6

Electrolyte Disorders

20 | Hyponatremia

SODIUM PHYSIOLOGY

INTRODUCTION

A basic understanding of physiology is essential for the proper approach and treatment of water balance and sodium balance disorders in clinical practice.

Water excess or deficit in the body leads to hyponatremia and hypernatremia. Therefore disorders of sodium concentration occur primarily due to water imbalance and not due to changes in total body sodium content. The below-mentioned equation will help to clarify the above statement.

$$\frac{\text{Serum Sodium}}{\text{Concentration}} = \frac{\text{Total Body Sodium}}{\text{Total Body Water}}$$

In the above equation, serum sodium concentration will decrease when total body water increases, leading to hyponatremia. Similarly, serum sodium concentration will increase when total body water decreases, leading to hypernatremia. So, to understand sodium disorders, we need to know about the physiology of water balance.

As serum osmolality is determined mainly by sodium salts (equation below) [1], the regulation of water balance is also discussed as the regulation of body fluid osmolality (osmoregulation). Normal serum osmolality is 275–290 mOsm/kg. Hyponatremia is usually associated with low serum osmolality.

Serum Osmolality (Calculated)

$$= 2 \, [Na^+] + \frac{Glucose}{18} + \frac{BUN}{2.8}$$

Where osmolality is in mOsm/kg, sodium in mEq/L, glucose in mg/dL, and blood urea nitrogen (BUN) in mg/dL.

WATER REGULATION

In a normal person, water is balanced by adjusting input and urine output, besides wide variations in water and salt intakes. Thirst and renal excretion of water are two primary mechanisms that control body water.

A. Response to water deficit

Increased water intake

In patients with water deprivation, water intake is regulated by thirst. The 4 major stimuli for thirst are [2]:

1. Increased extracellular fluid (ECF) osmolality: It is the most important stimulus for thirst. Increased concentration of sodium increases serum osmolality. Increased ECF osmolality by 1–2% stimulates the thirst center and increases thirst.

2. Hypovolemia: A decline in plasma volume of 10–15% stimulates thirst.

3. Hypotension: A fall in blood pressure stimulates specialized stretch baroreceptors located within the carotid sinus and aortic arch, increasing thirst independent of increased serum osmolality.

4. Increased angiotensin II: A fall in blood pressure activates the renin-angiotensin system (RAS) and increases the release of angiotensin II. Angiotensin II binds to the hypothalamus, stimulates thirst, and increases water intake. It also stimulates the release of antidiuretic hormone (ADH) by the posterior pituitary gland and increases renal water reabsorption.

Decreased water excretion

Antidiuretic hormone tightly regulates water excretion. ADH release increases due to increased plasma osmolality, blood pressure fall, and increased angiotensin II releases. ADH acts on the kidney at distal tubules and collecting duct. ADH increases water permeability by inserting aquaporin channels at the collecting duct with resultant increased water reabsorption. Under the influence of ADH, as much as 18 liters of water is reabsorbed in the collecting ducts. By increasing water reabsorption and decreasing urine output, ADH preserves body water.

B. Response to water excess

The combined effect of decreased ADH increases atrial natriuretic peptide (ANP), and thirst suppression controls water excess.

Decrease antidiuretic hormone

When the amount of water in the body increases, secretion of ADH will decrease, so water reabsorption by the collecting duct will decrease, and there will be increased excretion of dilute urine.

Increase atrial natriuretic peptide (ANP)

Volume expansion will also increase the secretion of atrial natriuretic peptide due to atrial stretching, promoting diuresis and natriuresis.

Decreased ADH and increased ANP will decrease water reabsorption, increase urine output, and maintain appropriate water in the body.

Thirst suppression

Excess body water suppresses thirst, decreases oral water intake, and prevents aggravation of water excess. Mechanisms by which thirst is suppressed are decreased plasma osmolality, increased blood volume, increased arterial blood pressure, and stomach distention.

SODIUM REGULATION

A. Physiological basis

- Sodium is the major ECF cation (serum sodium value 140 mEq/L ECF vs. 10 mEq/L intracellular).

- The total amount of sodium in an average adult is about 3,500 to 5,000 mEq.

- Sodium is distributed chiefly in ECF and is responsible for over 90% of ECF osmolality.

- The primary function of sodium is to control and regulate the ECF volume and maintain blood pressure.

- ECF volume is the reflection of total body sodium content (amount). The gain of sodium leads to water retention, causing an increase in extracellular fluid volume, blood volume, and blood pressure. So total body sodium content is high

in patients with anasarca. On the contrary, loss of sodium leads to water loss, causing extracellular fluid volume contraction, hypovolemia, and hypotension.

- Effective arterial blood volume (EABV, also called effective circulating volume) refers to the volume of blood in the arterial system that "effectively" perfuses tissues. EABV is a non-measurable, dynamic component of the ECF volume.

- The concept of EABV is helpful to understanding the regulation of sodium balance, and EABV normally changes in the same direction as changes in ECF volume (congestive heart failure (CHF) and cirrhosis are the exceptions in this relationship because the ECF volume is increased, but EABV reduces in these conditions).

- The daily sodium requirement is about 1 mEq/kg/day [3]. 1 gm of sodium chloride contains 17.1 mEq sodium.

- Excess salt is excreted chiefly by the kidney. Loss of sodium in sweat is poor (40–60 mEq/L) [4].

B. Regulatory mechanism of ECF volume

Sensors called vascular volume receptors or baroreceptors regulate sodium balance and control extracellular fluid volume by perceiving the changes in effective arterial blood volume. The most important volume receptors are located in the right atria, carotid sinus, and glomerular afferent arterioles (called juxtaglomerular cells). The mechanisms that play important roles in the regulation are renal sympathetic nerves, the renin-angiotensin-aldosterone system, natriuretic peptides, and antidiuretic hormone.

C. Response to sodium deficit

The various mechanisms by which the body counteracts ECF deficit are:

- **Renin-angiotensin-aldosterone system:** A sodium deficiency in the body will lead to hypovolemia. Reduced effective arterial blood volume activates renin secretion, resulting in increased angiotensin II and aldosterone levels.

  By acting on the kidney, angiotensin-II helps to increase sodium absorption at the proximal tubules and aldosterone at the collecting duct. In a state of sodium deficit, absorption of Na^+ under aldosterone control is so perfect that almost no urinary Na^+ loss occurs.

- **Sympathetic nervous system (SNS):** Increased renal sympathetic nerve activity leads to afferent and efferent arteriolar vasoconstriction, decreases glomerular filtration rate (GFR) and increases renal sodium reabsorption in proximal tubules.

- **Natriuretic peptides:** Inhibition of ANP and B-type natriuretic peptide (BNP) secretion due to ECF volume contraction prevents natriuretic peptide-dependent natriuresis and diuresis.

- **Antidiuretic hormone:** Increases ADH secretion by exerting its effects on the late distal tubule and collecting ducts, promoting water reabsorption.

- **Increased thirst and salt craving:** Hypovolemia, hypotension, and increased angiotensin II levels stimulate thirst and increase fluid intake. Angiotensin II and aldosterone stimulate salt appetite.

D. Response to sodium excess

The various mechanisms by which the body counteracts ECF volume expansion increases EABV, and restores euvolemia are:

- **Suppress renin-angiotensin-aldosterone system:** The excess sodium in the body causes ECF volume expansion suppressing the renin-angiotensin-aldosterone system and leading to urinary excretion of the excess body sodium.

- **Decreased renal sympathetic activity:** A decrease in renal sympathetic nerve activity results in the dilation of afferent arterioles, which in turn increases GFR and renal sodium excretion in the proximal tubules.

- **Releases of natriuretic peptides:** An increase in the secretion of ANP due to the expansion of ECF volume causes natriuresis and diuresis.

- **Suppress antidiuretic hormone secretion:** The increase in EABV decreases ADH secretion and promotes water excretion by decreasing sodium reabsorption from the collecting duct.

- **Abolish thirst and salt craving:** Suppressed angiotensin II levels diminish thirst and reduce fluid intake. Low angiotensin II and aldosterone levels suppress salt appetite.

Disorders of sodium balance - Hypovolemia and edema are two major disorders of sodium balance.

The regulation of water and sodium balance is summarized in Table 20.1.

HYPONATREMIA

INTRODUCTION

Hyponatremia is the most frequently encountered but often overlooked electrolyte disorder in clinical practice [5]. Hyponatremia is defined as serum sodium <135 mEq/L, which occurs

Table 20.1 Regulation of water and sodium balance		
	Water regulation (Osmoregulation)	**ECF volume (Sodium content regulation)**
Regulation of	The proportion of sodium to water (osmolality)	Total body sodium and water (ECF volume)
What is sensed?	Plasma osmolality	Effective circulating volume
Sensor	Hypothalamic osmoreceptors	Vascular volume receptors (carotid sinus, aortic arch, renal afferent arterioles, atria)
Effector pathways	Thirst, antidiuretic hormone	Renin-angiotensin-aldosterone system, sympathetic nervous system, ANP, ADH
Response	**Water excess, low plasma osmolality:** Inhibit ADH release, causing increased excretion of diluted urine Suppress thirst and reduce water intake **Net effect:** Excretion of excess water and correction of low osmolality	**Hypovolemia/ECF Na^+ deficit:** Increases renal absorption of sodium and water Increased thirst and salt craving Peripheral vasoconstriction **Net effect:** Retention of salt and water causing correction of hypovolemia
	Water deficit, high plasma osmolality: Stimulate thirst and water intake increases ADH release, causing water reabsorption **Net effect:** Retention of water and correction of high osmolality	**Hypervolemia/ECF Na^+ excess:** Increases renal loss of sodium and water Reduce thirst Peripheral vasodilatation **Net effect:** Excretion of excess salt and water causing correction of hypervolemia
Method to assess	Primarily laboratory evaluation	Primarily physical examination

in about 15% to 30% of hospitalized patients and about 7% of ambulatory patients [6–8]. Hyponatremia is associated with a longer hospital stay, readmission, and higher mortality [9–11]. Proper evaluation and investigations help to establish the etiology and various types of hyponatremia based on which treatment is planned.

Why is hyponatremia an important electrolyte disorder?

Hyponatremia is an important disorder, and every clinician should know about the approach and management of hyponatremia because:

- **Common:** Hyponatremia is the most common electrolyte disorder in both inpatients and outpatients.

- **Underdiagnosed:** Hyponatremia is often missed (due to vague symptoms) or misdiagnosed (confusion due to pseudohyponatremia or hypertonic hyponatremia).

- **Poorly assessed:** In hyponatremia, frequently insufficient diagnostic tests are ordered with resultant less precise therapy [12].

- **Confusing:** As a beginner, understanding the basic concept of hyponatremia can be confusing and complex. Electrolyte disorders such as hypokalemia or hypomagnesemia usually indicate a deficiency in potassium or magnesium and require supplementation. This simple understanding can be applied to many disorders with the prefix "hypo."

However, the development and treatment strategy of hyponatremia may be contrary to this common understanding.

"Hyponatremia suggests total body sodium deficiency, and all patients need sodium supplementation" is a wrong concept.

Hyponatremia usually means water excess.

Hyponatremia is a disorder of water and not sodium. Serum sodium reflects the relative proportion of sodium and water [13]. Therefore, hyponatremia tells us that there is a relative excess of water in relation to sodium rather than sodium deficiency.

- **Complex:** Managing hyponatremia is challenging due to the lack of a fixed treatment protocol (which varies based on symptoms and volume status for the same low serum sodium value) [14], differences in recommendations between American and European guidelines [5, 15], and the potential for detrimental effects

from inappropriate treatment (either too rapid or too slow) [16].

- **Harmful:** Hyponatremia can result in significant morbidity [11, 17], mortality, prolonged hospital stays, and increased hospital expenses [9].

CLASSIFICATION

For proper understanding, it is essential to know the classification of hyponatremia based on various parameters (Table 20.2).

ETIOLOGY

Hyponatremia can arise from multiple diseases, and it is characterized by hypoosmolality resulting from low serum sodium levels. Therefore, to establish the diagnosis of true hypotonic (hypoosmolar) hyponatremia, the first essential step in patients with hyponatremia is to exclude hyponatremia with normal or increased osmolality (Figure 20.1). The causes of true hypotonic hyponatremia are further classified based on the extracellular fluid volume as euvolemic, hypervolemic,

Table 20.2 Classification of hyponatremia		
1. Based on measured serum osmolality		
Hypotonic - true Low osmolality <280 mOsm/kg	**Isotonic** Normal osmolality 280–295 mOsm/kg	**Hypertonic** High osmolality >295 mOsm/kg
2. Based on the time of development		
Acute <48 hours	**Chronic** >48 hours	**Unknown**: Chronic
3. Based on the severity of sodium concentration		
Mild 130–135 mEq/L	**Moderate** 125–129 mEq/L	**Severe** <125 mEq/L
4. Based on the degree of symptoms		
Mild None, symptoms of chronic hyponatremia	**Moderate** Nausea, headache, confusion	**Severe** Vomiting, seizures, coma, death
5. Based on volume status		
Hypovolemic	**Hypervolemic**	**Euvolemic**

and hypovolemic hyponatremia (Figure 20.1), which are discussed in detail under the diagnostic approach to hyponatremia.

CLINICAL FEATURES

The severity of symptoms of hyponatremia depends upon the rate of onset (i.e., how fast hyponatremia develops), the severity of hyponatremia (i.e., mild, moderate, or severe), and its duration (acute or chronic hyponatremia - less or more than 48 hours).

Acute and severe hyponatremia is symptomatic, but chronic and mild hyponatremia is well tolerated and often has vague, nonspecific symptoms. Symptoms of acute hyponatremia are chiefly neurological, as summarized in Table 20.3 [13, 15, 18].

Why are symptoms of hyponatremia primarily neurogenic?

It is not the reduction of ECF sodium that gives rise to symptoms and signs of hyponatremia. Hyponatremia causes hypoosmolality of the ECF, resulting in water movement into cells (intracellular fluid or ICF), which causes cells to swell. This swelling has little impact on tissues such as skeletal muscles but increases the volume of brain cells, leading to neurological dysfunction [13, 18, 19].

Since the brain is enclosed in a rigid skull with a fixed volume, edema of brain cells compresses the brain parenchyma, increasing intracranial pressure (ICP) and causing neurological manifestations [20]. This increase in ICP can cause a decrease in cerebral blood flow, leading to hypoxic brain damage. In severe cases, the increase in ICP can lead to herniation of the brain, characterized by unequal or fixed dilated pupils, hypoventilation, cardiovascular instability, urinary or fecal incontinence, or respiratory arrest.

Chronic hyponatremia: Patients with mild chronic hyponatremia can be asymptomatic but may experience symptoms such as fatigue, attention deficits, memory loss, unsteady gait, recurrent unexplained falls, severe osteoporosis, increased bone fragility, and high fracture risk, which occur more commonly in the elderly [21–23].

A STEP-BY-STEP DIAGNOSIS

A simple stepwise approach to evaluate patients with hyponatremia is summarized.

Step 1: History and physical examination

A careful history in a patient with hyponatremia is helpful to determine the duration of hyponatremia (acute or chronic hyponatremia), identify underlying etiology (diarrhea, vomiting, etc.), underlying illness (CHF, cirrhosis, nephrotic syndrome, hypothyroidism, adrenal insufficiencies), and medications

Table 20.3 Manifestations of acute hyponatremia		
Severity	Serum sodium (mEq/L)	Symptoms
Mild	130–135	Usually asymptomatic, symptoms of chronic hyponatremia
Moderate	125–129	Nausea, malaise, mild lethargy, weakness, cramps, headache, confusion
Severe	<125	Vomiting, delirium, drowsiness, diminished reflexes, convulsions, coma, death

causing hyponatremia (diuretics, antihypertensives, antidepressants, or hypotonic IV fluids). Proper physical examination helps to establish hydration status (hypervolemia, euvolemia, or hypovolemia/dehydration). It also detects hyponatremia's serious signs or symptoms (such as vomiting, agitation, stupor, convulsion, loss of consciousness, coma, and cardio-respiratory distress, suggesting cerebral edema/cerebral herniation).

Subsequent major steps to establish the underlying cause of hyponatremia include conducting three crucial diagnostic tests: measuring serum osmolality, urinary osmolality, and urinary sodium concentration (urine Na) (as shown in Table 20.4), as well as assessing volume status (Figure 20.1).

Step 2: Measure serum osmolality

The aim is to clinch the diagnosis of true hypotonic hyponatremia and exclude hypertonic hyponatremia and Pseudohyponatremia. Normal serum osmolality is 275–290 mOsm/kg. True

Table 20.4 Major steps in the initial evaluation of hyponatremia
1. Serum osmolality
Low: True hyponatremia
Normal or elevated: Pseudohyponatremia or hypertonic hyponatremia
2. Urine osmolality
Low (<100 mOsm/kg): Diluted urine suggests primary polydipsia with normal water excretion, low solute intake (beer potomania syndrome), post TURP
High (>100 mOsm/kg): Conditions in which water excretion is impaired (Hypovolemia, SIADH, adrenal insufficiency)
3. Urine sodium concentration
<20 mEq/L: Hypovolemia, cirrhosis, congestive heart failure
>20 mEq/L: SIADH, adrenal insufficiency, or renal salt wasting (diuretics, renal disease, or hypoaldosteronism)

hypotonic hyponatremia is always associated with low serum osmolality.

In patients with hyponatremia, serum osmolality is measured using a freezing point depression osmometer, which

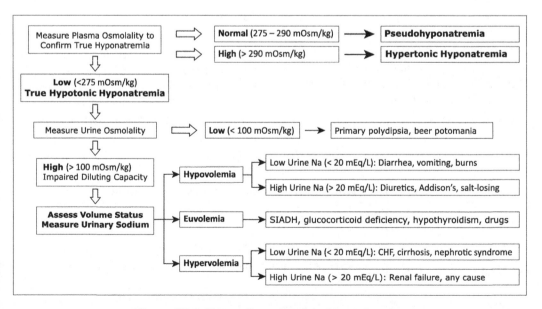

Figure 20.1 Diagnostic approach to hyponatremia.

is essential to confirm the diagnosis of true hypotonic hyponatremia and exclude pseudohyponatremia (isotonic hyponatremia) or translocational (hypertonic) hyponatremia [24].

Classification of hyponatremia based on measured serum osmolality, its etiology, and how it causes hyponatremia is summarized in Table 20.5:

- **Normal serum osmolality (POsm 275–290 mOsm/kg):** In patients with marked hyperlipidemia and hyperproteinemia, serum sodium concentration may appear spuriously low, a condition termed pseudohyponatremia [25]. Pseudohyponatremia, also known as isotonic hyponatremia, is a laboratory artifact caused by sodium measurement through less accurate indirect ion-specific electrode or flame photometry methods [26, 27]. While the sodium concentration in the aqueous portion of the serum is normal, the above techniques can also measure an increased nonaqueous portion of the serum (due to hyperlipidemia and hyperproteinemia), resulting in measurement errors.

To exclude pseudohyponatremia, measure serum sodium using the direct ion-specific electrode and always measure total cholesterol and triglycerides levels in patients with low serum sodium levels [28]. In hypertriglyceridemia, for every 500 mg/dL increase in serum triglyceride concentration (above 100 mg/dL), serum sodium will decrease by 1.0 mEq/L. In hyperproteinemia, for every 1 gm/dL increase in serum protein (above 8 gm/dL), serum sodium will decrease by 4.0 mEq/L (as shown in Table 20.6).

- **High serum osmolality (POsm >290 mOsm/kg):** Hypertonic hyponatremia occurs when there are osmotically active substances present in the plasma other than sodium (such as elevated glucose, mannitol, glycerol, glycine, sorbitol, or hyperosmolar radiocontrast agents). The high concentrations of these nonsodium solutes lead to hyperosmolality, which creates an osmotic gradient that causes a shift of water from the ICF to the ECF compartment. This translocation of water in the ECF compartment dilutes the sodium concentration, resulting in hyponatremia.

Hyperglycemia is the most common cause of hypertonic hyponatremia in hospitalized patients. For every 100 mg/dL increase in serum glucose concentration (above normal levels),

Table 20.5 Interpretation of measured serum osmolality in hyponatremia

Hyponatremia	Serum osmolality	Etiology	Mechanism
True hypotonic hyponatremia	Low <275 mOsm/kg	Multiple (Table 20.7)	Reduced ratio of sodium to water due to water excess or sodium deficit
Pseudo-hyponatremia	Normal 275–290 mOsm/kg	Severe hyperlipidemia and hyperproteinemia	An increased nonaqueous portion of the serum is responsible for falsely low Na+ concentration
Hypertonic or translocational hyponatremia	High >290 mOsm/kg	Hyperglycemia, mannitol, glycerol, glycine, or sorbitol	Hypertonicity shifts water from ICF to the ECF, causing hyponatremia due to dilution

Table 20.6 Equation and calculation of corrected sodium value in hyper and isotonic hyponatremia	
Hyperglycemia	**Equation:** For each 100 mg/dL increase in serum glucose concentration (above 100 mg/dL), serum sodium will fall by 1.6 mEq/L. The correction factor will be 2.4 when blood sugar is >400 mg/dL
	Example: Blood sugar 400 mg/dL and serum sodium 130 mEq/L
	Corrected Na$^+$ (mEq/L) = Measured Na$^+$ + 1.6 × [Glucose mg/dL–100/100] = 130 + 1.6 × [400–100/100] = 130 + 1.6 × [300/100] = 130 + 1.6 × 3 = 130 + 4.8 = 134.8 mEq/L
Hypertriglycer-idemia	**Equation:** For each 500 mg/dL increase in serum triglyceride concentration (above 100 mg/dL), serum sodium will fall by 1.0 mEq/L
	Example: Serum triglyceride 1200 mg/dL and serum sodium 130 mEq/L
	Corrected Na$^+$ (mEq/L) = Measured Na$^+$ + 1.0 × [Triglyceride mg/dL–100/500] = 130 + 1.0 × [1200–100/500] = 130 + 1.0 × [1100/500] = 130 + 1.0 × 2.2 = 130 + 2.2 = 132.2 mEq/L
Hyperprotein-emia	**Equation:** For every 1 gm/dL rise in serum protein (above 8 gm/dL), serum sodium will fall by 4.0 mEq/L
	Example: Serum protein 11 gm/dL and serum sodium 130 mEq/L
	Corrected Na$^+$ (mEq/L) = Measured Na$^+$ + 4.0 × [Protein gm/dL–8] = 130 + 4.0 × [11–8] = 130 + 4.0 × 3 = 130 + 12 = 142.0 mEq/L

serum sodium will decrease by 1.6 mEq/L. If the blood sugar is >400 mg/dL, the suggested formula will be a fall of 2.4 mEq/L in serum sodium for every 100 mg/dL increase in serum glucose concentration [29]. It is important to remember that in patients with severe hyperglycemia, the "normal value of serum sodium is actually elevated, which suggests hypernatremia. Refer to Table 20.6 to understand the formula, examples of calculating the expected fall in sodium, and determining serum sodium's actual or true value in patients with severe hyperglycemia.

- **Low serum osmolality (POsm <275 mOsm/kg):** A low value of serum osmolality confirms the diagnosis of true hypotonic hyponatremia, which is the most common form of hyponatremia.

Step 3: Measure urine osmolality

The aim is to assess the effect of ADH and differentiate hyponatremia due to the:

- **Increased ADH secretion**, causing impaired water excretion and resulting in high urine osmolality (ADH-dependent hypotonic hyponatremia).

- **ADH suppression** causing normal water excretion and resulting in low urine osmolality (ADH-independent hyponatremia).

Interpretation of measured urine osmolality (Figure 20.1) [1]

- Low urine osmolality (<100 mOsm/kg) with diluted urine suggests psychogenic polydipsia, low solute intake (beer potomania or tea and toast diet), or reset osmostat.

- High urine osmolality (>100 mOsm/kg) suggests conditions in which water excretion is impaired (hypovolemia, SIADH, adrenal insufficiency, etc.).

Step 4: Assess volume status

Based on the patient's extracellular fluid volume status, patients with hypotonic hyponatremia are classified into one of three categories (hypovolemic, hypervolemic, and euvolemic hyponatremia) [14], as shown in (Figure 20.1). This step is critical because the treatment plans differ significantly between the three categories.

Step 5: Urine sodium concentration

This step is essential in differentiating hyponatremia due to renal and extrarenal loss. The approach to hyponatremia based on the patient's volume status and urine sodium concentration is summarized in Table 20.7.

Step 6: Tests to clinch further details

Detailed evaluation and laboratory tests are necessary for further diagnostic workup and to establish the etiological diagnosis of hyponatremia:

- Serum uric acid and blood urea: Low values of both favor euvolemic hyponatremia, while both are high in hypovolemic hyponatremia [30].
- Blood sugar: To rule out hyperglycemia.
- Serum creatinine: To rule out renal failure.
- Serum protein: High in multiple myeloma and low in cirrhosis of the liver.
- Serum triglycerides: To rule out pseudohyponatremia.
- Serum potassium: High potassium suggests renal insufficiency, adrenal insufficiency with hypoaldosteronism (Addison's disease), or it can be an adverse effect of fixed-dose combinations of angiotensin receptor blockers (ARBs) with hydrochlorothiazide. Potassium can be low in hyponatremic patients with diuretics therapy, diarrhea, and vomiting.
- Thyroid function tests: To rule out hypothyroidism
- Adrenal functions: ACTH and ACTH stimulation tests to rule out Addison's disease.
- Acid-base disturbances: Metabolic alkalosis and hypokalemia suggest vomiting or diuretic therapy. In

Table 20.7 Classification of hyponatremia based on the volume status and urine sodium concentration		
	Urinary Na+ <20 mEq/L	**Urinary Na+ >20 mEq/L**
1. Hypovolemia Dry tongue, reduced skin turgor, tachycardia, low BP, or postural hypotension	Extra-renal losses: Diarrhea, vomiting, burns, pancreatitis	Renal losses: Diuretics, Addison's disease, cerebral salt wasting syndrome, salt-losing nephropathy
2. Euvolemic	Primary polydipsia, water intoxication, decreased solute intake	SIADH, glucocorticoid deficiency, hypothyroidism, drugs
3. Hypervolemic Edema, ascites, increased JVP, basal lung crackles	Congestive heart failure, cirrhosis, nephrotic syndrome	Renal failure, any cause

metabolic acidosis, the presence of hypokalemia suggests diarrhea, while the presence of hyperkalemia suggests adrenal insufficiency.

Step 7: Isotonic fluid challenge

When differentiation between hyponatremia due to volume depletion and SIADH is equivocal, the isotonic saline fluid challenge has a diagnostic and therapeutic role [5]. In patients with hypovolemia, normal saline administration will increase serum sodium levels and restore intravascular volume depletion [31]. But the reduction in serum sodium after saline infusion suggests the presence of SIADH.

ETIOLOGIES OF SPECIAL IMPORTANCE

Diuretics induced hyponatremia

Hyponatremia usually occurs with thiazides rather than loop diuretics. Thiazide-induced hyponatremia is common in older women with a low body mass [32].

Mechanism of thiazide induced hyponatremia [32–34]:

1. Thiazide blocks sodium chloride reabsorption at the distal convoluted tubule in the cortex, promoting sodium excretion in the urine, leading to diminished urine diluting ability, decreasing free water excretion, and resultant concentrated urine causing loss of sodium.

2. Thiazide-induced diuretic effects and renal sodium loss cause volume depletion, which stimulates ADH release, which in turn causes increased water retention and slight volume expansion.

3. Excessive fluid intake can occur due to increased thirst induced by thiazide.

So, Thiazide-induced hyponatremia is caused by the combination of urinary sodium loss from the diuretic effect, decreased free water excretion, increased water retention (due to hypovolemia-induced elevated ADH), and increased fluid intake.

In contrast, loop diuretics cause hypotonic renal losses (excretion of water in excess of sodium leading to hypotonic urine), so hyponatremia is infrequent. In fact, due to these effects, loop diuretics are used to treat euvolemic and hypervolemic hyponatremia [34].

SIADH

Syndrome of inappropriate antidiuretic hormone (SIADH) is the most common cause of euvolemic hyponatremia. SIADH is characterized by impaired water excretion leading to high urinary sodium, osmolality, and specific gravity despite low serum sodium and hypoosmolality. The diagnostic criteria of SIADH are summarized in Table 20.11.

Cerebral salt wasting (CSW)

The CSW occurs in acute neurological disorders (most commonly due to subarachnoid hemorrhage), characterized by inappropriate sodium loss in the urine causing hyponatremia and extracellular fluid volume depletion [35, 36]. Various mechanisms proposed to explain the natriuresis in CSW are increased release of brain atrial natriuretic peptides, impaired sympathetic tone to the kidney due to damage to the hypothalamus, and suppressed aldosterone level despite hypovolemia [37]. It is crucial to distinguish between CSW and SIADH as both can result in hyponatremia due to natriuresis in neurological disorders, but their treatment principles are exactly opposite, as summarized in Table 20.8 [38–41].

Exercise-associated hyponatremia (EAH)

The EAH is an acute, severe, and potentially life-threatening hyponatremia that can most commonly follow endurance exercise (e.g., marathon runners) [42–44]. ADH levels are high in such patients. Hyponatremia occurs due to excess free water consumption in athletes with impaired urinary water excretion due to persistent secretion of antidiuretic hormone (ADH) [45, 46].

MANAGEMENT

Early diagnosis and appropriate treatment reduce morbidity and mortality [47]. There is no fixed treatment protocol for patients with hyponatremia. Effective management of hypotonic hyponatremia depends on four major factors as shown in Figure 20.2) [48]:

- The severity of hyponatremia: Presence or absence of central nervous system symptoms such as lethargy, delirium, seizure, and coma.

Table 20.8 Difference between cerebral salt-wasting (CSW) and syndrome of inappropriate antidiuretic hormone (SIADH)

	CSW	SIADH
Mechanism	Excessive excretion of sodium and water by the kidney	Retention of water by kidney due to increased ADH
Similar features		
Intracranial diseases	Common	Common
Serum sodium concentration	Decreased	Decreased
Urinary sodium excretion	Increased	Increased
Serum uric acid	Decreased	Decreased
Initial fractional excretion of urate	High	High
Renal/adrenal/thyroid function	Normal	Normal
Different features		
Incidence	Rare	Common
ECF volume status	Hypovolemia	Euvolemia or hypervolemia
Postural hypotension	Present	Absent
Bodyweight	Decreased	Normal/slightly increased
Urine volume	High	Normal or low
BUN	Increased	Normal
Fractional excretion of urate after correction of hyponatremia	High	Normal
Brain natriuretic peptide level	Increased	Normal
Serum ADH	Normal	High
Treatment		
Effective measures	Salt and fluid supplementation, fludrocortisone	Fluid restriction, 3% NaCl, vaptans
Response to normal saline	Corrects hyponatremia	May worsen hyponatremia
Avoid	Fluid restriction, diuretics, vaptans	Normal saline, hypotonic fluids, liberal intake of fluids

- Duration of hyponatremia: acute (within 48 hours) or chronic (>48 hours).
- Volume status: Hypovolemia, hypervolemia or euvolemia.
- Etiology of hyponatremia.

A. Goal of therapy

1. Treat neurologic emergencies urgently

In acute hyponatremia with severe symptoms, prompt reduction of intracranial pressure is crucial to prevent life-threatening complications such as cerebral edema and brain herniation [49].

2. Avoid too slow or too fast correction

To increase the serum sodium concentration at a safe rate for appropriate correction of hyponatremia (to relieve symptoms and prevent fatal complications of cerebral edema) and to avoid rapid correction (thus reducing the risk of osmotic demyelination syndrome) [49–51].

3. Measures for individualized treatment

Treat the underlying cause, provide specific therapeutic measures, closely monitor the patient to ensure safe and effective correction, and take measures to prevent recurrence of hyponatremia.

B. Severely symptomatic hyponatremia

In severe symptomatic hyponatremia, to correct life-threatening or fatal complications from cerebral edema, urgent treatment is justified irrespective of biochemical degree (mild, moderate, or severe), timing (acute vs. chronic), and volume status [15].

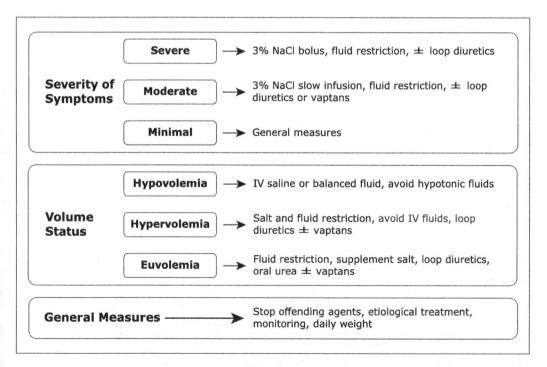

Figure 20.2 Management of Hyponatremia.

1. Hypertonic saline preferred agent

Hypertonic saline (typically 3% NaCl) is recommended for the urgent treatment of acute or symptomatic hyponatremia [5, 15].

In symptomatic patients (i.e., nausea, vomiting, headache, confusion, drowsiness, seizures, coma, respiratory arrest), a quick infusion of hypertonic saline (3% NaCl) in a peripheral vein is lifesaving [52–54]. Hypertonic saline increases the serum sodium concentration rapidly and reduces cerebral edema effectively.

2. Rate of administration

The infusion of a 100 mL bolus of 3% hypertonic saline intravenously over 10 minutes is recommended for initial treatment (American Guidelines 2013) [5]. However, if severe neurological symptoms persist, this bolus may be repeated twice (for a total dose of 300 mL). An alternative approach recommends 150 mL bolus infusions of 3% saline (to be given over 20 minutes), which may be repeated in symptomatic patients after measuring the serum sodium between infusions, as per European guidelines 2014 [15].

3. Bolus vs. slow continuous infusion

For treating severe hyponatremia, it is preferable to administer 3% NaCl using a rapid intermittent bolus (RIB) instead of a slow continuous infusion (SCI) due to the following reasons [55–58]:

- **Effectiveness:** The RIB method has a higher efficacy in achieving the sodium goal compared to SCI. This is because it raises serum sodium within minutes, which is more physiological and logical compared to the hours taken by SCI.
- **Safety:** The RIB method is safer than SCI since it poses a lesser risk of overcorrection and eliminates the need for therapeutic relowering treatment.
- **Convenience:** The RIB method is simple and user-friendly because there is no need for complicated calculations, making it a more convenient option.
- **Supported by guidelines:** Rapid intermittent bolus of 3% NaCl is recommended by American and European guidelines [5, 15] and the recent SALSA trial (2021) [58].

4. Sodium bicarbonate alternative agent

A 50 ml bolus of hypertonic bicarbonate (8.4% sodium bicarbonate) is an effective alternative option for treating acute symptomatic hyponatremia if hypertonic saline is not readily available [59, 60]. Each mL of 8.4% sodium bicarbonate solution contains 1 mEq of sodium. Therefore, 50 ml of hypertonic bicarbonate will provide 50 mEq of sodium, which is equivalent to sodium in 100 ml of 3% NaCl. Slow bicarbonate infusion (over 5–10 minutes) is recommended, and avoid bicarbonate in patients with metabolic alkalosis [61].

5. Loop diuretics

Loop diuretics are used along with hypertonic saline in patients with hypervolemic hyponatremia to increase free water excretion and avoid volume overload [5].

6. Initial correction goal

The goal of initial urgent treatment is to raise serum sodium by 4–6 mEq/L to reduce cerebral edema, improve clinical symptoms, and avoid the risk of brain herniation and neurological damage [5, 15].

C. Rate of correction

How rapidly hyponatremia should be corrected is a dilemma. The initial correction rate varies based on the severity of symptoms of hyponatremia [5, 15]. Severe hyponatremia (110–115 mEq/L) is potentially dangerous because it carries the risk of severe and potentially irreversible neurological damage, which can even be fatal. But on the other hand, too rapid correction of severe hyponatremia can produce osmotic demyelination syndrome (ODS), which can cause substantial morbidity and mortality. So, it is essential to balance the risk of hyponatremia against the risk of a correction. Dictum: Hyponatremia which develops quickly, should be treated fast, whereas hyponatremia, which develops slowly, should be corrected slowly.

1. Acute hyponatremia

In acute symptomatic hyponatremia, the rate of correction should not exceed 10 mEq/L over the first 24 hours. Subsequently, the daily rise should be 8 mEq/L for the patients at normal risk of ODS [15]. In patients at high risk of ODS, the correction rate should not exceed 8 mEq/L over 24 hours on any day [5]. The goal of correction of sodium is up to 130 mEq/L and not its normal value [15]. Therefore, while using hypertonic saline in acutely symptomatic patients, monitor serum sodium very closely (2–4 hourly) [15].

2. Chronic hyponatremia

In chronic hyponatremic patients with low risk for ODS, the rate of correction should not exceed 4–8 mEq/L over 24 hours, and in high-risk patients for ODS, it should not exceed 4–6 mEq/L over 24 hours [5].

3. Osmotic demyelination syndrome (ODS)

The ODS (formerly called central pontine myelinolysis-CPM) is an uncommon but serious and debilitating neurological complication that occurs due to overly rapid correction of serum sodium in patients with severe chronic hyponatremia [50, 62, 63]. Hyponatremic patients with hypokalemia, cirrhosis, alcoholism, malnutrition, older women on thiazide diuretics, and low initial serum sodium level (<115 mEq/L) are prone to develop ODS [64–66].

It is important to remember that symptoms of ODS don't occur immediately but are usually delayed by 2–6 days following rapid overcorrection [67]. ODS's clinical features are lethargy, dysarthria, dysphasia, flaccid paresis, coma, and "locked-in" syndrome [68]. MRI is the most preferred modality for the early diagnosis of ODSMRI is the most preferred modality for the early diagnosis of ODS. In patients with inadvertent overcorrection of hyponatremia, 5% dextrose and desmopressin are beneficial to re-lower the serum sodium to an acceptable level [69].

D. Chronic hyponatremia

Proper treatment is necessary for even asymptomatic chronic hyponatremia due to its potential to cause attention deficits, gait disturbances, and an increased risk of falls and fractures [70]. As chronic hyponatremia is a slow process, adaptive changes occur in the brain and carry a very low risk of cerebral herniation, unlike acute hyponatremia [20]. On the contrary, rapid correction of chronic hyponatremia carries the risk of osmotic demyelination syndrome, which can cause serious neurological deficits and death [62, 71]. Therefore, chronic hyponatremia should always be treated cautiously, aiming for gradual correction.

E. Treatment guidelines based on volume status

It is important to assess the volume status (hypovolemia, hypervolemia, or euvolemia) of each patient with hyponatremia, as the treatment protocol differs in all three groups (as summarized in Figure 20.2).

1. Hypovolemic hyponatremia [72–74]

These patients require fluid and salt supplementation to correct serum sodium and simultaneously restore intravascular volume. The administration of 0.9% normal saline or balanced crystalloid solution at 0.5–1.0 mL/kg per hour effectively corrects hypovolemic hyponatremia in most cases [15].

Restrict intake of simple water and low sodium-containing oral or intravenous (IV) fluids (dextrose solutions, 0.45% NaCl, all Isolyte solutions, etc.) because it may aggravate hyponatremia.

Diuretic-induced hyponatremia is treated by discontinuing diuretic therapy and supplementing with a combination of salt and potassium to restore the deficit. Cerebral salt wasting can be effectively treated by administering fludrocortisone.

2. Hypervolemic hyponatremia [75, 76]

Hyponatremia in congestive heart failure (CHF) and cirrhosis reflects the severity of underlying diseases and is usually asymptomatic. As supplementation of sodium may worsen fluid overload, it is challenging to treat hyponatremia in patients with edema.

The supplementation of salt carries the risk of fluid overload and therefore is generally avoided. The mainstays of therapy are salt restriction and fluid restriction (intake less than insensible losses plus urine output). Loop diuretics are first-line therapy that helps to excrete free water in hypervolemic hyponatremia, reduces edema, and corrects hyponatremia. The addition of a potassium-sparing diuretic (spironolactone) is helpful in the prevention of diuretic-induced hypokalemia and reduces edema in CHF and cirrhosis.

If fluid restriction and loop diuretics fail to correct hypervolemic hyponatremia effectively, vasopressin antagonists (vaptans) are used selectively as second-line therapy.

Edematous patients with acute severe symptomatic hyponatremia requiring rapid correction are cautiously treated by administering 3% NaCl along with fluid restriction and a high dose of furosemide [77].

In hyponatremic patients with renal failure, oliguria, and volume overload who are not responding to medical management, offering hemodialysis is an effective option.

3. Euvolemic hyponatremia

Identify and treat the underlying cause of euvolemic hyponatremia. Syndrome of inappropriate antidiuretic hormone (SIADH) is the most common cause of euvolemic hyponatremia. Various measures used in the treatment of SIADH are a fluid restriction, 3% NaCl or oral salt, loop diuretics, vaptans, and oral urea (discussed under the section on SIADH).

Pay attention and discontinue drugs that can cause SIADH. In euvolemic hyponatremia due to adrenal insufficiency, replace glucocorticoid at either maintenance or stress doses, considering the degree of intercurrent illness. Hypothyroidism-induced hyponatremia is treated with the replacement of thyroid hormone.

F. Formulas for estimating the rate of correction

1. Conventional formula

Sodium Requirement =
(Desired Na^+ - Actual Na^+) × Total Body Water

2. Adrogue-Madias formula

This most commonly used method directly calculates how much the serum sodium concentration will rise when 1 L of various intravenous fluids is given [72].

Change in Serum Sodium Concentration =
$$\frac{\text{Infusate Na / L} - \text{Serum Na}}{\text{Total Body Water (L)}} + 1$$

3. Formula for 3% saline

Administration of 1mL/kg of 3% NaCl (hypertonic saline) increases the serum Na^+ by 1mEq/L. 2 ml of 3% NaCl contains 1 mEq of sodium.

These methods serve only as a rough guide to estimating the change in serum sodium. The Adrogue formula carries a risk of inadvertent overcorrection [55]. Therefore, careful clinical assessment and close monitoring of electrolytes are mandatory in all patients, irrespective of the formulas used.

G. Vasopressin receptor antagonists (vaptans)

Newer agents, vasopressin receptor antagonists (often called the "vaptans"), are a valuable addition to treating dilutional hyponatremia. Tolvaptan

(selective V2 receptor antagonist for oral administration) and conivaptan (combined V1/V2 receptor antagonist for IV administration) are widely available agents.

Tolvaptan remains a second-line therapeutic option for ADH-dependent, hypervolemic (congestive heart failure or cirrhosis), and euvolemic hyponatremia (SIADH), refractory to primary treatment [78]. Cautious use of oral tolvaptan in selected patients with hypervolemic and euvolemic hyponatremia secondary to SIADH is safe and effective [78, 79]. See the treatment section of SIADH for further information about vaptans in hyponatremia.

H. General guidelines for all patients

1. Treat the underlying cause

Detection and elimination or treatment of specific underlying causes of hyponatremia are essential and effective in treating hyponatremia. Examples: Discontinuing offending drugs (like thiazide diuretics, antidepressant drugs such as serotonergic antidepressants -SSRIs, and antiepileptics), restricting water intake in patients with psychogenic polydipsia, replenishing depleted fluid volume, treating postoperative pain, treating hypothyroidism, and giving glucocorticoid replacement to patients with adrenal insufficiency.

Pseudohyponatremia is a laboratory artifact that requires no therapy. On the other hand, hypertonic (translocational) hyponatremia needs treatment of cause (e.g., correction of hyperglycemia or discontinuation of mannitol).

2. Restrict free water

Regardless of the patient's volume status, discontinue non-essential fluids

Table 20.9 Sodium concentration of IV fluids and solutions			
Solution	Na⁺ (mEq/L)	IV fluid	Na⁺ (mEq/L)
8.4% NaHCO₃	1000	Ringer's lactate	130
7.5% NaHCO₃	900	0.45% NaCl	77
5% NaCl	855	Isolyte-G	65
3% NaCl	513	Isolyte-M	40
0.9% NaCl	154	0.2% NaCl	34
PlasmaLyte	140	5% dextrose	0

and restrict intake of free water or hypotonic fluid because these solutions aggravate hyponatremia. Total fluid intake from oral and intravenous fluids should generally be less than 1.0 to 1.5 liter per day in hypervolemic or euvolemic patients [80].

3. Select the right fluid

The sodium concentration of various IV fluids is summarized in Table 20.9 for proper selection.

I. Monitoring

Serially re-evaluating the neurological status, vital signs, volume status, fluid balance, and electrolyte levels is important to monitor progress.

Step-down treatment intensity as symptoms resolve.

SYNDROME OF INAPPROPRIATE ANTIDIURETIC HORMONE SECRETION (SIADH)

SIADH is the most common cause of euvolemic hyponatremia. Inappropriate or excessive ADH secretion in SIADH leads to water retention due to impaired water excretion and high urinary sodium excretion, causing natriuresis with resultant dilutional hyponatremia.

ETIOLOGY

SIADH may be caused by increased hypothalamic secretion of ADH, ectopic ADH release (usually due to malignancy), enhancing effects of ADH (as with chlorpropamide), or ADH-like activity of administered medication [81]. The major causes of SIADH are summarized in Table 20.10).

PATHOGENESIS

1. In SIADH, increased ADH secretion is independent of normal osmotic or hemodynamic stimuli.

2. Because of increased ADH secretion, the kidney cannot excrete free water. Retention of water causes dilutional hyponatremia and progressive expansion of intracellular and extracellular fluids.

3. Expanded ECF volume leads to decreased secretion of aldosterone and increased secretion of atrial

Table 20.10 Common etiology of SIADH	
Central nervous system disorders	Stroke, trauma, subarachnoid hemorrhage, meningitis, encephalitis
Malignancies	Small-cell carcinoma of the lung, carcinoma of the gastrointestinal tract
Pulmonary diseases	Pneumonia, tuberculosis, acute respiratory failure, positive pressure ventilation
Drugs	Carbamazepine, oxcarbazepine, selective serotonin reuptake inhibitors (SSRI), chlorpropamide, cyclophosphamide, desmopressin (DDAVP), and other drugs
Miscellaneous	HIV infection, nausea, and postoperative pain

natriuretic peptide. These changes stimulate natriuresis with an isotonic loss of ECF, bringing ECF volume closer to its baseline volume.

4. The combined effect of natriuresis and water retention leads to inappropriately concentrated urine.

5. Natriuresis prevents the correction of hyponatremia besides routine salt supplementation (in the absence of fluid restriction).

6. In SIADH, increased renal blood flow due to volume expansion and the diuretic effect of ANP result in increased urine volume, preventing clinically evident signs of excess fluid volume.

The pathophysiology of hyponatremia in SIADH is summarized in Figure 20.3.

CLINICAL FEATURES

Signs and symptoms are related to the rapidity of water excess and the severity of hyponatremia.

The symptoms of acute severe hyponatremia are chiefly neurological. In chronic hyponatremia, common symptoms are attention deficits, unsteadiness, gait disturbances, and the risk of frequent falls (as discussed with clinical features of hyponatremia). Additionally, the patient will have characteristics related to the primary etiology.

DIAGNOSTIC CRITERIA

The diagnostic criteria of SIADH are summarized in Table 20.11 [82–84].

TREATMENT

The treatment of acute symptomatic or chronic asymptomatic patients in SIADH differs, as summarized in Table 20.12.

The aim of treatment is water restriction and to promote water excretion:

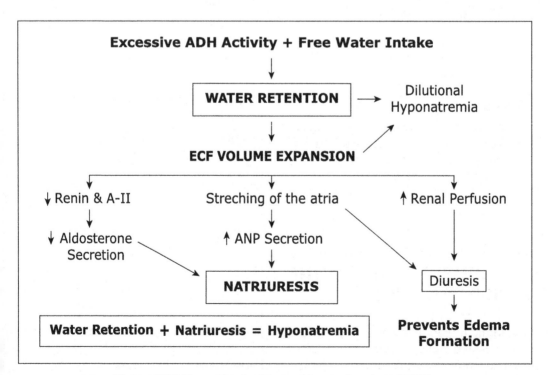

Figure 20.3 The pathophysiology of hyponatremia in SIADH.

Table 20.11 Essential and supporting diagnostic criteria of SIADH
Essential diagnostic criteria for SIADH
• Hypotonic hyponatremia (low serum osmolality <275 mOsm/kg H_2O)
• Clinical euvolemia. Exclude hypovolemia and hypervolemia
• Inappropriately concentrated urine (urinary osmolality high >100 mOsm/kg H_2O)
• Elevated urinary [Na^+] (>30 mEq/L) with normal dietary sodium intake
• Absence of adrenal insufficiency, hypothyroidism, renal disease with salt wastage, cirrhosis, or heart failure
• No recent use of diuretic agents
Supporting diagnostic criteria for SIADH
• Low serum uric acid (<4 mg/dL)
• Low blood urea nitrogen <10 mg/dL
• Fractional excretion of uric acid >10%
• Abnormal response to water load (excretion of <80% of a 20 mL/kg load in 4 h)
• Failure to improve or worsening of hyponatremia after 0.9% saline infusion
• Correction of hyponatremia with fluid restriction

1. Standard first-line therapy is water restriction.

2. If it fails or the patient remains symptomatic, we need a regimen that increases water excretion, i.e., diuretics, hypertonic saline, vaptans, oral urea, high protein diet, demeclocycline, lithium, etc.

Fluid restriction

Fluid restriction is the first-line therapy in treating mild to moderate chronic hyponatremia due to SIADH, which

Table 20.12 Treatment of SIADH
• Treat underlying etiology
• Acute: Water restriction, hypertonic saline, furosemide, avoid hypotonic fluids
• Chronic: Water restriction, high salt, furosemide, high protein diet, vaptans, oral urea, demeclocycline, lithium
Aim for a gradual rise of sodium to 130 mEq/L
Rate of rise of sodium 10 mEq/day in acute hyponatremia and 4–6 mEq in 24 hours in chronic hyponatremia

is the cheapest, least toxic, and most effective modality in many patients [5, 15]. According to the severity of hyponatremia, the daily fluid intake recommended in SIADH is less than 800 ml [72] or 500 mL below the 24-hour urine volume to achieve fluid restriction [5]. It is important to remember that fluid intake includes not only water but also all liquids consumed by drinking and all kinds of solutions administered intravenously. Negative water balance due to fluid restriction gradually raises the serum sodium concentration towards normal in SIADH.

Fluid restriction has limited effectiveness when used as a single treatment [85, 86] because of drawbacks such as very slow action (i.e., it takes several days) and poor patient compliance due to thirst [87]. Fluid restriction alone may not be adequate to correct hyponatremia in many patients and need second-line therapy [86, 87].

Factors that may predict poor response to fluid restriction are low urine volume (<1500 mL/d), the high osmolality of urine (>500 mOsm/ kg H_2O), and the Furst equation ratio >1 (sum of the urine Na^+ and K^+ concentrations exceeds the serum Na^+ concentration) [5, 88, 89].

In hyponatremic patients with subarachnoid hemorrhage, avoid fluid restriction because of the risk of cerebral vasospasm and resultant cerebral ischemia and infarction [90].

Hypertonic saline

In acute symptomatic hyponatremia, prompt administration of hypertonic saline may be lifesaving (for goal, dose, method, and rate of administration of hypertonic saline, see the section treatment of hyponatremia).

How does the NaCl concentration of IV solutions affect hyponatremia in SIADH?

In SIADH, abnormal fluid retention occurs due to ADH-mediated processes, while sodium excretion remains intact or normal. We know that maximum urine output is the direct function of solute excretion rate. So greater solute excretion results in more water loss.

Serum sodium will increase, and hyponatremia will improve only when the osmolality of the infused fluid (which is determined by electrolytes such as Na^+, K^+, Cl^-, etc.) is higher than that of the urine. Based on this information, we can predict the response to NaCl infusion by two factors:

1. Urinary osmolality (a reflection of the severity of SIADH).
2. Osmolality of the NaCl infusion (0.9% NaCl = 308 mOsm/kg and 3% NaCl = 1026 mOsm/kg).

If the urinary osmolality is greater than the osmolality of NaCl infusion, it leads to WATER RETENTION, and

aggravation of hyponatremia is the net end result. Conversely, if the osmolality of NaCl infusion is greater than the urinary osmolality, it leads to WATER EXCRETION, and correction of hyponatremia is the net end result.

What is the response of normal saline solution in SIADH?

Normal saline contains 154 mEq/L of sodium. The simple logic that infusion of normal saline will be helpful because it has a higher sodium concentration than the patient's serum sodium concentration is not correct in hyponatremic patients with SIADH. In fact, normal saline may make hyponatremia worse in SIADH. The response of 0.9% saline in SIADH depends upon the severity (urinary osmolality) of SIADH.

In severe SIADH with hyponatremia, urinary osmolality may be very high and fixed at 600 mOsm/kg. For example, if 1,000 ml of 0.9% NaCl is infused, it contains roughly 300 mOsm solutes (150 mOsm of each Na^+ and Cl^-). As urinary osmolality is 600 mOsm/kg, only in 500 ml of fluid all 300 mOsm of solutes will be excreted in urine (300 mOsm of each Na^+ and Cl^- in 500 ml of water equals 600 mOsm). So the end result is the retention of one-half (about 500 ml) of infused water. Such retention will lead to further dilution and reduction in the serum sodium concentration with worsening of hyponatremia (a process known as desalination) [91].

Why and how does 3% of NaCl correct hyponatremia in severe SIADH?

The osmolality of 3% NaCl is 1,026 mOsm/kg (513 mOsm of Na^+ and 513 mOsm of Cl^-), which is greater than the high urinary osmolality observed in severe SIADH (for example, 600 mOsm/kg). When 1,000 ml of 3% NaCl is infused, all NaCl is excreted in a larger volume of urine, approximately 1,700 ml. As a result, about 700 ml of abnormally retained water will be lost, leading to the correction of dilutional hyponatremia. Simultaneous fluid restriction and administration of furosemide may enhance the correction of hyponatremia.

Can we accurately predict change in serum sodium with 3% NaCl infusion using different formulas?

Different equations and formulas cannot predict serum sodium change reliably while infusing 3% NaCl [55, 92, 93]. The actual volume of hypertonic saline required to correct hyponatremia may be different than the calculated volume in clinical practice because:

1. Simultaneous fluid restriction corrects hyponatremia.

2. In a less severe form of SIADH, 3% NaCl excretes a greater volume of excess water.

3. Simultaneous administration of furosemide will reduce urinary osmolality, causing the excretion of a larger volume of free water.

4. The calculation cannot adjust for rapid changes in urinary composition.

So instead of using different equations, rely on frequent measurements of the serum sodium for correcting hyponatremia.

Loop diuretics

In SIADH, loop diuretics, by inhibiting sodium chloride reabsorption in the thick ascending limb of the loop of Henle, reduce renal medullary hypertonicity, impairs urinary concentration, and promote the excretion of less-concentrated, hypotonic urine, and increase free water excretion [94].

For the short-term treatment of moderate or profound SIADH hyponatremia, European guidelines recommended the administration of low-dose loop diuretics as second-line therapy [15]. Still, its use for the long-term treatment of SIADH is limited [95].

Furosemide is preferred in patients of SIADH of limited duration (i.e., pneumonia or drug-induced SIADH). It provides a greater benefit when administered twice a day (to achieve a urinary diluting effect throughout the day), combined with salt supplementation (oral or IV), particularly in SIADH patients with high urine osmolality (greater than 500 mOsm/kg) [72, 96, 97].

High solute intake

The oral intake of high solute (high-protein diet, oral salt tablets, or urea tablets) increases free-water excretion due to osmotic diuresis, achieves a negative water balance, and corrects hyponatremia in SIADH [98, 99].

Oral salt tablets

Administration of oral salt tabs as chronic maintenance therapy in SIADH restores urinary sodium losses and prevents negative sodium balance [100]. Oral salt is commercially available as 1 gm tablet of NaCl, which provides about 17 mEq of sodium. Oral salt tabs are usually combined with loop diuretics, and the dose commonly used is 6–9 gm per day in divided doses (e.g., 2–3 tablets three times per day) [97].

Oral urea

Oral urea is a safe and well-tolerated oral osmotic diuretic that increases urinary water excretion and effectively treats chronic hyponatremia [101–103].

In combination with fluid restriction, oral urea is emerging as front-line therapy for chronic hyponatremia due to its effectiveness, recommendations in European guidelines and current literature, and disadvantages of alternative therapeutic agent vaptans (e.g., high cost and potential risk of hepatotoxicity and osmotic demyelination) [15, 103–107]. Oral urea is available as 15 gm of per packet. Its usual dose ranges between 15–60 gm per day. Avoid the use of oral urea in patients with severe renal failure and cirrhosis with hepatic encephalopathy [108].

Vasopressin receptor antagonists - Tolvaptan

Vaptans increase water excretion by blocking aquaporin water channels in the kidneys (aquaresis). Selective water diuresis (without affecting sodium and potassium excretion) leads to loss of free water, which corrects hyponatremia in SIADH [78, 109].

Tolvaptan is used only in selective patients of SIADH when [110]:

- Persistent neurologic symptoms and serum sodium concentration below120 mEq/L despite adequate treatment with other measures.

- Hyponatremia is expected to last for a brief duration (e.g., pneumonia induced SIADH).

- Need to increase sodium for a specific reason (e.g., need for surgery).

Tolvaptan is frequently overused in the treatment of hyponatremia. Reasons to use tolvaptan in selected patients of SIADH are [111]:

- The potential risk of hepatotoxicity.

- Frequent adverse effects (thirst, urination frequency, fatigue).

- Risk of overly rapid correction of

hyponatremia (due to uncontrolled and unpredictable water loss).

- High cost.

Measures recommended for reducing the rate of complications of tolvaptan are [49, 112–116]:

- Cautious administration under close monitoring of electrolytes.

- Initiation of therapy in low dose (i.e., 7.5 mg a day).

- Avoiding it in patients with hypovolemic hyponatremia, severe neurologic symptoms (such as seizures or a markedly altered sensorium), liver disease (including cirrhosis), or inability to sense or respond to thirst.

- Avoiding concomitant use of diuretics or hypertonic saline solution.

- Discontinuation of fluid restriction before starting tolvaptan.

- Permit ad libitum fluid intake during the first 24–48 hours of treatment.

- Ensuring the availability of water so that patients can drink when thirsty.

- Avoiding its use for more than 30 days.

Demeclocycline and lithium

Both drugs act on collecting tubule cells and diminish their responsiveness to ADH, causing an increase in the free water excretion, leading to a rise in serum sodium concentration. Because of its unpredictable response and frequent side effects like nephrotoxicity and hepatotoxicity, the current literature recommends against using demeclocycline for hyponatremia secondary to SIADH [15, 117].

The use of lithium is almost abandoned in the management of SIADH-induced hyponatremia due to its high toxicity [15, 95].

REFERENCES

1. Rasouli M. Basic concepts and practical equations on osmolality: Biochemical approach. Clin Biochem. 2016;49(12):936–41.

2. McKinley MJ, Johnson AK. The physiological regulation of thirst and fluid intake. News Physiol Sci. 2004;19:1–6.

3. Intravenous Fluid Therapy in Adults in Hospital. London: National Institute for Health and Care Excellence, 2013 (https://www.nice.org.uk/guidance/cg174).

4. Turner MJ, Avolio AP. Does Replacing Sodium Excreted in Sweat Attenuate the Health Benefits of Physical Activity? Int J Sport Nutr Exerc Metab. 2016;26(4):377–89.

5. Verbalis JG, Goldsmith SR, Greenberg A, et al. Diagnosis, evaluation, and treatment of hyponatremia: expert panel recommendations. Am J Med. 2013;126(10 Suppl 1):S1–42.

6. Hawkins RC. Age and gender as risk factors for hyponatremia and hypernatremia. Clin Chim Acta. 2003;337(1–2):169–72.

7. Upadhyay A, Jaber BL, Madias NE. Incidence and prevalence of hyponatremia. Am J Med. 2006;119(7 Suppl 1):S30–S35.

8. Upadhyay A, Jaber BL, Madias NE. Epidemiology of hyponatremia. Semin Nephrol 2009;29(3):227–238.

9. Corona G, Giuliani C, Parenti G, et al. The Economic Burden of Hyponatremia: Systematic Review and Meta-Analysis. Am J Med. 2016;129(8):823–835.e4.

10. Tazmini K, Ranhoff AH. Electrolyte outpatient clinic at a local hospital - experience from diagnostics, treatment and follow-up. BMC Health Serv Res. 2020;20(1):154.

11. Wald R, Jaber BL, Price LL, et al. Impact of hospital-associated hyponatremia on selected outcomes. Arch Intern Med. 2010;170(3):294–302.

12. Hoorn EJ, van der Lubbe N, Zietse R. SIADH and hyponatraemia: why does it matter? NDT Plus. 2009; 2(Suppl_3):iii5–iii11.

13. Sterns RH. Disorders of plasma sodium--causes, consequences, and correction. N Engl J Med. 2015;372(1):55–65.

14. Adrogué HJ, Madias NE. The challenge of hyponatremia. J Am Soc Nephrol. 2012;23(7):1140–8.

15. Spasovski G, Vanholder R, Allolio B, et al. Clinical practice guideline on diagnosis and treatment of hyponatraemia. Eur J Endocrinol. 2014;170(3):G1–47.

16. Adrogué HJ. Consequences of inadequate management of hyponatremia. Am J Nephrol. 2005;25(3):240–9.

17. Waikar SS, Mount DB, Curhan GC. Mortality after hospitalization with mild, moderate, and severe hyponatremia. Am J Med. 2009;122(9):857–865.

18. Adrogue HJ, Madias NE. Hyponatremia. N Engl J Med. 2000;342(21):1581–9.

19. Fujisawa H, Sugimura Y, Takagi H, et al. Chronic Hyponatremia Causes Neurologic and Psychologic Impairments. J Am Soc Nephrol. 2016;27(3):766–780.

20. Gankam KF, Decaux G. Hyponatremia and the Brain. Kidney Int Rep. 2017;3(1):24–35.

21. Ayus JC, Moritz ML. Bone disease as a new complication of hyponatremia: moving beyond brain injury. Clin J Am Soc Nephrol. 2010;5(2):167–168.

22. Filippatos TD, Makri A, Elisaf MS, et al. Hyponatremia in the elderly: challenges and solutions. Clin Interv Aging. 2017;12:1957–1965.

23. Negri AL, Ayus JC. Hyponatremia and bone disease. Rev Endocr Metab Disord. 2017;18(1):67–78.

24. Faria DK, Mendes ME, Sumita NM. The measurement of serum osmolality and its application to clinical practice and laboratory: literature review. Jornal Brasileiro de Patologia e Medicina Laboratorial 2017;53(1):38–45.

25. Ball SG. How I approach hyponatremia. Clin Med. 2013;13:291–295.

26. Fortgens P, Pillay TS. Pseudohyponatremia revisited: a modern-day pitfall. Arch Pathol Lab Med 2011;135(4):516–9.

27. Goldwasser P, Ayoub I, Barth RH. Pseudohypernatremia and pseudohyponatremia: a linear correction, Nephrology Dialysis Transplantation 2015;30(2):252–257.

28. Filippatos TD, Liamis G, Christopoulou F, et al. Ten common pitfalls in the evaluation of patients with hyponatremia. Eur J Intern Med. 2016;29:22–5.

29. Hillier TA, Abbott RD, Barrett EJ. Hyponatremia: evaluating the correction factor for hyperglycemia. Am J Med. 1999;106(4):399–403.

30. Milionis HJ, Liamis GL, Elisaf MS. The hyponatremic patient: a systematic approach to laboratory diagnosis. CMAJ. 2002;166(8):1056–1062.

31. Weismann D, Schneider A, Höybye C. Clinical aspects of symptomatic hyponatremia. Endocr Connect. 2016;5(5):R35–R43.

32. Filippone EJ, Ruzieh M, Foy A. Thiazide-Associated Hyponatremia: Clinical Manifestations and Pathophysiology. Am J Kidney Dis. 2020;75(2):256–264.

33. Hix JK, Silver S, Sterns RH. Diuretic-associated hyponatremia. Semin Nephrol. 2011;31(6):553–66.

34. Liamis G, Filippatos TD, Elisaf MS. Thiazide-associated hyponatremia in the elderly: what the clinician needs to know. J Geriatr Cardiol. 2016;13(2):175–182.

35. Momi J, Tang CM, Abcar AC, et al. Hyponatremia-what is cerebral salt wasting? Perm J. 2010;14(2):62–65.

36. Yee AH, Burns JD, Wijdicks EFM. Cerebral salt wasting: pathophysiology, diagnosis, and treatment. Neurosurg Clin N Am. 2010;21(2):339–352.

37. Verbalis JG. The Curious Story of Cerebral Salt Wasting: Fact or Fiction? Clin J Am Soc Nephrol. 2020;15(11):1666–1668.

38. Maesaka JK, Imbriano L, Mattana J, et al. Differentiating SIADH from cerebral/renal salt wasting: failure of the volume approach and need for a new approach to hyponatremia. J Clin Med. 2014;3(4):1373–1385.

39. Oh JY, Shin JI. Syndrome of inappropriate antidiuretic hormone secretion and cerebral/renal salt wasting syndrome: similarities and differences. Front Pediatr. 2014;2:146.

40. Maesaka JK, Imbriano LJ, Miyawaki N. Determining Fractional Urate Excretion Rates in Hyponatremic Conditions and Improved Methods to Distinguish Cerebral/Renal Salt Wasting From the Syndrome of Inappropriate Secretion of Antidiuretic Hormone. Front Med (Lausanne). 2018;5:319.

41. Cui H, He G, Yang S, et al. Inappropriate Antidiuretic Hormone Secretion and Cerebral Salt-Wasting Syndromes in Neurological Patients. Front Neurosci. 2019;13:1170.

42. Almond CS, Shin AY, Fortescue EB, et al. Hyponatremia among runners in the Boston Marathon. N Engl J Med 2005;352(15):1550–6.

43. Hew-Butler T, Rosner MH, Fowkes-Godek S, et al. Statement of the Third International Exercise-Associated Hyponatremia Consensus Development Conference, Carlsbad, California, 2015. Clin J Sport Med 2015;25(4):303–320.

44. Bennett BL, Hew-Butler T, Rosner MH, et al. Wilderness Medical Society Clinical Practice Guidelines for the Management of Exercise-Associated Hyponatremia: 2019 Update. Wilderness Environ Med 2020;31(1):50–62.

45. Rosner MH. Exercise-Associated Hyponatremia. Trans Am Clin Climatol Assoc. 2019;130:76–87.

46. Hew-Butler T. Exercise-Associated Hyponatremia. Front Horm Res. 2019;52:178–189.

47. Corona G, Giuliani C, Verbalis JG, et al. Hyponatremia improvement is associated with a reduced risk of mortality: evidence from a meta-analysis. PLoS One. 2015;10(4):e0124105.

48. Goh KP. Management of Hyponatremia. Am Fam Physician. 2004;69(10):2387–2394.

49. Sterns RH. Treatment of Severe Hyponatremia. Clin J Am Soc Nephrol 2018;13(4):641–649.

50. Berl T. Treating hyponatremia: damned if we do and damned if we don't. Kidney Int. 1990;37(3):1006–18.

51. Giuliani C, Peri A. Effects of Hyponatremia on the Brain. J Clin Med. 2014;3(4):1163–1177.

52. Ayus JC, Caputo D, Bazerque F, e al. Treatment of hyponatremic encephalopathy with a 3%sodium chloride protocol: a case series. Am J Kidney Dis. 2015;65(3):435–442.

53. Ayus JC, Moritz ML. Misconceptions and Barriers to the Use of Hypertonic Saline to Treat Hyponatremic Encephalopathy. Front Med (Lausanne). 2019;6:47.

54. Metheny NA, Moritz ML. Administration of 3% Sodium Chloride Via A Peripheral Vein. J Infusion Nursing. 2021;44(2):94–102.

55. Mohmand HK, Issa D, Ahmad Z, et al. Hypertonic saline for hyponatremia: risk of inadvertent overcorrection. Clin J Am Soc Nephrol. 2007;2(6):1110–7.

56. Hoorn EJ, Zietse R. Diagnosis and treatment of hyponatremia: compilation of the guidelines. J Am Soc Nephrol. 2017;28(5):1340–1349.

57. Garrahy A, Dineen R, Hannon AM, et al. Continuous Versus Bolus Infusion of Hypertonic Saline in the Treatment of Symptomatic Hyponatremia Caused by SIAD. J Clin Endocrinol Metab 2019;104(9):3595–3602.

58. Baek SH, Jo YH, Ahn S, et al. Risk of Overcorrection in Rapid Intermittent Bolus vs Slow Continuous Infusion Therapies of Hypertonic Saline for Patients With Symptomatic Hyponatremia: The SALSA Randomized Clinical Trial. JAMA Intern Med. 2021;181(1):81–92.

59. Farkas J. Emergent treatment of hyponatremia or elevated ICP with bicarb ampules. PULMCrit September 7, 2015 (visit: https://emcrit.org/pulmcrit/emergent-treatment-of-hyponatremia-or-elevated-icp-with-bicarb-ampules/).

60. Hootman J, Alvarez A, Wilson J. Trick of the Trade: Sodium Bicarbonate for Acute Symptomatic Hyponatremia. Tox & Medications. 2020 (Visit: https://www.aliem.com/trick-of-trade-sodium-bicarbonate-symptomatic-hyponatremia/).

61. Farkas J. Hyponatremia. PULMCrit December 12, 2019 (Visit: https://emcrit.org/ibcc/hyponatremia/).

62. Sterns RH, Riggs JE, Schochet SS Jr. Osmotic demyelination syndrome following correction of hyponatremia. N Engl J Med. 1986;314(24):1535–42.

63. Lambeck J, Hieber M, Dreßing A, et al. Central Pontine Myelinosis and Osmotic Demyelination Syndrome. Dtsch Arztebl Int. 2019;116(35–36):600–606.

64. Berl T, Rastegar A. A patient with severe hyponatremia and hypokalemia: osmotic demyelination following potassium repletion. Am J Kidney Dis 2010;55(4):742–8.

65. Aratani S, Hara M, Nagahama M, et al. A low initial serum sodium level is associated with an increased risk of overcorrection in patients with chronic profound hyponatremia: a retrospective cohort analysis. BMC Nephrol. 2017;18(1):316.

66. George JC, Zafar W, Bucaloiu ID, et al. Risk Factors and Outcomes of Rapid Correction of Severe Hyponatremia. Clin J Am Soc Nephrol. 2018;13(7):984–992.

67. Sterns RH, Cappuccio JD, Silver SM, et al. Neurologic sequelae after treatment of severe hyponatremia: a multicenter perspective. J Am Soc Nephrol. 1994;4(8):1522–30.

68. Martin RJ. Central pontine and extrapontine myelinolysis: the osmotic demyelination syndromes. J Neurol Neurosurg Psychiatry. 2004;75 Suppl 3(Suppl 3):iii22–8.

69. Rafat C, Schortgen F, Gaudry S, et al. Use of desmopressin acetate in severe hyponatremia in the intensive care unit. Clin J Am Soc Nephrol. 2014;9(2):229–37.

70. Hoorn EJ, Rivadeneira F, van Meurs JB, et al. Mild hyponatremia as a risk factor for fractures: the Rotterdam Study. J Bone Miner Res. 2011;26(8):1822–1828.

71. Aegisdottir H, Cooray C, Wirdefeldt K, et al. Incidence of osmotic demyelination syndrome in Sweden: A nationwide study. Acta Neurol Scand 2019;140(5):342–349.

72. Adrogué HJ, Madias NE. Hyponatremia. N Engl J Med. 2000;342(21):1581–9.

73. Braun MM, Barstow CH, Pyzocha NJ. Diagnosis and management of sodium disorders: hyponatremia and hypernatremia. Am Fam Physician. 2015;91(5):299–307.

74. Mohottige D, Lehrich RW, Greenberg A. Hypovolemic Hyponatremia. Front Horm Res. 2019;52:93–103.

75. Yeates KE, Singer M, Morton AR. Salt and water: a simple approach to hyponatremia. CMAJ 2004;170(3):365–9.

76. Fortune BE, Garcia-Tsao G. Hypervolemic hyponatremia: Clinical significance and management. Clin Liver Dis. 2013;2(3):109–112.

77. Şorodoc V, Asaftei A, Puha G, et al. Management of Hyponatremia in Heart Failure: Practical Considerations. J Pers Med. 2023;13(1):140

78. Berl T, Quittnat-Pelletier F, Verbalis JG, et al. Oral tolvaptan is safe and effective in chronic hyponatremia. J Am Soc Nephrol. 2010;21(4):705–12.

79. Pose-Reino A, Runkle de la Vega I, de Jong-Laird A, et al. Real-World, Non-Interventional, Retrospective Study (SAMPLE) of Tolvaptan in Patients with Hyponatraemia Secondary to the Syndrome of Inappropriate Antidiuretic Hormone Secretion. Adv Ther. 2021;38(2):1055–1067.

80. Lee JJ, Kilonzo K, Nistico A, et al. Management of hyponatremia. CMAJ. 2014;186(8):E281–6.

81. Esposito P, Piotti G, Bianzina S, et al. The syndrome of inappropriate antidiuresis: pathophysiology, clinical management and new therapeutic options. Nephron Clin Pract. 2011;119(1):c62–73.

82. Schwartz WB, Bennett W, Curelop S, et al. A syndrome of renal sodium loss and hyponatremia probably resulting from inappropriate secretion of antidiuretic hormone. American Journal of Medicine 1957;23(4):529–542.

83. Janicic N, Verbalis JG. Evaluation and management of hypo-osmolality in hospitalized patients. Endocrinology and Metabolism Clinics of North America 2003;32(2):459–481.

84. Ellison DH, Berl T. Clinical practice. The syndrome of inappropriate antidiuresis. N Engl J Med 2007;356(20):2064–72.

85. Verbalis JG, Greenberg A, Burst V, et al. Diagnosing and Treating the Syndrome of Inappropriate Antidiuretic Hormone Secretion. Am J Med 2016;129(5):537.e9–537.e23.

86. Garrahy A, Galloway I, Hannon AM, et al. Fluid Restriction Therapy for Chronic SIAD; Results of a Prospective Randomized Controlled Trial. J Clin Endocrinol Metab. 2020;105(12):dgaa619.

87. Dineen R, Thompson CJ, Sherlock M. Hyponatraemia - presentations and management. Clin Med (Lond). 2017;17(3):263–269.

88. Furst H, Hallows KR, Post J, et al. The urine/plasma electrolyte ratio: a predictive guide to water restriction. Am J Med Sci. 2000;319(4):240–244.

89. Cuesta M, Ortolá A, Garrahy A, et al. Predictors of failure to respond to fluid restriction in SIAD in clinical practice; time to re-evaluate clinical guidelines? QJM. 2017;110(8):489–492.

90. Marupudi NI, Mittal S. Diagnosis and Management of Hyponatremia in Patients with Aneurysmal Subarachnoid Hemorrhage. J Clin Med. 2015;4(4):756–67.

91. Steele A, Gowrishankar M, Abrahamson S, et al. Postoperative hyponatremia despite near-isotonic saline infusion: a phenomenon of desalination. Ann Intern Med 1997;126(1):20–5.

92. Hanna RM, Yang WT, Lopez EA, et al. The utility and accuracy of four equations in predicting sodium levels in dysnatremic patients. Clin Kidney J 2016;9(4):530–9.

93. Sterns RH. Formulas for fixing serum sodium: curb your enthusiasm. Clin Kidney J 2016;9(4):527–9.

94. Schrier RW, Bansal S. Diagnosis and management of hyponatremia in acute illness. Curr Opin Crit Care. 2008;14(6):627–634.

95. Zietse R, van der Lubbe N, Hoorn EJ. Current and future treatment options in SIADH. NDT Plus. 2009;2(Suppl_3):iii12–iii19.

96. Decaux G. Treatment of the syndrome of inappropriate secretion of antidiuretic hormone by long loop diuretics. Nephron 1983;35(2):82–88.

97. Runkle I, Villabona C, Navarro A, et al. Treatment of hyponatremia induced by the syndrome of Inappropriate antidiuretic hormone secretion: a multidisciplinary spanish algorithm. Nefrologia. 2014;34(4):439–50.

98. Berl T. Impact of solute intake on urine flow and water excretion. J Am Soc Nephrol. 2008;19(6):1076–8.

99. Decaux G, Musch W. Estimated Daily Urine Volume and Solute Excretion from Spot Urine Samples to Guide the Therapy of Hyponatremia in SIADH. J Clin Med. 2019;8(10):1511.

100. Rondon-Berrios H, Berl T. Mild Chronic Hyponatremia in the Ambulatory Setting: Significance and Management. Clin J Am Soc Nephrol. 2015;10(12):2268–78.

101. Soupart A, Coffernils M, Couturier B, et al. Efficacy and tolerance of urea compared with vaptans for long-term treatment of patients with SIADH. Clin J Am Soc Nephrol. 2012;7(5):742–7.

102. Sterns RH, Silver SM, Hix JK. Urea for hyponatremia? Kidney Int 2015;87(2):268–270.

103. Rondon-Berrios H. Urea for chronic hyponatremia. Blood Purif 2020;49(1–2):212–218.

104. Rondon-Berrios H, Tandukar S, Mor MK, et al. Urea for the Treatment of Hyponatremia. Clin J Am Soc Nephrol. 2018;13(11):1627–1632.

105. Lockett J, Berkman KE, Dimeski G, et al. Urea treatment in fluid restriction refractory hyponatremia. Clin Endocrinol (Oxf) 2019;90(4):630–636.

106. Nervo A, D'Angelo V, Rosso D, et al. Urea in cancer patients with chronic SIAD-induced hyponatremia: Old drug, new evidence. Clin Endocrinol (Oxf) 2019;90(6):842–848.

107. Lerma EV, Rondon-Berrios H. Urea for the Treatment of Hyponatremia: An Old Treatment Offers Fresh Hope. Kidney News Online 2021;13(3):13–14.

108. Farkas J. Controlled aquaresis: Management of hypervolemic or euvolemic hyponatremia with oral urea. PULMCrit November 26, 2019 (Visit: https://emcrit.org/pulmcrit/aquaresis/).

109. Robertson GL. Vaptans for the treatment of hyponatremia. Nat Rev Endocrinol. 2011;7(3):151–61.

110. Seay NW, Lehrich RW, Greenberg A. Diagnosis and Management of Disorders of Body Tonicity-Hyponatremia and Hypernatremia: Core Curriculum 2020. Am J Kidney Dis. 2020;75(2):272–286.

111. Kim YC, Lee H. Light and Shadow in Oral Tolvaptan Treatment Kidney News Online 2021;13(3):14.

112. Tzoulis P, Waung JA, Bagkeris E, et al. Real-life experience of tolvaptan use in the treatment of severe hyponatraemia due to syndrome of inappropriate antidiuretic hormone secretion. ClinEndocrinol (Oxf). 2016;84(4):620–626.

113. Harbeck B, Lindner U, Haas CS. Low-dose tolvaptan for the treatment of hyponatremia in the syndrome of inappropriate ADH secretion (SIADH). Endocrine. 2016;53(3):872–873.

114. Verbalis JG, Adler S, Schrier RW, et al. Efficacy and safety of oral tolvaptan therapy in patients with the syndrome of inappropriate antidiuretic hormone secretion. Eur J Endocrinol 2011;164(5):725–32.

115. Morris JH, Bohm NM, Nemecek BD, et al. Rapidity of Correction of Hyponatremia Due to Syndrome of Inappropriate Secretion of Antidiuretic Hormone Following Tolvaptan. Am J Kidney Dis 2018;71(6):772–782.

116. Chatzimavridou-grigoriadou V, Al-othman S, Brabant G, et al. Clinical experience of the efficacy and safety of low dose tolvaptan therapy in a UK tertiary oncology setting. The Journal of Clinical Endocrinology & Metabolism. 2021:dgab131.

117. Miell J, Dhanjal P, Jamookeeah C. Evidence for the use of demeclocycline in the treatment of hyponatraemia secondary to SIADH: a systematic review. Int J Clin Pract. 2015;69(12):1396–1417.

21 | Hypernatremia

INTRODUCTION

Hypernatremia is an electrolyte disorder defined as an increase in plasma sodium concentration greater than 145 mEq/L, always results in hypertonicity (hyperosmolality), and usually occurs due to lack of water, loss of water, or primary sodium gain [1, 2].

Hypernatremia is a less frequent disorder (about 1%–3% of all hospitalized patients and 9% in critically ill patients) but carries significantly higher mortality (about 40–60%) [3–5]. HYPERNATREMIA IS USUALLY DUE TO WATER DEFICIT AND NOT SODIUM OVERLOAD.

Normal thirst is the most potent mechanism that effectively prevents hypernatremia. So, hypernatremia usually does not occur in healthy adults who can respond to thirst unless there is non-availability of water, restricted water intake, impaired thirst, or the patient cannot drink the water due to a comatose-confused state. Therefore, hypernatremia is seen chiefly in very young, very old, very sick, bed-ridden, or debilitated patients. A pure water deficit leading to hypernatremia is called dehydration.

ETIOLOGY

Common causes of hypernatremia classified based on volume status, water loss or salt gain, urinary sodium, and underlying etiologies are summarized in Table 21.1.

Table 21.1 Causes of hypernatremia		
ECF volume	**Urinary Na⁺**	**Examples**
Hypovolemia Loss of hypotonic fluid	<20 mEq/L	**Extrarenal loss** Gastrointestinal (GI) losses: Osmotic diarrhea, enterocutaneous fistula, protracted vomiting Dermal losses: Heat exposure, severe burns, severe exercise Respiratory losses: Febrile patients on a ventilator
	>20 mEq/L	**Renal loss** Loop diuretics, osmotic diuresis due to hyperglycemia, urea or mannitol, intrinsic renal diseases, post obstructive diuresis
Euvolemia Loss of pure water	<20 mEq/L	**Renal loss** Central diabetes insipidus: Lack of antidiuretic hormone (ADH) which can be idiopathic or due to head injury, surgery, or neoplasm Nephrogenic diabetes insipidus: Resistance to ADH, commonly due to chronic kidney disease, hypercalcemia, hypokalemia, lithium treatment, amphotericin B, and obstruction
	>20 mEq/L	**Extrarenal loss** Large respiratory or dermal insensible losses
Hypervolemia Hypertonic sodium gain	>20 mEq/L	Hypertonic infusion: Hypertonic saline or sodium bicarbonate (NaHCO₃) infusion, hypertonic enteral or parenteral feeding Other causes: Cushing syndrome, salt intoxication, soy sauce
Insufficient water intake: Lack of access to water, impaired thirst or altered consciousness are important coexisting factors which maintains hypernatremia		

CLINICAL FEATURES

The common presentation of hypernatremia is chiefly neurological, and sign symptoms depend upon the speed of onset, duration, severity, underlying etiology, and volume status [1].

CNS dysfunction

Early neurological symptoms of hypernatremia are extreme fatigue, muscular weakness, lethargy, cramps, nausea, malaise, and irritability.

In severe hypernatremia (i.e., sodium greater than 160 mEq/L), common symptoms are hyperthermia, headache, muscle twitching, altered mental status, confusion, delirium, focal neurological deficit, and occasionally coma. Convulsions are usually absent but can occur with aggressive rehydration or inadvertent sodium loading [1].

Chronic hypernatremia

In hypernatremia, hyperosmolality causes a shift of water from the intracellular space to the extracellular space leading to brain cell shrinkage. In chronic hypernatremia (>48 h), adaptive mechanisms increase the intracellular fluid (ICF) water, normalize brain parenchyma volume, and protect against brain dehydration and shrinkage. As adaptive mechanisms prevent brain shrinkage, symptoms in chronic hypernatremia are fewer and milder.

Acute hypernatremia

Severe symptoms typically occur in acute hypernatremia with serum sodium levels above 155–160 mEq/L [6]. In severe acute hypernatremia, significant brain shrinkage occurs due to a substantial shift of water out of the brain in the short term, which exerts traction on the venous sinuses [2]. As a result, it can cause intracerebral and subarachnoid hemorrhage, producing irreversible neurological damage or even death [1].

Patients with excessive sweating, diarrhea, or osmotic diuresis can cause volume depletion and resultant signs and symptoms. However, it is not easy to detect hypovolemia clinically, and orthostatic hypotension and tachycardia may be an early clue. Excessive thirst, dry sticky mucous membranes, and elevated body temperature are characteristic features of hypernatremia.

In hypernatremic patients, urine volume is low in hypovolemia and is high in diabetes insipidus or osmotic diuresis. Polyuria (persistent urine output of more than 100 mL/h) and excessive thirst are frequently the presenting symptoms of diabetes insipidus. Diabetes insipidus is characterized by diluted urine (low urine osmolality) even in the presence of hypernatremia due to insufficient production or response to antidiuretic hormone (ADH), presenting a mirror image of the syndrome of inappropriate antidiuretic hormone (SIADH).

Why are patients with hypertonic dehydration hemodynamically more stable than those with isotonic volume depletion with an equal volume of fluid losses?

Pure water loss leads to dehydration with hypernatremia (hypertonic dehydration), whereas proportionate combined loss of water and salt in isotonic volume depletion leads to hypovolemia and has normal serum sodium.

In isotonic volume depletion, fluid loss leads to a reduction only in extracellular

Table 21.2 Distribution of fluid loss in isotonic and pure water depletion

Reduction in	Loss of 1000 ml of fluid by	
	Isotonic loss	Pure water depletion
ICF volume	-	667 ml
ECF volume	1000 ml	333 ml
Intravascular volume	250 ml	83 ml

fluid (ECF) volume (and therefore the early reduction in intravascular volume), leading to hypotension and reduction in tissue perfusion. While in dehydration due to pure water depletion, there is a proportionate reduction in total body water (2/3 from intracellular fluid [ICF] and 1/3 from ECF). As ECF volume depletion (and therefore intravascular volume depletion, which is 1/4 of ECF) is much less, clinical features are lesser in pure water depletion.

Table 21.2 simplify how isotonic and pure water depletion are distributed in various fluid compartments.

DIAGNOSIS

Complete history, proper examination, and details of recent medications may provide a clue for the etiology of hypernatremia. However, if this preliminary evaluation clinches the etiological diagnosis in hypernatremia, laboratory studies for diagnosis may not be necessary (but frequent electrolyte checks are required to monitor therapy) [7].

Serum electrolytes, glucose, BUN, creatinine, urinary volume, osmolality and glycosuria, and response to vasopressin in diabetes insipidus are useful for the etiological diagnosis of hypernatremia. Interpretation of basic investigations used to evaluate patients with hypernatremia is outlined in Table 21.3.

Table 21.3 Interpretation of investigations in hypernatremia	
Plasma osmolality	• In hypernatremia, serum osmolality is always >290 mOsm/kg
Urinary osmolality	• >800 mOsm/kg: Small volume of concentrated urine is an appropriate renal response to hypernatremia. Hypovolemic hypernatremia due to GI, dermal, or respiratory losses in patients with impaired thirst or inability to access water. Hypervolemic hypernatremia due to salt overload
	• <800 mOsm/kg: Suggests a defect in renal water conservation
	• 300 to 800 mOsm/kg (intermediate value): Hypernatremia due to osmotic diuresis, partial central DI, central DI with volume depletion, partial nephrogenic DI
	• <300 mOsm/kg (inappropriately dilute urine): Complete forms of central or nephrogenic DI
Spot urinary Na⁺	• <20 mEq/L: Hypovolemic hypernatremia due to GI, dermal, or respiratory losses. Euvolemic hypernatremia due to central or nephrogenic DI
	• >20 mEq/L: Osmotic diuresis, infusion of hypertonic saline or $NaHCO_3$
Water restriction test	• Normally, urinary osmolality increases with water restriction
	• In central or nephrogenic DI, polyuria and diluted urine persist besides fluid restriction
Response to desmopressin	• Assess response to 10 µg intranasal administration of the vasopressin analog desmopressin (DDAVP) after careful restriction of water
	• Urinary osmolality will increase by at least 50% in central diabetes insipidus but lack of response in nephrogenic DI

MANAGEMENT

The therapeutic goals of hypernatremia treatment are as follows:

• Correcting volume depletion and shock promptly if present.

• Preventing ongoing excessive water loss by addressing the underlying causes and providing adequate water to prevent its recurrence of hypernatremia.

• Gradually and carefully correct the water deficit to lower the serum sodium level to the point where the patient becomes asymptomatic.

• Achieving a slow and gentle reduction of elevated serum sodium levels to prevent cerebral edema while avoiding symptoms resulting from brain shrinkage due to hypernatremia.

Two critical factors in determining a treatment plan are:

• ECF volume status.

• The severity of symptoms and the rate of development of hypernatremia.

Correction of the underlying causes

The initial step in management is to identify and address the specific etiology of hypernatremia. Managing the predisposing factors may involve treating conditions such as diabetes insipidus, hyperglycemia, hypokalemia, hypercalcemia, or diarrhea. Additionally, controlling fever, discontinuing offending medications like mannitol infusion, lactulose, diuretics, or drugs associated with nephrogenic diabetes insipidus, and withdrawing hypertonic tube feeds should be considered.

Treatment based on volume status

Hypernatremia can be divided into three groups based on volume status: hypovolemic, euvolemic, and hypervolemic, each requiring a different treatment approach.

A. Hypovolemic hypernatremia

1. In hemodynamically unstable patients: Correcting shock and restoring tissue perfusion is a priority, and for the prompt correction of hypotension, normal saline or Ringer's lactate (RL) is the fluid of choice, regardless of the degree of hypernatremia. A sodium concentration of 0.9% NaCl (154 mEq/L) is greater than the normal serum sodium (140 mEq/L) but is generally lower than the serum sodium concentration in hypernatremia. So, initial therapy with normal saline has the advantage of rapid correction of hypotension and avoiding unnecessary rapid fall of serum sodium.

2. In hemodynamically stable patients: After correcting the initial hypovolemia with isotonic fluids (normal saline, Ringer's lactate, or PlasmaLyte), restore the water deficit and ongoing losses with hypotonic solutions such as water by mouth or infusion of 5%-dextrose, 0.2% sodium chloride, or 0.45% sodium chloride. Correct about 50% of the water deficit in the first 24 hours; the remaining water deficit is restored over the next 48 hours.

B. Euvolemic hypernatremia

Euvolemic hypernatremia is often caused by diabetes insipidus (DI), which is the most common underlying condition. The primary treatment for central DI is desmopressin (DDAVP) administered through nasal spray (10–20 µg per 12–24 hours) or orally (0.1–0.8 mg orally per 12 hours). In cases of nephrogenic diabetes insipidus, treatment typically involves thiazide diuretics (such as hydrochlorothiazide, 25 mg once or twice daily), non-steroidal anti-inflammatory drugs (NSAIDs), reduced salt and protein intake, along with correcting underlying causes such as hypercalcemia or hypokalemia, or discontinuing precipitating drugs like lithium [8].

Supplementing with the potassium-sparing diuretic amiloride may provide an additive effect when combined with the thiazide diuretics and is useful, especially in the management of lithium-induced nephrogenic diabetes insipidus, using a dose of 2.5 to 10 mg per day [9, 10].

In nephrogenic diabetes insipidus, thiazide diuretics work by increasing urinary osmolality through enhanced sodium excretion compared to water and inducing a state of mild hypovolemia that stimulates increased water reabsorption in the proximal tubule, ultimately reducing polyuria [8, 11].

C. Hypervolemic hypernatremia

The administration of large amounts of hypertonic sodium-containing intravenous (IV) solutions, such as hypertonic saline or $NaHCO_3$ infusion, can lead to volume overload and hypernatremia, a condition that frequently occurs in the ICU. To manage hypervolemic hypernatremia effectively, discontinue causative medications, administer loop diuretics, and supplement hypotonic IV solutions or enteral water to facilitate sodium excretion while exercising caution to avoid volume overload when administering oral or IV hypotonic fluid [12].

Loop diuretics, by natriuresis, remove excess sodium from the body and, by achieving a net negative fluid balance, reduce volume overload [13]. Dialysis may be indicated in a few patients of hypervolemic hypernatremia with severe complications, such as oliguric renal failure and intractable fluid overload with dyspnea when the response to medical management is inadequate [14–16].

Treatment based on onset

Acute hypernatremia (<24 hours) is more symptomatic and requires rapid correction, whereas chronic hypernatremia (>48 hours) is less symptomatic and necessitates a slower correction approach.

Correction of hypertonicity

In the treatment of hypernatremia, correction of hypertonicity involves several key steps, as summarized below, including calculation of water deficit, selecting the appropriate type of replacement fluids, determining the rate of correction of hypernatremia, and addressing the route of fluid replacement.

A. Calculation of water deficit

Various formulas used in calculating fluid administration in hypernatremia are [1, 17]:

1. The standard formula used for the calculation of the free-water deficit.

   Free-Water Deficit =

   Current Total Body Water-TBW (L) × {(Serum [Na^+] ÷ 140) – 1}

2. The formula used to calculate the change in serum Na^+ with 1 liter of solution.

   Change in Serum Na^+ with 1 Liter of the Solution =

   (Solution Na^+ – Serum Na^+) ÷ (TBW [L] + 1)

3. The formula used to calculate the rough estimate of the volume of fluid to be administered.

- 3–4 ml x Body Weight (kg) x (Desired Na^+ Reduction [mEq/L])

In addition to the calculated volume of water deficit, ongoing and insensible losses should be replaced additionally. Correct the total fluid deficit over 48–72 hours.

B. The route of fluid replacement

The Best Route for fluid replacement is to provide free water to correct hypernatremia by oral administration or through a nasogastric tube utilizing the gut. It is challenging to correct large water deficits via the gastrointestinal tract alone, so the common strategy is to combine it with the IV fluid infusion.

C. Selecting the appropriate replacement fluids

- In cases where the patient is hypotensive, isotonic fluids such as normal saline or Ringer's lactate are the preferred choices, irrespective of the presence of hypernatremia.

- It is advisable to use oral water intake as the primary method for correcting hypernatremia whenever feasible.

- Most patients with severe hypernatremia require a large volume of fluids to meet their increased needs, and commonly used fluids to correct fluid deficit include dextrose 5%, 0.2%, or 0.45% saline. However, infuse 5% dextrose cautiously because its rapid administration in large volumes carries the risk of hyperglycemia even in non-diabetic patients. Hyperglycemia causes osmotic diuresis, leading to further loss of electrolyte-free water and aggravation of hypernatremia. If required, use insulin therapy to manage hyperglycemia. These precautions are crucial to safely correct hypernatremia without causing additional complications.

D. The rate of correction of hypernatremia

Strategy to correct hypernatremia differs between acute and chronic hypernatremia.

Acute hypernatremia: In cases of acute hypernatremia, it is advisable to correct the water deficit relatively rapidly to reduce the risk of cerebral edema; however, the precise safe rate of correction is not known [18, 19].

Chronic hypernatremia: To prevent the rapid correction of chronic hypernatremia and avoid the risk of cerebral edema, the traditional recommendation is to aim for a correction rate of 12 mEq/L over 24 hours [1]. A serum sodium correction rate greater than 0.5 mEq/L per hour carries the risk of cerebral edema leading to death or convulsion [20]. These complications were primarily documented in studies involving neonates [20].

However, growing evidence suggests that the traditional belief in the theoretical risk of cerebral edema and herniation with rapid correction of hypernatremia is not observed in adults [15, 18]. On the contrary, slower correction of hypernatremia has been associated with harmful effects, such as longer hospitalizations and worse outcomes, including excess mortality and neurologic damage [21–24].

Furthermore, Chauhan et al. (2019) did not find a higher risk of complications such as mortality, seizures, alterations of consciousness, or cerebral edema due to the rapid correction of hypernatremia in critically ill adult patients [25]. Recent evidence by Feigin et al. demonstrated significantly better survival rates without adverse neurological events, even with very rapid correction of severe hypernatremia [26]. This reinforces the changing trend to correct severe hypernatremia rapidly.

Monitoring

Different formulas used for the calculation cannot predict the fluid volume to be administered perfectly because of associated ongoing water losses via the GI tract, loss of variable quantity electrolyte-free water in the urine, and insensible losses [27, 28]. Close monitoring of the patient's clinical status, meticulous charting of fluid administered, urine output and weight, and serial monitoring of serum sodium (every 1–2 hours in acute hypernatremia and 6–8 hours in chronic hypernatremia) helps in the adjustment of fluid prescription and planning effective treatment plan.

REFERENCES

1. Adrogué HJ, Madias NE. Hypernatremia. N Engl J Med. 2000;342(20):1493–9.
2. Sterns RH. Disorders of plasma sodium--causes, consequences, and correction. N Engl J Med 2015;372(1):55–65.
3. Palevsky PM, Bhagrath R, Greenberg A. Hypernatremia in hospitalized patients. Ann Intern Med. 1996;124(2):197–203.
4. Funk GC, Lindner G, Druml W, et al. Incidence and prognosis of dysnatremias present on ICU admission. Intensive Care Med. 2010;36(2):304–11.
5. Muhsin SA, Mount DB. Diagnosis and treatment of hypernatremia. Best Pract Res Clin Endocrinol Metab. 2016;30(2):189–203.
6. Kim SW. Hypernatemia: successful treatment. Electrolyte Blood Press. 2006;4(2):66–71.
7. Braun MM, Barstow CH, Pyzocha NJ. Diagnosis and management of sodium disorders: hyponatremia and hypernatremia. Am Fam Physician. 2015;91(5):299–307.
8. Jessica MAA, Astrid CBG, Anusha K, et al. Management of Nephrogenic Diabetes Insipidus: An Overview. JOJ Urology & Nephrology. 2022;7(5):555722.
9. Lodin M, Dwyer J. The role of amiloride in managing patients with lithium-induced nephrogenic diabetes

insipidus Journal of Pharmacy Practice and Research 2017;47(5):389–392.

10. Danilo CR. Use of amiloride in lithium-induced nephrogenic diabetes insipidus. J Anal Pharm Res. 2018;7(3):286–287.

11. Mortensen LA, Bistrup C, Jensen BL, et al. A mini-review of pharmacological strategies used to ameliorate polyuria associated with X-linked nephrogenic diabetes insipidus. Am J Physiol Renal Physiol. 2020;319(5):F746–F753.

12. Nguyen MK, Kurtz I. Correction of hypervolaemic hypernatremia by inducing negative Na+ and K+ balance in excess of negative water balance: a new quantitative approach. Nephrol Dial Transplant. 2008;23(7):2223–7.

13. Morkos M, Fam M, Goel M, et al. Protracted acute hypervolemic hypernatremia unmasked after vasopressin therapy: case report, literature review, and proposed algorithmic approach. AACE Clin Case Rep. 2018;5(2):95–98.

14. Pazmiño PA, Pazmiño BP. Treatment of acute hypernatremia with hemodialysis. Am J Nephrol. 1993;13(4):260–265.

15. Nur S, Khan Y, Nur S, et al. Hypernatremia: correction rate and hemodialysis. Case Rep Med. 2014;2014:736073.

16. Rondon-Berrios H, Argyropoulos C, Ing TS, et al. Hypertonicity: Clinical entities, manifestations and treatment. World J Nephrol 2017;6(1):1–13.

17. Sterns RH, Silver SM. Salt and water: read the package insert. QJM. 2003;96(8):549–52.

18. Carlberg DJ, Borek HA, Syverud SA, et al. Survival of acute hypernatremia due to massive soy sauce ingestion. J Emerg Med 2013;45(2):228–31.

19. Farkas J. Hypernatremia & Dehydration in the ICU. IBCC [Internet]. June 25, 2021. Available from: https://emcrit.org/ibcc/hypernatremia/.

20. Bolat F, Oflaz MB, Güven AS, et al. What is the safe approach for neonatal hypernatremic dehydration? A retrospective study from a neonatal intensive care unit. Pediatr Emerg Care 2013;29(7):808–13.

21. Alshayeb HM, Showkat A, Babar F, et al. Severe hypernatremia correction rate and mortality in hospitalized patients. Am J Med Sci. 2011;341(5):356–60.

22. Bataille S, Baralla C, Torro D, et al. Under correction of hypernatremia is frequent and associated with mortality. BMC Nephrol. 2014;15:37.

23. Bohlouli B, Jackson TJ, Tonelli M, et al. Adverse outcomes associated with preventable complications in hospitalized patients with CKD. Clin J Am Soc Nephrol. 2017;12(5):799–806.

24. Ryu JY, Yoon S, Lee J, et al. Efficacy and safety of rapid intermittent bolus compared with slow continuous infusion in patients with severe hypernatremia (SALSA II trial): a study protocol for a randomized controlled trial. Kidney Res Clin Pract. 2022;41(4):508–520.

25. Chauhan K, Pattharanitima P, Patel N, et al. Rate of Correction of Hypernatremia and Health Outcomes in Critically Ill Patients. Clin J Am Soc Nephrol 2019;14(5):656–663.

26. Feigin E, Feigin L, Ingbir M, et al. Rate of Correction and All-Cause Mortality in Patients With Severe Hypernatremia. JAMA Netw Open. 2023;6(9):e2335415.

27. Lindner G, Schwarz C, Kneidinger N, et al. Can we really predict the change in serum sodium levels? An analysis of currently proposed formulae in hypernatremic patients. Nephrol Dial Transplant. 2008;23(11):3501–8.

28. Sterns RH. Formulas for fixing serum sodium: curb your enthusiasm. Clin Kidney J 2016;9(4):527–9.

22 | Hypokalemia

POTASSIUM

PHYSIOLOGICAL BASIS

Potassium (K^+) is a major intracellular cation and the second most abundant cation in the body (next to cation sodium). Total body potassium is about 3,500 mEq. Out of this, 98% of potassium is intracellular, and just 2% of potassium is extracellular. Thus, the normal serum potassium concentration is 3.5 to 5.0 mEq/L vs. an intracellular 140 to 150 mEq/L.

Potassium plays a crucial role in the following:

- Normal functioning of cells: Synthesis of DNA and protein, cell division and growth, enzyme function.

- Neuromuscular transmission: Maintaining cell membrane potential, cellular excitability, conduction of nerve impulses which help in maintaining skeletal, cardiac, and smooth muscle cell contraction.

- Regulate intracellular osmolality and cell volume.

- Maintain acid-base balance and regulate intracellular pH.

POTASSIUM HOMEOSTASIS

The average potassium intake is about 77 and 59 mEq per day in adult men and women, respectively [1]. 90% of potassium consumed is absorbed in the upper gastrointestinal (GI) tract, out of which kidneys excrete 90%, and the remaining 10% is excreted in the stool.

REGULATION OF SERUM POTASSIUM [2–6]

Internal potassium balance (transcellular K+ shift controlling its distribution) and external potassium balance (renal regulation controlling its excretion) are two defense mechanisms that tightly regulate the extracellular fluid (ECF) potassium concentration and maintain the plasma potassium level within narrow limits despite wide fluctuations in dietary K+ intake (K+ loading or depletion).

To minimize the transient change in plasma K+ concentrations, transcellular K+ shift (K+ shift between the ECF to intracellular fluid [ICF] compartments) occurs extremely fast (within minutes), which rapidly corrects abnormality in K+ concentration without changing the total amount of body potassium. This temporary correction in plasma K+ concentrations is followed by the excretion of potassium by the kidney, which is slow (occurs over several hours) but a definitive and effective mechanism for excreting extra potassium from the body.

A. Internal balance of potassium: transcellular shift

- The internal control regulates the intra/extracellular shift, which is a temporary mechanism to maintain a plasma concentration of potassium within the normal range.
- **Potassium shift from ICF to ECF:** To prevent a fall in plasma

potassium due to inadequate oral intake or abnormal potassium loss, potassium is shifted from the ICF to ECF. Critical factors responsible for this shift, leading to an increase in ECF potassium concentration, include metabolic acidosis, insulin deficiency (diabetes mellitus), plasma hyperosmolality, strenuous exercise, cell lysis, aldosterone deficiency (Addison's disease), alpha-adrenergic agonists, and beta-adrenergic blockade.

- **Potassium shift from ECF to ICF:** Conversely, to reduce ECF potassium concentration, potassium is shifted from the ECF to ICF. The important factors facilitating this shift include the effect of insulin, beta-adrenergic stimulation, aldosterone, metabolic alkalosis, and hypo-osmolality.

B. External potassium balance (renal and fecal excretion)

- The kidney excretes 90%, and stool eliminates 10% of the daily intake of potassium. Because of the robust capacity to excrete potassium, the kidney plays a vital role in maintaining the body's potassium content in a steady state.
- The healthy kidney can handle and excrete as high as 400 mEq of potassium per day without causing clinically significant hyperkalemia.
- In patients with very poor potassium intake, the kidney can lower 24-hour urinary potassium excretion to as low as 5–25 mEq/L/day, but it never approaches zero.
- Almost all filtered load of potassium is reabsorbed in the proximal tubule and loop of Henle. Urinary excretion of K+ ion is determined by its secretion at distal tubules and collecting duct.

C. Factors affecting renal excretion

Four major factors determining the excretion of potassium are:

- **Aldosterone:** Mechanisms by which aldosterone stimulates the urinary secretion of potassium are: (1) It stimulates the activity of the Na^+-K^+-ATPase in the distal nephron, which increases the reabsorption of sodium across the luminal membrane and, as a result, increases electronegativity of the lumen; (2) Increased luminal electrical gradient favors the urinary secretion of potassium; and (3) Direct effect of aldosterone on the luminal membrane is increased tubular K^+ permeability which leads to loss of K^+ in urine.

- **Distal delivery of Na^+ and water:** High delivery of sodium to the collecting duct (e.g., diuretics) and high flow of urine (e.g., osmotic diuresis) by lowering the luminal potassium concentration stimulate the secretion of potassium with resultant increased urinary loss of potassium.

- **High serum potassium levels:** Increase in plasma potassium concentration directly stimulate aldosterone secretion and promotes urinary potassium excretion.

- **Delivery of negatively charged ions to the collecting duct:** Increased lumen negativity due to anions such as bicarbonate markedly increases potassium excretion.

CORRELATION OF SERUM AND BODY POTASSIUM

It is important to remember that serum potassium rises proportionately whenever body potassium increases and may reach a dangerous level rapidly. But when there is a deficit in total body potassium, reduction in serum potassium is not proportionate because the K^+ shift from the intracellular compartment to ECF partly compensates for it. So, hyperkalemia suggests increased total body potassium, but the level of hypokalemia may underestimate the total body potassium deficit.

DISORDERS OF POTASSIUM CONCENTRATION

Disorders of potassium are hypokalemia and hyperkalemia.

HYPOKALEMIA

Hypokalemia is an electrolyte disorder characterized by persistent reduction of serum potassium (K^+) below 3.5 mEq/L. When serum potassium level is <2.5 mEq/L, hypokalemia is severe and life-threatening [5]. Hypokalemia is a common disorder, and its incidence is up to 21% in hospitalized patients and 2% to 3% in outpatients [7, 8].

ETIOLOGY

Common causes of hypokalemia are summarized in Table 22.1. Diuretics, vomiting, diarrhea, and hypomagnesemia are the most common causes of hypokalemia:

- **Diuretics:** Loop and thiazide diuretics are common cause of hypokalemia, and it occurs due to increase distal delivery of sodium and hypovolemia-induced increased aldosterone. The severity of hypokalemia is dose-dependent, and the incidence of hypokalemia is greater with thiazide diuretics than with loop diuretics.

- **Vomiting:** As the potassium content of gastric juice is low (less than 10 mEq/L, similar to that of plasma),

Table 22.1 Causes of hypokalemia
1. Poor intake (rarely the sole cause)
• Low dietary intake (malnutrition), anorexia nervosa, or potassium free intravenous (IV) fluids
2. Extrarenal loss/non-renal loss (Urinary potassium excretion <20–30 mEq/day)
• Vomiting, diarrhea, large nasogastric aspiration, laxatives, ureterosigmoidostomy, and excessive sweating
3. Renal loss (Urinary potassium excretion >20–30 mEq/day)
• Diuretics, osmotic diuresis, DKA, polyuria (e.g, post-ATN or post-obstructive diuresis)
• Mineralocorticoid excess (primary or secondary aldosteronism), cushing's syndrome, steroid therapy
• Magnesium deficiency, amphotericin B, Bartter's syndrome
• Renal tubular acidosis (RTA) types I or II
4. Redistribution (shift of K$^+$ into cell)
• Insulin release, beta-adrenergic agonist (e.g., salbutamol), metabolic alkalosis, hypokalemic periodic paralysis, refeeding syndrome
5. Pseudohypokalemia
• Delayed sample analysis in patients with high WBC count (e.g., acute myelogenous leukemia)

loss of gastric juice is not primarily responsible for hypokalemia. Hypokalemia in vomiting is chiefly due to a large amount of renal loss of potassium because of the combined effect of the stimulation of aldosterone secretion and metabolic alkalosis.

Hypovolemia-induced hyperaldosteronism leads to renal sodium and water reabsorption and potassium secretion with enhanced urinary potassium loss.

As plasma bicarbonate concentration is high in metabolic alkalosis, a large amount of bicarbonate is filtered in the proximal tubule.

As the amount of filtered bicarbonate exceeds the proximal tubular reabsorptive threshold, a large amount of bicarbonate is delivered in the distal nephron.

In the distal tubule, potassium secretion is stimulated due to the combined effect of hypovolemia-induced hyperaldosteronism, alkalemia, and increased distal delivery of bicarbonate, which results in increased urinary loss of K$^+$, leading to hypokalemia [9].

Metabolic alkalosis also contributes to hypokalemia by shifting ECF potassium into ICF.

• **Diarrhea:** In diarrhea, hypokalemia occurs due to loss of potassium-rich fluid (K$^+$ content 50–100 mEq/L). Diarrhea-induced hypovolemia activates RAAS, increases aldosterone secretion, and exacerbates potassium loss through the kidneys and colonic secretion.

As diarrheal fluid is rich in bicarbonate (HCO$_3$ content approximately 30 mEq/L), it can cause normal anion gap (hyperchloremic) metabolic acidosis. As acidosis shifts K$^+$ from ICF to ECF, the resultant rise in serum K$^+$ may mask hypokalemia or misguides clinicians to underestimate the severity of the potassium deficit in the body.

• **Hypomagnesemia:** Concomitant magnesium deficiency is a common cause of hypokalemia refractory to treatment by potassium. Magnesium deficiency occurs in more than 50% of clinically significant hypokalemia, and it occurs most frequently in patients receiving loop or thiazide diuretic therapy [5, 10].

CLINICAL FEATURES [5, 6]

- The clinical picture varies greatly according to the severity and rate at which hypokalemia develops and seldom occurs unless serum potassium is less than 3 mEq/L. The manifestation of hypokalemia varies from absent to life-threatening symptoms, which are mainly neuromuscular and cardiac.

- Fatigue, myalgia, leg cramps, and muscular weakness of the lower extremity.

- Smooth muscle involvement may result in constipation, ileus, or urinary retention.

- More severe hypokalemia leads to progressive weakness, ascending paralysis, hyporeflexia, hypoventilation (due to respiratory muscle involvement), and virtually complete paralysis. In addition, severe hypokalemia can cause life-threatening arrhythmias such as Torsades de pointes and ventricular tachycardia.

- In addition, severe hypokalemia can lead to even serious complications like rhabdomyolysis.

- Detrimental effects of hypokalemia on the cardiovascular system vary from mild asymptomatic ECG changes to lethal cardiac arrhythmias. Hypokalemia also triggers or worsens digitalis-associated arrhythmias.

- Hypokalemia can lead to metabolic acidosis, the low specific gravity of urine, and polyuria (due to the inability to concentrate the urine) [11].

- Hypokalemia can stimulate ammoniagenesis in the proximal tubule and can precipitate or aggravate hepatic encephalopathy in patients with hepatic failure.

ECG CHANGES [12–15]

Electrocardiogram (ECG) manifestations do not correlate well with the serum potassium level. Cardiac arrhythmia is a common presentation of hypokalemia, and the earliest ECG change in hypokalemia is a decrease in T wave amplitude. Different ECG changes with increased severity of hypokalemia are summarized in Table 22.2.

Hypokalemia causes ST depression which mimics ischemic heart diseases.

Hypokalemia is a nonischemic causes of ST depressions. Arrhythmias such as Torsades de pointes and ventricular tachycardia in severe hypokalemia can be life-threatening.

Table 22.2 Electrocardiographic changes of hypokalemia	
Potassium concentration	ECG manifestations
<3.5 mEq/L	Decrease in amplitude, flattening, or inversion of T-waves
<3.0 mEq/L	ST-segment depression, PR-interval prolongation, Q-T interval prolongation, prominent U waves (best seen in the mid-precordial-V2-V3 leads), tall P-wave, and premature ventricular beats
<2.5 mEq/L	Atrial fibrillation, atrial flutter, atrial tachycardia, ventricular and supraventricular tachyarrhythmias, Torsades de pointes (most classic), and ventricular fibrillation

DIAGNOSIS

Detailed history, meticulous examination, and appropriate tests help to establish the etiological diagnosis of hypokalemia [5, 16].

History

A detailed history may provide clues to the underlying cause of hypokalemia, such as GI losses (e.g., vomiting, diarrhea), polyuria in diabetes due to DKA, interventions causing K^+ shift to ICF (e.g., insulin, β-adrenergic agonists or $NaHCO_3$ therapy), medications (e.g., laxatives, loop or thiazide diuretics, antibiotics), and poor K^+ intake.

Physical examination

The blood pressure measurement is an essential step in assessing hypokalemia because high or normal blood pressure provides vital clues to the etiological diagnosis. If hypertension is present with hypokalemia, its common causes are primary aldosteronism (Conns Syndrome), Cushing's syndrome, renovascular disease, and the use of diuretics as an antihypertensive treatment [17]. Additionally, the physical exam also provides information about the volume status, cardiac arrhythmia, neurologic manifestations of hypokalemia, and signs suggestive of specific underlying disorders such as hyperthyroidism and Cushing's syndrome.

Laboratory evaluation

In addition to serum potassium, other tests such as sodium, chloride, magnesium, calcium, phosphate, glucose, arterial blood gas, anion gap, a complete blood count, BUN, creatinine, and serum osmolality are helpful to establish the etiological diagnosis of hypokalemia.

Additional diagnostic tests

In a few patients, the etiology of hypokalemia may not be apparent on primary evaluation, and such patients require further workup, as summarized in Figure 22.1 and 22.2. The two most important tests widely used for further diagnostic evaluation are the assessment of urinary potassium excretion and acid-base status.

Urinary potassium excretion [5, 18–20]

This is an important step to evaluate the etiology of hypokalemia which divides its causes into two broad groups, renal potassium losses and other causes of hypokalemia (extrarenal loss, transcellular shift, or decreased dietary intake).

The four methods used for the measurements of urinary potassium excretion are:

Spot urine potassium

- It is a simple and most commonly obtained test. It provides misleading results if the urine sodium is lower than 30 mEq/L and/or the urine osmolality is lower than the plasma osmolality (suggesting that the patient is polyuric).

24-hours urine potassium

- Measurement of potassium from the collection of 24-hour urine is the most accurate, gold-standard diagnostic tool, but it is cumbersome, impractical, and unsuitable for urgent diagnostic needs.

- Urinary potassium excretion below 25 to 30 mEq per day suggests appropriate renal conservation of potassium and indicates that the cause of hypokalemia can be extrarenal loss or transcellular shift.

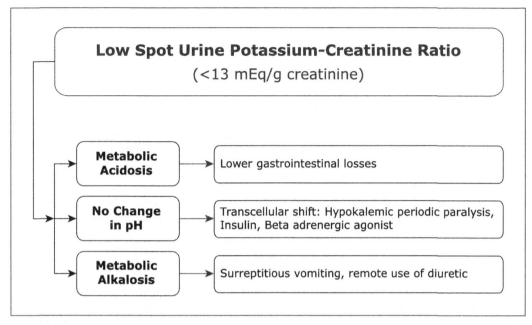

Figure 22.1 Approach to Hypokalemia with low urinary potassium excretion.

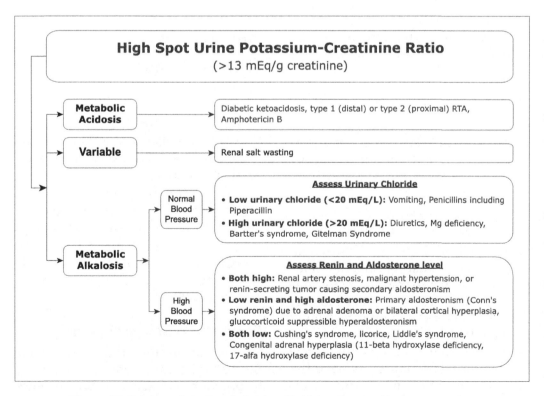

Figure 22.2 Approach to Hypokalemia with high urinary potassium excretion.

- The urinary potassium excretion >25 to 30 mEq per day on a 24-hour urine collection suggest urinary potassium wasting.

The spot urine potassium-to-creatinine ratio

- This is a rapid and reliable spot urine test to estimate potassium loss when collecting 24-hour urine is not feasible or available.

- As creatinine is excreted at a near-constant rate in urine, urine volume or urine osmolality variations do not affect the test result.

- The value of urine potassium-to-creatinine ratio is >13 mEq/g creatinine (1.5 mEq/mmol) usually indicates inappropriate renal wasting of potassium, and a ratio <13 mEq/g creatinine (1.5 mEq/mmol creatinine) suggests that hypokalemia is due to gastrointestinal losses, transcellular potassium shifts, remote use of diuretics, or decreased dietary intake.

Transtubular potassium gradient (TTKG)

- This is a semiquantitative index of the activity of the K$^+$ secretory process, which measures net K$^+$ secretion by the collecting duct.

- TTKG = Urine K$^+$/Serum K$^+$ × Serum Osmolality/Urine Osmolality.

- The value of TTKG >7 indicates renal potassium wasting and the value <3 suggests extrarenal potassium loss. The results of this test are inaccurate if the urine osmolality is lower than the serum osmolality or if urine sodium is <25 mEq/L. Recent literature does not recommend this test, and therefore not used for the diagnosis of hypokalemia [20–22].

Acid-base status

After differentiating renal potassium wasting and extrarenal cause of hypokalemia, the next step is the assessment of acid-base status. The acid-base status, blood pressure status, and the magnitude of renal potassium wasting further narrow the differential diagnosis when hypokalemia's etiology is unclear.

The causes of hypokalemia with low renal K$^+$ excretion (<25 mEq/day) are summarized in Figure 22.1.

In patients with high urinary K$^+$ excretion, associated acid-base disorders (metabolic acidosis or alkalosis), blood pressure status (normal or high), urinary chloride excretion (low or high), and measurement of the blood levels of renin and aldosterone are helpful in arriving at the etiological diagnosis of K$^+$ wasting with hypokalemia (Figure 22.2).

MANAGEMENT

Therapeutic goals

1. Prevention of hypokalemia.
2. To prevent life-threatening complications (cardiac arrhythmia and neuromuscular dysfunction such as diaphragmatic weakness and rhabdomyolysis).
3. To correct the potassium deficit and to raise serum potassium concentration to a safe level.
4. To treat underlying etiology, to reduce/discontinue the offending agent, and to minimize ongoing losses.

Prevention of hypokalemia

Normal potassium intake of about 50–100 mEq/day in adults is sufficient to prevent hypokalemia. But patients receiving digitalis, long-term diuretics, or large doses of steroids should receive a potassium-rich diet and supplement. Conditions where prevention of hypokalemia is of special importance, are digitalis therapy, hepatic failure, previous myocardial infarction or ischemic heart disease (IHD), and diabetes mellitus.

Reducing the loop or thiazide diuretics dosage, restricting sodium intake, and providing 20 mEq/day of potassium chloride are usually sufficient to prevent diuretic-induced hypokalemia or in patients with hyperaldosteronism [15, 23, 24].

In critical and postoperative patients with normal potassium and creatinine levels, administration of a maintenance dose of intravenous potassium prevents hypokalemia and is beneficial [25].

Replenishment of potassium deficit

A. Estimation of the potassium deficit

There is no fixed formula for calculating potassium deficit in hypokalemia, but 1 mEq/L fall in serum potassium = roughly 300–400 mEq total body potassium deficit [26]. However, it is important to remember that in hypokalemia with progressive potassium fall, the magnitude of total body potassium deficit increases exponentially (Table 22.3). Therefore, it may grossly underestimate the requirement of potassium.

Table 22.3 Total-body potassium deficit in the absence of a transcellular shift [6]			
Serum K^+ (mEq/L)	3.0	2.0	<2.0
Total K^+ deficit (mEq)	100–200	400–600	>600

B. Selection of treatment modality

Treatment selection based on the severity of hypokalemia is summarized below [5, 15, 26].

1. Borderline hypokalemia (3.5–3.9 mEq/L)

- Dietary potassium supplementation.
- Consider oral potassium chloride 20 mEq/day to prevent hypokalemia with diuretics or hyperaldosteronism.

2. Mild hypokalemia (3.0–3.4 mEq/L)

- Dietary potassium supplementation.
- The oral formulation of potassium.
- Intravenous potassium chloride (Inj. KCl) supplementation is recommended if the patient cannot tolerate oral formulations due to severe nausea, vomiting, abdominal distress, or nonfunctioning GI tract.

3. Moderate hypokalemia (2.5–2.9 mEq/L)

- Dietary potassium supplementation.
- The oral formulation of potassium (KCl 40 to 100 mEq/day).
- Intravenous route if unable to tolerate the oral form. Administer IV potassium at 10–20 mEq/h through the peripheral vein till K^+ reaches to normal level or oral supplementation of potassium is possible/safe. High-risk patients with life-threatening cardiac arrhythmias, severe neuromuscular dysfunction, digitalis toxicity, recent or ongoing cardiac ischemia, and advanced liver disease may need intravenous potassium supplementation.

4. Severe hypokalemia (<2.5 mEq/L)

- Intravenous potassium should be given with a central line at 20–40 mEq/h till K^+ reaches to normal level or the patient becomes asymptomatic.

C. Precautions before initiating potassium supplements

1. In oliguria-anuria, avoid or supplement K$^+$ cautiously.

2. Patients receiving potassium-sparing diuretics, ACE inhibitors, and patients with renal failure are at high risk of developing hyperkalemia, so potassium supplementation should be done cautiously.

3. Digitalis therapy: Potassium enters the cell at a slower rate in patients on digitalis due to the inhibitory effect of digitalis drugs on the Na$^+$-K$^+$-ATPase in the cell membrane, causing a risk of transient hyperkalemia with faster IV infusion of potassium. So, the rate of potassium infusion should be slower in such patients.

4. Continuous ECG monitoring and frequent serum potassium level estimation are advisable if the infusion rate is >20 mEq/hour in any patient.

D. How much potassium to give? How long to treat?

No fixed formula determines the amount of potassium to be administered to correct the potassium deficit. Therefore close monitoring of serum potassium and accordingly designing and modifying therapy is recommended.

When the average potassium deficit is about 200–400 mEq, the daily administration of 50–100 mEq of potassium slowly but adequately corrects the deficit.

Patients with severe hypokalemia or a high rate of ongoing losses may require larger doses of potassium supplementation and correct deficit slowly over days.

It may take weeks to correct severe potassium loss. However, if adequate dose and duration of potassium supplement fail to increase serum potassium level, it is important to exclude hypomagnesemia.

Oral potassium supplementation

A. Potassium-rich food

Fruit juices, coconut water, banana, dry fruits, chocolate, coffee, soup, potassium-rich salt substitutes, etc.

B. Oral potassium supplementation

- Oral potassium is a cheaper and safer mode of correcting hypokalemia as there is minimal risk of hyperkalemia in the presence of adequate renal function.

- In mild to moderate hypokalemia (serum potassium 3 to 3.5 mEq/L) with normal renal functions and without abnormal urinary potassium losses, the average dose of potassium chloride is 40 to 100 mEq/day (10–20 mEq, 2–5 times) along with the treatment of the underlying disorder (such as vomiting or diarrhea).

- Patients with severe or symptomatic hypokalemia need more rapid potassium replacement, which can be most easily done by IV replacement.

- Potassium chloride (KCl) 10% oral solution, available in the market, contains 20 mEq potassium per 15 ml oral solution (10 ml solution = 1gm KCl = 13.4 mEq of potassium).

- Potassium chloride tablets and capsules contain 8 mEq or 10 mEq of potassium per tablet.

- All oral potassium formulations (capsule, tablet, or liquid) may frequently cause GI irritation, abdominal discomfort, nausea, and diarrhea. Therefore, patients are advised to take potassium chloride solution with proper dilution in 100–250 mL of water, with or after food.

- Esophageal or small bowel erosion and stricture are uncommon side effects.

- Prefer to use intravenous potassium preparations instead of oral formulations in patients with severe hypokalemia (K+ <2.5 mEq/L), severe shock (absorption from the gut unpredictable), and patients unable to tolerate the oral formulations or is nothing by mouth (NPO).

Which oral potassium formulations are selected for supplementation?

Potassium chloride is a preferred formulation to correct hypokalemia with metabolic alkalosis [26].

Hypokalemia due to diuretic therapy or vomiting is associated with chloride depletion. Because potassium chloride corrects both deficits (i.e., potassium and chloride), it is a preferred and effective formulation.

As most potassium in food is almost entirely coupled with phosphate rather than chloride, dietary potassium has limited effectiveness in treating hypokalemia with chloride depletion [26].

Potassium citrate and bicarbonate are preferred in hypokalemic patients with normal anion gap metabolic acidosis (common causes are diarrhea or distal RTA) because of their alkalinizing effect.

Potassium citrate and bicarbonate tend to alkalinize the patient and would be more appropriate for treating hypokalemia associated with normal anion gap metabolic acidosis (common causes are diarrhea or distal RTA). The citrate is metabolized and converted into bicarbonate which improves acidosis.

IV potassium supplementation

A. Selection of IV potassium formulations

Potassium chloride and potassium phosphate are commercially available formulations:

- **Inj. potassium chloride (KCl)** is the most common IV formulation used in the treatment of hypokalemia. It is administered as a primary treatment and an adjunct to oral supplementation in the treatment of hypokalemia.

  Inj. potassium chloride 15%, 10 ml ampoule contains 20 mEq of potassium (Each ml of 15% KCl = 2 mEq of potassium).

- **Inj. potassium phosphate** is used in selected patients having hypophosphatemia along with hypokalemia (e.g., diabetes with ketoacidosis, alcohol abuse, and refeeding syndrome), as it corrects both disorders.

  Inj. potassium phosphate is available in 10 ml/15 ml/20 ml ampoules. Each ml of potassium phosphate contains 3 mmol Phosphate/mL and 4.4 mEq Potassium/mL.

B. Potassium containing IV fluids

- The potassium concentration of commonly used IV fluids is summarized in Table 22.4.

C. Indications

- IV potassium supplementation carries a higher risk of hyperkalemia compared to oral formulations. So, IV potassium supplementation should be reserved for severe hypokalemia (K+ <3 mEq/L) and patients who are symptomatic or unable to tolerate oral potassium.

Table 22.4 Potassium concentration of IV fluids					
IV fluid	**Isolyte-M**	**Isolyte- P**	**Isolyte- G**	**Isolyte- E**	**PlasmaLyte**	**RL Sterofundin**
Potassium (mEq/L)	35.0	20.0	17.0	10.0	5.0	4.0

D. Recommendations for administration

No rule is absolute, but common guidelines for IV potassium therapy are as follows [15, 24, 27, 28]:

- Avoid infusing at rate >10–20 mEq/hr.
- Avoid infusing at concentration >40 mEq/L.
- Avoid infusing total amount >240 mEq/day.
- Always monitor IV potassium therapy closely with frequent serum potassium estimation.
- Administration of K^+ in higher doses (>20 mEq/hour) or higher concentrations (>40 mEq/L) requires cardiac monitoring.
- Concentrated potassium infusion (>40 mEq/L) is administered via the central venous line using a volumetric infusion pump. Common local side effects of administrating of higher concentrations of IV potassium chloride into a peripheral vein are local pain, phlebitis, or venous thrombosis. Concentrated potassium infusion is indicated when the potassium requirement is high, or the patient needs fluid restriction.
- Never infuse undiluted inj. potassium chloride directly intravenously as a bolus form, as it can cause sudden hyperkalemia and instant death from cardiac arrest.
- Avoid adding potassium chloride to Isolyte-M because this fluid is rich in potassium (K^+ content 35 mEq/L).

- While preparing the potassium chloride drip, shake the solution well before use. Don't add potassium chloride in the hanging bottle because mixing will be improper.
- Remember that hypokalemia is safer than hyperkalemia, so avoid over-enthusiastic treatment.
- Rapid correction of hypokalemia with IV potassium administration can cause dangerous hyperkalemia even in potassium-depleted patients.

IV solutions for dilution

- Add KCl to normal saline or 0.45% saline to prepare potassium infusion. Avoid using dextrose-containing solutions as a diluent IV fluid because the administration of dextrose stimulates the release of insulin which shifts potassium intracellularly and exacerbates hypokalemia.

E. Special considerations

1. Metabolic acidosis in hypokalemia

When metabolic acidosis and severe hypokalemia coexist, replace potassium before correcting the acidosis. Treatment of acidosis with sodium bicarbonate may aggravate or precipitate hypokalemia due to ECF to ICF shift of potassium, which may be life-threatening in severe hypokalemia.

2. Hypomagnesemia in hypokalemia

Magnesium deficiency is the most common cause of hypokalemia refractory to treatment (particularly in patients receiving loop or thiazide diuretics). So always check magnesium in such patients and correct hypomagnesemia adequately (by oral or intravenous magnesium repletion) to facilitate more rapid correction of hypokalemia and reduce the risk of cardiac arrhythmia.

3. Hypokalemia in diabetic ketoacidosis

Why do patients of diabetic ketoacidosis (DKA) need potassium supplementation besides its normal serum level?

The normal value of serum potassium in DKA on presentation is common but deceptive. Serum potassium levels are high-normal or elevated in about 95% of patients hospitalized with hyperglycemic crises [29]. However, it is essential to remember that an adult patient with DKA, on average has about 3–5 mEq/kg/body weight potassium deficit and therefore needs potassium supplementation [30, 31]. In DKA, factors such as lack of insulin, acidosis, hyperglycemia, and hyperosmolality lead to the transcellular shift of potassium from the ICF to the ECF and raise the serum K^+ level besides its deficit in the body [30–32].

Why are patients of DKA prone to develop hypokalemia after initiation of therapy?

Hypokalemia can occur in about 50% of patients while managing hyperglycemic crises [33].

Mechanisms of the development of hypokalemia in DKA are [31]:

- **The shift of K^+ from ECF to ICF** due to insulin administration and correction of metabolic acidosis.
- **Loss of K^+** due to DKA-induced vomiting and hyperglycemia-induced diuresis.
- **Dilution** due to administration of IV fluids.

ADA guidelines for potassium supplementation in DKA [31]

- 3.3 to 5.2 mEq/L: Inj. KCl 20–30 mEq in each liter of IV fluid to be initiated after diuresis.
- <3.3 mEq/L: Inj. KCl 20–30 mEq in each liter of IV fluid, temporarily hold the administration of Insulin till K^+ >3.3 mEq/L.

The target of potassium supplementation in hypokalemia

In hypokalemia, the goal of K^+ supplementation is to achieve a serum potassium level of 4.0–5.0 mEq/L in most of the patients [34], 4.0–4.6 mEq/L in cardiac patients [15], and 4–5 mEq/L in patients with DKA [31]. In hypokalemic patients, once cardiac rhythm becomes normal, and the respiratory muscle strength is restored, potassium infusion is tapered gradually and discontinued, and the patient is shifted to oral potassium formulation.

Correction of the underlying causes and minimizing ongoing losses

Search and treat underlying causative etiology (e.g., Treatment of diarrhea, vomiting, and uncontrolled diabetes mellitus).

Upper GI losses: In vomiting or continuous nasogastric (NG) aspiration, the use of proton pump inhibitor (PPI) reduces hypokalemia. By inhibiting HCl secretion into the gastric lumen, PPIs reduce losses of hydrogen and chloride ions in the upper GI loss and, therefore, reduce hypochloremic metabolic alkalosis, resulting in lesser urinary loss of potassium [35].

K^+ loss due to diuretics: Measures suggested to reduce hypokalemia are discontinuing or reducing the dose of diuretics, K+ rich diet, supplementing oral formulation of potassium, correcting coexisting hypomagnesemia, co-administering mineralocorticoid receptor antagonist (spironolactone or eplerenone) or epithelial sodium channels (ENaC) inhibitor (amiloride). Additionally, treat the comorbid condition with drugs such as angiotensin-converting enzyme (ACE) inhibitors, angiotensin receptor blockers (ARBs), or beta-blockers which increase the serum potassium [8].

Use of spironolactone: In primary hyperaldosteronism, advanced heart failure, and in patients treated with thiazide or loop diuretics, supplementing spironolactone can effectively reduce hypokalemia.

Hypokalemic thyrotoxic periodic paralysis: Administration of oral propranolol (nonselective b-blocker) decreases the frequency and severity of attacks [36].

REFERENCES

1. U.S. Department of Agriculture, Agricultural Research Service. What We Eat in America, 2013–2014.

2. Rastegar A. Serum Potassium. In: Walker HK, Hall WD, Hurst JW, editors. Clinical Methods: The History, Physical, and Laboratory Examinations. 3rd edition. Boston: Butterworths; 1990. Chapter 195. Available from: https://www.ncbi.nlm.nih.gov/books/NBK307/.

3. Palmer BF. Regulation of potassium homeostasis. Clinical Journal of the American Society of Nephrology 2015;10(6):1050–1060.

4. Gumz ML, Rabinowitz L, Wingo CS. An Integrated View of Potassium Homeostasis. N Engl J Med. 2015;373(1):60–72.

5. Kardalas E, Paschou SA, Anagnostis P, et al. Hypokalemia: a clinical update. Endocr Connect. 2018;7(4):R135–R146.

6. Palmer BF, Clegg DJ. Physiology and Pathophysiology of Potassium Homeostasis: Core Curriculum 2019. Am J Kidney Dis. 2019;74(5):682–695.

7. Marti G, Schwarz C, Leichtle AB, et al. Etiology and symptoms of severe hypokalaemia in emergency department patients. European Journal of Emergency Medicine 2014;21(1):46–51.

8. Viera AJ, Wouk N. Potassium Disorders: Hypokalemia and Hyperkalemia. Am Fam Physician. 2015;92(6):487–95.

9. Aronson PS, Giebisch G. Effects of pH on potassium: new explanations for old observations. J Am Soc Nephrol. 2011;22(11):1981–1989.

10. Huang CL, Kuo E. Mechanism of hypokalemia in magnesium deficiency. J Am Soc Nephrol. 2007;18(10):2649–52.

11. Yalamanchili HB, Calp-Inal S, Zhou XJ, et al. Hypokalemic Nephropathy. Kidney Int Rep. 2018;3(6):1482–1488.

12. Levis JT. ECG diagnosis: hypokalemia. Perm J. 2012;16(2):57.

13. Kishimoto C, Tamaru K, Kuwahara H. Tall P waves associated with severe hypokalemia and combined electrolyte depletion. J Electrocardiol. 2014;47(1):93–4.

14. Wang X, Han D, Li G. Electrocardiographic manifestations in severe hypokalemia. J Int Med Res. 2020;48(1):300060518811058.

15. Krogager ML, Kragholm K, Thomassen JQ, et al. Update on management of hypokalaemia and goals for the lower potassium level in patients with cardiovascular disease: a review in collaboration with the European Society of Cardiology Working Group on Cardiovascular Pharmacotherapy, European Heart Journal - Cardiovascular Pharmacotherapy, 2021;pvab038.

16. Groeneveld JH, Sijpkens YW, Lin SH, et al. An approach to the patient with severe hypokalaemia: the potassium quiz. QJM. 2005;98(4):305–16.

17. Abcar AC, Kujubu DA. Evaluation of hypertension with hypokalemia. Perm J. 2009;13(1):73–76.

18. Jędrusik P, Symonides B, Wojciechowska E, et al. Diagnostic value of potassium level in a spot urine sample as an index of 24-hour urinary potassium excretion in unselected patients hospitalized in a hypertension unit. PLoS One. 2017;12(6):e0180117.

19. Palmer BF, Clegg DJ. The Use of Selected Urine Chemistries in the Diagnosis of Kidney Disorders. Clin J Am Soc Nephrol. 2019;14(2):306–316.

20. Grams ME, Hoenig MP, Hoorn EJ. Evaluation of Hypokalemia. JAMA. 2021;325(12):1216–1217.

21. Kamel K, Halperin M. Intrarenal urea recycling leads to a higher rate of renal excretion of potassium: an hypothesis with clinical implications. Curr Opin Nephrol Hypertens 2011;20(5):547–54.

22. Halperin ML. Assessing the renal response in patients with potassium disorders: a shift in emphasis from the TTKG to the urine K+/creatinine ratio. Afr J Nephrol. 2017;20(1):22–24.

23. Bourke E, Delaney V. Prevention of hypokalemia caused by diuretics. Heart Dis Stroke. 1994;3(2):63–7.

24. Cohn JN, Kowey PR, Whelton PK, et al. New Guidelines for Potassium Replacement in Clinical Practice: A Contemporary Review by the National Council on Potassium in Clinical Practice. Arch Intern Med. 2000;160(16):2429–2436.

25. Scotto CJ, Fridline M, Menhart CJ, Klions HA. Preventing hypokalemia in critically ill patients. Am J Crit Care. 2014;23(2):145–9.

26. Gennari FJ. Hypokalemia. N Engl J Med 1998;339(7):451–458.

27. Asmar A, Mohandas R, Wingo CS. A physiologic-based approach to the treatment of a patient with hypokalemia. Am J Kidney Dis. 2012;60(3):492–7.

28. Farkas J. Hypokalemia. Internet Book of Critical Care (IBCC) June 25, 2021. Visit: https://emcrit.org/ibcc/hypokalemia/.

29. Pasquel FJ, Tsegka K, Wang H, et al. Clinical outcomes in patients with isolated or combined diabetic ketoacidosis and hyperosmolar hyperglycemic state: a retrospective, hospital-based cohort study. Diabetes Care 2020;43(3):349–57.

30. Umpierrez GE, Murphy MB, Kitabchi AE. Diabetic Ketoacidosis and Hyperglycemic Hyperosmolar Syndrome. Diabetes Spectrum 2002;15(1):28–36.

31. Kitabchi AE, Umpierrez GE, Miles JM, et al. Hyperglycemic crises in adult patients with diabetes. Diabetes Care 2009;32(7):1335–1343.

32. Adrogué HJ, Lederer ED, Suki WN, Eknoyan G. Determinants of plasma potassium levels in diabetic keto-acidosis. Medicine (Baltimore) 1986;65(3):163–172.

33. Pasquel FJ, Lansang MC, Dhatariya K, et al. Management of diabetes and hyperglycaemia in the hospital. Lancet Diabetes Endocrinol. 2021;9(3):174–188.

34. Clase CM, Carrero JJ, Ellison DH, et al; Conference Participants. Potassium homeostasis and management of dyskalemia in kidney diseases: conclusions from a Kidney Disease: Improving Global Outcomes (KDIGO) Controversies Conference. Kidney Int. 2020;97(1):42–61.

35. Wainwright NJ, Azim A, Neary JD. Proton Pump Inhibition in the Management of Hypokalemia in Anorexia Nervosa with Self-Induced Vomiting. Canadian Journal of General Internal Medicine 2018;13(3):35–38.

36. Tella SH, Kommalapati A. Thyrotoxic Periodic Paralysis: An Underdiagnosed and Under-recognized Condition. Cureus. 2015;7(10):e342.

23 | Hyperkalemia

A serum potassium level greater than 5.5 mEq/L is considered hyperkalemia. The incidence of hyperkalemia is very low in the general population but increases in patients with chronic kidney disease (CKD), heart failure, diabetes and in patients receiving renin-angiotensin-aldosterone system inhibitor (RAASi) treatment [1–5]. Hyperkalemia is a potentially life-threatening electrolyte disorder associated with significantly increased hospitalizations, cardiovascular events, and all-cause mortality [6–9]. In addition, acute severe hyperkalemia is a potentially dangerous problem that can cause cardiac arrhythmias leading to cardiac arrest and death.

ETIOLOGY

The most common causes of hyperkalemia are renal dysfunction (acute or chronic), medication causing impaired potassium excretion, diabetes mellitus, cell lysis (rhabdomyolysis, tumor lysis syndrome, massive hemolysis), and pseudohyperkalemia [10]. The causes of hyperkalemia based on its mechanism of development are summarized in Table 23.1.

CKD is the most common risk factor for hyperkalemia, and hyperkalemia is the most common electrolyte disturbance in CKD [11, 12]. Furthermore, as CKD advances, the prevalence of hyperkalemia increases [3, 13].

Table 23.1 Causes of hyperkalemia
1. Increased potassium intake
• Intravenous (IV) fluid containing potassium
• High potassium-containing foods (rare unless underlying renal dysfunction)
• Potassium containing drugs
2. Tissue breakdown
• Bleeding into the soft tissue, gastrointestinal (GI) tract, or body cavities
• Haemolysis, rhabdomyolysis, tumor lysis syndrome
• Catabolic state
3. The shift of potassium out of cells
• Tissue damage (ischemia or shock), severe exercise
• Metabolic acidosis
• Poorly controlled diabetes due to insulin deficiency, hyperglycemia, and hyperosmolality
• Aldosterone deficiency
• Hyperkalemic periodic paralysis, succinylcholine
4. Impaired potassium excretion
• Acute kidney injury (AKI) or chronic kidney diseases
• Potassium-sparing diuretics, ACE inhibitors, ARBs, NSAIDs, heparin, cyclosporine
• Reduced tubular excretion: Addison's disease, hyporeninemic hypoaldosteronism (due to diabetic nephropathy, interstitial nephritis, type 4 renal tubular acidosis-RTA and NSAIDs), and amyloidosis
• Effective circulatory volume depletion
5. Pseudo hyperkalemia
• Hemolysis of blood samples
• Prolonged tourniquet use or fist clenching during sample collection
• Marked thrombocytosis, or leucocytosis

Drug-induced hyperkalemia

Various drugs interfere with potassium homeostasis and can cause hyperkalemia by affecting renal potassium excretion, inhibiting the renin-angiotensin-aldosterone system, or promoting the transcellular potassium shift from intracellular fluid (ICF) to extracellular fluid (ECF) compartment (Table 23.2. Drug-induced hyperkalemia) [10, 14, 15].

A. Drugs which impair renal potassium excretion

• **Potassium-sparing diuretics:** The common cause of hyperkalemia is potassium-sparing diuretics. By antagonizing the effect of aldosterone on the collecting tubule cells, it decreases renal potassium

excretion and causes hyperkalemia. Aldosterone antagonists (also called mineralocorticoid-receptor antagonists)

Table 23.2 Drug induced hyperkalemia
Drugs which impair renal potassium excretion
• Potassium-sparing diuretics
• ACE inhibitors, ARBs
• NSAIDs and COX-2 inhibitors
• Calcineurin inhibitors
• Heparin
• Trimethoprim
Drugs promoting transcellular potassium shift
• Nonselective beta blockers
• Digitalis
• Succinylcholine

such as spironolactone and eplerenone by competing and blocking aldosterone receptors, and ENaC inhibitors such as amiloride and triamterene by blocking epithelial sodium channels (ENaC) reduces the excretion of potassium and leads to hyperkalemia.

- **ACE inhibitors, ARBs:** Both drugs block the renin-angiotensin-aldosterone system (RAAS), which decreases the release of aldosterone, causing a reduction in urinary potassium excretion and leading to hyperkalemia, especially in renal-compromised patients. ACE inhibitors block the conversion of angiotensin I to angiotensin II, and angiotensin receptor blockers (ARBs) block the angiotensin's effect on angiotensin II receptors, causing a reduction in aldosterone secretion in the adrenal cortex.

- **NSAIDs and COX-2 inhibitors:** Reasons for developing hyperkalemia are decreased prostaglandin-mediated renin release leading to hyporeninemic hypoaldosteronism and reduced renal blood flow and gomerular filtration rate (GFR).

- **Calcineurin inhibitors (CNIs):** Cyclosporin or tacrolimus by decreasing synthesis of aldosterone, inhibiting basolateral Na^+-K^+-ATPase at the collecting duct, and inhibiting the luminal potassium channel, causes diminished secretion of potassium, leading to reduced urinary excretion of potassium.

- **Heparin:** Inhibits synthesis and reduces the release of aldosterone, causing hyperkalemia.

- **Trimethoprim:** The structure of trimethoprim is similar to the potassium-sparing diuretic amiloride, and it causes hyperkalemia by inhibiting epithelial sodium channels in the distal nephron.

B. Drugs promoting transcellular potassium shift

The shift of potassium from ECF into ICF is extremely fast; therefore, it is the effective defense mechanism that prevents hyperkalemia due to dietary potassium loading. Various drugs which affect this mechanism can cause hyperkalemia.

- **Nonselective beta-blockers (propranolol and labetalol):** These drugs inhibit the beta-2 mediated shift of potassium from ECF into ICF and increase the risk of hyperkalemia development.

- **Digitalis:** Hyperkalemia due to digitalis toxicity is dose-dependent. Inhibition of Na^+-K^+-ATPase pump due to digitalis causes blockade of entry of potassium into cells leading to hyperkalemia.

- **Succinylcholine:** Hyperkalemia occurs with succinylcholine due to the depolarization of skeletal muscle leading to a large efflux of potassium from muscle into plasma.

Diabetes is a common cause of hyperkalemia. Mechanisms of the development of hyperkalemia in diabetes are [16–22]:

- Hyporeninemic hypoaldosteronism (type 4 renal tubular acidosis).

- Transmembrane potassium shifts from ICF to ECF in DKA (due to lack of insulin, hyperosmolality, and acidosis).

- Reduced renal function.

- Other causes such as urinary tract obstruction, volume depletion, and coadministration of drugs such as ACEI, ARBs, nonselective beta-blockers, NSAIDs, and heparin.

Increased intake of potassium in diet rarely causes hyperkalemia unless patients have impaired renal function.

Pseudohyperkalemia (falsely elevated potassium concentrations, also known as spurious hyperkalemia or factitious hyperkalemia) is a common cause of high serum potassium laboratory reports which occurs in the absence of true hyperkalemia [23]. Suspect this laboratory artifact if the patient is asymptomatic, renal function is normal, electrocardiogram (ECG) changes of hyperkalemia are absent, and the cause for hyperkalemia is unexplained. This spurious hyperkalemia occurs due to increased potassium release from cells during sample collection (because of the use of tight tourniquets for a longer period, repeated fist-clenching, use of small-bore needles, and mechanical trauma during venipuncture) or after sample collection (because of hemolysis of blood, marked elevated platelet (>500,000/μL) or white blood cells (70,000/μL), high storage temperature or pressurized centrifugation) [15, 24–27].

To exclude pseudohyperkalemia, measure plasma potassium by carefully drawing blood [28]. Routinely blood is collected in a tube containing a clot activator to obtain a serum sample. But for obtaining a plasma sample, blood is collected in a tube containing heparin which prevents clotting.

In pseudohyperkalemia, serum potassium is higher than plasma potassium (difference greater than 0.4 mEq/L) when both samples are obtained simultaneously [29–31].

Reverse pseudohyperkalemia is a term used to describe the condition in which plasma potassium concentration is falsely elevated, and therefore the plasma potassium is greater than the serum potassium. Its common cause is extreme leucocytosis (e.g., chronic lymphocytic leukemia - CLL) [23, 32].

CLINICAL PRESENTATION

Hyperkalemia is associated with the risk of hospitalizations, ICU admissions, and when severe, it is a medical emergency because it can cause fatal cardiac arrhythmia and death (hence it is called a silent killer) [9, 33]. The correlation between the degree of hyperkalemia and the severity of symptoms is poor, but severe hyperkalemia with a rapid onset is always symptomatic. Hyperkalemia is often asymptomatic until serum potassium concentration is above 6.5 to 7.0 mEq/L. With the rise in serum potassium (S. K^+ ≥7.0 mEq/L), serious neuromuscular manifestations and cardiac conduction abnormalities are common.

Neuromuscular manifestations

Vague, generalized fatigue and muscular weakness are usually the first symptoms of hyperkalemia. Severe hyperkalemia can lead to hyporeflexia and gradual ascending muscle paralysis affecting the legs initially, subsequently trunk and arms, and at last, face and rarely respiratory muscles. With worsening, severe hyperkalemia can cause paralysis, but patients remain alert until cardiac arrest and death because muscles supplied by cranial nerves are usually spared. In hyperkalemia, the patient may complain of tingling around the lips (circumoral paresthesias), and fasciculations in the extremities. By reducing urinary ammonium excretion, hyperkalemia impairs the ability to excrete an acid load and may cause metabolic acidosis.

Cardiac manifestations

Usually, clinical cardiac signs or symptoms are absent. However, few patients may complain of palpitation, and bradycardia is an important clinical clue encountered in severe hyperkalemia. The correlation between the ECG changes and the severity of hyperkalemia is poor. The absence of ECG changes does not exclude hyperkalemia, and ECG changes usually occur when serum potassium levels are above 7.2 mEq/L [34–38]. It is important to remember that ECG changes of hyperkalemia correlate more with the development rate than the actual serum potassium level [15]. ECG changes occur early (potassium 6 to 7 mEq/L) with rapid onset hyperkalemia, while in chronic hyperkalemia ECG may be normal even with serum potassium concentrations >7 mEq/L. Progressive ECG changes of hyperkalemia need urgent attention and prompt management.

ECG changes

The ECG changes occurring in the usual sequence in hyperkalemia are [35, 39–41]:

- Tall, peaked T-waves: Narrow, pointy, prominent T-waves are the earliest manifestation of hyperkalemia.

- Absent P-waves: P wave widening/flattening, PR prolongation, and loss of P-waves.

- Widened QRS and sine waves: Progressive profound widening of QRS complex and ST-segment depression. In severe hyperkalemia, these changes merge with peaked T-waves forming a sine wave. The presence of a sine wave is a dangerous sign that predicts impending ventricular fibrillation and asystole, which can cause sudden death.

- The sine wave is an ominous sign that predicts imminent ventricular fibrillation and ultimately asystole leading to death.

- Bradycardia and arrhythmias: Severe hyperkalemia can cause sinus bradycardia, sinus arrest, slow junctional and ventricular escape rhythms, ventricular tachycardia or fibrillation, and asystole.

DIAGNOSIS OF HYPERKALEMIA

Clinical suspicion, serum potassium measurement, and characteristic ECG changes help to establish the diagnosis of hyperkalemia. If patients at high risk for hyperkalemia (e.g., renal failure, drugs like potassium-sparing diuretics, ACE inhibitors, or ARBs, etc.) present with recent onset of generalized fatigue and muscular weakness, suspect and exclude hyperkalemia. Serum potassium greater than 5.5 mEq/L is diagnostic. ECG changes suggestive of hyperkalemia provide a valuable clue for the diagnosis, but its absence does not exclude the presence of high potassium. Commonly reported ECG findings of hyperkalemia are summarized in Table 23.3 [41–43].

The recent classification of acute hyperkalemia severity based on the serum potassium level and ECG changes is summarized in Table 23.4 [41].

Table 23.3 ECG findings of hyperkalemia	
Serum potassium	**Common ECG findings**
5.5–6.5 mEq/L	Tall 'tented' narrow-based T-waves
6.5–7.0 mEq/L	Prolong PR interval, P-wave widening and loss, widening of QRS complex
7.0–9.0 mEq/L	Bradyarrhythmia, bizarre QRS complex, sine waves (QRS merges with T-waves)
>9.0 mEq/L	Atrioventricular dissociation, ventricular tachycardia or fibrillation, and cardiac standstill

Table 23.4 Classification of severity of acute hyperkalemia	
Severity of hyperkalemia	Serum K⁺ concentration and ECG changes of hyperkalemia
Mild	• Serum K^+ 5.0–5.9 mEq/L, No ECG changes
Moderate	• Serum K^+ 6.0–6.4 mEq/L, No ECG changes • Serum K^+ 5.0–5.9 mEq/L, ECG changes +
Severe	• Serum K^+ >6.5 mEq/L, No ECG changes • Serum K^+ 6.0–6.4 mEq/L, ECG changes +

DIAGNOSIS OF ETIOLOGY OF HYPERKALEMIA

With a thorough history and proper clinical examination, the clinician can establish the etiological diagnosis in most cases. However, relevant investigations are performed when the diagnosis is not clear.

When the patient is asymptomatic, ECG is normal, and clues for etiology are lacking, it is important to exclude pseudohyperkalemia.

One should remember that pseudohyperkalemia is caused by improper technique in drawing the blood, extravascular hemolysis, leucocytosis, and thrombocytosis [marked elevations in platelet or white blood cell counts].

History

Detailed history establishes the diagnosis of renal failure, drugs causing hyperkalemia, potassium-containing diet and dietary supplements, pseudohyperkalemia, and other common etiologies.

Examination

Assessment of vital signs and volume status to detect ECF volume depletion.

Vital signs, reduction in urine output, and assessment volume status help to detect ECF volume depletion. In addition, clinical evaluation should be done to assess the weakness of the respiratory and other muscles.

Laboratory evaluation

Common investigations performed in hyperkalemia to establish the etiological diagnosis are summarized in Table 23.5.

Urinary potassium excretion assessment

Two useful tests for evaluating urinary potassium excretion in cases of hyperkalemia are the transtubular potassium gradient (TTKG) and urine K⁺/creatinine ratio, which can be performed using a spot urine sample.

Transtubular potassium gradient

This test was earlier used to assess the renal potassium secretion by the cortical collecting duct, which indirectly reflects

Table 23.5 Investigations to establish the etiological diagnosis	
Test performed	Etiology to be diagnosed or excluded
Electrolytes	The basic test for diagnosis
CBC	Anemia, hemolysis, leukocytosis, leukemia, thrombocytopenia
ECG	Changes of hyperkalemia
Blood urea, creatinine	AKI or CKD
Creatine kinase (CPK)	Rhabdomyolysis
Arterial blood gas (ABG)	Normal anion gap hyperchloremic metabolic acidosis
Blood sugar	Diabetes
Plasma cortisol, ACTH stimulation test	Adrenal insufficiency

aldosterone activity in patients with hyperkalemia [44]. The low value of TTKG (<7) in patients with hyperkalemia may indicate hypoaldosteronism.

But in recent literature, TTKG was not found to be reliable and therefore is currently not recommended in evaluating hyperkalemia [45–47].

Measurement of urine K+/creatinine ratio

Current literature favors using K+/creatinine ratio in a spot urine sample to estimate potassium excretion rate in patients with hyperkalemia instead of using TTKG [46, 47]. This test is helpful in patients with acute hyperkalemia but is less useful in chronic hyperkalemia [47].

In patients with hyperkalemia, the urine K+/creatinine ratio >200 mEq/g or >20 mmol/mmol suggests an appropriate renal response and therefore provides a clue for the non-renal cause of hyperkalemia [46–48]. Conversely, low urine K+/creatinine ratio in hyperkalemia indicates a renal defect in K+ excretion (e.g., CKD, volume-depleted, or hyporeninemic hypoaldosteronism).

In chronic hyperkalemia, 24-hour urine collection is necessary to assess the renal excretion of potassium rather than spot urine K+/creatinine ratio because it avoids error due to diurnal variation in potassium ion excretion [49].

MANAGEMENT

How urgently and aggressively hyperkalemia needs to be treated is determined based on clinical status, ECG changes, and its degree of severity.

Goals

The goals of therapy are:
- To protect the heart by stabilizing the myocardium.

- To lower the serum potassium rapidly by shifting ECF potassium into ICF space in severe symptomatic hyperkalemia to reduce the risk of cardiac arrhythmias.
- To remove potassium from the body to correct hyperkalemia and reverse associated symptoms.
- To search and treat identifiable causes of hyperkalemia.

Emergency management for acute hyperkalemia

Always start the emergency management of acute hyperkalemia by administration of IV calcium gluconate for membrane stabilization. The second measure for emergency treatment is administering IV insulin plus dextrose to shift potassium from ECF to ICF. Subsequent measures for acute management are nebulized albuterol (salbutamol) and selective use of isotonic bicarbonate infusion in a patient with metabolic acidosis. As summarized in Table 23.6, acute management is followed by definite measures to remove potassium from the body and subsequent definitive measures. Temporary therapeutic measures like IV calcium, insulin with dextrose, nebulized albuterol, and IV bicarbonate are ineffective at removing potassium from the body and therefore are not preferred agents for non-emergencies management of stable, asymptomatic patients with chronic hyperkalemia.

Step 1 - Protect the heart

A. Injection calcium gluconate

Calcium gluconate injection is the first line and most rapid treatment available for life-threatening hyperkalemia, which reverses the ECG changes and reduces the risk of cardiac arrhythmia.

	Table 23.6 Treatment of hyperkalemia				
1. Emergency management for acute hyperkalemia					
	Medication	**Mechanism of action**	**Onset of action**	**Duration**	**Caution**
Step 1. Protect the heart	IV calcium (10 ml of 10%)	Cardiac membrane stabilization	Immediate	30–60 minutes	Avoid coadministration with bicarbonate as it will precipitate in the IV line. Risk of worsening of digitalis toxicity and hypercalcemia
Step 2. Redistribution	IV insulin plus dextrose (10 units + 50 ml of 50% dextrose)	Shift potassium from ECF to ICF	10–20 minutes	4–6 hours	High risk of hypoglycaemia, so closely monitor blood glucose
	Nebulized albuterol (salbutamol) (20 mg in 4 ml)		20–30 minutes	2–4 hours	Risk of tachycardia
	Isotonic bicarbonate (150 ml of NaHCO$_3$ in 1 L D5W)		4–6 hours	During infusion	Use selectively and not routinely, as it carries the risk of volume overload. Use only if metabolic acidosis
Step 3. Remove K⁺ from the body	IV furosemide (60–120 mg)	Potassium excretion in urine	15 minutes	2–3 hours	Correct hypovolemia simultaneously and avoid the volume depletion
	K⁺ binders: Patiromer, SZC or SPS	Increases GI excretion of potassium	2–24 hours	4–6 hours	
	Hemodialysis	Extracorporeal potassium elimination	Immediate	Few hours	
2. Subsequent management for chronic hyperkalemia					
Other measures	Restrict dietary potassium, treat identifiable causes, discontinue drugs that increase the serum potassium, correct hypovolemia, and continue gastrointestinal cation exchangers				
K⁺: Potassium, NaHCO$_3$⁻: Sodium bicarbonate, SPS: Sodium polystyrene sulfonate, SZC: Sodium zirconium cyclosilicate					

Calcium gluconate injection is available as a 10% solution in 10 ml ampoules. Every 10 ml or 1 gm of calcium gluconate solution contains 93 mg, 2.2 mmol, or 4.5 mEq elemental calcium. The usual dose is 10–20 ml (1–2 ampules) infused over 2 to 3 minutes via a large peripheral vein under continuous electrocardiographic monitoring.

Its cardioprotective effect begins within minutes but is short-lived (30–60 minutes). The dose can be repeated if the ECG changes persist after 5–10 minutes or cardiac abnormalities recur after initial improvement [50].

B. Injection calcium chloride

Calcium chloride injection is an

alternative salt containing three times higher calcium concentrations than calcium gluconate (13.6 mEq vs. 4.5 mEq Ca^{2+} in 10 ml of 10% solution). Every 10 ml of 10% calcium chloride solution contains 273 mg, 6.8 mmol, or 13.6 mEq elemental calcium. The advantage of this salt is the higher bioavailability of calcium. Therefore, a single dose of calcium chloride injection can be used in treating hyperkalemia rather than sequential doses of calcium gluconate. But the drawback of calcium chloride is irritation of veins and tissue necrosis on extravasation, and therefore needs a central venous line for its administration.

For the initial emergency treatment of hyperkalemia, calcium chloride or gluconate can be used as an equivalent dosage (10 ml, 1 gm of IV calcium chloride, or 30 ml, 3 gm of IV calcium gluconate) as per current recommendations [51].

Administration of calcium decreases membrane excitability and protects from cardiotoxicity in hyperkalemia.

It is important to remember that calcium does not lower serum potassium levels. Therefore it should not be used as a monotherapy but should be combined with other temporary and definitive measures [48].

Calcium may exacerbate or precipitate digitalis-induced arrhythmia because of hypercalcemia and, therefore, should be used cautiously and selectively for life-threatening hyperkalemia. To treat hyperkalemia in patients receiving digitalis, administer calcium IV slowly over 20 to 30 minutes as an infusion (10 mL of 10% calcium gluconate in 100 mL of dextrose 5%), avoiding acute hypercalcemia resultant aggravation of digitalis toxicity [52]. In human studies, the use of calcium in patients with digitalis toxicity was not associated with adverse outcomes [53, 54].

Step 2 - Redistribution

A. Insulin and glucose

- Insulin is used as a first measure for lowering potassium rapidly in emergency conditions because its effect is fast, reliable, dose-dependent, and reproducible [52]. In addition, this effect occurs even in patients with CKD-ESRD (end stage renal disease).

- Insulin shifts potassium into cells by enhancing the activity of the Na^+-K^+-ATPase pump in skeletal muscle, and glucose is co-administered to prevent hypoglycemia. Avoid using glucose without insulin in hyperkalemia because the release of endogenous insulin may be variable. In addition, hyperglycemia due to glucose increases plasma osmolality, which may acutely increase plasma potassium and worsen hyperkalemia.

- **Insulin administration:** 10 units of regular insulin with 25 gm of glucose is recommended to treat hyperkalemia. Two commonly used methods for administration are insulin bolus injection and insulin glucose infusion.

- **Insulin bolus injection:** For the urgent correction of hyperkalemia, 10 units of regular insulin is administered as a bolus injection, followed by 25 gm of glucose infusion (i.e., 50 ml of dextrose 50%, or 100 ml of dextrose 25%). In emergency conditions, insulin bolus injection may be preferred because it is easier to administer, and its potassium lowering effect is early and greater than insulin glucose infusion, but it carries a risk of hypoglycemia.

- **Insulin glucose infusion:** In this commonly used method, 10 units of regular insulin is added to 500 mL of dextrose 10% and infused slowly over 60 minutes. The advantage of this method is lesser chances of rebound hypoglycemia and lesser irritation of veins.

- **Insulin effect:** The potassium lowering effect of regular insulin begins in 10–15 minutes, peaks at 60 minutes, and may last for approximately 4 to 6 hours [52]. Therefore, the insulin dose is repeated every two to four hours in patients with persistent hyperkalemia. Regular insulin usually reduces plasma potassium concentration by about 0.5 to 1.2 mEq/L.

- **The onset of hypoglycemia:** Insulin-induced hypoglycemia usually occurs after 60 to 150 min (with a peak at 90 min) of administration [55]. To detect hypoglycemia in patients receiving regular insulin for hyperkalemia, monitor blood glucose every hour for about 5 to 6 hours due to the longer duration of insulin action compared to dextrose [56].

- **Risk factors for hypoglycemia:** In nondiabetic patients, lower pretreatment blood glucose level (<126 mg/dL or 7.0 mmol/L) is a major risk factor for hypoglycemia, but the risk of hypoglycemia is lesser in diabetic patients [57]. Patients with renal failure (AKI, stage 3–4 CKD, ESRD), low body weight, female sex, elderly and nondiabetic patients carry a higher risk of hypoglycemia [51]. In patients with severe renal failure, the risk of hypoglycemia is higher due to the longer half-life of insulin.

- **Strategies to reduce hypoglycemia:** Different strategies suggested to reduce the risk of hypoglycemia with insulin therapy, especially in patients at risk of developing hypoglycemia, are: (1) Using a lower dose of insulin (5 units instead of 10 units) [56, 58, 59]; (2) Providing weight-based intravenous insulin dose (0.1 units/kg up to a maximum 10 units) [60]; (3) Providing a larger dose of glucose (i.e., 50 gm instead of 25 gm) with insulin [61, 62]; (4) Administering insulin as an infusion (e.g., 4 hours) instead of a rapid IV bolus [56]; and (5) Administering a prolonged dextrose infusion (10% dextrose at 50 mL/hour for 5 hours) following administration of insulin [51].

- **Avoid glucose:** In hyperkalemic patients with hyperglycemia (serum glucose is ≥250 mg/dL or 14 mmol/L), avoid glucose administration and use insulin alone [63, 64].

- **Combine with beta-2 agonists:** The combined treatment of insulin with beta-2 agonists has synergistic potassium lowering effect, and such therapy also decreases the incidence of hypoglycemia [65–67].

B. Beta-adrenergic agonists

- Selective beta-2 agonists such as albuterol (also known as salbutamol) is a simple, potent, and safe but underutilized therapeutic modality for the emergency treatment of acute hyperkalemia [68, 69]. Therefore, always administer beta-2 agonists immediately after calcium and insulin for the urgent management of acute hyperkalemia.

- Beta-2 agonists, by activating Na^+-K^+-ATPase, promote the cellular uptake of potassium and effectively lower serum potassium level. Administration of albuterol (salbutamol) as a nebulized or intravenous, both forms effectively shift potassium from ECF to the ICF compartment [68, 70, 71].

- The effect of intravenous or nebulized salbutamol in hyperkalemia is dose-dependent [72]. The dose of salbutamol recommended is 10–20 mg in 4 ml of saline by nebulization over 10 minutes or 0.5 mg diluted in 100 mL of 5% dextrose infused over 10 to 15 minutes. In patients with ischemic heart disease, tachyarrhythmia, and open-angle glaucoma, use a lower dose (i.e., 10 mg) of salbutamol for nebulization [51].

- A common mistake in clinical practice is treating hyperkalemia with a low dose (2.5–5.0 mg) of salbutamol nebulization, a standard dose used for bronchodilation. However, it is essential to remember that the dose of salbutamol nebulization recommended for hyperkalemia is 10–20 mg, which is 4 to 8 times greater than the dose required for bronchodilation [73, 74].

- The onset of the effect of beta-2 agonist is about 20 to 30 minutes; the effect lasts for about 2 to 4 hours, and it lowers serum potassium level by 0.5 to 1.5 mEq/L.

- To manage hyperkalemia in the emergency department, the nebulized beta-2 agonist is an easy-to-use, rapid and preferred modality [70]; it lowers potassium like insulin [50] In addition, this therapy is without the risk of hypoglycemia and cumbersome frequent blood glucose monitoring in a busy emergency unit [75]. Beta-2 agonists also cause mild hyperglycemia and may provide partial protection against hypoglycemia due to insulin [51].

- Lesser side effects like tremors, increased heart rate, palpitations, and headache are an advantage of the nebulized form of beta-2 agonist over the intravenous route [68, 74].

- Insulin and beta-2 agonist exerts additive effect and reduces serum potassium by about 1.2 to 1.5 mEq/L [65, 66, 69, 76]. However, using the beta-2 agonists as monotherapy in severe hyperkalemia is discouraged [51, 71, 73, 77, 78].

C. Sodium bicarbonate

- Avoid routine use of sodium bicarbonate in treating hyperkalemia because of its limited efficiency in lowering potassium as a single agent or as a cotreatment [51, 52, 76, 79] and potential side effects.

- Sodium bicarbonate should be used only in a selected small group of hyperkalemia patients with metabolic acidosis who can tolerate the sodium load as a prolonged sodium bicarbonate isotonic infusion (e.g., 150 mEq of $NaHCO_3^-$ Three 50 ml ampoule of 8.4% $NaHCO_3^-$ in 1 L of dextrose 5%) rather than a bolus [50, 77, 80]. It is important to remember that in the absence of acidosis, bicarbonate is ineffective.

- Slow administration of isotonic bicarbonate over 4 to 6 hours lowers serum potassium in patients with metabolic acidosis by shifting potassium from ECF to ICF and promoting renal potassium excretion. However, the IV push of hypertonic bicarbonate is ineffective because increased serum osmolality shifts potassium from ICF to ECF and counteracts the potassium shift from ECF to ICF due to an increase in pH. Thus, the net effect will be no change in serum potassium concentration.

- As IV sodium bicarbonate lowers serum potassium slowly (i.e., it takes several hours), it is not recommended for acute hyperkalemia emergency treatment.

- Hypernatremia, hypocalcemia, and volume overload are common side effects of sodium bicarbonate. In addition, the injudicious use of a large amount of alkali can cause excessive calcium binding to albumin and provokes tetany. Avoid contact between calcium gluconate and sodium bicarbonate in the needle, syringe, or infusion set, as it will precipitate into chalky deposits.

- Patients with CKD-ESRD seldom respond to this therapy and may not tolerate the sodium load and the resultant volume expansion.

Step 3 - Remove potassium from the body

Diuretics, potassium binders, and hemodialysis are three primary modalities to remove potassium from the body.

A. Diuretics

- The strategy to administer potassium-wasting diuretics varies, considering the renal function and volume status.

- Normal renal function or mild renal dysfunction: Loop diuretic, often combined with thiazide diuretics for better efficacy, increases urine volume and enhances potassium excretion. In euvolemic or hypovolemic patients, normal saline or isotonic bicarbonate may be given along with diuretics to prevent volume depletion and facilitates further potassium elimination. Avoid the use of diuretics in hypovolemic or oliguric patients with hyperkalemia.

- Moderate renal impairment: Loop diuretics (e.g., furosemide, bumetanide) are the most effective agents in hyperkalemic patients with volume overload. In severe renal insufficiency, the effectiveness of diuretic therapy is limited.

- The dose of diuretics is adjusted according to the severity of the hyperkalemia and the degree of renal dysfunction.

B. Potassium binders

Sodium polystyrene sulphonate (keyxalate) has been widely used and the only available potassium binder for years, while patiromer and sodium zirconium cyclosilicate are two newer effective and safer potassium binders [81].

Newer potassium binders have emerged as an important treatment modality in medications induced chronic hyperkalemia, where despite dietary potassium restrictions, potassium levels remain high [82]. Administration of drugs like RAASi may cause hyperkalemia, but the continuation of these drugs has substantial benefits due to their cardioprotection, renoprotection, and mortality benefits [83].

Basic information about potassium binders is summarized in Table 23.7.

C. Sodium polystyrene sulphonate (SPS)

- Sodium polystyrene sulphonate is a polymeric cation-exchange resin used to manage hyperkalemia for the last 60 years [50]. Sodium polystyrene sulphonate in the large intestine exchanges sodium for potassium and promotes the fecal excretion of potassium [84, 85].

- Sodium polystyrene sulphonate is given orally or as an enema, which effectively lowers the serum

	Sodium polystyrene sulfonate (SPS)	Patiromer	Sodium zirconium cyclosilicate (SZC)
Table 23.7 Potassium binding agents to treat hyperkalemia			
Year of US FDA/ EMA approval	1958/NA	2015/2017	2018/2018
Site of action	Colon	Distal colon	Entire GI tract
Exchange ion for K+	Sodium	Calcium	Sodium and hydrogen
Mechanism of action	Sodium-potassium exchange resin	Calcium-potassium cation exchange also binds Mg^{2+}	Selectively binds potassium in exchange for Na^+ and H^+
Onset of action	Variable (hours to days)	7 hours	1 hour
Duration of activity	4–24 hours	12–48 hours	2.2–12 hours
Mode of administration	Oral suspension or enema	Oral suspension	Oral suspension
Sodium content	1500 mg or 65.25 mmol Na^+ per each 15 gm dose	None	800 mg or 34.8 mmol Na^+ per each 10 gm dose
Sorbitol content	20 gm in each 15 gm of SPS	4 gm in each 8.4 gm of oral suspension	None
Initial dose	Oral: 15 gm, 1–4 times daily Enema: 30 gm every 6 hr	Oral: 8.4 gm once daily	Oral: 10 gm 3 times daily Maintenance: 10 gm once daily
Separation with other medications	Avoid other medications 3 hr before or 3 hr after	Avoid other medications 3 hr before or 3 hr after	Avoid other medications 2 hr before or 2 hr after
Adverse effects	Nausea, vomiting, constipation, colonic necrosis	Constipation, nausea, flatulence, diarrhea, and abdominal pain	Fluid overload, edema, and hypokalemia

potassium in hyperkalemia, and this effect is dose-dependent [86, 87].

- Sodium polystyrene sulphonate is not a suitable agent for the emergency management of hyperkalemia because of its delayed onset of action (peak effect is observed after 4–6 hours of administration).

- When given orally, the usual dose is 15 gm mixed with 20 gm (100 ml 20%) of sorbitol administered 3–4 times daily. It can also be given as a retention enema consisting of 30 to 50 gm of resins mixed in 100 ml of warm water administered every 6 hours.

- As the addition of sorbitol to sodium polystyrene sulphonate increases the risk of colonic necrosis [88–90], US FDA in 2009 recommended against the concomitant use of sorbitol with sodium polystyrene sulphonate [91].

- Use sodium polystyrene sulphonate only in patients with normal bowel function. Avoid using sodium polystyrene sulphonate in patients with ileus, large or small bowel obstruction, severe constipation, or recent bowel surgery.

- Sodium polystyrene sulphonate can cause gastrointestinal side effects such as anorexia, nausea, vomiting, constipation, and diarrhea [90], and the incidence of these adverse effects is higher when prescribed as per-label doses [92].

- Sodium polystyrene sulphonate also carries the risk of serious GI adverse effects such as ulceration, bleeding, intestinal ischemia, and colonic necrosis [92, 93], especially when combined with sorbitol.

- Each gm of sodium polystyrene sulphonate binds with 1 mEq of potassium and releases 2–3 mEq of sodium. As sodium released is absorbed by the GI tract, sodium polystyrene sulphonate should be used cautiously in patients with congestive heart failure or volume overload.

D. Novel intestinal potassium binders

Patiromer and Sodium zirconium cyclosilicate (SZC; formerly ZS-9) are two new potassium binders that recently became available for the management of both chronic and acute hyperkalemia to fill the treatment gap and overcome the limitations of SPS [94–98]. Recent literature recommends using these newer agents because they are safer, effective, more palatable, free of severe side effects like intestinal necrosis, and are well documented [5, 50, 51, 74, 99–101].

Patiromer oral suspension is a sodium-free, nonabsorbable, potassium-binding ion-exchange resin that exchanges calcium for potassium in the distal colon and lowers serum potassium [67, 99].

Common adverse effects of Patiromer are hypomagnesemia and GI side effects such as constipation, nausea, flatulence, diarrhea, and abdominal pain.

The recommended initial dose is 8.4 gm per day, and the higher dose is adjusted up to 25.2 gm per day if necessary.

In treating chronic hyperkalemia (i.e., in chronic kidney disease or heart failure), patiromer is preferred over SZC because SZC exchanges potassium with sodium causing increased absorption of sodium with a resultant higher risk of edema [101].

Sodium zirconium cyclosilicate is a highly selective potassium binder available as a powder for suspension (in water) that exchanges sodium and hydrogen ions in exchange for potassium in the entire intestine [102, 103].

The common side effects of CZS are fluid overload, edema, constipation, headache, and hypokalemia occur in a few patients. The recommended initial dose is 10 gm administered orally three times a day for about 48 hours, and the maintenance dose is 10 gm once daily.

As the onset of action of sodium zirconium cyclosilicate is fast (i.e., 1 hour), it is recommended for the emergency management of acute life-threatening hyperkalemia for a more rapid reduction of serum potassium [95, 101].

Conclusion: Currently, literature favors the use of newer potassium binders, and the efficacy, as well as safety of sodium polystyrene sulfonate, is questioned [81]. However, sodium polystyrene sulfonate is widely used in managing hyperkalemia because newer potassium binders are not available everywhere and are expensive [104]. Furthermore, in recent systematic reviews and meta-analyses, the risk of intestinal necrosis with sodium polystyrene sulphonate is not statistically high [105].

E. Dialysis

- The most rapid, effective, and reliable method for lowering the plasma potassium concentration is hemodialysis (potassium removal rate 25–50 mEq/hour).

- Dialysis is used in selected patients with renal failure and those with severe life-threatening hyperkalemia unresponsive to standard medical modalities.

- Peritoneal dialysis removes potassium very slowly (potassium removal rate 5 mEq/hour) but effectively.

Monitoring

The need for continuous cardiac monitoring and the frequency of measurement of potassium concentration in hyperkalemia is based on the severity of the hyperkalemia and its clinical manifestations [50]. Therefore, during the emergency management of severe hyperkalemia, all patients need continuous cardiac monitoring and frequent estimation of potassium concentration (usually 2–4 hourly) to assess the effectiveness of therapy and modify the treatment plan.

Subsequent therapy or management for chronic Hyperkalemia

- Dietary potassium restriction: Avoid fruit juice, coconut water, and food rich in potassium.
- Discontinue drugs that increase serum potassium (Table 23.2).
- Discontinue potassium-containing medications or fluids.
- Potassium binders.

Specific etiological treatment

- Addison's diseases: Glucocorticoid (hydrocortisone) therapy.
- Hypoaldosteronism: Mineralocorticoid supplement (0.2 mg/day, fludrocortisone).
- Treatment of diabetic ketoacidosis.
- Correct metabolic acidosis: In hyperkalemia, correction of associated metabolic acidosis lowers serum

potassium. So treat chronic hyperkalemia with metabolic acidosis with sodium bicarbonate tablets or sodium citrate (Shohl's solution).

- Hyperkalemic periodic paralysis: Beta-agonist inhalation is effective as an acute potassium-lowering therapy, and diuretics and carbonic anhydrase inhibitors such as acetazolamide are effective for the chronic treatment of hyperkalemic periodic paralysis [106].
- Correct volume depletion. In hyperkalemic patients with hypovolemia, preferred fluids to correct fluid deficit are [80]:

  a. If bicarbonate is low, isotonic bicarbonate solution (150 mEq of sodium bicarbonate in a liter of D5W).

  b. If bicarbonate is normal, Ringer's lactate or PlasmaLyte are chosen. Administration of normal saline in a large volume may increase the serum potassium and therefore should be avoided.

- RAASi drugs: To avoid hyperkalemia, measure urea and electrolytes before starting ACE-I or ARB, use these drugs cautiously if the serum K^+ is >5.0 mEq/L and measure urea and electrolytes 1 week after initiation of these drugs or after each dose titration [107]. If serum K^+ is 5.5–5.9 mEq/L, reduce the dose of RAASi drugs by half and monitor potassium closely. If serum K^+ is >6.0 mEq/L, discontinue these drugs in patients without heart failure.

- As RAASi is beneficial in patients with heart failure with reduced ejection fraction (HFrEF) and renoprotective in proteinuria, CKD, and diabetic kidney disease, its advantages should be balanced against the potential risk of developing hyperkalemia [100]. Mineralocorticoid receptor antagonists (aldosterone receptor antagonists) such as spironolactone and eplerenone are recommended in patients with heart failure with reduced ejection fraction (HFrEF) because it causes diuresis, lower blood pressure, and protects the heart and other target organs such as kidney and blood vessels from deleterious effects of aldosterone and improves outcome [108]. In patients with heart failure, RAASi therapy reduces mortality and morbidity. Therefore, rather than discontinuing RAASi therapy in such patients, the goal is to lower potassium levels and allow them to continue RAASi therapy [83]. Lowering potassium levels by using newer potassium binders such as patiromer and sodium zirconium cyclosilicate may allow the continuation of RAASi therapy in patients with hyperkalemia [100].

REFERENCES

1. Nilsson E, Gasparini A, Ärnlöv J, et al. Incidence and determinants of hyperkalemia and hypokalemia in a large healthcare system. Int J Cardiol. 2017;245:277–284.

2. Betts KA, Woolley JM, Mu F, et al. The prevalence of hyperkalemia in the United States. Curr Med Res Opin. 2018;34(6):971–978.

3. Belmar Vega L, Galabia ER, Bada da Silva J, et al. Epidemiology of hyperkalemia in chronic kidney disease. Nefrologia (Engl Ed). 2019;39(3):277–286.

4. Kashihara N, Kohsaka S, Kanda E, et al. Hyperkalemia in real-world patients under continuous medical care in Japan. Kidney Int Rep. 2019;4(9):1248–60.

5. Palmer BF, Carrero JJ, Clegg DJ, et al. Clinical Management of Hyperkalemia. Mayo Clin Proc. 2021;96(3):744–762.

6. Kovesdy CP, Matsushita K, Sang Y, et al. CKD Prognosis Consortium. Serum potassium and adverse outcomes across the range of kidney function: a CKD Prognosis Consortium meta-analysis. Eur Heart J. 2018;39(17):1535–1542.

7. Hoppe LK, Muhlack DC, Koenig W, et al. Association of Abnormal Serum Potassium Levels with Arrhythmias and Cardiovascular Mortality: A Systematic Review and Meta-Analysis of Observational Studies. Cardiovasc Drugs Ther. 2018;32(2):197–21.

8. Cooper LB, Benson L, Mentz RJ et al. Association between potassium level and outcomes in heart failure with reduced ejection fraction: a cohort study from the Swedish Heart Failure Registry. Eur J Heart Fail 2020;22(8):1390–1398.

9. Hougen I, Leon SJ, Whitlock R, et al. Hyperkalemia and its Association with Mortality, Cardiovascular Events, Hospitalizations, and Intensive Care Unit Admissions in a Population-Based Retrospective Cohort. Kidney Int Rep. 2021;6(5):1309–1316.

10. Hunter RW, Bailey MA. Hyperkalemia: pathophysiology, risk factors and consequences. Nephrol Dial Transplant. 2019;34(Suppl 3):iii2–iii11.

11. Dunn JD, Benton WW, Orozco-Torrentera E, et al. The burden of hyperkalemia in patients with cardiovascular and renal disease. Am J Manag Care. 2015;21(15 Suppl):s307–15.

12. Seliger SL. Hyperkalemia in patients with chronic renal failure. Nephrol Dial Transplant. 2019;34(Suppl 3):iii12–iii18.

13. Einhorn LM, Zhan M, Hsu VD, et al. The frequency of hyperkalemia and its significance in chronic kidney disease. Arch Intern Med. 2009;169(12):1156–62.

14. Ben Salem C, Badreddine A, Fathallah N, et al. Drug-induced hyperkalemia. Drug Saf. 2014;37(9):677–92.

15. Palmer BF, Clegg DJ. Physiology and Pathophysiology of Potassium Homeostasis: Core Curriculum 2019. Am J Kidney Dis. 2019;74(5):682–695.

16. Adrogué HJ, Lederer ED, Suki WN, et al. Determinants of plasma potassium levels in diabetic ketoacidosis. Medicine (Baltimore) 1986;65(3):163–172.

17. Grande VJ, Macias Nunez JF, Miralles JM, et al. Hyporeninemic hypoaldosteronism in diabetic patients with chronic renal failure. Am J Nephrol 1988;8(2):127–37.

18. Uribarri J, Oh MS, Carroll HJ. Hyperkalemia in diabetes mellitus. J Diabet Complications. 1990;4(1):3–7.

19. Umpierrez GE, Murphy MB, Kitabchi AE. Diabetic Ketoacidosis and Hyperglycemic Hyperosmolar Syndrome. Diabetes Spectrum 2002;15(1):28–36.

20. Hollander-Rodriguez JC, Calvert JF Jr. Hyperkalemia. Am Fam Physician. 2006;73(2):283–90.

21. Kitabchi AE, Umpierrez GE, Miles JM, et al. Hyperglycemic crises in adult patients with diabetes. Diabetes Care 2009;32(7):1335–1343.

22. Palmer BF, Clegg DJ. Electrolyte and Acid-Base Disturbances in Patients with Diabetes Mellitus. N Engl J Med. 2015;373(6):548–59.

23. Asirvatham JR, Moses V, Bjornson L. Errors in potassium measurement: a laboratory perspective for the clinician. N Am J Med Sci. 2013;5(4):255–259.

24. Wiederkehr MR, Moe OW. Factitious hyperkalemia. Am J Kidney Dis 2000;36(5):1049–53.

25. Ismail A, Shingler W, Seneviratne J, et al. In vitro and in vivo haemolysis and potassium measurement. BMJ 2005;330(7497):949.

26. Smellie WS. Spurious hyperkalaemia. BMJ. 2007;334(7595):693–5.

27. Krogager ML, Kragholm K, Thomassen JQ, et al. Update on management of hypokalaemia and

goals for the lower potassium level in patients with cardiovascular disease: a review in collaboration with the European Society of Cardiology Working Group on Cardiovascular Pharmacotherapy. Eur Heart J Cardiovasc Pharmacother. 2021:pvab038.

28. Šálek T. Pseudohyperkalemia - Potassium released from cells due to clotting and centrifugation - a case report. Biochem Med (Zagreb). 2018;28(1):011002.

29. Sevastos N, Theodossiades G, Archimandritis AJ. Pseudohyperkalemia in serum: a new insight into an old phenomenon. Clin Med Res. 2008;6(1):30–32.

30. Jain AG, Tauseef A, Hasan SA, et al. Pseudohyperkalemia: To Treat or not to Treat. Cureus. 2018;10(11):e3570.

31. Mahto M, Kumar M, Kumar S, et al. Pseudohyperkalemia in Serum and Plasma: The Phenomena and Its Clinical Implications. Indian J Clin Biochem. 2021;36(2):235–238.

32. Avelar T. Reverse pseudohyperkalemia in a patient with chronic lymphocytic leukemia. Perm J. 2014;18(4):e150–152.

33. Montford JR, Linas S. How Dangerous Is Hyperkalemia? J Am Soc Nephrol 2017;28(11):3155–3165.

34. Martinez-Vea A, Bardají A, Garcia C, et al. Severe hyperkalemia with minimal electrocardiographic manifestations: a report of seven cases. J Electrocardiol. 1999;32(1):45–9.

35. Montague BT, Ouellette JR, Buller GK. Retrospective review of the frequency of ECG changes in hyperkalemia. Clin J Am Soc Nephrol. 2008;3(2):324–30.

36. Cohen R, Ramos R, Garcia CA, et al. Electrocardiogram manifestations in hyperkalemia. World Journal of Cardiovascular Diseases 2012;2:57–63.

37. Ryuge A, Nomura A, Shimizu H, et al. Warning: the ECG may be normal in severe hyperkalemia. Intern Med. 2017;56(16):2243–2244.

38. Yoon D, Lim HS, Jeong JC, et al. Quantitative Evaluation of the Relationship between T-Wave-Based Features and Serum Potassium Level in Real-World Clinical Practice. Biomed Res Int. 2018;2018:3054316.

39. Diercks DB, Shumaik GM, Harrigan RA, et al. Electrocardiographic manifestations: Electrolyte abnormalities. J Emerg Med. 2004;27(2):153–160.

40. Littmann L, Gibbs MA. Electrocardiographic manifestations of severe hyperkalemia. J Electrocardiol. 2018;51(5):814–817.

41. Clase CM, Carrero JJ, Ellison DH, et al. Potassium homeostasis and management of dyskalemia in kidney diseases: conclusions from a Kidney Disease: Improving Global Outcomes (KDIGO) Controversies Conference. Kidney Int. 2020;97(1):42–61.

42. Sood MM, Sood AR, Richardson R. Emergency management and commonly encountered outpatient scenarios in patients with hyperkalemia. Mayo Clin Proc. 2007;82(12):1553–61.

43. Campese VM, Adenuga G. Electrophysiological and clinical consequences of hyperkalemia. Kidney Int Suppl. 2016;6(1):16–19.

44. Choi MJ, Ziyadeh FN. The utility of the transtubular potassium gradient in the evaluation of hyperkalemia. J Am Soc Nephrol. 2008;19(3):424–6.

45. Kamel KS, Halperin M. Intrarenal urea recycling leads to a higher rate of renal excretion of potassium: an hypothesis with clinical implications. Curr Opin Nephrol Hypertens 2011;20(5):547–54.

46. Halperin ML. Assessing the renal response in patients with potassium disorders: a shift in emphasis from the TTKG to the urine K+/creatinine ratio. Afr J Nephrol. 2017;20(1):22–24.

47. Kamel KS, Halperin ML. Use of Urine Electrolytes and Urine Osmolality in the Clinical Diagnosis of Fluid, Electrolytes, and Acid-Base Disorders. Kidney Int Rep. 2021;6(5):1211–1224.

48. Palmer BF, Clegg DJ. Diagnosis and treatment of hyperkalemia. Cleve Clin J Med. 2017;84(12):934–942.

49. Kamel KS, Halperin ML. Fluid, Electrolyte, and Acid-Base Physiology - A Problem-Based Approach (5th ed.). Philadelphia: Elsevier; 2017:445–446.

50. Lindner G, Burdmann EA, Clase CM, et al. Acute hyperkalemia in the emergency department: a summary from a Kidney Disease: Improving Global Outcomes conference. Eur J Emerg Med. 2020;27(5):329–337.

51. Alfonzo A, Harrison A, Baines R, et al. Clinical practice guidelines: Treatment of Acute Hyperkalemia in Adults. UK Renal Association July 2020.

52. Mount DB. Disorders of potassium balance. In: Brenner and Rector's The Kidney, 11th ed, Yu A, Chertow G, Luyckx V, et al (Eds), W.B. Saunders & Company, Philadelphia 2020.p.573.

53. Fenton F, Smally AJ, Laut J. Hyperkalemia and digoxin toxicity in a patient with kidney failure. Ann Emerg Med 1996;28(4):440–441.

54. Levine M, Nikkanen H, Pallin DJ. The effects of intravenous calcium in patients with digoxin toxicity. J Emerg Med 2011;40(1):41–46.

55. Crnobrnja L, Metlapalli M, Jiang C, et al. The Association of Insulin-dextrose Treatment with Hypoglycemia in Patients with Hyperkalemia. Sci Rep. 2020;10(1):22044.

56. Moussavi K, Fitter S, Gabrielson SW, et al. Management of Hyperkalemia with Insulin and Glucose: Pearls for the Emergency Clinician. J Emerg Med. 2019;57(1):36–42.

57. Tee SA, Devine K, Potts A, et al. Iatrogenic hypoglycaemia following glucose-insulin infusions for the treatment of hyperkalaemia. Clin Endocrinol (Oxf) 2021;94(2):176–182.

58. LaRue HA, Peksa GD, Shah SC. A comparison of insulin doses for the treatment of hyperkalemia in patients with renal insufficiency. Pharmacotherapy 2017;37(12):1516–1522.

59. McNicholas BA, Pham MH, Carli K, et al. Treatment of hyperkalemia with a low-dose insulin protocol is effective and results in reduced hypoglycemia. Kidney Int Rep 2018;3(2):328–336.

60. Wheeler DT, Schafers SJ, Horwedel TA, et al. Weight-based insulin dosing for acute hyperkalemia results in less hypoglycemia. J Hosp Med. 2016;11(5):355–7.

61. Harel Z, Kamel KS. Optimal Dose and Method of Administration of Intravenous Insulin in the Management of Emergency Hyperkalemia: A Systematic Review. PLoS One. 2016;11(5):0154963.

62. Coca A, Valencia AL, Bustamante J, et al. Hypoglycemia following intravenous insulin plus glucose for hyperkalemia in patients with impaired renal function. PLoS ONE. 2017;12:0172961.

63. Li T, Vijayan A. Insulin for the treatment of hyperkalemia: a double-edged sword?. Clin Kidney J. 2014;7(3):239–241.

64. Viera AJ, Wouk N. Potassium Disorders: Hypokalemia and Hyperkalemia. Am Fam Physician. 2015;92(6):487–95.

65. Allon M, Copkney C. Albuterol and insulin for treatment of hyperkalemia in hemodialysis patients. Kidney Int. 1990;38(5):869–872.

66. Mahoney BA, Smith WA, Lo DS, et al. Emergency interventions for hyperkalaemia. Cochrane Database Syst Rev. 2005;2005(2):CD003235.

67. Dépret F, Peacock WF, Liu KD, et al. Management of hyperkalemia in the acutely ill patient. Ann Intensive Care. 2019;9(1):32.

68. Liou HH, Chiang SS, Wu S, et al. Hypokalemic effects of intravenous infusion or nebulization of salbutamol in patients with chronic renal failure: comparative study. Am J Kidney Dis. 1994;23(2):266–271.

69. Mount DB. Disorders of potassium balance. In: Brenner and Rector's The Kidney, 11th ed, Yu A, Chertow G, Luyckx V, et al (Eds), W.B. Saunders & Company, Philadelphia 2020.p.574.

70. McClure RJ, Prasad VK, Brocklebank JT. Treatment of hyperkalaemia using intravenous and nebulised salbutamol. Arch Dis Child 1994;70(2):126–128.

71. Batterink J, Cessford TA, Taylor RAI. Pharmacological interventions for the acute management of hyperkalaemia in adults. Cochrane Database Syst Rev 2015;CD010344.

72. Allon M, Dunlay R, Copkney C. Nebulised albuterol for acute hyperkalaemia in patients on haemodialysis. Ann Intern Med 1989;110(6):426–429.

73. Sterns RH, Grieff M, Bernstein PL. Treatment of hyperkalemia: something old, something new. Kidney Int. 2016;89(3):546–554.

74. Bianchi S, Aucella F, De Nicola L, et al. Management of hyperkalemia in patients with kidney disease: a position paper endorsed by the Italian Society of Nephrology. J Nephrol. 2019;32(4):499–516.

75. Montassier E, Legrand M, Rossignol P, et al. Hyperkalemia in the emergency department: Consider the use of nebulized salbutamol. Am J Emerg Med. 2019;37(5):1004.

76. Lim AKH, Crnobrnja L, Metlapalli M, et al. The Effect of Patient Factors and Cotreatments on the Magnitude of Potassium Lowering with Insulin-Glucose Treatment in Patients with Hyperkalemia. Epidemiologia. 2021;2(1):27–35.

77. Weisberg LS. Management of severe hyperkalemia. Crit Care Med. 2008;36(12):3246–3251.

78. Chalisey A, Ross C, Weavers N. Joint Trust Guideline for the management of hyperkalaemia in adults, James Paget University Hospitals and Norfolk and Norwich University Hospitals. 2018.

79. Geng S, Green EF, Kurz MC, et al. Sodium bicarbonate administration and subsequent potassium concentration in hyperkalemia treatment. Am J Emerg Med. 2021;50:132–135.

80. Farkas J. Hyperkalemia. The Internet Book of Critical Care. June 20, 2021. Visit: https://emcrit. org/ibcc/hyperkalemia/#Rx_severe_hyperkalemia:_ Temporizing_measures.

81. Esposito P, Conti NE, Falqui V, et al. New Treatment Options for Hyperkalemia in Patients with Chronic Kidney Disease. J Clin Med. 2020;9(8):2337.

82. Rakisheva A, Marketou M, Klimenko A, et al. Hyperkalemia in heart failure: Foe or friend? Clin Cardiol 2020;43(7):666–7.

83. Rosano GMC, Tamargo J, Kjeldsen KP, et al. Expert consensus document on the management of hyperkalaemia in patients with cardiovascular disease treated with renin angiotensin aldosterone system inhibitors: coordinated by the working group on cardiovascular pharmacotherapy of the European Society of Cardiology. Eur Heart J Cardiovasc Pharmacother. 2018;4(3):180–8.

84. Watson M, Abbott KC, Yuan CM. Damned if you do, damned if you don't: potassium binding resins in hyperkalemia. Clin J Am Soc Nephrol. 2010;5(10):1723–1726.

85. Chaitman M, Dixit D, Bridgeman MB. Potassium-binding agents for the clinical management of hyperkalemia. P T. 2016;41(1):43–50.

86. Lepage L, Dufour AC, Doiron J, et al. Randomized clinical trial of sodium polystyrene sulfonate for the treatment of mild hyperkalemia in CKD. Clin J Am Soc Nephrol. 2015;10(12):2136–2142.

87. Mistry M, Shea A, Giguère P, et al. Evaluation of Sodium Polystyrene Sulfonate Dosing Strategies in the Inpatient Management of Hyperkalemia. Ann Pharmacother 2016;50(6):455–62.

88. Dardik A, Moesinger RC, Efron G, et al. Acute abdomen with colonic necrosis induced by Kayexalate-sorbitol. South Med J. 2000;93(5):511–3.

89. McGowan CE, Saha S, Chu G, et al. Intestinal necrosis due to sodium polystyrene sulfonate (Kayexalate) in sorbitol. South Med J. 2009;102(5):493–497.

90. Harel Z, Harel S, Shah PS, et al. Gastrointestinal adverse events with sodium polystyrene sulfonate (Kayexalate) use: a systematic review. Am J Med. 2013;126(3):264.e9–24.

91. US Food and Drug Administration. Kayexalate (sodium polystyrene sulfonate, USP) powder approval letter (2009). US Food and Drug Administration website. https://www.accessdata.fda.gov/drugsatfda_ docs/appletter/2009/011287s022ltr.pdf. Accessed September 6, 2021.

92. Laureati P, Xu Y, Trevisan M, et al. Initiation of sodium polystyrene sulphonate and the risk of gastrointestinal adverse events in advanced chronic kidney disease: a nationwide study. Nephrol Dial Transplant. 2020;35(9):1518–1526.

93. Noel JA, Bota SE, Petrcich W, et al. Risk of hospitalization for serious adverse gastrointestinal events associated with sodium polystyrene sulfonate use in patients of advanced age. JAMA Intern Med. 2019;179(8):1025–1033.

94. Meaney CJ, Beccari MV, Yang Y, et al. Systematic Review and Meta-Analysis of Patiromer and Sodium Zirconium Cyclosilicate: A New Armamentarium for the Treatment of Hyperkalemia. Pharmacotherapy. 2017;37(4):401–411.

95. National Institute for Health and Care Excellence. Sodium zirconium cyclosilicate for treating hyperkalaemia. 2019. https://www.nice.org.uk/guidance/ta599/chapter/1-Recommendations (accessed 8 September 2021).

96. Rafique Z, Liu M, Staggers KA, et al. Patiromer for Treatment of Hyperkalemia in the Emergency Department: A Pilot Study. Acad Emerg Med 2020;27(1):54–60.

97. Peacock WF, Rafique Z, Vishnevskiy K, et al. Emergency Potassium Normalization Treatment Including Sodium Zirconium Cyclosilicate: A Phase II, Randomized, Double-blind, Placebo-controlled Study (ENERGIZE). Acad Emerg Med 2020;27(6):475–486.

98. National Institute for Health and Care Excellence. Patiromer for treating hyperkalaemia. National Institute for Health and Care Excellence 2020. https://www.nice.org.uk/guidance/ta623/chapter/1-Recommendations (Accessed 8 September 2021).

99. Campbell P, McKeveney P, Donegan K, et al. Practical guidance for the use of potassium binders in the management of hyperkalaemia in patients with heart failure and/or chronic kidney disease. Br J Hosp Med (Lond). 2021;82(4):1–11.

100. Morales E, Cravedi P, Manrique J. Management of Chronic Hyperkalemia in Patients with Chronic Kidney Disease: An Old Problem with News Options. Front Med (Lausanne). 2021;8:653634.

101. Shrestha DB, Budhathoki P, Sedhai YR, et al. Patiromer and Sodium Zirconium Cyclosilicate in Treatment of Hyperkalemia: A Systematic Review and Meta-Analysis. Curr Ther Res Clin Exp. 2021;95:100635.

102. Hoy SM. Sodium Zirconium Cyclosilicate: A Review in Hyperkalaemia [published correction appears in Drugs. 2019;79(5):591]. Drugs. 2018;78(15):1605–1613.

103. Spinowitz BS, Fishbane S, Pergola PE, et al. Sodium Zirconium Cyclosilicate among Individuals with Hyperkalemia: A 12-Month Phase 3 Study. Clin J Am Soc Nephrol. 2019;14(6):798–809.

104. Mount DB. Disorders of potassium balance. In: Brenner and Rector's The Kidney, 11th ed, Yu A, Chertow G, Luyckx V, et al (Eds), W.B. Saunders & Company, Philadelphia 2020.p.577.

105. Holleck JL, Roberts AE, Marhoffer EA, et al. Risk of Intestinal Necrosis with Sodium Polystyrene Sulfonate: A Systematic Review and Meta-analysis. J Hosp Med. 2021;16(8):489–494.

106. Statland JM, Fontaine B, Hanna MG, et al. Review of the Diagnosis and Treatment of Periodic Paralysis. Muscle Nerve. 2018;57(4):522–530.

107. Renal Association Clinical Practice Guidelines - Treatment of Acute Hyperkalaemia in Adults - July 2020. (https://ukkidney.org/sites/renal.org/files/RENAL%20ASSOCIATION%20HYPERKALAEMIA%20GUIDELINE%202020.pdf). Accessed on 19 August 2021.

108. Berbenetz NM, Mrkobrada M. Mineralocorticoid receptor antagonists for heart failure: systematic review and meta-analysis. BMC Cardiovasc Disord. 2016;16(1):246.

24 | Hypocalcemia

BASIC PHYSIOLOGY

Calcium (Ca) is essential for bone formation, neuromuscular function, and blood coagulation. If calcium intake is inadequate, it may impair bone mineralization in children and accelerate bone loss in adults.

Distribution

An average adult's body contains 20 to 25 gm/kg or 1.2 to 1.4 kg of calcium, so it is the most abundant cation in the body. Out of this, about 99% is present in the bone, 1% in the soft tissue cells, and 0.15% in the extracellular fluid (ECF). As serum calcium concentration constitutes less than 1% of the total body calcium, it is a poor marker of overall total body calcium content.

Serum calcium

The normal value is about 8.5 to 10.5 mg/dL (4.3 to 5.2 mEq/L, 2.2 to 2.6

mmol/L). The total ECF calcium exists in three forms:

1. Bound to proteins: About 40% of calcium is bound to protein (mainly albumin) which will not be diffusible and biologically active.
2. Free-ionized: 50% of calcium is in an ionized form which is diffusible and biologically active.
3. Bound to anions: 10% calcium is complexed with the anions of organic acids such as phosphate, bicarbonate, citrate, lactate, or sulfate phosphate. This form of calcium is diffusible but biologically inactive.

Ionized calcium

The ionized-free calcium is the physiologically active form, and its average standard value is 4.3 to 5.3 mg/dL (2.2–2.6 mEq/L, 1.16 to 1.31 mmol/L). The total serum calcium does not always reflect the ionized calcium level because it is affected by pH, protein, and phosphate levels. For example, hypoproteinemia reduces protein-bound and total serum calcium, but the ionized calcium remains unchanged. In such cases, hypocalcemia may be wrongly diagnosed.

Corrected total calcium

Hypoalbuminemia reduces total calcium concentration without affecting the ionized calcium concentration. Each 1 gm/dL fall in the serum albumin concentration will reduce the total calcium concentration by approximately 0.8 mg/dL (0.4 mEq/L, 0.2 mmol/L). In patients with hypoalbuminemia, corrected serum calcium concentration can be calculated using the following equation:

Corrected Calcium =
Measured Total Calcium (mg/dL) +
0.8 × (4.0 − Serum Albumin [gm/dL])

Current literature discourages the use of corrected calcium in practice because this formula overestimates ionized calcium in patients with hypoalbuminemia, with resultant inadequate treatment of hypocalcemia [1, 2]. When in a dilemma, measure ionized calcium to avoid confusion and the potential risk of withholding appropriate treatment [3].

REGULATION

Dietary intake of calcium from food is about 1.0 to 1.3 gm/day in adults. 30%–35% of dietary calcium intake is absorbed. Excess calcium from the body gets excreted through urine. Parathyroid hormone (PTH) and the active form of vitamin D (1,25-dihydroxy vitamin D3, calcitriol) increase serum calcium concentration, and calcitonin decreases serum calcium concentration.

These three hormones, along with the Ca^{2+} sensing receptor system, tightly regulate serum calcium within a very normal range (Table 24.1). Actions of these hormones on bone, intestine, and kidney achieve the fine control of serum calcium. Changes in the level of phosphorus also affect calcium levels.

Role of parathyroid hormone

The function of PTH is to raise serum calcium levels rapidly when plasma calcium concentration falls. Serum calcium regulates PTH secretion from the chief cells of the parathyroid gland by a negative feedback mechanism. A fall in calcium quickly leads to a rise in PTH secretion, which raises serum calcium within a short time.

PTH increases serum calcium and prevents hypocalcemia by three actions: (1) Increasing renal calcium reabsorption; (2) Rapid release of calcium from bone by stimulating

Table 24.1 Hormonal regulation of calcium (Ca²⁺) and phosphorous (PHO₄)			
	PTH	**1,25-dihydroxy vitamin D3**	**Calcitonin**
Stimulus for secretion	Low Ca^{2+}, high PHO_4, low calcitriol	Low Ca^{2+} and PHO_4, low PTH	High calcium
Effect on serum calcium	Increases rapidly	Increases	Decreases
Effect on serum phosphorous	Decreases	Increases	Decreases
Effect on bones	Increases bone resorption	Increases bone resorption (weak effect)	Decreases bone resorption
Effect on intestine	Increases production of calcitriol which indirectly increases intestinal Ca^{2+} and PHO_4 absorption	Increases intestinal calcium and phosphorous absorption	No direct effect
Effect on kidney	Increases urinary calcium reabsorption and decreases phosphorous reabsorption	Increases urinary reabsorption of calcium and phosphorous (weak effect)	Increases urinary excretion of Ca^{2+} and PHO_4

osteoclastic bone resorption; and (3) Promoting the conversion of vitamin D to its active form (1,25-dihydroxyvitamin D3 or calcitriol) and thereby by increasing intestinal calcium absorption.

An increase in PTH causes hypercalcemia and hypophosphatemia, and a decrease in PTH levels leads to hypocalcemia and hyperphosphatemia.

Role of vitamin D

Vitamin D increases serum calcium slowly, but its effect lasts for a longer period. The active form of vitamin D - Calcitriol (1,25-dihydroxy-vitamin D3), increases serum calcium by promoting intestinal calcium absorption, stimulating renal reabsorption of calcium, and increasing calcium release from the bone (resorption). Calcitriol is a potent suppressor of PTH.

Role of calcitonin

The action of calcitonin is just opposite to that of PTH. High serum calcium level stimulates calcitonin secretion from the parafollicular cells of the thyroid gland. A high level of this hormone reduces high plasma calcium levels by decreasing bone resorption. High calcitonin also promotes osteoblastic activity and facilitates bone formation.

Calcium sensing receptor (CaSR) system

CaSR is a Class C G-protein coupled receptor located in several organs, including the parathyroid gland and kidneys, which senses fluctuations in extracellular ionized calcium and mediates feedback inhibition of PTH secretion and thereby controls secretion of PTH [4].

A high calcium level activates CaSR, which suppresses PTH secretion, resulting in calcium reduction. On the contrary, a reduction in calcium inactivates CaSR, which promotes the secretion of PTH, causing a rise in calcium.

Effect of pH

The value of ionized serum calcium is inversely related to serum pH because calcium binding to albumin depends on the serum pH. Acidosis (low pH) increases ionized calcium due to decreased binding of calcium to albumin, while alkalosis (high pH) decreases ionized calcium due to increased calcium binding to albumin.

Effect of phosphate and magnesium level

In Hyperphosphatemia, phosphate binds to calcium, causing a reduction of ionized calcium and triggering PTH release. In hypomagnesemia, impaired secretion of PTH from parathyroid glands and resistance to the effect of PTH on bone and kidney leads to hypocalcemia.

HYPOCALCEMIA

INTRODUCTION

Hypocalcemia is defined as total serum calcium <8.5 mg/dL (<4.4 mEq/L or <2.2 mmol/L) with normal serum albumin or ionized calcium <4.3 mg/dL (<2.2 mEq/L, <1.1 mmol/L). Hypocalcemia is the commonly encountered electrolyte abnormalities in critically ill patients, and its symptoms are mild in most patients but can be life-threatening in severe cases.

ETIOLOGY

Common causes of hypocalcemia are hypoalbuminemia, acute kidney injury and chronic kidney disease (CKD), hypoparathyroidism, hypomagnesemia, vitamin D deficiency, sepsis, acute pancreatitis, removal or damage to

Table 24.2 Causes of hypocalcemia
1. **Hypoalbuminemia**
2. **Hypoparathyroidism**
• Postoperative/surgical (hungry bone syndrome)
• Post-radiation, infiltrative
• Functional in hypomagnesemia
• Autoimmune destruction, congenital, idiopathic
3. **Inadequate vitamin D**
• Vitamin D deficiency (nutritional, lack of exposure to sunlight)
• Malnutrition and malabsorption syndrome
• Liver disease, chronic kidney disease
4. **Resistance to vitamin D**
• Vitamin D resistance rickets
5. **Redistribution, complexation, or deposition of calcium**
• Multiple red blood transfusions
• Acute pancreatitis, rhabdomyolysis, fat embolism, tumor lysis syndrome
• Hyperphosphatemia
• Sodium bicarbonate infusion, respiratory alkalosis
6. **Miscellaneous**
• Sepsis, burns
• Drugs: Bisphosphonate, denosumab, cisplatin, cinacalcet, phenobarbitone, phenytoin, and parenteral phosphate administration

the parathyroid glands during thyroid surgeries, and others, as summarized in Table 24.2.

Postsurgical

The hungry bone syndrome is a condition seen post-parathyroidectomy or after thyroid surgery characterized by rapid, profound, and prolonged hypocalcemia along with hypophosphatemia and hypomagnesemia [5].

Severe hypocalcemia occurs in hungry bone syndrome due to a sudden decline in high PTH levels, causing [6, 7]:

1. Suppression of osteoclast-mediated bone resorption (so process to increase serum calcium stops).

2. Osteoblastic activity continues, which rapidly increases the calcium uptake by "calcium-starved" bones, leading to reduced serum calcium.

Vitamin D deficiency

A deficiency of Vitamin D is a common cause of hypocalcemia. Vitamin D deficiency occurs due to poor dietary intake, malabsorption, or inadequate exposure to sunlight. In renal or hepatic failure, vitamin D deficiency occurs due to poor conversion of vitamin D to the active form, calcitriol (1,25(OH)2D).

Acute pancreatitis

In acute pancreatitis, many reactive enzymes (e.g., lipase) are released, which causes autodigestion of mesenteric fat and releases free fatty acids. Released free fatty acids bind with calcium ions leading to hypocalcemia [8, 9].

CLINICAL FEATURES

- Symptoms of hypocalcemia vary with the degree of ionized calcium levels and rate of onset and are due to increased neuromuscular excitability (Table 24.3).

- Mild to moderate acute hypocalcemia (ionized serum calcium 4–4.5 mg/dL or 1–1.12 mmol/L) may present with the complaint of weakness, circumoral and distal extremity paresthesia, muscle cramps, tetany, and mental changes such as irritability, depression, and psychosis.

- Severe acute hypocalcemia (ionized serum calcium <4 mg/dL [<1 mmol/L]) may cause lethargy, confusion, laryngeal spasm, seizures, bradycardia, hypotension refractory to fluids and vasopressors due to loss of vascular tone, or reversible heart failure. As digitalis acts by increasing intracellular calcium, hypocalcemia can reduce the efficacy of digoxin.

- Chronic hypocalcemia is asymptomatic in most patients but may cause fatigue, irritability, anxiety, depression, dry skin, cataract formation, and osteopenia/osteoporosis.

Table 24.3 Severity of hypocalcemia and its symptoms									
	Normal value			Mild to moderate hypocalcemia			Severe hypocalcemia		
Calcium	mg/dL	mEq/L	mmol/L	mg/dL	mEq/L	mmol/L	mg/dL	mEq/L	mmol/L
Total	8.5–10.5	4.3–5.2	2.2–2.6	8.0–8.4	4.0–4.2	2.0–2.1	<8.0	<4.0	<2.0
Ionized	4.3–5.3	2.2–2.6	1.1–1.3	4.0–4.2	2.0–2.1	1.0–1.1	<4.0	<2.0	<1.0
Common symptoms	-			Weakness, paresthesia, muscle cramps, tetany, and mental changes			Laryngeal spasms, seizures, bradycardia, hypotension, and heart failure		

- Clinical tests: On physical examination patient may have increased deep tendon reflexes or signs of latent tetany (which is elicited by Chvostek's sign and Trousseau's sign). In hypocalcemia, Trousseau's hypocalcemia sign (carpopedal spasm) is relatively more specific than Chvostek's (facial twitch) sign [10].

- Chvostek's sign is a twitch of the facial muscles, which can be provoked by gentle tapping on the facial nerve about 2 cm anterior to the earlobe, just below the zygomatic arch, with the mouth slightly open.

- Trousseau's sign is the development of wrist flexion, metacarpophalangeal joint flexion, and hyperextended fingers and thumb flexion when a blood pressure cuff is inflated above systolic pressure for 3 minutes to occlude the brachial artery.

- The electrocardiogram (ECG) may show a prolonged QT interval (due to the long ST segment) in severe hypocalcemia.

DIAGNOSIS

A simple stepwise method to evaluate patients with hypocalcemia is summarized [11].

Step 1: History and examination

Detailed history and physical examination may give a clue for the underlying etiology of hypocalcemia. History regarding lack of sun exposure, nutrition, low-calcium diet, acute or chronic renal failure, liver failure, chronic diarrhea or intestinal disease (e.g., crohn's disease, sprue, chronic pancreatitis), and family history of hypocalcemia helps to establish the etiological diagnosis. In addition, a history of thyroid or parathyroid surgery is vital because postsurgical hypoparathyroidism

and resultant hypocalcemia are common [12]. On physical examination, look for neck scarring, hypotension, bony changes, etc.

Step 2: Confirm the diagnosis of true hypocalcemia

When serum albumin is low, it causes a reduction in the total calcium but does not affect the value of ionized calcium. So, the diagnosis of true hypocalcemia is established either by measuring the ionized calcium or by correcting the value of total calcium for serum albumin levels.

Step 3: Measure serum PTH

The normal physiological response to hypocalcemia is an increase in PTH. Therefore, if PTH is low or inappropriately normal in patients with hypocalcemia, it is diagnostic of hypoparathyroidism. Conversely, high PTH values in patients with hypocalcemia occur due to acute or chronic kidney disease, vitamin D deficiency, and pseudohypoparathyroidism.

Step 4: Measure serum phosphate, magnesium, and vitamin D status

These tests provide valuable help to narrow down etiological diagnosis further. Various tests used to determine the etiological diagnosis of hypocalcemia and their interpretation, common causes of hypocalcemia and tests for their differential diagnosis, and how to investigate hypocalcemia are summarized in Tables 24.4, 24.5, and Figure 24.1.

Step 5: Order other tests

Check liver and renal functions, and order further investigations based on history and clinical examination.

Table 24.4 Diagnosis of etiology hypocalcemia		
Tests	**Value**	**Interpretation**
Albumin	Low	Calculate corrected calcium
PTH	Low	Hypoparathyroidism, calcium-sensing defect (rare)
	N-Low	Hypomagnesemia
	High	Vitamin D deficiency or resistance, chronic kidney disease, pseudohypoparathyroidism
Phosphate	High	Hypoparathyroidism, rhabdomyolysis, tumor lysis, or renal failure
	Low	Severe malnutrition, Vitamin D deficiency
Magnesium	Low	Hypomagnesemia
	High	Renal failure
Vitamin D	Low	Vitamin D deficiency or inadequate vitamin D activation (e.g., renal failure, hypoparathyroidism)
Creatinine	High	Renal failure
Alkaline phosphatase	High	Osteomalacia, rickets, or osteoblastic bone metastases
Lipase	High	Pancreatitis
CPK	High	Rhabdomyolysis
pH	High	Alkalosis decreases ionized calcium
Other investigations		
Liver functions, 24-hour urinary calcium and phosphate, ECG, skeletal x-rays, renal ultrasonography, and bone mineral density by DXA.		

Table 24.5 Differential diagnosis of low ionized calcium				
	PTH	**Phosphate**	**Magnesium**	**Vitamin D**
Hypoparathyroidism	Low	High	Normal	Normal
Hypomagnesemia	Normal-low	Normal	Low	Normal
Vitamin D deficiency	High	Normal	Normal	Low
Chronic kidney disease (high creatinine)	High	High	Normal-high	Normal-low
Pseudohypoparathyroidism (PTH resistant)	High	High	Normal-high	Normal-low

MANAGEMENT

The treatment of hypocalcemia is determined based on the severity of symptoms, speed of onset, level of calcium, underlying etiology, and coexisting illness [10, 13].

A. Acute management

Emergency therapy

Severe symptomatic hypocalcemia (tetany, seizures, laryngospasm, arrhythmias, refractory hypotension, and ionized

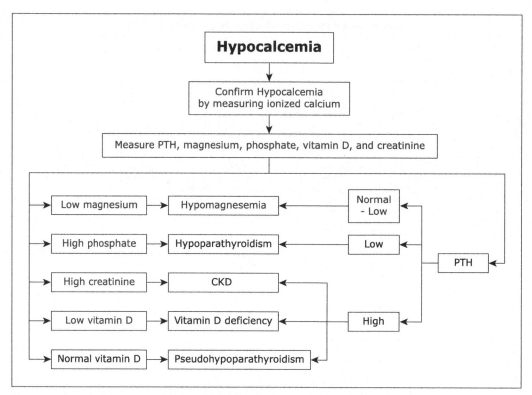

Figure 24.1 Approach to hypocalcemia.

calcium <4 mg/dL [<1 mmol/L]) should be treated as an emergency with a 10% calcium gluconate injection. Administer 10–20 ml of 10% calcium gluconate mixed in 50–100 mL of D5W (or normal saline) slowly over 10 minutes with ECG monitoring [10, 14]. Each ampule of 10% calcium gluconate injection provides 1 gm or 90 mg elemental calcium per 10 ml.

The effect of intravenous (IV) calcium bolus is for a short duration (raises serum calcium for 2 to 3 hours only). Therefore, continuous calcium infusion should follow the initial bolus to prevent rebound hypocalcemia.

Calcium gluconate infusion

Add 11 amps equal to 110 ml of calcium gluconate (990 mg elemental calcium) to 900 ml of D5W or normal saline to prepare calcium infusion. The calcium concentration of the drip will be 1 mg/ml.

In symptomatic patients with hypocalcemia, continuous calcium infusion may be infused at a rate of 0.5 mg to 1.5 mg/kg/hour. Monitor infusions of calcium closely because the rapid infusion of calcium carries the risk of hypotension, bradycardia, and cardiac arrhythmias.

Monitoring

The rate of administration should be adjusted by monitoring calcium every 4 to 6 hours to raise the serum calcium to avoid symptoms of hypocalcemia but to keep the serum calcium at the low-normal range (8.0–8.5 mg/dL), especially in hypoparathyroidism to minimize the hypercalciuria which can cause nephrolithiasis [15]. As the adjusted calcium formula does not adequately reflect ionized calcium concentrations, ionized calcium is the gold standard for monitoring [1, 11, 16].

Calcium chloride

Calcium chloride injection is a potent alternative to calcium gluconate for correcting hypocalcemia. The advantage of calcium chloride is a three times higher concentration of elemental calcium compared to calcium gluconate. Each ampule of 10% calcium chloride injection provides 273 mg, 13.6 mEq, or 6.80 mmol of elemental calcium per 10 ml. However, it is essential to note that calcium gluconate injection is the preferred and routinely used agent for symptomatic hypocalcemia due to the highly irritant nature of calcium chloride, which makes it unsuitable for infusion through a peripheral vein.

Massive transfusion

Hypocalcemia can occur during the administration of citrated blood products due to citrate and serum calcium chelation. The severity of hypocalcemia correlates with the number of packed red blood cells transfused [17]. Administration of 4 units of packed red blood cells + fresh frozen plasma is associated with a significantly higher risk of severe hypocalcemia [16]. The optimal calcium replacement strategy to avoid hypocalcemia after massive transfusion remains uncertain, but the common practice is to infuse 10 ml of 10% calcium gluconate after transfusing every 2–4 units of blood products is beneficial [18].

Precautions

Clinical situations and coexisting electrolyte abnormalities where administration of parenteral calcium needs extra caution are summarized:

1. Patients on digitalis therapy need continuous electrocardiographic monitoring during infusion of calcium because hypercalcemia aggravates digitalis toxicity and may provoke life-threatening cardiac arrhythmias.

2. Hypomagnesemia: If IV calcium fails to correct hypocalcemia and does not relieve tetany, rule out hypomagnesemia. If the serum magnesium level is <1.7 mEq/L, administer 2 gm (16 mEq) of magnesium sulfate intravenously as a 10% solution over 10–15 minutes, followed by 1 gm (8 mEq) in 100 ml infusion per hour to raise serum magnesium to a normal level. It's important to note that 2 ml of Injection 50% Magnesium Sulfate is equivalent to one gram or 8 mEq.

3. Hyperphosphatemia: Avoid the administration of calcium in patients with severe hyperphosphatemia (>6.5 mg/dL) because the resultant increased calcium-phosphorus product will precipitate in soft tissues. In patients of tumor lysis syndrome with hyperphosphatemia and hypocalcemia, avoid calcium or supplement it cautiously to prevent the precipitation of calcium phosphate salts and resultant metastatic calcification.

4. Metabolic acidosis: While treating metabolic acidosis with hypocalcemia (e.g., CKD), correct hypocalcemia before correction of acidosis because correction of acidosis reduces the ionized calcium and further aggravates hypocalcemia. Additionally, avoid coadministration of calcium and bicarbonate-containing solutions because of the risk of precipitation of calcium carbonate.

B. Long term management

Calcium supplementation

An asymptomatic patient with chronic mild hypocalcemia (ionized calcium levels >0.8 mmol/L) needs 1 to 3 gm per day of oral elemental calcium in 2–3 divided doses. Absorption of calcium is best when taken between meals.

Calcium carbonate is a commonly used preparation that is less expensive and well-tolerated. On the other hand, calcium citrate preparation has better bioavailability, but its cost is higher.

Vitamin D supplementation

Vitamin D supplementation is commonly recommended with calcium in hypocalcemia because vitamin D deficiency is common, and vitamin D promotes the absorption of calcium. Vitamin D should be replaced when the level of 25 hydroxyvitamin D is <20 ng/ml. Vitamin D2 (ergocalciferol) and D3 (cholecalciferol) are low-cost oral preparations commonly used to treat hypocalcemia due to vitamin D deficiency.

The dose varies depending on the level of deficiency, but usually, a capsule of ergocalciferol is given 50,000 IU weekly or monthly to correct the deficit, followed by 1,000–2,000 IU daily supplementation as a maintenance dose. The onset of action of vitamin D (ergocalciferol) is slow (about two weeks), but because of its long half-life and storage in fat, it carries a higher risk of vitamin D intoxication.

Activated vitamin D (calcitriol) is preferred in patients with abnormal vitamin D metabolism (renal or liver disease) and recommended dose of oral calcitriol is 0.25–1.0 mcg/day.

Amongst vitamin D preparations, calcitriol is the most potent and fastest acting preparation with the shortest duration of action. As calcitriol is short-acting, there is no risk of vitamin D intoxication. However, the higher cost is the disadvantage of calcitriol.

C. Treatment of underlying etiology

Identifying and treating the underlying cause of hypocalcemia is an essential part of treatment.

Hypoparathyroidism: In the treatment of hypocalcemia secondary hypoparathyroidism, calcium and vitamin D are the first line of conventional therapy.

Amongst vitamin D preparations, choose calcitriol or alfacalcidol rather than conventionally used practices such as ergocalciferol or cholecalciferol [10].

Additional valuable measures in the therapy of hypoparathyroidism are thiazide diuretics, phosphate binders, and a low-salt and low-phosphorus diet [19].

In patients of hypoparathyroidism with failure of conventional therapy, Recombinant human parathyroid hormone (1–84) is a newer therapeutic modality (approved in the USA and Europe) that improves health-related quality of life, but its use is limited due to high cost, black box warning for potential risk of osteosarcoma, and lack of availability in different parts of the world [20–23].

REFERENCES

1. Steen O, Clase C, Don-Wauchope A. Corrected calcium formula in routine clinical use does not accurately reflect ionized calcium in hospital patients. Can J Gen Int Med. 2016;11(3):14–21.

2. Lian IA, Asberg A. Should total calcium be adjusted for albumin? A retrospective observational study of laboratory data from central Norway. BMJ Open. 2018;8(4):e017703.

3. Kenny CM, Murphy CE, Boyce DS, et al. Things We Do for No Reason™: Calculating a "Corrected Calcium" Level. J Hosp Med. 2021;16(8):499–501.

4. Conigrave AD. The Calcium-Sensing Receptor and the Parathyroid: Past, Present, Future. Front Physiol. 2016;7:563.

5. Witteveen JE, van Thiel S, Romijn JA, et al. Hungry bone syndrome: still a challenge in the post-operative management of primary hyperparathyroidism: a

systematic review of the literature. Eur J Endocrinol. 2013;168(3):R45–53.

6. Kaya C, Tam AA, Dirikoç A, et al. Hypocalcemia development in patients operated for primary hyperparathyroidism: Can it be predicted preoperatively? Arch Endocrinol Metab. 2016;60(5):465–471.

7. Jain N, Reilly RF. Hungry bone syndrome. Curr Opin Nephrol Hypertens. 2017;26(4):250–255.

8. Kelly A, Levine MA. Hypocalcemia in the critically ill patient. J Intensive Care Med. 2013;28(3):166–77.

9. Ahmed A, Azim A, Gurjar M, et al. Hypocalcemia in acute pancreatitis revisited. Indian J Crit Care Med. 2016;20(3):173–177.

10. Cooper MS, Gittoes NJL. Diagnosis and management of hypocalcaemia. BMJ 2008;336:1298–1302.

11. Pepe J, Colangelo L, Biamonte F, et al. Diagnosis and management of hypocalcemia. Endocrine. 2020;69(3):485–495.

12. Kakava K, Tournis S, Papadakis G, et al. Postsurgical Hypoparathyroidism: A Systematic Review. In Vivo. 2016;30(3):171–9.

13. Augustine M, Horwitz MJ. Are You Sure the Patient Has Hypocalcemia? Hypocalcemia Endocrinology Metabolism, Endocrinology Adviser February 4, 2019. Accessed on 27 Nov 2021: https://www. endocrinologyadvisor.com/author/mara-j-horwitz-dsm/.

14. Walsh J, Gittoes N, Selby P. Society for Endocrinology Endocrine Emergency Guidance: Emergency management of acute hypocalcemia in adult patients. Endocr Connect. 2016;5(5):G9–G11.

15. Bove-Fenderson E, Mannstadt M. Hypocalcemic disorders. Best Pract Res Clin Endocrinol Metab. 2018;32(5):639–656.

16. Byerly S, Inaba K, Biswas S, et al. Transfusion-Related Hypocalcemia After Trauma. World J Surg. 2020;44(11):3743–3750.

17. Hall C, Nagengast AK, Knapp C, et al. Massive transfusions and severe hypocalcemia: An opportunity for monitoring and supplementation guidelines. Transfusion. 2021;61:S188–S194.

18. Kyle T, Greaves I, Beynon A, et al. Ionised calcium levels in major trauma patients who received blood en route to a military medical treatment facility. Emerg Med J. 2018;35(3):176–179.

19. Fong J, Khan A. Hypocalcemia: updates in diagnosis and management for primary care. Can Fam Physician. 2012;58(2):158–62.

20. Mannstadt M, Clarke BL, Vokes T, et al. Efficacy and safety of recombinant human parathyroid hormone (1–84) in hypoparathyroidism (REPLACE): a double-blind, placebo-controlled, randomised, phase 3 study. Lancet Diabetes Endocrinol 2013;1(4):275–83.

21. Vokes TJ, Mannstadt M, Levine MA, et al. Recombinant Human Parathyroid Hormone Effect on Health-Related Quality of Life in Adults with Chronic Hypoparathyroidism. J Clin Endocrinol Metab. 2018;103(2):722–731.

22. Mannstadt M, Clarke BL, Bilezikian JP, et al. Safety and efficacy of 5 years of treatment with recombinant human parathyroid hormone in adults with hypoparathyroidism. J Clin Endocrinol Metab. 2019;104(11):5136–5147.

23. Laurer E, Grünberger J, Naidoo U, et al. Recombinant human parathyroid hormone (1–84) replacement therapy in a child with hypoparathyroidism. Bone. 2021;144:115834.

25 | Hypercalcemia

Hypercalcemia is a less common disorder than hypocalcemia, occurring in about 0.6–7.5% of hospitalized and less than 1.0% of outpatients [1–6].

Hypercalcemia is defined as total serum calcium >10.5 mg/dL (>2.6 mmol/L) with normal serum albumin or ionized calcium >5.2 mg/dL (>1.3 mmol/L) [7].

When total serum calcium is >14.0 mg/dL (>3.5 mmol/L) or ionized calcium is >7.0 mg/dL (>1.7 mmol/L), it is considered severe hypercalcemia [7]. Early detection and prompt treatment of hypercalcemia are essential because it carries high morbidity and mortality [7, 8].

ETIOLOGY

Primary hyperparathyroidism and malignancy are the two most common causes of hypercalcemia in more than 90% of patients [7, 9]. In recent times, there has been a significant rise in hypercalcemia due to Vitamin D toxicity.

Mechanisms by which different etiologies cause hypercalcemia are enhanced bone resorption, increased intestinal absorption, or decreased renal calcium excretion (Table 25.1).

Primary hyperparathyroidism (PHPT)

This disorder is the most common cause of hypercalcemia in about 50%

Table 25.1 Causes of hypercalcemia
1. Increased bone resorption
• Primary hyperparathyroidism
• Secondary hyperparathyroidism
• Malignancy (lung, breast, kidney, multiple myeloma)
• Hyperthyroidism
• Lithium therapy
2. Increased intestinal absorption
• Vitamin D or vitamin A excess
• Milk-alkali syndrome
• Granulomatous disease (i.e. sarcoidosis, tuberculosis)
3. Decreased renal excretion
• Familial hypocalciuric hypercalcemia
• Thiazide diuretics
4. Miscellaneous causes
• Prolong immobilization
• Rhabdomyolysis (recovery stage)
• Parenteral nutrition

to 60% of ambulatory and 25% of hospitalized patients [10]. Primary hyperparathyroidism occurs in middle age (between 50 and 60 years) and is two to three times more common in women. It is characterized by an elevated PTH, hypercalcemia, hypophosphatemia, loss of cortical bone, and hypercalciuria. Hypercalcemia in this condition is usually mild, and in >80% of patients, it occurs due to a single parathyroid adenoma [7]. An abnormal, incompletely-regulated, high secretion of parathyroid hormone (PTH) from the parathyroid gland activates osteoclast, causing bone resorption and increasing intestinal calcium absorption, leading to hypercalcemia [11].

Familial hypocalciuric hypercalcemia (FHH) is a disorder of autosomal dominant inheritance and a rare cause of hypercalcemia characterized by mild hypercalcemia, low urinary calcium excretion, and inappropriately normal or elevated PTH [12].

The onset of hypercalcemia at an early age (before the age of 40) and hypocalciuria due to increased renal tubular reabsorption of calcium are features of FHH, in contrast to an average age of onset after 50 years and hypercalciuria in typical primary hyperparathyroidism [13].

Malignancy

Malignancy is the second commonest cause of hypercalcemia. It is the most common cause of inpatient hypercalcemia (accounts for up to 65%). It occurs in 20% to 30% of all cancer patients [14, 15]. Multiple myeloma and primary lung tumors (particularly squamous cell carcinoma), breast, and kidney are the most common malignancies causing hypercalcemia [16].

Malignancy-associated hypercalcemia can be severe, rapidly progressive, and, therefore, more symptomatic and fatal [17]. As PTH levels are typically low in malignancy, high calcium level in cancer patients is labeled as PTH-independent hypercalcemia. In malignancy, hypercalcemia occurs in approximately 80% of patients due to excessive PTH-related protein (PTHrP) secretion by the tumor, enhancing osteoclastic activity. In comparison, in other 20% of patients, hypercalcemia is due to metastasis which causes bone erosion due to osteolytic activities and the resultant release of skeletal calcium into the circulation.

Vitamin D toxicity

By increasing intestinal calcium absorption, vitamin D can cause hypercalcemia [18]. The incidence of hypercalcemia due to excessive vitamin D consumption (i.e., vitamin D toxicity) was previously less common, but it is currently growing [19]. The reason for this rising incidence is public awareness of the health benefits of vitamin D and, consequently, self-administration and consumption of vitamin D in doses higher than recommended [20, 21].

Hypervitaminosis D induced hypercalcemia is characterized by low PTH and hyperphosphatemia (seen commonly but not always) [22].

Milk alkali syndrome

This syndrome consists of a classic triad of hypercalcemia, metabolic alkalosis, and acute kidney injury that commonly occurs due to prolonged use of large quantities of calcium-containing antacids for peptic ulcer disease in the past or currently because of the increasing use of calcium carbonate for prevention or treatment of osteoporosis [23, 24].

Granulomatous diseases

In patients with granulomatous disease such as sarcoidosis, hypercalcemia occurs due to the overproduction of active vitamin D (calcitriol) through increased conversion of 25-hydroxy vitamin D to 1,25-dihydroxy vitamin D by macrophages. Due to high 1,25-dihydroxy vitamin D, intestinal calcium absorption increases, resulting in hypercalcemia and suppressed PTH.

Thiazide diuretics

By blocking the thiazide-sensitive NaCl transporter in the distal convoluted tubule, thiazides increase calcium reabsorption and reduce urinary calcium excretion with resultant hypercalcemia [25]. Thiazide-induced hypercalcemia is usually mild and transient (1 to 2 weeks). However, thiazides can unmask or aggravate hypercalcemia due to underlying primary hyperparathyroidism [26].

Immobilization

Prolonged immobilization can cause hypercalcemia due to decreased bone formation and a marked unopposed increase in bone resorption, which is more common in children, adolescents, and patients with underlying high bone turnover states such as thyrotoxicosis, Paget disease, or extensive fractures [27].

CLINICAL FEATURES

Variable clinical features can be:

1. Secondary to underlying disorders.

2. Secondary to hypercalcemia.

Clinical features of hypercalcemia are diverse and involve multiple organ systems, depending on the severity and rapidity of onset (Table 25.2). Mild hypercalcemia is generally asymptomatic. The signs and symptoms of hypercalcemia due to primary hyperparathyroidism are classically described with the old mnemonic "renal stones, painful bones, abdominal groans, psychic moans" to recall the symptoms [28].

Table 25.2 Severity of hypercalcemia and its symptoms					
Severity	**Mild**		**Moderate**		**Severe/Hypercalcemic crisis**
Calcium	mg/dL	mmol/L	mg/dL	mmol/L	mg/dL	mmol/L
Total	10.5–11.9	2.6–3.0	12.0–13.9	3.0–3.5	>14.0	>3.5
Ionized	5.4–6.0	1.3–1.50	6.0–7.0	1.5–1.7	>7.0	>1.7
Symptoms	Asymptomatic or mild symptoms like malaise, weakness, anxiety, and other vague symptoms.		Weakness, fatigue, depression, constipation, anorexia, nausea, polyuria, and shortened QT interval		Delirium, lethargy, confusion, stupor, coma, vomiting, peptic ulcer disease, pancreatitis, hypovolemia, AKI, and arrhythmias

Symptoms of hypercalcemia are [7]:

- **General:** Weakness, easy fatigability, malaise.
- **Central nervous system manifestations:** depression, lethargy, confusion, and stupor, which can progress to seizures, and coma.
- **Gastrointestinal manifestations:** Constipation, anorexia, nausea, and vomiting. Abdominal pain may result from severe hypercalcemia-induced peptic ulcer disease or pancreatitis. Hypercalcemia can cause peptic ulcer disease via stimulation of gastrin secretion. Mechanisms of the development of acute pancreatitis are deposition of calcium in pancreatic ducts, causing obstruction, and accelerated intrapancreatic conversion of trypsinogen to trypsin within the parenchyma, causing pancreatic damage [29].
- **Renal manifestations:** Polyuria and nocturia due to impaired renal concentration ability. When polyuria is severe, it can cause severe extracellular fluid (ECF) volume depletion leading to acute kidney injury (AKI). Prolonged hypercalcemia can cause nephrocalcinosis or stone formation and may present as renal colic and hematuria. It can also cause chronic kidney diseases.
- **Skeletal "Bones":** Bone pain, arthritis, osteoporosis, pathological fracture, osteitis fibrosa cystica in hyperparathyroidism.
- **Cardiac manifestations:** Hypercalcemia can cause hypertension and aggravate digitalis toxicity. Electrocardiogram (ECG) shows shortened QT interval and, in severe cases, arrhythmia like complete heart block leading to cardiac arrest.
- **Metastatic calcification:** Band keratopathy, red-eye syndrome, nephrocalcinosis, and vascular calcification.

DIAGNOSIS

It is important to remember that the most common causes of hypercalcemia are primary hyperparathyroidism and cancer (in about 90%), and vitamin D toxicity is its growing cause. Step by step, the proper workup of hypercalcemia is summarized.

Step 1: Confirm the diagnosis

Confirm the diagnosis of true hypercalcemia by measuring serum ionized calcium or using the corrected value of total calcium for albumin in case of hypoalbuminemia or hyperalbuminemia.

Step 2: History and physical examination

Detailed history and physical examination help to diagnose the underlying cause of hypercalcemia:

- Patients with primary hyperparathyroidism are usually asymptomatic. Generally, primary hyperparathyroidism is the etiology in asymptomatic outpatients with mild hypercalcemia (total serum calcium 11.0 mg/dL or lower), present for more than 6 months without apparent cause. Hypertension is common in primary hyperparathyroidism.
- In malignancy, symptoms bring the patient to the physician, and laboratory investigations diagnose hypercalcemia. Malignancy is often the cause in symptomatic patients with an abrupt onset of diseases and severe hypercalcemia (serum calcium 14 mg/dL or higher).
- Hypercalcemia with renal stone favors long duration, so malignancy is unlikely.

- The use of vitamin D, calcium, antacids, and lithium therapy may be the underlying cause of hypercalcemia.

- Elicit a family history of kidney stones or hypercalcemia in a parent or sibling.

Step 3: Measure serum PTH

The measurement of serum PTH levels is the first and most crucial test in the diagnostic approach to hypercalcemia, as shown in a flow diagram (Figure 25.1).

Suppression of PTH is a normal physiological response in hypercalcemia. Therefore, PTH level measurement helps to differentiate PTH-dependent hypercalcemia (with high PTH levels in primary hyperparathyroidism) from PTH-independent carcinoma (with low PTH levels in malignancy and other causes). Primary hyperparathyroidism is the most common cause of high or inappropriately normal PTH in patients not taking thiazides or lithium and the absence of advanced kidney disease.

Urinary calcium excretion helps further to narrow down the diagnosis of hypercalcemia with high PTH. In primary hyperparathyroidism, urinary calcium excretion is high, while low urinary calcium excretion occurs in familial hypocalciuric hypercalcemia (a rare disorder with the onset of hypercalcemia at a young age).

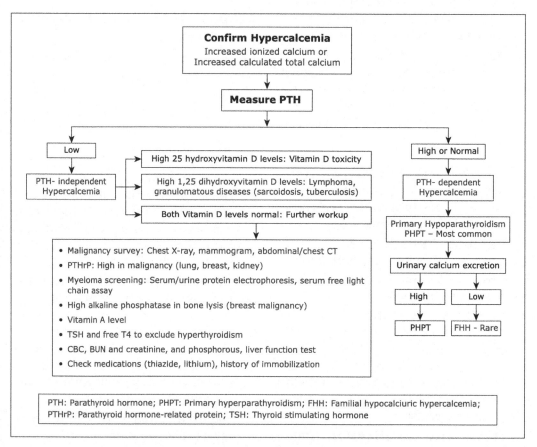

Figure 25.1 Diagnostic approach to hypercalcemia.

Step 4: Order other tests

In PTH-independent carcinoma, various tests are carried out to establish the etiological diagnosis, as shown in Figure 25.1. Based on the history and physical examination, investigations commonly performed are:

- Complete blood count (CBC) and erythrocyte sedimentation rate (ESR).
- Electrolytes such as sodium, potassium, magnesium, and phosphate.
- Renal, liver, and thyroid function tests, including alkaline phosphatase, total protein, and albumin.
- 25 hydroxyvitamin D, 1,25 dihydroxy vitamin D levels and parathyroid hormone-related protein (PTHrP) test (if available).
- Serum and urine protein electrophoresis and a skeletal survey.

Laboratory tests provide important clues such as:

- A low serum chloride, high serum HCO_3, and elevated BUN and creatinine are characteristics of milk-alkali syndrome causing PTH-independent hypercalcemia.
- In patients with high total protein with reversed albumin/globulin (A/G) ratio suspect multiple myeloma.
- Low plasma phosphate is found in primary hyperparathyroidism and humoral hypercalcemia of malignancy (elevated PTHrP), while high plasma phosphate associated with renal impairment suggests tertiary hyperparathyroidism.
- If the level of 1,25 dihydroxy vitamin D is high, a chest X-ray should be done to assess the presence of granulomatous disease (sarcoidosis, tuberculosis).
- In patients with osteolytic hypercalcemia, alkaline phosphatase increases due to bony metastases such as breast tumors.

MANAGEMENT

Treatment of hypercalcemia is determined based on the severity of hypercalcemia, presence of symptoms, underlying cause, and associated comorbidities. Initial treatment is planned to reduce serum calcium until the underlying cause is identified and treated:

- **Mild hypercalcemia (<12 mg/dL):** Asymptomatic patients do not require immediate treatment but need observation, correction of reversible factors like volume deficits, withdrawal of the offending agent like thiazide diuretics, and management of underlying causes.
- **Moderate hypercalcemia (12 to 14 mg/dL):** Symptoms dictate the therapeutic plan in moderate hypercalcemia. Patients with chronic moderate hypercalcemia without symptoms do not require urgent therapy but need the same precautions described for mild hypercalcemia. However, when the onset of moderate hypercalcemia is acute, patients are usually symptomatic and require more aggressive treatment as required for severe hypercalcemia.
- **Severe hypercalcemia (>14 mg/dL):** All patients with severe hypercalcemia, regardless of symptoms, require immediate treatment.

Five common strategies for the treatment of hypercalcemia are (Figure 25.2):

1. Enhancing renal excretion of calcium.
2. Reducing gastrointestinal absorption of calcium.
3. Inhibiting bone resorption.

4. Direct removal of calcium from the ECF.

5. Treatment of the underlying cause.

A. Selection of modality

For the emergency management of hypercalcemia, first-line therapy routinely administered are isotonic saline hydration, forced calciuresis (effect within 2–4 hours), and calcitonin (effect within 4–6 hours). Other modalities which slowly correct hypercalcemia are bisphosphonates (within 2 days), glucocorticoids (within 3 days), and denosumab (within 4 days). Hemodialysis corrects hypercalcemia immediately (effect within 1 hour), but it is only used in a few selected patients.

In the treatment of hypercalcemia, rapidly acting first-line measures, slowly working but more potent measures to lower serum calcium and specific treatment of underlying etiology are initiated simultaneously (Table 25.3).

B. Measures to increase urinary excretion

1. Isotonic saline hydration

The first, most important, and effective step to correct symptomatic hypercalcemia is the administration of normal saline at a rate of 200–300 mL/hour to correct hypovolemia. By expanding intravascular volume, intravenous (IV) normal saline increases natriuresis, reduces the sodium and calcium reabsorption in the renal tubule, and facilitates urinary calcium excretion. In the past, the administration of 4 to 6 L of intravenous normal fluid in the first 24 hours was recommended, but a large volume of IV fluid infusion is currently no longer recommended [30, 31].

In patients with severe hypercalcemia, poor oral intake, nausea, vomiting, and polyuria (due to nephrogenic diabetes insipidus) lead to volume deficit. Hypercalcemic patients with severe

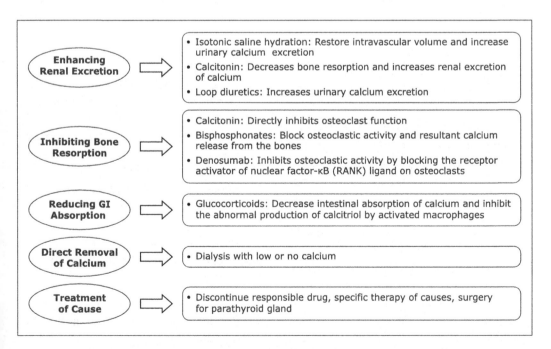

Figure 25.2 Treatment options for hypercalcemia.

		Table 25.3 Treatment of severe Hypercalcemia			
Treatment	**Route**	**Regimen**	**Onset of action**	**Duration of action**	**Adverse effects**
1. Measures to increase urinary excretion					
Normal saline	IV	200–300 mL/hour Initially, 100 to 150 mL/hour after rehydration for 1–5 days	2–4 hours	While infusing	Volume overload, exacerbate congestive heart failure
Furosemide	IV	20–40 mg every 12–24 hours after correction of hypovolemia	Minutes to hours	During therapy	Dehydration, hypokalemia, hypomagnesemia, may aggravate renal failure if given before adequate rehydration
2. Measures to inhibit bone resorption					
Calcitonin	IV	4–8 IU/kg intramuscular (IM) or SC every 6 to 12 hours for the first 48 hours only	4–6 hours	2–3 days	Flushing, nausea, hypersensitivity, rarely allergic reactions, tachyphylaxis
Pamidronate	IV	60 to 90 mg in 100–200 ml of saline or D5W over 2–4 hours as a single dose, repeated only after one week if necessary	1–3 days	2–4 weeks	Nephrotoxicity, transient flue like syndrome with fever, chills, and aches
Zoledronic acid	IV	4 mg in 50 ml saline or D5W over 15–30 minutes as a single dose, repeated only after one week if necessary	1–3 days	2–4 weeks	
Denosumab	SC	60 mg weekly for 4 weeks, followed by 60 mg monthly	4–10 days	1–4 months	Prolonged hypocalcemia, risk of infection, with long-term use risk of osteonecrosis of the jaw and atypical femoral fractures
3. Measures to decrease intestinal absorption					
Glucocorticoids	IV oral	Hydrocortisone 200–300 mg/day for 3–5 days Prednisolone 20–40 mg/day for additional 5–7 days	2–5 days	Days to weeks	Hyperglycemia, hypertension, hypokalemia, interfere with chemotherapy
4. Measures to remove calcium directly					
Hemodialysis	-	Variable	Immediately	During dialysis	Not significant

dehydration may require 1 to 2 L of fluid in the ED to replace the volume lost [32].

Once the volume deficit is adequately corrected, the rate of saline administration is adjusted to maintain the urine output at 100 to 150 mL/hour with close monitoring to avoid volume overload. To avoid fluid overload in a patient with underlying hypoalbuminemia, cardiac disease, or renal insufficiency, limit the rate of saline infusion to 75 to 150 mL/hour and consider the judicious use of furosemide [30].

Normal saline may not be a suitable fluid when metabolic acidosis is associated with hypercalcemia as its large volume infusion can aggravate acidosis. Balanced crystalloid PlasmaLyte is an excellent choice in such patients because it doesn't contain calcium and corrects acidosis [33]. Balanced crystalloid Ringer lactate is usually avoided in treating hypercalcemia because it contains calcium (3 mEq/L).

2. Furosemide

Traditionally, after volume expansion, a loop diuretic (furosemide) is co-administered with the large volume of saline because it causes increased urinary calcium excretion by blocking the sodium-potassium-chloride cotransport system in the thick ascending loop of Henle. However, in current literature, routine administration of furosemide in hypercalcemia with normal renal and cardiac functions is not preferred because of the potential risk of volume depletion and electrolyte abnormalities and the availability of much more specific and effective therapies for hypercalcemia [34, 35].

The use of furosemide in hypercalcemia is currently reserved for patients with impaired renal and cardiac functions carrying the risk of fluid overload. Please avoid the use of thiazide diuretics because it impairs urinary calcium excretion.

C. Measures to inhibit bone resorption

1. Calcitonin

This drug inhibits bone resorption by interfering with osteoclast activity and increases urinary calcium excretion [36].

Because of its rapid action (effect within 2 hours), it is useful for urgent therapy of severe hypercalcemia (serum calcium >14 mg/dL) or acute rise in serum calcium with life-threatening symptoms. However, calcitonin is not very potent (it can decrease serum calcium by no more than 1 to 2 mg/dL), and its effects are short-lived. Therefore it should not be used as a monotherapy and should be administered along with rehydration and saline diuresis. So, the role of calcitonin as an initial treatment is to decrease calcium rapidly while waiting for other treatment modalities like bisphosphonates to take effect.

Dose and administration: 4–8 IU/kg IM or SC every 6 to 12 hours. It is important to remember that in treating hypercalcemia, calcitonin in injectable form is preferred, and its nasal spray is not recommended because it is less effective [37]. Calcitonin is discontinued after 48 hours because of the development of tachyphylaxis after 24 to 48 hours due to receptor downregulation.

2. Bisphosphonates

These agents inhibit osteoclast-mediated bone resorption effectively and therefore are the most preferred and first choice in managing severe hypercalcemia (particularly for hypercalcemia of malignancy). As the onset of action of bisphosphonates is slow (approximately 48 to 72 hours), they should be started early, along with volume resuscitation and calcitonin. IV bisphosphonates are generally well tolerated and suitable for long-term treatment of hypercalcemia.

IV Pamidronate (30, 60, or 90 mg) or IV zoledronic acid (4 mg) are the two most widely used bisphosphonates for parenteral therapy. Zoledronic acid is about 100 to 850 times more potent than pamidronate in reversing hypercalcemia and therefore is the preferred agent [38].

Bisphosphonates are usually avoided in milk-alkali syndrome because of the risk of prolonged hypocalcemia [39] and should be used with caution in premenopausal women [40]. In patients with moderate renal insufficiency (GFR >30 mL/minute), dose reduction and an increase in infusion duration are necessary [41, 42], and bisphosphonates should be avoided in severe renal insufficiency [43]. As IV bisphosphonates may be nephrotoxic, serum creatinine level monitoring is recommended during therapy [44].

3. Denosumab

Denosumab is a humanized monoclonal antibody directed against receptor activator of nuclear factor-κB ligand (RANKL) on osteoclasts.

By binding and neutralizing RANKL on the cell surface of osteoclast precursors, denosumab inhibits the maturation, survival, and function of osteoclasts, thereby reducing bone resorption [45]. In treating hypercalcemia of malignancy, this drug is used when bisphosphonate failure, refractory hypercalcemia, or bisphosphonates are contraindicated (e.g., in patients with renal dysfunction) [46].

Denosumab, like bisphosphonates, is not immediately acting. The recommended dosage is 60 mg SC weekly for 4 weeks, followed by 60 mg monthly.

Other agents, such as gallium nitrate and plicamycin (mithramycin), which inhibit bone resorption, are no longer used because of their potential toxicity.

D. Measures to decrease intestinal absorption

1. Glucocorticoids

By reducing calcitriol (1,25-hydroxyvitamin D), glucocorticoids decrease intestinal calcium absorption, promote urinary excretion of calcium, and lower serum calcium.

Glucocorticoids are effective in hypercalcemia due to vitamin D intoxication, sarcoidosis, and malignancies (multiple myeloma, leukemia, Hodgkin's disease, etc.). However, they do not alter calcium levels in primary hyperparathyroidism, solid tumors, or in a normal person.

The onset of effect is about 2–4 days, the recommended dose is 200–300 mg/day of hydrocortisone or 20–40 mg/day of prednisolone, and it is usually given for about 3–7 days.

Alternative drugs like ketoconazole and hydroxylchloroquine inhibit the hydroxylation of 25-hydroxy vitamin D to 1,25-dihydroxy vitamin D and decrease the production of 1,25-dihydroxy vitamin D, correct calcitriol-induced hypercalcemia.

2. Phosphate

Oral phosphate inhibits calcium absorption by forming insoluble calcium phosphate in the gut. Phosphate infusion rapidly decreases the serum calcium level, but its use in hypercalcemia is discouraged because of the risks of the deposition of calcium phosphate products in tissues.

E. Measures to remove calcium directly

Dialysis

Hemodialysis or peritoneal dialysis with low calcium dialysate solution is the most potent, effective, and rapid method to lower plasma calcium levels in severe hypercalcemia. Avoid using calcium-free dialysate in severe hypercalcemia as it can cause hemodynamic instability [47].

Urgent hemodialysis is reserved for patients with [48–51]:

- Congestive heart failure, impaired renal function, or end-stage renal disease in which saline hydration is risky and diuretics are ineffective.
- Severe hypercalcemia when standard medical therapy fails or is contraindicated.
- Hypercalcemic crisis with severe life-threatening neurological or cardiovascular symptoms along with standard medical management.

Hemodialysis effectively lower calcium by removing calcium directly from the blood, but the effect is transit, so simultaneous administration of other medical measures is mandatory.

F. Specific treatment of underlying causes

- Discontinue drugs responsible.
- Specific treatment for malignancy, thyrotoxicosis, adrenal insufficiency, rhabdomyolysis, etc.
- Steroid therapy for hypercalcemia due to granulomas (e.g., sarcoidosis) or lymphoma.
- Primary hyperparathyroidism: Surgical treatment is the only curative therapy for this disorder. Parathyroidectomy is more cost-effective than drug therapy and indicated in all symptomatic patients and most asymptomatic patients with serum calcium levels greater than 1 mg/dL above normal, age <50 years, or end-organ disease (renal stones, nephrocalcinosis, impaired renal function, fragility fractures or osteoporosis with bone density T score >2.5) [52, 53].

- Calcimimetics (cinacalcet) may be used in the medical management of hypercalcemia due to parathyroid carcinoma or primary hyperparathyroidism. In addition, this drug is routinely used in treating secondary hyperparathyroidism in patients on renal replacement therapy. Cinacalcet is a calcium-sensing receptor agonist (also called a calcimimetic) that increases sensitivity and stimulates calcium-sensing receptors on the parathyroid gland. Negative feedback suppresses PTH secretion, leading to lower PTH of serum calcium. Cinacalcet is well-tolerated and is initiated at a dose of 30 mg once- or twice daily orally, with a maximum dose of 90 mg three-four times daily.
- Vitamin D toxicity: Stop vitamin D consumption, discontinue a calcium-rich diet, and increase salt and fluid intake. Patients with severe hypercalcemia may require saline hydration, corticosteroids, and bisphosphonate.

REFERENCES

1. Fisken RA, Heath DA, Somers S, et al. Hypercalcaemia in hospital patients: clinical and diagnostic aspects. Lancet. 1981;1(8213):202–7.

2. Dent DM, Miller JL, Klaff L, et al. The incidence and causes of hypercalcaemia. Postgrad Med J. 1987;63(743):745–750.

3. Lee CT, Yang CC, Lam KK, et al. Hypercalcemia in the emergency department. Am J Med Sci. 2006;331(3):119–23.

4. Lindner G, Felber R, Schwarz C, et al. Hypercalcemia in the ED: prevalence, etiology, and outcome. Am J Emerg Med. 2013;31(4):657–60.

5. Catalano A, Chilà D, Bellone F, et al. Incidence of hypocalcemia and hypercalcemia in hospitalized patients: Is it changing? J Clin Transl Endocrinol. 2018;13:9–13.

6. Korkut S, Polat Ö, Kazancı MH, et al. Hypercalcemia in the emergency department: prevalence, etiology, and mortality rate. Med J Bakirkoy 2020;16(2):143–7.

7. Carroll MF, Schade DS. A practical approach to hypercalcemia. Am Fam Physician. 2003;67(9):1959–66.

8. Mousseaux C, Dupont A, Rafat C, et al. Epidemiology, clinical features, and management of severe hypercalcemia in critically ill patients. Ann Intensive Care. 2019;9(1):133.

9. Renaghan ADM, Rosner M. Hypercalcemia: etiology and management. Nephrol Dial Transpl. 2018;33(6):549–551.

10. Khoury N, Carmichael KA. Evaluation and therapy of hypercalcemia. Mo Med. 2011;108(2):99–103.

11. Bilezikian JP. Primary Hyperparathyroidism. J Clin Endocrinol Metab. 2018;103(11):3993–4004.

12. Afzal M, Kathuria P. Familial Hypocalciuric Hypercalcemia. [Updated 2021 Jul 23]. In: StatPearls [Internet]. Treasure Island (FL): StatPearls Publishing; 2021 Jan-. Available from: https://www.ncbi.nlm.nih.gov/books/NBK459190/.

13. Marx SJ. Familial Hypocalciuric Hypercalcemia as an Atypical Form of Primary Hyperparathyroidism. J Bone Miner Res. 2018;33(1):27–31.

14. Lafferty FW. Differential diagnosis of hypercalcemia. J Bone Miner Res 1991;6(Suppl 2):S51–S59.

15. Stewart AF. Clinical practice. Hypercalcemia associated with cancer. N Engl J Med 2005;352(4):373–379.

16. Gastanaga VM, Schwartzberg LS, Jain RK, et al. Prevalence of hypercalcemia among cancer patients in the United States. Cancer Med 2016;5(8):2091–100.

17. Zagzag J, Hu MI, Fisher SB, et al. Hypercalcemia and cancer: Differential diagnosis and treatment. CA Cancer J Clin. 2018;68(5):377–386.

18. Tebben PJ, Singh RJ, Kumar R. Vitamin D-Mediated Hypercalcemia: Mechanisms, Diagnosis, and Treatment. Endocr Rev. 2016;37(5):521–547.

19. Taylor PN, Davies JS. A review of the growing risk of vitamin D toxicity from inappropriate practice. Br J Clin Pharmacol. 2018;84(6):1121–1127.

20. Marcinowska-Suchowierska E, Kupisz-Urbańska M, Łukaszkiewicz J, et al. Vitamin D Toxicity-A Clinical Perspective. Front Endocrinol (Lausanne). 2018;9:550.

21. Çağlar A, Tuğçe Çağlar H. Vitamin D intoxication due to misuse: 5-year experience. Arch Pediatr. 2021;28(3):222–225.

22. Nguyen T, Joe D, Shah AD. Forget the phosphorus: A case of hypervitaminosis D-induced symptomatic hypercalcemia. Clin Nephrol Case Stud. 2021;9:1–3

23. Medarov BI. Milk-alkali syndrome. Mayo Clin Proc. 2009;84(3):261–267.

24. Patel V, Mehra D, Ramirez B, et al. Milk-Alkali Syndrome as a Cause of Hypercalcemia in a Gentleman With Acute Kidney Injury and Excessive Antacid Intake. Cureus. 2021;13(2):e13056.

25. Grieff M, Bushinsky DA. Diuretics and disorders of calcium homeostasis. Semin Nephrol. 2011;31(6):535–541.

26. Griebeler ML, Kearns AE, Ryu E, et al. Thiazide-Associated Hypercalcemia: Incidence and Association With Primary Hyperparathyroidism Over Two Decades. J Clin Endocrinol Metab. 2016;101(3):1166–1173.

27. Tettero JM, van Eeghen E, Kooter AJ. Extreme hypercalcaemia caused by immobilisation due to acute spinal cord injury. BMJ Case Rep. 2021;14(6):e241386.

28. Myśliwiec J. Mnemonics for endocrinologists: hyperparathyroidism. Endokrynologia Polska 2012;63(6):504–505.

29. Ma YB, Hu J, Duan YF. Acute pancreatitis connected with hypercalcemia crisis in hyperparathyroidism: A case report. World J Clin Cases. 2019;7(16):2367–2373.

30. Legrand SB. Modern management of malignant hypercalcemia. Am J Hosp Palliat Care. 2011;28(7):515–517.

31. Maier JD, Levine SN. Hypercalcemia in the intensive care unit: a review of pathophysiology, diagnosis, and modern therapy. J Intensive Care Med. 2015;30(5):235–252.

32. Carrick AI, Costner HB. Rapid Fire: Hypercalcemia. Emerg Med Clin North Am. 2018;36(3):549–555.

33. Farkas J. Hypercalcemia Internet Book of Critical Care, June 25, 2021. https://emcrit.org/ibcc/hypercalcemia/ Accessed 20 Dec 2021.

34. LeGrand SB, Leskuski D, Zama I. Narrative review: furosemide for hypercalcemia: an unproven yet common practice. Ann Intern Med. 2008;149(4):259–63.

35. Mirrakhimov AE. Hypercalcemia of Malignancy: An Update on Pathogenesis and Management. N Am J Med Sci. 2015;7(11):483–493.

36. Austin LA, Heath H III. Calcitonin: physiology and pathophysiology. N Engl J Med. 1981;304(5):269–278.

37. O'Doherty DP, Bickerstaff DR, McCloskey EV, et al. A comparison of the acute effects of subcutaneous and intranasal calcitonin. Clin Sci (Lond). 1990;78(2):215–9.

38. Klezlova R, Meystre C. Hypercalcemia of malignancy management. Specialist Palliative Audit and Guideline Group May 2019 Visit: http://www.wmcares.org.uk/wp-content/uploads/SPAGG_Hypercalcaemia_Jan-2020-Final-Version.pdf Searched on 21 Dec 2021.

39. Wang M, Cho C, Gray C, et al. Milk-alkali syndrome: a 'quick ease' or a 'long-lasting problem'. Endocrinol Diabetes Metab Case Rep. 2020;2020:EDM20–0028.

40. Cohen A, Shane E. Treatment of premenopausal women with low bone mineral density. Curr Osteoporos Rep. 2008;6(1):39–46.

41. Miller PD. The kidney and bisphosphonates. Bone. 2011;49(1):77–81.

42. Palmer S, Tillman F 3rd, Sharma P, et al. Safety of Intravenous Bisphosphonates for the Treatment of Hypercalcemia in Patients With Preexisting Renal Dysfunction. Ann Pharmacother. 2021;55(3):303–310.

43. Miller PD, Jamal SA, Evenepoel P, et al. Renal safety in patients treated with bisphosphonates for osteoporosis: a review. J Bone Miner Res. 2013;28(10):2049–59.

44. Hirschberg R. Renal complications from bisphosphonate treatment. Curr Opin Support Palliat Care. 2012;6(3):342–7.

45. Hanley DA, Adachi JD, Bell A, et al. Denosumab: mechanism of action and clinical outcomes. Int J Clin Pract. 2012;66(12):1139–46.

46. Karuppiah D, Thanabalasingham G, Shine B, et al. Refractory hypercalcaemia secondary to parathyroid carcinoma: response to high-dose denosumab. Eur J Endocrinol. 2014;171(1):K1–5.

47. Camus C, Charasse C, Jouannic-Montier I, et al. Calcium free hemodialysis: experience in the treatment of 33 patients with severe hypercalcemia. Intensive Care Med. 1996;22(2):116–21.

48. Loh HH, Mohd Noor N. The Use of Hemodialysis in Refractory Hypercalcemia Secondary to Parathyroid Carcinoma. Case Rep Crit Care 2014;2014:140906.

49. Trabulus S, Oruc M, Ozgun E, et al. The Use of Low-Calcium Hemodialysis in the Treatment of Hypercalcemic Crisis. Nephron. 2018;139(4):319–331.

50. Marouço CN, Caeiro F, da Costa BM, et al. The use of hemodialysis in hypercalcemic crisis secondary to primary hyperparathyroidism. Port J Nephrol Hypert 2021;35(2):123–127.

51. Bentata Y, Benabdelhak M, Haddiya I, et al. Severe hypercalcemia requiring acute hemodialysis: A retrospective cohort study with increased incidence during the Covid-19 pandemic. Am J Emerg Med. 2022;51:374–377.

52. Wilhelm SM, Wang TS, Ruan DT, et al. The American Association of Endocrine Surgeons Guidelines for Definitive Management of Primary Hyperparathyroidism. JAMA Surg. 2016;151(10):959–968.

53. National Guideline Centre (UK). Hyperparathyroidism (primary): diagnosis, assessment and initial management. London: National Institute for Health and Care Excellence (UK); 23 May 2019 May. (NICE Guideline, No. 132.). Visit: https://www.nice.org.uk/guidance/ng132.

26 | Hypophosphatemia

SERUM PHOSPHATE AND HYPOPHOSPHATEMIA

Phosphorus is a vital component of all body tissues and plays an essential role in various body functions. The terms phosphate and phosphorus are commonly used interchangeably.

BASIC PHYSIOLOGY

- Phosphate is the most abundant intracellular anion, the second-largest mineral in the body after calcium, and comprises approximately 1% of the body weight.

- Distribution: Most (about 85%) of the body's phosphorus is found within bone and teeth as hydroxyapatite, and the rest is distributed in tissues throughout the body. As only 1% of total body phosphorus is found in the extracellular fluid (ECF), the value of serum phosphorus may not necessarily reflect total body phosphorus content. In addition, even a change in pH leads to a shift of phosphate (acidosis shifts phosphate from intracellular fluid (ICF) to ECF) and affects the value of serum phosphorus.

- Normal value: Normal serum phosphorus levels in adults range from 2.5 to 4.5 mg/dL (0.75 to 1.45 mmol/L). It is best measured in the fasting state since there is as much as 50% diurnal variation (lower value in the morning and higher at night and after meals). Clinically, serum phosphorus level reflects nutritional status.

- Function: Phosphorus plays a major role in bone formation and is involved in cellular energy metabolism for almost all cellular functions (e.g., cell membranes, phospholipids, nucleic acids, acid buffering, enzyme systems, the energy carrier ATP-adenosine triphosphate, etc.).

• Dietary intake: The daily dietary phosphate intake is about 1000 mg per day. Foods rich in phosphorous are animal proteins (meats, chicken, fish, and egg), dairy products (cheese, chocolate, ice cream, and condensed milk), dry fruits, and certain vegetables (carrot, corn, groundnut, fresh peas, and sweet potato).

• Regulation: Four key organs involved in phosphate homeostasis are the small intestine, kidneys, bones, and parathyroid glands that tightly maintain serum phosphate in the normal range.

• Intestine absorption: In the intestine, phosphate absorption is largely unregulated, so increased phosphate intake in the diet increases phosphate absorption. 1,25-Dihydroxy vitamin D also increases gut absorption of phosphate phosphaturic.

• Renal handling: Under the influence of dietary, metabolic, and hormonal factors, kidneys modify phosphate excretion or absorption and regulate serum phosphate levels. The major factors that control phosphate balance are parathyroid hormone (PTH), fibroblast growth factor 23 (FGF23), active vitamin D (calcitriol), and insulin.

• Factors that increase renal phosphorus excretion: Elevated PTH levels, fibroblast growth factor 23 (FGF 23), a high dietary phosphate intake, ECF volume expansion, metabolic acidosis, and hypokalemia by increasing renal phosphorus excretion, decreases serum phosphate. FGF 23 is a potent phosphaturic hormone produced by osteocytes in response to hyperphosphatemia, high PTH, and increased calcitriol.

• Factors that decrease renal phosphorus excretion: High vitamin D levels, insulin, low PTH levels, and low dietary phosphate by decreasing renal phosphorus excretion increases serum phosphate.

• Regulation by PTH, FGF-23, and vitamin D: PTH and FGF-23 decrease serum phosphorous levels by causing significant phosphate loss in urine. Vitamin D increases serum phosphorous levels by increasing chiefly renal and, to some extent, intestinal phosphorous absorption.

• Conditions that stimulate cellular phosphate uptake and reduce serum phosphate are alkalemia, insulin, refeeding syndrome, hungry bone syndrome, and dextrose infusion.

• Calcium and phosphate balance are closely related, and they react in opposite ways in the body (when blood calcium levels increase, phosphate levels decrease).

HYPOPHOSPHATEMIA

Hypophosphatemia is defined as a serum phosphorus level <2.5 mg/dL (or <0.80 mmol/L). Based on serum phosphorus level, hypophosphatemia is classified into mild (2–2.5 mg/dL or 0.65–0.81 mmol/L), moderate (1–2 mg/dL or 0.32–0.65 mmol/L), or severe (<1 mg/dL or 0.32 mmol/L) degree.

Hypophosphatemia is uncommon in the general population but occurs in up to 5% of hospitalized patients, with a higher incidence in patients with trauma, alcoholism, diabetic ketoacidosis, sepsis, or ICU patients [1], and carries high mortality in ICU patients [2].

ETIOLOGY

Important causes of hypophosphatemia can be classified into four major groups: (1) Decreased intestinal absorption or intake, (2) Increased renal losses, (3) Internal redistribution, and (4) Other causes, as summarized in Table 26.1.

The most common causes of hypophosphatemia are respiratory alkalosis, sepsis, diabetic ketoacidosis, and the postoperative period.

Acute respiratory alkalosis

Acute respiratory alkalosis is one of the most common causes of hypophos-

---

Table 26.1 Causes of hypophosphatemia

1. **Decreased intestinal absorption/intake**
   - Vitamin D deficiency
   - Vitamin D dependant rickets type I and II
   - Malabsorption, phosphate binding antacids
   - Poor intake due to chronic protein malnutrition
2. **Increased renal excretion**
   - Hyperparathyroidism (primary or secondary)
   - Vitamin D deficiency
   - Phosphaturic drugs (diuretics, theophylline, corticosteroids)
   - X-linked hypophosphatemic rickets
   - Volume expansion
   - Fanconi syndrome
3. **Intracellular shift of phosphate**
   - Acute respiratory alkalosis
   - Dextrose infusion
   - Insulin therapy/refeeding syndrome
   - Hungry bone syndrome
4. **Other causes**
   - Metabolic alkalosis
   - Phosphate removal by renal replacement therapies
   - Diabetic ketoacidosis

---

phatemia which usually occurs due to the number of conditions that produce hyperventilation, such as sepsis, liver failure, pain, acute salicylate poisoning, and in patients who are being overventilated while on ventilator support [3, 4]. In respiratory alkalosis, an increase in intracellular pH stimulates glycolysis which shifts phosphorus into the cells and decreases serum phosphorus levels.

Sepsis

The mechanism causing hypophosphatemia in sepsis is unclear. But sepsis is a common cause of hypophosphatemia and is associated with a marked increase in mortality [5–7].

Increased insulin secretion

In refeeding syndrome, diabetic ketoacidosis, or rapid dextrose infusions, a high insulin concentration shifts phosphorus intracellularly and causes hypophosphatemia [8–10]. Patients with chronic alcoholism, anorexia nervosa, and chronic malnutrition are at greater risk of developing hypophosphatemia during carbohydrate refeeding.

Diabetic ketoacidosis (DKA)

Hypophosphatemia is common in DKA [11], and important causes of its development in DKA are: (1) Intracellular shifting of phosphate due to insulin therapy, volume expansion due to fluid repletion, and correction of acidosis; and (2) Increased urinary phosphate excretion for a prolonged period due to hyperglycemia-induced osmotic diuresis [12–14].

Hungry bone syndrome

A sudden decline in high PTH levels following Parathyroidectomy in patients with preexisting osteopenia causes marked deposition of calcium and phosphate in bone, leading to significant hypocalcemia and hypophosphatemia is called the hungry bone syndrome [15].

In postoperative period

Multiple causes which can combinedly cause severe hypophosphatemia after surgery are the administration of glucose and antacids, volume expansion, respiratory alkalosis secondary to pain, perioperative catecholamine surge, prior diuretic use, and poor oral intake [16].

CLINICAL FEATURES

The severity and chronicity of hypophosphatemia determine clinical manifestations. Mild hypophosphatemia is usually asymptomatic, and a wide variety of symptoms are usually evident when plasma phosphate is below 1 mg/dL (0.32 mmol/L).

Clinical manifestations of hypophosphatemia are due to three biochemical abnormalities, which are:

- Impairs intracellular energy production due to a decrease in intracellular adenosine triphosphate (ATP), causing disruption of essential cellular functions in multiple organ systems leading to most symptoms.

- Reduction in erythrocyte 2,3-DPG (diphosphoglycerate) increases the affinity of hemoglobin for oxygen, resulting in decreased oxygen delivery to peripheral tissues, which is responsible for hematological symptoms.

- Prolonged defect in mineral metabolism causing musculoskeletal complaints, including deformities in chronic hypophosphatemia.

A. Acute hypophosphatemia

Muscular symptoms: Proximal muscle weakness is the most common symptom of hypophosphatemia. Other symptoms may include weak hand grip, slurred speech, dysphagia, and ileus. In addition, rhabdomyolysis may occur in patients with acute severe hypophosphatemia, commonly amongst alcoholics and patients receiving parenteral nutrition without phosphate supplementation [17].

Respiratory symptoms: In severe hypophosphatemia, respiratory failure can occur due to weakness of the diaphragm and respiratory muscles, which may cause hypoxia. Due to severe hypophosphatemia, failure to wean from ventilation resulting in prolonged ventilator dependency is common in the ICU [18].

Cardiac symptoms: Impaired myocardial contractility causing heart failure, increased requirement of vasoactive drug support following cardiac surgery, and cardiac arrhythmias are severe but uncommon manifestations.

Neurological symptoms: Severe hypophosphatemia may cause variable neurological symptoms such as paresthesia, altered mental status, confusion, and lethargy, which can progress to seizures or coma.

Hematological symptoms: Impaired function and decreased life span of all cell lineages. Red blood cell dysfunction causes tissue hypoxia and increased erythrocyte rigidity, predisposing hemolysis. Leukocyte dysfunction causes impaired phagocytosis and granulocyte chemotaxis leading to increased susceptibility to gram-negative sepsis.

Platelet dysfunction causes thrombocytopenia and petechial hemorrhages.

In clinical practice, suspect or anticipate hypophosphatemia and check phosphate levels before or during therapy in patients with refeeding syndrome, diabetic ketoacidosis, hyperosmolar hyperglycemic nonketotic syndrome, continuous renal replacement therapy (CRRT), and failure or difficulty to weaning from ventilation [19].

B. Chronic hypophosphatemia

Prolonged hypophosphatemia causes mineralization defects leading to pain in muscles and bones, rickets in children, osteomalacia in adults, and fractures.

DIAGNOSIS

A stepwise approach to hypophosphatemia is summarized [20, 21].

Step 1: History and physical examination

Detailed history and physical examination often provide clues for the etiology of hypophosphatemia. Attention should be paid to dietary intake,

alcoholism, diarrhea, medications, and IV fluids infused. The presence of skeletal deformities, bone pain, muscle weakness, and a history of nontraumatic fractures suggest chronic hypophosphatemia. Hypophosphatemia rickets in children is characterized by skeletal deformities (e.g., leg bowing) and short stature with bone pain.

Step 2: Basic investigations

To narrow down the differential diagnosis of hypophosphatemia, investigations commonly ordered are serum sodium, potassium, calcium, magnesium, PTH, vitamin D levels, alkaline phosphatase, serum protein, serum creatinine, and acid-base parameters (respiratory alkalosis). These test helps to diagnose many common causes (Figure 26.1).

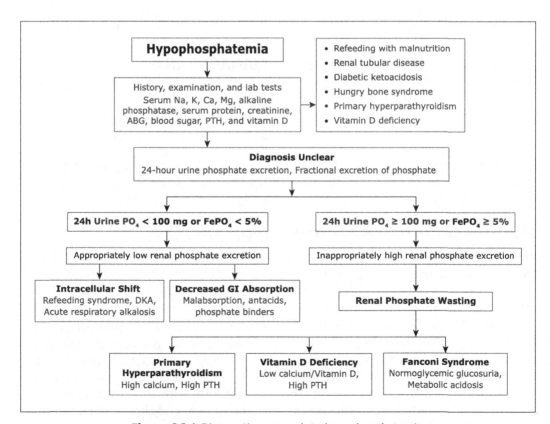

Figure 26.1 Diagnostic approach to hypophosphatemia.

Step 3: Measurement of urinary phosphate excretion

When the diagnosis is not clear, urinary phosphate excretion is measured either by a 24-hour urine collection (24h Urine PO_4) or by calculating the fractional excretion of filtered phosphate ($FePO_4$) from a random urine specimen. The usual response to hypophosphatemia is 24-hour urine phosphate excretion less than 100 mg or a $FePO_4$ less than 5 percent.

In patients with hypophosphatemia

A 24-hour urine phosphate excretion less than 100 mg or a $FePO_4$ less than 5 percent reflects appropriate low renal phosphate excretion, which can occur due to hypophosphatemia because of:

1. Intracellular shift of phosphate (e.g., refeeding syndrome, acute respiratory alkalosis).

2. Decreased intestinal absorption (e.g., malabsorption, chronic antacid therapy, phosphate binders).

A 24-hour urine phosphate excretion greater than or equal to 100 mg or a $FePO_4$ greater than or equal to 5 percent reflects renal phosphate wasting, which can occur due to hyperparathyroidism, Fanconi syndrome, vitamin D deficiency, and other causes.

Step 4: Measure serum PTH and vitamin D levels

In patients with renal phosphate wasting, serum calcium, PTH, and vitamin D levels help to diagnose hyperparathyroidism, vitamin D deficiency, or Fanconi syndrome:

- Primary hyperparathyroidism: High calcium with high PTH in patients with hypophosphatemia and renal phosphate wasting suggests hyperparathyroidism.

- Vitamin D deficiency: Low calcium with high PTH in patients with hypophosphatemia and renal phosphate wasting suggests vitamin D deficiency (serum 25-hydroxyvitamin D levels may be low or inappropriately normal).

- Fanconi syndrome: In a urine test, uricosuria, aminoaciduria, normoglycemic glucosuria, and phosphaturia are diagnostic.

Step 5: Other helpful tests

High serum creatine phosphokinase (CPK) level is suggestive of rhabdomyolysis.

In very few selected patients, Fibroblast Growth Factor 23 (FGF23) level is measured, and its high level is found in hereditary forms of hypophosphatemic rickets (X-linked hypophosphatemia-XLH) and oncogenic osteomalacia/tumor-induced osteomalacia (TIO).

MANAGEMENT

Treatment of hypophosphatemia depends on the severity (mild, moderate, or severe), symptoms (asymptomatic or severely symptomatic), onset (acute or chronic), coexisting problems requiring cautions (like renal failure, hypercalcemia, or hypocalcemia), and underlying condition [22].

Basic principles

- In mild cases, increased intake of dietary phosphorus may be adequate. Skim milk is an excellent source of phosphorus (900 mg/L).

- Oral phosphate repletion is safer and preferred over IV phosphate therapy and is administered in mild hypophosphatemia, asymptomatic patients with moderate hypophosphatemia, and chronic hypophosphatemia [20].

- IV phosphate administration is generally reserved for symptomatic moderate hypophosphatemia, severe acute hypophosphatemia, or patients unable to take oral phosphate preparations [20]. The goal of acute IV phosphate therapy in hypophosphatemia is to raise the serum phosphorus concentration to a safe range (>1.0 mg/dL) and correct the symptoms of hypophosphatemia. Subsequently, IV therapy is switched to oral phosphate therapy.

- Based on the severity of hypophosphatemia, the selection of route and dose of phosphate preparations is summarized in Table 26.2. Commonly used oral and IV phosphate preparations and their phosphate, sodium, and potassium content are outlined in Table 26.3.

- The usual dose for oral phosphate supplementation is 40–80 mmol daily in 3–4 divided doses (1–2 packets/ tablet of PHOS-NAK or K$^+$ PHOS Neutral 3–4 times daily). Limitations of oral phosphate preparations are unpredictable absorption and side effects like nausea, diarrhea, and abdominal pain.

- For IV administration, IV sodium or potassium phosphate preparations are diluted in either normal saline or 5% dextrose and infused slowly (usually, the rate should not exceed 7.5 mmol per hour) with serum phosphate monitoring every 12–24 hours. In patients with coexisting hypokalemia, potassium phosphate is preferred, while sodium sodium phosphate is chosen in patients with hyperkalemia.

- As magnesium deficiency often coexists with hypophosphatemia, look for it and treat it.

Precautions

Precautions required during phosphate replacement are:

- Hypercalcemia: Risk of increased calcium-phosphate product due to phosphate replacement in hypercalcemia, which may precipitate in tissues (calciphylaxis).

- Hypocalcemia: Risk of rapid lowering of calcium causing hypocalcemia due to IV phosphate infusion.

- Chronic kidney disease: Risk of developing hyperphosphatemia due to phosphate accumulation, so administer about 50% lower dose of phosphate.

- Diabetic ketoacidosis: Insulin therapy stimulate cellular phosphate uptake

Table 26.2 Treatment of hypophosphatemia					
Severity	Serum phosphate	Symptoms	Preferred route	Dose of oral phosphate	Dose-IV phosphate
Mild	2.0–2.5 mg/dL 0.65–0.81 mmol/L	Asymptomatic	Oral	40–80 mmol in 4–5 divided doses	0.08–0.16 mmol/kg
Moderate	1.0–2.0 mg/dL 0.32–0.65 mmol/L	Asymptomatic	Oral	40–80 mmol in 4–5 divided doses	0.16–0.32 mmol/kg
		Symptomatic	IV	Oral phosphate preparations are not preferred	0.32–1.0 mmol/kg
Severe	<1.0 mg/dL <0.3 mmol/L	Symptomatic			
Injection of sodium phosphate and potassium phosphate both provide 3 mmol of phosphates per milliliter					

Table 26.3 Oral and IV phosphate preparations

Preparation	Phosphate content	Sodium content	Potassium content
Oral preparation			
Skim milk (1 liter)	1.0 gm 32 mmol/L	28 mEq	38 mEq
PHOS-NAK powder (1 packet 1.5 gm)	250 mg 8.0 mmol	6.9 mEq 160 mg	7.1 mEq 280 mg
K-PHOS neutral tablet	250 mg 8.0 mmol	13.0 mEq 298 mg	1.1 mEq 45 mg
K-PHOS original tablet	114 mg 3.68 mmol	0	3.7 mEq 144 mg
K-Phos no. 2 tablet	250 mg 8.0 mmol	5.8 mEq 134 mg	2.3 mEq 88 mg
IV preparation			
Inj. sodium phosphate	3.0 mmol/mL	4.0 mEq	0
Inj. potassium phosphate	3.0 mmol/mL	0	4.4 mEq

and reduces serum phosphate causing hypophosphatemia. But the routine replacement of phosphate is not recommended because of the lack of benefits and the ability of normal dietary phosphate intake to correct it [11, 13]. However, phosphate replacement is necessary for selected patients with severe hypophosphatemia (serum phosphate concentration <1.0 mg/dL), cardiac dysfunction, hemolytic anemia, and/or respiratory depression [23, 24].

- Hypoparathyroidism: As hypocalcemia is common in patients with hypoparathyroidism, replace phosphate cautiously to avoid the aggravation of hypocalcemia.

Correction of underlying causes

- Vitamin D deficiency: Supplementation of vitamin D.
- Fanconi syndrome: Treated usually with oral phosphate, active vitamin D, administration of alkali, and fluid deficit correction.

- Hypophosphataemic rickets: Treated with a combination of high dose oral phosphate supplementation and calcitriol [25]. Recently, a monoclonal antibody targeted to FGF23 called burosumab has been approved to treat X-linked hypophosphatemia [26]. This novel therapy may be used in selected patients with disease refractory to conventional therapy, but cost and availability are major limitations [25].

REFERENCES

1. Gaasbeek A, Meinders AE. Hypophosphatemia: an update on its etiology and treatment. Am J Med. 2005;118(10):1094–1101.

2. Wang L, Xiao C, Chen L et al. Impact of hypophosphatemia on outcome of patients in intensive care unit: a retrospective cohort study. BMC Anesthesiol. 2019;19(1):86.

3. Halevy J, Bulvik S. Severe hypophosphatemia in hospitalized patients. Arch Intern Med. 1988;148(1):153–155.

4. O'Brien TM, Coberly L. Severe Hypophosphatemia in Respiratory Alkalosis. Adv Stud Med. 2003;3(6):345–348.

5. Barak V, Schwartz A, Kalickman I, et al. Prevalence of hypophosphatemia in sepsis and infection: the role of cytokines. Am J Med. 1998;104(1):40–7.

6. Khan AA, Mir AA, Vani ZA, et al. Significance of hypophosphatemia as an indicator of Gram negative sepsis. International Journal of Health and Clinical Research, 2021;4(10):63–66.

7. Shor R, Halabe A, Rishver S, et al. Severe hypophosphatemia in sepsis as a mortality predictor. Ann Clin Lab Sci. 2006;36(1):67–72.

8. Marinella MA. Refeeding syndrome and hypophosphatemia. J Intensive Care Med. 2005;20(3):155–9.

9. Kebler R, McDonald FD, Cadnapaphornchai P. Dynamic changes in serum phosphorus levels in diabetic ketoacidosis. Am J Med 1985;79(5):571–6.

10. Rasmussen A. Hypophosphatemia during postoperative glucose infusion. Acta Chir Scand. 1985;151(6):497–500.

11. van der Vaart A, Waanders F, van Beek AP, et al. Incidence and determinants of hypophosphatemia in diabetic ketoacidosis: an observational study. BMJ Open Diab Res Care 2021;9(1):e002018.

12. Wolfsdorf J, Craig ME, Daneman D, et al. Diabetic ketoacidosis in children and adolescents with diabetes. Pediatr Diabetes. 2009;10(12):118–33.

13. Ditzel J, Lervang HH. Disturbance of inorganic phosphate metabolism in diabetes mellitus: clinical manifestations of phosphorus-depletion syndrome during recovery from diabetic ketoacidosis. Diabetes Metab Syndr Obes. 2010;3:319–324.

14. Choi HS, Kwon A, Chae HW, et al. Respiratory failure in a diabetic ketoacidosis patient with severe hypophosphatemia. Ann Pediatr Endocrinol Metab. 2018;23(2):103–106.

15. Witteveen JE, van Thiel S, Romijn JA, et al. Hungry bone syndrome: still a challenge in the post-operative management of primary hyperparathyroidism: a systematic review of the literature. Eur J Endocrinol. 2013;168(3):R45–53.

16. Narayan A, Subramanian A. Severe hypophosphataemia: a rare cause of postoperative muscle weakness. BMJ Case Rep. 2018;2018:bcr2017221193.

17. Knochel JP, Barcenas C, Cotton JR, et al. Hypophosphatemia and rhabdomyolysis. J Clin Invest. 1978;62(6):1240–1246.

18. Zhao Y, Li Z, Shi Y, et al. Effect of hypophosphatemia on the withdrawal of mechanical ventilation in patients with acute exacerbations of chronic obstructive pulmonary disease. Biomed Rep 2016;4(4):413–416.

19. Farkas J. Hypophosphatemia. Internet Book of Critical Care, May 9, 2019. Visit: https://emcrit.org/ibcc/hypophos/ Accessed 1 January 2022.

20. Florenzano P, Cipriani C, Roszko KL, et al. Approach to patients with hypophosphataemia. Lancet Diabetes Endocrinol. 2020;8(2):163–174.

21. Imel EA, Econs MJ. Approach to the hypophosphatemic patient. J Clin Endocrinol Metab. 2012;97(3):696–706.

22. García Martín A, Varsavsky M, Cortés Berdonces M, et al. Phosphate disorders and clinical management of hypophosphatemia and hyperphosphatemia. Endocrinol Diabetes Nutr (Engl Ed). 2020;67(3):205–215.

23. Kitabchi AE, Umpierrez GE, Miles JM, et al. Hyperglycemic crises in adult patients with diabetes. Diabetes Care. 2009;32(7):1335–43.

24. Wolfsdorf JI, Allgrove J, Craig ME, et al. ISPAD Clinical Practice Consensus Guidelines 2014. Diabetic ketoacidosis and hyperglycemic hyperosmolar state. Pediatr Diabetes. 2014;15 Suppl 20:154–79.

25. Haffner D, Emma F, Eastwood DM, et al. Clinical practice recommendations for the diagnosis and management of X-linked hypophosphataemia. Nat Rev Nephrol. 2019;15(7):435–455.

26. Lyseng-Williamson KA. Burosumab in X-linked hypophosphatemia: a profile of its use in the USA. Drugs Ther Perspect 2018;34(11):497–506.

27 | Hyperphosphatemia

Hyperphosphatemia is defined as serum phosphate concentration greater than 4.5 mg/dL (1.45 mmol/L) in adults.

Renal excretion of phosphate is very effective, and therefore the person with normal renal function is unlikely to develop hyperphosphatemia because of increased phosphate intake. Therefore, Hyperphosphatemia is rare in the general population but commonly occurs in later stages of chronic kidney disease (CKD) with significantly impaired kidney function [1].

ETIOLOGY

Based on the mechanism of its development, the causes of hyperphosphatemia can be classified into four groups [1].

Decreased renal phosphate excretion

- Impaired renal phosphate excretion: Acute kidney injury (AKI) or chronic kidney disease with significant renal impairment are the most common cause of hyperphosphatemia [2].

- Increased renal tubular reabsorption: Hypoparathyroidism, vitamin D toxicity, acromegaly or thyrotoxicosis.

Transcellular shift

Transcellular shift from intracellular fluid (ICF) to extracellular fluid (ECF)

- Extensive cell destruction: Rhabdomyolysis, tumor lysis syndrome, or massive hemolysis.

- Severe acidosis: Severe lactic acidosis, diabetic acidosis and respiratory acidosis.

- Lack of insulin: Diabetic ketoacidosis (before treatment).

Acute massive phosphate load

Administration of phosphate-containing laxatives or enemas and IV or oral phosphate administration.

Spurious or pseudohypophosphatemia

The falsely elevated phosphate levels due to laboratory artifact (interference in phosphate assay) is a relatively rare condition seen in patients with hyperglobulinemia (e.g., multiple myeloma), hyperlipidemia, hyperbilirubinemia, and certain medications (e.g., amphotericin B and heparin) [3].

CLINICAL FEATURES

Hyperphosphatemia itself is usually asymptomatic, and presenting symptoms are related to:

1. Hypocalcemia: It is a common reason for clinical presentation in patients with hyperphosphatemia causing weakness, muscle cramps, paresthesia, tetany, positive Chvostek's sign and Trousseau's sign, laryngospasms, confusion, and seizure.

2. Metastatic calcification: In a few patients with severe chronic hyperphosphatemia, the high calcium-phosphate product increases the risk of calciphylaxis (the precipitation of calcium phosphate in tissues), resulting in soft-tissue and smaller blood vessels calcification leading to clinical manifestations such as cutaneous necrosis and skin ulceration.

Multiplication of the total calcium and phosphate (measured in mg/dL) determines the calcium-phosphate product. When the serum calcium-phosphorus product ($Ca^{2+} \times Pi$) is above 70 mg2/dL2, the risk of calciphylaxis is high.

In CKD, untreated chronic hyperphosphatemia carries risks of developing complications like secondary hyperparathyroidism, renal osteodystrophy, and metastatic calcification.

3. Symptoms of an underlying disease: More commonly, the patient presents with symptoms related to the underlying condition that causes hyperphosphatemia.

DIAGNOSIS

Step 1: History and physical examination

Detailed history and physical examination provide the clue for underlying etiology in many cases of hyperphosphatemia.

Step 2: Measure serum creatinine

Measure serum creatinine level first to assess renal function, as renal failure is the most common cause of hyperphosphatemia. If creatinine is high, a workup is necessary to differentiate between AKI and CKD.

Step 3: Further investigations

Further investigations are helpful if the diagnosis is unclear and for the complete assessment of patients with hyperphosphatemia:

- Complete blood count: Low hemoglobin in CKD and hemolysis.
- Electrolytes: To detect associated electrolyte disturbances.
- Blood glucose: To detect diabetic ketoacidosis.
- Serum calcium level: High levels in vitamin D intoxication (high Ca^{2+}, high PHO_4, low parathyroid hormone [PTH]). Low levels in hypoparathyroidism (low Ca^{2+}, high PHO_4, low PTH), and CKD (low Ca^{2+}, high PHO_4, high PTH).
- Vitamin D level: High levels in vitamin D intoxication (high PHO_4, high Ca^{2+}, low PTH).

- PTH: Low levels in hypoparathyroidism (low PTH, high PHO_4, low Ca^{2+}), and high levels in CKD (high PTH, high PHO_4, low Ca^{2+}).

- Uric acid: Tumor lysis syndrome is characterized by hyperuricemia, hyperphosphatemia, hypocalcemia, and hyperkalemia.

- Creatinine kinase: High levels in rhabdomyolysis.

- Lactate dehydrogenase: High levels in hemolysis.

- Fractional phosphate excretion: This test is helpful in assessing urinary phosphate excretion. Increased fractional excretion of phosphate (>15%) suggests excess phosphate load (e.g., rhabdomyolysis, excess use of a phosphate-containing laxative or enema use, or phosphate toxicity). In comparison, its decreased value (<15%) suggests impaired renal excretion of phosphate (e.g., renal failure, hypoparathyroidism, ECF volume depletion, and tumoral calcinosis).

- X-ray studies: Helps to detect defective bone development in chronic hyperphosphatemia and metastatic calcifications.

- Electrocardiogram (ECG) to detect a prolonged QT interval, a common ECG change in hypocalcemia.

MANAGEMENT

The treatment of hyperphosphatemia is planned according to etiology, severity, rapidity of onset, and kidney function.

A. Treatment of underlying etiology

As this is the most important and effective measure, no other therapies are often required to correct hyperphosphatemia (e.g., hyperphosphatemia in diabetic ketoacidosis usually improves rapidly with insulin administration and correction of metabolic acidosis). In addition to treating the cause, it is important to search for and remove exogenous phosphate supplementation of any form.

B. Acute Hyperphosphatemia

In patients with normal renal function, hyperphosphatemia usually resolves within 6 to 12 hours. In acute severe hyperphosphatemia with intact kidney functions, measures to increase the renal excretion of phosphate are:

- **Saline infusion:** Extracellular volume expansion with IV normal saline solution can increase urinary phosphate excretion significantly.

- **Loop diuretics:** Concomitant use of loop diuretics helps in renal phosphate excretion.

- **Acetazolamide:** The administration of acetazolamide also helps increase the urinary excretion of phosphate.

- **Hemodialysis:** Hemodialysis is the most effective therapy in the treatment of hyperphosphatemic patients with severely impaired renal function due to conditions like rhabdomyolysis or tumor lysis syndrome, where conservative measures are unsuccessful. It is also indicated in cases of severe symptomatic acute hypocalcemia, where treatment with injected calcium carries the risk of widespread soft tissue calcification in the presence of high phosphate levels.

C. Chronic hyperphosphatemia

Chronic hyperphosphatemia is common in chronic kidney disease and CKD patients receiving hemodialysis. These patients need due attention because of the risk of developing cardiovascular morbidity and mortality, vascular classification, secondary hyperparathyroidism, and hospitalization [4].

The treatment strategies recommended by KDOQI (2020) and KDIGO (2017) for chronic hyperphosphatemia are dietary restriction of phosphate, phosphate binders, and dialysis therapy [5, 6].

Dietary phosphate restriction

Restricting phosphate intake to about 800 to 1000 mg/d in the diet is frequently the first and important step in treating hyperphosphatemia [4, 6]. Avoid phosphorus-rich food like milk and dairy products (e.g., cheese, cottage cheese, ice cream), meat (especially organ meats), whole grains, processed foods, and carbonated beverages containing phosphoric acid.

Oral phosphate binders

Phosphate binders help to control hyperphosphatemia by reducing the absorption of dietary phosphate in the gastrointestinal tract. Oral phosphate binders are indicated when hyperphosphatemia increases persistently or progressively despite dietary phosphate restriction.

Oral phosphate binders are divided into three main types:

- Calcium-containing binders (calcium carbonate or calcium acetate).
- Non-calcium binders (sevelamer, lanthanum carbonate, or sucroferric oxyhydroxide).
- Aluminum-containing phosphate binders.

Appropriate phosphate binders are selected based on the patient's serum calcium level, cost, pill burden, iron stores, individual tolerability, and the drug's side effect profile [7, 8].

- **Calcium acetate and calcium carbonate** are the most widely used agents and are effective when administered with meals. The drawback of calcium-based binders is the risk of hypercalcemia and vascular calcification, so avoid it in patients with hypercalcemia, vitamin D intoxication, and Ca^{2+}-Phos product >66.

- **Sevelamer** is a calcium-free phosphate binder that corrects hyperphosphatemia as much as calcium-containing binders with advantages such as no risk of hypercalcemia, reduction in cardiovascular mortality, a significant decrease in serum total cholesterol and low-density lipoprotein cholesterol, and prevention and improvement in vascular calcification [9, 10]. However, drawbacks of sevelamer are high cost, increased pill burden, gastrointestinal intolerance such as nausea and constipation, and a recent large study that failed to demonstrate cardiovascular events or all-cause mortality benefits in dialysis and nondialysis CKD patients [11–14].

- **Lanthanum:** This non-calcium-based phosphate binder is available as a chewable tablet, an alternative treatment for hyperphosphatemia in patients with CKD. Lanthanum offers advantages such as a low pill burden, high efficacy (roughly twice as potent as calcium and sevelamer), and lower incidences of over-suppression of PTH levels [15, 16]. But limitations of this phosphate binder are its relatively high cost, concerns regarding possible toxicity from accumulation [17], and lack of superiority to prevent cardiovascular events. The recent landmark trial (2021) failed to demonstrate a significant difference in composite cardiovascular events when lanthanum carbonate is compared with calcium carbonate [18].

- **Aluminum hydroxide** is effective and well-tolerated, but its prolonged use is currently avoided due to the risk of aluminum toxicity causing adynamic bone disease, encephalopathy, microcytic anemia, and premature death [6].

- **Other phosphate binders:** Drugs like Sucroferric Oxyhydroxide, Ferric Citrate, Nicotinic Acid and Nicotinamide, Tenapanor, and Magnesium Carbonate are also used as phosphate binders.

Renal replacement therapies

In patients with CKD-ESRD on maintenance dialysis, conventional hemodialysis, and peritoneal dialysis, both remove phosphate. However, removing excess phosphate by standard dialysis therapy is inadequate to reduce serum phosphate concentration in the normal range.

For the effective removal of phosphate and better control of hyperphosphatemia, increased frequency and duration of hemodialysis or modality like hemodiafiltration are recommended [4].

REFERENCES

1. Leaf DE, Wolf M. A physiologic-based approach to the evaluation of a patient with hyperphosphatemia. Am J Kidney Dis. 2013;61(2):330–6.

2. García Martín A, Varsavsky M, Cortés Berdonces M, et al. Phosphate disorders and clinical management of hypophosphatemia and hyperphosphatemia. Endocrinol Diabetes Nutr (Engl Ed). 2020;67(3):205–215.

3. Liamis G, Liberopoulos E, Barkas F, et al. Spurious electrolyte disorders: a diagnostic challenge for clinicians. Am J Nephrol. 2013;38(1):50–7.

4. Vallée M, Weinstein J, Battistella M, et al. Multidisciplinary Perspectives of Current Approaches and Clinical Gaps in the Management of Hyperphosphatemia. Int J Nephrol Renovasc Dis. 2021;14:301–311.

5. Ikizler TA, Burrowes JD, Byham-Gray LD, et al. KDOQI clinical practice guideline for nutrition in CKD: 2020 update. Am J Kidney Dis. 2020;76(3):S1–S107.

6. Ketteler M, Block GA, Evenepoel P, et al. Executive summary of the 2017 KDIGO chronic kidney disease–mineral and bone disorder (CKD-MBD) guideline update: what's changed and why it matters. Kidney Int. 2017;92(1):26–36.

7. Sekar A, Kaur T, Nally JV, et al. Phosphorus binders: The new and the old, and how to choose. Cleve Clin J Med. 2018;85(8):629–638.

8. Ketteler M, Block GA, Evenepoel P, et al. Diagnosis, evaluation, prevention, and treatment of chronic kidney disease-mineral and bone disorder: synopsis of the kidney disease: Improving Global Outcomes 2017 Clinical Practice Guideline Update. Ann Intern Med. 2018;168(6):422–30.

9. Evenepoel P, Selgas R, Caputo F, et al. Efficacy and safety of sevelamer hydrochloride and calcium acetate in patients on peritoneal dialysis. Nephrol Dial Transplant. 2009;24(1):278–285.

10. Patel L, Bernard LM, Elder GJ. Sevelamer Versus Calcium-Based Binders for Treatment of Hyperphosphatemia in CKD: A Meta-Analysis of Randomized Controlled Trials. Clin J Am Soc Nephrol 2016;11(2):232–44.

11. Manns B, Klarenbach S, Lee H, et al. Economic evaluation of sevelamer in patients with end-stage renal disease. Nephrol Dial Transplant 2007;22(10):2867–78.

12. Chan S, Au K, Francis RS, et al. Phosphate binders in patients with chronic kidney disease. Aust Prescr. 2017;40(1):10–14.

13. Spoendlin J, Paik JM, Tsacogianis T, et al. Cardiovascular Outcomes of Calcium-Free vs Calcium-Based Phosphate Binders in Patients 65 Years or Older With End-stage Renal Disease Requiring Hemodialysis. JAMA Intern Med 2019;179(6):741–749.

14. Lioufas NM, Pascoe EM, Hawley CM, et al. Systematic Review and Meta-Analyses of the Effects of Phosphate-Lowering Agents in Nondialysis CKD. J Am Soc Nephrol. 2022;33(1):59–76.

15. Finn WF, SPD 405–307 Lanthanum Study Group. Lanthanum carbonate versus standard therapy for the treatment of hyperphosphatemia: safety and efficacy in chronic maintenance hemodialysis patients. Clin Nephrol 2006;65(3):191–202.

16. Zhao L, Liu A, Xu G. Safety and effectiveness of lanthanum carbonate for hyperphosphatemia in chronic kidney disease (CKD) patients: a meta-analysis. Ren Fail. 2021;43(1):1378–1393.

17. Drüeke TB. Lanthanum carbonate as a first-line phosphate binder: the "cons". Semin Dial. 2007;20(4):329–32.

18. Ogata H, Fukagawa M, Hirakata H, et al. Effect of Treating Hyperphosphatemia With Lanthanum Carbonate vs Calcium Carbonate on Cardiovascular Events in Patients With Chronic Kidney Disease Undergoing Hemodialysis: The LANDMARK Randomized Clinical Trial. JAMA. 2021;325(19):1946–1954.

28 | Hypomagnesemia

Disorder of magnesium, especially hypomagnesemia, is expected particularly in ICU patients and usually occurs due to renal and gastrointestinal (GI) losses. However, hypermagnesemia is a less frequent disorder than hypomagnesemia, and its most common cause is renal failure.

BASIC PHYSIOLOGY

- Magnesium is the fourth most common cation of the body (after Na^+, K^+, and Ca^{2+}), the second most common intracellular cation (after K^+), and the commonest intracellular divalent cation.

- **Distribution:** About 60% of body magnesium is in bones, 39% is within the cells, and only 1% is in extracellular fluid (ECF). Up to 40% of total plasma magnesium is protein-bound, 5–10% is in complex form, and about 50–55% is in a free, ionized form, which is a biologically active ion (like calcium).

- **Normal blood ranges:** The normal serum magnesium level is 1.7 to 2.1 mg/dL (0.70 to 0.85 mmol/L, 1.4 to 1.7 mEq/L), and their values in magnesium disorders are summarized in Table 28.1.

- As the clinical effects of magnesium disorders are determined primarily

Table 28.1 Interpretation of serum magnesium concentration

Hypomagnesemia			Normal range	Hypermagnesemia		
Severe	Moderate	Mild		Mild	Moderate	Severe
<1.0 mg/dL	1.0-1.5 mg/dL	1.6-1.9 mg/dL	1.7-2.1 mg/dL	4.8-7.2 mg/dL	7.2-12 mg/dL	>12 mg/dL
<0.5 mmol/L	0.4-0.6 mmol/L	0.7-0.8 mmol/L	0.70-0.85 mmol/L	2.0-3.0 mmol/L	3.0-5.0 mmol/L	>5 mmol/L
<0.8 mEq/L	0.8-1.2 mEq/L	1.4-1.6 mEq/L	1.4-1.7 mEq/L	4.0-6.0 mEq/L	6.0-10 mEq/L	>10 mEq/L
Conversion factors for serum magnesium: 1 mEq/L = 1.2 mg/dL = 0.5 mmol/L						

by tissue magnesium content, serum magnesium levels have limited diagnostic value.

- **Physiological function:** Magnesium is a cofactor in oxidative-phosphory-lation reactions in mitochondria and plays an important physiological role in over 600 enzymatic reactions [1]. Magnesium helps in physiological processes like glucose and fat metabolism, DNA and protein synthesis, and oxidative phosphorylation and plays a vital role in neuromuscular transmission, cardiovascular excitability, contraction of muscles, and secretion of parathyroid hormone (PTH) hormone [2].

- **Effect on serum calcium:** A change in magnesium concentration also affects serum calcium level because the release of parathyroid hormone and its effect on the target organ is regulated by magnesium. It is important to note that hypocalcemia due to suppressed PTH secretion or action occurs in hypomagnesemia [3, 4] and hypermagnesemia [5, 6]. But hypocalcemia is usually symptomatic in hypomagnesemia, and it is transient and may not be symptomatic in hypermagnesemia.

- **Recommended intake:** The daily magnesium intake recommended in adults is 400–420 mg for men and 310–320 mg for women.

- **Regulation:** Two major regulatory mechanisms of magnesium homeostasis are intestinal absorption and renal excretion. Considering the serum magnesium levels and dietary magnesium intake, coordination of function and dynamic balance between the intestinal and renal transport and bone exchange maintains the balance of magnesium [7]. Two distinctive features of

magnesium homeostasis, in contrast to other ions, are:

a. No single hormone plays a substantial role in magnesium homeostasis [8]. Because of the lack of specific endocrine control, this essential mineral is often termed the "orphan ion" [9].

b. 60% of body magnesium is stored in bones as bioapatite, which does not exchange readily with circulating magnesium. Due to the inability to mobilize the stored magnesium readily in the state of magnesium depletion, plasma magnesium concentration may fall.

- **Gastrointestinal absorption:** Approximately 30%–40% of dietary magnesium is absorbed. Absorption occurs primarily in the jejunum and ileum via a non-saturable passive paracellular pathway (90%), and smaller amounts are absorbed in the colon, mainly via a saturable active transcellular pathway (10%) involving TRPM6/7 (Transcellular teceptor potential channel melastatin member) channel proteins [10]. Gastrointestinal magnesium absorption increases with magnesium depletion, a low magnesium diet, and calcitriol, while a high magnesium diet and foods rich in calcium, phosphate, and fibers decrease GI absorption.

Kidney handling and excretion: The kidney plays a major role in regulating magnesium homeostasis [11]. Approximately 80 percent of the free and non-protein-bound magnesium ions are ultrafiltered at the glomerulus. Out of which, up to 96% of filtered magnesium is reabsorbed (15 to 25% in the proximal tubule, 60 to 70% in the thick ascending limb of the loop of Henle (TAL), and 5 to 10% in the distal tubule). So renal handling of magnesium transport differs from that of most other ions (i.e., the proximal tubule is not the major site of reabsorption, and the primary site of magnesium transport is the thick ascending limb of the loop of Henle).

Reabsorption of magnesium in thick ascending limbs of the loops of Henle occurs passively with calcium through paracellular tight junctions secondary to a lumen-positive electrochemical gradient. Conversely, magnesium reabsorption occurs in the distal convoluted tubule by an active transcellular process.

The kidney keeps serum magnesium in a narrow range by various factors regulating magnesium transport in the TAL and distal collecting tubules [7].

- **Factors increasing magnesium reabsorption:** Dietary magnesium restriction, hypomagnesemia, volume depletion, metabolic alkalosis, and hormones like a parathyroid hormone, calcitonin, glucagon, insulin, and aldosterone.

- **Factors increasing renal loss of magnesium (by decreasing reabsorption):** Loop diuretics, hypermagnesemia, hypercalcemia, fluid volume expansion, metabolic acidosis, hypokalemia, hypophosphatemia, and different diuretics like a magnesium-sparing diuretic (amiloride), osmotic diuretics, such as mannitol and urea, and thiazide diuretics.

HYPOMAGNESEMIA

Hypomagnesemia is defined as serum magnesium concentration less than 1.7 mg/dL (1.4 mEq/L or 0.7 mmol/L). Hypomagnesemia usually reflects magnesium deficiency (a state of decreased total body magnesium content). But serum magnesium concentration may not truly reflect total body magnesium content because serum magnesium represents only 0.3% of total body magnesium, and a major reservoir (60%) of body magnesium in bones does not readily exchange with ECF magnesium [12].

Hypomagnesemia is a common but underdiagnosed electrolyte abnormality. The incidence of hypomagnesemia ranges from 11% to 20% in hospitalized patients and 50–70% in critically ill patients, and this disorder is associated with greater morbidity and mortality rate [13–17]. Higher prevalence was observed in ICU patients with comorbid conditions such as chronic malnutrition, alcoholism, and diabetes [18].

ETIOLOGY

Common causes of hypomagnesemia are increased gastrointestinal losses (chronic diarrhea, malabsorption syndrome, prolonged nothing by mouth (NPO) or nasogastric suction in surgical patients), increased losses in urine (loop and thiazide diuretic use, aminoglycosides, acute tubular necrosis), malnutrition, alcohol consumption, intracellular shift (treatment of diabetic ketoacidosis, refeeding syndrome) and other conditions [19]. The causes of hypomagnesemia can be divided into four major categories: (1) Increased renal excretion, (2) Increased gastrointestinal losses, (3) Decreased intake, and (4) Intracellular shift (Table 28.2).

CLINICAL FEATURES

Clinical presentation of hypomagnesemia is nonspecific, and symptoms in patients with hypomagnesemia depend on its severity, coexisting electrolyte abnormalities (hypocalcemia and hypokalemia), and underlying causative problems. Mild degrees of hypomagnesemia are usually asymptomatic, and

Table 28.2 Causes of hypomagnesemia

A. Increased renal excretion
- Loop, thiazide and osmotic diuretics
- Hyperaldosteronism, hyperparathyroidism, hyperthyroidism
- Hypercalcemia
- Volume expansion
- Drugs: Aminoglycosides, cisplatin, amphotericin B
- Chronic tubulointerstitial disease
- Post obstructive diuresis, recovery from acute tubular necrosis
- Diabetic ketoacidosis
- Gitelman syndrome and Bartter syndrome

B. Increased gastrointestinal losses
- Malabsorption, chronic diarrhea, laxative abuse
- Protracted vomiting or prolonged nasogastric aspiration
- Small bowel bypass surgery, acute pancreatitis
- Proton pump inhibitor (PPI)
- Vitamin D deficiency

C. Decreased intake
- Starvation or prolonged malnutrition
- Magnesium deficient PN or IV fluids
- Chronic alcoholism

D. Intracellular shift
- Treatment of diabetic ketoacidosis
- Refeeding syndrome
- Hungry bone syndrome

symptoms are commonly seen in severe hypomagnesemia (serum magnesium concentration falls below 1.2 mg/dL, 1.0 mEq/L, or 0.5 mmol/L). Because hypomagnesemia causes hypocalcemia and hypokalemia, the clinical picture is a combined presentation of all three electrolyte abnormalities, and manifestations are mostly related to neuromuscular and cardiovascular systems:

- **General symptoms:** Anorexia, nausea, vomiting, and weakness.

- **Neuromuscular manifestations:** They are similar to hypocalcemia and include lethargy, confusion, headache, depression, tremor, cramps, tingling and numbness, fasciculations, insomnia, ataxia, tetany with positive trousseau and chvostek signs, and seizures.

- **Cardiovascular manifestations:** Hypertension, tachycardia, and electrocardiogram (ECG) abnormalities like widening of QRS complex, peaked T-waves, prolonged PR and QT intervals, and atrial and ventricular arrhythmia. Patients with severe hypomagnesemia carry the risk of life-threatening ventricular arrhythmia such as Torsades de pointes. In addition, digitalis toxicity may be precipitated or aggravated by hypomagnesemia.

Associated abnormalities

- Hypocalcemia: Magnesium deficiency decreases PTH secretion and end-organ resistance to PTH, leading to hypocalcemia [3, 4]. If hypocalcemic patients do not respond to calcium or vitamin-D replacement, think of hypomagnesemia and correct it.

- Hypokalemia: Magnesium deficiency enhances renal excretion of potassium. The prevalence of hypokalemia in patients with hypomagnesemia may be as high as 40–60% [20]. In addition, hypomagnesemia aggravates hypokalemia and makes it refractory to treatment [21]. So, when hypokalemia does not respond to K+ replacement, rule out associated magnesium deficiency and correct it.

- Diabetes (DM): Hypomagnesemia is common in diabetes mellitus (occurs in about 13.5 to 47.7% of type 2 DM) and is associated with insulin resistance and impaired glycometabolic control [9, 22].

- Hypomagnesemia also increases the risk of hypertension, cardiovascular disease, and vascular calcification [23, 24]. In addition, hypomagnesemia is also associated with hypercalciuria and nephrolithiasis [25].

DIAGNOSIS

As hypomagnesemia may be asymptomatic, a high index of suspicion is essential for the diagnosis. Suspect hypomagnesemia and check serum magnesium levels in clinical situations such as chronic diarrhea, chronic alcoholism, malnutrition, and long-term hospitalization. In addition, if hypokalemia, hypocalcemia, or cardiac arrhythmias do not respond to standard therapy, think of hypomagnesemia.

Step 1: History and physical examination

A proper history and physical examination usually establish the causes of hypomagnesemia in most patients.

Step 2: Routinely ordered investigations

Serum calcium, phosphate, albumin, electrolytes, creatinine, glucose levels, and acid-base measurement are important investigations routinely ordered to establish the etiological diagnosis of hypomagnesemia.

Step 3: Urinary magnesium excretion

When the diagnosis is not clear, measurement of 24-hour urinary magnesium excretion or fractional excretion of magnesium (FEMg) in spot urine helps to differentiate renal and nonrenal causes of hypomagnesemia [25]. Out of these two methods, a 24-hour urinary magnesium excretion measurement is preferred over a FEMg from a spot urine sample because magnesium excretion varies with dietary intake and diurnal circadian rhythm [26].

$$FEMg = [(UMg \times PCr) / (PMg \times UCr \times 0.7)] \times 100$$

Where U and P refer to the urine and plasma concentrations of magnesium (Mg) and creatinine (Cr):

- 24-hour urinary magnesium excretion <10 mg or FEMg <2%: It suggests nonrenal causes of hypomagnesemia such as poor intake, gastrointestinal losses, or a shift of magnesium into cells.

- 24-hour urinary magnesium excretion >10–30 mg or FEMg >3% (with normal kidney function): It suggests renal magnesium wasting due to drugs such as loop or thiazide diuretics, aminoglycosides, or cisplatin, Bartter syndrome, Gitelman syndrome, and familial hypomagnesemia with hypercalciuria.

MANAGEMENT

The correction of hypomagnesemia is planned for an individual patient based on the degree of hypomagnesemia, the urgency of the clinical situation, renal function, hemodynamic stability, coexisting electrolyte abnormalities (such as hypocalcemia and hypokalemia), and the underlying cause of the disorder.

A. Correct underlying problems

Search and correct underlying etiology and coexisting electrolyte abnormalities such as hypocalcemia and hypokalemia. A drug like amiloride reduces the urinary excretion of magnesium and may be useful in patients with hypomagnesemia due to renal magnesium wasting.

B. Basic principles of therapy

- Intravenous magnesium sulfate is the most useful therapeutic agent. IV magnesium administration is the preferred modality in treating hypomagnesemia because it is highly effective, well-tolerated, readily available, and inexpensive. IV magnesium is recommended in patients with severe (serum magnesium <1 mg/dL) symptomatic (seizures, tetany, or life-threatening arrhythmias, or severe neuromuscular irritability) hypomagnesemia, or mild hypomagnesemia when oral magnesium replacement is not tolerable [12, 27].

- Infusion of magnesium at a slower rate for a prolonged period is crucial and beneficial: Rapid magnesium infusion increases serum magnesium levels abruptly and inhibits renal absorption leading to up to 50% loss of magnesium in the urine despite the presence of a total body deficit [28]. Additionally, administered magnesium distributes slowly with the intracellular compartment, and therefore restoration of intracellular magnesium occurs gradually over a few days [27].

- Because of significant renal loss and slow intracellular distribution, to correct hypomagnesemia adequately and replenish body magnesium stores effectively [29, 30], administer IV magnesium at a slower rate (i.e., at a rate not exceeding 1 gm/hour) as an infusion and administer IV magnesium for a prolonged period (i.e., at least 2 days after the serum magnesium level becomes normal).

- Magnesium infusion is generally well tolerated and safe. The risk of hypermagnesemia while replacing recommended dosages of IV magnesium in patients with normal kidney function is minimal because of the ability of kidneys to excrete excess magnesium effectively.

- A low magnesium level suggests magnesium depletion, but normo-magnesemia does not exclude hypomagnesemia. Do not always rely on serum magnesium levels. The magnesium in ECF is just 1% of total body magnesium, and therefore, normomagnesemia does not reflect actual body magnesium status or exclude hypomagnesemia [27]. Because of this reason, even in normomagnesemia, consider empirical magnesium therapy in patients at risk of magnesium deficiency or clinical presentation is consistent with hypomagnesemia [29].

- Recheck serum magnesium several hours after magnesium supplementation: It is important to remember that rise in serum magnesium levels following magnesium replacement is quick but temporary (i.e., just for a few hours), and therefore a measurement of magnesium too soon after magnesium repletion may be artificially high and can be misleading.

- Keep serum magnesium in the safe range during magnesium therapy. Aims of magnesium therapy in symptomatic patients is to raise serum magnesium above 1.5 mg/dL and maintain it below 3 mg/dL by proper monitoring [27, 31].

- Monitoring: During magnesium therapy, measure serum magnesium levels 6 to 12 hourly in hemodynamically unstable patients, daily in stable hospitalized patients, and at least weekly after discharge. Continuous cardiac monitoring is recommended in severe symptomatic hypomagnesemia with tetany, arrhythmias, or seizures receiving IV magnesium infusion.

- Dose in renal failure: In patients with impaired kidney function, avoid or reduce the dose of IV magnesium by 50% or more, and monitor serum magnesium levels frequently to avoid hypermagnesemia [32].

- Replace magnesium in unexplained hypocalcemia and/or hypokalemia. In the presence of hypomagnesemia, hypokalemia and hypocalcemia do not recover without magnesium supplementation.

C. Replacement of magnesium

The severity of hypomagnesemia and clinical manifestations determines the route and the rate of magnesium supplementation, as summarized in Table 28.3 [32–34]. Magnesium supplementation aims to raise the serum magnesium and correct symptoms of hypomagnesemia while avoiding magnesium toxicity [27].

1. Mild hypomagnesemia (Serum magnesium 1.6–1.9 mg/dL, 0.7 to 0.8 mmol/L or 1.4 to 1.6 mEq/L)

Diet: Increase intake of magnesium-rich food (e.g., green leafy vegetables, beef, seafood, nuts, etc.).

Oral magnesium therapy: Oral magnesium supplementation is the first-line therapy for chronic mild hypomagnesemia with minimal or no symptoms. It is also used to replace ongoing magnesium losses and add-on therapy after an initial IV magnesium supplementation.

Various oral magnesium prepara-

tions are available commercially, but sustained-release formulations are preferred. The usual dose of oral magnesium recommended in a patient with adequate kidney functions and severe hypomagnesemia is 240–1000 mg of elemental magnesium. Patients with mild hypomagnesemia need half of this dose (120 to 500 mg, 5 to 20 mmol, or 10 to 40 mEq of elemental magnesium) and to provide it, supplement magnesium oxide 400 mg (240 mg of elemental magnesium per tablet) 2–3 times/day [30].

The major dose-limiting side effect of oral magnesium replacement is diarrhea which can worsen hypomagnesemia. Therefore, if diarrhea occurs, reduce the oral dose.

IV therapy: Needs about 1 to 2 gm of magnesium sulfate, which is infused slowly over 1 to 2 hours. Patients with mild hypomagnesemia require IV magnesium if oral magnesium is not tolerated or appropriate and mild symptoms are present. If IV administration is not feasible, intramuscular administration of 1 gm of magnesium every 6 hours for 4 doses is recommended.

2. Moderate hypomagnesemia (Serum magnesium 1.0–1.5 mg/dL, 0.4 to 0.6 mmol/L or 0.8 to 1.2 mEq/L)

IV therapy: Administer 2–4 gm of magnesium sulfate IV intermittently over 4 to 12 hours (at a maximum rate of 1 gm/hr) [32].

"Rules of thumb": Each 1 gm (8 mEq) of IV magnesium will raise the serum magnesium concentration by 0.15 mEq/L and effectively correct mild to moderate hypomagnesemia [35].

Diet and oral therapy: In addition to IV supplementation, provide magnesium rich food and oral magnesium preparations in higher doses if tolerated.

3. Severe hypomagnesemia (Serum magnesium less than 1.0 mg/dL, 0.4 mmol/L or 0.8 mEq/L)

a. Hemodynamically unstable patients: Initially, 2 gm magnesium (diluted in 50 mL of D5W or normal saline) is infused rapidly as a bolus over 2–15 min with subsequent continuous magnesium infusion [33, 34].

b. Hemodynamically stable patients: Initially, 1 to 2 gm magnesium (diluted in 100 mL of D5W or normal saline) is infused slowly over one hour with subsequent continuous magnesium infusion.

Subsequent infusion: Administer 4 to 8 gm of magnesium diluted in 250–1,000 mL of D5W or normal saline as a continuous infusion over 12 to 24 hours for 3 to 5 days to keep the magnesium level above 1.5 mg/dL [12].

Parenteral magnesium therapy

- Magnesium sulfate 50% solution, available as a 2 ml ampoule, provides 1 gm of magnesium sulfate or 4 mmol/8 mEq of elemental magnesium (Each mL contains: 500 mg magnesium sulfate or 2 mmol/48 mEq of elemental magnesium).

Table 28.3 Management of hypomagnesemia		
A. Treatment of underlying disease		
B. Replacement of magnesium		
Severity	**Magnesium level**	**Recommended therapy**
Mild hypomagnesemia	1.6–1.9 mg/dL 0.7–0.8 mmol/L 1.4–1.6 mEq/L	Diet: Increase intake of magnesium rich food Oral therapy: Magnesium oxide 400 mg 2–3 times/day IV/IM therapy: 1 gm of magnesium sulfate infused over 1 to 2 hours or given intramuscularly every 6 hours for 4 doses
Moderate hypomagnesemia	1.0–1.5 mg/dL 0.4–0.6 mmol/L 0.8–1.2 mEq/L	2 to 4 gm of magnesium sulfate infused over 4 to 12 hours
Severe symptomatic hypomagnesemia	<1.0 mg/dL <0.4 mmol/L <0.8 mEq/L	A. Hemodynamically unstable patients 2 gm magnesium sulfate infused as a bolus over 2–15 min followed by a continuous infusion
		B. Hemodynamically stable patients 1 to 2 gm of magnesium sulfate infused over one hour, followed by a continuous infusion
		Subsequent continuous infusion: 4 to 8 gm of magnesium sulfate diluted in 250–1000 mL of D5W or normal saline infused over 12 to 24 hours
Torsades de pointes	-	1 to 2 gm of magnesium sulfate diluted in more than 10 ml of saline or D5W is pushed initially over 15 minutes, followed by a continuous 0.5 to 1 gm/hr magnesium sulfate infusion
Maintenance dose of IV magnesium	-	30 to 60 mg/kg/day or 1–3 gm/day magnesium sulfate in parenteral nutrition
Magnesium sulfate 50%, 1 ampoule (2 ml) = 1 gm of magnesium sulfate = 4 mmol magnesium = 8 mEq magnesium		
If kidney function is impaired, reduce the dose of IV magnesium by 50% or more		

- Conversion relationships: 240 mg magnesium sulfate = 1 mmol or 2 mEq of elemental magnesium.

- Always dilute the 50% magnesium sulfate solution and mix thoroughly before use. To administer magnesium sulfate solution via a peripheral vein, dilute concentrated magnesium sulfate solutions to a concentration of 20% (200 mg/mL) or less. For example, to prepare 20% magnesium sulfate solution, in 2 ml of 50% magnesium sulfate, add 3 ml of D5W or normal saline (Two parts of 50% magnesium sulfate solution and three parts of diluent).

- The osmolarity of magnesium sulfate 50% solution is very high (4060 mOsmol/L) and therefore carries the risk of tissue damage and necrosis if it extravasates into the surrounding tissue.

- Precautions: Magnesium is avoided or used with caution in patients with severe renal failure, myasthenia gravis, cardiac ischemia, and heart block (For further information, please refer to Chapter 12 "Magnesium Sulfate").

- Monitoring: While administering IV magnesium, closely monitor heart rate, blood pressure, respiratory rate, patellar reflex, urine output, and oxygen saturation (SpO_2) to avoid its serious adverse effects (For further information, please refer to Chapter 12 "Magnesium Sulfate").

- Discontinue IV administration of magnesium if respiratory rate is less than 12 breaths/minute, knee jerk is absent, urine output is less than 25 mL/hour or less than 100 mL over 4 hours, and diastolic blood pressure decreases more than 15 mmHg below the baseline.

- Antidote: Administer 10% calcium gluconate 10 ml IV slowly over 5–10 minutes to antagonize the serious neuromuscular and cardiovascular effects of magnesium therapy [36].

REFERENCES

1. de Baaij JH, Hoenderop JG, Bindels RJ. Magnesium in man: implications for health and disease. Physiol Rev. 2015;95(1):1–46.
2. Jahnen-Dechent W, Ketteler M. Magnesium basics. Clin Kidney J. 2012;5(1):i3–i14.
3. Fatemi S, Ryzen E, Flores J, et al. Effect of experimental human magnesium depletion on parathyroid hormone secretion and 1,25-dihydroxyvitamin D metabolism. J Clin Endocrinol Metab 1991;73(5):1067–72.
4. Lindsay AL, Bazydlo, Needham M, et al. Calcium, Magnesium, and Phosphate, Laboratory Medicine 2014;45(1):e44–e50.
5. Eisenbud E, LoBue CC. Hypocalcemia after therapeutic use of magnesium sulfate. Arch Intern Med 1976;136(6):688–91.
6. Rodríguez-Ortiz ME, Canalejo A, Herencia C, et al. Magnesium modulates parathyroid hormone secretion and upregulates parathyroid receptor expression at moderately low calcium concentration. Nephrol Dial Transplant. 2014;29(2):282–9.
7. Blaine J, Chonchol M, Levi M. Renal control of calcium, phosphate, and magnesium homeostasis. Clin J Am Soc Nephrol. 2015;10(7):1257–1272.
8. Swaminathan R. Magnesium metabolism and its disorders. Clin Biochem Rev. 2003;24(2):47–66.
9. Yee J. Magnesium: An Important Orphan. Adv Chronic Kidney Dis. 2018;25(3):217–221.
10. Schuchardt JP, Hahn A. Intestinal Absorption and Factors Influencing Bioavailability of Magnesium-An Update. Curr Nutr Food Sci. 2017;13(4):260–278.
11. Curry JN, Yu ASL. Magnesium Handling in the Kidney. Adv Chronic Kidney Dis. 2018;25(3):236–243.
12. Martin KJ, González EA, Slatopolsky E. Clinical consequences and management of hypomagnesemia. J Am Soc Nephrol. 2009;20(11):2291–5.
13. Wong ET, Rude RK, Singer FR, et al. A high prevalence of hypomagnesemia and hypermagnesemia in hospitalized patients. Am J Clin Pathol. 1983;79(3):348–352.
14. Limaye CS, Londhey VA, Nadkart MY, et al. Hypomagnesemia in critically ill medical patients. J Assoc Physicians India. 2011;59:19–22.
15. Cheungpasitporn W, Thongprayoon C, Qian Q. Dysmagnesemia in Hospitalized Patients: Prevalence and Prognostic Importance. Mayo Clin Proc. 2015;90(8):1001–10.
16. Cheungpasitporn W, Thongprayoon C, Chewcharat A, et al. Hospital-Acquired Dysmagnesemia and In-Hospital Mortality. Med Sci (Basel). 2020;8(3):37.
17. M Kumar A, Naik MK. Prevalence of admission hypomagnesemia in critically ill patients International Journal of Health and Clinical Research, 2021;4(2):129–133.

18. Van Laecke S. Hypomagnesemia and hypermagnesemia. Acta Clin Belg. 2019;74(1):41–47.

19. Liamis G, Liberopoulos E, Alexandridis G, et al. Hypomagnesemia in a department of internal medicine. Magnes Res. 2012;25(4):149–58.

20. Whang R, Ryder KW. Frequency of hypomagnesemia and hypermagnesemia. Requested vs routine. JAMA 1990;263(22):3063–4.

21. Huang CL, Kuo E. Mechanism of hypokalemia in magnesium deficiency. J Am Soc Nephrol. 2007;18(10):2649–52.

22. Pham PC, Pham PM, Pham SV, et al. Hypomagnesemia in patients with type 2 diabetes. Clin J Am Soc Nephrol. 2007;2(2):366–73.

23. Chrysant SG, Chrysant GS. Association of hypomagnesemia with cardiovascular diseases and hypertension. Int J Cardiol Hypertens. 2019;1:100005.

24. Ter Braake AD, Shanahan CM, de Baaij JHF. Magnesium Counteracts Vascular Calcification: Passive Interference or Active Modulation? Arterioscler Thromb Vasc Biol. 2017;37(8):1431–1445.

25. Assadi F. Hypomagnesemia: an evidence-based approach to clinical cases. Iran J Kidney Dis. 2010;4(1):13–19.

26. Tucker BM, Pirkle JL Jr, Raghavan R. Urinary Magnesium in the Evaluation of Hypomagnesemia. JAMA. 2020;324(22):2320–2321.

27. Velissaris D, Karamouzos V, Pierrakos C, et al. Hypomagnesemia in Critically Ill Sepsis Patients. J Clin Med Res. 2015;7(12):911–8.

28. Agus ZS. Hypomagnesemia. J Am Soc Nephrol. 1999;10(7):1616–22.

29. Hansen BA, Bruserud Ø. Hypomagnesemia in critically ill patients. J Intensive Care. 2018;6:21.

30. Chonchol M, Smogorzewski MJ, Stubbs JR, et al. Disorders of Calcium, Magnesium, and Phosphate Balance. In: Brenner and Rector's The Kidney, 11th ed, Yu A, Chertow G, Luyckx V, et al (Eds), W.B. Saunders & Company, Philadelphia 2020.p.603.

31. Fulop T. Hypomagnesemia treatment & management. Updated Oct 30, 2020. Available at https://emedicine.medscape.com/article/2038394-treatment#d10 (accessed 18 January 2022).

32. Kraft MD, Btaiche IF, Sacks GS, et al. Treatment of electrolyte disorders in adult patients in the intensive care unit. Am J Health Syst Pharm. 2005;62(16):1663–82.

33. Neumar RW, Otto CW, Link MS, et al. Part 8: adult advanced cardiovascular life support: 2010 American Heart Association guidelines for cardiopulmonary resuscitation and emergency cardiovascular care. Circulation. 2010;122(18 Suppl 3):S729–67.

34. Tzivoni D, Banai S, Schuger C, et al. Treatment of torsade de pointes with magnesium sulfate. Circulation. 1988;77(2):392–7.

35. Hammond DA, Stojakovic J, Kathe N, et al. Effectiveness and Safety of Magnesium Replacement in Critically Ill Patients Admitted to the Medical Intensive Care Unit in an Academic Medical Center: A Retrospective, Cohort Study. J Intensive Care Med. 2019;34(11–12):967–972.

36. McDonnell NJ, Muchatuta NA, Paech MJ. Acute magnesium toxicity in an obstetric patient undergoing general anaesthesia for caesarean delivery. Int J Obstet Anesth. 2010;19(2):226–31.

29 | Hypermagnesemia

Hypermagnesemia is an uncommon electrolyte disorder defined as serum magnesium concentration above 2.6 mg/dL (1.1 mmol/L, or 2.14 mEq/L). As a normal kidney can effectively excrete magnesium load, hypermagnesemia is rarely seen in clinical practice if renal function is normal.

ETIOLOGY

Hypermagnesemia is frequently iatrogenic and almost always occurs either due to impaired excretion of magnesium in acute kidney injury (AKI) or chronic kidney disease (CKD) or the administration of magnesium in a large amount [1–4].

Common causes are:

- Renal failure: AKI or CKD patients receiving magnesium-containing antacids, laxatives, or IV fluids [3, 5, 6].
- Excessive magnesium intake: Treatment of preeclampsia or eclampsia with IV magnesium sulfate, aggressive treatment of hypomagnesemia with IV magnesium, intake of large amounts of magnesium salts as cathartics or antacids, and use of rectal magnesium sulfate enemas.
- Compartment shift or leak: Diabetic ketoacidosis untreated, tumor lysis

syndrome, acute rhabdomyolysis, hemolysis, and severe burns.

- Miscellaneous causes: Milk-alkali syndrome and impaired renal excretion of magnesium due to primary hyperparathyroidism, adrenal insufficiency, and hypothyroidism.

CLINICAL FEATURES [7, 8]

Symptoms of hypermagnesemia are chiefly neuromuscular, cardiac, and related to hypocalcemia, which varies as per the magnesium level and, in severe form, can be serious and potentially fatal, as summarized in Table 29.1.

Neuromuscular manifestations: Hypermagnesemia inhibits acetylcholine release from the neuromuscular endplate, causing the blockage of neuromuscular transmission leading to a neuromuscular symptom. It includes muscular weakness, lethargy, loss of deep tendon jerks, muscular paresis leading to respiratory depression, respiratory failure, and quadriparesis. In addition, due to smooth-muscle paralysis, hypermagnesemia may present as paralytic ileus or urinary retention.

Cardiovascular manifestations: As magnesium blocks extracellular and intracellular calcium channels and intra-

Table 29.1 Clinical features of hypermagnesemia			
Magnesium levels			Clinical effects
mg/dL	mEq/L	mmol/L	
2.5–5.0	2.1–4.2	1.05–2.1	Clinically asymptomatic
5.0–7.0	4.2–5.8	2.1–2.9	Nausea, vomiting, flushing, weakness, lethargy, drowsiness, confusion, and impaired deep tendon (patellar) reflexes
7.0–12.0	5.8–10.0	2.9–5.0	Loss of deep tendon reflexes, transient hypocalcemia, confusion, somnolence, paralytic ileus, bladder paralysis, bradycardia, hypotension, hypoventilation, and ECG changes (P-Q interval prolongation, widen QRS complex)
>12.0	>10.0	>5.0	Muscle flaccid paralysis, respiratory failure, complete heart block, and cardiac arrest

cellular potassium channels needed for repolarization, hypermagnesemia impairs cardiovascular function. Hypotension due to peripheral vasodilatation is often refractory to volume expansion and vasopressors, which is one of the earliest manifestations of hypermagnesemia [9]. In addition, due to conduction defects, hypermagnesemia causes bradycardia and cardiac asystole in severe cases.

Electrocardiogram (ECG) changes: Due to generalized depression of cardiac conduction, ECG abnormalities seen are prolonged PR, QRS, and QT intervals with sinus bradycardia, atrioventricular block, and lastly, complete heart block in more severe cases.

Hypocalcemia: Hypermagnesemia causes transient and asymptomatic hypocalcemia due to decreased secretion of parathyroid hormone (PTH) and end-organ resistance of PTH.

DIAGNOSIS

- Serum magnesium and ECG are two basic tests essential to diagnose the disorder and its severity.

- Detailed history and examination help to establish the diagnosis of the clinical disorder responsible for hypermagnesemia.

- The first step in approaching hypermagnesemia patients is obtaining creatinine (to assess renal function) and electrolytes, including K^+, Ca^{2+}, and phosphorus (to detect coexisting electrolyte abnormalities).

- This evaluation is very important because renal failure is the most common cause of hypermagnesemia, and hypocalcemia is a common concurrent disorder.

- Other investigations performed selectively based on the clinical evaluation are creatinine kinase, uric acid, LDH, PTH, thyroid function tests, blood sugar, and serum acetone which helps to exclude rhabdomyolysis, tumor lysis syndrome, hemolysis, hyperparathyroidism, hypothyroidism, and diabetic ketoacidosis, respectively.

MANAGEMENT

Treatment of hypermagnesemia is determined based on magnesium concentration, the severity of symptoms, renal function, and underlying etiology.

Eliminate exogenous sources: Stop magnesium-containing antacids and laxatives and discontinue magnesium-containing IV fluids.

Prevention and precautions

1. Avoid using magnesium-containing medications for the long term in patients with kidney failure.

2. Monitor serum magnesium closely in patients receiving parenteral magnesium.

3. In patients with preeclampsia, discontinue infusion if respiratory rate is <12 breaths/minute, deep tendon reflexes are absent, and urine output is <25 mL/hour or <100 mL over 4 hours.

Temporary antidote: 10% calcium gluconate, 10 ml (1 gm) IV is infused slowly over 5–10 minutes and can be repeated after 5 minutes if there is no improvement in symptomatic patients [9, 10]. Calcium inhibits the effect of high magnesium on neuromuscular and cardiac function without changing the magnesium level.

Forced saline diuresis: If renal function is normal, high-volume saline infusion (e.g., 150 mL/hour) followed by furosemide for diuresis will enhance renal excretion of magnesium and correct hypermagnesemia [11].

Hemodialysis: In patients with severe kidney diseases, hemodialysis is an effective and preferred treatment modality to remove excess magnesium and correct severe symptomatic hypermagnesemia [2].

Emergency supportive treatment: Patients with impaired respiration may need mechanical ventilation, and a temporary pacemaker may be necessary for significant bradyarrhythmias.

REFERENCES

1. Jahnen-Dechent W, Ketteler M. Magnesium basics. Clin Kidney J. 2012;5(Suppl 1):i3–i14.

2. Alaini A, Roldan CA, Servilla K, et al. Near death by milk of magnesia. BMJ Case Rep. 2017;2017:bcr2016218260.

3. Wakai E, Ikemura K, Sugimoto H, et al. Risk factors for the development of hypermagnesemia in patients prescribed magnesium oxide: a retrospective cohort study. J Pharm Health Care Sci. 2019;5:4.

4. Mori H, Suzuki H, Hirai Y, et al. Clinical features of hypermagnesemia in patients with functional constipation taking daily magnesium oxide. J Clin Biochem Nutr. 2019;65(1):76–81.

5. Wyskida K, Witkowicz J, Chudek J, et al. Daily magnesium intake and hypermagnesemia in hemodialysis patients with chronic kidney disease. J Ren Nutr 2012;22(1):19–26.

6. Khairi T, Amer S, Spitalewitz S, et al. Severe Symptomatic Hypermagnesemia Associated with Over-the-Counter Laxatives in a Patient with Renal Failure and Sigmoid Volvulus. Case Rep Nephrol. 2014;2014:560746.

7. Topf JM, Murray PT. Hypomagnesemia and hypermagnesemia. Rev Endocr Metab Disord. 2003;4(2):195–206.

8. Kraft MD, Btaiche IF, Sacks GS, et al. Treatment of electrolyte disorders in adult patients in the intensive care unit. Am J Health Syst Pharm. 2005;62(16):1663–82.

9. Mordes JP, Swartz R, Arky RA. Extreme hypermagnesemia as a cause of refractory hypotension. Ann Intern Med. 1975;83(5):657–658.

10. McDonnell NJ, Muchatuta NA, Paech MJ. Acute magnesium toxicity in an obstetric patient undergoing general anaesthesia for caesarean delivery. Int J Obstet Anesth. 2010;19(2):226–31.

11. Ishida Y, Tabuchi A. Severe Hypermagnesemia with Normal Renal Function Can Improve with Symptomatic Treatment. Case Rep Emerg Med. 2020;2020:2918249.

Part 7

Acid-Base Disorders

30 | Basic Understanding and Approach to Acid-Base Disorders

Arterial blood gas (ABG) measurements are a crucial diagnostic test in medicine, providing vital insights for diagnosing acid-base disorders and guiding life-saving treatments in critically ill patients. Acid-base disorders frequently manifest in critically ill patients and can also serve as initial indicators of underlying diseases, such as Kussmaul's breathing presenting in diabetic ketoacidosis or renal failure.

To clearly understand the subject and its approach, this chapter outlines basic terminology, the physiology of pH regulation, compensation in various acid-base disorders, and the diagnostic approach.

UNDERSTANDING BASIC TERMINOLOGY

Basic terminology used to discuss acid-base disorders and their values in simple acid-base disorders are summarized below (Table 30.1).

pH: pH represents the concentration of free hydrogen ions (H^+). It has an inverse relationship with H^+ ion concentration. The normal value of pH in arterial blood is 7.4 (7.35–7.45).

Acid, acidemia and acidosis

- A decrease in pH indicates an increase in H^+ ion concentration.
- An acid is a substance that can donate H^+ ions or, when added to a solution, increase the H^+ ion concentration, thereby lowering the pH.
- An acidemia, which refers to "acid blood," is characterized by a blood pH below normal (pH <7.35) and an increased H^+ ion concentration.
- Acidosis is an abnormal process or disease that reduces pH (pH <7.35) due to an increase in acid or a decrease in alkali.

Base, alkalemia and alkalosis

- An increase in pH signifies a decrease in H^+ ion concentration.
- A base is a substance that can accept H^+ ions or, when added to a solution, reduces the H^+ ion concentration, thereby raising the pH.
- Alkalemia, which refers to "alkaline blood," is characterized by a blood pH above normal (pH>7.45) and decreased H^+ ion concentration.
- Alkalosis is an abnormal process or disease that increases pH due to a decrease in acid or an increase in alkali.

Metabolic acidosis is defined by bicarbonate (HCO_3) levels <22 mEq/L and a pH <7.35.

Metabolic alkalosis is defined by HCO_3 levels >26 mEq/L and a pH >7.45.

Respiratory acidosis is defined by partial pressure of carbon dioxide ($PaCO_2$) >45 mm of Hg and a pH <7.35.

Respiratory alkalosis is defined by $PaCO_2$ <35 mm of Hg and a pH >7.45.

SIMPLE ACID-BASE DISORDER

Acid-base disorders can be divided into simple acid-base disorders or mixed acid-base disorders. A simple acid-base disorder is a primary disturbance in the body's acid-base balance characterized by the presence of just one disorder, such as either acidosis or alkalosis. Acidosis and alkalosis are further divided

Table 30.1 Summary of acid-base terminology and their values	
Clinical terminology	**Criteria**
Normal pH	7.4 (7.35–7.45)
Acidemia	pH <7.35 (low pH)
Alkalemia	pH >7.45 (high pH)
Normal HCO_3	24 (22 - 26) mEq/Lw
Metabolic acidosis	HCO_3 <22 mEq/L and low pH
Metabolic alkalosis	HCO_3 >26 mEq/L and high pH
Normal $PaCO_2$	40 (35–45) mm of Hg
Respiratory acidosis	$PaCO_2$ >45 mm of Hg and low pH
Respiratory alkalosis	$PaCO_2$ <35 mm of Hg and high pH
Anion gap (AG)	8 to 16 mEq/L

into metabolic disorders (characterized by decreased or increased HCO_3^-) or respiratory disorders (characterized by decreased or increased pCO_2).

Four primary acid-base disorders are defined depending on initial disturbances:

If the initial disturbance affects HCO_3:

1. Metabolic acidosis: The primary change is a fall in HCO_3.

2. Metabolic alkalosis: The primary change is a rise in HCO_3.

If the initial disturbance affects $PaCO_2$:

3. Respiratory acidosis: The primary change is a rise in $PaCO_2$.

4. Respiratory alkalosis: The primary change is a fall in $PaCO_2$.

When you see "Metabolic," think of a primary change in HCO_3, and when you see "Respiratory," think of a primary change in $PaCO_2$. The characteristics of primary acid-base disorders are summarized in Table 30.2.

Metabolic disorders

Primary metabolic disorders are characterized by disturbances in HCO_3^- concentration, with metabolic acidosis typically involving a decrease and metabolic alkalosis involving an increase in HCO_3^- concentration).

- Metabolic acidosis is defined by HCO_3 levels <22 mEq/L and a pH <7.35. If the underlying disorder causes excess loss of bicarbonate (i.e., diarrhea) or excess accumulation

of acid (i.e., diabetic ketoacidosis or lactic acidosis), or bicarbonate is not generated (i.e., renal tubular acidosis), it leads to decrease in blood bicarbonate levels and a subsequent decrease in pH, resulting in metabolic acidosis.

- Metabolic alkalosis is defined by HCO_3 levels >26 mEq/L and a pH >7.45. Mechanisms that can lead to metabolic alkalosis include: (1) Excessive loss of hydrogen ions, as seen in cases of vomiting; (2) Increased generation of HCO_3, as occurs in salicylate poisoning; (3) Failure of renal excretion of bicarbonate, which can occur in conditions such as hypovolemia, hypokalemia, and hypochloremia due to the use of loop or thiazide diuretics. These mechanisms contribute to an elevation in blood bicarbonate levels and a subsequent increase in pH, ultimately resulting in metabolic alkalosis.

Respiratory disorders

Primary respiratory disorders are characterized by disturbances in $PaCO_2$ concentration, with respiratory acidosis involving an increase in $PaCO_2$ and respiratory alkalosis involving a decrease in $PaCO_2$:

- Respiratory acidosis is defined by $PaCO_2$ >45 mm of Hg and a pH <7.35. If the underlying disorders (CNS or respiratory) cause hypoventilation

Table 30.2 Characteristics of primary acid-base disorders				
Basic disorder	**H+**	**pH**	**Primary change**	**Secondary change**
Metabolic acidosis	High	Low	Low HCO_3	Low $PaCO_2$
Metabolic alkalosis	Low	High	High HCO_3	High $PaCO_2$
Respiratory acidosis	High	Low	High $PaCO_2$	High HCO_3
Respiratory alkalosis	Low	High	Low $PaCO_2$	Low HCO_3

or reduced CO_2 excretion, it leads to retained $PaCO_2$ (hypercapnia) and a fall in pH, resulting in respiratory acidosis.

- Respiratory alkalosis is defined by $PaCO_2 < 35$ mm of Hg and a pH > 7.45. If the underlying disorder leads to inappropriately high hyperventilation, CO_2 is washed out, causing low $PaCO_2$ (hypocapnia), a rise in pH, and respiratory alkalosis.

Mixed acid-base disorder: A mixed acid-base disorder is a complex disruption of the body's acid-base balance characterized by the simultaneous presence of more than one acid-base disorder.

BASIC PHYSIOLOGY OF ACID-BASE REGULATION

It is essential to understand the importance of pH regulation, the variables that can affect pH, and the regulatory systems that maintain pH in response to insults caused by various factors and disorders [1, 2].

A. Importance of pH regulation

Precisely maintaining pH within a narrow range of 7.35 to 7.45 is crucial. pH plays a vital role in normal cellular enzymatic reactions and the regulation of ionic concentrations. Any pH alteration can lead to cardiac arrhythmias. Extreme pH values falling below 7.2 or exceeding 7.55 can be potentially life-threatening due to the disruption of essential cellular enzymatic reactions and physiological processes.

Basic physiology of acid-base regulation

The body maintains pH within a normal range despite variations in dietary intake of acid, alkali, and endogenous acid production.

Endogenous acid production

Usually, when food is metabolized, two types of acids are added to extracellular fluid:

1. Volatile acid in the form of carbonic acid (H_2CO_3) determines the level of CO_2 in the blood ($PaCO_2$) and is excreted by the lung. About 22,000 mEq volatile acid is produced daily.

2. Nonvolatile (fixed) acids (like sulfuric and phosphoric acids) are produced by dietary and endogenous protein catabolism, roughly at the rate of 1 mEq/kg. The kidneys excrete them.

B. Acid-base regulation

Three major regulatory systems are responsible for maintaining pH within a narrow range: buffers for immediate effects, the lungs, which act rapidly by eliminating CO_2, and the kidneys, which act slowly but have the most potent buffering effect.

The Henderson-Hasselbalch Equation describes the correlation of metabolic and respiratory regulations, which maintains pH.

$$pH = 6.1 + \log HCO_3/0.3 \times PaCO_2 = pK + Kidney/Lung$$

1. **Buffers:** Buffers are chemical systems that can either release or accept H^+ ions. They play a crucial role in minimizing pH changes caused by the introduction of acids or bases and provide immediate defense against shifts in acidity. Buffers act quickly but have limited buffering capacity. The most important buffers include bicarbonate, phosphate, proteins, hemoglobin, and bone bicarbonate.

2. **Respiratory regulation:** The lungs regulate $PaCO_2$ by excreting volatile acids, which help to maintain Blood pH.

In metabolic acidosis, characterized by a low serum HCO_3 level, the respiratory compensatory mechanism increases the rate and depth of breathing due to low pH, reducing pCO_2. This alteration in the serum HCO_3 to pCO_2 ratio, resulting from the decrease in pCO_2 levels due to hyperventilation, contributes to the normalization of blood pH.

Conversely, in metabolic alkalosis, characterized by a high serum HCO_3 level, the respiratory compensatory mechanism is hypoventilation, which increases pCO_2. Resultant pCO_2 shifts in the same direction as the serum HCO_3 (both high), prevents the change in the serum HCO_3 to pCO_2 ratio, and brings the high pH level towards normal.

Respiratory regulation acts rapidly; response starts in about 30 minutes, is usually complete within 12 to 24 hours, and has greater buffering power than chemical buffers.

3. **Renal regulation:** The role of the kidney is to maintain plasma HCO_3 concentration and, thereby, pH regulation. It has the most powerful buffering system, which starts within hours and takes 5-6 days for peak effect. The kidney regulates HCO_3 by excreting nonvolatile-fixed acids by following three main mechanisms:

   - Excretion of H^+ ions by tubular secretion.
   - Reabsorption of filtered bicarbonate ions.
   - Production of new HCO_3 ions.

How the kidney responds to acid-base disorders and regulates pH:

- In cases of metabolic acidosis with an acid load, normal kidneys can significantly increase net acid excretion (by more than 10 times). This increased excretion of H^+ ions, coupled with bicarbonate regeneration, contributes to the correction of plasma HCO_3 levels towards the normal range.

- Conversely, when there is a primary increase in plasma HCO_3 (i.e., metabolic alkalosis), there will be increased renal HCO_3 excretion in the urine.

- In respiratory acidosis, where there is an increase in $PaCO_2$, the kidneys respond by increasing hydrogen ion secretion and retaining bicarbonate ions (HCO_3^-). This helps to increase plasma HCO_3^- concentration, which in turn raises the blood pH towards normal.

- Similarly, in respiratory alkalosis, characterized by decreased $PaCO_2$, the kidneys excrete more bicarbonate ions, reducing plasma HCO_3^- concentration and lowering the blood pH towards normal.

COMPENSATION IN ACID-BASE DISORDERS

A. Understanding compensation

The body's response to neutralize the effect of the initial insult on pH homeostasis is called compensation.

To understand compensation, first of all, it is essential to remember that pH is maintained by the ratio of $HCO_3/PaCO_2$ (Henderson-Hasselbalch equation).

To maintain normal pH, primary metabolic disorders (primary change in HCO_3) lead to compensatory respiratory responses (secondary change in $PaCO_2$).

Example: Metabolic acidosis (Fall in HCO_3) leads to low pH. Low pH stimulates the respiratory center, causing hyperventilation.

Hyperventilation leads to CO_2 washout and decreased $PaCO_2$. So, low HCO_3 leads to compensatory low $PaCO_2$, which returns a ratio of $PaCO_2/HCO_3$ towards normal. This compensation keeps pH within a normal range as far as possible.

Similarly, to maintain normal pH, primary respiratory disorders (primary change in $PaCO_2$) lead to compensatory metabolic (renal) responses (secondary change in HCO_3).

B. Same direction rule

From the above discussion (as well as Table 30.2), we can conclude that in each acid-base disorder, the compensatory changes are in the same direction as the primary changes. Decreased HCO_3 leads to decreased $PaCO_2$, and increased HCO_3 leads to increased $PaCO_2$ (i.e., up yields up, down yields down).

This principle is commonly referred to as the "Same Direction Rule" of compensation.

C. Determine the expected compensation

Calculating expected compensation helps determine the body's ability to compensate for existing disorders. To evaluate acid-base disorders, understanding the formula that calculates the expected compensation for simple acid-base disorders is crucial. Comparison of calculated and actual values helps to confirm the diagnosis of simple disorders, and the significant differences between these are indicative of the presence of a mixed acid-base disorder. Table 30.3 lists equations that will help to calculate expected compensation in all 4 simple acid-base disorders [3, 4].

1. Response to metabolic acidosis

In metabolic acidosis, respiratory compensation leads to a reduction in $PaCO_2$, which is commonly calculated by Winter's formula:

Expected $PaCO_2$ =
(1.5 x Serum HCO_3) + 8

Table 30.3 Prediction of compensation for simple acid-base disorders				
Disorder	Primary change	Expected compensation	Upper limit of compensation	Compensation time
Metabolic acidosis	pH <7.35 HCO_3 <22 mEq/L	Expected $PaCO_2$ = (1.5 x serum HCO_3) + 8 or = HCO_3 + 15	$PaCO_2$ up to 10 mm Hg	Respiratory compensation starts within 30 minutes and complete within 12–24 hrs
Metabolic alkalosis	pH >7.45 HCO_3 >26 mEq/L	Increase in $PaCO_2$ = 0.7 × (Measured HCO_3 − 24)	$PaCO_2$ up to 55 mm Hg	Starts within a few minutes, complete within 24–36 hrs
Respiratory acidosis	pH <7.35 $PaCO_2$ >45 mm of Hg	**Acute:** Increase in HCO_3 = 0.1 × (Measured $PaCO_2$ − 40) **Chronic:** Increase in HCO_3 = 0.4 × (Measured $PaCO_2$ − 40)	HCO_3 up to 40 mEq/L	Renal compensation begins within hours and complete within 2–5 days
Respiratory alkalosis	pH >7.45 $PaCO_2$ <35 mm of Hg	**Acute:** Fall in HCO_3 = 0.2 × (40 - Measured $PaCO_2$) **Chronic:** Fall in HCO_3 = 0.4 × (40 − Measured $PaCO_2$)	HCO_3 up to 10-12 mEq/L	

2. Response to metabolic alkalosis

In metabolic alkalosis, respiratory compensation leads to an increase in $PaCO_2$. The compensatory increase in $PaCO_2$ (in mm Hg) is usually about 0.6 to 0.7 mm Hg for each 1 mEq/L increase in HCO_3 (up to approximately 55 mm Hg):

Increase in $PaCO_2$ =
    0.7 × (Measured HCO_3 − 24)

3. Response to respiratory acidosis

In respiratory acidosis, metabolic compensation leads to an increase in HCO_3. Renal compensation is slower, resulting in a minor increase in HCO_3 in acute respiratory acidosis and a more significant increase in chronic respiratory acidosis.

Acute respiratory acidosis: In acute respiratory acidosis, the compensatory increase in HCO_3 is usually about 0.1 mEq/L for each 1 mm Hg increase in $PaCO_2$:

Expected Increase in HCO_3 =
    0.1 × (Measured $PaCO_2$ − 40)

Chronic respiratory acidosis: In chronic respiratory acidosis, the compensatory increase in HCO_3 is usually about 0.4−0.5 mEq/L for each 1 mm Hg increase in $PaCO_2$:

Expected Increase in HCO_3 =
    0.4 × (Measured $PaCO_2$ − 40)

4. Response to respiratory alkalosis

In respiratory alkalosis, metabolic compensation leads to a reduction in HCO_3. The expected decrease in HCO_3 will be small in acute respiratory alkalosis but more pronounced in chronic respiratory alkalosis.

Acute respiratory alkalosis: In acute respiratory alkalosis, the compensatory reduction in HCO_3 is usually about 0.2 mEq/L for each 1 mm Hg increase in $PaCO_2$:

Expected Fall in HCO_3 =
    0.2 × (40 − Measured $PaCO_2$)

Chronic respiratory alkalosis: In chronic respiratory alkalosis, the compensatory reduction in HCO_3 is usually about 0.4 mEq/L for each 1 mm Hg increase in $PaCO_2$:

Expected Fall in HCO_3 =
    0.4 × (Measured $PaCO_2$ − 40)

D. Importance of calculation and checking compensation

Calculating compensation based on formulas is valuable in simple acid-base disorders for the following reasons:

1. Useful in differentiating between simple and mixed disorders.

2. When the calculated or expected change matches the actual value, it suggests a simple disorder.

3. If the actual value differs significantly from the predicted value, it may indicate a mixed disorder.

4. Compensation always follows the "Same Direction Rule." If the changes are in opposite directions, it could indicate a mixed disorder.

MIXED ACID-BASE DISORDER

Definition: A mixed acid-base disorder is defined as the independent coexistence of more than one primary acid-base disorder.

Mixed disorders often occur in critically ill patients. The most common mixed disorder is a combination of mixed metabolic and respiratory acidosis. The most detrimental mixed disorders involve a combination of mixed metabolic with respiratory acidosis and mixed metabolic with respiratory alkalosis.

Different mixed acid-base disorders and their common causes are summarized in Table 30.4.

Triple mixed disorders

1. High AG metabolic acidosis + Metabolic alkalosis + Respiratory alkalosis

Example: A patient with heavy alcohol intake (high AG metabolic acidosis due to alcoholic ketoacidosis), with vomiting (metabolic alkalosis), who subsequently develops superimposed respiratory alkalosis due to sepsis or liver disease.

2. High AG metabolic acidosis + Metabolic alkalosis + respiratory acidosis

Example: A patient with COPD and hypercapnia (respiratory acidosis) who develops metabolic alkalosis due to diuretics or vomiting subsequently develops superimposed high anion gap metabolic acidosis from conditions such as sepsis, hypotension, or hypoxemia.

3. High AG metabolic acidosis + Normal AG metabolic acidosis + Respiratory alkalosis

Example: A diabetic patient experiences an acute bronchial asthma attack, resulting in respiratory alkalosis. Concurrently, he developed diabetic ketoacidosis, characterized by high anion gap metabolic acidosis. Additionally, the patient encounters an episode of diarrhea, leading to normal anion gap metabolic acidosis.

Important: Remember that primary respiratory acidosis and respiratory alkalosis cannot coexist. The lungs can only create one primary disturbance characterized by either high or low CO_2 levels. Additionally, a primary respiratory disorder cannot have a compensatory respiratory response simultaneously.

Table 30.4 Common mixed acid base disorders

Disorders	Common causes
1. Metabolic acidosis Respiratory acidosis **(Low pH, low HCO$_3$, high PaCO$_2$)**	a. Cardiac arrest (hypoventilation + lactic acidosis) b. Shock with respiratory failure c. Diabetic ketoacidosis with respiratory diseases
2. Metabolic acidosis Respiratory alkalosis **(Normal pH, low HCO$_3$, low PaCO$_2$)**	a. Salicylate intoxication b. Gram-negative sepsis c. Liver failure
3. Metabolic alkalosis Respiratory acidosis **(Normal pH, high HCO$_3$, high PaCO$_2$)**	a. COPD with diuretics b. Metabolic alkalosis with severe hypokalemia and respiratory weakness leads to hypoventilation
4. Metabolic alkalosis Respiratory alkalosis **(High pH, high HCO$_3$, low PaCO$_2$)**	a. Liver failure with vomiting b. Patient on ventilator with continuous nasogastric aspiration
5. Metabolic acidosis Metabolic alkalosis **(Near normal pH and HCO$_3$)**	a. Diabetic ketoacidosis with vomiting b. Vomiting with severe volume depletion causing lactic acidosis
6. Respiratory acidosis Respiratory alkalosis	• Do not co-exist

DIAGNOSIS OF ACID-BASE DISORDERS

To establish the diagnosis of acid-base disorders, commonly used approach for evaluation includes:

1. History and physical examination

2. Primary investigations

3. Obtaining a blood gas analysis

4. Selecting the appropriate method for interpreting an acid-base disorder

5. Interpretation of basic investigations and,

6. A step-by-step diagnostic approach

A. Comprehensive history, physical examination

Careful history and examination can provide clues for underlying clinical disorders. As underlying disorders provide clues for possible acid-base disorders, it is essential to have basic knowledge of clinical diseases causing them (Table 30.5). On this basis, existing underlying clinical problems should alert the clinician to the likelihood of an acid-base disorder. For example, conditions like diarrhea may lead to metabolic acidosis, while vomiting may result in metabolic alkalosis, highlighting the importance of history and clinical

Table 30.5 Clinical problems that may cause acid base disorders	
Clinical disorder	**Expected acid-base disorder**
Cardiovascular system	
Congestive heart failure	Respiratory alkalosis
Shock	High AG metabolic acidosis
Central nervous system	
Coma	Respiratory acidosis or alkalosis
Seizures	Metabolic acidosis, respiratory alkalosis
Endocrine system	
Diabetic ketoacidosis	High AG metabolic acidosis
Hyperaldosteronism	Metabolic alkalosis
Gastrointestinal system	
Diarrhea	Normal AG metabolic acidosis
Vomiting	Metabolic alkalosis
Renal system	
Renal failure (acute or chronic)	High AG metabolic acidosis
Renal tubular acidosis	Normal AG metabolic acidosis
Respiratory system	
Tachypnea, hyperventilation	Respiratory alkalosis
Chronic hypoventilation	Respiratory acidosis
Miscellaneous causes	
Diuretic use (excessive)	Metabolic alkalosis
Salicylate poisoning	High AG acidosis, respiratory alkalosis
Sepsis and septic shock	Lactic acidosis

assessment in evaluating acid-base imbalances.

B. Primary investigations

These initial tests are crucial for evaluating patients comprehensively. Although they don't directly reveal underlying disorders or acid-base issues, they are essential for identifying various associated problems, which is vital for proper patient management. Key investigations include checking serum levels of sodium, potassium, chloride, HCO_3, and anion gap. Additional relevant investigations are complete blood count (CBC), urine analysis, urinary electrolytes, blood sugar, and renal function tests.

C. Obtaining a blood gas analysis

In determining the appropriateness of obtaining arterial blood gases, there is no precise guideline that dictates when to order this test. The decision should be made following a thorough evaluation of each patient.

1. Selective use of ABG

Blood gas analysis, which requires arterial puncture (a painful procedure with a small risk of arterial occlusion) and is relatively expensive, should not be routinely performed. Except in emergencies, it is advisable to order non-invasive primary blood tests first, such as electrolytes and HCO_3. Based on their results and considering clinical findings, if there are no significant acid-base disturbances, ABG is typically not required.

Indications of ABG

- In emergencies involving critically unstable patients where a significant acid-base disorder is suspected, an ABG is immediately necessary.

- If the patient's history, physical examination, and serum electrolytes suggest severe or progressive acid-base disorders.

- For patients with significant respiratory distress due to acute respiratory diseases or exacerbations of chronic respiratory diseases, ABG analysis is essential for detecting and monitoring oxygenation, ventilation, and acid-base disturbances.

2. Contraindications of ABG

- An abnormal modified Allen's test, local infection, distorted anatomy, peripheral vascular disease, active Raynaud disease, and arteriovenous fistulas.

- Relative contraindications involve impaired coagulation, such as anticoagulation therapy, thrombolytic therapy, known coagulopathies, or low platelet count (<50), which may increase the risk of complications like bleeding and hematoma formation during the procedure.

3. Method for collecting arterial blood gases

Radial artery puncture technique

1. Begin by performing the modified Allen's test.

2. Clean the site (local anesthesia is optional).

3. Use a 21-gauge needle with a syringe.

4. Flush the syringe and needle with heparin.

5. Palpate the artery with one hand and insert the needle at a 45-degree angle.

6. Collect 2-4 ml of blood, preferably without aspiration.

7. After withdrawing the syringe, apply firm pressure at the puncture site.

Special precautions

1. Collect blood in a low-friction syringe under arterial pressure. Avoid pulling (suctioning) the syringe, as it may affect both $PaCO_2$ and PaO_2 values.

2. Use a heparinized syringe to prevent blood clotting, but be cautious not to use excessive heparin, which can dilute the sample.

3. If the sample contains an air bubble, tap it to the surface and expel it from the syringe. Air bubbles can lead to increased PaO_2 and decreased $PaCO_2$.

4. If laboratory analysis is expected to be delayed for more than a few minutes, refrigerate the sample by placing the capped syringe in a glass of ice water. This precaution prevents red blood cells (RBC) metabolism at room temperature, which can produce lactic acid and potentially acidify the sample".

4. Arterial vs. venous blood gases

Venous blood gases are increasingly used as an alternative to arterial blood gases for pH, pCO_2, and HCO_3 assessment in various clinical situations, including emergency services and ICUs, due to small and relatively constant arteriovenous differences. The Role of VBGs in clinical practice is summarized below [5–13]:

Convenience: VBG is a valuable alternative in the intensive care unit and the emergency department as it consumes less time, is less painful and easy to collect, is less invasive with a decrease in needle stick injuries, and makes blood gas evaluation easier in hypotensive settings.

Effectiveness: VBG offers an effective option for assessing non-critical oxygenation and conducting acid-base screening, making it valuable in clinical situations involving chronic respiratory conditions, uremic and diabetic ketoacidosis (DKA) patients, trauma cases with limited arterial access for initial ED assessment, as well as in the evaluation, early resuscitation, and treatment response assessment of shock, and for routine testing.

Correlation with ABG: When utilizing peripheral VBG for clinical decision-making, it is essential to remember that in comparison to ABG:

- Venous pH tends to be approximately 0.02 to 0.04 pH units lower.

- Venous serum HCO_3 concentration is about 2 to 3 mEq/L higher.

- Venous pCO_2 is typically about 3 to 8 mmHg higher, as summarized in Table 30.6.

Simultaneous SpO_2 monitoring: The combination of finger pulse oximetry monitoring with peripheral VBG provides accurate information on acid-base, ventilation, and oxygenation, simplifying

Table 30.6 Normal adult arterial and venous blood gases values		
Parameters	**Arterial sample values**	**Venous sample values**
pH	7.4 (7.35-7.45)	7.37 (7.33-7.42)
$PaCO_2$/$PvCO_2$	40 (35-45) mm Hg	46 (41-51) mm Hg
HCO_3	22-26 mEq/L	24-28 mEq/L
Oxygen saturation	93-98%	65-75%
Partial pressure of O_2 (PO_2)	95-100 mm Hg	35-40 mm Hg

and enhancing clinical assessment in critically ill patients and individuals with respiratory disorders such as COPD exacerbations, potentially decreasing the need for routine ABG tests.

ABG is mandatory and superior to VBG: In post-cardiac arrest or neurotrauma patients, ABG is crucial for managing pCO_2. For patients with poor peripheral perfusion due to severe shock, severe acidosis, severe hypoxemia, or ARDS, ABG, specifically PaO_2, is needed for meticulous oxygenation assessment.

D. Selecting the appropriate method for interpreting an acid-base disorder

Selecting the appropriate method for interpreting an acid-base disorder involves choosing between the traditional Henderson–Hasselbalch method using carbonic acid/bicarbonate and the physicochemical approach, known as the Stewart approach [14].

The Stewart's approach is chiefly used by intensivists because it offers the benefit of a more comprehensive and precise analysis of acid-base disorders by considering factors like strong ion difference and weak acids, which the traditional bicarbonate-centered approach may overlook [15–18]. However, there is no advantage to using this more complicated method, as it does not significantly improve diagnostic or therapeutic abilities in critically ill patients [19].

Current literature favors the use of the physiological approach because

no significant differences have been found when utilizing Stewart's method [20–22], and the traditional approach is simpler, more practical, and can be easily applied at the bedside [2, 4, 19, 23, 24].

E. Interpretation of basic investigations

It is important to remember that ABG and serum electrolytes should be performed simultaneously for the correct interpretation of acid-base disorders.

1. pH
Normal value: 7.4 (7.35 to 7.45).

Low pH (<7.35): Suggests acidosis/acidemia.

High pH (>7.45): Suggests alkalosis/alkalemia.

Normal pH: It suggests either the absence of disorders or the presence of mixed disorders (i.e., metabolic acidosis with respiratory alkalosis, metabolic acidosis with metabolic alkalosis, and metabolic alkalosis with respiratory acidosis).

pH is determined by and inversely related to H^+ concentration. The relation between pH and corresponding H^+ ion concentration (nmol/L) is as follows (Table 30.7).

Equation which defines relationship between H^+, HCO_3 and $PaCO_2$ is:

$$H^+ = 24 \times (PaCO_2/HCO_3)$$

2. Bicarbonate (mEq/L)
Normal value: 24 (22–26) mEq/L.

Table 30.7 pH value and corresponding H⁺ ion concentration									
pH	6.9	7.0	7.1	7.2	7.3	7.4	7.5	7.6	7.7
H⁺ (nmol/L)	125	100	80	64	51	40	32	25	20
H⁺ falls by 20% for each 0.1 pH unit increment									

Low (<22 mEq/L): Metabolic acidosis (primary change) or respiratory alkalosis (secondary change).

High (>26 mEq/L): Metabolic alkalosis (primary change) or respiratory acidosis (secondary change).

Normal HCO$_3$: Does not exclude acid-base disorders. Acute respiratory disturbances or mixed disorders (metabolic acidosis with metabolic alkalosis) can give normal HCO$_3$.

3. PaCO$_2$ (mm of Hg)

Normal value: 40 (35–45) mm of Hg.

High PaCO$_2$ (>45): Respiratory acidosis (primary change) or metabolic alkalosis (secondary change).

Low PaCO$_2$ (<35): Respiratory alkalosis (primary change) or metabolic acidosis (secondary change).

Normal PaCO$_2$: Does not exclude acid-base disorders. Mixed disorders like metabolic acidosis with metabolic alkalosis can have normal PaCO$_2$.

4. Anion gap (AG)

The anion gap (AG) is a critical parameter in the interpretation of acid-base disorders as it provides valuable insights into the classification of metabolic acidosis and the diagnosis of hidden or complex mixed acid-base disorders [25–27].

Anion Gap (AG)

$$= Na^+ - (Cl^- + HCO_3^-)$$
$$= 12 \pm 2 \text{ mEq/L (Normal Value)}$$

The charge difference between an unmeasured anion and a cation is termed the anion gap. Important unmeasured anions are anionic protein, phosphate, sulfate, and organic acids. Important unmeasured cations are calcium, magnesium, and potassium. Increased anion chiefly reflects an increase in the unmeasured anion.

Albumin normally accounts for the majority of the anion gap. Therefore, in cases of hypoalbuminemia, when serum albumin levels are low, it can lead to an artificially lower calculated anion gap. In hypoalbuminemia, for every 1 gm/dL decline in serum albumin, add 2.5 mEq/L to the AG to obtain the corrected value of the anion gap [26, 28].

Corrected Anion Gap =
  Measured AG +
  2.5 × [4 - Serum Albumin (gm/dL)]

Importance of anion gap (AG)

To classify metabolic acidosis: AG is a crucial parameter to classify metabolic acidosis into two groups: high AG metabolic acidosis (e.g., lactic acidosis and diabetic ketoacidosis) and normal AG metabolic acidosis (e.g., in conditions like diarrhea) (Table 30.8). This classification

Table 30.8 Classification of metabolic acidosis based on anion gap	
Anion gap <12	**Anion gap >12**
Normal AG metabolic acidosis	**High AG metabolic acidosis**
Renal tubular acidosis	Lactic acidosis
Diarrhea	Ketoacids (diabetic, alcohol, starvation)
Ureterogastrointestinal fistulas	Toxic ingestions (methanol, ethylene glycol, or salicylates)
Renal failure	Sepsis
Large volume infusion of normal saline	Renal failure

based on AG helps in the appropriate management of metabolic acidosis.

To detect hidden metabolic acidosis: In mixed disorders like metabolic acidosis with metabolic alkalosis, pH, HCO_3, and pCO_2, all basic screening parameters to detect acid-base disorders are normal. Only the measurement of AG provides a clue to detect underlying hidden disorders. High AG in cases with pH, HCO_3, and pCO_2 suggests underlying metabolic acidosis with metabolic alkalosis. So, always calculate the anion gap in ABG interpretation, irrespective of pH status [24].

To identify mixed or triple acid-base disorders: In cases of high AG metabolic acidosis, further evaluation using the formula based on the anion gap may help in revealing coexisting disorders that may not be immediately evident [4].

In high AG metabolic acidosis, compare the rise in AG (calculated AG-12) with the fall in HCO_3 (24-measured HCO_3):

- It is important to remember that usually, the fall in HCO_3 equals the rise in anion gap. So, the equal value of both suggests uncomplicated/pure high AG metabolic acidosis.

- If the rise in anion gap is significantly greater (>5 mmol/L) than the fall in HCO_3, consider the possibility of superimposed metabolic alkalosis.

Explanation of this diagnostic clue: In cases of superimposed metabolic alkalosis, extra bicarbonate is added. This extra bicarbonate leads to a smaller decrease in HCO_3, which is why the value of "rise in the anion gap" becomes relatively greater compared to the value of "fall in HCO_3":

- Conversely, if the rise in anion gap is significantly lesser (<5 mmol/L) than the fall in HCO_3, consider the

possibility of superimposed normal AG metabolic acidosis.

Explanation of this diagnostic clue: In cases of superimposed normal AG metabolic acidosis, there is an additional loss of bicarbonate. This extra loss of bicarbonate leads to a more substantial decrease in HCO_3 compared to the increase in the anion gap, resulting in a significantly lower value of "rise in anion gap" relative to the value of "fall in HCO_3".

Two other methods, similar to the above-discussed approach, are used in clinical practice to evaluate high anion gap metabolic acidosis and reveal potential superimposed metabolic alkalosis or normal AG metabolic acidosis: (1) Comparing the delta anion gap with the delta HCO_3 and (2) Using the delta ratio [29].

Delta Ratio =
(Change in AG) / (Change in HCO_3)

Interpretation of delta ratio [30]

- Delta ratio 0.8–1.2: Uncomplicated/pure high AG metabolic acidosis.

- Delta ratio <0.8: Superimposed normal AG metabolic acidosis in high AG metabolic acidosis.

- Delta ratio >1.2: Superimposed metabolic alkalosis in high AG metabolic acidosis.

5. Serum potassium

Normal value: 3.5 to 5.5 mEq/L.

Low potassium: Metabolic alkalosis (e.g., vomiting, diuretic use), respiratory alkalosis (excessive carbon dioxide losses due to hyperventilation shift potassium into cells), and normal AG metabolic acidosis (e.g., diarrhea, distal renal tubular acidosis-RTA).

High potassium: Metabolic acidosis due to renal failure, Type-4 RTA, DKA, or respiratory acidosis.

6. Pulse oximetry

Pulse oximetry measures the O_2 saturation of arterial hemoglobin, with a normal range of 96–100%. A saturation of less than 90% suggests significant tissue hypoxia, corresponding to a PaO_2 of less than 60%. It is a valuable tool for screening hypoxemia but does not provide information about $PaCO_2$ levels. It's important to note that hypercapnia can occur even when O_2 saturation is 100%.

7. Osmolal gap

The serum osmolal gap is a diagnostic tool useful for identifying unexplained high anion gap metabolic acidosis, particularly when toxic alcohol ingestion is suspected.

The formula to calculate the osmolar gap:

Osmolal Gap =
    Measured − Calculated Osmolality

Where:

Calculated Osmolality

$$= 2 \times Na^+ + \frac{Glucose\ (mg/dL)}{18} + \frac{BUN\ (mg/dL)}{2.8}$$

The normal value of the osmolal gap is usually <10 mOsm/kg, and an osmolal gap exceeding >10 mOsm/kg is regarded as significant. In cases of anion gap metabolic acidosis, major causes of a significant osmolal gap include ingestion of ethylene glycol or methanol, and infusion of propylene glycol.

8. Urinary anion gap

The urinary anion gap (UAG) is a valuable diagnostic tool used to differentiate between gastrointestinal and renal causes of hyperchloremic metabolic acidosis, which helps narrow down the diagnosis of normal AG metabolic acidosis [31–33]. UAG is useful for differentiation between gastrointestinal and renal causes of hyperchloremic acidosis. Usually, UAG is zero or has a positive value.

The urinary anion gap is calculated using the following equation where the concentrations are expressed in mEq/L:

Urinary Anion Gap =
    Urinary ($Na^+ + K^+$) − Urinary Cl^-

Positive urinary anion gap (>20): In cases of normal AG metabolic acidosis, a positive UAG indicates impaired or normal renal ammonium (acid) excretion. Common underlying causes include distal renal tubular acidosis (Type 1 RTA), hyperkalemic renal tubular acidosis (Type 4 RTA) in hypoaldosteronism, and moderate kidney dysfunction.

Negative urinary anion gap (<20): In cases of normal AG metabolic acidosis, a negative UAG results from increased ammonium excretion (i.e., >80 mEq/L). Common contributing factors include severe diarrhea, proximal (Type 2) RTA (often associated with hypophosphatemia, hyperuricemia, and renal glucosuria), NH_4Cl administration, carbonic anhydrase inhibitor therapy, and advanced stages of chronic kidney disease.

The reliability of the urinary anion gap diminishes in the presence of polyuria, when urine pH is greater than 6.5, or when urinary ammonium is excreted alongside an anion other than chloride, such as keto acids, acetylsalicylic acid, D-lactic acid, or significant amounts of penicillin [4].

9. Other investigations

Various investigations commonly performed to establish the etiological diagnosis of acid-base disorders are blood levels of lactate, ketones, and salicylates.

DIAGNOSIS OF ACID-BASE DISTURBANCES: A STEP-BY-STEP APPROACH

Although the interpretation of the diagnosis of acid-base disturbances may seem complex to beginners, a step-by-step approach makes it easy to identify both simple and mixed disorders.

Step 1: Is there an acid-base disorder?

Look at $PaCO_2$ and HCO_3 to determine whether they are in a normal range. If abnormal, go to step 2. If normal, either there is no acid-base disorder, or in critical-sick patients, rule out mixed acid-base disorders (step 5).

Step 2: Is there acidosis or alkalosis?

Look at the pH (normal value between 7.35 and 7.45):

- If pH is <7.35, it suggests acidosis/ acidemia.
- If pH is >7.45, it suggests alkalosis/ alkalemia.

Step 3: What is the primary acid-base disorder?

Determine the primary defect from the pH, HCO_3, and $PaCO_2$:

A. If the pH is low (<7.35), the patient has acidemia, which may be either:

1. Metabolic acidosis:
Characterized by a low HCO_3

2. Respiratory acidosis:
Characterized by high $PaCO_2$

B. If the pH is high (>7.45), the patient has alkalemia, which may be either:

1. Metabolic alkalosis:
Characterized by high HCO_3

2. Respiratory alkalosis:
Characterized by low $PaCO_2$

Step 4: Determine the presence of mixed acid-base disorder

Whether the disorder is simple or mixed is judged by the following steps:

A. Check the direction of changes.

As per the "rule of the same direction," in simple acid-base disorders, HCO_3 and $PaCO_2$ change from normal in the same direction. If these changes are in the opposite direction, it suggests mixed disorder.

B. Compare expected compensation with actual value.

If the actual value is either more or less as compared to the calculated expected compensation, it suggests mixed disorder.

C. Check the anion gap (AG)

In certain mixed disorders, pH, $PaCO_2$, and HCO_3 are normal, and the only clue to an acid-base disorder may be an increased anion gap. So, always determine the anion gap when interpreting ABG results, regardless of the pH level.

D. Compare a fall in HCO_3 with an increase in plasma anion gap in high AG metabolic acidosis:

1. In high AG metabolic acidosis, a rise in the plasma AG (AG-12) matches with a fall in serum HCO_3 (24-HCO_3). Rise in AG = Fall in HCO_3.

2. If the rise in AG exceeds the fall in HCO_3 (Rise in AG > Fall in HCO_3), it suggests coexisting metabolic alkalosis.

3. If the increase in AG is lesser than the fall of HCO_3 (Rise in AG

< Fall in HCO_3), it suggests loss of HCO_3 (diarrhea), causing non-AG metabolic acidosis.

Step 5: Clinical correlation and to establish etiological diagnosis

In the final step of diagnosing acid-base disturbances through a step-by-step approach, it's vital to meticulously correlate the ABG findings with the patient's clinical presentation to pinpoint the underlying cause. Additional investigations are ordered based on clinical judgment. In cases of high anion gap metabolic acidosis, measuring the serum osmolal gap can assist in detecting unexplained toxic alcohol poisoning. Similarly, for normal AG metabolic acidosis, assessing the urinary anion gap helps differentiate between gastrointestinal and renal origins of hyperchloremic metabolic acidosis. This comprehensive assessment ensures a precise diagnosis and guides appropriate treatment strategies.

EXAMPLES OF ACID-BASE DISORDERS

Case 1: A 15-year-old boy is brought from an examination hall in an apprehensive state with a complaint of tightness of the chest. pH 7.54, HCO_3 21 mEq/L, $PaCO_2$ 21 mm Hg.

Interpretation: The high pH indicates alkalosis. The low $PaCO_2$ suggests respiratory alkalosis:

- The low HCO_3 indicates compensation (following the "same direction rule").
- Expected acute compensation (fall in HCO_3) in respiratory alkalosis will be:

Fall in HCO_3 =
$0.2 \times$ Fall in $PaCO_2 = 0.2 \times (40-21)$
$= 0.2 \times 19 = 3.8$

So, the expected HCO_3 will be 24–3.8 = 20.2 mEq/L, which closely matches the actual HCO_3 of 21 mEq/L, suggesting a simple acid-base disorder.

Therefore, the patient has primary respiratory alkalosis due to anxiety.

Case 2: A patient with poorly controlled IDDM missed his insulin for three days. pH 7.1, HCO_3 8 mEq/L, $PaCO_2$ 20 mm Hg Na^+ 140 mEq/L, Cl^- 106 mEq/L, and urinary ketones +++.

Interpretation: The low pH indicates acidosis. The low HCO_3 suggests metabolic acidosis, and the low $PaCO_2$ indicates compensation (following the "same direction rule").

- Expected compensation (fall in $PaCO_2$) will be:

$PaCO_2$ =
$HCO_3 \times 1.5 + 8 = 8 \times 1.5 + 8$
$= 12 + 8 = 20$

So, the expected $PaCO_2$ matches the actual $PaCO_2$ at 20 mm Hg, suggesting a simple acid-base disorder.

- The anion gap is 26 (AG = Na^+ - (Cl^- + HCO_3) = 140 - (106 + 8) = 140 - 114 = 26, which is high, suggesting high anion gap metabolic acidosis. The presence of urinary ketones suggests diabetic ketoacidosis.

Therefore, the patient has high anion gap metabolic acidosis due to DKA.

Case 3: ABG of a patient with CHF on furosemide is as follows: pH 7.48, HCO_3 34 mEq/L, $PaCO_2$ 48 mm Hg.

Interpretation: The high pH indicates alkalosis. The high HCO_3 suggests metabolic alkalosis:

- The high $PaCO_2$ indicates compensation (following the "same direction rule").

- Expected compensation (rise in $PaCO_2$) will be:

  Rise in $PaCO_2$ =

  $0.7 \times$ Rise in HCO_3 = $0.7 \times (34-24)$ = $0.7 \times 10 = 7.0$

So, the expected $PaCO_2$ will be 40 + 7.0 = 47.0 mm Hg, which closely matches the actual $PaCO_2$ at 48 mm Hg, suggesting a simple acid-base disorder.

Therefore, the patient has primary metabolic alkalosis due to diuretics.

Case 4: Following sleeping pills ingestion, the patient presented in a drowsy state with sluggish respiration, having a respiratory rate of 4/min. pH 7.1, HCO_3 28 mEq/L, $PaCO_2$ 80 mm Hg, PaO_2 42 mm Hg.

Interpretation: The low pH indicates acidosis. The high $PaCO_2$ suggests respiratory acidosis. The low PaO_2, indicating hypoxemia, supports the diagnosis of respiratory failure and acidosis:

- The high HCO_3 also suggests compensation (following the "same direction rule").

- Expected acute compensation (rise in HCO_3) will be:

  Rise in HCO_3 =

  $0.1 \times$ Rise in $PaCO_2$ = $0.1 \times (80 - 40)$ = $0.1 \times 40 = 4$ mEq/L

So, the expected HCO_3 matches the actual HCO_3 at 28 mEq/L, suggestive of a simple acid-base disorder.

Therefore, the patient has primary respiratory acidosis due to respiratory failure caused by sleeping pills.

Case 5: A patient with severe diarrhea complains of difficulty in breathing. pH 7.1, HCO_3 14 mEq/L, $PaCO_2$ 44 mm Hg, and K^+ 2.0 mEq/L.

Interpretation: The low pH indicates acidosis. The low HCO_3 suggests metabolic acidosis:

- The low HCO_3 also and high $PaCO_2$ suggests that changes are in opposite direction.

- Although $PaCO_2$ is expected to decrease due to compensation, the actual $PaCO_2$ is high, indicating the presence of associated respiratory acidosis. The very low K^+ level, causing weakness of respiratory muscles, is the underlying cause of respiratory failure, leading to respiratory acidosis.

Therefore, this patient has a mixed disorder, including metabolic acidosis with respiratory acidosis.

Case 6: ABG of a patient with shock on ventilatory support for the last 4 hours is pH 7.48, HCO_3 14 mEq/L, $PaCO_2$ 22 mm Hg.

Interpretation: The high pH indicates alkalosis. The low $PaCO_2$ suggests respiratory alkalosis, which an increased respiratory rate and high tidal volume on the ventilator can cause:

- The low HCO_3 also suggests compensation (following the "same direction rule").

- Expected acute compensation (fall in HCO_3) will be:

  Fall in HCO_3 =

  $0.2 \times$ Fall in $PaCO_2$ = $0.2 \times (40 - 22)$ = $0.2 \times 18 = 3.6$ mEq/L

So, the expected HCO_3 would be $24 - 3.6 = 20.4$ mEq/L. However, the actual value of HCO_3 is lower (14 vs. 20.4 mEq/L), suggesting the presence of additional metabolic acidosis, which could be attributed to shock-induced lactic acidosis.

Therefore, the patient has a mixed disorder, including respiratory alkalosis with metabolic acidosis.

Case 7: A known case of COPD develops severe vomiting. pH 7.4, HCO_3 36 mEq/L, $PaCO_2$ 60 mm Hg.

Interpretation: The pH is normal, indicating that the patient either has no disorder or has a mixed acid-base disorder.

- However, the abnormal values of HCO_3 and $PaCO_2$ suggest the presence of mixed disorders.

- The high HCO_3 indicates the presence of metabolic alkalosis (which can occur due to vomiting), while the high $PaCO_2$ is suggestive of respiratory acidosis (which can occur due to COPD). Metabolic alkalosis is expected to increase the pH, while respiratory acidosis is expected to decrease the pH.

- The normal pH can be explained as the result of opposite changes caused by both primary disorders.

Therefore, the patient has a mixed disorder, including respiratory acidosis with metabolic alkalosis.

Case 8: A case of hepatic failure experiences persistent vomiting. pH 7.54, HCO_3 38 mEq/L, $PaCO_2$ 44 mm Hg.

Interpretation: The high pH indicates alkalosis. The high HCO_3 suggests metabolic alkalosis (due to vomiting).

- The high $PaCO_2$ suggests compensation (following the "same direction rule").

- Expected compensation (rise in $PaCO_2$) will be:

Rise in $PaCO_2$ =

$0.7 \times$ Rise in $HCO_3 = 0.7 \times (38-24)$
$= 0.7 \times 14 = 9.8$

So, the expected $PaCO_2$ would be $40 + 9.8 = 49.8$ mm Hg. However, the actual value of $PaCO_2$ is lower than the expected $PaCO_2$ (44 vs. 49.8 mm Hg), suggesting the presence of additional respiratory alkalosis, which can be attributed to hepatic failure.

Therefore, the patient has a mixed disorder, including metabolic alkalosis with respiratory alkalosis.

Case 9: A patient with poorly controlled IDDM presents with severe vomiting. pH 7.4, HCO_3 24 mEq/L, $PaCO_2$ 40 mm Hg Na^+ 136 mEq/L, Cl^- 84 mEq/L, and urinary ketones +++.

Interpretation: The pH, HCO_3, and $PaCO_2$ values are within the normal range:

- However, the elevated anion gap is 16 (AG = $Na^+ - (Cl^- + HCO_3)$ = $136 - (84 + 24) = 136 - 108 = 28$), suggesting high anion gap metabolic acidosis. The presence of urinary ketones suggests diabetic ketoacidosis.

- Despite the high anion gap metabolic acidosis, normal pH and HCO_3, indicates the coexistence of metabolic alkalosis.

- Therefore, the patient has a mixed disorder, including diabetic ketoacidosis and metabolic alkalosis.

This case illustrates a unique scenario where the anion gap is elevated, indicating a mixed disorder, despite the pH, HCO_3, and $PaCO_2$ being within the normal range.

Case 10: A patient presents with a history of abdominal pain, vomiting, oliguria, and shock. Their blood gas analysis reveals the following values: pH = 7.46, HCO_3 = 20 mEq/L, pCO_2 = 29 mm Hg, Na^+ = 126 mEq/L, K^+ = 4.0 mEq/L, and Cl^- = 79 mEq/L.

Interpretation: The patient's blood gas analysis reveals a complex acid-base disorder:

- The elevated pH suggests alkalosis.

- The low $PaCO_2$ indicates respiratory alkalosis.

- The low HCO_3 also indicates compensation, following the "same direction rule."

Expected acute compensation (fall in HCO_3) in respiratory alkalosis would be:

Fall in HCO_3 =

$0.2 \times$ Fall in $PaCO_2 = 0.2 \times (40-29)$ $= 0.2 \times 11 = 2.2$ mEq/L

So, the expected HCO_3 should be $24-2.2 = 21.8$ mEq/L. However, the actual value of HCO_3 is slightly lower at 20.0 mEq/L, suggesting the possibility of additional metabolic acidosis.

The high anion gap (AG) is calculated as 27 (AG = Na^+ - (Cl^- + HCO_3)) = 126 - (79 + 20) = 126 - 99 = 27), confirming the presence of additional high anion gap metabolic acidosis.

To further analyze the high anion gap metabolic acidosis, we compare the "Rise AG" with the "Fall in HCO_3":

- Rise in AG = 27 − 12 = 15

- Fall in HCO_3 = 24 − 20 = 4. The "Rise in AG" is greater than the "Fall in HCO_3", suggesting the presence of metabolic alkalosis in addition to the existing acid-base disturbances.

Therefore, the patient has a mixed acid-base disorder, including respiratory alkalosis, high anion gap metabolic acidosis, and metabolic alkalosis.

This case highlights how using a systematic approach, including the assessment of the anion gap and comparison of Rise AG with Fall in HCO_3, can make it easier and more accurate to solve complex cases involving acid-base disturbances.

REFERENCES

1. Ayers P, Dixon C. Simple acid-base tutorial. JPEN J Parenter Enter Nutr. 2012;36(1):18-23.

2. Adrogué HJ, Gennari FJ, Galla JH, et al. Assessing acid-base disorders. Kidney Int. 2009;76(12):1239–1247.

3. Adrogué HJ, Madias NE. Secondary responses to altered acid-base status: the rules of engagement. J Am Soc Nephrol 2010;21(6):920–3.

4. Berend K, de Vries AP, Gans RO. Physiological approach to assessment of acid-base disturbances. N Engl J Med. 2014;371(15):1434–1445.

5. Malatesha G, Singh NK, Bharija A, et al. Comparison of arterial and venous pH, bicarbonate, PCO2 and PO2 in initial emergency department assessment. Emerg Med J. 2007;24(8):569–71.

6. Kim BR, Park SJ, Shin HS, et al. Correlation between peripheral venous and arterial blood gas measurements in patients admitted to the intensive care unit: a single-center study. Kidney Res Clin Pract. 2013;32(1):32–8.

7. Byrne AL, Bennett M, Chatterji R, et al. Peripheral venous and arterial blood gas analysis in adults: are they comparable? A systematic review and meta-analysis. Respirology 2014;19(2):168–175.

8. McKeever TM, Hearson G, Housley G, et al. Using venous blood gas analysis in the assessment of COPD exacerbations: a prospective cohort study. Thorax 2016;71(3):210–5.

9. Zeserson E, Goodgame B, Hess JD, et al. Correlation of Venous Blood Gas and Pulse Oximetry With Arterial Blood Gas in the Undifferentiated Critically Ill Patient. J Intensive Care Med 2018;33(3):176–181.

10. Schütz N, Roth D, Schwameis M, et al. Can Venous Blood Gas Be Used as an Alternative to Arterial Blood Gas in Intubated Patients at Admission to the Emergency Department? A Retrospective Study. Open Access Emerg Med. 2019;11:305–312.

11. Erdoğan YK, Karakuş A. Can venous blood gas be used instead of arterial blood gas in emergency department?. Interdisciplinary Medical Journal. 2023;14(49):74–78.

12. Prasad H, Vempalli N, Agrawal N, et al. Correlation and agreement between arterial and venous blood gas analysis in patients with hypotension-an emergency department-based cross-sectional study. Int J Emerg Med. 2023;16(1):18.

13. Saberian L, Sharif M, Aarabi M, et al. Arterial Versus Venous Blood Gas Analysis Comparisons, Appropriateness, and Alternatives in Different Acid/Base Clinical Settings: A Systematic Review. Cureus. 2023;15(7):e41707.

14. Kimura S, Shabsigh M, Morimatsu H. Traditional approach versus Stewart approach for acid-base disorders: Inconsistent evidence. SAGE Open Med. 2018;6:2050312118801255.

15. Morgan TJ. The Stewart approach--one clinician's perspective. Clin Biochem Rev. 2009;30(2):41–54.

16. Magder S, Emami A. Practical approach to physical-chemical acid-base management. Stewart at the bedside. Ann Am Thorac Soc. 2015;12(1):111–7.

17. Story DA. Stewart Acid-Base: A Simplified Bedside Approach. Anesth Analg. 2016;123(2):511–5.

18. Rubin DM. Stewart's approach to quantitative acid-base physiology should replace traditional bicarbonate-centered models. J Appl Physiol (1985). 2021;130(6):2019–2021.

19. Masevicius FD, Dubin A. Has Stewart approach improved our ability to diagnose acid-base disorders in critically ill patients? World J Crit Care Med. 2015;4(1):62–70.

20. Maria V, Francesca B, Shirin D, et al. Comparison between bicarbonate-based and Stewart methods to assess metabolic acid-base disorders in internistic patients. A pilot study International Journal of Medicine 2017;5(2):234–238.

21. Paliwal R, Pakavakis A, Divatia JV, et al. Utility of Stewart's Approach to Diagnose Missed Complex Acid–Base Disorders as Compared to Bicarbonate-anion Gap-based Methodology in Critically Ill Patients: An Observational Study. Indian J Crit Care Med 2022;26(1):23–32.

22. Gopaldas JA. Revisiting Stewart's Approach toward Assessment of Unidentified or Complex Acid–Base Disorders. Indian J Crit Care Med 2022;26(1):5–6.

23. Kurtz I, Kraut J, Ornekian V, et al. Acid-base analysis: a critique of the Stewart and bicarbonate-centered approaches. Am J Physiol Renal Physiol. 2008;294(5):F1009–31.

24. Achanti A, Szerlip HM. Acid-Base Disorders in the Critically Ill Patient. Clin J Am Soc Nephrol. 2023;18(1):102–112.

25. Emmett M. Anion-gap interpretation: the old and the new. Nat Clin Pract Nephrol. 2006;2(1):4–5.

26. Kraut JA, Madias NE. Serum anion gap: its uses and limitations in clinical medicine. Clin J Am Soc Nephrol. 2007;2(1):162–74.

27. Reddy P. Clinical utility of anion gap in deciphering acid-base disorders. Intl J Clin Pract. 2009;63(10):1516–1525.

28. Figge J, Jabor A, Kazda A, et al. Anion gap and hypoalbuminemia. Crit Care Med 1998;26(11):1807–1810.

29. Seifter JL. Anion-gap metabolic acidemia: case-based analyses. Eur J Clin Nutr. 2020;74(1):83–86.

30. Tucker AM, Johnson TN. Acid-base disorders: A primer for clinicians. Nutr Clin Pract. 2022;37(5):980–989.

31. Berend K. Review of the Diagnostic Evaluation of Normal Anion Gap Metabolic Acidosis. Kidney Dis (Basel). 2017;3(4):149–159.

32. Batlle D, Ba Aqeel SH, Marquez A. The Urine Anion Gap in Context. Clin J Am Soc Nephrol. 2018;13(2):195–197.

33. Uribarri J, Oh MS. The Urine Anion Gap: Common Misconceptions. J Am Soc Nephrol. 2021;32(5):1025–1028.

31 | Metabolic Acidosis

Metabolic acidosis is a frequently encountered acid-base disorder in critical care patients, demanding meticulous attention and effective management due to its potential for serious consequences.

DEFINITION

It is characterized by a fall in plasma HCO_3 and a fall in pH (below 7.35). The $PaCO_2$ is reduced secondarily by hyperventilation, and this compensatory mechanism minimizes the fall in pH.

ETIOLOGY

Metabolic acidosis can result from the loss of HCO_3 via the gastrointestinal (GI) tract or kidneys, overproduction of endogenous nonvolatile acids, ingestion or infusion of acid or potential acids, and failure of H^+ excretion by the kidney.

Calculation of anion gap (AG) is extremely helpful in narrowing etiological diagnosis:

Anion Gap (AG)
$$= Na^+ - (Cl^- + HCO_3^-)$$
$$= 12 \pm 2 \text{ (Normal Value)}$$

Metabolic acidosis can be classified into two groups based on the anion gap: high anion gap acidosis (e.g., lactic acidosis, ketoacidosis, ingested toxins, and acute or chronic renal impairment) and normal anion gap acidosis (e.g., diarrhea, renal tubular acidosis, or large volume saline administration). Table 31.1 summarizes the causes of metabolic acidosis classified based on the anion gap, their mechanisms of development, and how acidosis occurs in each cause.

The mnemonic "GOLDMARK" is helpful for remembering the causes of high anion gap metabolic acidosis (Table 31.2) [1].

Lactic acidosis

Lactic acidosis is one of the most common causes of high anion gap metabolic acidosis, often seen in ICU patients who have critical illness or

	Table 31.1 Common causes of metabolic acidosis	
	Normal anion gap (6-12 mEq) metabolic acidosis (NAGMA)	
1.	**GI loss of bicarbonate**	**Diarrhea:** Due to loss of bicarbonate rich stool. Colonic secretion of HCO_3 in exchange for chloride causes hyperchloremia.
		Laxative abuse: Due to laxative induced diarrhea.
		External pancreatic or small-bowel drainage: Due to losses of bicarbonate rich fluid.
		Urinary diversion: Due to exchange for urinary chloride by colonic secretion of HCO_3 and the reabsorption of urinary ammonium.
2.	**Renal loss of bicarbonate**	**Renal tubular acidosis:** Due to impaired renal tubules' ability to excrete hydrogen ions as ammonium or inadequate reabsorption of filtered HCO_3^-.
		Acute and chronic kidney failure: Due to impaired renal ammonia production and secretion, and thus limiting H^+ ion excretion.
		Acetazolamide: By enhancing renal excretion of bicarbonate due to its carbonic anhydrase inhibitor effect.
3.	**Addition of acid**	**Hyperalimentation:** Due to the excessive supplementation of chloride-containing lysine and arginine in parenteral nutrition, as well as the addition of hydrochloric acid to amino acid parenteral nutrition (PN) mixtures to lower the pH.
4.	**Dilution**	**Normal saline:** Excessive administration of chloride rich and buffer free saline causes dilution of the serum bicarbonate leading to hyperchloremic acidosis.
	High anion gap (>12 mEq) metabolic acidosis (HAGMA)	
1.	**Increased production of endogenous acids**	**Lactic acidosis:** Due to the overproduction of lactic acid in sepsis, shock, hypoxia, and medication like metformin.
		Ketoacidosis: Due to accumulation of ketoacids in uncontrolled diabetes mellitus, excessive intake of alcohol or prolong starvation.
2.	**Addition of exogenous acids**	**Toxins:** Due to ingestion of certain toxins such as methanol, ethylene glycol, and salicylates.
		Ethanol: Due to excessive alcohol consumption.
3.	**Failure to excrete acid**	**Renal failure:** Decreased renal acid excretion and accumulation of sulfuric and phosphoric acid in severe kidney dysfunction.

Table 31.2 Mnemonic for causes of high anion gap metabolic acidosis: "GOLDMARK"	
G	Glycols (ethylene glycol and propylene glycol)
O	Oxoproline
L	L-lactate
D	D-lactate
M	Methanol
A	Aspirin (salicylates)
R	Renal failure (uremia)
K	Ketoacidosis (diabetic/alcoholic/starvation)

multiorgan failure. It occurs either due to the excessive production or reduced clearance of lactic acid, often seen in conditions such as sepsis, shock, or severe hypoxia. When the lactate production rate exceeds its hepatic clearance, increased blood lactate levels result in acidosis. Usually, plasma lactate levels range from 0.5 to 1.5 mEq/L, and lactic acidosis is generally defined when lactate levels exceed 4–5 mEq/L. Severe lactic acidosis is associated with high mortality.

There are two primary subtypes of lactic acidosis:

Type A: Lactic acidosis - inadequate oxygen delivery: This subtype is typically caused by significantly inadequate tissue oxygenation, resulting from severe hypoxemia or decreased perfusion. It leads to an increased peripheral generation of lactate and the subsequent accumulation of lactic acid.

Common triggers for this type of lactic acidosis include:

- Reduced tissue oxygen delivery due to severe hypoxemia or anemia.
- Tissue hypoperfusion, which can result from cardiogenic, septic, or hemorrhagic shock, cardiopulmonary arrest, or regional hypoperfusion such as mesenteric or limb ischemia.
- Anaerobic muscular activity, often associated with seizures or generalized convulsions.

Type B: Lactic acidosis - altered cellular metabolism: Type B Lactic Acidosis, characterized by increased lactate production due to impaired cellular and/or mitochondrial metabolism, is caused by various medical conditions, medications, or toxins and is not related to impaired tissue oxygenation. Common conditions that trigger type B lactic acidosis include:

- Medical conditions such as diabetes, thiamine deficiency, severe infection, liver disease, short bowel syndrome, and malignancies like leukemia or lymphoma.
- Medications like metformin, antiretroviral drugs causing mitochondrial dysfunction in HIV therapy, salicylates, or isoniazid.
- Toxins such as chronic severe alcoholism, ethylene glycol, methanol, or propylene glycol poisoning.

Ketoacidosis: Diabetic and alcoholic ketoacidosis are two common causes of high anion gap metabolic acidosis, often necessitating hospitalization. In both these disorders, the pathophysiology of ketoacidosis is similar, involving insulin deficiency, increased levels of counterregulatory hormones such as glucagon, cortisol, or catecholamines, and lipolysis, which leads to an increase in the formation of acidic ketones, particularly b-hydroxybutyrate acid [2].

Diabetic ketoacidosis

The most common cause of ketoacidosis is diabetic ketoacidosis (DKA), which usually occurs in patients with uncontrolled type 1 diabetes.

DKA usually occurs when insulin is missed or is inadequate and is commonly precipitated by an intercurrent illness that increases insulin requirements, such as an infection, trauma, surgery, emotional stress, myocardial ischemia, gastroenteritis, or pancreatitis. The combined effect of insulin deficiency (causing increased lipolysis) and increased levels of counterregulatory hormones like glucagon (causing accelerated hepatic fatty acid oxidation and ketogenesis) results in high AG metabolic acidosis.

Diabetic ketoacidosis is characterized by the triad of hyperglycemia (blood glucose concentration of >200 mg/dL), metabolic acidosis (venous pH <7.3 and serum bicarbonate <18 mmol/L), and ketonemia or ketonuria. The routinely performed urine test for ketones detects less common ketones like acetoacetate and acetone. However, it may not identify the main ketone, beta-hydroxybutyrate, which can lead to an unreliable diagnosis of DKA and an underestimation of the degree of ketosis. Therefore, if available, the preferred test to diagnose DKA is the direct measurement of serum β-hydroxybutyrate, which can resolve this issue.

Patients with DKA are always volume depleted, and correcting this hypovolemia with a large volume of saline can cause the development of hyperchloremic normal anion gap metabolic acidosis during the recovery phase of DKA.

Alcoholic ketoacidosis

Alcoholic ketoacidosis predominantly affects malnourished individuals who consume substantial quantities of alcohol over a short period. Common symptoms include nausea, vomiting, abdominal pain, and severe fluid depletion, often necessitating hospitalization. Diagnostic criteria consist of a low pH (<7.3), reduced serum bicarbonate levels (<15 mEq/L), an elevated anion gap (>14), and are frequently associated with hypokalemia, hypomagnesemia, and hypophosphatemia.

It is important to differentiate between two important causes of ketoacidosis: alcohol-induced and diabetes-induced. Blood glucose levels within the low to normal range favor alcoholic ketoacidosis, while hyperglycemia indicates diabetic ketoacidosis. When distinguishing between alcoholic and diabetic ketoacidosis is confusing or difficult, a lower HbA1c level can provide a valuable clue for diagnosing alcoholic ketoacidosis.

Salicylate (aspirin) poisoning

A common presentation of salicylate toxicity includes a mixed acid-base disorder characterized by:

1. **Respiratory alkalosis** due to direct stimulation of the medullary respiratory center.
2. **High anion gap (AG) metabolic acidosis** resulting from interference with cellular metabolism.

The most common clinical features of salicylate poisoning include symptoms such as tinnitus, nausea, vomiting, hyperventilation, tachycardia, noncardiogenic pulmonary edema, altered mental status, seizures, and coma.

Renal tubular acidosis

The three major types of renal tubular acidosis (RTA) differ primarily in their underlying causes, biochemical abnormalities, mechanism of development, and the specific renal tubules affected (Table 31.3).

Type 1 RTA (distal RTA)

- Cause: Impaired hydrogen ion secretion in the distal tubules of the kidneys, often due to a defect in the H^+-ATPase pump or H^+/K^+ exchanger.
- Result: Inability to acidify urine properly, leading to metabolic acidosis.
- Lab feature: Inappropriately high urine pH (alkaline urine with pH >5.5), hypokalemia, and decreased urinary ammonium excretion.

- Clinical features: Nephrolithiasis, nephrocalcinosis, and metabolic bone disease.

Type 2 RTA (proximal RTA)

- Cause: Impaired bicarbonate reabsorption in the proximal tubules of the kidneys, leading to profound loss of bicarbonate into the urine.
- Result: Loss of bicarbonate in the urine, resulting in metabolic acidosis.
- Lab features: Urinary pH is acidic (pH <5.5) when bicarbonate levels

Table 31.3 Comparison of different types of renal tubular acidosis			
	Hyperchloremic normal AG metabolic acidosis		
	Distal RTA (Type 1)	**Proximal RTA (Type 2)**	**Hyperkalemic RTA (Type 4 RTA)**
Serum potassium	**Hypokalemic RTA**		**Hyperkalemic RTA**
Incidence	Rare	Rare	Common
Metabolic acidosis	Severe	Moderate	Mild
Serum HCO_3	Can be significantly low (<10 mEq/L)	Usually 12 to 20 mEq/L	Usually >17 mEq/L
Primary defect	Impaired distal H^+ excretion	Reduced proximal HCO_3 reabsorption (bicarbonate wasting)	Reduced aldosterone secretion or aldosterone resistance
Fractional HCO_3 excretion	<5%	>10–15%	5–10%
Urine pH	Always >5.3	Low (<5.5)	Variable, usually >5.3
Urine anion gap	Positive (>20 mEq/L)	Negative	Positive (>20 mEq/L)
Urine NH_4^+	Low	Low	Low
Urine citrate	Low	High/normal	Low/normal
Urine Ca^{2+}/Cr ratio	High	Normal	Normal
Renal stones/ nephrocalcinosis	Yes	No	No
Bone diseases	Often present	Common	Absent
Kidney function	Usually, normal	Usually, normal	CKD is common
Causes	Sjögren's syndrome, SLE, RA, amphotericin B toxicity	Multiple myeloma, acetazolamide, Fanconi syndrome	Diabetic nephropathy, chronic interstitial nephritis, adrenal insufficiency, K^+ sparing diuretics
Alkali requirement	1 to 3 mEq/kg/day	Large 10 to 15 mEq/kg/day	1 to 3 mEq/kg/day
Response	Responds promptly	Poor response	Moderate response

are low, and when serum bicarbonate increases due to bicarbonate therapy, urine pH becomes alkaline (pH >5.5). A common characteristic feature is hypokalemia. In cases where type 2 RTA is associated with Fanconi syndrome, additional features include glycosuria, generalized aminoaciduria, and phosphaturia.

Type 4 RTA (hyperkalemic RTA)

- Cause: Impaired secretion of potassium ions in the distal tubules or collecting ducts, often due to hypoaldosteronism or resistance to aldosterone.
- Result: Hyperkalemia, which is disproportionate to the reduction in glomerular filtration rate and mild metabolic acidosis.
- Key feature: High urinary pH, high serum potassium, and kidney function may be compromised.

CLINICAL FEATURES

Clinical presentation in metabolic acidosis is primarily due to:

- Manifestations depend on the underlying disorder.
- Manifestations of metabolic acidosis depend on its rapidity of onset and severity.

The clinical presentation of metabolic acidosis depends on various changes in pulmonary, cardiovascular, neurological, metabolic, and other aspects.

Pulmonary changes: Kussmaul's breathing (rapid, deep, labored breathing at a consistent pace) suggests the presence of metabolic acidosis. This compensatory hyperventilation is due to increased depth and frequency of breathing resulting from the body's attempt to eliminate excess carbon dioxide and correct the acid-base imbalance. In acute metabolic acidemia, hyperventilation for a prolonged period can lead to respiratory muscle fatigue, decreased diaphragmatic contractility, and even respiratory failure and cyanosis.

Cardiovascular changes: When severe acidemia (pH <7.2) is present, there is an increased susceptibility to cardiac arrhythmias and a decreased response to inotropes, possibly leading to secondary hypotension. The reduced blood pressure in these patients results from depressed myocardial contractility and arterial vasodilatation induced by the low pH.

Neurological changes: It ranges from anxiety, headache, confusion, lethargy, and drowsiness to coma.

Metabolic changes: Severe acidemia can lead to hyperkalemia, hyperphosphatemia, and shifts of potassium and phosphorus from the intracellular to the extracellular compartment. Chronic acidemia, as with renal failure, can cause stunted growth and rickets in children, bone demineralization, and fractures due to osteomalacia in adults.

Other changes: Severe acidosis can cause nonspecific symptoms such as anorexia, nausea, vomiting, and muscle weakness, especially in infants and young children.

DIAGNOSIS

History

Proper history elicitation provides clues for the presence of metabolic acidosis and underlying etiology:

- Kussmaul's breathing is the most important diagnostic presentation.
- Pre-existing diabetes, renal failure, and recurrent renal stones provide a clue to the presence as well as the cause of acidosis.

- Lactic acidosis can be suspected in patients with hypotension, shock, cardiac failure, and septicemia.
- Order toxicology panel in high AG metabolic acidosis with suspected drug or toxic ingestion.

Investigations

A. Confirm the diagnosis: Obtain arterial blood gases, and low HCO_3, low pH, and compensatory fall in $PaCO_2$ will confirm the diagnosis.

B. To establish the etiological diagnosis: To establish the etiological diagnosis of metabolic acidosis, commonly ordered investigations include measuring the anion gap, serum electrolytes, blood sugar, renal function tests, serum lactate levels, and assessing the levels of salicylates. Additionally, urinary examination for pH, ketones, and the presence of oxalate crystals can also be very useful in diagnosing the underlying cause of metabolic acidosis. The choice of tests ordered for each patient should be individualized based on their history and clinical evaluation:

1. **Calculate serum anion gap (AG) to classify metabolic acidosis:** Always order serum electrolytes along with ABG, as it is essential to calculate AG [Anion Gap = Na^+ - (Cl^- + HCO_3)]. Based on anion gap, metabolic acidosis is divided in to two groups: Normal AG (e.g., diarrhea, GI fistulas, urinary diversion, renal tubular acidosis, acetazolamide, and large volume saline infusion), and high AG metabolic acidosis (e.g., lactic acidosis, ketoacidosis toxic alcohol ingestion, renal failure).

2. **Calculate urinary anion gap to evaluate normal AG metabolic acidosis**

   Urinary Anion Gap (UAG) =
   Urinary (Na^+ + K^+) − Urinary Cl^-

The urinary anion gap reflects the kidney's ability to excrete NH_4Cl and is helpful in differentiating between gastrointestinal and renal causes of normal anion gap (hyperchloremic) metabolic acidosis. Normally, UAG is zero or has a positive value.

Negative urinary anion gap (<20) indicates that in normal AG metabolic acidosis, renal acidification remains unaffected, and NH_4Cl excretion increases appropriately in response to acidosis, potentially due to causes such as gastrointestinal HCO_3 loss (e.g., diarrhea), proximal (Type 2) RTA, or carbonic anhydrase inhibitor therapy.

Positive urinary anion gap (>20) indicates impaired NH_4Cl excretion in normal AG metabolic acidosis, which can occur due to distal renal tubular acidosis (Type 1 RTA) or renal failure (with impaired NH_4Cl excretion).

3. **Calculate osmolal gap to evaluate further high AG metabolic acidosis:** The serum osmolal gap is a diagnostic tool useful for identifying unexplained high anion gap metabolic acidosis, particularly when toxic alcohol ingestion is suspected.

   Osmolal Gap =
   Measured − Calculated Osmolality

   The normal osmolal gap value is typically <10 mOsm/kg, and a significantly higher osmolal gap indicates potential ingestion of ethylene glycol, methanol, or exposure to propylene glycol.

4. **Detect coexisting acid-base disorders**
   a. Calculate expected pCO_2 and compare it with the actual value of pCO_2: To detect coexisting

acid-base disorders, calculate the expected pCO_2 using Winter's formula:

Expected $PaCO_2$ = $(1.5 \times Serum\ HCO_3) + 8$

In cases of simple metabolic acidosis, the calculated and actual pCO_2 values will be the same.

- If the actual pCO_2 value is greater than the calculated pCO_2, it suggests the presence of coexisting respiratory acidosis.

- If the actual pCO_2 value is lower than the calculated pCO_2, it suggests the presence of coexisting respiratory alkalosis.

b. In high AG metabolic acidosis,

Compare rise in AG with the fall in HCO_3

Where,

The rise in AG (or Delta AG) = Calculated AG-12

and,

The fall in HCO_3 (or Delta HCO_3) = 24-measured HCO_3

- It is important to remember that the fall in HCO_3 equals the rise in anion gap in uncomplicated/pure high AG metabolic acidosis.

- If the rise in anion gap is significantly greater (>5 mmol/L) than the fall in HCO_3, consider the possibility of superimposed metabolic alkalosis.

- Conversely, if the rise in anion gap is significantly lesser (<5 mmol/L) than the fall in HCO_3, consider the possibility of superimposed normal AG metabolic acidosis.

TREATMENT

Treatment of metabolic acidosis includes:

1. **Specific management of underlying disorder:** As a rule, meticulously treat the underlying disorder, which is the most critical measure and may be the only required treatment for mild to moderate acidosis. Providing attention to special measures for the given etiology of metabolic acidosis is very important and will be discussed later.

2. **General measures:** Important measures to consider are as follows:

   Fluid replacement: Adequate fluid resuscitation is crucial to correct dehydration, improve organ perfusion, and restore acid-base balance. Preferred IV fluids include balanced solutions like Ringer's lactate, which not only correct hypovolemia but also contain buffers that help correct acidosis. Isotonic bicarbonate solution (e.g., dextrose 5% 850 ml with $NaHCO_3$ 150 mEq/L) is a useful option for providing fluid replacement and for simultaneously correcting severe metabolic acidosis.

   Correction of electrolyte imbalances: In patients with metabolic acidosis, monitoring and correcting electrolyte imbalances, especially potassium, is essential to prevent complications. Metabolic acidosis can result in elevated potassium levels that mask underlying hypokalemia. Conversely, correcting this imbalance can shift potassium from the extracellular and intracellular compartments, potentially worsening the pre-existing hypokalemia, which can be harmful.

   Supportive care: As the administration of sodium bicarbonate can increase CO_2 production, it is vital to assess and ensure adequate ventilation before administering sodium bicarbonate in metabolic acidosis. Administer empiric antibiotics after obtaining samples for cultures and sensitivities in patients with suspected sepsis. Additionally, ensure the provision of proper nutrition, identify and manage precipitating factors, and closely monitor the patient.

3. **Alkali therapy:** The administration of sodium bicarbonate is an essential part of managing metabolic acidosis, but indications, goals, routes, and dosages vary significantly between acute and chronic metabolic acidosis.

Alkali therapy in acute metabolic acidosis

It's important to note that the use of bicarbonate therapy in acute metabolic acidosis is carefully considered, and treatment decisions should be based on a thorough evaluation of the patient's condition, the underlying etiology, and the potential risks and benefits associated with bicarbonate administration. The role of sodium bicarbonate in acute metabolic acidosis is controversial [3, 4], and bicarbonate therapy should be used selectively and not routinely in all such patients [4].

To ensure the optimal administration of bicarbonate, it is important to consider the following factors:

• Indications of bicarbonate therapy.

• Benefits of providing bicarbonate therapy.

• Rationale for using bicarbonate therapy selectively in specific patients.

• Precautions while administering bicarbonate therapy.

• Volume of bicarbonate to be infused.

• Administering bolus vs. infusion.

• Goals of bicarbonate therapy.

Indications of bicarbonate therapy

Common indications of bicarbonate therapy in metabolic acidosis are:

• **Normal AG metabolic acidosis:** Reasonable indications to use bicarbonate therapy in normal anion gap (hyperchloremic) metabolic acidosis (NAGMA) is pH <7.2 [3] or serum HCO_3 below 16–18 mEq/L [5]. As the loss of large quantities of bicarbonate is the most common cause of hyperchloremic metabolic acidosis, replacing bicarbonate is beneficial and hastens recovery [6, 7].

• **Lactic acidosis:** Lactic acidosis is the most common cause of high anion gap metabolic acidosis. In lactic acidosis, the role of bicarbonate therapy is controversial, it should not be used routinely, and is reserved for selected patients with life-threatening severe metabolic acidosis (pH<7.1) [2, 8–10]. The 2021 Surviving Sepsis Campaign Guidelines discourage the use of sodium bicarbonate therapy to improve hemodynamics or reduce vasopressor requirements in adults with septic shock and hypoperfusion-induced lactic acidemia [2].

• **Lactic acidosis with acute kidney injury:** In patients with lactic acidosis with severe acute kidney injury, even with less severe metabolic acidosis (pH 7.1 to 7.2), bicarbonate therapy is recommended [11–14]. Bicarbonate therapy is beneficial in this subgroup of patients with lactic acidosis and severe acute kidney injury and reduces 28-day mortality and the need for dialysis [11, 12, 15].

- **Diabetic ketoacidosis (DKA):** In DKA, bicarbonate's role is controversial and is rarely indicated. Bicarbonate therapy is used very selectively in patients with extremely severe acidosis with arterial pH less than 6.9 (recommendation by the American Diabetes Association) [16]. In recent literature, the role of bicarbonate in DKA has been discouraged [13, 17, 18].

- **Metabolic acidosis with hyperkalemia:** Sodium bicarbonate should be used in patients with hyperkalemia associated with metabolic acidosis as it reduces serum potassium levels by facilitating the shift of potassium from the extracellular fluid (ECF) to the intracellular fluid (ICF).

Benefits of providing bicarbonate therapy

The proposed major benefits of bicarbonate therapy in acute metabolic acidosis are as follows:

1. **Correction of hyperventilation:** In acute metabolic acidosis, correcting compensatory hyperventilation is crucial because prolonged compensatory hyperventilation in this condition can lead to exhaustion and, if left uncorrected for the long term, may result in respiratory failure.

2. **Improvement in cardiac function and oxygen delivery:** Bicarbonate therapy is used to treat common harmful effects of severe metabolic acidosis (pH<7.1), such as decreased cardiac contractility [19] and cardiac output due to myocardial depression, vasodilatation, impaired responsiveness to catecholamines, and a higher risk of cardiac arrhythmias [20]. Sodium bicarbonate leads to the correction of a low pH, restoring cardiovascular function to normal, improved cardiac output, higher mean arterial pressure, and subsequently enhanced oxygen delivery [21].

3. **Reduced need for renal replacement therapy:** In AKI, treating acute metabolic acidosis with sodium bicarbonate is associated with a reduced need for renal replacement therapy (RRT) in the ICU [11].

The rationale for using bicarbonate therapy selectively in specific patients

In acute metabolic acidosis due to lactic acidosis, bicarbonate therapy is given in selected patients, aimed for only partial correction, and not recommended routinely.

Major reasons to avoid or use bicarbonate therapy judiciously in lactic acidosis are:

A. Bicarbonate therapy can be harmful.

B. Mild to moderate lactic acidosis may be beneficial and may not be harmful.

C. No strong evidence of benefits.

A. Bicarbonate therapy can be harmful

Major potential complications due to bicarbonate therapy in patients with lactic acidosis are [22]:

1. **Risk of hypernatremia and ECF volume expansion:** Risk of hypernatremia and volume overload, especially in congestive heart failure or renal failure (100 ml of 7.5% and 8.4% $NaHCO_3$ provides 89 and 100 mEq of sodium, respectively). The sodium content of 150 ml of 8.4% $NaHCO_3$ is roughly similar to that of 1000 ml of 0.9% saline and 300 ml of 3% hypertonic saline.

As osmolality of 7.5% $NaHCO_3$ and 8.4% $NaHCO_3$ are very high (1786 mOsm/L and 2000 mOsm/L, respectively), large volume bolus administration can lead to hyperosmolar states.

2. **Increased lactate production:** Intracellular acidosis by reducing the activity of the rate-limiting enzyme phosphofructokinase inhibits lactic acid production. Administration of bicarbonate increases pH and may increase lactic acid production due to the removal of acidotic inhibition [23].

3. **An increase in $PaCO_2$ and paradoxical intracellular acidosis:** Bicarbonate infusion leads to worsening of intracellular pH (so-called paradoxical acidosis) [3, 24, 25] due to the following metabolic changes:

   - The reaction of sodium bicarbonate with hydrogen ions forms water and carbon dioxide.

   - Adequate perfusion transports carbon dioxide from the tissue bed into circulation and is subsequently transferred to the lung, where adequate ventilation removes it from the body.

   - Bicarbonate infusion induces a large generation of carbon dioxide and may lead to a transient rise in carbon dioxide. Inadequate perfusion and poor ventilation can impair the effective removal of carbon dioxide, resulting in a further rise in carbon dioxide.

   - CO_2 diffuses across the cell membrane faster than HCO_3. So, high carbon dioxide concentration will lead to increased CO_2 transfer into the intracellular compartment with resultant intracellular hypercapnic acidosis.

   - Therefore, if the elevated pCO_2 is not effectively eliminated through increased ventilation, bicarbonate infusion may lead to paradoxical intracellular acidosis.

4. **Central nervous system (CNS) acidosis:** Mechanism of CNS acidosis due to bicarbonate administration in metabolic acidosis are [26, 27]:

   - Bicarbonate does not cross the blood-brain barrier readily, but CO_2 generated due to bicarbonate infusion crosses the blood-brain barrier readily and aggravates CNS acidosis.

   - Compensatory hyperventilation occurs in metabolic acidosis. A rise in the serum pH due to bicarbonate administration slows down this drive for hyperventilation with a resultant increase in systemic pCO_2, increased pCO_2 transfer in the brain and CSF, and worsening of CNS acidosis.

   - Paradoxical CNS acidosis can cause cerebral edema with adverse neurological outcomes.

5. **Hypokalemia:** Bicarbonate administration increases the pH, which will shift potassium intracellularly and can lead to hypokalemia.

6. **Ionized hypocalcemia:** The binding of calcium to albumin is pH-dependent. Bicarbonate administration can lead to abrupt onset alkalosis in patients with metabolic acidosis, which reduces ionized calcium concentration by increasing calcium binding to albumin [28]. The rapid decline in the ionized calcium may contribute to decreased cardiac output, hypotension, and reduced catecholamine responsiveness [28].

7. **Overshoot or rebound alkalosis:** Administer bicarbonate judiciously

in lactic acidosis to avoid the risk of overshoot or rebound alkalosis. During the recovery phase in lactic acidosis, the risk of rebound alkalosis is due to the combined effect of the infused bicarbonate and the conversion of endogenous "potential" bicarbonate (lactate) into bicarbonate.

8. **Decreased myocardial contractility:** Use of bicarbonate decreases vasomotor tone and myocardial contractility [22].

B. Mild to moderate lactic acidosis may be beneficial and may not be harmful

There is a growing body of supporting evidence against the use of bicarbonate when the degree of acidosis is mild (pH 7.30–7.36, serum HCO_3 >20 mEq/L) to moderate (pH 7.20–7.29, serum HCO_3 10–19 mEq/L) [3].

1. **Mild to moderate metabolic acidosis may be beneficial:** Literature supporting the beneficial effect of mild to moderate metabolic acidosis (pH fell from 7.40 to 7.20) is growing [3, 4, 25, 29]. Suggested beneficial effects of mild to moderate metabolic acidosis are increased tissue oxygen delivery [30], greater blood flow to tissues due to vasodilatation of vessels, and increased myocardial contractility due to increased ionized calcium [19].

2. **The harmful effect of metabolic acidosis only in a severe degree of acidosis:** The deleterious effect of metabolic acidosis is restricted only to patients with pH less than 7.2 (i.e., in severe metabolic acidosis and not in mild to moderate acidosis when pH fell from 7.40 to 7.20) in various studies and review literature [4, 25, 31–34].

Cardiovascular dysfunction in metabolic acidosis is pH-dependent [4]. Cardiac output increased when systemic pH fell from 7.40 to 7.20, but cardiac output inevitably falls with further worsening of pH (i.e., pH falls below 7.1–7.2) [4, 19].

3. **Guidelines do not recommend the use of bicarbonate in mild to moderate metabolic lactic acidosis:** Surviving Sepsis Guidelines [14] and French Guidelines [13] do not recommend the use of sodium bicarbonate in mild to moderate metabolic lactic acidosis.

C. No strong evidence of benefits

Strong evidence supporting the benefits of bicarbonate in metabolic lactic acidosis is lacking:

1. **No benefit in various human studies:** Bicarbonate therapy failed to show significant benefits on mortality, morbidity, vasopressor requirements, and hemodynamic variables in metabolic lactic acidosis in several human studies [28, 35–38]. Recent two trials (Jaber et al. 2018 and Zhang et al. 2018) also failed to demonstrate a mortality benefit in patients with metabolic lactic acidosis in the absence of acute kidney injury [11, 12]. Studies suggesting the benefits of bicarbonate in lactic acidosis are very few and small and, therefore, have little consideration [39–41].

2. **No benefit in the current literature:** Recent systematic data and reviews do not provide robust recommendations supporting the beneficial effects of intravenous bicarbonate therapy in metabolic lactic acidosis [2, 4, 42, 43]. The 2021 Surviving Sepsis Campaign Guidelines discourage the use of sodium bicarbonate therapy to

improve hemodynamics or reduce vasopressor requirements and do not provide specific recommendations regarding the pH threshold for using sodium bicarbonate [14].

3. **Recent literature suggesting some benefits:** A systematic review conducted by Fujii et al. in 2019 on the biochemical effects of intravenous sodium bicarbonate in acute metabolic acidosis demonstrated an increase in pH, serum bicarbonate, base excess, serum sodium, and $PaCO_2$ during and after the administration of intravenous sodium bicarbonate [42]. The retrospective observational study conducted by Fujii et al. in 2021 was the first to demonstrate the beneficial effect of bicarbonate therapy, showing that it could lead to a faster resolution of acid–base derangements and PaO_2/FiO_2 ratio, as well as higher mean arterial pressure in acidotic vasopressor-dependent patients [21]. Additionally, the recent small study by Huang et al. (2023) demonstrated reduced ICU and hospital mortality with sodium bicarbonate therapy for septic patients with acute moderate lactic acidosis [44].

Conclusion: Although it may appear theoretically attractive, avoiding bicarbonate therapy routinely in less severe lactic acidosis (pH 7.1 or higher) is crucial due to the lack of evidence supporting its benefits and potential for harm. However, its careful use may benefit selected patients with acute kidney injury and severe lactic acidosis (pH <7.1). To conclude, reserve bicarbonate therapy for patients with clear benefits and avoid its routine use.

Administering bolus vs. infusion

Administering bicarbonate therapy as a bolus provides rapid correction of acidemia. However, giving sodium bicarbonate infusion as an isotonic mixture in 5% dextrose is preferable rather than as a hypertonic bolus. Bicarbonate infusion offers more controlled correction of acidemia and minimizes the risk associated with hypertonic bolus such as sodium overload and related complications, such as pulmonary edema and hypernatremia.

Volume of bicarbonate to be infused

The empirical formula commonly used to calculate the dose of bicarbonate (mEq/L) required to correct metabolic acidosis based on the body weight (kg) is:

Bicarbonate Dose =
$$0.5 \times \text{Weight (kg)} \times \text{Desired } \Delta HCO_3$$

Desired ΔHCO_3 =
$$\text{Targeted } HCO_3 - \text{Serum } HCO_3$$

Usually, 50% of the dose is replaced over the initial 3 to 4 hours and the remainder over 8 to 24 hours. It is important to remember that this is a rough guideline used to plan an initial therapy, and it should be constantly modified based on serial monitoring of serum bicarbonate level and arterial pH. Because of its limitations, many authorities prefer to employ an empirical approach rather than relying on formula-based calculations [45].

Goals of bicarbonate therapy

In metabolic acidosis, bicarbonate is administered judiciously to raise the pH to a safe level to reduce the risk of life-threatening complications of acidosis. However, overcorrection should be avoided to minimize the potential complications of bicarbonate infusion and an "overshoot" metabolic alkalosis. The most critical parameters to determine therapeutic goals are the serum anion gap, the severity of metabolic acidosis, and coexisting electrolyte abnormalities.

The goals of bicarbonate therapy in metabolic acidosis are:

- Normal anion gap (hyperchloremic) metabolic acidosis: Raise pH above 7.2 and slowly increase the plasma bicarbonate level to 22 mEq/L.
- Lactic acidosis: In high anion gap metabolic acidosis, maintain the arterial pH up to 7.1–7.2 and increase the bicarbonate level up to 10–12 mEq/L. Caution: Do not raise the blood pH to greater than 7.20.
- Lactic acidosis with acute kidney injury: Maintain the arterial pH above 7.3.
- Diabetic ketoacidosis: Raise the arterial pH only up to 7.0.

Precautions while administering IV bicarbonate therapy [3, 46]

Precautions while administering IV bicarbonate therapy include establishing a proper large IV line, monitoring electrolyte levels, avoiding IV boluses (except in emergencies), and administering rapid or large-volume infusions cautiously to prevent circulatory overload [3, 46]. (For more details see Chapter 14 on "Sodium Bicarbonate").

Alkali therapy in chronic metabolic acidosis

Advanced chronic kidney disease, diarrhea, and the different types of renal tubular acidosis are the most common causes of chronic metabolic acidosis.

A. Benefits

The benefits of alkali therapy in chronic metabolic acidosis are:

1. **Respiratory symptom relief:** In patients with metabolic acidosis accompanied by compensatory hyperventilation, bicarbonate therapy can provide relief from respiratory muscle fatigue and dyspnea. This is achieved by correcting the acidosis and reducing the need for hyperventilation.

2. **Improvement in muscle wasting and weakness:** Chronic metabolic acidosis can have detrimental effects on muscle function and metabolism, leading to muscle wasting and reduced energy production. Alkali therapy can restore acid-base balance and mitigate these adverse effects by enhancing muscle function and metabolic processes [47, 48].

3. **Prevention of bone demineralization:** Chronic metabolic acidosis can negatively impact bone health by inhibiting osteoblast activity, reducing bone formation, and increasing osteoclast activity. This results in elevated bone resorption, leading to bone loss and a higher risk of fractures [47, 49, 50]. Alkali therapy minimizes the degree of negative calcium balance, prevents bone resorption, and may help reduce the adverse impact on bone health.

4. **Slow down kidney disease progression:** In patients with chronic kidney disease (CKD), chronic metabolic acidosis increases the risk of progressing to kidney failure, accelerating the development of end-stage renal disease (ESRD) that may require renal replacement therapy. While using sodium bicarbonate to correct acidosis in CKD patients is generally considered safe and may slow the progression of kidney failure [51–57], more data is needed to support these benefits [58, 59].

5. **Reduction of urinary calcium excretion:** In patients with chronic

distal (type 1) RTA, chronic metabolic acidosis is associated with increased urinary calcium excretion, leading to a higher risk of nephrocalcinosis and formation of calcium-containing kidney stones. Alkali therapy can benefit such patients by correcting acidosis and reducing calcium excretion [60].

B. Alkali agents and their composition

The primary alkali agents for treating chronic metabolic acidosis are sodium bicarbonate ($NaHCO_3$) and citrate salts.

Sodium bicarbonate is the preferred agent for correcting chronic metabolic acidosis in chronic kidney diseases. 1 gm of $NaHCO_3$ provides 11.5 mEq of HCO_3 and is commonly administered at a dose of 0.5 to 1 mEq/kg/day.

Citrate salts are available as potassium citrate and/or mixtures of citric acid with sodium citrate. In the case of renal tubular acidosis, potassium citrate is preferred to treat chronic metabolic acidosis as it corrects both hypokalemia and acidosis and helps in preventing nephrocalcinosis and nephrolithiasis. However, this agent carries a risk of hyperkalemia in CKD patients.

Citrate salts: The composition of commonly used citrate-containing formulations are:

- Potassium citrate and citric acid USP oral solution, each mL provides 2 mEq of potassium ion and is equivalent to 2 mEq of bicarbonate.
- Potassium citrate-sodium citrate-citric acid solution offers 1 mEq of potassium ion and 1 mEq of sodium ion, equivalent to 2 mEq of bicarbonate.
- Shohl's solution contains 100 mg/mL of sodium citrate and 66.8 mg/mL of citric acid, with each 1 mL delivering 1 mEq of both bicarbonate and sodium.

The requirement for citrate salts varies in each patient, depending on the severity of acidosis. The starting dose is usually 50 to 100 mEq per day, and this dosage is adjusted based on the response to therapy and the rate of ongoing losses of bicarbonate, monitored through electrolytes and bicarbonate levels.

Treatment of metabolic acidosis in specific situations

A. Conditions associated with high anion gap metabolic acidosis

1. Lactic acidosis

Treatment of lactic acidosis includes:

The therapy aims to achieve adequate perfusion and oxygenation, which helps reduce lactic acid production and its clearance from the body.

The first and most crucial step in the management of lactic acidosis is to detect underlying causes and effectively eliminate or treat them, which in many cases may be the only required therapy.

The Surviving Sepsis Campaign Guidelines [14] recommend early crystalloid resuscitation with balanced solutions and timely use of vasopressors, specifically choosing noradrenaline to target a mean arterial pressure (MAP) of 65 mmHg.

Septicemia and septic shock are common and serious causes of tissue hypoperfusion leading to lactic acidosis, requiring a comprehensive evaluation, including sending blood cultures and a focused search for an anatomic source. The administration of broad-spectrum antibiotics within the first hour of sepsis recognition is of utmost importance [14].

Bicarbonate therapy should be used judiciously, considering potential risks, such as:

- Enhanced lactate production due to stimulation of phosphofructokinase activity, which can exacerbate lactic acidosis.

- An increase in carbon dioxide production and the possibility of paradoxical intracellular acidosis.

- Other complications, including the risk of hypernatremia, ECF volume expansion, hypocalcemia, hypokalemia, overshoot, or rebound alkalosis, among others.

Administration of $NaHCO_3$ may be beneficial only in selected patients with severe acidemia (pH less than 7.1) and should be given for partial correction only. However, in patients with severe acute kidney injury, the administration of $NaHCO_3$ can be beneficial even for cases of less severe acidosis (i.e., pH 7.1 to 7.2), as it reduces the need for dialysis and offers survival benefits [11].

The preferred mode of administration is isotonic sodium bicarbonate infusion rather than a hypertonic bolus.

Before administering sodium bicarbonate, ensure adequate ventilation to prevent the accumulation of carbon dioxide, and closely monitor for hypokalemia and hypocalcemia, correcting them as needed.

Dialytic therapy can be lifesaving in critical situations with refractory severe lactic acidosis, as it not only rapidly eliminates excess lactate but also reduces the risk of volume overload, hypernatremia, hypocalcemia, and the removal of associated toxins [34].

2. Diabetic ketoacidosis

The mainstay for managing DKA is the adequate replacement of IV fluids and electrolytes, insulin therapy, and addressing precipitating factors.

The administration of sodium bicarbonate is not recommended in adult patients with DKA with pH ≥6.9 due to possible clinical harm and lack of sustained benefits [17, 61–65]. However, it is recommended in a few patients with severe DKA who have pH <6.9, which can compromise cardiac contractility, presence of shock, or have Severe, life-threatening hyperkalemia (serum potassium >6.5–7 mEq/L) [3, 16, 65].

For patients with a pH ≤6.9, ADA recommends administering 100 mEq of sodium bicarbonate (two ampules) diluted in 400 ml of sterile water (an isotonic solution) with 20 mEq of potassium chloride (KCl) to be infused at a rate of 200 ml/h until the venous pH is >7.0 [16].

3. Alcoholic ketoacidosis

Alcoholic Ketoacidosis (AKA) is diagnosed clinically, and its treatment comprises thiamine supplementation, glucose administration, fluid resuscitation, and electrolyte supplementation [66–68].

Thiamine (vitamin B1) supplementation: It is essential to administer 200 mg of thiamine prophylactically together with glucose to avoid the development of Wernicke's encephalopathy, but thiamine should not delay the administration of dextrose.

Dextrose and saline supplementation: Provide glucose to correct hypoglycemia. Dextrose administration stimulates insulin secretion while inhibiting glucagon secretion, effectively suppressing ketone body production. This not only corrects ketoacidosis but also supports the regeneration of bicarbonate through the metabolism of retained ketones.

Before infusing dextrose solutions, it is important to exclude severe hypokalemia and hyperglycemia. Correcting severe hypokalemia before infusing dextrose solutions is crucial because dextrose can stimulate insulin secretion, causing potassium to shift from the extracellular fluid to the intracellular fluid and potentially worsening hypokalemia. In some cases of alcoholic ketoacidosis with severe hyperglycemia, insulin administration may be necessary. Such patients require infusion of only saline without dextrose.

Intravenous resuscitation with balanced crystalloids (e.g., Ringer's lactate or PlasmaLyte) or normal saline helps correct hypovolemia by replenishing intravascular volume, which is often depleted due to vomiting, urinary sodium loss, and reduced fluid intake [68].

Electrolyte replacement: Hypokalemia, hypomagnesemia, and hypophosphatemia are common in patients with alcoholic ketoacidosis, which needs to be diagnosed and treated appropriately. These patients may also require supplementation of potassium, phosphate, and magnesium. Oral or IV potassium phosphate is recommended to correct hypokalemia with hypophosphatemia.

In undernourished alcoholic patients, normal electrolyte reports should be viewed cautiously because disorders like hypokalemia, hypophosphatemia, and thiamine deficiency may become apparent 12 to 24 hours after glucose administration.

Sodium bicarbonate supplementation: Administration of bicarbonate is usually unnecessary, even in patients with severe acidemia (i.e., pH <7.0),

because supportive management alone corrects it quickly.

Alcohol cessation: Encourage the patient to stop alcohol consumption to prevent further episodes of AKA.

4. Salicylate (aspirin) poisoning

The treatment of salicylate (Aspirin) poisoning involves several key steps [69–71]:

Gastric lavage: If the ingestion is recent, consider vigorous gastric lavage by administering activated charcoal to reduce drug absorption.

Supportive care: Provide general supportive care, including monitoring vital signs, ensuring adequate oxygenation, and maintaining a patent airway.

Fluid resuscitation: Correct dehydration and maintain electrolyte balance by administering intravenous Ringer's lactate or normal saline to correct hypotension and decrease extracellular fluid volume, ensuring adequate renal perfusion and urine output. In cases of severe intoxication, patients may have fluid deficits as high as 4 to 6 liters.

Alkalinization: In moderate or severe salicylate toxicity, administering IV sodium bicarbonate to alkalinize the urine is the mainstay of treatment. Raising urine pH from 6.5 to 7.5 and maintaining continuous urine output through infusing an isotonic bicarbonate solution (150 ml containing 132 mmol of sodium bicarbonate in 1 liter of 5% dextrose) can increase total salicylate excretion more than fivefold by effectively 'trapping' salicylate anions in the renal tubules.

Additionally, the lipid-soluble form of salicylic acid can easily penetrate the blood-brain barrier, but bicarbonate infusion raises the pH, reducing the lipid-soluble form in cases of moderate or severe salicylate toxicity, preventing the diffusion of salicylates into the CNS. This intervention can help prevent or alleviate CNS symptoms.

It's worth noting that even when coexisting respiratory alkalosis is present, it is not a contraindication for administering sodium bicarbonate, and patients should receive it.

Provide glucose and potassium: Administer glucose in adequate amounts due to the potential risk of hypoglycemia and reduced brain glucose levels, even in the presence of normal plasma glucose [72].

Ensure adequate potassium supplementation since hypokalemia is commonly observed in salicylate toxicity and is likely to worsen during vigorous alkaline diuresis.

Hemodialysis: Hemodialysis is recommended in severe salicylate toxicity with persistently high salicylate levels (>100 mg/dL), severe acidosis, marked neurological symptoms, organ dysfunction, or severely impaired kidney function, as well as in cases of fluid overload [73]. It effectively removes salicylates and corrects acid-base imbalances.

5. Renal failure

In patients with chronic kidney disease, correcting metabolic acidosis through oral alkali replacement, such as sodium bicarbonate supplementation, to maintain serum bicarbonate levels at approximately the normal value (25 mEq/L) helps prevent muscle catabolism and wasting, bone demineralization, the development of rickets or osteomalacia, and slows down the progression of chronic kidney disease.

B. Conditions associated with normal anion gap (hyperchloremic) metabolic acidosis

1. GI loss of bicarbonate

In the management of non-renal causes of normal anion gap metabolic acidosis resulting from gastrointestinal losses such as diarrhea, the most crucial measures include correcting hypovolemia, addressing hypokalemia, and managing metabolic acidosis. In cases of severe acidosis, correcting the acidosis by supplementing $NaHCO_3$ by intravenous or oral administration is necessary.

2. Renal tubular acidosis

Renal tubular acidosis is a group of renal disorders characterized by defects in distal H^+ excretion or reduced bicarbonate reabsorption (bicarbonate wasting).

Management of RTA is summarized below [74, 75]:

Treatment of distal (type 1) renal tubular acidosis

Distal (type 1) renal tubular acidosis is characterized by hypokalemic hyperchloremic metabolic acidosis, and its treatment involves potassium supplementation and alkali therapy to correct hypokalemia and achieve a normal serum bicarbonate concentration (22 to 24 mEq/L) [76–78].

Benefits of using oral alkali supplements like potassium citrate in the treatment of distal RTA, which corrects both metabolic acidosis and hypokalemia, include:

• Positive effects on bone health: Potassium citrate helps mitigate symptoms and prevent complications associated with chronic acidosis, such as bone demineralization, nephrocalcinosis, and kidney stone formation. Additionally, it diminishes calcium losses linked to bone buffering in children, thereby improving bone density, preventing rickets, and restoring normal growth rates.

- Correction of hypokalemia: Potassium citrate supplementation provides potassium and corrects its depletion.
- Prevention of chronic kidney disease: It corrects metabolic acidosis and prevents the progressive loss of kidney function.

Dose: 1–2 mEq/kg/day potassium citrate or sodium bicarbonate is usually sufficient. Regular follow-up and monitoring of serum bicarbonate levels are essential to adjust the dose.

Treatment of proximal (type 2) renal tubular acidosis

The primary goal in managing proximal RTA is identifying and addressing underlying treatable disorders, such as multiple myeloma, carbonic anhydrase inhibitor use, and vitamin D deficiency.

Therapeutic measures include administering high doses of alkali to correct acidosis (preventing bony deformities and promoting growth), potassium (to address hypokalemia), and phosphate (to correct hypophosphatemia) [75].

Usually, approximately 80-90% of filtered bicarbonate is reabsorbed in the proximal tubule, but in proximal RTA, there is reduced proximal HCO_3 reabsorption, leading to significant bicarbonate wasting. Treating proximal RTA is particularly challenging because ingested alkali is promptly excreted in the urine due to its defective proximal tubular absorption, resulting in poor effectiveness in raising serum bicarbonate levels.

Dose: Large amounts of oral alkali (10-15 mEq/kg/day) are required to treat proximal RTA because of significant urinary loss.

When a high dose of alkali is ineffective or poorly tolerated, adding 12.5 to 25 mg of thiazide diuretics can be beneficial. These diuretics induce volume depletion and reduce extracellular volume, leading to increased bicarbonate reabsorption in the proximal tubule and enhancing the overall effectiveness of alkali therapy.

Administering potassium salts is necessary to correct hypokalemia caused by increased urinary potassium losses associated with alkali therapy.

Supplementing vitamin D and correcting hypophosphatemia can help improve bone health and prevent complications like rickets or osteomalacia.

Treatment of hyperkalemic (type 4) renal tubular acidosis

The management of type 4 RTA includes:

- Correcting metabolic acidosis by providing 1 to 3 mEq/kg/day of potassium-free alkali.
- Addressing hyperkalemia using various measures, such as dietary potassium restriction, low-dose fludrocortisone (0.1 mg per day) for patients with aldosterone deficiency without hypertension, heart failure, or edema, as well as the use of loop diuretics (1 to 2 mg/kg/day) and, if necessary, cation-exchange resin.

REFERENCES

1. Mehta AN, Emmett JB, Emmett M. GOLD MARK: an anion gap mnemonic for the 21st century. Lancet. 2008;372(9642):892.

2. Achanti A, Szerlip HM. Acid-Base Disorders in the Critically Ill Patient. Clin J Am Soc Nephrol. 2023;18(1):102–112.

3. Kraut JA, Madias NE. Treatment of acute metabolic acidosis: a pathophysiologic approach. Nat Rev Nephrol. 2012;8(10):589–601.

4. Forni LG, Hodgson LE, Se lby NM. The Janus faces of bicarbonate therapy in the ICU: not sure! Intensive Care Med. 2020;46(3):522–524.

5. Farkas J. Non-anion-gap metabolic acidosis (NAGMA) PulmCrit September 19, 2019 https://emcrit.org/ibcc/nagma/#treatment.

6. Sabatini S, Kurtzman NA. Bicarbonate therapy in severe metabolic acidosis. J. Am. Soc. Nephrol. 2009;20(4):692–695.

7. Adeva-Andany MM, Fernández-Fernández C, Mouriño-Bayolo D, et al. Sodium bicarbonate therapy in patients with metabolic acidosis. ScientificWorldJournal. 2014;2014:627673.

8. Boyd JH, Walley KR. Is there a role for sodium bicarbonate in treating lactic acidosis from shock? Curr Opin Crit Care. 2008;14(4):379–83.

9. Velissaris D, Karamouzos V, Ktenopoulos N, et al. The use of sodium bicarbonate in the treatment of acidosis in sepsis: a literature update on a long term debate. Crit Care Res Pract. 2015;2015:605830.

10. Ghauri S, Javaeed A, Mustafa K, et al. Bicarbonate therapy for critically ill patients with metabolic acidosis: a systematic review. Cureus 2019;11(3):e4297.

11. Jaber S, Paugam C, Futier E, et al. Sodium bicarbonate therapy for patients with severe metabolic acidaemia in the intensive care unit (BICAR-ICU): a multicentre, open-label, randomised controlled, phase 3 trial. Lancet. 2018;392(10141):31–40.

12. Zhang Z, Zhu C, Mo L, et al. Effectiveness of sodium bicarbonate infusion on mortality in septic patients with metabolic acidosis. Intensive Care Med 2018;44(11):1888–1895.

13. Jung B, Martinez M, Claessens YE, et al. Diagnosis and management of metabolic acidosis: guidelines from a French expert panel. Ann Intensive Care. 2019;9(1):92.

14. Evans L, Rhodes A, Alhazzani W, et al. Surviving sepsis campaign: international guidelines for management of sepsis and septic shock 2021. Crit Care Med 2021;49(11):e1063–143.

15. Matyukhin I, Patschan S, Ritter O, et al. Etiology and management of acute metabolic acidosis: An Update. Kidney Blood Press Res. 2020;45(4):523–531.

16. Kitabchi AE, Umpierrez GE, Miles JM, et al. Hyperglycemic crises in adult patients with diabetes. Diabetes Care 2009;32(7):1335–43.

17. Duhon B, Attridge RL, Franco-Martinez AC, et al. Intravenous sodium bicarbonate therapy in severely acidotic diabetic ketoacidosis. Ann Pharmacother. 2013;47(7–8):970–5.

18. Patel MP, Ahmed A, Gunapalan T, et al. Use of sodium bicarbonate and blood gas monitoring in diabetic ketoacidosis: A review. World J Diabetes. 2018;9(11):199–205.

19. Wildenthal K, Mierzwiak DS, Myers RW, et al. Effects of acute lactic acidosis on left ventricular performance. Am J Physiol 1968;214(6):1352–1359.

20. Kraut JA, Madias NE. Metabolic acidosis: pathophysiology, diagnosis and management. Nat Rev Nephrol. 2010;6(5):274–85.

21. Fujii T, Udy AA, Nichol A, et al. Incidence and management of metabolic acidosis with sodium bicarbonate in the ICU: An international observational study. Crit Care. 2021;25(1):45.

22. Rudnick MR, Blair GJ, Kuschner WG, Barr J. Lactic Acidosis and the Role of Sodium Bicarbonate: A Narrative Opinion. Shock. 2020;53(5):528–536.

23. Rachoin JS, Weisberg LS, McFadden CB. Treatment of lactic acidosis: appropriate confusion. J Hosp Med 2010;5(4):E1–7.

24. Kraut JA, Kurtz I. Treatment of acute non-anion gap metabolic acidosis. Clin Kidney J. 2015;8(1):93–9.

25. Kimmoun A, Novy E, Auchet T, et al. Hemodynamic consequences of severe lactic acidosis in shock states: from bench to bedside. Crit Care. 2015;19(1):175.

26. Sing RF, Branas CA, Sing RF. Bicarbonate therapy in the treatment of lactic acidosis: medicine or toxin? J Am Osteopath Assoc. 1995;95(1):52–7.

27. Abeysekara S, Zello GA, Lohmann KL, et al. Infusion of sodium bicarbonate in experimentally induced metabolic acidosis does not provoke cerebrospinal fluid (CSF) acidosis in calves. Can J Vet Res. 2012;76(1):16–22.

28. Cooper DJ, Walley KR, Wiggs BR, et al. Bicarbonate does not improve hemodynamics in critically ill patients who have lactic acidosis: a prospective, controlled clinical study. Ann Intern Med 1990;112(7):492–498.

29. Gehlbach BK, Schmidt GA. Bench-to-bedside review: treating acid-base abnormalities in the intensive care unit-the role of buffers. Crit Care. 2004;8(4):259–65.

30. Handy JM, Soni N. Physiological effects of hyperchloraemia and acidosis. Br J Anaesth 2008;101(2):141–150.

31. Al Alawi AM, Al Flaiti A, Falhammar H. Lactation Ketoacidosis: A systematic review of case reports. Medicina (Kaunas). 2020;56(6):299.

32. Kraut JA, Kurtz I. Use of base in the treatment of severe acidemic states. Am. J. Kidney Dis. 2001;38(4):703–727.

33. Jung B, Rimmele T, Le Goff C, et al. Severe metabolic or mixed acidemia on intensive care unit admission: incidence, prognosis and administration of buffer therapy. A prospective, multiple-center study. Crit Care Lond Engl. 2011;15(5):R238.

34. Kraut JA, Madias NE. Lactic Acidosis: Current treatments and future directions. Am J Kidney Dis. 2016;68(3):473–82.

35. Mathieu D, Neviere R, Billard V, et al. Effects of bicarbonate therapy on hemodynamics and tissue oxygenation in patients with lactic acidosis: a prospective, controlled clinical study. Crit Care Med 1991;19(11):1352–6.

36. Stacpoole PW, Wright EC, Baumgartner TG, et al. Natural history and course of acquired lactic acidosis in adults. Am J Med. 1994;97(1):47–54.

37. Kim HJ, Son YK, An WS. Effect of sodium bicarbonate administration on mortality in patients with lactic acidosis: a retrospective analysis. PLoS One 2013;8(6):e65283.

38. Ahn S, Kim YJ, Sohn CH, et al. Sodium bicarbonate on severe metabolic acidosis during prolonged cardiopulmonary resuscitation: a double-blind,

randomized, placebo-controlled pilot study. J Thorac Dis. 2018;10(4):2295–2302.

39. Fang ZX, Li YF, Zhou XQ, et al. Effects of resuscitation with crystalloid fluids on cardiac function in patients with severe sepsis. BMC Infect Dis. 2008;8:50.

40. El-Solh AA, Abou Jaoude P, Porhomayon J. Bicarbonate therapy in the treatment of septic shock: a second look. Intern Emerg Med 2010;5(4):341–47.

41. Chen XF, Ye JL, Zhu ZY. The use of sodium bicarbonate in stages in treating hypoperfusion induced lactic acidemia in septic shock [Article in Chinese]. Zhonghua Wei Zhong Bing Ji Jiu Yi Xue. 2013;25(1):24–7.

42. Fujii T, Udy A, Licari E, et al. Sodium bicarbonate therapy for critically ill patients with metabolic acidosis: a scoping and a systematic review. J Crit Care 2019;51:184–191.

43. Lo KB, Garvia V, Stempel JM, et al. Bicarbonate use and mortality outcome among critically ill patients with metabolic acidosis: A meta analysis. Heart Lung. 2020;49(2):167–174.

44. Huang S, Yang B, Peng Y, et al. Clinical effectiveness of sodium bicarbonate therapy on mortality for septic patients with acute moderate lactic acidosis. Front Pharmacol. 2023;13:1059285.

45. Wiederkehr M, Emmett M, Sterns RH, et al. Bicarbonate therapy in lactic acidosis. In: UpToDate, Post TW (Ed), Wolters Kluwer. https://www.uptodate.com (Accessed on November 12, 2023).

46. Australian Product Information - Sodium Bicarbonate 8.4% (Sodium Bicarbonate) Injection BP." [Internet]. Date of Revision: 09 February 2021. Available from: https://medsinfo.com.au/api/documents/Sodium_Bicarbonate_PI?format=pdf.

47. Melamed ML, Raphael KL. Metabolic Acidosis in CKD: A Review of Recent Findings. Kidney Med. 2021;3(2):267–277.

48. Wang XH, Mitch WE, Price SR. Pathophysiological mechanisms leading to muscle loss in chronic kidney disease. Nat Rev Nephrol. 2022;18(3):138–152.

49. Bushinsky DA, Krieger NS. Effects of acid on bone. Kidney Int. 2022;101(6):1160–1170.

50. Levy RV, McMahon DJ, Agarwal S, et al. Comprehensive Associations between Acidosis and the Skeleton in Patients with Kidney Disease. J Am Soc Nephrol 2023;34(4):668–681.

51. Kraut JA, Madias NE. Adverse Effects of the Metabolic Acidosis of Chronic Kidney Disease. Adv Chronic Kidney Dis. 2017;24(5):289–297.

52. Di Iorio BR, Bellasi A, Raphael KL, et al. Treatment of metabolic acidosis with sodium bicarbonate delays progression of chronic kidney disease: the UBI Study. J Nephrol. 2019;32(6):989–1001.

53. Hultin S, Hood C, Campbell KL, et al. A Systematic Review and Meta-Analysis on Effects of Bicarbonate Therapy on Kidney Outcomes. Kidney Int Rep. 2020;6(3):695–705.

54. Kim HJ, Ryu H, Kang E, et al. Metabolic Acidosis Is an Independent Risk Factor of Renal Progression in Korean Chronic Kidney Disease Patients: The KNOW-CKD Study Results. Front Med (Lausanne). 2021;8:707588.

55. Asahina Y, Sakaguchi Y, Kajimoto S, et al. Association of Time-Updated Anion Gap With Risk of Kidney Failure in Advanced CKD: A Cohort Study. Am J Kidney Dis. 2022;79(3):374–382.

56. Vincent-Johnson A, Scialla JJ. Importance of Metabolic Acidosis as a Health Risk in Chronic Kidney Disease. Adv Chronic Kidney Dis. 2022;29(4):329–336.

57. Beynon-Cobb B, Louca P, Hoorn EJ, et al. Effect of Sodium Bicarbonate on Systolic Blood Pressure in CKD: A Systematic Review and Meta-Analysis. Clin J Am Soc Nephrol. 2023;18(4):435–445.

58. Hu MK, Witham MD, Soiza RL. Oral bicarbonate therapy in non-haemodialysis dependent chronic kidney disease patients: a systematic review and meta-analysis of randomised controlled trials. J Clin Med. 2019;8(2):208.

59. BiCARB study group. Clinical and cost-effectiveness of oral sodium bicarbonate therapy for older patients with chronic kidney disease and low-grade acidosis (BiCARB): a pragmatic randomised, double-blind, placebo-controlled trial. BMC Med. 2020;18(1):91.

60. Alexander RT, Cordat E, Chambrey R, et al. Acidosis and Urinary Calcium Excretion: Insights from Genetic Disorders. J Am Soc Nephrol. 2016;27(12):3511–3520.

61. Hale PJ, Crase J, Nattrass M. Metabolic effects of bicarbonate in the treatment of diabetic ketoacidosis. Br Med J (Clin Res Ed). 1984;289(6451):1035–8.

62. Okuda Y, Adrogue HJ, Field JB, et al. Counterproductive effects of sodium bicarbonate in diabetic ketoacidosis. J Clin Endocrinol Metab. 1996;81(1):314–20.

63. Viallon A, Zeni F, Lafond P, et al. Does bicarbonate therapy improve the management of severe diabetic ketoacidosis? Crit Care Med. 1999;27(12):2690–3.

64. Chua HR, Schneider A, Bellomo R. Bicarbonate in diabetic ketoacidosis – a systematic review. Ann Intensive Care 2011;1(1):23.

65. Gil-Olivares F, Manrique H, Castillo-Bravo, et al. Management of glycemic crises in adult patients With diabetes mellitus: evidence-based clinical Practice guideline clinical Rev. Fac. Med. Hum. January 2021;21(1):50–64.

66. Palmer BF, Clegg DJ. Electrolyte Disturbances in Patients with Chronic Alcohol-Use Disorder. N Engl J Med 2017;377(14):1368–1377.

67. Kraut JA, Mullins ME. Toxic Alcohols. N Engl J Med. 2018;378(3):270–280.

68. Long B, Lentz S, Gottlieb M. Alcoholic Ketoacidosis: Etiologies, Evaluation, and Management. J Emerg Med. 2021;61(6):658–665.

69. American College of Medical Toxicology. Guidance document: management priorities in salicylate toxicity. J Med Toxicol. 2015;11(1):149–52.

70. Shively RM, Hoffman RS, Manini AF. Acute salicylate poisoning: risk factors for severe outcome. Clin Toxicol (Phila). 2017;55(3):175–180.

71. Palmer BF, Clegg DJ. Salicylate Toxicity. N Engl J Med 2020;382(26):2544–2555.

72. Thurston JH, Pollock PG, Warren SK, et al. Reduced brain glucose with normal plasma glucose in salicylate poisoning. J Clin Invest 1970;49(11):2139–45.

73. Juurlink DN, Gosselin S, Kielstein JT, et al. Extracorporeal Treatment for Salicylate Poisoning: Systematic Review and Recommendations From the EXTRIP Workgroup. Ann Emerg Med. 2015;66(2):165–81.

74. Palmer BF, Kelepouris E, Clegg DJ. Renal Tubular Acidosis and Management Strategies: A Narrative Review. Adv Ther. 2021;38(2):949–968.

75. Reddy S, Kamath N. Clinical approach to renal tubular acidosis in children. Karnataka Paediatr J 2020;35(2):88–94.

76. Watanabe T. Improving outcomes for patients with distal renal tubular acidosis: recent advances and challenges ahead. Pediatric Health Med Ther. 2018;9:181–190.

77. Lopez-Garcia SC, Emma F, Walsh SB, et al. Treatment and long-term outcome in primary distal renal tubular acidosis. Nephrol Dial Transplant 2019;34(6):981–991.

78. Giglio S, Montini G, Trepiccione F, et al. Distal renal tubular acidosis: a systematic approach from diagnosis to treatment. J Nephrol. 2021;34(6):2073–2083.

32 | Metabolic Alkalosis

Metabolic alkalosis is the most common acid-base disorder, typically developing after hospitalization in critically ill patients, but it is not most frequently present upon admission, unlike metabolic acidosis [1, 2].

DEFINITION

Metabolic alkalosis is a primary acid-base disorder characterized by an increase in serum HCO_3 (>26 mEq/L), a high pH (>7.45), and a compensatory increase in $PaCO_2$ due to alveolar hypoventilation. Hypochloremia and hypokalemia are commonly encountered electrolyte imbalances in metabolic alkalosis.

Respiratory compensation: Hypoventilation, which occurs as a respiratory compensation in metabolic alkalosis, is a relatively slow process compared to the hyperventilation response that occurs in metabolic acidosis. Hypoventilation-induced hypoxia is a limiting factor for compensatory mechanisms in metabolic alkalosis because severe hypoxia (PO_2

<60 mm Hg) is a potent stimulus to increase alveolar ventilation, offsetting this protective respiratory response.

Comparison with chronic respiratory acidosis: Increased HCO_3 and increased $PaCO_2$ are also features of chronic respiratory acidosis, but the differentiating feature is a low pH.

PATHOGENESIS [3–5]

For a proper understanding of the pathogenesis of metabolic alkalosis, it is important to know the two distinct phases involved in sustaining metabolic alkalosis: 1. Generation of metabolic alkalosis and 2. Maintenance of metabolic alkalosis, as summarized in Table 32.1.

Generation of metabolic alkalosis

Mechanisms leading to the primary increase in plasma HCO_3 can involve one or more of the following:

- Gastrointestinal (GI) loss of hydrogen ion: Due to conditions like vomiting,

Table 32.1 Generation and maintenance factors of metabolic alkalosis

Generation factors	Maintenance factors
• GI loss of H+ ion	• Hypovolemia
• Renal loss of H+ ion	• Hypochloremia
• Exogenous HCO_3 load	• Hypokalemia
• Endogenous alkali gain	• Aldosterone excess
• Hypokalemia	• Reduced GFR/ kidney failure
• Post-hypercapnic	

nasogastric suction, or congenital chloride-losing diarrhea.

- Renal loss of hydrogen ion: It includes the use of diuretics, primary hyperaldosteronism, Bartter syndrome, and Gitelman syndrome.

- Exogenous HCO_3 load: Due to the administration of HCO_3, balanced crystalloids containing buffers, blood products containing citrate as an anticoagulant, and the development of milk-alkali syndrome.

- Endogenous alkali gain: This is due to rebound alkalosis during the recovery phase of conditions like diabetic ketoacidosis (DKA) or lactic acidosis.

- Hypokalemia: Hypokalemia commonly occurs in metabolic alkalosis due to increased urinary potassium excretion driven by volume depletion-stimulated high aldosterone levels or mineralocorticoid excess. In hypokalemic patients, K+ shifts from the intracellular fluid (ICF) to the extracellular fluid (ECF) to maintain and increase serum potassium levels. As a compensatory mechanism to maintain electroneutrality, H+ shifts from the ECF to the ICF, leading to the development of metabolic alkalosis.

- Post-hypercapnic: Chronic hypercapnia triggers a compensatory increase in bicarbonate levels. When mechanical ventilation is started, CO_2 drops quickly, but the slower decrease in bicarbonate levels can lead to metabolic alkalosis as the elevated bicarbonate effect persists.

Maintenance of metabolic alkalosis

Under normal circumstances, excess bicarbonate generated by any process is rapidly excreted in the urine. However, metabolic alkalosis persists when the kidneys fail to eliminate and retain excess bicarbonate, leading to its maintenance. The contributing factors are summarized below [3–5].

Hypovolemia: Reduced filtration of HCO_3^- at the glomerulus due to ECF volume contraction and increased reabsorption of HCO_3^- in both the proximal and distal tubules due to hypovolemia prevent the renal excretion of bicarbonate, resulting in the maintenance of metabolic alkalosis.

Hypochloremia: Chloride depletion reduces chloride delivery to the collecting tubules, limiting bicarbonate excretion and promoting increased bicarbonate reabsorption. Hypochloremia, even without volume depletion, enhances bicarbonate reabsorption by this mechanism. Therefore, hypochloremia plays a role in sustaining metabolic alkalosis by enhancing bicarbonate reabsorption and decreasing bicarbonate secretion within the distal tubule.

Hypokalemia: Hypokalemia actively maintains metabolic alkalosis through the following mechanisms in both volume-depleted and volume-expanded states:

- Hypokalemia drives hydrogen ions intracellularly, facilitating the movement of potassium out of cells in exchange for hydrogen ions in the extracellular fluid, which helps sustain metabolic alkalosis.

- By stimulating the apical H^+/K^+ ATPase in the collecting duct, hypokalemia increases potassium reabsorption and promotes hydrogen ion secretion.

- Hypokalemia stimulates renal ammonia genesis, leading to new HCO_3 generation, and enhances the excretion of hydrogen ions into the urine, further contributing to the persistence of metabolic alkalosis.

- Hypokalemia also increases proximal tubular reabsorption of filtered HCO_3.

Aldosterone excess or increased mineralocorticoid activity: Excess aldosterone promotes metabolic alkalosis by enhancing sodium reabsorption in renal tubules in exchange for K^+ and H^+ secretion. This increased H^+ secretion into the collecting duct results in greater bicarbonate reabsorption, sustaining the alkalotic state. Excess aldosterone also increases K^+ secretion, resulting in hypokalemia, further contributing to the maintenance of metabolic alkalosis, as discussed.

Reduced glomerular filtration rate (GFR)/kidney failure: Impaired kidney function leads to reduced filtration of HCO_3, which plays a role in sustaining metabolic alkalosis.

ETIOLOGY [4–8]

Metabolic alkalosis is characterized by an excessive concentration and content of

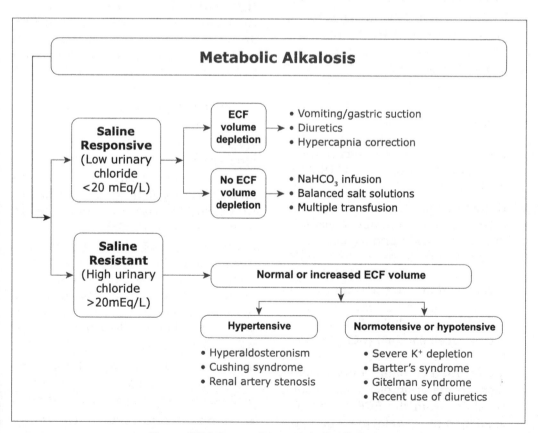

Figure 32.1 Approach to metabolic alkalosis.

bicarbonate in the body, with its most important causes being loss of gastric secretions (e.g., vomiting), diuretics, hypokalemia, and aldosterone excess. The most useful factors in determining the etiology of metabolic alkalosis are ECF volume, blood pressure, urinary chloride concentration, and serum potassium. Urinary chloride concentration differentiates metabolic alkalosis into two major groups: saline-responsive and saline-resistant metabolic alkalosis (Figure 32.1).

Saline-responsive metabolic alkalosis is a more commonly encountered cause of metabolic alkalosis, usually associated with signs of extracellular volume contraction (contraction alkalosis), and its most frequent causes are loss of gastric secretions and diuretic therapy. Hypotension, orthostatic fall of blood pressure, and hypokalemia are the most common associated features.

Saline-resistant metabolic alkalosis is a less common form of metabolic alkalosis, associated with either euvolemia or hypervolemia in contrast to extracellular volume contraction in saline-responsive metabolic alkalosis. The presence or absence of hypertension helps to determine the causes of saline-resistant metabolic alkalosis.

Chloride-resistant metabolic alkalosis with hypertension suggests overactivation of the RAAS system, and assessment of plasma renin and aldosterone levels are useful in further differentiating its causes, such as hyperaldosteronism, Cushing syndrome, and renal artery stenosis. Saline-resistant metabolic alkalosis without hypertension is less common, and it should raise suspicion of underlying conditions such as Bartter syndrome, Gitelman syndrome, severe potassium depletion, or recent diuretic use as potential causes.

CLINICAL FEATURES

Metabolic alkalosis rarely causes specific manifestations, and signs and symptoms can vary depending on its severity and are usually related to the underlying cause or associated volume, potassium, or magnesium depletion. Elevated pH in metabolic alkalosis leads to the binding of calcium ions to albumin, resulting in hypocalcemia, which can lead to neuromuscular symptoms.

Patients with mild to moderate metabolic alkalosis (serum HCO_3 <40 mEq/L, pH <7.50) are usually asymptomatic, but symptoms become evident when metabolic alkalosis is severe (serum HCO_3 >45 mEq/L, pH >7.55) [9]. Common features include [3–5]:

CNS symptoms: Alkalemia can increase neuromuscular excitability secondary to hypocalcemia, leading to paresthesia, light headache, tetany, carpopedal spasm, confusion, and seizures.

CVS symptoms: Hypotension and cardiac arrhythmias are common presentations, usually related to hypovolemia, hypokalemia, and hypomagnesemia rather than the alkalemia itself.

Respiratory abnormalities: In moderate to severe metabolic alkalosis, compensatory hypoventilation may cause hypoxia in patients with preexisting lung disease. This reduction in the respiratory drive can impair the weaning process from mechanical ventilation and make extubation difficult.

Other symptoms: Weakness, muscle cramps, and postural dizziness result from hypovolemia, while muscle weakness and polyuria are due to hypokalemia. Metabolic alkalosis can also precipitate hepatic encephalopathy in susceptible individuals by elevating ammonia production.

DIAGNOSIS

Three key steps for approaching metabolic alkalosis include confirming the diagnosis (e.g., primary metabolic or primary respiratory acidosis), establishing the etiological diagnosis (e.g., vomiting, diuretics, primary hyperaldosteronism, etc.), and identifying any coexisting acid-base disorders (e.g., metabolic acidosis, respiratory acidosis, or respiratory alkalosis).

A. Confirm diagnosis

Increased serum HCO_3 (>26 mEq/L), with high pH (>7.45), confirms the diagnosis of metabolic alkalosis. However, even in primary respiratory acidosis, increased HCO_3 and increased $PaCO_2$ are present, with low pH as the distinguishing feature. So, always obtain a blood gas to differentiate these disorders, with arterial blood gas considered the gold standard and venous blood gas offering a more convenient and acceptable alternative.

B. Establishing the etiological diagnosis

In most cases, a detailed patient history can provide valuable clues for establishing the etiological diagnosis of metabolic alkalosis; however, when the cause is unclear, a systematic and stepwise further evaluation becomes essential.

Physical examination: A thorough physical examination should include the presence of hypertension and extracellular fluid (ECF) volume status, especially assessing postural changes in pulse and blood pressure.

Laboratory tests: Check serum potassium, sodium, chloride, calcium, magnesium, blood urea nitrogen (BUN), and creatinine to detect associated disorders. Obtain urinary chloride concentration, plasma renin, and aldosterone levels for further workup to establish the etiological diagnosis of metabolic alkalosis.

Based on urinary chloride concentration, metabolic alkalosis is divided into two groups: saline-responsive (chloride-responsive) and saline-resistant (chloride-resistant) metabolic alkalosis, which are very useful in narrowing down the etiological diagnosis. Figure 32.1 summarizes the etiological differential diagnosis of metabolic alkalosis based on urinary chloride concentration and extracellular fluid volume status.

Table 32.2 Approach to metabolic alkalosis with high urinary chloride (Chloride-resistant alkalosis)		
High blood pressure		
Low renin High aldosterone	High renin High aldosterone	Low renin Low aldosterone
Primary hyperaldosteronism	Secondary aldosteronism	Apparent mineralocorticoid excess
Adenoma Bilateral adrenal hyperplasia Carcinoma	Malignant hypertension, renal artery stenosis, renin-secreting tumor	Licorice, Cushing syndrome, Liddle syndrome, Congenital adrenal hyperplasia
Normal or low blood pressure		
Recent use of diuretics, severe K^+ depletion, Bartter or Gitelman syndromes, hypomagnesemia		

Metabolic alkalosis with low urinary chloride: Common causes of saline-responsive metabolic alkalosis (urine chloride <20 mEq/L) are vomiting, nasogastric suction, diuretic therapy, post-hypercapnia syndrome, and Exogenous HCO_3 load.

Metabolic alkalosis with high urinary chloride: Saline-resistant metabolic alkalosis (urine chloride >20 mEq/L) can be further evaluated into two groups based on blood pressure measurement: patients with hypertension and those who are normotensive or hypotensive, as summarized in Table 32.2.

Metabolic alkalosis with high urinary chloride and hypertension: To establish the etiology of metabolic alkalosis with hypertension, measurement of renin and aldosterone is essential.

Metabolic alkalosis having high urinary chloride without hypertension: To establish the etiology of metabolic alkalosis in individuals with normal or low blood pressure, it is useful to elicit the history of recent use of thiazides or loop diuretics and perform blood tests to measure serum potassium and magnesium levels. In the absence of causes like diuretics, severe hypokalemia, and hypomagnesemia, suspect causes such as Bartter syndrome and Gitelman syndrome.

Both Bartter syndrome and Gitelman syndrome are genetic disorders characterized by metabolic alkalosis, reduction of the extracellular fluid volume, normal or low blood pressure, hypokalemia, high renin, and secondary hyperaldosteronism, and shared symptoms such as polyuria and polydipsia. However, the differentiating features of these disorders are that Bartter syndrome typically presents in infancy, has more severe symptoms, and is associated with hypercalciuria and usually normal serum magnesium levels. In contrast, Gitelman syndrome usually occurs later in life, presents milder symptoms, and is characterized by hypocalciuria and low serum magnesium levels.

C. Identifying coexisting acid-base disorders

Two steps for detecting coexisting acid-base disorders include calculating respiratory compensation and evaluating the anion gap:

1. Calculating compensation: The formula used to calculate respiratory compensation is:

   Expected increase in $PaCO_2$ = 0.7 × Rise in HCO_3 (Measured HCO_3 – 24)

   If the actual value of pCO_2 is higher than the calculated expected value, it suggests coexisting respiratory acidosis.

   In contrast, if the actual value of pCO_2 is lower than the calculated expected value, it suggests coexisting respiratory alkalosis.

2. Calculating anion gap: If the anion gap $[Na^+ - (Cl^- + HCO_3)]$ is high (i.e., greater than 20 mEq/L) in patients with metabolic alkalosis, it suggests coexisting high anion gap metabolic acidosis.

MANAGEMENT

Treatment of underlying cause

Treatment of the underlying cause is generally sufficient to correct metabolic alkalosis in most cases. However, specific therapy may be indicated in symptomatic or moderate to severe alkalosis.

Saline (chloride/volume) responsive alkalosis

- The aim of therapy is adequate correction of hypovolemia, hypochloremia, hypokalemia, and hypomagnesemia.

- Provide saline with potassium: IV normal saline with potassium chloride is the preferred solution for correcting hypovolemia in metabolic alkalosis because it corrects both hypochloremia and hypokalemia. Optimal correction of hypovolemia effectively expands the extracellular fluid volume, enhances renal sodium bicarbonate excretion, and corrects metabolic alkalosis.

- Inhibition of gastric acid secretion: Treatment with H2 inhibitors or, more effectively, with proton pump inhibitors reduces gastric acid secretion, minimizes further loss of H^+, and prevents or reduces metabolic alkalosis resulting from vomiting or nasogastric suction [10, 11]. Octreotide effectively controls hypergastrinemia and reduces gastric H^+ secretion in Zollinger–Ellison syndrome [12].

- Discontinue diuretics: Diuretics-induced metabolic alkalosis efforts should be made to hold or decrease the dose of diuretics. However, in cases of heart failure or liver cirrhosis with edema, where diuretics are necessary, it can be challenging to manage diuretic-induced metabolic alkalosis. Measures useful in such patients are dose reduction of diuretics, KCl supplementation, adding a K^+ sparing diuretic, such as spironolactone, or combining carbonic anhydrase inhibitors with loop and/or thiazide diuretics.

- Avoid exogenous alkali: To prevent excessive alkalinization, avoid or discontinue the use of exogenous alkali sources, including $NaHCO_3$ infusions, balanced crystalloids with lactate or acetate buffers, and citrate-containing blood products that can generate bicarbonate.

- Rare use of hydrochloric acid: In rare cases, when severe metabolic alkalosis (pH >7.55) with profound clinical symptoms is refractory to standard treatment or other treatments are contraindicated, the infusion of diluted hydrochloric acid (HCl) can be used to reduce plasma HCO_3 concentration rapidly [13]. Due to HCl's highly corrosive nature, diluted HCl solution must be given cautiously via a central line to prevent accidental extravasation, resulting in severe irritation, thrombophlebitis, and tissue necrosis [14].

As diluted HCl solution is not available commercially, it needs to be formulated by the pharmacist. Commercially, hydrochloric acid is available as a 1 normal (1 N) solution. To prepare HCl infusion for clinical use, mix 100 mL of 1 N hydrochloric acid with 900 mL of normal saline, dextrose 5%, or sterile water [15]. This customized HCl infusion contains 0.1 normal HCl and provides 100 mEq/L of H^+. To achieve the clinical goal of delivering 10 mEq/hour of H^+, administer 100 mL of this pre-mixed solution slowly over an hour [13].

Calculation of dose of HCl:

H^+ Ion Deficit (mEq) =

0.3 × Body Weight (kg) × (Measured − Desired HCO_3 [mEq/L])

Rate of HCl administration: The safe infusion rate of HCl is 0.1 to 0.2 mEq/kg/hour.

The goal of administering HCl in cases of severe metabolic alkalosis is to partially correct HCO_3 levels, aiming to reduce HCO_3 to a safe bicarbonate level, e.g., 35 mEq/L or lower [16].

- Dialysis therapy: Dialysis therapy with a low bicarbonate bath may be considered in a few patients with severe metabolic alkalosis unresponsive to standard treatment or acetazolamide, particularly in cases of volume overload, profound electrolyte abnormalities, and renal failure [17, 18].

- Post-hypercapnic metabolic alkalosis: When initiating mechanical ventilatory support in chronic hypercapnia, there can be a risk of developing metabolic alkalosis because the rapid decrease in pCO_2 occurs concurrently with the slower decline in elevated HCO_3 levels, allowing the unopposed effect of elevated HCO_3 to lead to post-hypercapnic metabolic alkalosis. Important treatment measures for post hypercapnic metabolic alkalosis include reducing minute ventilation by decreasing respiratory rate or tidal volume, correcting hypovolemia and hypokalemia, and considering the supplementation of Acetazolamide [19]. Acetazolamide enhances urinary bicarbonate excretion and helps in the correction of post-hypercapnic metabolic alkalosis.

Saline (chloride/volume) resistant metabolic alkalosis

Saline-resistant metabolic alkalosis is characterized by an increased aldosterone effect and requires therapy with aldosterone antagonists. It is important to remember that this condition with volume expansion does not benefit from rehydration therapy. Basic management includes specific treatment of underlying causes, blockage of Na^+ reabsorption with aldosterone antagonists aiming to enhance NaCl excretion and K^+ retention, Acetazolamide to increase urinary bicarbonate excretion, aggressive correction of hypokalemia, and dietary sodium restriction.

Etiological treatment: The specific treatment of underlying causes includes surgical removal of the pituitary tumor or adrenal adenoma in Cushing's syndrome, discontinuing licorice intake, using potassium-sparing diuretics (such as spironolactone, eplerenone, amiloride, and triamterene) to treat primary mineralocorticoid excess and primary hyperaldosteronism, and utilizing Indomethacin for the treatment of Bartter syndrome.

Correction of hypokalemia: Hypokalemia occurs in nearly all saline-resistant alkalosis, and correction of potassium deficiency is essential to reduce the severity of metabolic alkalosis [4]. A diet rich in potassium should be encouraged. Potassium should also be supplemented either orally or intravenously, judiciously considering the severity of hypokalemia. Potassium-sparing diuretics, such as aldosterone receptor antagonists (e.g., spironolactone and eplerenone) and epithelial sodium channel (ENaC) inhibitors (e.g., amiloride and triamterene), help correct hypokalemia by increasing sodium excretion while decreasing potassium excretion. Correction of hypokalemia helps in the resolution of metabolic alkalosis and reduces the severity of hypertension.

Acetazolamide: Acetazolamide inhibits the enzyme carbonic anhydrase in the proximal tubule, leading to the blockade of renal acidification, increased urinary bicarbonate excretion, and a consequent reduction in blood pH due to bicarbonaturia. Patients with metabolic alkalosis with volume overload, such as those with diuretic-resistant heart failure who cannot tolerate volume expansion with normal saline, can be treated with acetazolamide [20]. Acetazolamide is commonly prescribed at daily doses ranging from 250 to 500 mg, usually taken once or twice a day. As acetazolamide can cause hypokalemia, which can aggravate metabolic alkalosis, it is essential to monitor potassium levels carefully and aggressively correct hypokalemia [21].

Spironolactone: Spironolactone corrects hypokalemia through its aldosterone antagonism and potassium-sparing effect, which in turn contributes to the correction of alkalosis. Spironolactone is useful for treating saline-resistant metabolic alkalosis in cases associated with primary or secondary hyperaldosteronism, as well as in patients with volume overload conditions such as congestive heart failure [4]. During spironolactone therapy, careful monitoring of serum potassium levels is crucial to prevent life-threatening hyperkalemia.

Amiloride: Amiloride corrects hypokalemia by blocking sodium channels in the distal renal tubules, distinguishing it from the aldosterone receptor antagonist effect of spironolactone. Amiloride is not commonly used in the treatment of metabolic alkalosis, but it is the preferred treatment for metabolic alkalosis associated with Liddle syndrome, whereas spironolactone is ineffective in such cases [22].

REFERENCES

1. Webster NR, Kulkarni V. Metabolic alkalosis in the critically ill. Crit Rev Clin Lab Sci. 1999;36(5):497–510

2. Mæhle K, Haug B, Flaatten H, et al. Metabolic alkalosis is the most common acid-base disorder in ICU patients. Crit Care. 2014;18(2):420

3. Emmett M. Metabolic Alkalosis: A Brief Pathophysiologic Review. Clin J Am Soc Nephrol. 2020;15(12):1848–1856

4. Do C, Vasquez PC, Soleimani M. Metabolic Alkalosis Pathogenesis, Diagnosis, and Treatment: Core Curriculum 2022. Am J Kidney Dis. 2022;80(4):536–551

5. Krishnan N, Alpern RJ. Metabolic Alkalosis. Nephrology Self-Assessment Program. 2022;20(2):145–146

6. Galla JH. Metabolic alkalosis. J Am Soc Nephrol 2000;11(2):369–375

7. Khanna A, Kurtzman NA. Metabolic alkalosis. J Nephrol 2006;19 Suppl 9:S86–96

8. Gillion V, Jadoul M, Devuyst O, et al. The patient with metabolic alkalosis. Acta Clin Belg. 2019;74(1):34–40

9. Tinawi M. Pathophysiology, Evaluation, and Management of Metabolic Alkalosis. Cureus. 2021;13(1):e12841

10. Eiro M, Katoh T, Watanabe T. Use of a proton-pump inhibitor for metabolic disturbances associated with anorexia nervosa. N Engl J Med. 2002;346(2):140

11. Kirsch BM, Sunder-Plassmann G, Schwarz C. Metabolic alkalosis in a hemodialysis patient-- successful treatment with a proton pump inhibitor. Clin Nephrol 2006;66(5):391–4

12. Mozell EJ, Cramer AJ, O'Dorisio TM, et al. Long-term efficacy of octreotide in the treatment of Zollinger-Ellison syndrome. Arch Surg. 1992;127(9):1019–24

13. Guffey JD, Haas CE, Crowley A, et al. Hydrochloric Acid Infusion for the Treatment of Metabolic Alkalosis in Surgical Intensive Care Unit Patients. Ann Pharmacother. 2018;(6):522–526

14. Buchanan IB, Campbell BT, Peck MD, et al. Chest wall necrosis and death secondary to hydrochloric acid infusion for metabolic alkalosis. South Med J. 2005;98(8):822–824

15. Hydrochloric Acid (HCL). In: IV Dilutions Medication Reference and Infusion Guidelines. GlobalRxPh: The Clinician's Ultimate Reference. [Internet]. Available from: https://globalrph.com/dilution/hydrochloric-acid-hcl/

16. Achanti A, Szerlip HM. Acid-Base Disorders in the Critically Ill Patient. Clin J Am Soc Nephrol. 2023;18(1):102–112

17. Huber L, Gennari FJ. Severe metabolic alkalosis in a hemodialysis patient. Am J Kidney Dis 2011;58(1):144–149

18. Lisawat P, Gennari FJ. Approach to the hemodialysis patient with an abnormal serum bicarbonate concentration. Am J Kidney Dis 2014;64(1):151–5

19. Yi Y. Post-Hypercapnic Alkalosis: A Brief Review. Electrolyte Blood Press. 2023;21(1):18–23

20. Peixoto AJ, Alpern RJ. Treatment of severe metabolic alkalosis in a patient with congestive heart failure. Am J Kidney Dis. 2013;61(5):822–7

21. Ellison DH. Clinical pharmacology in diuretic use. Clin J Am Soc Nephrol. 2019;14(8):1248–1257

22. Enslow BT, Stockand JD, Berman JM. Liddle's syndrome mechanisms, diagnosis and management. Integr Blood Press Control. 2019;12:13–22

33 | Respiratory Acid–Base Disorders

Respiratory acidosis and respiratory alkalosis are the two primary respiratory acid-base disorders commonly encountered in clinical practice, both resulting from primary changes in pCO_2 due to various disorders.

RESPIRATORY ACIDOSIS

Definition

Respiratory acidosis, also known as primary hypercapnia, is a clinical disorder characterized by a primary elevation in the $PaCO_2$ (>45 mmHg) leading to a reduction in pH (<7.35) and variable compensatory increase in the plasma HCO_3 concentration.

Respiratory acidosis occurs when the effective alveolar ventilation (CO_2 excretion by the lung) fails to keep pace with the rate of CO_2 production. Acute respiratory acidosis occurs rapidly within <48 hours, while chronic respiratory acidosis develops slowly over days to weeks (>48 hours).

Renal (metabolic) compensation

Respiratory acidosis leads to renal compensation through increased urinary H^+ secretion, resulting in acidic urine. This gradual process leads to a rise in plasma HCO_3 levels, mitigating acidosis. Because renal compensation is a slow process, the compensatory increase in HCO_3 is small in acute respiratory acidosis. In contrast, in chronic respiratory acidosis, the compensatory rise in HCO_3 is more substantial over time due to robust and prolonged renal compensation.

Acute respiratory acidosis: Every 10 mm of Hg rise in $PaCO_2$ causes 1 mEq/L rise in HCO_3 and 0.1 fall in pH.

Chronic respiratory acidosis: Every 10 mm Hg rise in $PaCO_2$ causes a 4 mEq/L rise in HCO_3 and a 0.03 fall in pH.

Serum HCO_3 usually does not exceed 38 mEq/L due to compensation. If HCO_3 is >38 mEq/L, think of concomitant metabolic alkalosis.

Respiratory acidosis vs. metabolic alkalosis

Increased $PaCO_2$ and increased HCO_3 characterize both disorders, but pH is low in respiratory acidosis, and pH is high in metabolic alkalosis.

Relation between high $PaCO_2$ (hypercapnia) and low PaO_2 (hypoxemia) [1]

1. In most cases, hypoxemia occurs earlier and is more prominent than hypercapnia because alveolar diffusion of CO_2 is 20 times faster than O_2.

2. All patients with hypercapnia who are breathing room air are also hypoxic.

3. In patients with hypoventilation, oxygen therapy corrects hypoxemia, but hypercapnia persists.

4. In chronic hypercapnia, hypoxemia serves as the primary stimulus to respiration. Therefore, rapid and excessive correction of hypoxemia with uncontrolled oxygen can diminish the hypoxic stimulation of ventilation, potentially resulting in extreme hypercapnia and neurological symptoms.

Etiology

Respiratory acidosis occurs due to an accumulation of carbon dioxide (CO_2) as a result of inadequate exhalation of CO_2 due to hypoventilation, impaired lung function or iatrogenic causes as summarized in Table 33.1.

Clinical features

Clinical features of respiratory acidosis can vary depending on [2, 3]:

Table 33.1 Mechanism and causes of respiratory acidosis (hypercapnia)
A. Reduced ventilation
• CNS depression: Drugs (anesthesia, sedative), infection, stroke
• Neuromuscular impairment: Myopathy, myasthenia gravis, polymyositis
• Muscular: Hypokalemia, hyperkalemia
• Airway obstruction: Severe asthma or laryngospasm, airway blockage due to foreign body, aspiration
• Miscellaneous: Chest wall disorders, severe kyphoscoliosis, obstructive sleep apnea, obesity hypoventilation syndrome
B. Defects in CO_2 transport
• Decreased lung perfusion: Pulmonary embolism or heart failure
• Pulmonary diseases: Abnormal gas exchange in COPD, emphysema, ARDS, interstitial lung diseases, severe pneumonitis, pneumothorax, massive pleural effusion
C. Iatrogenic
• Hypoventilation due to improper settings of mechanical ventilation
D. Increased CO_2 production
• Rare, unless ventilation is fixed in fever, shivering, increased physical activity

- The characteristics of the underlying primary disorder.

- The severity and rapidity of onset of hypercapnia is a major determinant of symptoms. The severity of hypoxemia also plays a role in clinical presentation, as hypercapnic patients are hypoxic when breathing room air.

The clinical features of respiratory acidosis are as follows:

Central nervous system manifestations: The predominant symptoms of respiratory acidosis are neurological, resulting from cerebral vasodilation, which can lead to increased intracranial pressure, neuronal dysfunction due to acidemia, and CNS depression due to hypercapnia.

Anxiety and headache typically present early, and as pCO_2 levels rise, patients can develop severe symptoms, including confusion, somnolence, obtundation, and coma, also known as "CO_2 narcosis. Other neuromuscular symptoms often seen are twitching, tremors, myoclonus, and seizures. Prolonged or severe respiratory acidosis may lead to increased intracranial pressure, which may cause papilloedema.

Lipid soluble CO_2 crosses blood brain barrier rapidly, compared to HCO_3. So fall in CSF pH is greater in respiratory acidosis as compared to metabolic acidosis. So CNS manifestations are more with acute respiratory acidosis and less with acute metabolic acidosis.

Cardiovascular manifestations: Hypercapnia can result in systemic vasodilation, reduced myocardial contractility, and potentially lead to cardiac arrhythmias, cardiovascular instability, and even death.

Diagnosis

A comprehensive diagnostic approach, including a detailed medical history, a thorough physical examination, and a battery of tests, is performed to establish the diagnosis of primary respiratory acidosis, determine its underlying causes, detect any associated mixed acid-base disorders, and differentiate between acute and chronic forms of respiratory acidosis.

A. History

It is essential to elicit a history regarding fever, the presence of respiratory symptoms like shortness of breath and cough, any pre-existing pulmonary or nonpulmonary conditions that may contribute to the development of respiratory acidosis, and a medication history.

B. Physical examination

Physical examination should be performed thoroughly to:

- Assess respiratory rate, pattern, and distress, check for the presence of cyanosis, and evaluate the patient's volume status.

- Auscultate the lungs to evaluate for bilateral adequate air entry, wheezing, and crepitations.

- Conduct a neurological exam to identify neurological causes of respiratory acidosis and assess symptoms, including confusion, lethargy, and altered sensorium, which can occur in respiratory acidosis.

C. Investigations

Various tests aim to detect respiratory acidosis, assess its severity, and search for underlying causative etiology:

1. Laboratory tests: a. Arterial blood gas analysis is essential to confirm the diagnosis of respiratory acidosis, determine its severity, classify respiratory acidosis as acute, acute-on-chronic,

Table 33.2 Interpretations of arterial blood gas analysis in respiratory acidosis	
Parameters	**Interpretations**
Elevated pCO$_2$ (>45 mmHg) and low pH (<7.35)	These values suggest the presence of respiratory acidosis
	A greater increase in pCO$_2$ and a more significant decrease in pH suggest more severe acidosis
Compensatory changes in serum bicarbonate levels	In acute respiratory acidosis, for every 10 mmHg rise in PaCO$_2$, there is a 1 mEq/L rise in HCO$_3^-$ levels
	In chronic respiratory acidosis, this compensatory mechanism becomes more pronounced, with every 10 mmHg rise in PaCO$_2$ resulting in a 4 mEq/L increase in HCO$_3^-$ levels over time
Serum bicarbonate levels beyond expectations	A serum bicarbonate level lower than normal (moving in the opposite direction) suggests the presence of coexisting metabolic acidosis
	Conversely, a serum bicarbonate level higher than expected in the context of respiratory acidosis (HCO$_3$>38 mEq/L) suggests the presence of coexisting metabolic alkalosis
Anion gap (AG)	High AG suggests the presence of coexisting high AG metabolic acidosis
Serum pH levels	A pH below 7.35 suggests respiratory acidosis, and the severity of acidosis is greater with a lower pH level
	In acute respiratory acidosis, there is an abrupt decrease in pH, with approximately a 0.08 reduction for every 10 mm Hg increase in PaCO$_2$
	In chronic respiratory acidosis, the compensatory increase in HCO$_3$ leads to a less significant pH reduction, with an approximate 0.03 decrease for every 10 mm Hg rise in PaCO$_2$

or chronic, and detect the presence of associated mixed disorders (Table 33.2). Arterial blood gas analysis also guides treatment decisions, including oxygen therapy and mechanical ventilation, based on the severity of the respiratory failure. It also facilitates monitoring of treatment response, allowing for necessary ventilation adjustments.

2. Other laboratory tests: Various laboratory tests commonly performed in respiratory acidosis are complete blood count (CBC), serum electrolytes (including Ca^{2+}, Mg^{2+}, and phosphate), thyroid function tests, and creatinine kinase:

- In patients with chronic hypercapnia and respiratory acidosis, persistent hypoxemia can lead to polycythemia, which is characterized by elevated hemoglobin and hematocrit levels.

- Hypophosphatemia, hyperkalemia, and hypokalemia can result in muscle weakness, including severe weakness of respiratory muscles, which can contribute to its development or delayed recovery.

- Hypochloremia reflects chronic hypercapnia. In chronic respiratory acidosis, increased renal bicarbonate retention is a normal adaptation that results in elevated chloride ion excretion in the urine, leading to hypochloremia.

- Thyroid function tests are recommended for obese patients to detect hypothyroidism, which can contribute to obstructive sleep apnea (OSA) and hypoventilation during sleep.

3. Radiologic studies: Perform radiological imaging, such as X-ray, computed tomography, or magnetic resonance imaging of the chest, to identify the underlying causes that affect respiration and ventilation, potentially leading to respiratory acidosis.

In patients with respiratory acidosis caused by neurological problems leading to hypoventilation, consider diagnostic brain imaging studies such as computerized tomography (CT) scanning and magnetic resonance imaging (MRI).

4. Pulmonary function tests: Pulmonary function tests are performed for the diagnosis of obstructive lung disease and the assessment of the severity of the disease.

Treatment

Treatment strategies for respiratory acidosis vary depending on the severity, rate of onset, and underlying etiology. Along with hypercapnia, hypoxia usually occurs in respiratory acidosis, but not always, and careful treatment of both is essential considering their interrelationship.

General measures

- The primary goal of therapy is to promptly identify and treat the underlying cause. Treatment of underlying etiology is essential; at times, only treatment is required. This may involve antibiotics for respiratory infections, β2-agonists, and other bronchodilator therapy for severe bronchoconstriction or treatment for neuromuscular diseases.

- Establish a patent airway and restore adequate oxygenation.

- If a patient with chronic hypercapnia develops a sudden increase in $PaCO_2$, search for the aggravating factor. Vigorous treatment of pulmonary infection, bronchodilator therapy, and removal of secretions

can offer considerable benefits in such patients.

Oxygen therapy

The role of oxygen therapy in correcting hypoxia in respiratory acidosis (hypoxemic hypercapnic respiratory failure) resembles a 'double-edged sword' and thus requires careful titration. In acute respiratory acidosis, the major threat to life is significant hypoxia rather than hypercapnia or acidosis. So, oxygen supplementation is essential to ensure adequate oxygenation, and it should never be withheld or withdrawn in the presence of high or rising $PaCO_2$ [4].

However, it's important to note that hypoxemia (when PaO_2 decreases below 80 mm Hg) is an essential stimulus for respiration [5]. Injudicious therapy can lead to the suppression of the hypoxia-driven respiratory drive, causing a drastic reduction in alveolar ventilation and aggravation of hypercapnia [6]. Mechanisms other than the abolition of the 'hypoxic drive' in the development of oxygen-induced hypercapnia include the loss of hypoxic vasoconstriction and the occurrence of absorption atelectasis, both of which contribute to an increase in dead-space ventilation and the Haldane effect [7].

Considering potential benefits and risks, oxygen therapy should be initiated cautiously in chronic hypercapnia cases. Initiate treatment with the lowest possible concentration and gradually increase it to achieve a SpO_2 of 88% to 92% or a PaO_2 of 60 to 70 mmHg [8–11]. The usual practice for controlled oxygen therapy involves administering oxygen at a low flow rate, such as 2 L/min via nasal cannula, with gradual increments of 1 L/min every 10 to 15 minutes, targeting an oxygen saturation of 88% to 92%. Exceeding this range is unnecessary and not recommended because liberal oxygen administration is associated with increased mortality [12].

Ventilatory support

Two commonly used options for ventilatory support in respiratory acidosis are noninvasive ventilation (NIV) and invasive mechanical ventilation. The choice between these two modalities depends on various factors, including the severity of the hypoxemia and hypercapnia, the underlying cause, and the patient's clinical status [11]. It's important to note that asymptomatic or stable patients with chronic respiratory acidosis can tolerate hypercapnia well and may not require ventilatory support.

1. Noninvasive ventilation (NIV)

- NIV, by delivering positive pressure ventilation via a mask or nasal interface, reduces the breathing workload and plays a crucial role in improving oxygenation and correcting hypercapnia without the need for intubation, thus avoiding the complications associated with invasive mechanical ventilation.

- It is often preferred for patients with mild to moderate respiratory acidosis who are conscious, cooperative, and able to protect their airways.

- Common indications for NIV in respiratory acidosis include acute exacerbations of chronic obstructive pulmonary disease (COPD), respiratory failure from cardiogenic pulmonary edema, obstructive sleep apnea, and neuromuscular disorders.

2. Invasive mechanical ventilation

Invasive mechanical ventilation necessitates the use of artificial airways, such as an endotracheal tube or tracheostomy tube, and is commonly used under the following circumstances:

- Hemodynamically unstable, severely symptomatic patients with progressive worsening of hypoxia and hypercapnia.

- Profound loss of consciousness, coupled with excessive secretions in individuals who cannot protect their airways.

- Initiation of mechanical ventilation if the patient exhibits signs of muscle fatigue before respiratory failure becomes critical.

- Transition to invasive mechanical ventilation in cases where NIV fails to adequately correct respiratory acidosis or those who cannot tolerate NIV.

3. Correction of hypercapnia and post hypercapnic alkalosis

Initiating mechanical ventilatory support in chronic hypercapnia carries the risk of developing metabolic alkalosis, as the rapid decrease in pCO_2 occurs concurrently with the slower decline in elevated HCO_3 levels, allowing the unopposed effect of elevated HCO_3 to lead to sudden, substantial alkalemia and marked rise in pH. This leads to post-hypercapnic alkalosis, which can be detrimental. To minimize the risk of "overshoot" alkalemia, lowering the $PaCO_2$ gradually by reducing minute ventilation through adjustments in respiratory rate or tidal volume is essential [2].

4. Target PaCO2 on mechanical ventilator

In patients with chronic respiratory acidosis on ventilatory support, the target $PaCO_2$ is usually the patient's prior stable level, not a "normal" $PaCO_2$ of 40 mm of Hg. In contrast, in acute respiratory acidosis, the target $PaCO_2$ should be at the normal level.

Alkali therapy

Avoid administering alkali therapy in cases of simple respiratory acidosis, but consider it in certain patients with associated metabolic acidosis (i.e., mixed respiratory and metabolic acidosis), permissive hypercapnia, or severe bronchospasm [13, 14]. Alkali therapy administration restores bronchial musculature responsiveness to beta-adrenergic agonists by reducing calcium availability to bronchial smooth muscle, ultimately alleviating bronchoconstriction [14].

Administering $NaHCO_3$ is contraindicated in respiratory acidosis because it can lead to the production of carbon dioxide as sodium bicarbonate reacts with hydrogen ions, and poor ventilation may impair its removal, further exacerbating hypercapnia [15].

Respiratory stimulants: Medications such as medroxyprogesterone, acetazolamide, and theophylline, which have been utilized in the past as respiratory stimulants, have not demonstrated effectiveness in the treatment of hypercapnic states.

RESPIRATORY ALKALOSIS

Respiratory alkalosis is a frequently encountered disorder in critically ill patients; however, it rarely has life-threatening clinical adverse effects [16].

Definition

Respiratory alkalosis, also known as primary hypocapnia, is a clinical disorder characterized by a low $PaCO_2$ (<35mm of Hg) leading to an increase in pH (>7.45) and compensatory reduction in the plasma HCO_3 concentration.

Respiratory alkalosis occurs when hyperventilation reduces the $PaCO_2$ (hypocapnia) and increases pH. It occurs when respiratory disturbance causes excessive pulmonary CO_2 elimination (hyperventilation) that exceeds the metabolic production of CO_2 by the tissues. Acute respiratory alkalosis occurs rapidly within <48 hours, while chronic respiratory alkalosis develops slowly over days (>48 hours).

Renal (metabolic) compensation

In respiratory alkalosis, renal compensation starts after 2–6 hours of sustained hypocapnia and is usually completed in 36 to 72 hours. This compensation involves a decreased renal excretion of ammonium and titratable acid and a reduction in the renal reabsorption of filtered HCO_3, leading to an increased urinary loss of HCO_3. Notably, in respiratory alkalosis, renal compensation is primarily triggered by reduced $PaCO_2$ levels rather than the alkalosis itself.

Acute respiratory alkalosis: Every 10 mm Hg fall in $PaCO_2$ causes a 2 mEq/L fall in HCO_3 and a 0.1 rise in pH.

Chronic respiratory alkalosis: Every 10 mm of Hg fall in $PaCO_2$ causes a 4-5 mEq/L fall in HCO_3 and a 0.03 rise in pH.

The serum bicarbonate usually does not fall below 16 mEq/L unless a concomitant metabolic acidosis is present.

Etiology

Respiratory alkalosis is a frequently encountered acid-base disorder, often manifesting during normal pregnancy or in individuals living at high altitudes. Important causes of respiratory alkalosis are summarized in Table 33.3.

Clinical features

The clinical features of respiratory alkalosis vary with severity, rate of onset, and underlying disorders. Symptoms are more pronounced in acute respiratory alkalosis but tend to be milder or non-significant in chronic respiratory alkalosis. In acute hypocapnia, symptoms

Table 33.3 Causes of respiratory alkalosis
A. Hypoxemia   • Living at a high altitude, severe anemia, and hypotension
B. Pulmonary disorders   • Asthma, pneumonia, pulmonary embolism, pulmonary edema, ARDS, pulmonary fibrosis, and pneumothorax
C. Central nervous system stimulation   • Pain, anxiety fever, and disorders of the CNS such as cerebrovascular accident (infarction, hemorrhage), head injury, or tumor
D. Underlying serious illness   • Liver failure, sepsis
E. Medications and hormones   • Salicylate, nicotine, and xanthines   • Pregnancy (due to increased progesterone)
F. Iatrogenic causes   • Aggressive mechanical ventilation, vigorous physical activities

are related to decreased oxygen delivery to the brain and heart due to vasoconstriction, which reduces cerebral and coronary blood flow, along with the shifting of the oxygen-hemoglobin dissociation curve to the left, resulting in diminished oxygen availability to the tissues [2, 17].

Respiratory alkalosis may be the only clue of underlying causes like sepsis and hepatic failure. In cases of extreme hypocapnia with a $PaCO_2$ level below 20–25 mm Hg, the mortality rate is high [18].

Common features seen in acute respiratory alkalosis include the following [17, 19]:

- **Hyperventilation:** Rapid and deep breathing or shortness of breath are characteristic symptoms of acute respiratory alkalosis.

- **Central nervous system effects:** Symptoms include feelings of dizziness, lightheadedness, mental confusion, disorientation, and seizures.

- **Cardiovascular effects:** These include palpitations, shortness of breath, chest wall tightness, cardiac arrhythmias, and ischemic electrocardiogram (ECG) changes, especially in patients with ischemic heart diseases.

- **Metabolic effects:** Severe alkalosis increases calcium binding to albumin, resulting in acute hypocalcemia. Hypocalcemia can cause symptoms such as tetany, perioral and distal extremity tingling and numbness, and muscle cramps.

- **Potassium shift:** Alkalosis causes extracellular potassium ion shifts into cells, resulting in hypokalemia, leading to muscle weakness or irregular heart rhythms.

Diagnosis

A detailed medical history, a thorough physical examination, and various laboratory tests help establish the diagnosis of primary respiratory alkalosis and its underlying causes and assist in detecting any associated mixed acid-base disorders.

A. History

It is essential to elicit a history regarding various causes of respiratory alkalosis, including respiratory, cardiac, or hepatic disorders, sepsis, and the use of drugs like salicylates, as well as factors such as pain and anxiety.

B. Physical examination

Hyperventilation is the characteristic finding of acute respiratory alkalosis, often accompanied by mild tachycardia and carpopedal spasms in severe cases.

C. Investigations

Arterial blood gas analysis: It is essential to obtain ABGs to establish the diagnosis of respiratory alkalosis, characterized by an increase in pH (>7.45) and a low $PaCO_2$ (<35 mm Hg).

Check compensation: In respiratory alkalosis, the reduction of serum bicarbonate is a compensatory response. In acute respiratory alkalosis, the expected decrease in HCO_3 is 2 mEq/L for every 10 mm Hg decrease in $PaCO_2$, while in chronic respiratory alkalosis, the reduction in HCO_3 is 4-5 mEq/L.

To confirm a diagnosis of simple respiratory alkalosis and rule out mixed disorders, it is crucial to compare the actual value of HCO_3 with the expected or calculated value. In cases of simple respiratory alkalosis, these two values match.

However, if the serum bicarbonate level exceeds the expected or calculated value of HCO_3, it suggests the presence of coexisting metabolic alkalosis. Conversely, if the serum bicarbonate level falls below the expected or calculated value of HCO_3, it indicates the possible presence of coexisting metabolic acidosis.

If the value of the serum bicarbonate level is greater than the normal level (>24 mEq/L), and there's a rise in HCO_3 instead of a compensatory fall (moving in the opposite direction), it suggests the presence of coexisting metabolic alkalosis.

Anion gap (AG): The presence of coexisting high AG suggests the presence of coexisting high AG metabolic acidosis.

Serum chemistry: Commonly performed laboratory tests include a complete blood count to exclude infection or detect anemia, serum electrolytes to identify hypocalcemia, hypophosphatemia, and hypokalemia, liver function tests to search for hepatic failure, urea and creatinine to assess renal status, and thyroid function tests to rule out hyperthyroidism.

Other tests: Additional tests are often performed based on clinical evaluation and may include imaging studies such as chest x-rays and CT scans of the chest, pulmonary function tests, cultures of blood or sputum, and measurements of theophylline and salicylate drug levels.

Treatment

The approach to treatment of respiratory alkalosis varies based on the duration of the disease (acute vs. chronic), the severity of symptoms, the patient's clinical status, and the underlying causes. Respiratory alkalosis, an especially chronic entity with few symptoms, needs no active interventions or direct treatment. However, it is advisable to avoid rapid correction of severe respiratory alkalosis due to the potential risks of cerebral and pulmonary reperfusion injury [15]:

- The first and most crucial step in managing respiratory alkalosis involves establishing the diagnosis of the underlying cause and initiating appropriate treatment.

- Discontinuation of causative medications, such as salicylates, is essential.

- Since hypoxemia is a common cause of hyperventilation, O_2 supplementation is essential, along with identifying and treating the underlying cause.

- In the absence of hypoxemia, traditional therapy includes

rebreathing into a paper bag. This method increases the concentration of CO_2 in inhaled air, subsequently raising pCO_2 levels. However, using a paper bag for breathing should be avoided because it may not correct pCO_2 and can cause significant hypoxemia and, therefore, be harmful [20].

- Anxiety-induced hyperventilation may respond to reassurance alone, but severe cases may require additional treatments, such as behavioral therapy, calming techniques, sedatives, antidepressants, and, in some instances, beta-blockers.

- When managing respiratory alkalosis during mechanical ventilation, adjusting ventilatory settings, including decreasing tidal volume and/or reducing the respiratory rate, can help reduce CO_2 excretion.

- Before climbing to high altitudes, pre-treatment with oral acetazolamide for at least two days can help minimize hyperventilation symptoms associated with altitude sickness (acute mountain sickness) [21].

REFERENCES

1. Sarkar M, Niranjan N, Banyal PK. Mechanisms of hypoxemia. Lung India. 2017;34(1):47–60.

2. Palmer BF, Clegg DJ. Respiratory Acidosis and Respiratory Alkalosis: Core Curriculum 2023. Am J Kidney Dis. 2023;82(3):347–359.

3. Adrogué HJ, Madias NE. Management of Life-Threatening Acid–Base Disorders. N Engl J Med. 1998;338(1):26–34.

4. Boatright JE, Jensen MQ. Therapeutic Gases: Management and Administration. In: Hess DR, MacIntyre NR, Galvin WF, editors. Respiratory Care: Principles and Practice, 4th edition. Jones & Bartlett Learning, LLC, an Ascend Learning Company; 2021. Chapter 14, pages 285–320.

5. Theerawit P, Soipetkasem P. An importance of respiratory drive and effort during mechanical ventilation: Respiratory drive and effort in respiratory failure. Clin Crit Care [Internet]. 2023;31(1):2023:e0001.

6. Rocker G. Harms of over oxygenation in patients with exacerbation of chronic obstructive pulmonary disease. CMAJ. 2017;189(22):E762–E763.

7. Sarkar M, Madabhavi I, Kadakol N. Oxygen-induced hypercapnia: physiological mechanisms and clinical implications. Monaldi Arch Chest Dis. 2023;93(3):2399.

8. O'Driscoll BR, Howard LS, Earis J, et al. BTS guideline for oxygen use in adults in healthcare and emergency settings. Thorax 2017;72(Suppl 1):ii1–ii90.

9. Echevarria C, Steer J, Wason J, et al. Oxygen therapy and inpatient mortality in COPD exacerbation. Emerg Med J. 2021;38(3):170–7.

10. Barnett A, Beasley R, Buchan C, et al. Thoracic Society of Australia and New Zealand Position Statement on Acute Oxygen Use in Adults: 'Swimming between the flags'. Respirology. 2022;27(4):262–276.

11. Fujishima S. Guideline-based management of acute respiratory failure and acute respiratory distress syndrome. J Intensive Care. 2023;11(1):10.

12. Austin MA, Wills KE, Blizzard L, et al. Effect of high flow oxygen on mortality in chronic obstructive pulmonary disease patients in prehospital setting: randomized controlled trial. BMJ 2010;341:c5462.

13. Adrogué HJ, Madias NE. Alkali Therapy for Respiratory Acidosis: A Medical Controversy. Am J Kidney Dis. 2020;75(2):265–271.

14. Chand R, Swenson ER, Goldfarb DS. Sodium bicarbonate therapy for acute respiratory acidosis. Curr Opin Nephrol Hypertens. 2021;30(2):223–230.

15. Quade BN, Parker MD, Occhipinti R. The therapeutic importance of acid-base balance. Biochem Pharmacol. 2021;183:114278.

16. Sanghavi S, Albert TJ, Swenson ER. ACID-BASE BALANCE. In: Broaddus VC, Ernst JD, King TE Jr, editors. Murray & Nadel's Textbook of Respiratory Medicine. Seventh Edition. Elsevier - Health Sciences Division; 2021. Chapter 12, page 166.

17. Laffey JG, Kavanagh BP. Hypocapnia. N Engl J Med. 2002;347(1):43–53.

18. Mazzara JT, Ayres SM, Grace WJ. Extreme hypocapnia in the critically ill patient. Am J Med. 1974;56(4):450–6.

19. Foster GT, Varizi ND, Sassoon CS. Respiratory alkalosis. Respir Care. 2001;46(4):384–91.

20. Callaham M. Hypoxic hazards of traditional paper bag rebreathing in hyperventilating patients. Ann Emerg Med 1989;18(6):622–8.

21. Burtscher M, Gatterer H, Faulhaber M, et al. Acetazolamide pre-treatment before ascending to high altitudes: when to start? Int J Clin Exp Med. 2014;7(11):4378–83.

Part 8

Fluid Therapy in Medical Disorders

34 | Gastrointestinal Losses and Upper GI Bleeding

INTRODUCTION

Loss of gastrointestinal (GI) secretions and hematemesis are frequently encountered problems in clinical practice. Several gastrointestinal disorders lead to loss of GI secretions causing electrolytes and acid-base disturbances. The composition of gastrointestinal secretions and potential disturbances due to their losses are summarized in Table 34.1 [1–3], which will help plan its management.

The most common disorders, vomiting, diarrhea, and hematemesis, will be discussed.

VOMITING

Vomiting or nasogastric suction is a common problem in clinical practice causing loss of fluid and electrolytes. Therefore, it is necessary to understand the basic pathophysiology of hypovolemia and electrolytes and acid-base

Table 34.1 Composition of gastrointestinal secretions and potential disturbances due to losses							
Secretion or type of loss	pH	Common disturbances	Na⁺ mEq/L	K⁺ mEq/L	Cl⁻ mEq/L	HCO₃⁻ mEq/L	H⁺ mEq/L
Saliva	6.0–7.0	-	40	20	40	30	
Stomach or vomiting	1.5–3.5	Metabolic alkalosis, hypokalemia, hypochloremia	20–60	14	140	-	60–80
Bile	7.0–8.0	Metabolic acidosis	145	5.0	105	30	-
Pancreas	7.0–8.8	Metabolic acidosis	125–138	8.0	56	85	-
Jejunal loss via stoma or fistula	7.0–8.0	Metabolic acidosis	140	5.0	135	8.0	-
Ileal loss new	7.5–8.0	Metabolic acidosis	110–140	5.0	75–125	0–30	-
Ileal loss adapted	7.5–8.0	Metabolic acidosis	50–100	5.0	25–75	0–30	
Colon or diarrhea	7.5–8.5	Metabolic acidosis, hypokalemia	30–140	9.0–30	90	20–33	-

abnormalities due to upper GI losses and the proper selection of IV fluids to correct it.

FLUID AND ELECTROLYTE ABNORMALITIES

Which fluid and electrolyte abnormalities commonly occur due to vomiting and why?

Gastric juice contains approximately: Sodium (Na⁺) 20–60 mEq/L, chloride (Cl⁻) 140 mEq/L, potassium (K⁺) 14 mEq/L, and hydrogen ions (H⁺) 60–80 mEq/L [2].

So, vomiting (or nasogastric-NG suction) leads to hypokalemic, hypochloremic metabolic alkalosis with hypovolemia. Due to the loss of HCl containing gastric juice, the first abnormalities usually occur in vomiting are hypochloremia with metabolic alkalosis, and hypokalemia occurs subsequently. The pathogenesis of these abnormalities is summarized below (Figure 34.1).

- **Hypovolemia:** Due to loss of fluids, extracellular fluid (ECF) volume decreases.

- **Hypokalemia:** Vomiting or NG suction because of loss of fluid and sodium (20–40 mEq/L) causes hypovolemia, leading to increased aldosterone secretion. Aldosterone increases sodium reabsorption and stimulates potassium's urinary secretion in the distal nephron.

Vomiting or NG suction causes metabolic alkalosis with resultant bicarbonaturia. In addition, increased sodium bicarbonate delivery to the cortical collecting tubule increases lumen negativity and markedly increases urinary potassium excretion.

The combined effect of secondary hyperaldosteronism (due to hypovolemia) and renal bicarbonaturia leads to greater potassium loss in urine, causing hypokalemia (Figure 34.1).

So, hypokalemia due to vomiting or NG suction occurs chiefly due to significant loss of potassium in urine and only partly due to direct gastric juice loss (the potassium concentration in gastric secretions is just 5 to 10 mEq/L).

- **Metabolic alkalosis:** Metabolic alkalosis in upper gastrointestinal loss is multifactorial:
  - Gastric juice is acidic. Therefore, H^+ ions are lost during upper gastrointestinal loss, leading to alkalosis. Normally, this H^+ ion secreted in the stomach is reabsorbed distally in the intestine, so no acid-base disturbance occurs.
  - Hypovolemia (due to fluid deficit) will lead to greater reabsorption of bicarbonate (HCO_3) in proximal tubules of the kidney, leading to alkalosis.
  - During severe upper GI loss, there may be a state of severe potassium depletion. So in the kidney's collecting duct, high aldosterone will secrete H^+ ion (instead of potassium), leading to aciduria and aggravation of metabolic alkalosis. Urinary loss of H^+ ion in metabolic alkalosis is "paradoxical aciduria".

- **Hypochloremia:** As gastric juice is rich in hydrochloric acid (about 140 mEq/L chloride), vomiting will lead to a major loss of chloride, causing hypochloremia.

- **Urinary electrolytes:** Abnormalities of urinary electrolytes in patients with vomiting are summarized in Table 34.2.

- In patients with vomiting or nasogastric suction, the spot urine chloride concentration is persistently low due to hypovolemia and hypochloremia.

- In the early stage, urinary potassium will be high, and urinary bicarbonate will be high (alkaline urine).

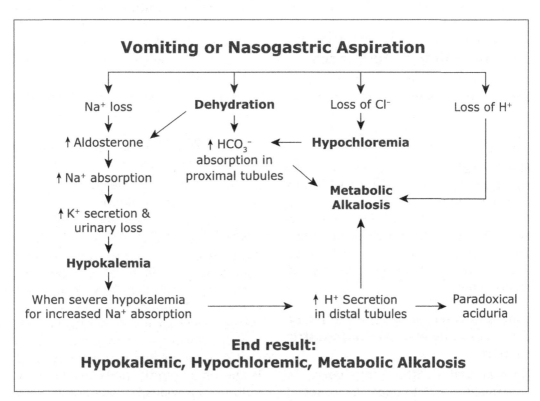

Figure 34.1 Fluid and electrolyte abnormalities in vomiting.

Table 34.2 Variation in urinary electrolytes with vomiting				
Time	Potassium	Chloride	HCO$_3$	pH
Day 1–3	Increased	Decreased	Increased	>6.5 Alkaline
Late	Decreased	Decreased	Decreased	<5.5 Aciduria

- If vomiting or gastric suction persists, during the later volume-depleted stage, absorption of sodium and bicarbonate increases, so urinary bicarbonate excretion decreases. In patients with severe hypokalemia, aldosterone increases sodium reabsorption and urinary hydrogen secretion, causing acidic urine.

MANAGEMENT

A. Etiological treatment

Search and treat the specific cause of vomiting to prevent or aggravate disturbances.

B. Correction of hypovolemia and electrolyte disturbances

The most preferred IV fluid to correct deficit due to vomiting is normal saline plus potassium infusion [1, 4], and in a few patients, multi electrolytes solution Isolyte-G is used.

Normal saline: 0.9% NaCl is used with the addition of potassium to restore previous and ongoing losses. Even 5% Dextrose with 0.9% NaCl Solution can be used to provide calories additionally. The volume of saline to be infused is determined as per the severity of hypovolemia.

Why is normal saline an effective IV fluid in treating vomiting/nasogastric suction?

Normal saline effectively corrects abnormalities due to upper GI losses in the following ways (Figure 34.2):

- It corrects the deficit of fluid and so increases ECF volume and decreases bicarbonate reabsorption by proximal tubules. So, reducing renal bicarbonate reabsorption and thereby increasing renal excretion corrects metabolic alkalosis.

- Correction of volume and sodium deficit will decrease aldosterone secretion. Easy availability of sodium at distal tubules and decreased aldosterone level will lead to reduced potassium and H+ ion secretion at distal tubules. So it will prevent further hypokalemia and alkalosis. However, additional potassium supplementation is necessary to correct already existing hypokalemia.

- The maximum chloride concentration (154 mEq/L) in normal saline corrects hypochloremia. Increased chloride in the collecting duct will permit an increased rate of Cl$^-$/HCO$_3$ exchange. It favors bicarbonate secretion, which will correct metabolic alkalosis.

So normal saline corrects all biochemical abnormalities caused by vomiting or continuous nasogastric aspiration (except potassium deficit).

Isolyte-G: This is the specific fluid used to replace upper GI loss. Because it contains ammonia (70 mEq/L), high chloride (154 mEq/L), potassium (17 mEq/L), and sodium (63 mEq/L) content, it corrects hydrogen, chloride, potassium and sodium losses, respectively. This is the only commercially available IV fluid that provides H+ ions and directly corrects metabolic alkalosis.

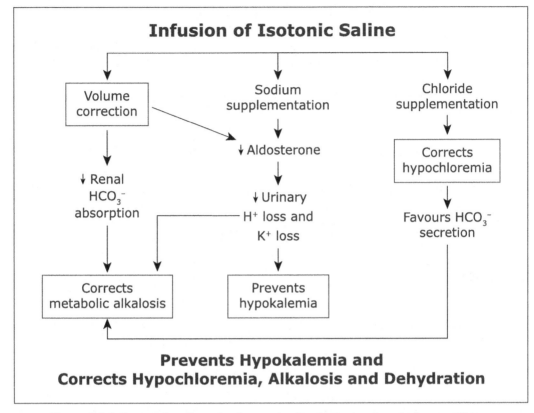

Figure 34.2 Summarizes the role of normal saline in the treatment of upper GI loss.

Balanced crystalloids: As lactate in Ringer's lactate (RL) and acetate in PlasmaLyte are converted into bicarbonate, it may worsen alkalosis and therefore are, not preferred.

Potassium supplementation: When oral potassium supplementation is not possible or is inadequate, potassium is provided by the IV route. Usually, 20–40 mEq/L potassium chloride is added to saline to restore previous and ongoing potassium losses. In patients with shock, oliguria, or renal failure, potassium supplementation should be done cautiously or avoided.

How to assess the efficacy of fluid therapy in upper GI loss?

Besides clinical criteria and urine output monitoring, two crucial parameters for determining the effectiveness of fluid therapy are urinary pH and chloride. Acidic urine suggests the need for more vigorous fluid replacement, while alkaline urine indicates a positive response to adequate fluid therapy. Increased urine chloride concentration signifies the correction of extracellular fluid volume depletion and adequate chloride replacement.

C. Fluid selection for gastric irrigation

Which fluid is ideal for gastric irrigation? Why?

Normal saline is ideal for gastric irrigation (especially in patients with electrolyte disturbances, hypovolemia, and hemodynamically unstable patients). However, avoid the use of plain water for irrigation. Plain water draws more gastric secretions into the stomach to make the fluid isotonic for absorption. Removal of these electrolytes containing fluid can further deplete fluid and electrolytes.

For the above reason, in patients with continuous nasogastric aspiration, it is essential to restrict the ice chips given by mouth. Nasogastric suctioning of water administered in the form of ice chips can cause loss of fluid and electrolytes from the stomach.

DIARRHEA

When diarrhea is severe, homeostasis of the body (e.g., kidney and other organs) fail to maintain the equilibrium of fluid, electrolytes, and acid base, causing various abnormalities [1].

Alterations in serum chemistries may vary depending on the specific characteristics of diarrhea, its severity, and the treatment administered, as summarized in Table 34.3 [3]. The composition of diarrheal stool is influenced by the type of diarrhea, which can be categorized as follows [3]:

1. Secretory diarrhea is characterized by stool that is rich in electrolytes, with sodium (Na^+) levels ranging from 100 to 130 mEq/L, chloride (Cl^-) levels between 90 and 100 mEq/L, potassium (K^+) levels of 9 to 30 mEq/L, and bicarbonate (HCO_3^-) levels ranging from 20 to 33 mEq/L.

2. Osmotic diarrhea results in watery stool with lower electrolyte content, featuring sodium (Na^+) levels between 10 and 36 mEq/L, chloride (Cl^-) levels ranging from 2 to 10 mEq/L, potassium (K^+) levels of 9 to 30 mEq/L, and bicarbonate (HCO_3^-) levels between 2 and 7 mEq/L.

3. Congenital chloride diarrhea leads to stool that is rich in chloride (Cl^-), with sodium (Na^+) levels exceeding 100 mEq/L, chloride (Cl^-) levels over 90 mEq/L, and potassium (K^+) levels exceeding 10 mEq/L.

These variations in stool composition contribute to the different electrolyte abnormalities observed in acute diarrheal illnesses, such as hyponatremia, hypokalemia, and metabolic acidosis [5–11].

The causes and mechanism of the development of volume, fluid,

Table 34.3 Characteristics of diarrheal fluids and electrolyte abnormalities

Type of diarrhea	Causes of diarrhea	Characteristics of diarrhea	Composition of diarrhea (mEq/L)	Common abnormalities
Secretory diarrhea	Cholera, escherichia coli, or clostridioides difficile	Electrolyte-rich diarrheal fluid with high Na^+, Cl^-, K^+, and HCO_3	Na^+ 100–130, Cl^- 90–100, K^+ 9–30, and HCO_3 20–33	Hyponatremia, hypokalemia, and metabolic acidosis
Osmotic diarrhea	Lactulose, magnesium sulfate, sorbitol, or polyethylene glycol (PEG)	Electrolyte poor watery diarrhea with low Na^+, Cl^-, K^+, and HCO_3	Na^+ 10–36, Cl^- 2–10, K^+ 9–30, and HCO_3 2–7	Hypokalemia, and hypernatremia
Congenital chloride diarrhea	Defect in the apical Cl^-/HCO_3 exchanger	Watery diarrhea with high chloride	Na^+ >100, Cl^- >90, and K^+ >10	Metabolic alkalosis with hypochloremia, and hypokalemia

electrolytes, and acid-base abnormalities in diarrhea are summarized below:

A. Hypovolemia: Loss of fluid in diarrhea occurs due to:

- Secretory diarrhea: Abnormally increased fluid secretion into the small bowel due to GI infections like E. coli, Vibrio cholera, or rotavirus.

- Osmotic diarrhea: Decreased fluid absorption due to the presence of osmotically active, poorly absorbed solutes in the bowel lumen (e.g., lactulose, magnesium sulfate, sorbitol, or polyethylene glycol-PEG) or malabsorption of glucose or lactate in children.

- Additional loss of water due to associated vomiting or fever.

B. Sodium disturbances: Diarrhea causes loss of sodium, resulting in sodium deficit in all patients, but the proportion of sodium loss compared to water loss will decide serum sodium concentration and type of dehydration. In severe diarrhea, hyponatremia is common, while hypernatremia occurs in very few patients [3, 9, 10].

- In most cases of diarrhea, water loss and sodium loss are in the same proportion, leading to isotonic dehydration- hypovolemia.

- Marked volume depletion due to the loss of a large volume of electrolyte-rich fluid (e.g., secretory diarrhea) stimulates antidiuretic hormone secretion. Usually, adult patients with diarrhea who drink a large amount of water or hypotonic fluids or receive hypotonic IV fluids (e.g., 5%-dextrose) may develop hyponatremia.

- Significant loss of electrolyte poor diarrheal fluid in patients with large volume osmotic diarrhea causes a net loss of water more than the loss of sodium (deficit of water is greater than the deficit of sodium), leading to hypernatremia and hypertonic (hypernatremic) dehydration. Thirst is a robust mechanism that prevents the development of hypernatremia. So, hypernatremia is uncommon in awake and alert patients who can respond to thirst and have access to water.

C. Hypokalemia: In diarrhea, hypokalemia is a common electrolyte disorder [3, 9, 10].

- Hypokalemia occurs because fluid lost in diarrhea is rich in potassium. (Normally, 8–15 mEq potassium ions are excreted in stool daily, while much greater loss occurs with diarrhea).

- When the diarrheal loss is significant, severe hypovolemia occurs, leading to secondary hyperaldosteronism. High aldosterone stimulates the renal reabsorption of sodium and increases urinary and intestine secretion of potassium, which aggravates hypokalemia.

- In patients with hypokalemia due to diarrhea, the actual serum potassium concentration may be misleading due to metabolic acidosis and losses of water and sodium. In patients with diarrhea, serum potassium may be normal (or even high) despite the loss of total exchangeable body potassium and a low potassium concentration in cells. Diarrhea induced metabolic acidosis shifts potassium from the intracellular fluid to the ECF compartment and causes normal (or even high) serum potassium, even in a state of potassium deficit in the body.

D. Metabolic acidosis: Normal AG metabolic acidosis is a common disorder in patients with severe diarrhea. Fluid secreted distal to pylorus is rich in bicarbonate. Therefore, when a large volume of diarrheal fluid containing high concentrations of bicarbonate is secreted in the gut and excreted, it leads to normal AG metabolic acidosis.

- High AG metabolic acidosis: In a few patients, large-volume diarrhea causes severe hypovolemia with hypotension and decreases tissue perfusion leading to lactic acidosis or renal failure resulting in high AG metabolic acidosis. The inability of the kidneys to compensate for the loss of bicarbonate leads to the rapid worsening of acidosis.

E. Hyperchloremia: Hyperchloremia is common in diarrhea-induced normal AG metabolic acidosis patients.

- The ileal and colonic mucosa possesses a luminal Cl^-/HCO_3^- exchanger capable of reabsorbing chloride in exchange for bicarbonate

[1, 12, 13]. So, during diarrhea, when more bicarbonate is secreted into the intestinal lumen, more chloride is absorbed from the intestine, causing hyperchloremia along with normal AG metabolic acidosis. Furthermore, in an attempt to increase sodium absorption (to maintain ECF volume) from the intestine and kidney, simultaneous chloride absorption by the NaCl transporter will also aggravate hyperchloremia.

How hypokalemic hyperchloremic metabolic acidosis occurs in patients with diarrhea is summarized in Figure 34.3.

MANAGEMENT

A. Etiological treatment

Search and treat the specific cause of diarrhea to prevent or aggravate disturbances.

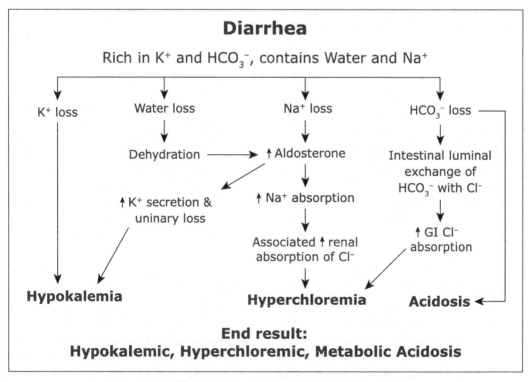

Figure 34.3 Fluid and electrolyte abnormalities in diarrhea.

B. Correction of hypovolemia and electrolyte disturbances

The goals of fluid therapy include:

1. Correcting dehydration.
2. Correction of sodium deficit (which indirectly prevents potassium loss and chloride retention).
3. Treating hypokalemia and metabolic acidosis.

It is crucial to manage both conditions simultaneously and with precision. If metabolic acidosis is treated without potassium supplementation in a patient with hypokalemia, the correction of acidosis may lead to potentially dangerous hypokalemia. Conversely, administering potassium without addressing acidosis can result in dangerous hyperkalemia.

Selection of fluids for treating diarrheal deficits:

Fluid and electrolyte losses caused by diarrhea can be replaced orally or intravenously. Oral rehydration therapy, a specially formulated solution, is the preferred initial choice for oral supplementation. An intravenous route is usually needed for rehydration in a few patients with severe diarrhea where Ringer's lactate solution is used.

1. Oral rehydration therapy (ORT)

As oral rehydration therapy is easily available, simple to use, and safe, it is a preferred method of fluid replacement. Losses due to diarrhea can be effectively corrected by oral rehydration solutions (ORS). Readily available ORS provides sodium, potassium, chloride and bicarbonate along with glucose, which effectively corrects fluid and electrolyte abnormalities and provides calories.

- Oral rehydration therapy is based on the principle that the intestine actively absorbs glucose, and sodium is carried with it. Glucose enhances sodium and secondary water transport across the upper intestine's mucosa, even in the presence of infective diarrhea.

- Avoid correction of losses due to diarrhea totally with electrolyte-free solutions (i.e., water, glucose water, tea, soft drinks, or commercially available fruit drinks). As it provides only fluid but lacks electrolytes, it can cause hyponatremia and is ineffective in correcting hypovolemia. For a detailed discussion on ORT, please refer to Chapter 50 "Oral Rehydration Therapy".

2. Intravenous fluid therapy

IV fluid therapy is indicated when rapid blood volume correction is required for severe dehydration and shock, the inability of the patient to take ORS due to persistent vomiting, or ORT fails to correct volume depletion due to greater losses. But ORS should be given as soon as the patient on IV fluid can drink.

The preferred IV fluids to correct losses due to diarrhea are Ringer's lactate and normal saline [14, 15]. But no IV fluid is ideal because they all are deficient in some of the electrolytes required to correct the abnormalities found in patients with severe diarrhea-induced hypovolemia.

To ensure adequate electrolyte replacement, some patients may need supplementation of potassium and/or bicarbonate to IV fluids.

a. Ringer's lactate solution: The World Health Organization (WHO) recommends Ringer lactate as the preferred IV fluid to correct dehydration due to severe diarrhea [16]. Compared to normal saline solution, Ringer's lactate demonstrated better clinical response and more rapid correction of hypokalemia, serum bicarbonate concentration, and serum pH [17–20].

RL is the preferred solution because it provides the following:

- An adequate concentration of sodium (130 mEq/L).
- An adequate (28 mEq/L) bicarbonate (by hepatic conversion of lactate) for correcting metabolic acidosis.
- Potassium.

However, it is essential to remember that the potassium concentration of RL is low (just 4 mEq/L) and does not contain glucose. So, the patient with diarrhea receiving RL needs glucose supplementation (oral or IV) to meet caloric requirements and prevent hypoglycemia. In addition, such patients may require additional potassium supplementation to correct hypokalemia and, at times, bicarbonate supplementation to correct acidosis.

b. Normal saline: It effectively corrects hypovolemia and provides sodium and water. The limitation of normal saline is that it does not contain potassium (requires to correct potassium deficit) and lacks base (requires to correct metabolic acidosis). In addition, as normal saline is rich in chloride (154 mEq/L compared to 100 mEq/L serum sodium), its infusion in large volumes carries the risk of hyperchloremic metabolic acidosis [21]. Hyperchloremia also carries a risk of acute kidney injury due to increased renal vasoconstriction leading to decreased renal blood flow and decreased glomerular filtration [22, 23].

Besides the lack of potassium, saline, by supplying sodium and water adequately, suppresses aldosterone and prevents further urinary loss of potassium. Similarly, normal saline does not correct metabolic acidosis directly, but adequate correction of hypovolemia will improve renal perfusion, permitting renal correction of metabolic acidosis.

C. Avoid hypotonic fluids

Hyponatremia is common in severe diarrhea, so hypotonic fluids like Isolyte M, Isolyte P, and 5% dextrose are usually avoided. Likewise, IV fluids free of electrolytes, such as 5% or 10% dextrose, are not acceptable and harmful because they not only fail to correct hypovolemia and electrolyte abnormalities but also carry the risk of hyponatremia.

In addition, rapid large volume replacement of 5% dextrose can cause hyperglycemia leading to osmotic diuresis and further fluid loss. However, a small group of patients in whom hypernatremic dehydration occurs due to diarrhea may need hypotonic fluids.

UPPER GASTROINTESTINAL BLEEDING

Upper gastrointestinal bleeding is the most commonly encountered gastrointestinal emergency requiring hospitalization, accounting for over half a million admissions annually in the USA [24–26]. The most important causes of upper GI bleeding (bleeding proximal to the ligament of Treitz at the duodenojejunal junction) are peptic ulcer disease (about 47%), esophageal varices due to portal hypertension, acute erosive gastritis, gastric cancer bleeding, lower esophageal tear (Mallory-Weiss syndrome), and others [27–29].

COMMON PRESENTATIONS

Common presentations of acute upper gastrointestinal bleeding are [30]:

- Hematemesis: Overt bleeding with vomiting of fresh blood or coffee-ground material.
- Melena: Black, tarry stools due to degradation of blood when blood passes through the GI tract, and melena may develop after losing as little as 50–100 ml of blood.
- Hematochezia: Fresh red or maroon blood per rectum, which occurs in a few patients with acute massive upper GI bleed (usually >1000 mL) with rapid blood transit through the intestines.
- Other symptoms: Epigastric pain, weakness, dizziness, orthostatic hypotension, and in severe cases syncope, dizziness, and shock.

MANAGEMENT

Treatment of acute upper GI bleeding must begin with the initial assessment of the patient's hemodynamic status, resuscitation, and stabilization. Subsequently, further evaluation is done to search for underlying etiology and plan specific therapy accordingly.

A. Initial assessment

1. Hemodynamic assessment

Hemodynamic status should be assessed immediately by measuring heart rate, blood pressure, and postural changes:

- Resting tachycardia usually suggests mild to moderate hypovolemia (loss of less than 15% of total blood volume) [31].
- Supine hypotension (systolic blood pressure less than 100 mm Hg) usually suggests severe life-threatening acute bleeding (loss of approximately 40% of total blood volume) [32].
- The patient may be stable (normal heart rate and blood pressure in the supine position) even with significant blood loss. So always look for postural hypotension (fall in systolic blood pressure (SBP) >20 mm Hg and/or increase in heart rate of >20 beats/min when moving from supine to standing), which suggests a loss of 15% or more of total blood volume [31].

2. Basic laboratory investigations

Blood is sent immediately, and investigations commonly performed are:

- Complete blood cell (CBC) count: It is important to remember that fall in hemoglobin supports the diagnosis of upper GI bleeding, but normal hemoglobin does not exclude blood loss because even after significant bleeding, hemoglobin may be normal in the early stage until hemodilution occurs. It is important to remember that the hemoglobin level is not a reliable indicator of the severity of acute GI loss. In patients with an active upper GI bleed, monitor hemoglobin levels serially (every 2–8 hours), depending upon the severity of the bleeding.
- Coagulation parameters (international normalized ratio [INR] and partial thromboplastin time): Helps to detect coagulopathy in patients with liver dysfunction or receiving anticoagulants.
- Blood group and cross-matching of at least two units of blood if a significant bleed is suspected.
- Metabolic profile (liver enzymes (AST, ALT), albumin, creatinine, and blood urea nitrogen).

3. History and evaluation

Detailed history may provide a clue for the severity of blood loss, help to establish a source of bleeding, and the presence of medical comorbidities (malignancy, chronic obstructive pulmonary disease, coronary artery disease, etc.). Particular attention should be given to the history of medications such as anticoagulants (heparin, warfarin, and newer oral anticoagulants such as dabigatran, rivaroxaban, and apixaban), antiplatelet agents (clopidogrel and aspirin), and NSAIDs.

B. Treatment

1. Stabilization

- **Intravenous access:** For all patients with significant bleeding, the first step is inserting at least two large-bore peripheral catheters (18 gauge or larger) or urgently establishing central access to IV fluid resuscitation.

- **Fluid resuscitation:** The first and most crucial step in managing upper GI bleeding in an emergency is fluid resuscitation. Patients with active bleeding should be administered at least 500 mL of readily available crystalloid fluids (normal saline or Ringer's lactate) to maintain adequate blood pressure [31]. In major upper GI bleeding, rapid infusion of crystalloids helps to correct shock and achieve hemodynamic stability until blood is received. If hypotension persists or worsens, increase the fluid infusion rate, and start vasopressors for temporary support. Current evidence does not support the use of colloids for resuscitation due to the potential risk of kidney injury, coagulopathy, anaphylaxis, and no benefits over crystalloids [33].

- **General support:** Patients with significant upper GI blood loss may need [31, 34].

Oxygen: Patients with hypoxia may require oxygen supplementation by nasal cannula to keep SpO_2 ≥94% to enhance the oxygen-carrying capacity of the blood.

Nil by mouth: The patient should be kept nil by mouth (to prepare for urgent endoscopy).

A foley catheter should be inserted (to monitor the urine output).

Intubation: Some patients who are at a high risk of aspiration, such as those with altered mental status, massive bleeding, or anticipated massive bleeding, may need endotracheal intubation to protect the airway and prevent bronchoaspiration.

2. Blood transfusion

In acute upper gastrointestinal bleeding, blood transfusion can be lifesaving. In acute upper GI bleed, the clinician should decide the need for blood transfusion based on clinical presentation, vital signs, the severity of bleeding from nasogastric aspirate, initial hemoglobin level, rate of fall in hemoglobin, and associated comorbid conditions.

When to transfuse?

Strategy for hemodynamically unstable patients

When the patient with active upper GI bleed is hemodynamically unstable and clinical signs of hemorrhagic shock (tachycardia, hypotension, altered consciousness, pallor, coldness, etc.) are present, it is essential to begin the blood transfusion without delay and before the hemoglobin result.

In patients with massive bleeding, blood transfusion should not be withheld based on their hemoglobin level because hemoglobin drops with time as hemoglobin equilibrates with the extravascular fluid.

Symptomatic or hemodynamically unstable actively bleeding patients should be transfused urgently, even at higher hemoglobin levels [35].

Strategy for hemodynamically stable patients

Red blood cells (RBC) transfusion is recommended if the hemoglobin level is <7 gm/dL for hemodynamically stable hospitalized adult patients [26].

In patients with acute upper GI bleeding, a restrictive RBC transfusion threshold (hemoglobin level <7 gm/dL), as compared to a liberal threshold (most commonly hemoglobin level 9.0 gm/dL to 10.0 gm/dL), improves outcomes significantly, as shown in various studies [36, 37], reviews [38–40], and therefore is currently recommended [26, 41–43].

High-risk patients (e.g., pre-existing cardiovascular disease, older adults) with upper GI bleeding need blood transfusion at a higher value of hemoglobin (<8 gm/dL) [26, 43].

What should be the goal of transfusion?

Red-cell transfusions aim to raise hemoglobin which helps to achieve hemodynamic stability and improve the delivery of oxygen to tissues.

The goal of blood transfusion is to maintain hemoglobin between 8–9 gm/dL in stable patients [43].

Avoid over-transfusion because it may be as dangerous as under-transfusion [44]. Over-transfusion (e.g., hemoglobin >9 gm/dL) increases the risk of rebleeding and mortality and therefore is detrimental [36, 45–48], especially in patients with variceal bleeding [36, 49–51].

In patients with variceal bleeding, over transfusion increases portal venous pressure due to blood volume expansion, leading to further bleeding or predisposing the patient to rebleeding [52–55].

If the patient is hemodynamically stable and active bleeding is absent, to avoid over transfusion, administer just one unit of packed red blood cells (PRBCs) at a time, followed by an appropriate evaluation to justify additional units [56]. Each unit of packed red blood cells roughly increases 1 gm of hemoglobin.

How to treat coagulation disorders?

Patients with active upper GI bleeding with INR greater than 2.5 are traditionally treated with fresh frozen plasma transfusion and vitamin K administration.

Current literature favors the use of prothrombin complex concentrate (PCC) over fresh frozen plasma (FFP) to treat severe coagulopathy because it contains significantly higher amounts of the clotting factors than FFP, requiring low drug volume and more rapid onset, better safety, and convenience [43, 57, 58]. Still, cost and availability are major limiting factors [59].

Platelet transfusion: When the platelet count is <50,000 in actively bleeding patients, platelet transfusion is indicated. Platelet transfusion is also traditionally considered in GI bleeding with platelet dysfunction due to antiplatelet drugs with normal platelet counts, but this benefit is not supported in recent studies [60].

Massive transfusion protocol: Massive blood transfusion is defined as administering 10 units of red cells within 24 hours or three units of red cells within one hour [61]. The goal of massive transfusion protocol is to avoid common complications associated with massive transfusions like dilutional coagulopathy, acidosis, and hypothermia.

The massive transfusion protocol is designed to deliver a balanced transfusion with PRBCs, platelets, and fresh frozen plasma in a ratio approximating whole blood. Current literature suggests the infusion of one unit of plasma, one unit of platelets, and one unit of red blood cells (1:1:1 ratio) [62].

3. Medications

Proton pump inhibitor (PPI): In patients with upper GI bleeding, PPIs are used in pre-endoscopy and post-endoscopy phases.

Pre-endoscopy phase: Administration of IV PPIs (esomeprazole or pantoprazole, 80 mg IV bolus) immediately after initiating fluid resuscitation and before endoscopy facilitate the clot in peptic lesions, downstage the endoscopic lesion and reduces the need for endoscopic hemostatic treatment at index endoscopy [25, 42, 43, 57, 63–65]. However, although the administration of PPIs is standard practice, pre-endoscopy PPIs are without benefits in rebleeding, surgery, or mortality [64, 65]. Therefore, data supporting the routine use of PPIs before endoscopy are conflicting [26, 44].

Post-endoscopy phase: The risk of rebleeding is highest in the first 72 hours post-endoscopy in upper GI bleeding. So high-dose (8 mg/h) PPI therapy is recommended as a continuous infusion for 72 hours post-endoscopy to reduce the risk of rebleeding in patients with peptic ulcers [26, 42, 43]. In the absence of bleeding, after 3 days, PPI is switched to an oral route and given twice daily for 14 days, followed by a once-daily dose for four to eight weeks in patients with peptic ulcer bleeding [42, 43].

The use of antacids and H+ 2-receptor antagonists is not recommended in patients with acute upper GI bleeding.

Prokinetics: The administration of prokinetics like erythromycin and metoclopramide before endoscopy may improve endoscopic visualization of gastric mucosa by increasing gastric emptying.

Erythromycin: In patients with acute upper GI bleeding, using erythromycin before upper GI endoscopy is beneficial to improve visualization, reduce the need for the second endoscopy, and may shorten the length of hospital stay [66–71], and therefore is recommended [26, 43].

A single intravenous dose of erythromycin (250 mg intravenously over 20 to 30 minutes), given 30 to 120 minutes before endoscopy, is safe, generally well-tolerated, and cost-effective [43, 72]. However, as IV erythromycin can prolong the QT interval, it should be avoided in patients with prolonged QTc intervals.

Metoclopramide: Evidence supporting the use of the prokinetic agent metoclopramide in upper GI bleed is scanty [69, 73–75]; therefore, its use is not recommended [26, 43].

Vasoactive medications: Vasoactive drugs (e.g., terlipressin, somatostatin, or its analogues octreotide and vapreotide) should be initiated as soon as the bleeding is suspected in patients of cirrhosis with esophageal varices [49, 76–79], but these drugs are not recommended in non-variceal upper gastrointestinal hemorrhage (e.g., peptic ulcer bleeding) [42, 43, 80]. Vasoactive medications significantly improve the control of bleeding, causing reduced transfusion requirements, shortening hospital stays, and reducing in-hospital mortality [81, 82].

Vasoactive drugs, by inhibiting glucagon release, cause splanchnic vasoconstriction, reduce gastroduodenal mucosal blood flow, and reduce GI bleeding [83].

Terlipressin is a widely used vasoactive drug in practice. As terlipressin was not available in the United States before September 2022, the somatostatin analogue drug octreotide was mainly used.

Antibiotics: In all cirrhotic patients with acute GI bleeding (from varices or other causes), short-term antibiotics should be administered, as it reduces the risk of infections, rebleeding, all-cause mortality, and length of hospitalization [49, 84, 85]. The usual first choice is ceftriaxone 1 gm IV daily for seven days because most infections are due to gram-negative bacteria and have been found to be superior to norfloxacin [50]. However, recent literature suggests using quinolones and β-lactams either alone or in combination as prophylactic antibiotics due to their beneficial effects in cirrhotic patients with upper GI bleeding [86].

Tranexamic acid: Tranexamic acid is traditionally used in upper GI bleeding to prevent ongoing fibrinolysis. But current literature does not recommend the use of tranexamic acid in treating upper GI bleeding because of the lack of benefits and possible increased risk of venous thromboembolism [87, 88].

4. Placement of nasogastric tube

Nasogastric lavage (NGL) seems to be a logical procedure. Its routine use was recommended in predicting high-risk lesions and evaluating suspected upper GI bleeding [89]. But currently, nasogastric aspiration/lavage is not recommended in patients with acute upper GI bleeding [43, 90, 91]. Its drawbacks are that insertion is painful and uncomfortable, negative aspirate does not exclude upper GI blood loss, does not affect rebleeding rates or mortality, and can be harmful [89–94]. However, in selected patients, it may be helpful to differentiate the source of bleeding (upper or lower GI tract) or clean particulate matter, fresh blood, and clots from the stomach before emergency endoscopy [42, 95–98].

5. Endoscopy

In upper GI bleeding, endoscopy is the most effective diagnostic tool for localization of the exact bleeding site, helps in risk stratification, and plays a crucial role in the therapeutic management of high-risk and active bleeding.

Timing of endoscopy

- In upper GI bleeding, early endoscopy (≤24 hours from the time of patient presentation, usually between 12–24 hours) following adequate hemodynamic resuscitation is strongly recommended by various guidelines [26, 42–44, 57, 76, 79, 99, 100]. Timely performed endoscopy reduces transfusion requirements, rebleeding, mortality, need for surgery, hospital stay, and costs [101–107].

- Avoid delayed endoscopy (>24 hours) because it is associated with higher mortality and longer stay in the hospital [107, 108].

- Recent evidence does not favor urgent (≤12 hours) upper GI endoscopy compared to early endoscopy because of conflicting results [43, 109, 110].

- Emergent endoscopy (performed ≤6 hours from the time of patient presentation) is not recommended because of the lack of benefits [43, 103, 111–114] or the possibility of worse outcomes [108].

Indications and methods of endoscopy

- It is essential to perform an endoscopy after initiating appropriate resuscitation, stabilizing hemodynamic status [78], and optimally managing comorbid conditions.

- Endoscopic therapy is recommended in high-risk patients for persistent or recurrent bleeding, such as ulcers with active spurting or oozing and nonbleeding visible vessels in patients with upper GI bleeding [26, 42, 43, 57].

- Endoscopic methods to control upper GI bleeding due to non-variceal bleeding are sclerosant injection (e.g., epinephrine or absolute ethanol), thermal therapies (e.g., bipolar electrocoagulation, heater probe), or endoscopic clips [78]. The endoscopic method of choice is variceal band ligation to control esophageal variceal bleeding [76].

6. Specific treatment

With proper evaluation, establish the diagnosis of the underlying etiology and decide on further treatment plans accordingly.

7. Risk factors

The glasgow blatchford score (GBS) is currently recommended as a reliable and easy tool to stratify patients with upper gastrointestinal bleeding into a higher or lower risk of poor outcome, which helps clinicians to ascertain the urgency of investigations, predicting clinical outcome and helps to decide management plan [43, 57, 115, 116].

In upper GI bleeding, parameters such as GBS ≥8–12, persistent bloody vomiting, bloody gastric aspiration, tachycardia, hypotension, and comorbidities like cirrhosis are high-risk patients and are associated with poor outcomes [78].

8. Monitoring

Patients with acute upper GI bleeding should be closely observed with frequent hemodynamic measurements, hourly urine output, the occurrence of hematemesis, hematochezia, or persistent melena, and every two to eight hourly monitoring of hemoglobin.

REFERENCES

1. Gennari FJ, Weise WJ. Acid-base disturbances in gastrointestinal disease. Clin J Am Soc Nephrol. 2008;3(6):1861–8.

2. National Clinical Guideline Centre (UK). Intravenous Fluid Therapy: Intravenous Fluid Therapy in Adults in Hospital [Internet]. London: Royal College of Physicians (UK); 2013.

3. Do C, Evans GJ, DeAguero J, et al. Dysnatremia in Gastrointestinal Disorders. Front. Med. 2022;9:892265.

4. National Collaborating Centre for Women's and Children's Health (UK). Diarrhoea and Vomiting Caused by Gastroenteritis: Diagnosis, Assessment and Management in Children Younger than 5 Years. London: RCOG Press; 2009. (NICE Clinical Guidelines, No. 84.) 5, Fluid management. Available from: https://www.ncbi.nlm.nih.gov/books/NBK63837/.

5. Shah GS, Das BK, Kumar S, et al. Acid base and electrolyte disturbance in diarrhoea. Kathmandu Univ Med J (KUMJ). 2007;5(1):60–62.

6. Onyiriuka AN, Iheagwara EC. Serum electrolyte profiles ofunder-five Nigerian children admitted for severe dehydration due to acute diarrhea. Niger J Heal Sci 2015;15(1):14–17.

7. Dhyani A, Ameta P, Patel JB, et al. Clinical profile of children with diarrhoea admitted in pediatric intensive care unit of Bal Chikitsalay, M.B. Hospital, RNT Medical College, Udaipur, Rajasthan, India. Int J ContempPediatr2016;3(4):1371–1374.

8. Dastidar RG, Konar N. A Study of Electrolyte Disturbances in a Child Presenting with Acute Gastroenteritis, with Special Emphasis on Hyponatremic Dehydration-A Hospital based CrossSectional Study. Pediatr Ther 2017;7(2):322.

9. Gopchade A. Electrolyte Disturbances in Children Presenting with Acute Diarrhea: A Prospective Cohort Study. JMSCR 2019;7(9):777.

10. Tayab MA, Hoq MA. Acid-base and Electrolyte Disturbances in Children Presenting with Acute Watery Diarrhoea in Emergency Observation and Referral Unit of Dhaka Shishu (Children) Hospital. Dhaka Shishu (Children) Hospital Journal, 2021;36(2):120–124.

11. Riaz L, Hussain MK, Javed M, et al. Challenges and Complications Associated with Sodium, Potassium Imbalances and Preventive Measures in Children Under-Five with Acute Gastroenteritis. Pak Armed Forces Med J 2022;72(Suppl-1):S64–67.

12. Kiela PR, Ghishan FK. Physiology of Intestinal Absorption and Secretion. Best Pract Res Clin Gastroenterol. 2016;30(2):145–159.

13. Nagami GT. Hyperchloremia - Why and How. Nefrologia. 2016;36(4):347–53.

14. Mahajan V, Sajan SS, Sharma A, et al. Ringer's lactate vs normal saline for children with acute diarrhea and severe dehydration: A double blind randomized controlled trial. Indian Pediatr 2012;49(1):963–68.

15. Naseem M, Dubey AP, Mishra TK, et al. Effect of Rehydration with Normal Saline versus Ringer Lactate on Serum Sodium Level of Children with Acute Diarrhea and Severe Dehydration: A Randomized Controlled Trial. Indian Pediatr. 2020;57(6):519–522.

16. World Health Organization. The treatment of diarrhoea: a manual for physicians and other senior health workers, 4th rev. World Health Organization. 2005. https://apps.who.int/iris/handle/10665/43209.

17. Mahalanabis D, Brayton JB, Mondal A, et al. The use of Ringer's lactate in the treatment of children with cholera and acute noncholera diarrhoea. Bull World Health Organ. 1972;46(3):311–9.

18. Cieza JA, Hinostroza J, Huapaya JA, et al. Sodium chloride 0.9% versus Lactated Ringer in the management of severely dehydrated patients with choleriform diarrhoea. J Infect Dev Ctries. 2013;7(7):528–32.

19. Rasheed S, Rafique S, Hussain A, et al. Comparison of outcome between Ringer's lactate and normal saline fluid replacement in pediatric patients with acute watery diarrhoea. PAFMJ. 2020;70(Suppl-1):S101–05.

20. Shaikh B, Ghoto IS, Langah AU, et al. A Randomized Double Blind Controlled Trial of Ringers Lactate versus Normal Saline among Pediatric Patients with Acute Severe Diarrhea. PJMHS 2022;16(3):281–282.

21. Lobo DN, Awad S. Should chloride-rich crystalloids remain the mainstay of fluid resuscitation to prevent "pre-renal" acute kidney injury? con. Kidney International. 2014;86(6):1096–1105.

22. Heng Li, Sun SR, Yap JQ, et al. 0.9% saline is neither normal nor physiological. J Zhejiang Univ Sci B. 2016;17(3):181–187.

23. Yunos NM, Bellomo R, Glassford N, et al. Chloride-liberal vs. Chloride-restrictive intravenous fluid administration and acute kidney injury: an extended analysis. Intensive Care Med 2015;41:257–64.

24. Kamboj AK, Hoversten P, Leggett CL. Upper Gastrointestinal Bleeding: Etiologies and Management. Mayo Clin Proc. 2019;94(4):697–703.

25. Cañamares-Orbís P, Lanas Arbeloa Á. New Trends and Advances in Non-Variceal Gastrointestinal Bleeding-Series II. J Clin Med. 2021;10(14):3045.

26. Laine L, Barkun AN, Saltzman JR, et al. ACG Clinical Guideline: Upper Gastrointestinal and Ulcer Bleeding. Am J Gastroenterol. 2021;116(5):899–917.

27. Tielleman T, Bujanda D, Cryer B. Epidemiology and risk factors for upper gastrointestinal bleeding. Gastrointest Endosc Clin N Am. 2015;25(3):415–428.

28. Wuerth BA, Rockey DC. Changing Epidemiology of Upper Gastrointestinal Hemorrhage in the Last Decade: A Nationwide Analysis. Dig Dis Sci. 2018;63(5):1286–1293.

29. Oakland K. Changing epidemiology and etiology of upper and lower gastrointestinal bleeding. Best Pract Res Clin Gastroenterol 2019;42–43:101610.

30. Wilkins T, Wheeler B, Carpenter M. Upper Gastrointestinal Bleeding in Adults: Evaluation and Management. Am Fam Physician. 2020 Mar 1;101(5):294–300. Erratum in: Am Fam Physician. 2021;103(2):70.

31. Cappell MS, Friedel D. Initial management of acute upper gastrointestinal bleeding: from initial evaluation up to gastrointestinal endoscopy. Med Clin North Am 2008;92(3):491–509.

32. Kupfer Y, Cappell MS, Tessler S. Acute gastrointestinal bleeding in the intensive care unit. The intensivist's perspective. Gastroenterol Clin North Am 2000;29(2):275–307.

33. Elsayed IAS, Battu PK, Irving S. Management of acute upper GI bleeding. BJA Education 2017;17(4):117–123.

34. Dinesen L, Benson M. Managing acute upper gastrointestinal bleeding in the acute assessment unit. Clin Med (Lond). 2012;12(6):589–593.

35. Hernandez-Gea V, Berbel C, Baiges A, et al. Acute variceal bleeding: risk stratification and management (including TIPS). Hepatol Int 2018;12:81–90.

36. Villanueva C, Colomo A, Bosch A. Transfusion for acute upper gastrointestinal bleeding. N Engl J Med. 2013;368(14):1362–3.

37. Jairath V, Kahan BC, Gray A, et al. Restrictive versus liberal blood transfusion for acute upper gastrointestinal bleeding (TRIGGER): A pragmatic, open-label, cluster randomised feasibility trial. Lancet 2015;386(9989):137–44.

38. Carson JL, Stanworth SJ, Roubinian N, et al. Transfusion thresholds and other strategies for guiding allogeneic red blood cell transfusion. Cochrane Database Syst Rev 2016;10:CD002042.

39. Odutayo A, Desborough MJR, Trivella M et al. Restrictive versus liberal blood transfusion for gastrointestinal bleeding: a systematic review and meta-analysis of randomised controlled trials. Lancet Gastro-enterol Hepatol 2017;2(5):354–360.

40. Carson JL, Stanworth SJ, Dennis JA, et al. Transfusion thresholds for guiding red blood cell transfusion. Cochrane Database Syst Rev 2021;12(12):CD002042.

41. Carson JL, Guyatt G, Heddle NM, et al. Clinical practice guidelines from the AABB: Red blood cell transfusion thresholds and storage. JAMA 2016;316(19):2025–35.

42. Barkun AN, Almadi M, Kuipers EJ, et al. Management of nonvariceal upper gastrointestinal bleeding: Guideline recommendations from the

International Consensus Group. Ann Intern Med 2019;171(11):805–822.

43. Gralnek IM, Stanley AJ, Morris AJ, et al. Endoscopic diagnosis and management of nonvariceal upper gastrointestinal hemorrhage (NVUGIH): European Society of Gastrointestinal Endoscopy (ESGE) Guideline - Update 2021. Endoscopy. 2021;53(3):300–332.

44. NICE Guidelines 2012. Acute Upper Gastrointestinal Bleeding in over 16s management Clinical guideline [CG141] (https://www.nice.org.uk/guidance/cg141).

45. Restellini S, Kherad O, Jairath V, et al. Red blood cell transfusion is associated with increased rebleeding in patients with nonvariceal upper gastrointestinal bleeding. Aliment Pharmacol Ther 2013;37(3):316–322.

46. Stokes A, Thompson C, Clegg A, et al. The influence of a simple blood transfusion policy on overtransfusion in acute upper gastrointestinal haemorrhage. Clin Med (Lond) 2015;15(4):325–9.

47. Subramaniam K, Spilsbury K, Ayonrinde OT, et al. Red blood cell transfusion is associated with further bleeding and fresh-frozen plasma with mortality in nonvariceal upper gastrointestinal bleeding. Transfusion 2016;56(4):816–26.

48. Chen YC, Hsiao CT, Lin LC, et al. The association between red blood cell transfusion and outcomes in patients with upper gastrointestinal bleeding. Clin Transl Gastroenterol 2018;9(3):138.

49. Garcia-Tsao G, Abraldes JG, Berzigotti A, et al. Portal hypertensive bleeding in cirrhosis: Risk stratification, diagnosis, and management: 2016 practice guidance by the American Association for the study of liver diseases. Hepatology. 2017;65(1):310–335.

50. European Association for the Study of the Liver. EASL Clinical Practice Guidelines for the management of patients with decompensated cirrhosis. J Hepatol. 2018;69(2):406–460.

51. Liu P, Hum J, Jou J, et al. Transfusion strategies in patients with cirrhosis. Eur J Haematol. 2020;104(1):15–25.

52. Boyer JL, Chatterjee C, Iber FL, et al. Effect of plasma-volume expansion on portal hypertension. N Engl J Med. 1966;275(14):750–755.

53. McCormick PA, Jenkins SA, McIntyre N, et al. Why portal hypertensive varices bleed and bleed: a hypothesis. Gut 1995;36(1):100–103.

54. Castaneda B, Morales J, Lionetti R, et al. Effects of blood volume restitution following a portal hypertensive-related bleeding in anesthetized cirrhotic rats. Hepatology. 2001;33(4):821–825.

55. Farkas J. PulmCrit- Coagulopathy management in the bleeding cirrhotic: Seven pearls and one crazy idea. EMCrit Blog. http://emcrit.org/pulmcrit/coagulopathy-bleeding-cirrhotic-inr/. Accessed 5 June 2022.

56. Heyes J, Kelly PA, Monaghan K, et al. A single unit transfusion policy reduces red cell transfusions in general medical in-patients. QJM 2017;110(11):735–739.

57. Sung JJ, Chiu PW, Chan FKL, et al. Asia-Pacific working group consensus on non-variceal upper gastrointestinal bleeding: an update 2018. Gut 2018;67(10):1757–1768.

58. Abraham NS, Barkun AN, Sauer BG, et al. American College of Gastroenterology-Canadian Association of Gastroenterology Clinical Practice Guideline: Management of Anticoagulants and Antiplatelets during Acute Gastrointestinal Bleeding and the Periendoscopic Period. Am J Gastroenterol. 2022;117(4):542–558.

59. Munlemvo DM, Tobias JD, Chenault KM, et al. Prothrombin Complex Concentrates to Treat Coagulation Disturbances: An Overview with a Focus on Use in Infants and Children. Cardiol Res. 2022;13(1):18–26.

60. Cohn SM, Jimenez JC, Khoury L, et al. Inability to Reverse Aspirin and Clopidogrel-induced Platelet Dysfunction with Platelet Infusion. Cureus. 2019;11(1):e3889.

61. Savage SA, Sumislawski JJ, Zarzaur BL, et al. The new metric to define large-volume hemorrhage: results of a prospective study of the critical administration threshold. J Trauma Acute Care Surg 2015;78(2):224–9.

62. Holcomb JB, Tilley BC, Baraniuk S, et al. Transfusion of Plasma, Platelets, and Red Blood Cells in a 1:1:1 Vs a 1:1:2 Ratio and Mortality in Patients with Severe Trauma: The Proppr Randomized Clinical Trial. JAMA 2015;313(5):471–82.

63. Lau JY, Leung WK, Wu JC, et al. Omeprazole before endoscopy in patients with gastrointestinal bleeding. N Engl J Med. 2007;356(16):1631–40.

64. Sreedharan A, Martin J, Leontiadis GI, et al. Proton pump inhibitor treatment initiated prior to endoscopic diagnosis in upper gastrointestinal bleeding. Cochrane Database Syst Rev. 2010;2010(7):CD005415.

65. Kanno T, Yuan Y, Tse F, et al. Proton pump inhibitor treatment initiated prior to endoscopic diagnosis in upper gastrointestinal bleeding. Cochrane Database Syst Rev. 2022;1(1):CD005415.

66. Bai Y, Guo JF, Li ZS. Meta-analysis: erythromycin before endoscopy for acute upper gastrointestinal bleeding. Aliment Pharmacol Ther 2011;34(2):166–171.

67. Szary NM, Gupta R, Choudhary A, et al. Erythromycin prior to endoscopy in acute upper gastrointestinal bleeding: a meta-analysis. Scand J Gastroenterol 2011;46(7–8):920–924.

68. Theivanayagam S, Lim RG, Cobell WJ et al. Administration of erythromycin before endoscopy in upper gastrointestinal bleeding: a metaanalysis of randomized controlled trials. Saudi J Gastroenterol 2013;19(5):205–210.

69. Barkun AN, Bardou M, Martel M, et al. Prokinetics in acute upper GI bleeding: a meta-analysis. Gastrointest Endosc 2010;72(6):1138–1145.

70. Rahman R, Nguyen DL, Sohail U, et al. Pre-endoscopic erythromycin administration in upper gastrointestinal bleeding: an updated metaanalysis and systematic review. Ann Gastroenterol 2016;29(3):312–317.

71. Na HK, Jung HY, Seo DW, et al. Erythromycin infusion prior to endoscopy for acute nonvariceal upper gastrointestinal bleeding: A pilot randomized controlled trial. Korean J Intern Med 2017;32(6):1002–1009.

72. Winstead NS, Wilcox CM. Erythromycin prior to endoscopy for acute upper gastrointestinal haemorrhage: a cost–effectiveness analysis. Aliment Pharmacol Ther 2007;26(10):1371–1377.

73. Daram S, Johnson W, Abrasley C, et al. A double blind randomized study to evaluate the use of metoclopramide before endoscopy for upper gastrointestinal bleeding. Am J Gastroenterol 2010;105(Suppl 1):S508.

74. Daram SR, Garretson R. Erythromycin is preferable to metoclopramide as a prokinetic in acute upper GI bleeding. Gastrointest Endosc 2011;74(1):234.

75. Estes DJ, Berera S, Deshpande AR, et al. Re-Visiting Metoclopramide to Optimize Visualization with Gastrointestinal Bleeding - Mobilizing Existing Data. Clin Endosc. 2019;52(5):516–517.

76. Tripathi D, Stanley AJ, Hayes PC, et al. U.K. guidelines on the management of variceal haemorrhage in cirrhotic patients. Gut 2015;64(11):1680–704.

77. de Franchis R, Baveno VI Faculty. Expanding consensus in portal hypertension: report of the Baveno VI Consensus Workshop: Stratifying risk and individualizing care for portal hypertension. J Hepatol 2015;63(3):743–52.

78. Stanley AJ, Laine L. Management of acute upper gastrointestinal bleeding. BMJ. 2019;364:l536.

79. Yoshiji H, Nagoshi S, Akahane T, et al. Evidence-based clinical practice guidelines for Liver Cirrhosis 2020. J Gastroenterol. 2021;56(7):593–619.

80. Riha HM, Wilkinson R, Twilla J, et al. Octreotide added to a proton pump inhibitor versus a proton pump inhibitor alone in nonvariceal upper-gastrointestinal bleeds. Ann Pharmacother 2019;53(8):794–800.

81. Wells M, Chande N, Adams P, et al. Meta-analysis: vasoactive medications for the management of acute variceal bleeds. Aliment Pharmacol Ther 2012;35(11):1267–78.

82. Zhou X, Tripathi D, Song T, et al. Terlipressin for the treatment of acute variceal bleeding: a systematic review and meta-analysis of randomized controlled trials. Medicine (Baltimore). 2018;97(48):e13437.

83. Bolognesi M, Di Pascoli M, Verardo A, et al. Splanchnic vasodilation and hyperdynamic circulatory syndrome in cirrhosis. World J Gastroenterol. 2014;20(10):2555–2563.

84. Wong YJ, Tan CK, Lin Yii YL, et al. Antibiotic prophylaxis in cirrhosis patients with upper gastrointestinal bleeding: An updated systematic review and meta-analysis. Portal Hypertension & Cirrhosis 2022;1(3):167–177.

85. Tandon P, Abraldes JG, Keough A, et al. Risk of bacterial infection in patients with cirrhosis and acute variceal hemorrhage, based on childPugh class, and effects of antibiotics. Clin Gastroenterol Hepatol. 2015;13(6):1189–96.e2.

86. Gao Y, Qian B, Zhang X, et al. Prophylactic antibiotics on patients with cirrhosis and upper gastrointestinal bleeding: A meta-analysis. PLoS One. 2022;17(12):e0279496.

87. Bennett C, Klingenberg SL, Langholz E, et al. Tranexamic acid for upper gastrointestinal bleeding. Cochrane Database Syst Rev 2014;2014(11):CD006640.

88. HALT-IT Trial Collaborators. Effects of a high-dose 24-h infusion of tranexamic acid on death and thromboembolic events in patients with acute gastrointestinal bleeding (HALT-IT): an international randomised, double-blind, placebo-controlled trial. Lancet 2020;395(10241):1927–1936.

89. Aljebreen AM, Fallone CA, Barkun AN. Nasogastric aspirate predicts high-risk endoscopic lesions in patients with acute upper-GI bleeding. Gastrointest Endosc. 2004;59(2):172–8.

90. Rockey DC, Ahn C, de Melo SW Jr. Randomized pragmatic trial of nasogastric tube placement in patients with upper gastrointestinal tract bleeding. J Investig Med. 2017;65(4):759–764.

91. Karakonstantis S, Tzagkarakis E, Kalemaki D, et al. Nasogastric aspiration/lavage in patients with gastrointestinal bleeding: a review of the evidence. Expert Rev Gastroenterol Hepatol 2018;12(1):63–72.

92. Palamidessi N, Sinert R, Falzon L, et al. Nasogastric aspiration and lavage in emergency department patients with hematochezia or melena without hematemesis. Acad Emerg Med. 2010;17(2):126–32.

93. Huang ES, Karsan S, Kanwal F, et al. Impact of nasogastric lavage on outcomes in acute GI bleeding. Gastrointest Endosc 2011;74(5):971–80.

94. Pallin DJ, Saltzman JR. Is nasogastric tube lavage in patients with acute upper GI bleeding indicated or antiquated? Gastrointest Endosc. 2011;74(5):981–4.

95. Laine L, Jensen DM. Management of patients with ulcer bleeding. Am J Gastroenterol. 2012;107(3):345–60;quiz 361.

96. Gené E, Calvet X. Nasogastric intubation in patients with upper gastrointestinal bleeding? Gastroenterol Hepatol. 2016;39(8):497–9.

97. Gong EJ, Hsing LC, Seo HI, et al. Selected nasogastric lavage in patients with nonvariceal upper gastrointestinal bleeding. BMC Gastroenterol. 2021;21(1):113.

98. Saltzman JR. Approach to acute upper gastrointestinal bleeding in adults. In: UpToDate, Post TW (Ed), UpToDate, Waltham, MA. (Accessed on June 1, 2022).

99. Dai JY, Yin L, Xu J, et al. Expert consensus on emergency diagnosis and treatment procedures for acute upper gastrointestinal bleeding. J Acute Dis 2020;9(6):231–43.

100. Kim JS, Kim BW, Kim DH, et al. Guidelines for Nonvariceal Upper Gastrointestinal Bleeding. Gut Liver. 2020;14(5):560–570.

101. Spiegel BM, Vakil NB, Ofman JJ. Endoscopy for acute nonvariceal upper gastrointestinal tract hemorrhage: is sooner better? A systematic review. Arch Intern Med 2001;161(11):1393–404.

102. Cooper GS, Kou TD, Wong RC. Use and impact of early endoscopy in elderly patients with peptic ulcer hemorrhage: A population-based analysis. Gastrointest Endosc 2009;70(2):229–35.

103. Laursen SB, Leontiadis GI, Stanley AJ, et al. Relationship between timing of endoscopy and mortality in patients with peptic ulcer bleeding: A nationwide cohort study. Gastrointest Endosc 2017;85(5):936–944.e3.

104. Garg SK, Anugwom C, Campbell J, et al. Early esophagogastroduodenoscopy in upper gastrointestinal bleeding: a nationwide study. Endosc Int Open 2017;5(5):E376–E386.

105. Xia XF, Chiu PWY, Tsoi KKF, et al. The effect of off-hours hospital admission on mortality and clinical outcomes for patients with upper gastrointestinal hemorrhage: a systematic review and meta-analysis of 20 cohorts. United European Gastroenterol J. 2018;6(3):367–381.

106. Siau K, Hodson J, Ingram R, et al. Time to endoscopy for acute upper gastrointestinal bleeding: results from a prospective multicentre trainee-led audit. United European Gastroenterol J 2019;7(2):199–209.

107. Jeong N, Kim KS, Jung YS, et al. Delayed endoscopy is associated with increased mortality in upper gastrointestinal hemorrhage. Am J Emerg Med. 2019;37(2):277–280.

108. Guo CLT, Wong SH, Lau LHS, et al. Timing of endoscopy for acute upper gastrointestinal bleeding: a territory-wide cohort study. Gut. 2021:gutjnl-2020-323054.

109. Jairath V, Kahan BC, Logan RF, et al. Outcomes following acute nonvariceal upper gastrointestinal bleeding in relation to time to endoscopy: results from a nationwide study. Endoscopy. 2012;44(8):723–30.

110. Lim LG, Ho KY, Chan YH, et al. Urgent endoscopy is associated with lower mortality in high-risk but not low-risk nonvariceal upper gastrointestinal bleeding. Endoscopy 2011;43(4):300–6.

111. Targownik LE, Murthy S, Keyvani L, et al. The role of rapid endoscopy for high-risk patients with acute nonvariceal upper gastrointestinal bleeding. Can J Gastroenterol. 2007;21(7):425–9.

112. Tai CM, Huang SP, Wang HP, et al. High-risk ED patients with nonvariceal upper gastrointestinal hemorrhage undergoing emergency or urgent endoscopy: a retrospective analysis. Am J Emerg Med. 2007;25(3):273–8.

113. Lau JYW, Yu Y, Tang RSY, et al. Timing of endoscopy for acute upper gastrointestinal bleeding. N Engl J Med 2020;382(14):1299–1308.

114. Kim J, Gong EJ, Seo M, et al. Timing of endoscopy in patients with upper gastrointestinal bleeding. Sci Rep 2022;12:6833.

115. Laursen SB, Hansen JM, Schaffalitzky de Muckadell OB. The Glasgow Blatchford score is the most accurate assessment of patients with upper gastrointestinal hemorrhage. Clin Gastroenterol Hepatol 2012;10(10):1130–1135.e1.

116. Tham J, Stanley A. Clinical utility of pre-endoscopy risk scores in upper gastrointestinal bleeding. Expert Rev Gastroenterol Hepatol. 2019;13(12):1161–1167.

35 | Ascites in Cirrhosis

INTRODUCTION

The term ascites is defined as a pathologic fluid accumulation in the peritoneal cavity. The most common cause of ascites is decompensated cirrhosis which accounts for about 80% of the cases.

In patients with cirrhosis, ascites is the most common complication, which suggests the progression of diseases from a compensated to a decompensated stage [1]. About 60% of patients with compensated cirrhosis develop ascites within 10 years of its diagnosis [2]. Development of ascites in cirrhotic patients carries a poor prognosis as the five-year survival rate is significantly low in decompensated cirrhosis with ascites compared with compensated cirrhosis (about 30% vs. 80%) [1, 3].

Refractory ascites (RA) is defined as ascites that cannot be mobilized or recurs after large volume paracentesis (LVP) despite dietary sodium restriction and diuretic therapy. Refractory ascites is one of the most serious signs of the decompensated stage in liver cirrhosis which is associated with poor survival [4].

PATHOPHYSIOLOGY

In cirrhosis of the liver, the development of ascites is determined by four major factors: portal hypertension, splanchnic vasodilatation, renal sodium and water retention, and hypoalbuminemia.

A. **Portal hypertension:** The development of intrahepatic portal hypertension plays a crucial role in ascites formation. The normal value of portal pressure (pressure gradient between the hepatic and portal vein) is approximately <5 mm Hg. However, a portal pressure of usually >12 mmHg is required for ascites to develop. Without elevated portal pressure, ascites or edema do not occur.

Portal hypertension occurs in liver cirrhosis because of both increased resistance to portal blood flow (increase in intrahepatic resistance due to distortion of the hepatic vascular architecture) and increased portal venous inflow (due to splanchnic vasodilatation). This increased portal hypertension increases hydrostatic pressure within the hepatic sinusoids, causing excessive fluid transudation into the peritoneal space, leading to ascites.

Portal hypertension occurs in liver cirrhosis because of both an increase in resistance to portal blood flow (increase in intrahepatic resistance due to distortion of the hepatic vascular architecture) and an increase in portal venous inflow (due to splanchnic vasodilatation). Due to increased portal hypertension, hydrostatic pressure increases within the hepatic sinusoids, leading to excess transudation of fluid into the peritoneal space and causing ascites.

B. **Splanchnic vasodilatation:** In portal hypertension, the increased production of the local vasodilator nitric oxide (NO) in splanchnic and systemic arteries plays a significant role in the pathogenesis of ascites. Elevated nitric oxide levels lead to splanchnic vasodilation, which, in turn, increases portal venous blood inflow. This increased blood inflow aggravates portal hypertension, contributing to ascites formation.

Both these abnormalities, portal hypertension, and NO-induced splanchnic vasodilatation, contribute to increased splanchnic lymph production, ultimately leading to the development of ascites.

C. **Renal retention of sodium and water:** Cirrhosis-related increased NO production leads to systemic vasodilation, resulting in the redirection of blood from the systemic circulation into the spleen, causing extracellular fluid volume contraction. This leads to the underfilling of the arterial circulation, reduced effective arterial blood volume, renal vasoconstriction, and resultant activation of the renin-angiotensin-aldosterone system and hyperaldosteronism.

Hyperaldosteronism, in turn, leads to sodium retention, causing fluid accumulation and expansion of the extracellular fluid volume, ultimately resulting in peripheral edema and ascites formation.

As cirrhosis worsens, NO production further increases, leading to a marked reduction in systemic vascular resistance, more pronounced vasodilation, and further activation of the renin-angiotensin-aldosterone and sympathetic nervous systems. Increased aldosterone level exacerbates sodium retention, contributing to the development of refractory ascite.

D. **Hypoalbuminemia:** In cirrhosis, hypoalbuminemia occurs because of decreased albumin synthesis due to hepatocellular dysfunction. Reduced plasma oncotic pressure due to hypoalbuminemia shifts fluid from the vascular compartment into the peritoneal cavity, further contributing to ascites development.

MANAGEMENT

A. Goal of therapy

The goals of therapy are:

- To decrease ascitic fluid volume and reduce associated symptoms like abdominal discomfort, bloating, and shortness of breath.

- To reduce ascitic fluid volume at a safe rate to avoid electrolyte disorders and intravascular volume depletion.

- To diagnose and treatment of underlying causes to slow down the progression of diseases.

- To avoid aggravating factors like intake of alcohol and harmful drugs.

B. Salt restriction

- The first step in the management of ascites is the salt restriction [3, 5–7].

- Dietary sodium restriction is not indicated in cirrhotic patients without ascites.

- Traditionally, strict salt restriction (<2 gm/day) is recommended to reduce sodium and water retention and the resultant ascitic fluid volume. But the strict salt restriction is difficult to follow, impairs appetite, leads to reduced caloric intake, compromises nutritional status, and is therefore discouraged [3, 5, 8, 9].

- Additionally, such a rigid salt restriction can lead to higher adverse effects like acute kidney injury (AKI), hyponatremia, hepatic encephalopathy, or hepatorenal syndrome [7, 10].

- So the current recommendation for moderate uncomplicated ascites is to avoid excess salt intake and permit moderate salt restriction (no more than 5–6.5 gm or 80–120 mmol sodium/day), which can be followed by choosing a less salt-containing diet with avoidance of commercial processed and preprepared salt reach meals [3, 5, 6].

C. Fluid restriction and bed rest

Restriction of fluid is inappropriate in all patients with ascites. However, fluid restriction is required in a few ascitic patients with moderate or severe hyponatremia (serum sodium ≤125 mmol/L) [11]. In contrast, avoid fluid restriction in patients with fever, sepsis, bleeding, or azotemia.

D. Diuretics

Diuretic therapy is a second step in managing cirrhosis with ascites (in combination with salt restriction), which is highly effective in controlling water retention [7]. Potassium-sparing diuretics (spironolactone) and loop diuretics (furosemide) are widely used agents. Combined therapy (spironolactone + furosemide) is very successful if faster diuresis is needed [6].

Spironolactone: Compared to loop diuretics, spironolactone is more effective as a monotherapy in managing cirrhotic ascites [12]. The recommended initial dose of spironolactone is 100 mg/day (given once a day in the morning due to its long half-life), gradually increasing to 400 mg/day depending on clinical response [11]. As its onset of effect is slow (about 3–4 days), the dose is increased cautiously stepwise at an interval of at least 72 hours [3, 11]. The response rate of spironolactone is 95%, and it has additional benefits of cardioprotective and renoprotective via nonepithelial mineralocorticoid receptor blockade [13]. Spironolactone is a potent aldosterone antagonist, the common side effects of which are hyperkalemia and painful gynecomastia.

Diuretics combination therapy: In patients with long-standing, severe, or recurrent ascites, and if faster diuresis is needed, start a combination of oral spironolactone and furosemide [3, 6, 11]. To shorten the time to mobilize moderate ascites, a combination of diuretics is better than monotherapy or sequential diuretics therapy (i.e., spironolactone alone, followed by adding furosemide) [14]. For combination therapy, oral spironolactone and furosemide are used in a ratio of 100:40 mg per day, which maintains normokalemia and achieves diuresis in >90% of cirrhotic ascites.

Furosemide: The oral loop diuretics furosemide is usually initiated in a dose of 20–40 mg/dL and is subsequently increased gradually every few days up to a maximum of 160 mg/d. Furosemide may be preferred over spironolactone in ascitic patients with hyperkalemia and renal parenchymal disease. Common complications of furosemide are hypokalemia, hyponatremia, hypovolemia leading to renal dysfunction, and hypochloremic metabolic alkalosis.

In patients with weak responses to furosemide, torasemide can be used. The dose of diuretics should be reduced once ascites resolve and discontinued in patients who develop complications like severe hyponatremia (serum sodium < 125 mEq/L), development of AKI, aggravation of hepatic encephalopathy, severe hypokalemia, or the development of severe cramps [3]. Diuretic therapy aims to achieve a weight loss of 0.5 kg/day in patients without edema and 1 kg/day in edematous patients [3].

E. Large volume paracentesis (LVP)

Indications: Repeated large-volume paracentesis (defined as a paracentesis of >5 L) with albumin infusion is recommended as a first-line treatment in patients with large volume, diuretic-resistant, or refractory ascites, which effectively reduces symptoms of a tense abdomen [5, 6, 11].

Contraindications: Common contraindications to paracentesis are abdominal skin infection, severe coagulopathy, severe bowel distension, pregnancy, and uncooperative patient.

Safety: LVP is a preferred therapeutic modality because it is safe, carries a low risk of complications, shortens hospital stay, effectively mobilizes edema, and is associated with a lower risk of electrolyte abnormalities, renal dysfunction, and hemodynamic disturbance compared with continued diuretic use [7, 11, 15, 16]. Even in patients with an international normalized ratio (INR)>1.5 and platelet count <50,000/µl, performing LVP carries a very low risk of local complications [17]. Ultrasound guidance is recommended for performing LVP because it improves the success rates of the procedure and reduces the risk of local complications like bleeding [6, 18, 19].

Volume and frequency of fluid removal: Standard recommended for LVP is the amount of ascites removal per session to be more than 5 L (but less than 8 L) [3, 6, 20, 11]. The minimum dose of diuretics should be administered after LVP to prevent re-accumulation of ascites [3]. The frequency of LVP depends on compliance with dietary salt restriction and the rapidity at which the ascites reaccumulate. With proper salt restriction, patients with refractory ascites may need LVP of about 8 liters every two weeks.

Risk: Paracentesis of more than 5 L of ascites at one time without a plasma expander can lead to serious complications like paracentesis induced circulatory dysfunction (PICD) characterized by like renal impairment, increased incidence of hepatorenal syndrome (HRS), dilutional hyponatremia, hepatic encephalopathy, and reduces survival [16].

Plasma volume expansion to prevent PICD: During LVP, infusion of albumin is preferred over other volume expanders (e.g., dextran, gelatin, hydroxyethyl starch, and hypertonic saline) to prevent paracentesis-induced circulatory dysfunction (PICD) [21, 22].

During LVP, the replacement of 6–8 gm of albumin for every liter of ascites removed is recommended, which effectively expands plasma volume and prevents paracentesis-induced abrupt hemodynamic changes (circulatory dysfunction) [6, 11, 20, 23, 24] and may prevent the associated morbidity [25].

F. Drugs in ascites

In patients of cirrhosis with ascites, avoid medications such as non-steroidal anti-inflammatory drugs (NSAIDs), angiotensin-converting enzyme inhibitors (ACEIs), angiotensin II receptor blockers (ARBs), beta-blockers (propranolol), and aminoglycosides [3].

NSAIDs are contraindicated in patients with cirrhosis and ascites because of the risk of acute kidney injury, hepatorenal syndrome, and gastrointestinal hemorrhage [26]. In addition, NSAIDs by inhibiting renal prostaglandin synthesis, can cause acute renal failure, hyponatremia, and diuretic resistance [27].

The use of angiotensin-converting-enzyme inhibitors and angiotensin-receptor blockers in persons with cirrhosis with ascites is not recommended because they can induce arterial hypotension, causing a higher risk of renal failure and increased mortality [3, 11, 28–30].

Avoid or discontinue using non-selective beta-blockers (e.g., propranolol) in decompensated cirrhosis with refractory ascites and in patients whose blood pressure is declining because of the risk of worsening of renal function and decreased survival [3, 11, 28, 30–32].

Aminoglycosides are potentially nephrotoxic antibiotics, so they carry the risk of AKI and, therefore, should be avoided in cirrhotic patients for treating bacterial infections [3, 11].

G. Other measures

Bed rest, alcohol abstinence, management of underlying liver disease, transjugular intrahepatic portosystemic shunts (TIPS), automated pumps, and liver transplantation are other measures required in cirrhotic patients with ascites.

Bed rest: Bed rest was previously recommended but is currently no longer advocated due to a lack of evidence that it is beneficial [3, 33, 34].

Alcohol abstinence: Long-term abstinence from alcohol is recommended as it improves the prognosis of alcoholic cirrhosis [5].

TIPS: Transjugular intrahepatic portosystemic shunt (TIPS) has emerged as a crucial therapeutic option in difficult-to-treat patients with refractory ascites (diuretic-resistant ascites, requiring very frequent paracentesis or intolerant of paracentesis), without access to liver transplantation [3, 7, 35, 36].

TIPS is an artificial communication (side-to-side shunt) between the portal and the hepatic vein, which decompresses the portal system and can convert diuretic-resistant ascites back to diuretic-sensitive ascites. A higher rate of hepatic encephalopathy is a major adverse consequence of TIPS [37]. Common contraindications of TIPS are age >70 years, severe pulmonary hypertension, severe systolic or diastolic dysfunction, severe tricuspid regurgitation, serum bilirubin >3 mg/dL, low platelet count, current hepatic encephalopathy, active infection or hepatorenal syndrome [3, 6].

In recent studies, TIPS demonstrated better control of ascites than paracentesis, increased survival, and lowered the risk of mortality and hepatic encephalopathy compared to other treatment modalities (e.g., paracentesis) in refractory ascites [38, 39]. Because of these benefits, current guidelines recommend using TIPS for patients with refractory ascites without access to liver transplantation [3, 5–7].

Automated pumps (ALFA PUMP): Automated low flow ascitic pumps are recommended only in selected patients with recurrent or refractory ascites in whom TIPS is contraindicated [6, 40].

In this modality, a medical device transfers ascitic fluid to the bladder, eliminating it with urine, reducing the need for repeated paracentesis, and improving the quality of life in patients with medically untreatable ascites [40–44].

Liver transplantation: The most appropriate and the only curative option for decompensation liver diseases with refractory ascites is liver transplantation. But lack of facility, absolute organ shortage, and cost are major limiting factors for liver transplantation.

MONITORING

In patients with ascites with cirrhosis, it is important to monitor:

- Daily body weight: Measuring weight daily at the same time helps to assess diuretics' efficacy. Furthermore, adjusting the dose of diuretics to achieve a weight loss of 0.5 kg/day in patients without edema and 1 kg/day in edematous patients helps to prevent their adverse effects [3, 11].

- Laboratory monitoring: Periodic serum electrolyte concentrations measurement helps detect diuretics-induced electrolyte disorders.

- Spot urine sodium (Na^+)/K^+ ratio: The ratio is >1, which suggests a response to therapy, and the patient should lose fluid weight. The ratio ≤1 indicates insufficient natriuresis and needs an increment in the diuretics doses.

REFERENCE

1. D'Amico G, Garcia-Tsao G, Pagliaro L. Natural history and prognostic indicators of survival in cirrhosis. A systematic review of 118 studies. J Hepatol 2006;44(1):217–31.

2. Ginès P, Quintero E, Arroyo V, et al. Compensated cirrhosis: natural history and prognostic factors. Hepatology 1987;7(1):122–8.

3. European Association for the Study of the Liver. EASL Clinical Practice Guidelines for the management of patients with decompensated cirrhosis. J Hepatol. 2018;69(2):406–460.

4. Zhao R, Lu J, Shi Y, et al. Current management of refractory ascites in patients with cirrhosis. J Int Med Res 2018;46(3):1138–1145.

5. Yoshiji H, Nagoshi S, Akahane T, et al. Evidence-based clinical practice guidelines for Liver Cirrhosis 2020. J Gastroenterol. 2021;56(7):593–619.

6. Aithal GP, Palaniyappan N, China L, et al. Guidelines on the management of ascites in cirrhosis. Gut. 2021;70(1):9–29.

7. Baiges A, Hernández-Gea V. Management of Liver Decompensation in Advanced Chronic Liver Disease: Ascites, Hyponatremia, and Gastroesophageal Variceal Bleeding. Clin Drug Investig. 2022;42(Suppl 1):25–31.

8. Gauthier A, Levy VG, Quinton A, et al. Salt or no salt in the treatment of cirrhotic ascites: a randomised study. Gut 1986;27(6):705–9.

9. Morando F, Rosi S, Gola E, et al. Adherence to a moderate sodium restriction diet in outpatients with cirrhosis and ascites: A real-life cross-sectional study. Liver Int. 2015;35(5):1508–1515.

10. Reynolds TB, Lieberman FL, Goodman AR. Advantages of treatment of ascites without sodium restriction and without complete removal of excess fluid. Gut. 1978;19(6):549–53.

11. Biggins SW, Angeli P, Garcia-Tsao G, et al. Diagnosis, Evaluation, and Management of Ascites, Spontaneous Bacterial Peritonitis and Hepatorenal Syndrome: 2021 Practice Guidance by the American Association for the Study of Liver Diseases. Hepatology. 2021;74(2):1014–1048.

12. Pérez-Ayuso RM, Arroyo V, Planas R, et al. Randomized comparative study of efficacy of furosemide versus spironolactone in nonazotemic cirrhosis with ascites. Relationship between the diuretic response and the activity of the renin-aldosterone system. Gastroenterology. 1983;84(5 Pt 1):961–8.

13. Slotki IN, Skorecki K. Disorders of Sodium Balance. In: Brenner and Rector's The Kidney, 11th ed, Yu A, Chertow G, Luyckx V, et al (Eds), W.B. Saunders & Company, Philadelphia 2020.p.437.

14. Angeli P, Fasolato S, Mazza E, et al. Combined versus sequential diuretic treatment of ascites in non-azotaemic patients with cirrhosis: results of an open randomised clinical trial. Gut 2010;59(1):98–104.

15. Ginés P, Arroyo V, Quintero E, et al. Comparison of paracentesis and diuretics in the treatment of cirrhotics with tense ascites. Results of a randomized study. Gastroenterology 1987;93(2):234–241.

16. Alsebaey A, Rewisha E, Waked I. Paracentesis-induced circulatory dysfunction: are there albumin alternatives? Egypt Liver Journal 2020;10:39.

17. Lin CH, Shih FY, Ma MH, et al. Should bleeding tendency deter abdominal paracentesis? Dig Liver Dis. 2005;37(12):946–51.

18. Mercaldi CJ, Lanes SF. Ultrasound guidance decreases complications and improves the cost of care among patients undergoing thoracentesis and paracentesis. Chest. 2013;143(2):532–538.

19. Cho J, Jensen TP, Reierson K, et al. Recommendations on the Use of Ultrasound Guidance for Adult Abdominal Paracentesis: A Position Statement of the Society of Hospital Medicine. J Hosp Med. 2019;14:E7–E15.

20. Runyon BA, AASLD Practice Guidelines Committee. Management of adult patients with ascites due to cirrhosis: an update. Hepatology 2009;49(6):2087–2107.

21. Moreau R, Valla DC, Durand-Zaleski I, et al. Comparison of outcome in patients with cirrhosis and ascites following treatment with albumin or a synthetic colloid: a randomised controlled pilot trial. Liver Int 2006;26(1):46–54.

22. Bernardi M, Caraceni P, Navickis RJ, et al. Albumin infusion in patients under-going large-volume paracentesis: a meta-analysis of randomized trials. Hepatology 2012;55(4):1172–1181.

23. Ginès P, Titó L, Arroyo V, et al. Randomized comparative study of therapeutic paracentesis with and without intravenous albumin in cirrhosis. Gastroenterology. 1988;94(6):1493–502.

24. Bernardi M, Angeli P, Claria J, et al. Albumin in decompensated cirrhosis: new concepts and perspectives. Gut 2020;69(6):1127–38.

25. Tan HK, James PD, Wong F. Albumin may prevent the morbidity of paracentesis-induced circulatory dysfunction in cirrhosis and refractory ascites: a pilot study. Dig Dis Sci 2016;61(10):3084–3092.

26. Dwyer JP, Jayasekera C, Nicoll A. Analgesia for the cirrhotic patient: a literature review and recommendations. J Gastroenterol Hepatol. 2014;29(7):1356–60.

27. Elia C, Graupera I, Barreto R, et al. Severe acute kidney injury associated with non-steroidal anti-inflammatory drugs in cirrhosis: a case-control study. J Hepatol 2015;63(3):593–600.

28. Pariente EA, Bataille C, Bercoff E, et al. Acute effects of captopril on systemic and renal hemodynamics and on renal function in cirrhotic patients with ascites. Gastroenterology 1985;88(5 Pt 1):1255–1259.

29. Albillos A, Lledó JL, Rossi I, et al. Continuous prazosin administration in cirrhotic patients: effects on portal hemodynamics and on liver and renal function. Gastroenterology 1995;109(4):1257–1265.

30. Korean Association for the Study of the Liver (KASL). KASL clinical practice guidelines for liver cirrhosis: Ascites and related complications. Clin Mol Hepatol. 2018;24(3):230–277.

31. Llach J, Ginès P, Arroyo V, et al. Prognostic value of arterial pressure, endogenous vasoactive systems, and renal function in cirrhotic patients admitted to the hospital for the treatment of ascites. Gastroenterology 1988;94(2):482–7.

32. Sersté T, Melot C, Francoz C, et al. Deleterious effects of beta-blockers on survival in patients with cirrhosis and refractory ascites. Hepatology. 2010;52(3):1017–22.

33. Moore KP, Aithal GP. Guidelines on the management of ascites in cirrhosis. Gut. 2006;55 Suppl 6(Suppl 6):vi1–vi12.

34. Runyon BA; AASLD Practice Guidelines Committee. Management of adult patients with ascites due to cirrhosis: Update 2012. Hepatology. Visit: https://www.aasld.org/sites/default/files/2019-06/141020_Guideline_Ascites_4UFb_2015.pdf.

35. García-Pagán JC, Saffo S, Mandorfer M, et al. Where does TIPS fit in the management of patients with cirrhosis? JHEP Rep. 2020;2(4):100122.

36. Boike JR, Thornburg BG, Asrani SK, et al. North American Practice-Based Recommendations for Transjugular Intrahepatic Portosystemic Shunts in Portal Hypertension. Clin Gastroenterol Hepatol. 2021:S1542–3565(21)00749–7.

37. Copelan A, Kapoor B, Sands M. Transjugular intrahepatic portosystemic shunt: indications, contraindications, and patient work-up. Semin Intervent Radiol. 2014;31(3):235–242.

38. Bureau C, Thabut D, Oberti F, et al. Transjugular intrahepatic portosystemic shunts with covered stents increase transplant-free survival of patients with cirrhosis and recurrent ascites. Gastroenterology. 2017;152(1):157–163.

39. Will V, Rodrigues SG, Berzigotti A. Current treatment options of refractory ascites in liver cirrhosis - A systematic review and meta-analysis. Dig Liver Dis. 2022 8:S1590–8658(21)00894-X.

40. Aagaard NK, Malago M, De Gottardi A, et al. Consensus care recommendations for alfapump® in cirrhotic patients with refractory or recurrent ascites. BMC Gastroenterol. 2022;22(1):111.

41. Bureau C, Adebayo D, Chalret de Rieu M, et al. Alfapump® system vs. large volume paracentesis for refractory ascites: A multicenter randomized controlled study. J Hepatol 2017;67(5):940–949.

42. Stepanova M, Nader F, Bureau C, et al. Patients with refractory ascites treated with alfapump® system have better health-related quality of life as compared to those treated with large volume paracentesis: the results of a multicenter randomized controlled study. Qual Life Res 2018;27(6):1513–1520.

43. Lepida A, Marot A, Trépo E, et al. Systematic review with meta-analysis: automated low-flow ascites pump therapy for refractory ascites. Aliment Pharmacol Ther. 2019;50(9):978–987.

44. Wong F, Bendel E, Sniderman K, et al. Improvement in quality of life and decrease in large volume paracentesis requirements with the automated low flow ascites pump. Liver Transpl. 2020;26(5):651–61.

36 | Hepatic Encephalopathy

INTRODUCTION

Hepatic encephalopathy (HE) is a potentially reversible condition characterized by a spectrum of neurological or psychiatric abnormalities ranging from subclinical alterations to coma, which occurs as one of the many complications of decompensated liver disease or portosystemic shunting [1]. About 30 to 45% of patients with cirrhosis develop overt hepatic encephalopathy [2], which is associated with significant morbidity, mortality, high healthcare cost, and a huge burden on patients and their caregivers [3, 4].

PATHOPHYSIOLOGY

The pathophysiology of HE is poorly understood, it is often multifactorial, and different abnormalities may be present at the same time, leading to the development of HE [5].

The various pathogenetic mechanisms proposed in the development of HE are [5, 6]:

- Neurotoxins (Ammonia, benzo-diazepines, benzodiazepine-like compounds such as gamma-am-inobutyric acid, and manganese deposition within the basal ganglia).

- Alteration in neurotransmission due to increased GABA - neurotransmitters and serotonin activity in HE.

- False neurotransmitters such as tyramine, octopamine, and beta-phenylethanolamines may compete with the normal catecholamine neurotransmitters.

- Altered brain energy due to impaired hepatic gluconeogenesis in the terminal stages of liver failure.

- The systemic inflammatory response may exacerbate the harmful effects of hyperammonaemia on the brain [7].

- Alterations of the blood-brain barrier contribute to an increased influx of varieties of neurotoxic substances into the brain, which may contribute to HE.

Ammonia produced from the breakdown of dietary protein by gut bacteria plays a major role in the pathogenesis of HE. Increased production or impaired excretion leads to the accumulation of ammonia [8].

The raised ammonia levels cross the blood-brain barrier (BBB) readily, which, together with inflammation, leads to astrocyte swelling, alterations in neurotransmitters, and brain edema causing HE [8, 9].

CLASSIFICATION

Hepatic encephalopathy is broadly classified based on four factors: etiology, clinical features, frequency, and precipitating factors, as summarized in Table 36.1 [1]. The most common

subtype of HE is type C (due to cirrhosis and portal hypertension). Classification of HE helps to plan out a proper therapeutic strategy.

MANAGEMENT

A. Basic principles

The principles of treatment of HE can be broadly divided into:

1. Supportive care.
2. Identification and treatment of the precipitating causes.
3. Specific Firstline therapy.
4. Alternative or additional therapy.
5. Emerging or experimental therapy.

The treatment of hepatic encephalopathy is summarized in Table 36.2 [1, 9–13].

B. Nutrition

In hepatic encephalopathy, the goals of nutritional therapy are to ensure appropriate nutritional support, improve protein-calorie malnutrition, prevent

Table 36.1 Classification of hepatic encephalopathy			
A. According to the underlying disease			
Type A	Type B		Type C
Due to ALF	Due to portosystemic bypass or shunting		Due to cirrhosis and portal hypertension
B. According to the severity of manifestations			
Convert	Overt		
Grade I	Grade II	Grade III	Grade IV
Change in behavior, mild confusion, slurred speech, disordered sleep	Lethargy, moderate confusion	Marked confusion (stupor), incoherent, sleeping but arousable	Coma
C. According to the time course			
Episodic HE	Recurrent HE (bouts occur within 6 months or less)		Persistent HE (behavioral alternations always present)
D. According to precipitating factors			
Spontaneous or precipitated			

Table 36.2 Treatment of hepatic encephalopathy	
A. Supportive care	**B. Identification and treatment of the precipitating causes**
Airway management to prevent aspiration	Infections
IV fluids to correct dehydration and AKI	Gastrointestinal bleeding
Adequate nutrition	Diuretics overdose
Empirical antibiotics, if indicated	Acid-base and electrolyte disturbances
Antiepileptic drugs if seizures	Constipation
	Avoid sedatives, tranquilizers, narcotics, NSAIDs, and alcohol
C. Specific firstline therapy	**D. Alternative or additional therapy**
Lactulose and lactitol	Polyethylene glycol (PEG)
Oral antibiotic: Rifaximin	L-ornithine-L-aspartate (LOLA)
Embolization of portosystemic shunt	Branched-chain amino acids
	Prebiotics and probiotics
	Other antibiotics: Neomycin, metronidazole, and oral vancomycin
E. Emerging or experimental therapy	
Agents modifying gut flora	**Ammonia scavenging agents**
Fecal microbiota transplantation (FMT)	Ornithine phenylacetate, phenylbutyrate, and sodium benzoate
Nutrition, supplementation	
Zinc	**Other modalities**
Acetyl-L-carnitine	Albumin and albumin dialysis
Neurotransmitter modulation	GABA-A antagonist
Flumazenil	Glycerol phenylbutyrate
Dopamine agonists	Peritoneal dialysis liposomes

skeletal muscle degradation, and avoid catabolism by providing [14, 15]:

1. Adequate calories: At least 35 kcal/kg body weight per day energy intake is necessary for nonobese patients with HE. Compared to energy requirements in normal adults (20–30 kcal/kg/d), supplement calories in higher amounts (35–40 kcal/kg ideal body weight/day or more than 200 gm of carbohydrate per day) is recommended in cirrhotic patients to spare protein metabolism [1, 16].

Approximately 50–60% of non-protein energy requirements should be provided as carbohydrates. As patients with alcoholism and cirrhosis carry the risk for Wernicke's encephalopathy, empirical parenteral administration of large doses of thiamine simultaneously or before any glucose administration is prudent.

2. Protein intake: As the metabolism of dietary proteins produces ammonia, protein restriction was advised for patients with HE in the past.

However, protein restrictions can lead to muscle loss, cachexia, and increased mortality in HE [17, 18], and benefit occurs with normal to high protein intake [14]. So, current recommendations are to avoid protein restriction [19] and to provide 1.2–1.5 gm/kg of protein per day [1, 16], which helps to prevent sarcopenia, reverse minimal HE, and slow the development of overt HE [14]. In addition, vegetable and dairy proteins are preferred over meat and fish because they are better tolerated and improve nitrogen balance and mental status [16, 20, 21].

3. Small frequent meals: Consumption of more frequent small meals evenly distributed throughout the day and complex carbohydrate-containing snacks before bedtime should be encouraged [1, 16, 19, 22]. Administration of small frequent meals helps to avoid prolonged periods of fasting and prevents gluconeogenesis, minimizes protein catabolism and resultant ammonium production.

4. Branched-chain amino acids (BCAAs): Oral BCAAs supplementation has beneficial effects on symptoms and signs of HE and is recommended in selected patients with HE who cannot achieve adequate protein intake or are severely intolerant to protein [1, 23]. But BCAAs are not used as a first-line treatment in HE, and patient compliance is poor because of unpalatable taste, associated adverse gastrointestinal symptoms, cost, and lack of benefits for quality of life or mortality [15].

5. Zinc supplementation: In cirrhotic patients, zinc deficiency is common [24], which occurs due to decreased intake and absorption, the restricted diet of animal-origin protein, and treatment with diuretics [25]. Zinc deficiency can lead to anorexia, immune system dysfunction, and dysgeusia and may increase the risk of HE because zinc participates in ammonia detoxification [15, 26].

Oral zinc supplementation (600 mg/d) may be beneficial during the treatment of HE, but in the absence of strong evidence, its routine use cannot be justified [13, 27–30].

C. Fluid and electrolyte management

1. Avoid hypoglycemia: In cirrhosis, hypoglycemia is common and harmful [31]. It occurs more frequently in patients with malnourishment and sepsis. Patients with decompensated cirrhosis with HE are more prone to hypoglycemia due to deficient glycogen storage, hepatic resistance to glucagon, and decreased glycogenolysis.

Supplementation of either oral glucose (200 gm/day approximately) or continuous infusion of 10%, 20%, 25%, or 50% dextrose is necessary to avoid hypoglycemia.

Frequent blood sugar monitoring should be conducted to rule out hypoglycemia and to avoid hyperglycemia.

2. Metabolic alkalosis: In cirrhotic patients, metabolic alkalosis can occur due to [32–35]: (1) Secondary hyperaldosteronism (effective hypovolemia, loop diuretics, vomiting, nasogastric suction, diarrhea due to overuse of lactulose, etc.); (2) Hypoalbuminemia (as albumin is a weak acid, its loss or reduction can cause metabolic alkalosis); (3) Hypokalemia; (4) Lactate clearance; and (5) Ingestion of large doses of nonabsorbable antacids.

The loop diuretics lead to bicarbonate retention with chloride depletion, increased aldosterone secretion, and increased urinary excretion of potassium, which increases ammonia production and can consequently contribute to hyperammonemia [33].

Metabolic alkalosis promotes the conversion of harmless ionized ammonium (NH_4^+) to toxic un-ionized ammonia (NH_3). This increase in ammonia, which has increased blood-brain barrier permeability, readily crosses the BBB and accumulates in the central nervous system (CNS), predisposing the development of hepatic encephalopathy. Therefore, in patients with metabolic alkalosis, all precautions should be taken to correct precipitant causes, such as avoiding loop diuretic overdosing, choosing to use aldosterone antagonists, and treating hypovolemia, hypokalemia, and vomiting.

3. Correction of hypokalemia: Common causes of hypokalemia are loop diuretics, gastrointestinal losses (vomiting/diarrhea), secondary hyperaldosteronism, alkalemia, hypomagnesemia due to chronic malnutrition, terlipressin therapy, and refeeding syndrome [32–34]. Hypokalemia increases production and reduces the removal of ammonia which may contribute to hepatic encephalopathy [36]. In the treatment of early HE, higher potassium levels (5.4–5.5 mEq/L) had much better survival, and lesser episodes of HE compared to patients with the lowest normokalemia (serum K^+ 3.4–3.5 mEq/L) [37]. In patients of HE with hypokalemia, discontinue furosemide if serum potassium is <3 mEq/L [38], add potassium-sparing diuretics such as spironolactone, aggressively correct hypokalemia, and treat causative factors.

4. Hyponatremia: Hyponatremia is the most common electrolyte imbalance in patients with HE, which is associated with increased morbidity and mortality [38]. In cirrhotic patients, hyponatremia is chiefly hypervolemic or dilutional. However, in less than 10% of patients, hyponatremia is hypovolemic (e.g., prolonged negative sodium balance because of excessive diuretic use,

vomiting, or diarrhea, particularly from lactulose) [39, 40].

Hyponatremia needs attention because it aggravates cerebral edema in HE. Hypovolemic hyponatremia with serum sodium <130 mEq/L, is treated with volume expansion with saline solution and when serum sodium is <125 mEq/L, discontinue diuretics [38]. Hypervolemic hyponatremia is usually treated with fluid restricted to 1,000 ml/day. Treatment of severe and symptomatic hyponatremia is discussed in detail in the Chapter on 20 "Hyponatremia".

5. Selection of IV fluids: When patients need administration of IV fluids, basic principles are:

- **Avoid 5% dextrose:** Glucose-containing fluid is preferred to avoid hypoglycemia, but avoid 5% dextrose, as it is hypotonic. Hypotonic fluid can cause hyponatremia which may aggravate cerebral edema.

- **Avoid Isolyte-G:** The ammonium chloride content of this solution gets converted into H^+ and urea by the liver, and available H^+ corrects metabolic alkalosis, which is beneficial in HE. However, this conversion is defective in severe liver failure, resulting in an accumulation of ammonium chloride, which may be detrimental.

- **Use Ringer's lactate (RL) cautiously:** RL contains lactate, which gets converted into bicarbonate by the liver. This can aggravate pre-existing metabolic alkalosis, which can be harmful in hepatic encephalopathy. Furthermore, in severe liver failure, the liver may not be able to convert lactate to bicarbonate effectively, which leads to an increased level of lactate in the blood.

- **Preferred fluids:** To provide adequate calories, 10%, 20%, 25%, or 50% dextrose solutions are preferred. To provide maintenance requirements of sodium, and correct hypovolemic hyponatremia, hypovolemic shock, and metabolic alkalosis, IV normal saline or dextrose saline are chosen in HE.

- To treat hypokalemia, when peripheral administration of potassium is needed, use saline (and not dextrose solutions) as a vehicle to dilute and infuse potassium chloride (1 amp of 15% inj. KCl contains 20 mEq of potassium). However, an oral potassium supplement is preferred if feasible.

D. Medical therapy

Lactulose and rifaximin are the two most important specific therapeutic measures used in the treatment of HE.

1. Lactulose: A nonabsorbable disaccharide lactulose is the first-line therapy to treat HE because it effectively improves clinical recovery, decreases mortality, and prevents the recurrence of HE [1, 10, 41, 42].

Lactulose is usually administered orally (or via nasogastric tube) but may be given as an enema to patients at risk for aspiration. The usual initial dose of lactulose is 25 mL every 1–2 hours, which is adjusted to achieve at least two soft or loose bowel movements per day.

The most important mechanisms by which lactulose reduces intestinal ammonia production and absorption are:

- Decrease in the pH. The breakdown of lactulose to lactic acid by the bacterial flora causes acidic intraluminal pH. Acidic pH facilitates the conversion of ammonia (absorbable form) to ammonium (nonabsorbable form),

causing decreased plasma ammonia concentration.

- Laxative effect: The nonabsorbable disaccharide lactulose increases intraluminal osmolality and gas formation, reducing transit time and less time for ammonia absorption. Lactitol, a synthetic disaccharide composed of lactose and sorbitol, is similar to lactulose and is beneficial in the management of overt hepatic encephalopathy [43].

2. Rifaximin: A gut-restricted oral antibiotic, rifaximin is recommended as a first-line treatment for the treatment of HE [1, 10].

Rifaximin provides beneficial effects in patients with HE by reducing the bacterial content of the bowel and playing a role in gut barrier repair leading to improvement in the survival rate, a significant reduction in the rate of hospitalization, and prolonged remission from HE [44–49].

The combination of rifaximin and lactulose is recommended [1] because it provides additional benefits in terms of significantly increased clinical efficacy, more chances to have complete resolution of HE, and decreased mortality, and therefore is superior to lactulose monotherapy [50–53].

REFERENCES

1. Vilstrup H, Amodio P, Bajaj J, et al. Hepatic encephalopathy in chronic liver disease: 2014 Practice Guideline by the American Association for the Study of Liver Diseases and the European Association for the Study of the Liver. Hepatology. 2014;60(2):715–35.

2. Romero-Gómez M, Boza F, García-Valdecasas MS, et al. Subclinical hepatic encephalopathy predicts the development of overt hepatic encephalopathy. Am J Gastroenterol 2001;96(9):2718–23.

3. Kabaria S, Dalal I, Gupta K, et al. Hepatic Encephalopathy: A Review. EMJ Hepatol. 2021;9(1):89–97.

4. García-Martínez R, Diaz-Ruiz R, Poncela M. Management of Hepatic Encephalopathy Associated

with Advanced Liver Disease. Clin Drug Investig. 2022;42(Suppl 1):5–13.

5. Elwir S, Rahimi RS. Hepatic Encephalopathy: An Update on the Pathophysiology and Therapeutic Options. J Clin Transl Hepatol. 2017;5(2):142–151.

6. Ferenci P. Hepatic encephalopathy. Gastroenterol Rep (Oxf). 2017;5(2):138–147.

7. Shawcross DL, Davies NA, Williams R, et al. Systemic inflammatory response exacerbates the neuropsychological effects of induced hyperammonaemia in cirrhosis. J Hepatol. 2004;40(2):247–54.

8. Jaffe A, Lim JK, Jakab SS. Pathophysiology of Hepatic Encephalopathy. Clin Liver Dis. 2020;24(2):175–188.

9. Häussinger D, Dhiman RK, Felipo V, et al. Hepatic encephalopathy. Nat Rev Dis Primers. 2022;8(1):43.

10. Montagnese S, Russo FP, Amodio P, et al. Hepatic encephalopathy 2018: A clinical practice guideline by the Italian Association for the Study of the Liver (AISF). Dig Liver Dis. 2019;51(2):190–205.

11. Hasan LZ, Wu GY. Novel Agents in the Management of Hepatic Encephalopathy: A Review. J Clin Transl Hepatol. 2021;9(5):749–759.

12. Bajaj JS, O'Leary JG, Lai JC, et al. Acute-on-Chronic Liver Failure Clinical Guidelines. Am J Gastroenterol. 2022;117(2):225–252.

13. Hoilat GJ, Suhail FK, Adhami T, et al. Evidence-based approach to management of hepatic encephalopathy in adults. World J Hepatol 2022;14(4):670–681.

14. Maharshi S, Sharma BC, Sachdeva S, et al. Efficacy of nutritional therapy for patients with cirrhosis and minimal hepatic encephalopathy in a randomized trial. Clin Gastroenterol Hepatol 2016;14(3):454–460.e3.

15. Faccioli J, Nardelli S, Gioia S, et al. Nutrition Assessment and Management in Patients with Cirrhosis and Cognitive Impairment: A Comprehensive Review of Literature. J. Clin. Med. 2022;11(10):2842.

16. Amodio P, Bemeur C, Butterworth R, et al. The nutritional management of hepatic encephalopathy in patients with cirrhosis: International Society for Hepatic Encephalopathy and Nitrogen Metabolism Consensus. Hepatology 2013;58(1):325–36.

17. Córdoba J, López-Hellín J, Planas M, et al. Normal protein diet for episodic hepatic encephalopathy: results of a randomized study. J Hepatol. 2004;41(1):38–43.

18. Maharshi S, Sharma BC, Srivastava S. Malnutrition in cirrhosis increases morbidity and mortality. J Gastroenterol Hepatol. 2015;30(10):1507–13.

19. Plauth M, Bernal W, Dasarathy S, et al. ESPEN guideline on clinical nutrition in liver disease. Clin Nutr. 2019;38(2):485–521.

20. Bianchi GP, Marchesini G, Fabbri A, et al. Vegetable versus animal protein diet in cirrhotic patients with chronic encephalopathy. A randomized cross-over comparison. J Intern Med. 1993;233(5):385–92.

21. Merli M, Iebba V, Giusto M. What is new about diet in hepatic encephalopathy. Metab Brain Dis. 2016;31(6):1289–1294.

22. Tsien CD, McCullough AJ, Dasarathy S. Late evening snack: exploiting a period of anabolic opportunity in cirrhosis. J Gastroenterol Hepatol. 2012;27(3):430–41.

23. Gluud LL, Dam G, Les I, et al. Branched-chain amino acids for people with hepatic encephalopathy. Cochrane Database Syst Rev. 2017;2017(5):CD001939.

24. Katayama K, Kawaguchi T, Shiraishi K, et al. The Prevalence and Implication of Zinc Deficiency in Patients With Chronic Liver Disease. J Clin Med Res. 2018;10(5):437–444.

25. Silva M, Gomes S, Peixoto A, et al. Nutrition in Chronic Liver Disease. GE Port J Gastroenterol. 2015;22(6):268–276.

26. Loomba V, Pawar G, Dhar KL, et al. Serum zinc levels in hepatic encephalopathy. Indian J Gastroenterol. 1995;14(2):51–53.

27. Takuma Y, Nouso K, Makino Y, et al. Clinical trial: oral zinc in hepatic encephalopathy. Aliment Pharmacol Ther. 2010;32(9):1080–90.

28. Chavez-Tapia NC, Cesar-Arce A, Barrientos-Gutiérrez T, et al. A systematic review and meta-analysis of the use of oral zinc in the treatment of hepatic encephalopathy. Nutr J. 2013;12:74.

29. Shen YC, Chang YH, Fang CJ, et al. Zinc supplementation in patients with cirrhosis and hepatic encephalopathy: a systematic review and meta-analysis. Nutr J. 2019;18(1):34.

30. Fallahzadeh MA, Rahimi RS. Hepatic Encephalopathy and Nutrition Influences: A Narrative Review. Nutr Clin Pract. 2020;35(1):36–48.

31. Hung TH, Tseng CW, Tsai CC, et al. Prognosis of hypoglycemia episode in cirrhotic patients during hospitalization. BMC Gastroenterol. 2021;21(1):319.

32. Scheiner B, Lindner G, Reiberger T, et al. Acid-base disorders in liver disease. J Hepatol. 2017;67(5):1062–1073.

33. Jiménez JV, Carrillo-Pérez DL, Rosado-Canto R, et al. Electrolyte and Acid-Base Disturbances in End-Stage Liver Disease: A Physiopathological Approach. Dig Dis Sci. 2017;62(8):1855–1871.

34. Musso CG, Juarez R, Glassock RJ. Water, electrolyte, acid-base, and trace elements alterations in cirrhotic patients. Int Urol Nephrol. 2018;50(1):81–89.

35. Katopodis P, Pappas EM, Katopodis KP. Acid-base abnormalities and liver dysfunction. Ann Hepatol. 2022;27(2):100675.

36. Mikkelsen ACD, Thomsen KL, Vilstrup H, et al. Potassium deficiency decreases the capacity for urea synthesis and markedly increases ammonia in rats. Am J Physiol Gastrointest Liver Physiol. 2021;320(4):G474–G483.

37. Zavagli G, Ricci G, Bader G, et al. The importance of the highest normokalemia in the treatment of early hepatic encephalopathy. Miner Electrolyte Metab. 1993;19(6):362–7.

38. European Association for the Study of the Liver. EASL Clinical Practice Guidelines for the management of patients with decompensated cirrhosis. J Hepatol. 2018;69(2):406–460.

39. Fortune B, Cardenas A. Ascites, refractory ascites and hyponatremia in cirrhosis. Gastroenterol Rep (Oxf). 2017;5(2):104–112.

40. Alukal JJ, John S, Thuluvath PJ. Hyponatremia in Cirrhosis: An Update. Am J Gastroenterol. 2020;115(11):1775–85.

41. Sharma BC, Sharma P, Agrawal A, et al. Secondary prophylaxis of hepatic encephalopathy: an open-label randomized controlled trial of lactulose versus placebo. Gastroenterology. 2009;137(3):885–91, 891.e1.

42. Gluud LL, Vilstrup H, Morgan MY. Non-absorbable disaccharides vs placebo/no intervention and lactulose vs lactitol for the prevention and treatment of hepatic encephalopathy in people with cirrhosis. Cochrane Database Syst Rev. 2016;4:CD003044.

43. Morgan MY, Hawley KE, Stambuk D. Lactitol versus lactulose in the treatment of chronic hepatic encephalopathy. A double-blind, randomised, crossover study. J Hepatol. 1987;4(2):236–44

44. Bass N, Mullen K, Sanyal A, et al. Rifaximin treatment in HE. N Engl J Med. 2010;362(12):1071–1081.

45. Sanyal A, Younossi ZM, Bass NM, et al. Randomised clinical trial: rifaximin improves health-related quality of life in cirrhotic patients with hepatic encephalopathy - a double-blind placebo-controlled study. Aliment Pharmacol Ther. 2011;34(8):853–61.

46. Eltawil KM, Laryea M, Peltekian K, et al. Rifaximin vs. conventional oral therapy for hepatic encephalopathy: a meta-analysis. World J Gastroenterol 2012;18(8):767–77.

47. Kimer N, Krag A, Møller S, et al. Systematic review with meta-analysis: the effects of rifaximin in hepatic encephalopathy. Aliment Pharmacol Ther 2014;40(2):123–32.

48. Bajaj JS, Barrett AC, Bortey E, et al. Prolonged remission from hepatic encephalopathy with rifaximin: results of a placebo crossover analysis. Aliment Pharmacol Ther 2015;41(1):39–45.

49. Patel VC, Lee S, McPhail MJW, et al. Rifaximin-α reduces gut-derived inflammation and mucin degradation in cirrhosis and encephalopathy: RIFSYS randomised controlled trial. J Hepatol 2022;76(2):332–342.

50. Sharma BC, Sharma P, Lunia MK, et al. A randomized, double-blind, controlled trial comparing rifaximin plus lactulose with lactulose alone in treatment of overt hepatic encephalopathy. Am J Gastroenterol. 2013;108(9):1458–1463.

51. Hudson M, Schuchmann M. Long-term management of hepatic encephalopathy with lactulose and/or rifaximin: a review of the evidence. Eur J Gastroenterol Hepatol. 2019;31(4):434–450.

52. Wang Z, Chu P, Wang W. Combination of rifaximin and lactulose improves clinical efficacy and mortality in patients with hepatic encephalopathy. Drug Des Devel Ther. 2018;13:1–11.

53. Fu J, Gao Y, Shi L. Combination therapy with rifaximin and lactulose in hepatic encephalopathy: A systematic review and meta-analysis. PLoS ONE 2022;17(4):e0267647.

37 | Hepatorenal Syndrome

Kidney failure is the most frequent organ failure in patients with acute or chronic liver disease, with a frequency of 20–50% in hospitalized cirrhotic patients [1–3].

Hepatorenal syndrome (HRS) is a life-threatening complication and one of many causes of acute kidney injury in patients with acute or chronic liver disease. HRS frequently occurs in hospitalized patients and is associated with a high mortality rate (about 32 to 37%) [4–6], readmission rate (about 23%) [5], hospital and health care costs [6, 7], and longer stay in hospital [4].

The most common precipitating factors of HRS are gastrointestinal bleeding, large volume paracentesis, diuretics, non-steroidal anti-inflammatory drugs (NSAIDs), spontaneous bacterial peritonitis, and other infections [5, 8].

DEFINITIONS AND TYPES OF HEPATORENAL SYNDROME

Hepatorenal syndrome is a specific cause of acute kidney injury (AKI) frequently encountered in advanced cirrhosis characterized by rapidly progressive renal failure, which occurs without apparent pathologic abnormalities in the kidneys [9].

Hepatorenal syndrome is traditionally classified into Type 1 and Type 2 HRS based on the severity of diseases reflected by the rapidity of decline in kidney function [10]. Type 1 (HRS-1) is a serious form of AKI that occurs in advanced cirrhosis with ascites.

Type 1 HRS is characterized by a rapid and progressive reduction in renal function (a 2-fold increase of serum creatinine to at least 2.5 mg/dL or a decrease of creatinine clearance by 50% to less than 20 mL/min within 2 weeks) [11], and has a poor prognosis (median survival only 8 to 12 weeks) [12]. Type 2 HRS is a less severe form of kidney function impairment that is slowly progressive and clinically characterized by ascites resistant to diuretics [11] and has a median survival of about 6 months [12].

The traditional classification of HRS-1 and HRS-2 has recently been reclassified (Type 1 HRS renamed as HRS-acute kidney injury (HRS-AKI), and HRS-2 renamed as HRS-NAKI (that is, non-AKI) [13–15]. Diagnostic features of HRS-AKI as recommendations by the International Club of Ascites (2019) are summarized in Table 37.1 [13].

PATHOGENESIS

The pathogenesis of HRS is multifactorial, complex, and poorly understood. However, two major mechanisms that interact and contribute to the development of HRS-AKI are the combination of hemodynamic abnormalities and systemic inflammation [3].

A. Hemodynamic abnormalities: The "splanchnic arterial vasodilation theory" is the main hypothesis in the pathophysiology of HRS [16]. Essential components of the pathogenesis of neurohormonal cascade in HRS are:

- **Vasodilatation:** In portal hypertension, increased intrahepatic vascular tone promotes the release of vasodilatory substances like nitric oxide and prostaglandins, which cause arterial vasodilatation in the splanchnic and systemic circulation.

- **Activation of vasoconstrictors:** Systemic and splanchnic vasodilation reduces effective arterial blood volume and systemic arterial pressure, which triggers the carotid and aortic arch baroreceptors and activates three powerful vasoconstrictor systems (renin-angiotensin-aldosterone system, vasopressin release, and activation of the sympathetic nervous system).

- **Renal vasoconstriction:** Activation of vasoconstrictor systems increases arterial pressure and kidney vasoconstriction. In advanced stages of cirrhosis, synthesis of vasodilator factors is more pronounced with further vasodilatation of systemic and splanchnic and resultant worsening of hypotension [17]. Vasoconstrictor systems are further activated [18] to combat severe hypotension and achieve optimal arterial pressure, which is compatible with life. As renal circulation is very sensitive to the vasoconstrictive effects of these vasoconstrictors, it causes a marked reduction in renal perfusion and the development of HRS-AKI [19].

Table 37.1 Diagnostic criteria of HRS-AKI
1. Presence of cirrhosis and ascites
2. Presence of AKI (increase in serum creatinine >0.3 mg/dL within 48 hours, or >50% increase in serum creatinine from baseline in 3 months)
3. Lack of improvement of serum creatinine (decrease of creatinine ≤0.3 mg/dL of baseline) after at least 48 hr of diuretic withdrawal and volume expansion with albumin (1 gm/kg body weight/day for 2 d)
4. Absence of shock (septic, cardiogenic, distributive)
5. Exclusion of current or prior treatment with nephrotoxic drugs
6. Absence of proteinuria ≥500 mg/day, microhematuria, or structural abnormalities on ultrasonography

- **Cardiac dysfunction:** In cirrhotic patients with systemic vasodilation, cardiac output increases initially. But with the progression of liver disease, cardiac output decreases, further reducing impaired renal blood flow and contributing to the development of hepatorenal syndrome [20, 21].

B. Systemic inflammation: According to this new theory, in portal hypertension, gut permeability increases, causing bacterial translocation from the gut to mesenteric lymph nodes, which triggers a systemic inflammatory response with the release of pro-inflammatory cytokine [18]. Three different mechanisms by which systemic inflammation causes organ dysfunction, and failure are [22–24]: (1) Nitric oxide production in splanchnic arterioles due to systemic inflammation accentuates the preexisting splanchnic vasodilation and stimulates endogenous vasoconstrictor systems causing renal hypoperfusion; (2) Activation of immune cells resulting in tissue damage; and (3) Metabolic alterations.

DIAGNOSIS

In patients with cirrhosis, renal dysfunction can occur due to HRS and many other causes for the development of AKI in cirrhotic patients, such as hypovolemia (gastrointestinal [GI] bleeding, use of diuretics or GI losses), medications (drug-induced or contrast-induced nephropathy), infections, intrinsic renal disease, and obstructive uropathy [25]. In cirrhotic patients with HRS, multiple causes that can potentially lead to AKI can coexist and overlap [26].

While evaluating AKI in patients with liver disease, it is important to remember that hepatorenal syndrome is the cause of AKI in about 15–43% [27, 28], AKI frequently occurs due to hypovolemia in 27–50% of all cases, and acute tubular necrosis (ATN) in about 14–35%.

As hepatorenal syndrome (HRS-AKI) is a diagnosis of exclusion, it is essential to exclude other potential causes of kidney injury in patients with liver disease [15, 18]. So detailed history, clinical assessment, laboratory assessments, and abdominal imaging should be performed to exclude different causes of AKI, such as prerenal AKI (hypovolemia), acute tubular necrosis (hypovolemic shock, infection, or nephrotoxic agents), and other causes (abdominal compartment syndrome, glomerulonephritis, acute interstitial nephritis, and obstructive uropathy) [29, 30]. Differentiating ATN and HRS-AKI may be difficult, and in such patients, the role of urinary biomarkers is promising and may prove helpful [31, 32].

PREVENTION

As HRS carries a poor prognosis, it is better to prevent than treat it. Measures to prevent HRS are:

- Avoid using nephrotoxic drugs (such as NSAIDs, aminoglycosides, amphotericin, ACE-I, angiotensin receptor blockers, or radiographic dye), and use diuretics and laxatives judiciously.

- Early detection and prompt treatment of coexisting infections and antibiotic prophylaxis in patients with increased risk of spontaneous bacterial peritonitis are effective measures to prevent AKI-HRS [28].

- Correct intravascular volume depletion, which may occur due to excessive diuretic use, diarrhea due to lactulose, variceal bleeding, and large volume paracentesis without albumin administration).

- IV albumin infusion: In patients with spontaneous bacterial peritonitis, the

IV administration of albumin reduces the risk of both kidney function impairment and mortality [33–35].

- In patients with spontaneous bacterial peritonitis, albumin is started together with antibiotics. The recommended dose of IV albumin to prevent HRS is 1.5 gm/kg within 6 hours of detection of infection (on the first day) and a second dose of 1 gm/kg after 48 hours of the first dose (on the third day).

- During large volume paracentesis, replacing 6–8 gm of albumin for every liter of ascites removed reduces the risk of HRS-AKI [14, 30, 36, 37].

- Antibiotics prophylaxis: In patients with advanced cirrhosis, administration of oral norfloxacin (or alternative trimethoprim-sulfamethoxazole if norfloxacin is unavailable) decreases the one-year probability of spontaneous bacterial peritonitis, delays the development of HRS, and improves survival [38]. Rifaximin also reduced the incidence of HRS-AKI in cirrhotic patients [39, 40].

- Early diagnosis and prompt management of gastrointestinal bleeding.

- Pentoxifylline: Due to its protective effect against oxidative renal cell injury, pentoxifylline (1200 mg/day) is found to reduce the risk of HRS-AKI in alcoholic hepatitis and may be an effective prophylaxis [41–44]. However, larger studies are needed to validate the efficacy [45, 46].

- As HRS is a common complication in acute alcohol hepatitis, early detection and treatment of alcoholic hepatitis, alcohol abstinence, and proper nutritional supplementation are essential [47].

MANAGEMENT

HRS requires early and aggressive therapy because, besides all therapeutic advances, the outcome of HRS is poor.

The goals of management of hepatorenal syndrome are:

- Identify and treat reversible factors.

- To correct hypovolemia and avoid volume overload.

- To achieve a higher mean arterial blood pressure (rise in MAP ≥10–15 mmHg from baseline) is the most effective approach for better perfusion of the kidneys [29, 48, 49].

- Reversal of hemodynamic disturbances and acute kidney injury.

- To stabilize the patient, provide renal replacement therapy if necessary, and prolong survival until candidates undergo liver transplantation.

Three primary treatment options for managing HRS are general measures, pharmacological therapy, and non-pharmacological therapy.

A. General measures

- Meticulous evaluation to diagnose underlying precipitating factors and their early treatment.

- Volume expansion. The first step in managing AKI in cirrhosis is volume expansion (with crystalloids or intravenous albumin). As prerenal AKI is the most common cause of renal failure in cirrhotic patients, it is essential to correct hypovolemia immediately by replacing fluids, considering the cause and severity of the fluid loss [14, 18, 50]. Normal saline infusion is preferred to correct hypovolemia due to vomiting or the excess dose of diuretics. Blood or blood products effectively correct hypovolemia and anemia due to gastrointestinal bleeding. The reversal of AKI in 48 hours with volume expansion favors prerenal AKI [50].

- Assessing the volume status of cirrhotic patients can be challenging due to the complexity of the condition. At times it can be challenging to correct hypovolemia optimally in these patients because they may have intravascular volume depletion despite the presence of ascites or peripheral edema. Additionally, over-infusing fluids can worsen existing conditions such as ascites, pleural effusion, heart failure, or respiratory failure [51].

- To determine the best approach for volume assessment and fluid management, a careful history, detailed clinical examination, laboratory tests, X-ray-based imaging, and point-of-care ultrasound should be used [52].

- Stop β-blockers in patients with low or borderline blood pressure [14]. Discontinue nephrotoxic drugs (as discussed in prevention).

- Stop diuretics and avoid the temptation to use diuretics to increase urine output in severe AKI in HRS [14]. Diuretic therapy in HRS can lead to volume depletion and further reduction of effective circulating volume, which can aggravate renal hypoperfusion and may trigger or worsen HRS [53, 54]. In addition, it is essential to discontinue spironolactone in HRS as it carries the risk of life-threatening hyperkalemia.

- As spontaneous bacterial peritonitis is a main triggering factor of AKI-HRS, its prompt treatment with albumin and antibiotics helps in preventing AKI-HRS [28, 33, 34]. But the administration of albumin is not recommended in patients of HRS with non-spontaneous bacterial peritonitis infections [55, 56].

- Always search for the presence of electrolyte disorders (such as hyponatremia, hyperkalemia, hypokalemia, etc.) or acid-base disorders (such as respiratory alkalosis, metabolic alkalosis, and metabolic acidosis) and treat them [51].

- Etiology-driven management of AKI.

- Measure vitals, urine output, fluid balance, and daily weight and closely monitor patients.

B. Pharmacological therapy

Combined therapy with albumin and a vasopressor is recommended as the first line of treatment for HRS-AKI and should be started as soon as possible [14, 18, 30, 57].

Albumin

In cirrhotic patients with AKI, administering albumin is important for both diagnostic and therapeutic purposes [18, 58].

It is essential to differentiate AKI-HRS from prerenal AKI because AKI occurs due to prerenal AKI in about half of patients with AKI in cirrhosis.

Renal recovery within 48 hours after administration of albumin (along with removing risk factors and discontinuing diuretics) favors the diagnosis of prerenal AKI, and failure in improvement in renal function suggests the diagnosis of AKI-HRS [15].

IV Albumin is recommended for volume resuscitation in prerenal AKI regardless of the etiology or severity of prerenal azotemia [52].

Effects: Albumin infusion increases oncotic pressure, effectively expands circulating volume, improves hemodynamics and cardiac output, increases renal perfusion, and enhances renal recovery.

In addition to volume expanding effects in HRS, other benefits of albumin proposed in current literature are [37, 58, 59] antioxidant and anti-inflammatory effects [60, 61], positive cardiac inotropic effects [62], improvement in the autoregulation of renal perfusion [63], preservation of the integrity of endothelial glycocalyx [64], and stabilization of endothelial function [65].

Dose: Recommended dose of albumin is 1 gm/kg/d (up to 100 gm/d) for two consecutive days, preferably given in divided doses (e.g., 25 gm every 6 hourly) [13, 14]. Subsequently, the dose may decrease to 20–40 gm daily. However, as per the recent ATTIRE trial (2021), tailoring albumin therapy to raise serum albumin to 3.0 gm/dL or more is not beneficial in reducing infection, kidney dysfunction, or death [66].

Combination therapy: It is important to remember that instead of albumin alone, combination therapy of albumin with vasoconstrictor therapy is more effective [67–70]. Therefore all guidelines recommend albumin with vasoconstrictor, the adjunct therapy for HRS-AKI [3, 14, 30, 57]. This combination therapy significantly improves renal function in HRS and reduces mortality compared with no treatment or albumin alone [15, 71, 72].

Duration of treatment: Albumin plus vasoconstrictor therapy should be continued until serum creatinine reduces to a value within 0.3 mg of the baseline value of serum creatinine [15].

Combination therapy is discontinued within 14 days if patients do not respond or respond partially [15].

Adverse effect: The major concern of albumin infusion in HRS is the significant risk of volume overload, especially pulmonary edema [66, 70].

So, before administration, it is essential to assess volume status and avoid albumin infusion in patients with volume overload.

As albumin increases preload and terlipressin increases afterload, the combined treatment carries the risk of precipitation of pulmonary edema [29].

Vasoconstrictors

Administration of IV albumin, combined with vasoconstrictors such as IV terlipressin, noradrenaline, or oral midodrine plus octreotide initiated as soon as the diagnosis of HRS is suspected. The combination therapy helps in the reversal of hemodynamic disturbances, restoration of effective circulating volume, and improvement in renal perfusion.

Terlipressin

According to international guidelines, terlipressin, a synthetic vasopressin analog, is recommended as the first and most preferred vasoconstrictor for managing HRS [14, 18, 25, 30, 57, 73, 74]. This is because it has been shown to improve renal function in 24–44% of patients in various studies [68–70, 75–79] and meta-analyses [69, 71, 72, 80–83], making it an effective treatment option for HRS. In addition, potent vasoconstrictor terlipressin is also found to reduce short-term mortality and hospital cost in various studies [71, 72, 81, 84, 85]. But the effect on mortality is controversial as survival benefits are lacking in other literature [69, 70, 76, 80].

Mechanism of action: Terlipressin has a high affinity for V1 receptors. V1 receptors are predominantly located in the splanchnic bed and systemic vascular smooth muscle, while V2 receptors are found more commonly in the kidney. Because of its selective effect, terlipressin causes splanchnic vessels and extrarenal vasoconstriction, which improves effective circulating volume and renal perfusion pressures.

Indications: In HRS, initiate terlipressin at early stages of AKI (i.e., serum creatinine >1.5 mg/dL), as there is a higher likelihood of a positive response to treatment when initiated at an earlier stage. However, avoid using terlipressin in milder forms of HRS-AKI (i.e., serum creatinine <1.5 mg/dL) as they are typically benign and potentially reversible with fluid expansion alone. Terlipressin should also be avoided in patients with advanced renal dysfunction (i.e., serum creatinine >5.0 mg/dL or higher).

Dose: Initial dosage of terlipressin in HRS is 1–2 mg/12 h by continuous IV infusion or 0.5–1.0 mg/4–6 h by IV boluses, and the dose is progressively increased as per need [14]. In the absence of response, the dose of continuous IV terlipressin infusion should be increased stepwise from 2 mg/day to a maximum of 12 mg/d according to the change in urine output and serum creatinine [74, 86]. One ampoule (8.5 ml solution) contains 1 mg terlipressin acetate.

Route: Administration of terlipressin by continuous IV infusion is preferred over IV boluses because infusion is better tolerated, and the requirement of effective doses is lower [87].

Poor response: Response to terlipressin is poor in HRS-AKI patients with higher total serum bilirubin [88], higher serum creatinine [89], underlying chronic kidney disease (CKD) with significant structural kidney injury, presence of severe bacterial infections [90], and failure to achieve an increase in the mean arterial pressure and cardiac output [73].

Contraindications: As terlipressin causes extrarenal vasoconstriction, it is usually avoided in HRS patients with coronary artery disease, cerebral or peripheral vascular diseases, cardiac arrhythmias, asthma, chronic obstructive pulmonary disease, and elderly patients [91].

Adverse effects: Common adverse effects of terlipressin are abdominal pain, nausea, diarrhea (due to gastrointestinal smooth muscle spasm), coronary or peripheral vascular ischemic complications, and respiratory adverse events. Serious side effects like dyspnea and respiratory distress occur because of terlipressin-induced pulmonary vasoconstriction and cardiac overload because of increased afterload due to terlipressin and preload due to albumin [74, 92].

Measures suggested to reduce respiratory adverse events of terlipressin are judicious use of albumin and careful attention to respiratory distress, monitoring pulse oximetry, and frequent chest radiographs or point of care ultrasound [93].

Terlipressin was introduced first time in the year 1990 and was widely used worldwide subsequently. But due to respiratory adverse events [70] and the lack of mortality benefits [94], it was not approved by the FDA and therefore was unavailable. However, recently, in September 2022, the US FDA approved the use of terlipressin for the treatment of hepatorenal syndrome in adults [95].

Norepinephrine (Noradrenaline)

In a country like the USA, where terlipressin was unavailable till recently (September 2022), norepinephrine (plus albumin) was a preferred agent and considered a first-line treatment for HRS [52]. Early studies and meta-analyses have shown equal effectiveness of terlipressin plus albumin and norepinephrine plus albumin in reversing HRS [96–101], but in a recent study, terlipressin plus albumin was associated with a higher HRS reversal rate in patients with acute on chronic liver failure [102].

The advantages of norepinephrine are that it is significantly cheaper than terlipressin and is widely available with fewer side effects [78, 96, 100, 101, 103]. In addition, physicians use norepinephrine routinely and are very familiar with its use because it is the most standard drug for augmenting sepsis circulation.

But the requirements of the central venous catheter for its administration and the need for ICU or close monitoring for potential adverse effects such as arrhythmia and ischemia may offset the cost-benefit of this drug [103–105].

Mechanism of action: Alpha-adrenergic agonist norepinephrine by nonselective systemic vasoconstriction improves the mean arterial pressure and renal perfusion in HRS.

Dose: The dose of norepinephrine varies from 0.5 to 3 mg/h in HRS. Norepinephrine is usually started at an initial dose of 1 mg/hour by continuous infusion and is gradually increased to maintain the mean arterial blood pressure to ensure renal perfusion [106].

Midodrine and octreotide

In the USA, until now, the combination of midodrine and octreotide is routinely used to treat HRS-1 in general wards because terlipressin was not available in the USA, and norepinephrine cannot be administered outside of the intensive care unit [52]. But as compared to terlipressin and norepinephrine, the combination of midodrine and octreotide has shown low rates of renal recovery in HRS [72, 107, 108].

Therefore, midodrine and octreotide having much lower efficacy than terlipressin, are not preferred in ICU patients and are used in general wards only when terlipressin is unavailable [14, 30].

The combination of midodrine and octreotide plus albumin is the most effective therapy for increasing serum sodium in dilutional hyponatremia associated with HRS [83].

Midodrine is an orally available alpha-adrenergic agonist which causes systemic vasoconstriction and improves renal perfusion. Midodrine is usually started at a dose of 5–7.5 mg thrice daily orally, which can be increased maximum up to 15 mg three times daily as needed [109]. Synthetic somatostatin octreotide is potent splanchnic vasoconstriction which is given either as a continuous infusion (usual initial dose 50 mcg/h) or subcutaneously (usual dose 100–200 mcg/8 h) [109]. The combination of octreotide and midodrine is beneficial in HRS, but midodrine as a monotherapy does not improve renal function.

The selection of vasoconstrictors with albumin in hepatorenal syndrome based on treatment setup (in the intensive care unit or ward) is summarized in Table 37.2.

C. Non-pharmacological therapy

When patients do not respond to the above pharmacological measures,

Table 37.2 Vasoconstrictor with albumin in hepatorenal syndrome				
Albumin To all patients (expands intravascular volume)				
Choice of vasoconstrictors				
	Setup	Firstline drugs	Class	Route
Terlipressin available	ICU	Terlipressin	Vasopressin analog	IV
	Wards			
Terlipressin not available	ICU	Norepinephrine	Alpha agonist	IV
	Wards	Midodrine and octreotide	Alpha agonist Somatostatin analog	Oral and SQ
Duration of therapy: About 1–2 weeks				
Goal: To raise mean arterial pressure by 10–15 mm of Hg, reduction of serum creatinine <1.5 mg/dL				

treatment options are dialysis, transjugular intrahepatic portosystemic shunt (TIPS), liver transplantation, or simultaneous liver-kidney transplantation.

Renal replacement therapy (RRT)

The use of RRT in patients with HRS is controversial [110–112]. HRS patients with failure of medical treatment but the possibility of improvement in kidney or liver function or patients who are eligible for liver transplantation are usually offered RRT [52]. Common indications of RRT in HRS-AKI are worsening renal function, electrolyte disturbances, or increasing volume overload besides optimum vasoconstrictor therapy [30].

Transjugular intrahepatic portosystemic shunt

TIPS may be used as a salvage therapy when medical management fails. When the intrahepatic stent is connected between the portal vein and the hepatic vein, it redirects portal blood into the systemic circulation, which decompresses the portal system and increases systemic venous return leading

to the return of more blood to the heart, causing increased cardiac output and improvement in arterial and renal perfusion. In a recent meta-analysis, it was found that TIPS can improve serum creatinine levels, urine volume, and urinary sodium excretion [113].

However, TIPS is not routinely recommended in patients with AKI-HRS because: (1) In clinical practice, its use is very limited (contraindicated in HRS with severe liver failure or severe hepatic encephalopathy) [14]; (2) It is associated with complications such as procedure-related bleeding, worsening of liver function, or development of hepatic encephalopathy [114]; and (3) Its role of in HRS is not precisely defined [115] and data supporting its use are insufficient [30].

Liver transplantation

Liver transplantation is the only curative treatment and therapy of choice for both types of HRS. But unfortunately, this most effective modality is available to a small fraction of the affected patients, and many patients die before a donor liver can be obtained.

Simultaneous liver-kidney transplantation (SLKT)

SLKT is usually recommended in patients with HRS-AKI when kidney function is not expected to recover post-liver transplantation (e.g., AKI associated with dialysis ≥6 weeks and glomerular filtration rate [GFR] ≤25 mL/min for more than 6 weeks or presence of underlying advanced CKD or CKD requiring dialysis) [116, 117].

REFERENCE

1. Garcia-Tsao G, Parikh CR, Viola A. Acute kidney injury in cirrhosis. Hepatology. 2008;48(6):2064–77.

2. Tandon P, James M, Abraldes J, et al. Relevance of New Definitions to Incidence and Prognosis of Acute Kidney Injury in Hospitalized Patients with Cirrhosis: A Retrospective Population-Based Cohort Study. PLoS One 2016;11(8):e0160394.

3. Bajaj JS, O'Leary JG, Lai JC, et al. Acute-on-Chronic Liver Failure Clinical Guidelines. Am J Gastroenterol. 2022;117(2):225–252.

4. Pant C, Jani BS, Desai M, et al. Hepatorenal syndrome in hospitalized patients with chronic liver disease: results from the Nationwide Inpatient Sample 2002–2012. J Investig Med 2016;64(1):33–38.

5. Jamil K, Huang X, Hayashida D, et al. The Hepatorenal Syndrome Patient Pathway: Retrospective Analysis of Electronic Health Records. Curr Ther Res Clin Exp. 2022;96:100663.

6. Jamil K, Huang X, Lovelace B, et al. The burden of illness of hepatorenal syndrome (HRS) in the United States: a retrospective analysis of electronic health records. J Med Econ. 2019;22(5):421–429.

7. Rice JP, Skagen C, Said A. Liver transplant outcomes for patients with hepatorenal syndrome treated with pretransplant vasoconstrictors and albumin. Transplantation, 2011;91(10):1141–7.

8. Low G, Alexander GJ, Lomas DJ. Hepatorenal syndrome: aetiology, diagnosis, and treatment. Gastroenterol Res Pract. 2015;2015:207012.

9. Durand F, Graupera I, Ginès P, et al. Pathogenesis of hepatorenal syndrome: implications for therapy. Am J Kidney Dis 2016;67(2):318–328.

10. Arroyo V. New treatments for hepatorenal syndrome. Liver Transplantation. 2000;6(3):287–289.

11. Arroyo V, Gines P, Gerbes AL, et al. Definition and diagnostic criteria of refractory ascites and hepatorenal syndrome in cirrhosis. International Ascites Club. Hepatology 1996;23(1):164–176.

12. Ng CK, Chan MH, Tai MH, et al. Hepatorenal syndrome. Clin Biochem Rev. 2007;28(1):11–17.

13. Angeli P, Garcia-Tsao G, Nadim MK, et al. News in pathophysiology, definition and classification of hepatorenal syndrome: A step beyond the International Club of Ascites (ICA) consensus document. J Hepatol. 2019;71(4):811–822.

14. European Association for the Study of the Liver. EASL Clinical Practice Guidelines for the management of patients with decompensated cirrhosis. J Hepatol. 2018;69(2):406–60.

15. Angeli P, Garcia-Tsao G, Nadim MK, et al. News in pathophysiology, definition and classification of hepatorenal syndrome: a step beyond the International Club of Ascites (ICA) consensus document. J Hepatol 2019;71(4):811–22.

16. Schrier RW, Arroyo V, Bernardi M, et al. Peripheral arteriolar vasodilation hypothesis: a proposal for the initiation of renal sodium and water retention in cirrhosis. Hepatology 1988;8(5):1151–1157.

17. Francoz C, Durand F, Kahn JA, et al. Hepatorenal Syndrome. Clin J Am Soc Nephrol. 2019;14(5):774–781.

18. Morelli MC, Rendina M, La Manna G, et al. Position paper on liver and kidney diseases from the Italian Association for the Study of Liver (AISF), in collaboration with the Italian Society of Nephrology (SIN). Dig Liver Dis. 2021;53(Suppl 2):S49–S86.

19. Neong SF, Adebayo D, Wong F. An update on the pathogenesis and clinical management of cirrhosis with refractory ascites. Expert Rev Gastroenterol Hepatol 2019;13(4):293–305.

20. Krag A, Bendtsen F, Henriksen JH, et al. Low cardiac output predicts development of hepatorenal syndrome and survival in patients with cirrhosis and ascites. Gut. 2010;59(1):105–10.

21. Kazory A, Ronco C. Hepatorenal Syndrome or Hepatocardiorenal Syndrome: Revisiting Basic Concepts in View of Emerging Data. Cardiorenal Med. 2019;9(1):1–7.

22. Albillos A, Lario M, Alvarez-Mon M. Cirrhosis-associated immune dysfunction: distinctive features and clinical relevance. J Hepatol 2014;61(6):1385–1396.

23. Bernardi M, Moreau R, Angeli P, et al. Mechanisms of decompensation and organ failure in cirrhosis: From peripheral arterial vasodilation to systemic inflammation hypothesis. J Hepatol 2015;63(5):1272–84.

24. Arroyo V, Angeli P, Moreau R, et al. The systemic inflammation hypothesis: towards a new paradigm of acute decompensation and multiorgan failure in cirrhosis. J Hepatol 2021;74(3):670–685.

25. Terra C, Mattos ÂZ, Pereira G, et al. Recommendations of the Brazilian society of hepatology for the management of acute kidney injury in patients with cirrhosis. Arq Gastroenterol. 2018;55(3):314–320.

26. Velez JCQ, Therapondos G, Juncos LA. Reappraising the spectrum of AKI and hepatorenal syndrome in patients with cirrhosis. Nat Rev Nephrol 2020;16(3):137–155.

27. Ginès P, Schrier RW. Renal failure in cirrhosis. N Engl J Med 2009;361(13):1279–1290.

28. Ginès P, Solà E, Angeli P, et al. Hepatorenal syndrome. Nat Rev Dis Primers 2018;4(1):23.

29. Velez JCQ. Hepatorenal Syndrome Type 1: From Diagnosis Ascertainment to Goal-Oriented Pharmacologic Therapy. Kidney360. 2021;3(2):382–395.

30. Biggins SW, Angeli P, Garcia-Tsao G, et al. Diagnosis, Evaluation, and Management of Ascites, Spontaneous Bacterial Peritonitis and Hepatorenal Syndrome: 2021 Practice Guidance by the American Association for the Study of Liver Diseases. Hepatology. 2021;74(2):1014–1048.

31. Pozzoli S, Simonini M, Manunta P. Predicting acute kidney injury: current status and future challenges. J Nephrol. 2018;31(2):209–223.

32. Lee HA, Seo YS. Current knowledge about biomarkers of acute kidney injury in liver cirrhosis. Clin Mol Hepatol. 2022;28(1):31–46.

33. Salerno F, Navickis RJ, Wilkes MM. Albumin infusion improves outcomes of patients with spontaneous bacterial peritonitis: a meta-analysis of randomized trials. Clin Gastroenterol Hepatol 2013;11(2):123–30.e1.

34. Sort P, Navasa M, Arroyo V, et al. Effect of intravenous albumin on renal impairment and mortality in patients with cirrhosis and spontaneous bacterial peritonitis. N Engl J Med 1999;341(6):403–9.

35. Salerno F, Gerbes A, Ginès P, et al. Diagnosis, prevention and treatment of hepatorenal syndrome in cirrhosis. Gut. 2007;56(9):1310–8.

36. Bernardi M, Caraceni P, Navickis RJ, et al. Albumin infusion in patients undergoing large-volume paracentesis: a meta-analysis of randomized trials. Hepatology. 2012;55(4):1172–81.

37. Bernardi M, Angeli P, Claria J, et al. Albumin in decompensated cirrhosis: new concepts and perspectives. Gut 2020;69(8):1127–38.

38. Fernández J, Navasa M, Planas R, et al. Primary prophylaxis of spontaneous bacterial peritonitis delays hepatorenal syndrome and improves survival in cirrhosis. Gastroenterology 2007;133(3):818–24.

39. Dong T, Aronsohn A, Gautham Reddy K, et al. Rifaximin decreases the incidence and severity of acute kidney injury and hepatorenal syndrome in cirrhosis. Dig Dis Sci 2016;61(12):3621–6.

40. Flamm SL, Mullen KD, Heimanson Z, et al. Rifaximin has the potential to prevent complications of cirrhosis. Therap Adv Gastroenterol 2018;11:1756284818808030.

41. Akriviadis E, Botla R, Briggs W, et al. Pentoxifylline improves short-term survival in severe acute alcoholic hepatitis: a double-blind, placebo-controlled trial. Gastroenterology. 2000;119(6):1637–1648.

42. Tyagi P, Sharma P, Sharma BC, et al. Prevention of hepatorenal syndrome in patients with cirrhosis and ascites: a pilot randomized control trial between pentoxifylline and placebo. Eur J Gastroenterol Hepatol 2011;23(3):210–217.

43. Ozturk H, Cetinkaya A, Firat TS, et al. Protective effect of pentoxifylline on oxidative renal cell injury associated with renal crystal formation in a hyperoxaluric rat model. Urolithiasis 2019;47(5):415–424.

44. Lee YS, Kim HJ, Kim JH, et al. Treatment of severe alcoholic hepatitis with corticosteroid, pentoxifylline, or dual therapy: a systematic review and meta-analysis. J Clin Gastroenterol. 2017;51(4):364–377.

45. Whitfield K, Rambaldi A, Wetterslev J, et al. Pentoxifylline for alcoholic hepatitis. Cochrane Database Syst Rev 2009;2009(4):CD007339.

46. Stine JG, Wang J, Cornella SL, et al. Treatment of Type-1 hepatorenal syndrome with pentoxifylline: a randomized placebo controlled clinical trial. Ann Hepatol 2018;17(2):300–6.

47. Tariq R, Singal AK. Management of Hepatorenal Syndrome: A Review. J Clin Transl Hepatol. 2020;8(2):192–199.

48. Velez JC, Nietert PJ. Therapeutic response to vasoconstrictors in hepatorenal syndrome parallels increase in mean arterial pressure: a pooled analysis of clinical trials. Am J Kidney Dis. 2011;58(6):928–38.

49. Velez JC, Kadian M, Taburyanskaya M, et al. Hepatorenal Acute Kidney Injury and the Importance of Raising Mean Arterial Pressure. Nephron. 2015;131(3):191–201.

50. Russ KB, Stevens TM, Singal AK. Acute Kidney Injury in Patients with Cirrhosis. J Clin Transl Hepatol. 2015;3(3):195–204.

51. Velasco JAVR, García-Jiménez ES, Aldana-Ledesma JM, et al. Evaluation and management of emergencies in the patient with cirrhosis Rev Gastroenterol Méx. 2022;87(2):198–215.

52. Cullaro G, Kanduri SR, Velez JCQ. Acute Kidney Injury in Patients with Liver Disease. Clin J Am Soc Nephrol. 2022:CJN.03040322.

53. Piano S, Angeli P. Dopamine and Furosemide for the Treatment of Hepatorenal Syndrome: A Reappraisal or Just Smoke and Mirrors? J Clin Exp Hepatol. 2015;5(4):273–5.

54. Dundar HZ, Yılmazlar T. Management of hepatorenal syndrome. World J Nephrol. 2015;4(2):277–86.

55. Leao GS, Neto GJ, Jotz RF, et al. Albumin for cirrhotic patients with extraperitoneal infections: a meta-analysis. J Gastroenterol Hepatol. 2019;34(12):2071–2076.

56. Zaccherini G, Tufoni M, Bernardi M. Albumin administration is efficacious in the management of patients with cirrhosis: a systematic review of the literature. Hepat Med 2020;12:153–72.

57. Aithal GP, Palaniyappan N, China L, et al. Guidelines on the management of ascites in cirrhosis. Gut 2021;70(1):9–29.

58. Tufoni M, Zaccherini G, Caraceni P, et al. Albumin: Indications in chronic liver disease. United European Gastroenterol J. 2020;8(5):528–535.

59. Valerio C, Theocharidou E, Davenport A, et al. Human albumin solution for patients with cirrhosis and acute on chronic liver failure: Beyond simple volume expansion. World J Hepatol 2016;8(7):345–354.

60. Arroyo V, García-Martinez R, Salvatella X. Human serum albumin, systemic inflammation, and cirrhosis. J Hepatol. 2014;61(2):396–407.

61. Fernández J, Clària J, Amorós A, et al. Effects of albumin treatment on systemic and portal hemodynamics and systemic inflammation in patients with decompensated cirrhosis. Gastroenterology 2019;157(1):149–162.

62. Bortoluzzi A, Ceolotto G, Gola E, et al. Positive cardiac inotropic effect of albumin infusion in rodents

with cirrhosis and ascites: molecular mechanisms. Hepatology 2013;57(1):266–276.

63. Garcia-Martinez R, Noiret L, Sen S, et al. Albumin infusion improves renal blood flow autoregulation in patients with acute decompensation of cirrhosis and acute kidney injury. Liver Int. 2015;35(2):335–43.

64. Aldecoa C, Llau JV, Nuvials X, et al. Role of albumin in the preservation of endothelial glycocalyx integrity and the microcirculation: a review. Ann Intensive Care. 2020;10(1):85.

65. Zhang WJ, Frei B. Albumin selectively inhibits TNF alpha-induced expression of vascular cell adhesion molecule-1 in human aortic endothelial cells. Cardiovasc Res 2002;55(4):820–9.

66. China L, Freemantle N, Forrest E, et al. A randomized trial of albumin infusions in hospitalized patients with cirrhosis. N Engl J Med. 2021;384(9):808–817.

67. Ortega R, Gines P, Uriz J, et al. Terlipressin therapy with and without albumin for patients with hepatorenal syndrome: results of a prospective, nonrandomized study. Hepatology. 2002;36(4 Pt 1):941–948.

68. Martín-Llahí M, Pépin MN, Guevara M, et al. Terlipressin and albumin vs albumin in patients with cirrhosis and hepatorenal syndrome: a randomized study. Gastroenterology 2008;134(5):1352–1359.

69. Boyer TD, Sanyal AJ, Wong F, et al. Terlipressin plus albumin is more effective than albumin alone in improving renal function in patients with cirrhosis and hepatorenal syndrome type 1. Gastroenterology 2016;150(7):1579–1589.e2.

70. Wong F, Pappas SC, Curry MP, et al. Terlipressin plus Albumin for the Treatment of Type 1 Hepatorenal Syndrome. N Engl J Med. 2021;384(9):818–828.

71. Gluud LL, Christensen K, Christensen E, et al. Systematic review of randomized trials on vasoconstrictor drugs for hepatorenal syndrome. Hepatology 2010;51(2):576–84.

72. Facciorusso A, Chandar AK, Murad MH, et al. Comparative efficacy of pharmacological strategies for management of type 1 hepatorenal syndrome: a systematic review and network meta-analysis. Lancet Gastroenterol Hepatol. 2017;2(2):94–102.

73. Arora A, Kumar A, Prasad N, et al. INASL-ISN Joint Position Statements on Management of Patients with Simultaneous Liver and Kidney Disease. J Clin Exp Hepatol. 2021;11(3):354–386.

74. Qi X, Bai Z, Zhu Q, et al. Practice guidance for the use of terlipressin for liver cirrhosis-related complications. Therap Adv Gastroenterol. 2022;15:17562848221098253.

75. Moreau R, Durand F, Poynard T, et al. Terlipressin in patients with cirrhosis and type 1 hepatorenal syndrome: a retrospective multicenter study. Gastroenterology 2002;122(4):923–930.

76. Sanyal AJ, Boyer T, Garcia-Tsao G, et al. A randomized, prospective, double-blind, placebo-controlled trial of terlipressin for type 1 hepatorenal syndrome. Gastroenterology 2008;134(5):1360–1368.

77. Sanyal AJ, Boyer TD, Frederick RT, et al. Reversal of hepatorenal syndrome type 1 with terlipressin plus albumin vs. placebo plus albumin in a pooled analysis of the OT-0401 and REVERSE randomised clinical studies. Aliment Pharmacol Ther. 2017;45(11):1390–1402.

78. Best LM, Freeman SC, Sutton AJ, et al. Treatment for hepatorenal syndrome in people with decompensated liver cirrhosis: a network meta-analysis. Cochrane Database Syst Rev. 2019;9(9):CD013103.

79. Moore K, Jamil K, Verleger K, et al. Real-world treatment patterns and outcomes using terlipressin in 203 patients with the hepatorenal syndrome. Aliment Pharmacol Ther. 2020;52(2):351–358.

80. Gifford FJ, Morling JR, Fallowfield JA. Systematic review with meta-analysis: vasoactive drugs for the treatment of hepatorenal syndrome type 1. Aliment Pharmacol Ther 2017;45(5):593–603.

81. Allegretti AS, Israelsen M, Krag A, et al. Terlipressin versus placebo or no intervention for people with cirrhosis and hepatorenal syndrome. Cochrane Database Syst Rev 2017;6(6):CD005162.

82. Nanda A, Reddy R, Safraz H, et al. Pharmacological Therapies for Hepatorenal Syndrome: A Systematic Review and Meta-Analysis. J Clin Gastroenterol. 2018;52(4):360–367.

83. Wang L, Long Y, Li KX, et al. Pharmacological treatment of hepatorenal syndrome: a network meta-analysis. Gastroenterol Rep 2019;8(2):111–118.

84. Sridharan K, Sivaramakrishnan G. Vasoactive agents for hepatorenal syndrome: a mixed treatment comparison network meta-analysis and trial sequential analysis of randomized clinical trials. J Gen Intern Med 2018;33(1):97–102.

85. Terres AZ, Balbinot RS, Muscope ALF, et al. Evidence-based protocol for diagnosis and treatment of hepatorenal syndrome is independently associated with lower mortality. Gastroenterol Hepatol 2022;45(1):25–39.

86. Facciorusso A. Hepatorenal Syndrome Type 1: Current Challenges and Future Prospects. Ther Clin Risk Manag. 2019;15:1383–1391.

87. Cavallin M, Piano S, Romano A, et al. Terlipressin given by continuous intravenous infusion versus intravenous boluses in the treatment of hepatorenal syndrome: a randomized controlled study. Hepatol Baltim Md. 2016;63(3):983–992.

88. Piano S, Schmidt HH, Ariza X, et al. Association between grade of acute on chronic liver failure and response to terlipressin and albumin in patients with hepatorenal syndrome. Clin Gastroenterol Hepatol Off Clin Pract J Am Gastroenterol Assoc. 2018;16(11):1792–1800.e3.

89. Boyer TD, Sanyal AJ, Garcia-Tsao G, et al. Predictors of response to terlipressin plus albumin in hepatorenal syndrome (HRS) type 1: relationship of serum creatinine to hemodynamics. J Hepatol. 2011;55(2):315–321.

90. Rodríguez E, Elia C, Solà E. Terlipressin and albumin for type-1 hepatorenal syndrome associated with sepsis. J Hepatol. 2014;60(5):955–961.

91. Sarin SK, Sharma P. Terlipressin: an asset for hepatologists! Hepatology. 2011;54(2):724–8.

92. Buccheri S, Da BL. Hepatorenal Syndrome: Definitions, Diagnosis, and Management. Clin Liver Dis. 2022;26(2):181–201.

93. Pichler RH, Swenson ER, Leary PJ, et al. Terlipressin: Hopes Fulfilled or Dashed? CJASN 2022;17(1):140–142.

94. Belcher JM, Parada XV, Simonetto DA, et al. Terlipressin and the Treatment of Hepatorenal Syndrome: How the CONFIRM Trial Moves the Story Forward. Am J Kidney Dis. 2022;79(5):737–745.

95. FDA Approved Drug Products: TERLIVAZ (terlipressin) for injection, for intravenous use (https://www.accessdata.fda.gov/drugsatfda_docs/label/2022/022231s000lbl.pdf).

96. Alessandria C, Ottobrelli A, Debernardi-Venon W, et al. Noradrenalin vs terlipressin in patients with hepatorenal syndrome: a prospective, randomized, unblinded, pilot study. J Hepatol. 2007;47(4):499–505.

97. Sharma P, Kumar A, Shrama BC, et al. An open label, pilot, randomized controlled trial of noradrenaline versus terlipressin in the treatment of type 1 hepatorenal syndrome and predictors of response. Am J Gastroenterol. 2008;103(7):1689–1697.

98. Singh V, Ghosh S, Singh B, et al. Noradrenaline vs. terlipressin in the treatment of hepatorenal syndrome: a randomized study. J Hepatol 2012;56(6):1293–1298.

99. Junior APN, Farias AQ, D' Albuquerque LAC, et al. Terlipressin versus norepinephrine in the treatment of hepatorenal syndrome: a systematic review and meta-analysis. PloS One. 2014;9(9):e107466.

100. Goyal O, Sidhu SS, Schgal N, et al. Noradrenaline is as effective as terlipressin in hepatorenal syndrome type 1: a prospective, randomized trial. J Assoc Physicians India. 2016;64(9):30–35.

101. Saif RU, Dar HA, Sofi SM, et al. Noradrenaline versus terlipressin in the management of type 1 hepatorenal syndrome: a randomized controlled study. Indian J Gastroenterol. 2018;37(5):424–429.

102. Arora V, Maiwall R, Rajan V, et al. Terlipressin is superior to noradrenaline in the management of acute kidney injury in acute on chronic liver failure. Hepatology 2020;71(2):600–610.

103. Ghosh S, Choudhary NS, Sharma AK, et al. Noradrenaline vs terlipressin in the treatment of type 2 hepatorenal syndrome: a randomized pilot study. Liver Int 2013;33(8):1187–93.

104. Subedi A, Suresh Kumar VC, Subedi AS, et al. A Review of Hepatorenal Syndrome. Cureus. 2021;13(7):e16084.

105. Bera C, Wong F. Management of hepatorenal syndrome in liver cirrhosis: a recent update. Therap Adv Gastroenterol. 2022;15:17562848221102679.

106. Gupta K, Rani P, Rohatgi A, et al. Noradrenaline for reverting hepatorenal syndrome: a prospective, observational, single-center study. Clin Exp Gastroenterol. 2018;11:317–324.

107. Cavallin M, Kamath PS, Merli M, et al. Terlipressin plus albumin versus midodrine and octreotide plus albumin in the treatment of hepatorenal syndrome: A randomized trial. Hepatology 2015;62(2):567–574.

108. Mahmoud EIED, Abdelaziz DH, Abd-Elsalam S, et al. Norepinephrine is more effective than midodrine/octreotide in patients with hepatorenal syndrome-acute kidney injury: a randomized controlled trial. Front Pharmacol 2021;12:675948.

109. Simonetto DA, Gines P, Kamath PS. Hepatorenal syndrome: pathophysiology, diagnosis, and management. BMJ. 2020;370:m2687.

110. Nadim MK, Kellum JA, Davenport A, et al. Hepatorenal syndrome: the 8th International Consensus Conference of the Acute Dialysis Quality Initiative (ADQI) Group. Crit Care. 2012;16(1):R23.

111. Velez JCQ. Patients with Hepatorenal Syndrome Should Be Dialyzed? PRO. Kidney360. 2020;2(3):406–409.

112. Wadei HM. Patients with Hepatorenal Syndrome Should Be Dialyzed? CON. Kidney360. 2020;2(3):410–412.

113. Song T, Rössle M, He F, et al. Transjugular intrahepatic portosystemic shunt for hepatorenal syndrome: A systematic review and meta-analysis. Dig Liver Dis 2018;50(4):323–330.

114. Suhocki PV, Lungren MP, Kapoor B, et al. Transjugular intrahepatic portosystemic shunt complications: prevention and management. Semin Intervent Radiol. 2015;32(2):123–32.

115. Allaire M, Walter A, Sutter O, et al. TIPS for management of portal-hypertension-related complications in patients with cirrhosis. Clin Res Hepatol Gastroenterol. 2020;44(3):249–263.

116. Formica RN, Aeder M, Boyle G, et al. Simultaneous Liver-Kidney Allocation Policy: A Proposal to Optimize Appropriate Utilization of Scarce Resources. Am J Transplant. 2016;16(3):758–766.

117. Colliou É, Del Bello A, Milongo D, et al. Kidney failure after liver transplantation. Transplantology 2021;2(3):315–335.

38 | Acute Pancreatitis

INTRODUCTION

Acute pancreatitis (AP) is a common gastrointestinal tract disease that occurs due to cellular injury and inflammation of the pancreas and is characterized by the abrupt onset of deep epigastric pain and elevated levels of lipase or amylase levels in the blood [1, 2]. Acute pancreatitis is increasing globally; it is one of the most common gastrointestinal causes of hospitalization in the United States and is associated with significant morbidity, mortality, and substantial health care cost [3–5].

CAUSES

The most common causes of acute pancreatitis are gallstones (about 42%) and chronic alcohol use (about 21%), while less frequent causes are hypertriglyceridemia, post-endoscopic retrograde cholangiopancreatography, hypercalcemia, trauma, infection, and idiopathic [6, 7].

DIAGNOSIS

The diagnosis of acute pancreatitis requires at least two of the following three criteria: (1) Typical abdominal pain (acute onset severe, persistent, epigastric, and left upper quadrant abdominal pain); (2) Threefold elevation in pancreatic enzymes activity (serum lipase and serum amylase); and (3) Imaging (computerized tomography [CT], magnetic resonance imaging [MRI], ultrasound) findings that are consistent with acute pancreatitis [8].

CLASSIFICATION

Based on pathological changes, onset, and severity, acute pancreatitis is classified in Table 38.1 [3, 8–16].

MANAGEMENT

Treatment of acute pancreatitis should be individualized depending on the severity of the disease, causative etiology, presence of complications of

Table 38.1 Classification of acute pancreatitis (AP)	
A. Based on the type of morphological changes	
Interstitial pancreatitis	Occurs in about 80–90% of AP, and this self-limiting mild form of AP is characterized by edema and inflammation of the pancreas and peripancreatic tissues but without pancreatic necrosis
Necrotizing pancreatitis	Occurs in about 5–10% of AP, and this severe form of AP is characterized by necrosis of more than 30% of the pancreatic gland and the peripancreatic tissue
B. Based on the clinical course	
Early phase	The early phase of AP usually lasts for about one week but may extend into the second week
Late phase	The late phase of acute pancreatitis occurs 1–2 weeks after the onset of the condition and is only seen in patients with moderate or severe acute pancreatitis. It is characterized by the development of local complications, such as peripancreatic fluid collections, necrotic collections, pancreatic pseudocysts, and walled-off necrosis, or by systemic signs of inflammation
C. Based on the severity	
Mild	Mild pancreatitis is the most common form of AP (around 80%), which is characterized by the absence of organ failure and no local or systemic complications, has a self-limiting course, usually resolves in the first week, and carries low mortality (<1–3%)
Moderate	Transient organ failure (such as pulmonary failure, renal failure, cardiovascular dysfunction, and gastrointestinal dysfunction) which resolves within 48 h, with local complications (such as peripancreatic fluid collections, pseudocyst, and acute necrotic collections) or systemic complications (exacerbation of co-morbid diseases such as coronary artery disease, chronic kidney disease or chronic lung diseases)
Severe	Persistent single or multiple organ failure (longer than 48 h) with or without local complications. It occurs in 15–20% of cases of AP and is associated with significantly high morbidity and mortality (up to 50%)

severe acute pancreatitis, and coexisting disorders. Management of acute pancreatitis is divided into three broad categories:

A. Initial medical management

B. Endoscopy therapy

C. Surgical therapy

A. Initial medical management

As no specific medication can effectively treat acute pancreatitis, the management of this condition typically focuses on supportive measures and addressing any complications that may arise. These may include control of pain, appropriate fluid and electrolyte replacement, nutrition supplementation, and antibiotics [17].

1. Control of pain

Severe abdominal pain is the common presentation, distressing symptom, and the leading reason for hospital admission. Therefore, early and effective relief of pain is a clinical priority. Furthermore, optimum pain relief treatment in acute pancreatitis helps reduce stress response, sympathetic-induced vasoconstriction, and pulmonary complications. Therefore, a multimodal analgesic approach is suggested for pain management in acute pancreatitis using opiates, non-steroidal anti-inflammatories (NSAIDs), paracetamol, metamizole, and epidural analgesia.

In a recent meta-analysis, non-steroidal anti-inflammatory drugs and paracetamol are found to be effective in controlling pain in patients with acute pancreatitis [18]. As NSAIDs are equally effective as opioids, they can be effectively used as an opiate-sparing alternative during the first 24 h [19]. In patients with mild acute pancreatitis, NSAIDs and opioids are equally effective in reducing the need for rescue analgesia [20]. But avoid the use of NSAIDs in patients with acute kidney injury [15].

Opioids are safe and effective in managing pain due to acute pancreatitis [21], and frequently used parenteral opioids are buprenorphine, pethidine, morphine, and fentanyl [22]. However, the use of opioids like morphine is discouraged in acute pancreatitis because it may cause spasms in Oddi's sphincter [23] and may worsen the severity of acute pancreatitis [24]. In addition, IV paracetamol, dexketoprofen, and tramadol are not superior to each other in pain management [25].

Epidural analgesia used infrequently very effectively reduces pain within the first 24 h [19]. Therefore, epidural analgesia is a valuable option for patients with acute pancreatitis requiring high doses of opioids for a prolonged period to control pain.

2. Fluid resuscitation

Fluid therapy is the first line of therapy that may play a critical role in managing acute pancreatitis.

Goals: Fluid resuscitation aims to achieve hemodynamic stability, improve perfusion of the pancreatic microcirculation, avoid pancreatic ischemia, and limit progression to pancreatic necrosis.

Rationale: Hypovolemia and hypotension are very common in severe acute pancreatitis, which occurs from multiple factors such as nausea, vomiting, low fluid intake, and third-space losses (pancreatic edema, peripancreatic edema, and paralytic ileus) due to increase vascular permeability, increased respiratory losses, fever, and diaphoresis [9]. The rationale for early hydration is to provide optimal fluid volume to correct severe intravascular depletion, improve tissue perfusion and prevent resultant multiorgan failure.

Optimal time: The timing of fluid resuscitation is crucial in patients with acute pancreatitis. Early IV hydration (i.e., within the first 12 to 24 hours after symptoms begin) is most helpful. In contrast, the delay in fluid resuscitation (i.e., after 24 hours of onset) may not be as beneficial [9].

Major guidelines recommend that IV fluids should be given to a patient with acute pancreatitis as soon as possible (the best time to start is immediately after the diagnosis of acute pancreatitis while the patient is still in the emergency department). Administrating IV fluids in the early stage, without waiting for hemodynamic worsening, helps to prevent hypovolemia and hypoperfusion and optimize tissue perfusion targets [9, 12, 15, 26]. In addition, early fluid resuscitation by maintaining the microcirculation reduces the risk of necrotizing pancreatitis [15] and reduces SIRS, decreases organ failure, lowers the rate of admission to the ICU, shortens the length of hospital stay, and diminishes in-hospital mortality [10, 27–29].

Aggressive vs. conservative fluid therapy: Controversy exists regarding the optimal rate, type, and duration of fluid administration in severe acute pancreatitis [30]. Various studies during the last decade demonstrated that aggressive fluid administration during the first 24 hours of acute pancreatitis corrects hypovolemia and hypotension, improves microcirculation, and prevents necrosis, resulting in rapid clinical recovery and reduction in morbidity and mortality [29, 31–34]. Because of these advantages, aggressive fluid therapy was recommended in acute pancreatitis in several publications [3, 35] and guidelines [9].

However, recent studies have shown that prolonged aggressive fluid therapy in patients with severe acute pancreatitis can have negative effects. Aggressive fluid therapy may increase the risk of acute kidney injury, pulmonary edema, and respiratory failure. It may also lead to the need for intubation, mechanical ventilation, and abdominal compartment syndrome, which can increase morbidity and mortality [36–41].

Recent guidelines (American Gastroenterological Association - AGA Guidelines 2018) [2], meta-analysis (Gad et al. 2020, Liao et al. 2022) [42, 43], randomized trial (WATERFALL trial 2022) [44], and several publications [7, 45, 46] have endorsed the detrimental effect of early aggressive fluid resuscitation and provided strong evidence against using aggressive fluid regimen routinely in acute pancreatitis.

Rate of fluid infusion: For initial treatment in acute pancreatitis, goal-directed administration of crystalloid solution at a rate of 5–10 mL/kg per hour (250–500 ml per hour) until resuscitation goals are reached was recommended in ACG (American College of Gastroenterology) and IAP/APA (International Association of Pancreatology and the American Pancreatic Association) 2013 guidelines [9, 10]. In patients with acute pancreatitis having severe hypovolemia and hypotension, aggressive fluid resuscitation at a rate of 20 mL/kg IV fluid bolus over 30 minutes, followed by 3 mL/kg/hr, was previously recommended [47].

According to the recent WATERFALL Clinical Trial (NEJM 2022), early aggressive fluid resuscitation was found to be associated with a significantly higher risk of fluid overload compared to moderate fluid resuscitation. Specifically, the risk of fluid overload was 20.5% in the aggressive fluid resuscitation group, compared to only 6.3% in the moderate fluid resuscitation group. Therefore, the trial recommended using moderate fluid resuscitation instead of aggressive fluid resuscitation [44].

As per the moderate fluid resuscitation regimen, hypovolemic patients with acute pancreatitis should receive a 10 mL/kg fluid bolus (instead of 20 mL/kg), while normovolemic patients should receive Ringer's lactate (RL) at a rate of 1.5 mL/kg/hr (instead of the aggressive 3 mL/kg/hr).

Hypovolemic patients may require additional 10 mL/kg RL boluses if urine output is <0.5 mL/kg/hr or systolic blood pressure <90 mm Hg.

A moderate fluid resuscitation regimen not only provides fluid at a slow rate but also provides a lesser total volume of infused fluid (6.6 vs. 8.3 liters for aggressive fluid resuscitation) [48], which reduces the risk of fluid overload.

After initial stabilization, it is essential to individualize and adjust the rate of fluid infusion based on age, weight, cardiac or renal comorbidities, the severity of the disease, and frequent reassessment of the volume, hemodynamic and mental status, and urine output to avoid volume overload and associated detrimental effects [15].

When patients with acute pancreatitis present after 24 hours of the onset of pain, a similar outcome is observed using nonaggressive versus aggressive hydration [49].

Choice of IV fluids: Normal saline, Ringer's lactate, and hydroxyethyl starch are frequently used for resuscitation in acute pancreatitis. Crystalloids are preferred over colloids, and the most commonly used crystalloids are normal saline and Ringer's lactate.

RL preferred: The current trend is to prefer Ringer's lactate to normal saline for fluid resuscitation in acute pancreatitis because of:

- Improved outcomes with its use, such as the lesser need for intensive care and reduced length of hospitalization [50–53].

- Improvement in the systemic inflammatory response and C-reactive protein was demonstrated in acute pancreatitis with the use of Ringer's lactate in different studies [47, 54–57].

- Guidelines by the American College of Gastroenterology and the International Association of Pancreatology have chosen Ringer's lactate as the best fluid for initial fluid resuscitation in acute pancreatitis [9, 10].

Still, this difference was not observed in recent studies [50, 51, 53, 58]. Furthermore, there was no difference in the incidence of organ failure and mortality while comparing both fluids [50, 53, 58].

Advantages of choosing RL over normal saline: Reasons for selecting RL over normal saline in acute pancreatitis include the following:

- In the SMART trial (2018), balanced crystalloid compared to saline reduced the rate of the composite outcome of death from any cause, new renal-replacement therapy, or persistent renal dysfunction in patients [59].

- Evidence supports the benefits of Ringer's lactate in acute pancreatitis [50–52].

- The administration of a large volume of normal saline can cause hyperchloremic metabolic acidosis and acute kidney failure [59–61].

- Normal saline-induced acidosis also increases the risk of developing inflammation and development of acute pancreatitis [62].

- Lactate in RL is converted into bicarbonate in the liver, which provides a potential protective impact on pancreatic tissue [62].

- Calcium in Ringer's lactate binds with excess nonesterified fatty acid (NEFA) like linoleic acid, preventing hypocalcemia and reducing early systemic inflammation [56].

Hydroxyethyl starch: Current literature does not support the use of hydroxyethyl starch in severe acute pancreatitis [2] due to evidence suggesting the possible risk of multiple organ failure and lack of benefits [63–65].

Monitoring: Patients with acute pancreatitis need close monitoring in the first 24 to 48 hours to optimize fluid replacement to achieve adequate tissue perfusion and avoid volume overload.

Frequently monitoring vital signs, urine output measurement, and laboratory markers such as hemoglobin, hematocrit, blood urea nitrogen, creatinine, and lactate are helpful in monitoring fluid administration.

The infusion rate should be continuously monitored and adjusted to achieve a goal of mean arterial pressure of 65–85 mmHg, a heart rate of <120 beats/min, and urine volume >0.5–1 mL/kg/hr [10].

As hypoxia is common (occurs in about 50–60% of patients) in acute pancreatitis [66], monitor oxygen saturation closely. In patients with acute pancreatitis who have hypoxia, oxygen should be administered as needed to maintain an arterial oxygen saturation of greater than 95% [67].

The use of central venous pressure is avoided for assessing volume responsiveness in acute pancreatitis because increased intra-abdominal pressure affects the value of central venous pressure [68].

3. Electrolyte and metabolic disorders

Common disorders encountered in patients with severe acute pancreatitis are hypocalcemia, hypomagnesemia, hypochloremic contraction alkalosis, and hyperglycemia.

Hypocalcemia: In patients with severe acute pancreatitis, hypocalcemia is common. It is a valuable marker for predicting severity in acute pancreatitis, the magnitude of the hypocalcemia correlates with the degree of illness, and the presence of hypocalcemic tetany predicts a poor prognosis [69, 70]. Hypocalcemia may occur due to a decrease in nonionized calcium, usually caused by loss of albumin from the circulation due to tissue inflammation and third space losses. These hypocalcemic patients with low total serum calcium (but normal albumin-corrected serum calcium or ionized calcium) are asymptomatic and do not require specific therapy.

In contrast, a reduction in ionized serum calcium (with low total and albumin-corrected serum calcium) may cause neuromuscular irritability and therefore needs attention. Reduction in ionized serum calcium occurs due to the deposition of calcium within the area of

fat necrosis, metabolic abnormalities involving inhibition of parathyroid hormone (PTH) secretion, refractoriness of bone to stimulation by PTH, and associated hypomagnesemia [71]. Such symptomatic patients should be treated with parenteral administration of calcium gluconate without hypomagnesemia. As hypercalcemia is one of the underlying causes of acute pancreatitis, it is essential to monitor calcium levels carefully and use calcium gluconate only in patients with severe acute or symptomatic hypocalcemia.

Hypomagnesemia: Factors contributing to the development of hypomagnesemia in acute pancreatitis are vomiting, urinary loss of magnesium, or magnesium deposition in fat necrosis [72]. Magnesium should be replaced intravenously, which helps in restoring the serum calcium level to normal.

Hypochloremic contraction alkalosis: Persistent vomiting can lead to this disorder in acute pancreatitis. Normal saline with potassium chloride supplementation is preferred to correct this disorder.

Hyperglycemia: Common causes of hyperglycemia in acute pancreatitis are uncontrolled pre-existing diabetes mellitus (DM), parenteral nutritional therapy, damage to the pancreas due to severe attack of acute pancreatitis causing loss of islet mass and hypoinsulinemia, and stress-induced increased gluconeogenesis and decreased glucose utilization [73].

The incidence of DM is high in patients with severe acute pancreatitis, alcoholic acute pancreatitis, and acute necrotizing pancreatitis [74]. Although the incidence of DM is as high as 40% in patients with severe acute pancreatitis, the risk following even in mild acute pancreatitis is around 15% [74].

The prevalence of new-onset DM after the first attack of acute pancreatitis was found to be high (37% in meta-analysis in 2014) [75], and this incidence is increasing rapidly (51% in meta-analysis in 2019) [76].

Tu J et al. found impaired glucose tolerance as high as 60% while following a first attack of acute pancreatitis for 5 years [77]. So, physicians should be aware of the risk of acute pancreatitis related diabetes and should closely follow every patient after acute pancreatitis to screen for DM and impaired glucose metabolism [78, 79].

Hospitalized patients of acute pancreatitis complicated by hyperglycemia or pre-existing diabetes need close blood glucose monitoring, and cautious administration of short-acting insulin is preferred to control hyperglycemia.

4. Nutrition

Timely adequate nutrition plays a crucial role in managing severe acute pancreatitis. Various aspects of nutrition in patients with acute pancreatitis are discussed in detail in the "Nutrition Considerations in Pancreatitis," part of the Chapter 56 on "Parenteral Nutrition in Specific Diseases," but the summary of important considerations are:

- The concept of "Pancreatic Rest" is outdated, detrimental, and should be abandoned [2, 17, 80, 81].
- Compared to parenteral nutrition (PN), oral or enteral nutrition (EN) has demonstrated multiple benefits like lower cost, shorter length of stay, and fewer complications [82–86].
- Recent guidelines recommend early initiation of oral feeding (within 24 hours) in patients with mild acute pancreatitis, as tolerated, because of benefits such as shorter length of stay, fewer complications, and

lower costs for patients with acute pancreatitis [2, 87, 88].
- EN is safer, more effective, and preferred in the early phases of severe acute pancreatitis than parenteral nutrition.
- The early EN (<48 h) had significant benefits over the delayed EN [89, 90].
- EN is a cheaper, safer, and the most preferred modality where feeding is provided directly into the stomach via a nasogastric tube (NG) or post-pyloric region by a nasojejunal tube (NJ).
- Nasogastric aspiration: Selected patients of acute pancreatitis with significant ileus, abdominal distension, or persistent vomiting needs nasogastric aspiration.

5. Antibiotics

To prescribe prophylactic antibiotics routinely to patients with acute pancreatitis is a common mistake in practice [91–93]. In fact, the injudicious use of antibiotics increases the risk of hospital-acquired infections rather than offering any benefit [94, 95].

Well-designed trials [96–98] and meta-analyses [99–101] performed to assess the advantage of antibiotic prophylaxis in acute pancreatitis failed to demonstrate any benefits. Because of this strong evidence, guidelines recommend against the routine use of prophylactic antibiotics in patients with mild and severe acute pancreatitis to prevent pancreatic or peripancreatic infections [2, 9, 10, 15, 26].

Prompt administration of IV antibiotics is recommended to treat infected pancreatic, peripancreatic, or associated extrapancreatic infections (e.g., cholangitis, catheter-acquired infections, urinary tract infections, or pneumonia) [9, 10, 15, 26, 102].

Parameters that suggest the presence of infected necrosis are:

- Overt clinical signs of sepsis (fever, hypotension, shock besides adequate resuscitation, or organ dysfunction) and increasing WBC counts.
- High serum procalcitonin (PCT) [103].
- The presence of gas in the retroperitoneal area.
- Patients who deteriorate or fail to improve after 7–10 days of hospitalization.

Antibiotics are selected either empirically or based on initial CT-guided fine needle aspiration (FNA) for gram stain and sensitivity of cultured organisms; appropriate antibiotics are chosen [9].

Drugs like meropenem Imipenem, clindamycin, piperacillin, fluoroquinolones, and metronidazole are usually preferred in acute pancreatitis because of their adequate tissue penetration and bactericidal properties in infected pancreatic necrosis [102, 104].

6. Other drugs

Drugs like Octreotide, H2 receptor blockers, anticholinergic drugs, and glucagon have no role in patients with acute pancreatitis.

B. Endoscopic retrograde cholangiopancreatography (ERCP)

Urgent ERCP (within 24 hours) and stone extraction are indicated in patients with severe acute pancreatitis resulting from gallstones who have acute cholangitis (e.g., fever, jaundice, right upper quadrant pain) or progressive jaundice due to bile duct obstruction. As gallstones are the most common cause (about 42%) of acute pancreatitis, early detection of gallstone (biliary) pancreatitis and urgent ERCP with endoscopic sphincterotomy and stone extraction can be life-saving.

C. Surgical therapy

Cholecystectomy: In patients with mild gallstone (biliary) acute pancreatitis, the recurrence rate of acute pancreatitis is high (22% at 5 years); if cholecystectomy is not performed [105, 106]. In patients with gallstone-induced mild acute pancreatitis, it is generally recommended to perform a cholecystectomy during the index (i.e., first) hospital admission [15]. Early cholecystectomy (within 24 to 48 hours of hospital admission) is safe, shortens the overall length of hospital stay, reduces readmissions due to attacks of acute pancreatitis, and lowers biliary complications [107–111].

In patients with severe biliary acute pancreatitis, elective cholecystectomy is delayed for several months until active inflammation and resorption or stabilization of fluid collections are resolved [15].

Local complications of severe acute pancreatitis, such as acute necrotic collection, pancreatic pseudocyst, and walled-off necrosis, are treated conservatively but may need surgical treatment.

The infected acute necrotic collection is a frequent local complication of severe acute pancreatitis, associated with higher mortality and morbidity. Treatment options for patients who do not respond to conservative management are percutaneous drainage/debridement, endoscopic drainage, and surgical debridement.

REFERENCES

1. Johnson CD, Besselink MG, Carter R. Acute pancreatitis. BMJ. 2014;349:g4859.

2. Crockett SD, Wani S, Gardner TB, et al. American Gastroenterological Association Institute Clinical Guidelines Committee. American Gastroenterological Association Institute Guideline on Initial Management of Acute Pancreatitis. Gastroenterology. 2018;154(4):1096–1101.

3. Forsmark CE, Vege SS, Wilcox CM, et al. Acute pancreatitis. N Engl J Med 2016;375(20):1972–1981.

4. Peery AF, Crockett SD, Murphy CC, et al. Burden and Cost of Gastrointestinal, Liver, and Pancreatic Diseases in the United States: Update 2018. Gastroenterology. 2019;156(1):254–272.e11.

5. Petrov MS, Yadav D. Global epidemiology and holistic prevention of pancreatitis. Nat Rev Gastroenterol Hepatol. 2019;16(3):175–184.

6. Zilio MB, Eyff TF, Azeredo-Da-Silva ALF, et al. A systematic review and meta-analysis of the aetiology of acute pancreatitis. HPB (Oxford). 2019;21(3):259–267.

7. Boxhoorn L, Voermans RP, Bouwense SA, et al. Acute pancreatitis. Lancet 2020;396(10252):726–734.

8. Banks PA, Bollen TL, Dervenis C, et al. Classification of acute pancreatitis--2012: revision of the Atlanta classification and definitions by international consensus. Gut. 2013;62(1):102–11.

9. Tenner S, Baillie J, DeWitt J, et al. American College of Gastroenterology guideline: management of acute pancreatitis. Am J Gastroenterol 2013;108(9):1400–1415.

10. Working Group IAP/APA Acute Pancreatitis Guidelines. IAP/APA evidence-based guidelines for the management of acute pancreatitis. Pancreatology. 2013;13(4 suppl 2):e1–15.

11. Phillip V, Steiner JM, Algül H. Early phase of acute pancreatitis: Assessment and management. World J Gastrointest Pathophysiol. 2014;5(3):158–68.

12. Yokoe M, Takada T, Mayumi T, et al. Japanese guidelines for the management of acute pancreatitis: Japanese Guidelines 2015. J Hepatobiliary Pancreat Sci. 2015;22(6):405–32.

13. Greenberg JA, Hsu J, Bawazeer M, et al. Clinical practice guideline: management of acute pancreatitis. Can J Surg. 2016;59(2):128–140.

14. Boumitri C, Brown E, Kahaleh M. Necrotizing Pancreatitis: Current Management and Therapies. Clin Endosc. 2017;50(4):357–365.

15. Leppäniemi A, Tolonen M, Tarasconi A, et al. 2019 WSES guidelines for the management of severe acute pancreatitis. World J Emerg Surg 2019;14:27.

16. Seppänen H, Puolakkainen P. Classification, Severity Assessment, and Prevention of Recurrences in Acute Pancreatitis. Scandinavian Journal of Surgery. 2020;109(1):53–58.

17. Lakananurak N, Gramlich L. Nutrition management in acute pancreatitis: Clinical practice consideration. World J Clin Cases. 2020;8(9):1561–1573.

18. Nelson AD, Lugo-Fagundo NS, Mahapatra SJ, et al. A Systematic Review and Meta-analysis of Opioids vs Nonopioids in Acute Pancreatitis. Gastro Hep Advances 2022;1(1):83–92.

19. Thavanesan N, White S, Lee S, et al. Analgesia in the Initial Management of Acute Pancreatitis: A Systematic Review and Meta-Analysis of Randomised Controlled Trials. World J Surg. 2022;46(4):878–890.

20. Cai W, Liu F, Wen Y, et al. Pain Management in Acute Pancreatitis: A Systematic Review and Meta-Analysis of Randomised Controlled Trials. Front Med (Lausanne). 2021;8:782151.

21. Basurto Ona X, Rigau Comas D, Urrútia G. Opioids for acute pancreatitis pain. Cochrane Database Syst Rev. 2013;(7):CD009179.

22. Stigliano S, Sternby H, de Madaria E, et al. Early management of acute pancreatitis: a review of the best evidence. Digestive and Liver Disease. 2017;49(6):585–594.

23. Meng W, Yuan J, Zhang C, et al. Parenteral analgesics for pain relief in acute pancreatitis: a systematic review. Pancreatology. 2013;13(3):201–206.

24. Barlass U, Dutta R, Cheema H, et al. Morphine worsens the severity and prevents pancreatic regeneration in mouse models of acute pancreatitis. Gut 2017;67:600–602.

25. Gülen B, Dur A, Serinken M, et al. Pain treatment in patients with acute pancreatitis: a randomized controlled trial. Turk J Gastroenterol 2016;27(2):192–6.

26. Li F, Cai S, Cao F, et al. Guidelines for the diagnosis and treatment of acute pancreatitis in China (2021). Journal of Pancreatology. 2021;4(2):67–75.

27. Gardner TB, Vege SS, Pearson RK, et al. Fluid resuscitation in acute pancreatitis. Clin Gastroenterol Hepatol. 2008;6(10):1070–6.

28. Talukdar R, Swaroop Vege S. Early management of severe acute pancreatitis. Curr Gastroenterol Rep 2011;13(2):123–30.

29. Warndorf MG, Kurtzman JT, Bartel MJ, et al. Early fluid resuscitation reduces morbidity among patients with acute pancreatitis. Clin Gastroenterol Hepatol. 2011;9(8):705–709.

30. Haydock MD, Mittal A, Wilms HR, et al. Fluid therapy in acute pancreatitis: anybody's guess. Ann Surg 2013;257(2):182–188.

31. Gardner TB, Vege SS, Chari ST, et al. Faster rate of initial fluid resuscitation in severe acute pancreatitis diminishes in-hospital mortality. Pancreatology 2009;9(6):770–776.

32. Wall I, Badalov N, Baradarian R, et al. Decreased morbidity and mortality in patients with acute pancreatitis related to aggressive intravenous hydration. Pancreas 2011;40(4):547–50.

33. Buxbaum JL, Quezada M, Da B, et al. Early aggressive hydration hastens clinical improvement in mild acute pancreatitis. Am J Gastroenterol 2017;112(5):797–803.

34. Yamashita T, Horibe M, Sanui M, et al. Large Volume Fluid Resuscitation for Severe Acute Pancreatitis is Associated with Reduced Mortality: A Multicenter Retrospective Study. J Clin Gastroenterol. 2019;53(5):385–391.

35. Fisher JM, Gardner TB. The "golden hours" of management in acute pancreatitis. Am J Gastroenterol. 2012;107(8):1146–1150.

36. Mao EQ, Tang YQ, Fei J, et al. Fluid therapy for severe acute pancreatitis in acute response stage. Chin Med J (Engl) 2009;122(2):169–73.

37. Mao EQ, Fei J, Peng YB, et al. Rapid hemodilution is associated with increased sepsis and mortality among patients with severe acute pancreatitis. Chin Med J (Engl) 2010;123(13):1639–44.

38. de-Madaria E, Soler-Sala G, Sánchez-Paya J, et al. Influence of fluid therapy on the prognosis of acute pancreatitis: a prospective cohort study. Am J Gastroenterol 2011;106(10):1843–50.

39. Ye B, Mao W, Chen Y, et al. Aggressive Resuscitation Is Associated with the Development of Acute Kidney Injury in Acute Pancreatitis. Dig Dis Sci. 2019;64(2):544–552.

40. Li L, Jin T, Wen S, et al. Early rapid fluid therapy is associated with increased rate of noninvasive positive-pressure ventilation in Hemoconcentrated patients with severe acute pancreatitis. Dig Dis Sci. United States. 2020;65(9):2700–11.

41. Messallam AA, Body CB, Berger S, et al. Impact of early aggressive fluid resuscitation in acute pancreatitis. Pancreatology. 2021;21(1):69–73.

42. Gad MM, Simons-Linares CR. Is aggressive intravenous fluid resuscitation beneficial in acute pancreatitis? A meta-analysis of randomized control trials and cohort studies. World J Gastroenterol. 2020;26(10):1098–1106.

43. Liao J, Zhan Y, Wu H, et al. Effect of aggressive versus conservative hydration for early phase of acute pancreatitis in adult patients: A meta-analysis of 3,127 cases. Pancreatology. 2022;22(2):226–234.

44. E de-Madaria JL, Buxbaum P, Maisonneuve A, et al. Aggressive or Moderate Fluid Resuscitation in Acute Pancreatitis. N Engl J Med 2022;387:989–1000.

45. Argaiz ER, de Moraes AG. Acute pancreatitis. Lancet. 2021;397(10271):279.

46. Boxhoorn L, Voermans RP, van Santvoort HC, et al. Acute pancreatitis. Lancet. 2021;397(10271):280.

47. Wu BU, Hwang JQ, Gardner TH, et al. Lactated Ringer's solution reduces systemic inflammation compared with saline in patients with acute pancreatitis. Clin Gastroenterol Hepatol. 2011;9(8):710–717.e1.

48. Gardnet TB. Fluid Resuscitation in Acute Pancreatitis - Going over the WATERFALL. N Engl J Med 2022;387(11):1038–1039.

49. Cuéllar-Monterrubio JE, Monreal-Robles R, González-Moreno EI, et al. Nonaggressive Versus Aggressive Intravenous Fluid Therapy in Acute Pancreatitis With More Than 24 Hours From Disease Onset: A Randomized Controlled Trial. Pancreas. 2020;49(4):579–583.

50. Aziz M, Ahmed Z, Weissman S, et al. Lactated Ringer's vs normal saline for acute pancreatitis: An updated systematic review and meta-analysis. Pancreatology. 2021;21(7):1217–1223.

51. Lee A, Ko C, Buitrago C, et al. Lactated Ringers vs Normal Saline Resuscitation for Mild Acute Pancreatitis: A Randomized Trial. Gastroenterology. 2021;160(3):955–957.e4.

52. Chen H, Lu X, Xu B, et al. Lactated Ringer Solution Is Superior to Normal Saline Solution in Managing Acute Pancreatitis: An Updated Meta-analysis of Randomized Controlled Trials. J Clin Gastroenterol 2022;56(2):e114–e120.

53. Guzmán-Calderón E, Diaz-Arocutipa C, Monge E. Lactate Ringer's Versus Normal Saline in the Management of Acute Pancreatitis: A Systematic Review and Meta-Analysis of Randomized Controlled Trials. Dig Dis Sci. 2022;67(8):4131–4139.

54. de-Madaria E, Herrera-Marante I, González-Camacho V, et al. Fluid resuscitation with lactated Ringer's solution vs normal saline in acute pancreatitis: a triple-blind, randomized, controlled trial. United European Gastroenterol J. 2018;6(1):63–72.

55. Iqbal U, Anwar H, Scribani M. Ringer's lactate versus normal saline in acute pancreatitis: a systematic review and meta-analysis. J Dig Dis. 2018;19(6):335–341.

56. Khatua B, Yaron JR, El-Kurdi B, et al. Ringer's Lactate Prevents Early Organ Failure by Providing Extracellular Calcium. J Clin Med 2020;9(1):263.

57. Karki B, Thapa S, Khadka D, et al. Intravenous Ringers lactate versus normal saline for predominantly mild acute pancreatitis in a Nepalese Tertiary Hospital. PLoS One. 2022;17(1):e0263221.

58. Zhou S, Buitrago C, Foong A, et al. Comprehensive meta-analysis of randomized controlled trials of lactated Ringer's versus normal saline for acute pancreatitis. Pancreatology 2021;21(8):1405–1410.

59. Semler MW, Self WH, Wanderer JP, et al. Balanced Crystalloids versus Saline in Critically Ill Adults. N Engl J Med. 2018;378(9):829–839.

60. Kellum JA. Saline-induced hyperchloremic metabolic acidosis. Crit Care Med 2002;30(1):259–261.

61. Reid F, Lobo DN, Williams RN, et al. (Ab)normal saline and physiological Hartmann's solution: a randomized double-blind crossover study. Clin Sci (Lond) 2003;104(1):17–24.

62. Bhoomagoud M, Jung T, Atladottir J, et al. Reducing extracellular pH sensitizes the acinar cell to secretagogue-induced pancreatitis responses in rats. Gastroenterology 2009;137(3):1083–1092.

63. Du XJ, Hu WM, Xia Q, et al. Hydroxyethyl starch resuscitation reduces the risk of intra-abdominal hypertension in severe acute pancreatitis. Pancreas 2011;40(8):1220–1225.

64. Myburgh JA, Finfer S, Bellomo R, et al. Hydroxyethyl starch or saline for fluid resuscitation in intensive care. N Engl J Med 2012;367(20):1901–1911.

65. Zhao G, Zhang JG, Wu HS, et al. Effects of different resuscitation fluid on severe acute pancreatitis. World J Gastroenterol 2013;19(13):2044–2052.

66. Browne GW, Pitchumoni CS. Pathophysiology of pulmonary complications of acute pancreatitis. World J Gastroenterol. 2006;12(44):7087–96.

67. Takeda K, Takada T, Kawarada Y, et al. JPN Guidelines for the management of acute pancreatitis: medical management of acute pancreatitis. J Hepatobiliary Pancreat Surg. 2006;13(1):42–7.

68. Huber W, Umgelter A, Reindl W, et al. Volume assessment in patients with necrotizing pancreatitis: a comparison of intrathoracic blood volume index, central venous pressure, and hematocrit, and their correlation to cardiac index and extravascular lung water index. Crit Care Med. 2008;36(8):2348–54.

69. Gutiérrez-Jiménez AA, Castro-Jiménez E, Lagunes-Córdoba R. Total serum calcium and corrected calcium as severity predictors in acute pancreatitis. Rev Gastroenterol Mex 2014;79(1):13–21.

70. Chhabra P, Rana SS, Sharma V, et al. Hypocalcemic tetany: a simple bedside marker of poor outcome in acute pancreatitis. Ann Gastroenterol. 2016;29(2):214–20.

71. Ahmed A, Azim A, Gurjar M, et al. Hypocalcemia in acute pancreatitis revisited. Indian J Crit Care Med. 2016;20(3):173–7.

72. Hersh T, Siddiqui DA. Magnesium and the pancreas. Am J Clin Nutr. 1973;26(3):362–366.

73. Xiu F, Stanojcic M, Diao L, et al. Stress hyperglycemia, insulin treatment, and innate immune cells. Int J Endocrinol. 2014;2014:486403.

74. Zhi M, Zhu X, Lugea A, et al. Incidence of New Onset Diabetes Mellitus Secondary to Acute Pancreatitis: A Systematic Review and Meta-Analysis. Frontiers in physiology. 2019;10:637.

75. Das SL, Singh PP, Phillips AR, et al. Newly diagnosed diabetes mellitus after acute pancreatitis: a systematic review and meta-analysis. Gut. 2014;63(5):818–31.

76. Liu QP, Hu CL, Chen NW. New-Onset Diabetes Mellitus After the First Attack of Acute Pancreatitis: A Systematic Review and Meta-Analysis. Iran Red Crescent Med J. 2019;21(7):e91740.

77. Tu J, Yang Y, Zhang J, et al. Effect of the disease severity on the risk of developing new-onset diabetes after acute pancreatitis. Medicine (Baltimore). 2018;97(22):e10713.

78. Hart PA, Bradley D, Conwell DL, et al. Diabetes following acute pancreatitis. Lancet Gastroenterol Hepatol. 2021;6(8):668–675.

79. Richardson A, Park WG. Acute pancreatitis and diabetes mellitus: a review. Korean J Intern Med. 2021;36(1):15–24.

80. Uomo G. Pancreatic rest or not? The debate on the nutrition in acute pancreatitis continues. JOP. 2013;14(2):216–7.

81. Rininnella, E, Annetta MG, Serricchio M et al. Nutritional support in acute pancreatitis: from physiopathology to practice: an evidence-based approach. Eur Rev Med Pharmacol Sci 2017;21(2):421–432.

82. Al-Omran M, Albalawi ZH, Tashkandi MF, et al. Enteral versus parenteral nutrition for acute pancreatitis. Cochrane Database Syst Rev 2010;2010(1):CD002837.

83. Vaughn VM, Shuster D, Rogers MAM, et al. Early versus delayed feeding in patients with acute pancreatitis: a systematic review. Ann Intern Med. 2017;166(12):883–892.

84. Li W, Liu J, Zhao S, et al. Safety and efcacy of total parenteral nutrition versus total enteral nutrition for patients with severe acute pancreatitis: a meta-analysis. J Int Med Res 2018;46(9):3948–3958.

85. Wu P, Li L, Sun W. Efficacy comparisons of enteral nutrition and parenteral nutrition in patients with severe acute pancreatitis: a meta-analysis from randomized controlled trials. Biosci Rep 2018;38(6):BSR20181515.

86. Yao H, He C, Deng L, et al. Enteral versus parenteral nutrition in critically ill patients with severe pancreatitis: a meta-analysis. Eur J Clin Nutr 2018;72(1):66–68.

87. National Institute for Health and Care Excellence. Pancreatitis (NICE guideline NG104). 2018. www.nice.org.uk/guidance/ng104.

88. Arvanitakis M, Ockenga J, Bezmarevic M, et al. ESPEN guideline on clinical nutrition in acute and chronic pancreatitis. Clin Nutr. 2020;39(3):612–631.

89. Guo QH, Tian XY, Qin YL, et al. Immediate enteral nutrition can accelerate recovery and be safe in mild acute pancreatitis: A meta-analysis of randomized controlled trials. Heliyon. 2022;8(2):e08852.

90. Yao Q, Liu P, Peng S, et al. Effects of immediate or early oral feeding on acute pancreatitis: a systematic review and metaanalysis. Pancreatology. 2022;22(2):175–184.

91. Vlada AC, Schmit B, Perry A, et al. Failure to follow evidence-based best practice guidelines in the treatment of severe acute pancreatitis. HPB (Oxford) 2013;15(10):822–7.

92. Sun E, Tharakan M, Kapoor S, et al. Poor compliance with ACG guidelines for nutrition and antibiotics in the management of acute pancreatitis: a North American survey of gastrointestinal specialists and primary care physicians. JOP 2013;14(3):221–7.

93. Parniczky A, Lantos T, Toth EM, et al. Antibiotic therapy in acute pancreatitis: from global overuse to evidence based recommendations. Pancreatology. 2019;19(4):488–99.

94. Nakaharai K, Morita K, Jo T, et al. Early prophylactic antibiotics for severe acute pancreatitis: a population-based cohort study using a nationwide database in Japan. J Infect Chemother 2018;24(9):753–758.

95. Horibe M, Sanui M, Sasaki M, et al. Impact of antimicrobial prophylaxis for severe acute pancreatitis on the development of invasive candidiasis: a large retrospective multicenter cohort study. Pancreas. 2019;48(4):537–43.

96. Isenmann R, Runzi M, Kron M, et al. Prophylactic antibiotic treatment in patients with predicted severe acute pancreatitis: a placebo-controlled, double blind trial. Gastroenterology. 2004;126(4):997–1004.

97. Dellinger EP, Tellado JM, Soto NE, et al. Early antibiotic treatment for severe acute necrotizing pancreatitis: randomized, double-blind, placebo-controlled study. Ann Surg. 2007;245(5):674–83.

98. Mandal AK, Chaudhary S, Shrestha B, et al. Efficacy of prophylactic use of ciprofloxacin and metronidazole in mild and moderately severe acute pancreatitis. JNMA J Nepal Med Assoc 2017;56(206):207–210.

99. Jafri NS, Mahid SS, Idstein SR, et al. Antibiotic prophylaxis is not protective in severe acute pancreatitis: a systemic review and meta-analysis. Am J Surg 2009;197(6):806–813.

100. Villatoro E, Bassi C, Larvin M. Antibiotic therapy for prophylaxis against infection of pancreatic necrosis in acute pancreatitis. Cochrane Database Syst Rev. 2010;(5):CD002941.

101. Lim CL, Lee W, Liew YX, et al. Role of antibiotic prophylaxis in necrotizing pancreatitis: a meta-analysis. J Gastrointest Surg 2015;19(3):480–91.

102. Mourad MM, Evans R, Kalidindi V, et al. Prophylactic antibiotics in acute pancreatitis: endless debate. Ann R Coll Surg Engl 2017;99(2):107–112.

103. Mofidi R, Suttie SA, Patil PV, et al. The value of procalcitonin at predicting the severity of acute pancreatitis and development of infected pancreatic necrosis: systematic review. Surgery. 2009;146(1):72–81.

104. Manes G, Rabitti PG, Menchise A, et al. Prophylaxis with meropenem of septic complications in acute pancreatitis: a randomized, controlled trial versus imipenem. Pancreas. 2003;27(4):e79–83.

105. van Baal MC, Besselink MG, Bakker OJ, et al. Dutch Pancreatitis Study Group. Timing of cholecystectomy after mild biliary pancreatitis: a systematic review. Ann Surg. 2012;255(5):860–866.

106. Hwang SS, Li BH, Haigh PI. Gallstone pancreatitis without cholecystectomy. JAMA Surg. 2013;148(9):867–872.

107. Uhl W, Müller CA, Krähenbühl L, et al. Acute gallstone pancreatitis: timing of laparoscopic cholecystectomy in mild and severe disease. Surg Endosc 1999;13(11):1070–6.

108. Aboulian A, Chan T, Yaghoubian A, et al. Early cholecystectomy safely decreases hospital stay in patients with mild gallstone pancreatitis: a randomized prospective study. Ann Surg 2010;251(4):615–9.

109. da Costa DW, Bouwense SA, Schepers NJ, et al. Same-admission versus interval cholecystectomy for mild gallstone pancreatitis (PONCHO): a multicentre randomised controlled trial. Lancet 2015;386(10000):1261–1268.

110. Laswi H, Attara B, Kwei R, et al. Readmissions after Biliary Acute Pancreatitis: Analysis of the Nationwide Readmissions Database. Gastroenterology Research 2022;15(4):188–199.

111. Lyu Y, Cheng Y, Wang B, et al. Safety of early same-admission laparoscopic cholecystectomy for acute mild biliary pancreatitis. A retrospective study for acute pancreatitis. Wideochir Inne Tech Maloinwazyjne. 2022;17(1):150–155.

39 | Fluid Therapy in Bronchial Asthma, ARDS, and in Mechanical Ventilation

Fluid therapy in common respiratory disorders such as acute respiratory distress syndrome, bronchial asthma, and patients receiving mechanical ventilation is discussed.

BRONCHIAL ASTHMA

In patients with bronchial asthma, important aspects of fluid therapy, electrolyte disorders, and acid-base disorders are discussed.

Fluid therapy

Adequate hydration protects the lung epithelium and helps in promoting effective mucociliary clearance [1, 2]. In dehydration, cough is significantly more prevalent, even in healthy individuals [3]. Poor oral intake during illness, increased work of breathing due to airway obstruction, increased insensible fluid losses due to hyperventilation, cold sweat during an asthma attack, and fluid loss due to associated fever all contribute to the loss of body water and sodium chloride during an asthma attack [4].

Proper hydration is essential because dehydration worsens respiratory symptoms and lung function in patients with bronchial asthma [5].

Dehydration carries problems such as:

1. Thickened secretions, which can lead to mucus plugging and airway obstruction.

2. Stimulates the production of inflammatory markers like histamine that leads to airway obstruction via smooth muscle contraction, bronchial secretion, and airway mucosal edema [6, 7].

So, maintaining adequate hydration through fluid therapy is crucial in the treatment of bronchial asthma, and neglecting to keep patients with status asthmatics well-hydrated is poor practice [8]. However, administering IV fluids cautiously is crucial during acute asthma exacerbation since excessive fluid administration can exacerbate fluid overload, leading to further deterioration of gas exchange and lung function, and potentially worsening clinical outcomes [9].

Electrolyte abnormalities

Hypokalemia, hypomagnesemia, hypophosphatemia, and hypocalcemia are frequently seen abnormalities in patients with bronchial asthma [10–12]. These electrolyte abnormalities can cause cardiac arrhythmias, affect the excitability of airway smooth muscles, and in severe cases, worsen respiratory failure, necessitating attention [11].

Hypokalemia is the earliest electrolyte disturbance in asthma, which may result from the use of ß2 agonists (such as salbutamol), aminophylline, or steroid therapy [13, 14].

Hypocalcemia can occur in bronchial asthma due to long-term beta-agonist therapy and underlying vitamin D deficiency [11, 12], which can be harmful [15, 16].

Hypomagnesemia is the most common electrolyte abnormality in bronchial asthma [10, 11, 17]. Hypomagnesemia may increase neuromuscular excitability, increase susceptibility to bronchospasm and can even cause paradoxical bronchoconstriction especially after inhaled beta 2 agonists (i.e., salbutamol) [18].

Administration of IV magnesium sulfate as an adjunct therapy is recommended in severe acute asthma exacerbations with inadequate response to standard intensive initial treatment [19–21]. However, routine use of IV magnesium sulfate is not recommended. Administration of a single dose of magnesium sulfate (2 gm infused over 20 min) is safe.

Acid-base disorders

In bronchial asthma, hypoxemia and respiratory alkalosis are frequently seen acid-base abnormalities, while respiratory acidosis, normal anion gap (AG) metabolic acidosis, and increased AG acidosis are less common acid-base abnormalities that occur in severe cases [22, 23].

In severe cases of bronchial asthma, it is crucial to order an ABG analysis because it evaluates the lungs' ability to deliver oxygen to the blood and eliminate carbon dioxide, helping to diagnose acid-base disorders early [23]. ABG analysis is usually performed in cases of severe asthma with a high likelihood of respiratory failure (such as when pretreatment SaO_2 <90%), inadequate response to treatment (as evidenced by falls in SaO_2 or peak expiratory flow rate failing to improve to 40-45% of predicted), or when symptoms fail to improve [24].

Early recognition and management of acid-base disorders through ABG analysis can guide their timely management, prevent complications, and improve outcomes in severe asthmatic patients.

Hypoxemia

In patients with bronchial asthma, hypoxemia (low PaO_2 levels) is a common complication resulting from various factors, including airway obstruction, respiratory muscle fatigue, and ventilation-perfusion (V/Q) mismatch [22].

Respiratory alkalosis

During an acute attack in patients with bronchial asthma, respiratory alkalosis is the most common acid-base abnormality which occurs due to hyperventilation [22, 25, 26].

Respiratory acidosis

Severe asthma can result in a significant obstruction of the airways, which can cause alveolar hypoventilation and impair CO_2 elimination, leading to increased pCO_2 (hypercapnia) and respiratory acidosis [22, 27]. Furthermore, prolonged periods of increased respiratory muscle workload can cause respiratory muscle fatigue, resulting in inadequate ventilation and contributing to the development of hypercapnia and respiratory acidosis. While respiratory acidosis is an uncommon complication (seen in only 4.65% of patients), it is a life-threatening condition that can cause respiratory failure and arrest if left untreated [26]. Therefore, this ominous disorder requires early recognition and treatment.

The treatment of hypoxemia, respiratory alkalosis, and respiratory acidosis in bronchial asthma depends on the underlying cause and may include medications such as bronchodilators, corticosteroids, other anti-inflammatory medications, oxygen therapy, or mechanical ventilation, as well as lifestyle modifications.

Metabolic acidosis

Bronchial asthma with more severe airflow obstruction is associated with two types of metabolic acidosis: normal anion gap metabolic acidosis, which is a common occurrence, and increased AG acidosis, which is less common [22, 26, 28].

Normal anion gap metabolic acidosis: In asthmatic patients with respiratory alkalosis and chronic hypocapnia, the kidneys compensate by excreting bicarbonate in the urine. This compensatory renal loss of bicarbonate leads to a decrease in the plasma bicarbonate concentration, resulting in a normal anion gap (hyperchloremic) metabolic acidosis [22, 28]. Patients with severe asthma who develop normal anion gap metabolic acidosis are at an increased risk of developing respiratory failure, requiring more frequent invasive mechanical ventilation support and a higher rate of admission to the intensive care unit [22, 28]. Since renal compensation for respiratory alkalosis and chronic hypocapnia is a slow process, normal anion gap metabolic acidosis indicates a chronic rather than the acute disorder.

Increased AG metabolic acidosis: Lactic acidosis or increased AG metabolic acidosis is common in acute, severe asthma, and its causes are multifactorial, including [22, 29]:

1. Respiratory muscle fatigue: Due to prolonged and increased work of breathing, the oxygen demands of respiratory muscles increases. An increased workload leads to an increase in lactic acid production through anaerobic metabolism in respiratory muscles, resulting in high blood lactate levels.

2. Tissue hypoxia: In bronchial asthma, tissue hypoxia occurs due

to decreased tissue oxygenation caused by heart-lung interactions reducing cardiac output, leading to severe hypoperfusion, hypoxemia, and increased energy needs of respiratory muscles due to increased workload.

3. Liver congestion and dysfunction causing impaired lactate clearance.

4. High doses of β2 agonist therapy can increase lactate production, which can cause salbutamol-induced lactic acidosis (SILA) [30–32]. SILA is a rare but known side effect of inhaled salbutamol, and clinicians should promptly recognize and manage it, remembering that increasing the dose of salbutamol can exacerbate the condition [33]. SILA typically resolves within 24-48 hours after discontinuing β2-agonist therapy.

Why is it important to detect and treat metabolic acidosis in bronchial asthma?

Early diagnosis and optimal treatment of metabolic acidosis are necessary for bronchial asthma, as it can cause adverse effects such as decreased cardiac output, reduced effectiveness of β-agonists, and stimulation of ineffective rapid, shallow ventilation.

Simple clue for easy diagnosis of metabolic acidosis: High serum chloride concentration in serum electrolytes in severe bronchial asthma patients can indicate normal anion gap metabolic acidosis and aid in identifying high-risk asthmatics [28]. Similarly, in severe bronchial asthma, a high serum lactate level suggests the presence of high anion gap metabolic acidosis.

Treatment of metabolic acidosis in bronchial asthma

The treatment of metabolic acidosis in bronchial asthma involves addressing the underlying cause of the condition, which may include correcting fluid and electrolyte imbalances, administering bronchodilators, and ensuring adequate oxygenation.

In addition, bicarbonate replacement therapy may be necessary in cases where the acidosis is severe or persistent, which results in an improvement in respiration [34]. This involves administering intravenous sodium bicarbonate to increase the pH and neutralize excess acid in the body.

Close monitoring of a patient's response to treatment, including ABG measurements as needed, is crucial to adjusting therapy and achieving optimal outcomes, while also preventing potential complications of alkali therapy, such as fluid overload, hyperosmolarity, and rebound alkalosis.

ACUTE RESPIRATORY DISTRESS SYNDROME

Acute respiratory distress syndrome (ARDS) is a common and life-threatening clinical condition characterized by increased pulmonary capillary permeability that causes acute onset of non-cardiogenic protein-rich pulmonary edema, which often progresses to respiratory failure, leading to hypoxemia and requiring mechanical ventilation.

Sepsis, trauma, pneumonia, multiple transfusions, and aspiration of gastric contents are common causes of ARDS [35]. ARDS carries a significant morbidity and high mortality rate ranging from 30% to 45% [36–38].

Why fluid therapy is important in patients with ARDS?

In the management of ARDS, fluid therapy plays a crucial role in maintaining hemodynamic stability, optimizing oxygenation, and preventing further lung injury. However, optimizing fluid therapy in ARDS is challenging because the goal is to achieve euvolemia while simultaneously avoiding both hypovolemia and positive fluid balance, which requires balancing a liberal versus conservative fluid strategy approach [39].

Here are some key principles to consider when administering fluid therapy in patients with ARDS.

Avoid fluid overload

Hypotension is common in patients with ARDS, often arising from sepsis or trauma, both of which commonly cause hypotension. Liberal fluid management or standard care improves hypotension, cardiac function, and end-organ perfusion. However, these treatments can also result in a positive fluid balance. In addition to correcting hypotension, critically ill patients with ARDS in the ICU may require intravenous fluid administration for maintenance requirements, nutrition, as diluents for various medications and inotropes, and to ensure patency of the IV line. The cumulative administration of a large volume of fluid, combined with oliguria, increases the risk of fluid overload.

In ARDS, the combined effect of increased vascular permeability and fluid overload can be dangerous, as it can result in worsening pulmonary edema, reduced lung compliance, and an increased risk of ventilator-induced lung injury. In addition, several studies have found that liberal fluid management induced fluid overload is associated with longer mechanical ventilation times, prolonged hospital or ICU stays, and increased mortality rates [40–43].

Therefore, avoiding fluid overload in patients with ARDS is essential

to improve outcomes and enhance recovery.

Use conservative fluid management

In ARDS, conservative fluid management aims to maintain a slightly negative fluid balance and prevent fluid overload. The landmark FACTT (Fluid and Catheter Treatment Trial 2006) study and other studies have demonstrated benefits, such as improved lung function, shorter duration of mechanical ventilation, less organ dysfunction, and a trend towards less renal replacement therapy in ARDS [44–46]. Due to its safety and benefits, recent guidelines recommend conservative fluid management for patients with ARDS [47].

Choose the right fluid regimen wisely

The strategy for administering fluids should be determined based on the patient's clinical status and the administration time, as both inadequate and excessive fluid infusions can be harmful.

To obtain the best benefits of fluid administration, it is crucial to clearly understand when to administer IV fluids and how much to administer. Providing adequate IV fluids in the early phase, avoiding fluid boluses in the majority of cases, and giving IV fluids conservatively in the later stage reduce mortality in patients with sepsis and ARDS [48]. In addition, the restrictive use of fluids, coupled with earlier administration of vasopressors if necessary, helps to achieve the initial target for mean arterial pressure (MAP) more quickly and reduces the risk of fluid overload [49].

Use diuretics

Diuretics serve as an effective pharmacological adjuvant therapy for removal of excess fluid and maintaining euvolemia in patients with ARDS [50]. Therefore, it is crucial to closely monitor the intake and output chart and administer diuretics as necessary to prevent fluid overload. When combined with fluid restriction, diuretics effectively reduce hydrostatic pressure, increase serum oncotic pressure, and decrease the risk of developing pulmonary edema [51].

Although diuretics have demonstrated advantages such as reducing positive fluid balance, improving lung compliance and oxygenation, and shortening the time on mechanical ventilation, early studies did not find any mortality benefits [44, 52]. However, a recent study has shown that the early use of diuretics in ARDS leads to lower hospital mortality rates [53, 54]. Despite these benefits, caution should be exercised to avoid excessive diuresis, as it can result in hypovolemia and electrolyte imbalances.

Choice of IV fluids

In ARDS, fluid therapy should be individualized, and the choice of IV fluids varies:

a. **Crystalloids:** Crystalloid fluids are the preferred choice for the initial resuscitation of patients with ARDS. Although data from ARDS patients is lacking to establish a clear preference, suggestions to use balanced crystalloids such as Ringer's lactate solution and PlasmaLyte rather than normal saline are based on studies of critically ill and septic patients [55–58].

b. **Colloids:** In ARDS, routine use of natural colloids like albumin or synthetic colloids like starches is not recommended [59]. Avoid the use of synthetic colloids (gelatins, starches, and dextran) in ARDS due to its well documented adverse effects [60, 61].

c. **Albumin:** Albumin may improve intravascular oncotic pressure and reduce interstitial edema, but the benefits of albumin therapy in ARDS are still controversial. In patients with ARDS and hypoalbuminemia, co-administration of albumin and diuretics has been found to increase urine output, improve pulmonary function and oxygenation, and improve hemodynamic stability [62–64]. Therefore, this treatment approach may be used selectively.

In conclusion, fluid therapy is an essential component of the management of ARDS. Careful fluid balance monitoring, avoiding fluid overload, and individualizing fluid therapy are crucial in preventing further lung injury and improving outcomes.

FLUID THERAPY IN MECHANICAL VENTILATION

Fluid management in a patient on a ventilator is an essential aspect of critical care management. Adequate fluid management is crucial in maintaining optimal cardiovascular and respiratory function and ensuring adequate tissue perfusion.

What care should be taken before initiating positive pressure ventilation in volume-depleted patients, and why?

Before starting ventilation, it is crucial to understand the significance of correcting hypovolemia.

Assess the patient's fluid status and correct hypovolemia before initiating mechanical ventilation. Volume-depleted patients are at risk of developing hypotension on initiating positive pressure ventilation due to several factors.

Hemodynamic effect of mechanical ventilation

Venous blood flows passively from the low-pressure venous system into the right atrium, right ventricle, and finally to the lungs.

A. **Effect of normal inspiration on venous return:** During normal spontaneous inspiration, intrathoracic pressure (ITP) decreases, which accelerates the return of the venous blood flow to the heart and lungs.

B. **Effect of positive pressure ventilation on venous return and cardiac output:** In the patient on positive pressure mechanical ventilation, ITP will increase during inspiration (effect opposite to normal inspiration on ITP). Increased intrathoracic pressure will reduce the systemic venous return.

Since the cardiac output is heavily dependent on venous return, positive pressure ventilation can actually have a detrimental effect on cardiac output. Furthermore, this type of ventilation can elevate pressure levels in the lungs, which in turn can compress pulmonary blood vessels and cause a decrease in blood flow to the right side of the heart. Ultimately, this decrease can lead to hypotension and a decrease in cardiac output.

Furthermore, positive pressure ventilation can also increase the pressure in the abdominal cavity, decreasing venous return to the heart and reducing cardiac output.

C. **Clinical importance:** In euvolemic patients with normal cardiac function, positive pressure ventilation increases ITP, resulting in decreased venous return and left ventricular stroke volume. However, the reduction in venous return is more pronounced in cases of hypovolemia or decreased venous tone (such as sepsis or hypoglycemia). Therefore, positive pressure ventilation may lead to severe hypotension in patients with hypovolemia, acute hemorrhage, or spinal shock.

D. **Prevention of hemodynamic abnormalities:** Correct hypovolemia before initiating positive pressure ventilation. It is important to closely monitor these patients and adjust the ventilator settings to prevent hemodynamic compromise.

Management

Achieving hemodynamic stability during ventilation initiation can be facilitated by correcting hypovolemia through optimal IV fluid replacement, early use of vasopressors in low vasomotor tone states, and smaller tidal volume ventilation. Additionally, avoid large tidal volume or excessively high levels of positive end-expiratory pressure (PEEP), because it will further reduce venous return as well as cardiac output and blood pressure.

A. Strategies for administering the correct fluid volume

Appropriate fluid management is essential in the treatment of critically ill patients on a ventilator and may require large volumes of fluid to provide hemodynamic support and maintain adequate organ perfusion, provide maintenance need, replace ongoing losses, ensure appropriate caloric/protein intake, and as a vehicle for drug delivery [65]. However, administering the appropriate volume of fluid can be challenging because both fluid overload and dehydration can be harmful.

Positive fluid balance in patients on a ventilator is associated with negative consequences such as a higher risk of ventilator-associated events, delayed weaning from the ventilator, longer time on mechanical ventilation, a longer length of ICU stay, higher mortality, and increased healthcare costs [41, 66–72].

Conservative fluid strategies are beneficial for patients on a ventilator as they help prevent volume overload and provide benefits such as decreased ventilator-associated events, reduced extubation failure, increased number of ventilator-free days, and decreased length of ICU stay, especially in patients with acute respiratory distress syndrome [46, 65, 73–75].

Strategies that help to avoid positive (cumulative) fluid balance and volume overload are [71, 76]:

- Fluid resuscitation is a lifesaving intervention for critically ill patients, but it is crucial to avoid overzealous use of intravenous fluids and to slow down the rate of infusion once resuscitation goals have been achieved.

- To prevent volume overload, adopt a more restrictive approach to fluid administration in the later phases immediately after early fluid resuscitation. To provide the maintenance needs, consider administering lower volumes of IV fluids or avoiding them altogether, considering the patient's volume status and other sources of fluid intake. Optimize fluid intake by using dynamic measures to assess fluid responsiveness rather than static measures such as central venous pressure.

- It is essential to minimize the volume of fluid used as a vehicle for drug delivery and to maintain the patency of indwelling intravascular catheters (recently termed fluid creep) [65]. This is important because the volume

of fluid used as drug diluents is a significant source of water, sodium, and chloride, and is often overlooked as a source of fluid administered to ICU patients [77].

- Early use of vasopressors (norepinephrine) to achieve a target arterial pressure and limit the volume of fluid to be infused [49].

B. Use diuretics

If the patient has evidence of fluid overload or impaired cardiac function, consider using diuretics to remove excess fluid. The conservative strategy of fluid management and diuretics at the initial phase improves lung function and helps to shorten the duration of mechanical ventilation without increasing the risk of nonpulmonary-organ failures and acute kidney injury [44].

Using furosemide in higher doses, and starting furosemide earlier, help significantly in achieving an overall negative fluid balance [52]. Diuretic-based de-resuscitation provides beneficial effects on clinical outcomes such as lower in-hospital mortality and higher ICU-free days in mechanically ventilated critically ill patients with volume overload [78]. Furosemide is a commonly used diuretic in critically ill patients.

C. Look for electrolyte disturbances

In patients receiving mechanical ventilation, the incidence of electrolyte imbalances is high [79, 80]. Electrolyte disorders such as hypokalemia, hypocalcemia, hypomagnesemia, and hypophosphatemia are frequently observed in patients on mechanical ventilation and are known to increase the duration of mechanical ventilation as well as prolong the stay in the ICU [79, 81].

1. **Hypophosphatemia:** The most common cause of hypophosphatemia in patients on a ventilator is redistribution, which arises from intracellular phosphorus shifting due to respiratory alkalosis caused by overventilation, sepsis, or Beta 2 agonist therapy.

   Severe hypophosphatemia can cause muscle weakness, which may result in a prolonged duration of mechanical ventilation or failure to wean from it [82, 83]. Therefore, correcting hypophosphatemia and malnutrition is essential for improving the strength of respiratory muscles.

2. **Hypokalemia:** Hypokalemia can occur due to treatment with steroids, diuretics, and beta 2 agonists. Hypokalemia can cause weakness of the respiratory muscles, potentially leading to longer durations of mechanical ventilation [84]. In severe cases, hypokalemia can even result in respiratory paralysis.

3. **Hypocalcemia:** It is a common disorder among ventilated patients, which is caused by a combination of factors, such as magnesium deficiency, respiratory alkalosis, and drugs like aminoglycosides, heparin, and theophylline. Hypocalcemia increases the risk of acute respiratory failure and the need for mechanical ventilation [85].

4. **Hypomagnesemia:** It can occur due to therapy with diuretics and antibiotics such as aminoglycosides. Hypomagnesemia causes muscle weakness and respiratory failure, which can make it challenging to wean patients off the ventilator [86]. Correcting hypokalemia and hypocalcemia can be difficult unless hypomagnesemia is addressed first.

To avoid a prolonged period of mechanical ventilation and achieve early and successful weaning, it is essential to routinely check and regularly monitor serum electrolyte levels and correct any imbalances early and optimally.

D. Look for acid-base disturbances

Patients receiving mechanical ventilation may develop respiratory alkalosis, respiratory acidosis, and post-hypercapnic alkalosis.

1. **Respiratory alkalosis:** To correct hypoxemia, patients on a mechanical ventilator may receive hyperventilation, which can lead to the washout of $PaCO_2$ and often cause respiratory alkalosis. If required, the respiratory alkalosis in such patients can be reversed by a reduction in minute ventilation, which involves lowering the tidal volume and/or respiratory rate.

2. **Respiratory acidosis:** In patients on a mechanical ventilator, setting a lower respiratory rate and tidal volume can lead to inadequate ventilation. A resultant accumulation of carbon dioxide (hypercapnia) can cause respiratory acidosis.

   Permissive hypercapnia is a ventilation strategy used in patients with acute respiratory distress syndrome, where low tidal volume and low airway pressure ventilation strategies are used to reduce the risks of lung injury [87]. Respiratory acidosis resulting from permissive hypercapnia is a deliberate increase in arterial carbon dioxide tension that occurs during mechanical ventilation and is commonly accepted in patients with ARDS in order to minimize the risk of further lung injury [88].

3. Post-hypercapnic alkalosis: It is a frequently overlooked complication that can occur in patients with chronic hypercapnia following intubation and mechanical ventilation [89].

In chronic respiratory acidosis (as in COPD), renal compensation leads to an elevated plasma HCO_3 due to increased urinary H^+ secretions, resulting in increased $PaCO_2$, increased HCO_3, and near-normal, acidic pH.

When these patients are intubated and ventilated, $PaCO_2$ levels decrease quickly and return to normal rapidly, but the correction of the elevated bicarbonate (renal compensation) is slow. This state of almost normal $PaCO_2$ but persistent metabolic alkalosis is called 'post-hypercapnic alkalosis'.

REFERENCES

1. Kalhoff H. Mild dehydration: a risk factor of broncho-pulmonary disorders? Eur J Clin Nutr. 2003;57(2):S81–7.

2. Åstrand AB, Hemmerling M, Root J, et al. Linking increased airway hydration, ciliary beating, and mucociliary clearance through ENaC inhibition. Am J Physiol Lung Cell Mol Physiol. 2015;308(1):L22–32.

3. Zanasi A, Mazzolini M, Fontana GA, et al. Alterations in the Hydration Status Affect Coughing in Otherwise Normal School Children. World Wide J. Multidiscip. Res. Dev. 2021;7(3):78–82.

4. Nievas IF, Anand KJ. Severe acute asthma exacerbation in children: a stepwise approach for escalating therapy in a pediatric intensive care unit. J Pediatr Pharmacol Ther. 2013;18(2):88–104.

5. Stookey JD, Brass B, Holliday A, et al. What is the cell hydration status of healthy children in the USA? Preliminary data on urine osmolality and water intake. Public Health Nutr. 2012;15(11):2148–56.

6. Moloney ED, Griffin S, Burke CM, et al. Release of inflammatory mediators from eosinophils following a hyperosmolar stimulus. Respir Med. 2003;97(8):928–32.

7. Yamauchi K, Ogasawara M. The Role of Histamine in the Pathophysiology of Asthma and the Clinical Efficacy of Antihistamines in Asthma Therapy. Int J Mol Sci. 2019;20(7):1733.

8. Sheldon JM. Intravenous use of fluids in bronchial asthma. JAMA. 1949;139(8):506–507

9. Kantor DB, Hirshberg EL, McDonald MC, et al. Fluid Balance Is Associated with Clinical Outcomes and Extravascular Lung Water in Children with Acute Asthma Exacerbation. Am J Respir Crit Care Med. 2018;197(9):1128–1135.

10. Alamoudi OS. Electrolyte disturbances in patients with chronic, stable asthma: effect of therapy. Chest. 2001;120(2):431–6.

11. Mohammad HA, Abdulfttah MT, Abdulazez AO, et al. A study of electrolyte disturbances in patients with chronic stable asthma and with asthma attacks. Egypt J Chest Dis Tuberc. 2014;63:529–34.

12. Das A, Patil S, Nair G, et al. Electrolyte disturbances in patients with acute exacerbation of bronchial asthma. JMSCR. 2018;6(9):315–319.

13. Hung CH, Chu DM, Wang CL, et al. Hypokalemia and salbutamol therapy in asthma. Pediatr Pulmonol. 1999;27(1):27–31.

14. Tsai WS, Wu CP, Hsu YJ, et al. Life-threatening hypokalemia in an asthmatic patient treated with high-dose hydrocortisone. Am J Med Sci. 2004;327(3):152–5.

15. Jain N, Kumari K, Roy S, et al. Hypocalcaemia-induced acute exacerbation of bronchial asthma: An unusual cause of a common disorder. Indian J Anaesth. 2020;64(9):820–821.

16. Kumari A, Nangrani K, Dolkar T, et al. Hypocalcemia Induced Bronchospasm. Cureus. 2022;14(6):e26339.

17. Kılıç H, Kanbay A, Karalezlı A, et al. The Relationship between Hypomagnesemia and Pulmonary Function Tests in Patients with Chronic Asthma. Med Princ Pract. 2018;27(2):139–144.

18. Vittal BG, Rudresha BM, Aliya N, et al. A study of serum electrolyte levels during nebulised salbutamol therapy. J. Clin. Diagn. Res. 2010;4(6):3460–3464

19. Kew KM, Kirtchuk L, Michell CI. Intravenous magnesium sulfate for treating adults with acute asthma in the emergency department. Cochrane Database of Systematic Reviews 2014;28(5):CD010909.

20. Griffiths B, Kew KM, Normansell R. Intravenous magnesium sulfate for treating children with acute asthma in the emergency department. Paediatr Respir Rev. 2016;20:45–47.

21. Su Z, Li R, Gai Z. Intravenous and nebulized magnesium sulfate for treating acute asthma in children: a systematic review and meta-analysis. PediatrEmerg Care. 2018;34(6):390–395.

22. Vasileiadis I, Alevrakis E, Ampelioti S, et al. Acid-Base Disturbances in Patients with Asthma: A Literature Review and Comments on Their Pathophysiology. J Clin Med. 2019;8(4):563.

23. Dias E, Shetty VP. A Study on Initial Arterial Blood Gas in Acute Asthmatic Children in Karnataka India. Acta Scientific Paediatrics 2023;6(1):14–16.

24. McFadden ER Jr. Acute severe asthma. Am J Respir Crit Care Med. 2003;168(7):740–59

25. McFadden ER, Lyons HA. Arterial blood gas tension in asthma. NEJM 1968;278(19):1027–1032.

26. Bagrecha M, Yannawar A, Gaikwad N, et al. A Prospective Study of Arterial Blood Gases in Bronchial Asthma in a Tertiary Care Hospital. MSCR 2019;7(12):82–86.

27. Shigemura M, Homma T, Sznajder JI. Hypercapnia: An Aggravating Factor in Asthma. J Clin Med. 2020;9(10):3207.

28. Rashid AO, Azam HM, DeBari VA, et al. Non-anion gap acidosis in asthma: clinical and laboratory features and outcomes for hospitalized patients. Ann Clin Lab Sci. 2008;38(3):228–34.

29. Mountain RD, Heffner JE, Brackett NC Jr, et al. Acid-base disturbances in acute asthma. Chest. 1990;98(3):651–5.

30. Liedtke AG, Lava SAG, Milani GP, et al. Selective ß2-adrenoceptor agonists and relevant hyperlactatemia: systematic review and meta-analysis. J Clin Med 2019;9(1):71.

31. Phoophiboon V, Singhagowinta P, Boonkaya S, et al. Salbutamol-induced lactic acidosis in status asthmaticus survivor. BMC Pulm Med. 2021;21(1):23.

32. Ruman-Colombier M, Rochat Guignard I, Di Paolo ER, et al. Prevalence and risk factors of lactic acidosis in children with acute moderate and severe asthma, a prospective observational study. Eur J Pediatr. 2021;180(4):1125–1131.

33. Kho SS, Nyanti LE, Muhammad NA, et al. The more you give, the worse it gets. Breathe 2021;17(3):210083

34. Bouachour G, Tirot P, Varache N, et al. Metabolic acidosis in severe acute asthma. Effect of alkaline therapy [French]. Rev Pneumol Clin. 1992;48(3):115–9.

35. Garber BG, Hébert PC, Yelle JD, et al. Adult respiratory distress syndrome: a systemic overview of incidence and risk factors. Crit Care Med. 1996;24(4):687–695.

36. Villar J, Blanco J, Kacmarek RM. Current incidence and outcome of the acute respiratory distress syndrome. Curr Opin Crit Care 2016;22(1):1–6.

37. Ma´ca J, Jor O, Holub M, et al. Past and present ARDS mortality rates: a systematic review. Respir Care 2017;62(1):113–22.

38. Wang Y, Zhang L, Xi X, et al. The Association Between Etiologies and Mortality in Acute Respiratory Distress Syndrome: A Multicenter Observational Cohort Study. Front Med (Lausanne). 2021;8:739596.

39. Vignon P, Evrard B, Asfar P, et al. Fluid administration and monitoring in ARDS: which management? Intensive Care Med. 2020;46(12):2252–2264.

40. Silversides JA, Fitzgerald E, Manickavasagam US, et al. Deresuscitation of Patients With Iatrogenic Fluid Overload Is Associated With Reduced Mortality in Critical Illness. Crit Care Med 2018;46(10):1600–1607.

41. Van Mourik N, Metske HA, Hofstra JJ, et al. Cumulative fluid balance predicts mortality and increases time on mechanical ventilation in ARDS patients. An observational cohort study. PLoS ONE 2019;14(10):e0224563.

42. Ho KS, Kohli P, Herrera Y, et al. Go Easy with the Fluids? Increased Mortality in Acute Respiratory Distress Syndrome with Hypervolemia. European Respiratory Journal 2020;56:3442.

43. Hu W, Zhang S, He Z, et al. Impact of Time-Varying Intensity of Mechanical Ventilation on 28-Day Mortality Depends on Fluid Balance in Patients With Acute Respiratory Distress Syndrome: A Retrospective Cohort Study. Front Med (Lausanne). 2022;9:906903.

44. National Heart, Lung, and Blood Institute Acute Respiratory Distress Syndrome (ARDS) Clinical Trials Network, Wiedemann HP, Wheeler AP, et al. Comparison of two fluid-management strategies in acute lung injury. N Engl J Med. 2006;354(24):2564–2575.

45. Grissom CK, Hirshberg EL, Dickerson JB, et al. Fluid management with a simplified conservative protocol for the acute respiratory distress syndrome*. Crit Care Med. 2015;43(2):288–95.

46. Silversides JA, Major E, Ferguson AJ, et al. Conservative fluid management or deresuscitation for patients with sepsis or acute respiratory distress syndrome following the resuscitation phase of critical illness: a systematic review and meta-analysis. Intensive Care Med. 2017;43(2):155–70.

47. Griffiths MJD, McAuley DF, Perkins GD, et al. Guidelines on the management of acute respiratory distress syndrome. BMJ Open Respir Res. 2019;6(1):e000420.

48. Murphy CV, Schramm GE, Doherty JA, et al. The importance of fluid management in acute lung injury secondary to septic shock. Chest 2009;136(1):102–109.

49. Shi R, Hamzaoui O, De Vita N, et al. Vasopressors in septic shock: which, when, and how much? Ann Transl Med. 2020;8(12):794.

50. Munshi L, Rubenfeld G, Wunsch H. Adjuvants to mechanical ventilation for acute respiratory distress syndrome. Intensive Care Med. 2016;42(5):775–8.

51. Casey JD, Semler MW, Rice TW. Fluid Management in Acute Respiratory Distress Syndrome. Semin Respir Crit Care Med. 2019;40(1):57–65.

52. Cinotti R, Lascarrou JB, Azais MA, et al. Diuretics decrease fluid balance in patients on invasive mechanical ventilation: the randomized-controlled single blind, IRIHS study. Crit Care. 2021;25(1):98.

53. Seitz KP, Caldwell ES, Hough CL. Fluid management in ARDS: an evaluation of current practice and the association between early diuretic use and hospital mortality. J Intensive Care. 2020;8:78.

54. Zhang R, Chen H, Gao Z, et al. The Effect of Loop Diuretics on 28-Day Mortality in Patients with Acute Respiratory Distress Syndrome. Front. Med. 2021;8:740675.

55. Semler MW, Self WH, Wanderer JP, et al. SMART investigators and the Pragmatic Critical Care Research Group: Balanced crystalloids versus saline in critically ill adults. N Engl J Med 2018;378(9):829–839.

56. Brown RM, Wang L, Coston TD, et al. Balanced crystalloids versus saline in sepsis. A secondary analysis of the SMART clinical trial. Am J Respir Crit Care Med. 2019;200(12):1487–1495.

57. Hammond NE, Zampieri FG, Di Tanna GL, et al. Balanced Crystalloids versus Saline in Critically Ill Adults — A Systematic Review with Meta-Analysis. NEJM Evid 2022;1(2).

58. Beran A, Altorok N, Srour O, et al. Balanced Crystalloids versus Normal Saline in Adults with Sepsis: A Comprehensive Systematic Review and Meta-Analysis. J Clin Med. 2022;11(7):1971.

59. Keddissi JI, Youness HA, Jones KR, et al. Fluid management in Acute Respiratory Distress Syndrome: A narrative review. Can J Respir Ther. 2019;55:1–8.

60. Myburgh JA, Finfer S, Bellomo R, et al. Hydroxyethyl Starch or Saline for Fluid Resuscitation in Intensive Care. N Engl J Med 2012;367(20):1901–11.

61. Zarychanski R, Abou-Setta AM, Turgeon AF, et al. Association of hydroxyethyl starch administration with mortality and acute kidney injury in critically ill patients requiring volume resuscitation: A systematic review and meta-analysis. JAMA 2013;309(7):678–88.

62. Martin GS, Mangialardi RJ, Wheeler AP, et al. Albumin and furosemide therapy in hypoproteinemic patients with acute lung injury. Crit Care Med. 2002;30(10):2175–2182.

63. Martin GS, Moss M, Wheeler AP, et al. A randomized, controlled trial of furosemide with or without albumin in hypoproteinemic patients with acute lung injury. Crit Care Med. 2005;33(8):1681–1687.

64. Itagaki Y, Yoshida N, Banno M, et al. Efficacy of albumin with diuretics in mechanically ventilated patients with hypoalbuminemia: A systematic review and meta-analysis. Medicine (Baltimore). 2022;101(37):e30276.

65. Langer T, D'Oria V, Spolidoro GCI, et al. Fluid therapy in mechanically ventilated critically ill children: the sodium, chloride and water burden of fluid creep. BMC Pediatr. 2020;20(1):424.

66. Upadya A, Tilluckdharry L, Muralidharan V, et al.. Fluid balance and weaning outcomes. Intensive Care Med 2005;31(12):1643–7.

67. Flori HR, Church G, Liu KD, et al. Positive fluid balance is associated with higher mortality and prolonged mechanical ventilation in pediatric patients with acute lung injury. Crit Care Res Pract. 2011;2011:854142.

68. Ingelse SA, Wiegers HM, Calis JC, et al. Early Fluid Overload Prolongs Mechanical Ventilation in Children With Viral-Lower Respiratory Tract Disease. Pediatr Crit Care Med. 2017;18(3):e106–e111.

69. Samaddar S, Sankar J, Kabra SK, et al. Association of Fluid Overload with Mortality in Critically-ill Mechanically Ventilated Children. Indian Pediatr. 2018;55(11):957–961.

70. Wang W, Zhu S, He Q, et al. Fluid Balance and Ventilator-Associated Events Among Patients Admitted to ICUs in China: A Nested Case-Control Study. Crit Care Med. 2022;50(2):307–316.

71. Arrahmani I, Ingelse SA, van Woensel JBM, et al. Current Practice of Fluid Maintenance and Replacement Therapy in Mechanically Ventilated Critically Ill Children: A European Survey. Front Pediatr. 2022;10:828637.

72. Wrzosek A, Drygalski T, Garlicki J, et al. The volume of infusion fluids correlates with treatment outcomes in critically ill trauma patients. Front. Med. 2023;9:1040098.

73. Wiedemann HP. A perspective on the fluids and catheters treatment trial (FACTT). Fluid restriction is superior in acute lung injury and ARDS. Cleve Clin J Med. 2008;75(1):42–8.

74. Klompas M. Ventilator-Associated Events: What They Are and What They Are Not. Respir Care. 2019;64(8):953–961.

75. Li T, Zhou D, Zhao D, et al. Association between fluid intake and extubation failure in intensive care unit patients with negative fluid balance: a retrospective observational study. BMC Anesthesiol. 2022;22(1):170.

76. Ogbu OC, Murphy DJ, Martin GS. How to avoid fluid overload. Curr Opin Crit Care. 2015;21(4):315–21.

77. Van Regenmortel N, Verbrugghe W, Roelant E, et al. Maintenance fluid therapy and fluid creep impose more significant fluid, sodium, and chloride burdens than resuscitation fluids in critically ill patients: a retrospective study in a tertiary mixed ICU population. Intensive Care Med. 2018;44(4):409–17.

78. Bissell BD, Laine ME, Thompson et al. Impact of protocolized diuresis for de-resuscitation in the intensive care unit. Critical care. 2020;24(1):70.

79. Vora CS, Karnik ND, Gupta V, et al. Clinical Profile of Patients Requiring Prolonged Mechanical Ventilation and their Outcome in a Tertiary Care Medical ICU. J Assoc Physicians India. 2015;63(10):14–9.

80. Kamdar PK, Kakaiya RR. A study of electrolytes imbalance in mechanically ventilated Patients. International Journal of Scientific Research 2020;9(1):64–67.

81. Morganroth ML, Grum CM. Weaning from Mechanical Ventilator. J Intensive Care Med 1988;3:109–120.

82. Zhao Y, Li Z, Shi Y, et al. Effect of hypophosphatemia on the withdrawal of mechanical ventilation in patients with acute exacerbations of chronic obstructive pulmonary disease. Biomed Rep. 2016;4(4):413–416.

83. Wang L, Xiao C, Chen L, et al. Impact of hypophosphatemia on outcome of patients in intensive care unit: a retrospective cohort study. BMC Anesthesiol. 2019;19(1):86.

84. Javdan Z, Talakoub R, Honarmand A, et al. The predicting ability of serum potassium to assess the duration of mechanical ventilation in critically ill patients. Adv Biomed Res. 2015;4:133.

85. Thongprayoon C, Cheungpasitporn W, Chewcharat A, et al. Serum ionised calcium and the risk of acute respiratory failure in hospitalised patients: a single-centre cohort study in the USA. BMJ Open. 2020;10(3):e034325.

86. Kumar S, Honmode A, Jain S, et al. Does magnesium matter in patients of Medical Intensive Care Unit: A study in rural Central India. Indian J Crit Care Med. 2015;19(7):379–83.

87. Bigatello LM, Patroniti N, Sangalli F. Permissive hypercapnia. Curr Opin Crit Care. 2001;7(1):34–40.

88. Morales-Quinteros L, Camprubí-Rimblas M, Bringué J, et al. The role of hypercapnia in acute respiratory failure. Intensive Care Med Exp. 2019;7(1):39.

89. Banga A, Khilnani GC. Post-hypercapnic alkalosis is associated with ventilator dependence and increased ICU stay. COPD. 2009;6(6):437–40.

40 Diabetic Ketoacidosis and Hyperosmolar Hyperglycemic State

Diabetic ketoacidosis (DKA) and hyperosmolar hyperglycemic state (HHS) are serious and potentially life-threatening metabolic complications of diabetes mellitus (DM). While DKA is a common hyperglycemic emergency with a low mortality rate, characterized by hyperglycemia and ketoacidosis, HHS, on the other hand, is less common, characterized by hyperglycemia and hyperosmolality without ketoacidosis, but has a high mortality rate.

DIABETIC KETOACIDOSIS

Diabetic ketoacidosis is a medical emergency that can be life-threatening if not treated promptly. DKA is one of the common complications of type-I diabetes mellitus (IDDM) associated with significant fluid and electrolyte imbalance.

DEFINITION

Diabetic ketoacidosis is characterized by the triad of [1, 2]:

1. Hyperglycemia: Blood glucose concentration of >200 mg/dL or 11.0 mmol/L.

2. Metabolic acidosis: Venous pH <7.3 and serum bicarbonate <18 mmol/L [1] (or 15 mmol/L [2]).

3. Ketonemia or ketonuria: Capillary ketones >3 mmol/L or urine ketones ++ ("moderate or large").

If a facility to measure blood beta-hydroxybutyrate (BOHB) concentration is available, it is a more precise and sensitive test to diagnose DKA [3].

The urine test for ketones is not a reliable means of diagnosing DKA because it can only detect less common ketones like acetoacetate and acetone, and it may not identify the main ketone beta-hydroxybutyrate that is present in DKA [4]. As a result, although the urine ketone stick test is easily accessible and relatively inexpensive, it does not correlate well with the ketone concentration in the blood plasma. While a positive urine ketone stick test may support the diagnosis of DKA, a negative result cannot rule out DKA and may potentially mislead clinicians.

Euglycemic DKA, which presents with near-normal or mildly elevated glucose levels in some DKA patients, can lead to diagnostic challenges and delay treatment, resulting in poorer outcomes [5]. The common causes of euglycemic DKA include using sodium-glucose cotransporter-2 inhibitors, prolonged fasting or a very low-calorie diet, chronic alcohol consumption, pregnancy, and insulin pump use [6].

Based on venous pH and serum bicarbonate level, the severity of DKA is subdivided into three groups (Table 40.1) [1].

The anion gap (AG) is included in the diagnostic criteria by the American Diabetes Association (ADA), and a high anion gap is an important indicator of the presence of DKA [7].

PATHOPHYSIOLOGY

Diabetic ketoacidosis can frequently lead to fluid and electrolyte imbalances such as dehydration, metabolic acidosis, potassium imbalance, hypophosphatemia, hypomagnesemia, and sodium imbalance. A rough deficit of body water and electrolytes is summarized in Table 40.2 [8, 9].

A. Diabetic ketoacidosis: DKA is caused by an absolute or relative deficiency of insulin combined with insulin resistance, along with the effect of counter-regulatory hormones such as catecholamines, glucagon, growth hormone, and cortisol [7].

This hormonal imbalance leads to three significant metabolic changes:

- Firstly, hyperglycemia occurs due to increased hepatic glucose production (accelerated gluconeogenesis), breakdown of glycogen into glucose (glycogenolysis), and reduced glucose utilization in the peripheral tissues.

- Secondly, there is an increase in proteolysis (breakdown of proteins) and a decrease in protein synthesis.

- Finally, there is an increase in lipolysis (breakdown of fats), resulting in ketone production.

When insulin is deficient, it results in an increased lipolysis, which in turn releases free fatty acids into the circulation. This causes an increase in plasma free fatty acids (FFA), leading to an elevation in hepatic free fatty acids. This process triggers the production of ketone bodies. Glucagon is the primary hormone responsible for inducing ketogenesis by increasing fatty acid oxidation in the liver.

Table 40.1 The severity of diabetic ketoacidosis			
	Mild	**Moderate**	**Severe**
Blood glucose	>11 mmol/L (200 mg/dL)		
Venous pH	<7.3	<7.2	<7.1
Serum bicarbonate	<18 mmol/L	<10 mmol/L	<5.0 mmol/L

Table 40.2 Approximate total body water and electrolytes deficits in DKA					
	Water	**Sodium**	**Potassium**	**Chloride**	**Phosphorus**
Deficits/kg	100 mL/kg	7.0–10 mEq/kg	3.0–5.0 mEq/kg	3.0–5.0 mEq/kg	1.0 mmol/kg
Total deficits	5–7 litres	500–700 mmol	200–350 mmol	200–350 mmol	350–500 mmol

The combined effect of insulin deficiency (causing increased lipolysis) and high glucagon levels (causing accelerated hepatic fatty acid oxidation and ketogenesis) results in ketonemia and an increased anion gap metabolic acidosis. Various factors can precipitate DKA, such as inadequate or discontinuation of insulin, an irregular diet, infection, trauma, surgery, emotional stress, myocardial ischemia, and others.

B. Metabolic acidosis: In DKA, there is an excessive mobilization of fat to supply energy. This process results in the formation of large amounts of ketone bodies, such as B-hydroxy butyric acid and acetoacetic acid. Bicarbonate buffer is utilized to counterbalance the acidic nature of these ketoacids, which causes a decrease in serum bicarbonate levels, leading to metabolic acidosis. Additionally, due to the high levels of ketones, the anion gap is also high.

Furthermore, in DKA, severe dehydration causes hypoperfusion leading to impaired renal function. This, in turn, further contributes to metabolic acidosis.

C. Dehydration: Major reasons for dehydration/hypovolemia in DKA are hyperglycemia-induced osmotic diuresis, vomiting, and reduced oral intake.

The primary cause is hyperglycemia-induced osmotic diuresis, which occurs when the renal threshold for glucose, approximately 196 mg/dL, is surpassed [10]. When glucose levels become elevated in DKA, glycosuria results,

which leads to the excretion of large amounts of water and electrolytes, resulting in volume depletion and dehydration.

Additionally, the hyperosmolality caused by hyperglycemia in DKA causes water to move out of cells, leading to intracellular (ICF) dehydration and extracellular fluid (ECF) expansion. This exacerbates the diuresis and further worsens hypovolemia.

As dehydration and volume depletion progress, renal blood flow decreases, and the kidneys' ability to excrete glucose is reduced, further exacerbating hyperglycemia [9].

Vomiting in DKA causes loss of water and electrolytes, which, when combined with reduced oral intake due to altered sensorium, can further aggravate hypovolemia.

D. Potassium imbalance: In DKA, total body potassium reserves are always substantially depleted, and the average deficit is about 3–5 mEq/kg or 200–350 mmol of potassium [8, 9]. Common causes of potassium depletion in DKA are increased urinary losses of potassium (due to both hyperglycemia-induced osmotic diuresis and the excretion of ketoacid anion salts), vomiting due to DKA, poor oral intake due to anorexia and associated hypomagnesemia.

Careful interpretation of serum potassium is crucial in DKA as there is a poor correlation between serum potassium and total body potassium deficit. Besides total body potassium deficit in most patients with DKA, on presentation, serum potassium is normal in the majority, low in less than 5% of patients, and high in as many as one-third of patients [11].

Hyperkalemia is frequently seen in patients with DKA despite substantial total body potassium deficits. Mechanisms of the development of hyperkalemia in DKA on presentation besides its deficit in the body are [7, 12–14]:

- **The shift of potassium from ECF to ICF:** Administration of short acting IV insulin and correction of metabolic acidosis during treatment shifts K^+ from ECF to ICF and reduces serum potassium levels.

- **Hypovolemia and prerenal failure** due to polyuria secondary to hyperglycemia can result in hyperkalemia.

Change in serum potassium concentration after therapy

Following treatment initiation, over 50% of DKA patients who initially had normal or high potassium levels will rapidly develop hypokalemia [15, 16]. Mechanisms of the development of hypokalemia after initiation of therapy in DKA are [7]:

- **The shift of potassium from ECF to ICF:** Administration of short acting IV insulin and correction of metabolic acidosis during treatment shifts K^+ from ECF to ICF and reduces serum potassium levels.

- **Loss of potassium** due to the persistence of DKA-induced vomiting and uncontrolled hyperglycemia-induced diuresis.

- **Dilution and volume expansion** due to the administration of IV fluids can decrease serum potassium concentrations.

E. Sodium imbalance: In DKA, hyponatremia is common, and hypernatremia is much less common electrolyte disturbances.

Hyponatremia: Important mechanisms that can contribute to the development of hyponatremia in DKA include [17]:

- Hypertonic or translocational hyponatremia: The hyperosmolar status caused by hyperglycemia in DKA shifts water from the intracellular to the extracellular space, resulting in a dilutional effect and hyponatremia.

- Dilutional hyponatremia due to the administration of hypotonic fluids used to correct dehydration in DKA.

- Urinary sodium loss due to hyperglycemia-induced osmotic diuresis.

- Greater water intake and excessive loss or reduced sodium intake due to nausea and vomiting.

Corrected sodium in DKA: Hyperglycemia in DKA shifts water from ICF to ECF, causing serum sodium to decrease by 1.6 mEq/L for every 100 mg/dL increase in serum glucose concentration (above normal levels). It's essential to remember that in severe hyperglycemia cases, the "normal" sodium level is actually elevated, indicating hypernatremia and severe volume depletion.

To choose the suitable sodium concentration of fluids for patients with DKA, it is crucial to know the corrected sodium value.

The formula to calculate the corrected sodium value is:

$$\text{Corrected Na}^+ \text{ (mEq/L)} = \text{Measured Na}^+ + 1.6 \times \frac{\text{Glucose (mg/dL)} - 100}{100}$$

For example, to calculate the corrected sodium value in hyperglycemia, please refer to Chapter 20 on "Hyponatremia."

Hypernatremia: Hyperglycemia-induced osmotic diuresis leading to hypotonic renal water losses and water deficit from inadequate water intake causes hypernatremia in DKA.

F. Other losses: In addition to the loss of water, sodium, and potassium, there is a loss of phosphorous and magnesium.

Hypophosphatemia: Causes of hypophosphatemia in DKA are a shift of phosphate from ECF to ICF due to metabolic acidosis, hyperglycemia-induced osmotic diuresis causes phosphaturia and poor oral intake of phosphate-containing diet [18, 19].

Hypomagnesemia: In DKA, hypomagnesemia occurs frequently, and its most important cause is excessive urinary magnesium loss.

Fluid replacement is a critical aspect of management because DKA leads to the significant fluid deficit (i.e., 100 mL/kg or about 5 to 7 liters).

TREATMENT

To successfully manage DKA, it is necessary to provide comprehensive treatment that corrects fluid deficits, replaces electrolytes, administers insulin therapy, and offers supportive care while identifying and treating precipitating factors and minimizing the risks of complications.

To effectively treat DKA, it is crucial to closely monitor the patient's clinical status (e.g., hydration and neurological status), chart vital signs (e.g., heart rate, blood pressure, temperature, and respiratory rate) and therapeutic interventions meticulously, and serially measure laboratory parameters such as glucose, serum electrolytes, urea and creatinine, pH, serum or urine ketones, and anion gap.

A. Fluid replacement

Administering appropriate fluid replacement should be the first and most important therapeutic measure in DKA and should begin before starting insulin therapy [1, 2].

The goals of fluid replacement in DKA are:

- To restore circulatory volume effectively and achieve hemodynamic stability and adequate tissue perfusion.

- To enhance renal filtration and promote the elimination of glucose and ketones from the blood, which improves glycemic control and reduces ketosis independent of insulin.

- To correct electrolyte imbalances.

Basic principles

Important basic principles to be followed in the management of DKA are outlined below:

- Fluid replacement is a critical aspect of managing DKA because the condition can result in a significant fluid deficit, usually around 100 mL/kg or approximately 5 to 7 liters.

- The rate of fluid replacement should be based on the patient's clinical status. In the past, there was a concern that rapid fluid replacement could lead to cerebral edema. However, this is no longer a significant risk, and clinicians should not restrict fluid administration unnecessarily [1, 20].

- The sodium content of intravenous fluids should be determined based on the patient's serum sodium concentration and any changes in it due to treatment.

- The decision on when and how much potassium to add to IV fluids in DKA is based on the serum potassium concentration.

- Switching to 5% to 10% dextrose-containing fluids is recommended when the blood sugar level drops to 200–250 mg/dL (11–14 mmol/L) or below to prevent hypoglycemia. In DKA, hyperglycemia improves first, and ketosis resolves later.

- When administering fluid replacement, caution should be exercised to avoid iatrogenic fluid overload, particularly in patients with kidney or heart failure and in elderly people.

Rate of fluid replacement

The rate at which fluid is infused for the initial and subsequent replacement differs:

1. **Initial fluid replacement:** The rate of initial fluid replacement is decided on the basis of clinical and hydration status [1, 2, 21–24].

   a. Hypovolemic shock: If a patient presents with hypotension (systolic BP <90 mmHg) and exhibits signs of shock, such as a weak, thready pulse with low volume and tachycardia, it is recommended to administer 20 mL/kg boluses of isotonic crystalloids as quickly as possible through a large bore cannula to restore circulatory volume rapidly. After administering the initial bolus, the patient should be reassessed. If shock persists or more fluid is needed to restore adequate circulation, additional boluses of 10 mL/kg may be administered.

   Once the systolic blood pressure exceeds 90mmHg, it is recommended to administer one liter of 0.9% sodium chloride within the next 60 minutes. It is important not to deduct the fluid bolus from the total fluid

deficit while calculating the overall fluid requirement.

   b. Hypovolemia without shock: In patients with DKA who are clinically dehydrated but without shock, it is recommended to administer 10 mL/kg of isotonic crystalloids as an intravenous bolus over 30 minutes [1, 21, 23]. Administer a second bolus of 10 mL/kg of crystalloid if needed to restore adequate circulation after clinical reassessment, and then subtract these initial bolus volumes from the total fluid deficit [21].

2. **Subsequent fluid management:** Subsequent fluid therapy aims to calculate the total fluid requirement, which is the sum of fluid deficit and maintenance fluid requirements, and replace the estimated total fluid over 48 hours [1, 22–24]. When calculating the replacement fluid volume, it is crucial to not subtract resuscitation boluses for shock and to avoid adding urinary losses [23]. Nonetheless, it is essential to subtract the volume of fluid initially infused as a bolus for non-shocked patients from the estimated fluid deficit. To calculate the fluid deficit, assume 5% dehydration for mild to moderate DKA (blood pH 7.1 or above) and 10% dehydration for severe DKA (blood pH below 7.1).

Usually, most patients need isotonic crystalloids at 150–200 ml/hr for subsequent fluid management.

Selecting the right fluid for replacement

Choosing the right fluid for replacement is essential in treating DKA effectively. When selecting a crystalloid for fluid replacement, it is crucial to consider the appropriate sodium concentration of the IV fluid based on the corrected serum sodium value, the buffer content of the crystalloid, and the dextrose content based on blood sugar levels.

1. Crystalloids vs. colloids for resuscitation

Recent guidelines on diabetic ketoacidosis recommend using crystalloids instead of colloids for resuscitation, as colloids may be associated with an increased risk of mortality and morbidity [1, 2].

2. Normal saline vs. balanced crystalloid solutions for resuscitation

The current controversy revolves around selecting either normal saline or balanced crystalloids (such as Ringer's lactate and PlasmaLyte) for resuscitation in cases of DKA.

Normal saline: For resuscitation in DKA, normal saline is a widely used and preferred IV fluid because [2]:

- Readily available, low cost, and decades of clinical experience.

- The fluid of choice for resuscitation in DKA, as recommended by most textbooks and clinical guidelines [1, 7, 21–25].

- In some countries, pre-mixed solutions of normal saline and varying potassium concentrations (e.g., 20 mEq/L or 40 mEq/L) are available commercially, which comply with National Patient Safety Agency (NPSA) recommendations.

The limitations or disadvantages of large-volume administration of normal saline are [26]:

- The chloride content in normal saline is high, at 154 mEq/L. Therefore, administering large volumes of saline may result in hyperchloremic metabolic acidosis. This condition can worsen high anion gap metabolic acidosis induced by DKA.

- Additionally, hyperchloremia carries the risk of acute kidney injury.

Balanced crystalloids: The rationales for using balanced crystalloids such as Ringer's lactate and PlasmaLyte for resuscitation in DKA are:

a. Various trials have demonstrated the benefits of balanced crystalloids [27–29], such as the faster resolution of metabolic acidosis in DKA [30–33], lower total cost, and lower rates of cerebral edema [34].

b. Recent systematic reviews and meta-analyses have demonstrated earlier and faster resolution of acidosis with balanced crystalloids [35, 36].

c. Saline may be associated with a longer resolution time for DKA and hospital stay compared to balanced crystalloids [37].

d. Several recent studies suggest the use of balanced crystalloids in DKA [38–42], and its use is also included in recent guidelines for treating DKA [2, 43, 44].

Thus, normal saline was preferred and recommended in DKA only because the evidence for the superiority of balanced crystalloids was inadequate in the past.

The limitation or disadvantage of balanced crystalloids is insufficient potassium if used alone (i.e., Ringer's lactate contains 4 mEq/L potassium, and PlasmaLyte contains 5 mEq/L potassium), and the lack of commercial availability of a balanced solution with adequate pre-mixed potassium [2].

3. Selection for subsequent fluid therapy based on corrected serum sodium concentration

After hypovolemia is corrected with initial fluid replacement, select the appropriate IV fluid based on the value of the corrected serum sodium concentration. The ADA guidelines recommend the continuation of normal saline if the corrected serum sodium level is below 135 mEq/L, indicating the presence of hyponatremia. However, in the majority of patients with normal or high sodium levels, the IV fluid is switched to 0.45% NaCl, which is usually infused at a rate of 250 to 500 mL/hour to provide electrolyte-free water [7].

4. Addition of dextrose solution

In treating DKA, a 5% to 10% dextrose solution is added to IV fluids once blood sugar levels reduced to less than 200–250 mg/dL (11–14.0 mmol/L) to avoid hypoglycaemia [25]. Hyperglycemia typically improves earlier than ketoacidosis during DKA treatment [7]. Therefore, adding dextrose to IV fluids allows for the continued administration of insulin until the resolution of ketoacidosis while avoiding the risk of hypoglycemia.

When administering fluid replacement to patients with euglycemic DKA, it is important to include dextrose solution from the beginning, alongside continuous insulin infusion. The insulin is used to correct ketoacidosis, while the dextrose solution helps prevent hypoglycemia and accelerates the clearance of ketosis. If, despite the addition of dextrose 5%, the patient's ketoacidosis persists, it may be necessary to shift to dextrose 10% in order to provide a greater amount of dextrose.

B. Insulin therapy

Insulin plays a critical role in treating DKA by reducing blood glucose levels, diminishing ketone production, resolving ketoacidosis, and correcting electrolyte disturbances [2].

The basic principle of administering insulin in DKA are [1, 2, 23]:

- Always start short-acting intravenous insulin one hour after administering intravenous fluids once the initial rehydration bolus is complete.

- Delaying insulin therapy in patients with DKA who have serum potassium levels below 3.3 mEq/L is critical to avoid life-threatening hypokalemia, which can occur due to insulin-induced intracellular shifts of potassium. It is essential to simultaneously infuse potassium while administering insulin when potassium levels range from 3.3 to 5.3 mEq/L.

- In the management of severe DKA, the use of a continuous fixed rate intravenous insulin infusion (FRIII) via an infusion pump is preferred over subcutaneous insulin due to its short half-life, rapid onset of action, and ease of titration.

- The standard insulin infusion preparation protocol is diluting 50 units of regular (soluble) insulin in 50 ml of 0.9% saline. The infusion is then administered at a dosage of 0.05 to 0.1 units per kilogram of body weight per hour.

- The current literature recommends low-dose insulin infusion (less than 0.1 units/kg/hr) rather than standard-dose insulin infusion (≥0.1 units/kg/hr) due to similar efficacy and a more favorable safety profile [45]. In addition, with low-dose continuous fixed rate intravenous insulin infusion, blood sugar reduction is smoother, and there is less risk of developing hypokalemia and hypoglycemia.

- Administering insulin through intravenous bolus doses is generally not recommended because of the potential risks of shock and exacerbation of hypokalemia.

However, a bolus (stat) dose of intramuscular insulin (0.1 unit/kg) may be given initially if there is an expected delay in setting up an insulin infusion.

- Once blood sugar levels are reduced to 200–250 mg/dL (11–14 mmol/L), and ketonemia is present, adding a 10% dextrose infusion and reducing the insulin infusion rate to 0.05 units/kg/hr can prevent hypoglycemia.

- Once blood ketoacidosis is resolved and the patient can eat and drink normally, consider switching from intravenous to subcutaneous insulin administration.

C. Potassium supplementation

In DKA, it is crucial to remember that all patients with severe DKA will have a total body potassium deficit, regardless of their serum potassium levels on presentation (low, normal, or high), as discussed in the pathophysiology. Therefore, all DKA patients require potassium supplementation. However, the timing for initiation, the amount of infusion, and the decision to discontinue potassium supplementation all depend on the serum potassium level.

The treatment plan based on the initial serum potassium levels within the first 24 hours [1, 2, 21, 23, 24, 43]:

- If the serum potassium level is high, greater than 5.3 mEq/L, delay K+ supplementation initially. Monitor the serum potassium level hourly and add 40 mEq/L potassium chloride once the serum potassium level is below 5.5 mEq/L and there is a history of passing urine.

- If the serum potassium level is normal, between 3.3 to 5.3 mEq/L, add potassium chloride 40 mEq/L to each liter of IV fluid to be initiated after diuresis.

- If the serum potassium level is low, between 2.5 to 3.3 mEq/L, add potassium chloride 40 mEq/L to each liter of IV fluid. Temporarily hold the insulin administration until the potassium level is above 3.3 mEq/L, and monitor the serum potassium level hourly.

Potassium supplementation in DKA aims to achieve and maintain a serum potassium level of 4.0–5.0 mEq/L [7].

When administering intravenous boluses for resuscitation in the initial phase, it's essential to avoid adding potassium to the infusion as it's typically infused rapidly. If the maximum rate of potassium replacement is insufficient to resolve hypokalemia, the insulin infusion rate may need to be reduced.

Supplementing potassium entirely as potassium chloride carries the risk of hyperchloremic metabolic acidosis. Options to decrease chloride load include administering a 50:50 mixture of 20 mEq/L potassium chloride and 20 mmol/L potassium phosphate or adding potassium chloride to other low chloride-containing fluids, such as 0.45% sodium chloride with 5% glucose, Ringer's lactate, or PlasmaLyte.

D. Treatment of metabolic acidosis

The mainstay for correcting high AG metabolic acidosis in DKA is the adequate replacement of IV fluids and insulin. Due to the lack of benefits, routine replacement of bicarbonate in DKA is not recommended [33]. Moreover, excessive bicarbonate administration in DKA carries potential risks such as a paradoxical increase in cerebrospinal fluid acidosis, cerebral edema, hypokalemia, delay in the resolution of ketosis, and post-treatment metabolic alkalosis.

Bicarbonate therapy is indicated in a few patients with DKA who have [7]:

- Severe metabolic acidosis (pH ≤6.9), which can compromise cardiac contractility.
- DKA associated with shock.
- Severe, life-threatening hyperkalemia (serum potassium >6.5–7 mEq/L).

For patients with a pH ≤6.9, ADA recommends administering 100 mEq of sodium bicarbonate (two ampules) diluted in 400 ml of sterile water (an isotonic solution) with 20 mEq of potassium chloride (KCl) to be infused at a rate of 200 ml/h until the venous pH is >7.0 [7].

E. Correction of hypophosphatemia

The routine use of phosphate supplements in DKA has not demonstrated any benefits, and as a result, current guidelines do not recommend their routine replacement [1, 2, 7, 21]. In addition to a lack of efficacy, phosphate administration is not without risk, as it may lead to hyperphosphatemia and hypocalcemia. However, severe hypophosphatemia can have serious consequences such as respiratory and skeletal muscle weakness, respiratory failure, rhabdomyolysis, impaired myocardial contractibility, and cardiac arrhythmias.

Phosphate replacement therapy is reserved for a few patients with severe hypophosphatemia (<1 mg/dL [0.32 mmol/L]) and significant symptoms [1].

A safe and effective method of providing phosphate without a significant risk of hypocalcemia is to combine the addition of 20 mEq/L of potassium phosphate with 20 mEq/L of potassium chloride in one liter of intravenous fluid [1]. It is essential to closely monitor serum calcium levels during phosphate administration to ensure early diagnosis of secondary hypocalcemia.

IDENTIFY AND TREAT PRECIPITATING FACTORS

80% of cases of DKA are caused by either insufficient insulin or an infection. A careful history and examination can help diagnose the precipitating factor for DKA, which in turn enables specific treatment planning.

AVOIDANCE OF THERAPY RELATED COMPLICATIONS

Care should be taken to avoid treatment-related complications:

1. Hypoglycemia
2. Hypokalemia and hyperkalemia
3. Cerebral edema
4. Hyperchloremic acidosis

Symptomatic cerebral edema in adult patients with DKA is relatively uncommon, and its possible causes are an idiosyncratic response to the metabolic injury and subsequent treatment [2].

MONITORING OF TREATMENT

To effectively treat DKA, it is crucial to monitor the following closely:

- Patient's clinical status, including hydration levels and neurological function.
- Chart vital signs (e.g., heart rate, blood pressure, temperature, and respiratory rate), urine output.
- Meticulously maintain a flow chart of therapeutic interventions, including the time and amount of insulin, fluid, and electrolytes administered.
- Monitor laboratory parameters serially such as glucose, serum electrolytes, urea and creatinine, pH, serum or urine ketones, and anion gap.

Urine output: Assessing urine output is a common way to determine fluid status in the body. In general, good urine output indicates adequate fluid replacement and proper hydration. However, urine output alone may not be a reliable indicator in patients with DKA.

DKA can cause osmotic diuresis due to hyperglycemia, resulting in high urine output even in the presence of a volume deficit. Therefore, additional parameters must be considered to assess hydration accurately in DKA cases.

Below are the most common laboratory parameters used to monitor treatment and their clinical implications summarized:

1. Blood Glucose

Effective therapy can reduce blood glucose levels, so monitoring blood glucose levels every hour is essential. When blood glucose falls below 200–250 mg/dL, insulin should be continued, but in a lesser dose, and glucose infusion should be added until ketosis disappears to avoid hypoglycemia.

2. Serum potassium and sodium

Adequate fluid and insulin therapy can effectively reduce serum potassium levels, while administering potassium-containing IV fluids increase serum potassium levels. Monitoring potassium levels every 2–4 hours is vital to assess changes in serum potassium concentration and plan therapeutic strategies accordingly.

Additionally, monitoring sodium levels serially every 2–4 hours is essential. Calculating the value of corrected serum sodium concentration and monitoring changes in sodium concentration with therapy will guide selecting the appropriate sodium concentration of IV fluid, such as normal saline versus half (0.45%) saline.

3. Serum and urine ketone measurement

The detection and serial monitoring of ketonemia or ketonuria are essential for diagnosing DKA and planning and adjusting its treatment in affected patients.

DKA is characterized by the accumulation of three ketone bodies: acetoacetate, beta-hydroxybutyrate, and acetone. Of these, beta-hydroxybutyrate is the most abundant ketone in DKA. Usually, the ratio of beta-hydroxybutyrate to acetoacetate is 1, but in DKA, this ratio increases to 7–10. Therefore, the detection of both acetoacetate and beta-hydroxybutyrate is more specific for the diagnosis of DKA.

Three commonly used methods for measuring ketones are urine ketone testing, semiquantitative serum ketone testing, and direct measurement of serum beta-hydroxybutyrate. The benefits and limitations of each of these tests are summarized below [4, 46].

a. Urine ketone testing

This is the most widely available bedside technique for measuring ketones in DKA. The urine dipstick test is a quick and easy-to-perform method. However, this test only measures aceto-acetic acid, not beta-hydroxybutyrate, the most abundant ketone. As a result, this test has lower sensitivity and specificity for diagnosing DKA.

It is crucial to note that the urine ketone test's results cannot be solely relied upon to modify therapy as it reflects the average urine ketone concentration since the last void. Therefore, timely treatment modification based solely on the test report is not possible. Furthermore, a significant issue with this test is the delay in obtaining a urine sample due to dehydration, which is usually present in patients with DKA.

Finally, it is important to note that after initiating treatment, blood β-hydroxybutyrate is oxidized to acetoacetate, which can cause urine ketone readings to rise. The presence of ketones in urine can potentially give a false impression and misguide clinicians that the condition is not improving, even though blood β-hydroxybutyrate concentrations are reducing and ketoacidosis is resolving.

b. Semiquantitative serum ketone testing

For many years, the major methodology used to detect high levels of blood ketoacid and acetone has been testing with nitroprusside. This method offers greater accuracy compared to urine ketone testing. However, it primarily measures acetoacetate and not beta-hydroxybutyrate. As a result, it is less sensitive than the direct measurement of the serum beta-hydroxybutyrate approach.

c. Direct measurement of serum beta-hydroxybutyrate

For measuring ketones in DKA, this is the most accurate and sensitive method. It involves using a laboratory assay to measure the blood concentration of beta-hydroxybutyrate, a predominant ketone in DKA. Recent guidelines favor diagnosing and managing hospitalized patients based on point-of-care or near-patient testing (bedside monitoring) [2, 23]. However, this method is more expensive and time-consuming than the other two methods and unavailable everywhere.

4. pH and anion gap

The measurement of venous blood gases (VBG) and the calculation of anion gap are valuable tests for diagnosing and managing DKA. VBG is particularly useful for assessing the status of metabolic acidosis. In DKA, VBG is preferred over arterial blood gas (ABG) measurement because both techniques yield almost similar pH results, and VBG avoids the pain, discomfort, and potential complications associated with repeated arterial punctures [47–50].

When bedside facilities for measuring ketones through blood beta-hydroxybutyrate estimations are not available, the anion gap measurement can serve as a practical alternative test for detecting the presence of ketones. Tracking changes in anion gap levels can also help in monitoring the response to treatment and resolution of ketosis.

The formula used to calculate anion gap in DKA is:

AG =
   Calculated Sodium –
      [Chloride + Bicarbonate]

The normal value for AG is 12 ± 2 mEq/L, whereas, in DKA, its value is typically greater than 16 mEq/L (usually 20–30 mEq/L). An increased pH and normalization of the previously increased anion gap levels indicate a positive response to therapy.

SUPPORTIVE TREATMENT

Supportive treatment is discussed later, along with treatment of hyperglycemic, hyperosmolar nonketotic coma.

HYPEROSMOLAR HYPERGLYCEMIC STATE (HHS)

Hyperosmolar hyperglycemic state (HHS), also known as a hyperosmotic hyperglycemic nonketotic state (HHNK), is a less common but more serious acute complication of diabetes mellitus compared to DKA. The mortality rate for

HHS is high, ranging from 5–20%, which is 10 times higher than that of patients with DKA, particularly in older patients and when accompanied by coma [51].

PRESENTATION

HHS occurs over a longer interval, typically days or weeks, and fluid losses, dehydration, and hyperglycemia are usually more pronounced than DKA.

The condition is often characterized by weakness, polyuria, and polydipsia and usually occurs in patients who cannot drink sufficient water to compensate for urinary fluid loss. It is more common in older and obese patients with type 2 diabetes who experience severe dehydration and hyperglycemia without developing ketoacidosis.

Hypotension, tachycardia, and altered mental status are common clinical findings in patients with HHS. However, clinical symptoms may be mild at an early stage, and diagnosis may be delayed. Neurological symptoms such as lethargy and confusion typically occur when the serum osmolality exceeds 310 mOsm/kg, while convulsions and coma are observed when osmolality exceeds 320–330 mOsm/kg.

HHS is often triggered by infections, cerebrovascular events, myocardial infarction, or drug therapy, such as glucocorticoids, thiazide diuretics, phenytoin, and β-blockers. Non-compliance to treatment can also contribute to the development of HHS.

Table 40.3 summarizes the differentiation of pathophysiology,

Table 40.3 Differences between DKA and HHS		
	DKA	**HHS**
Primary abnormality	Ketoacidosis	Hypertonicity
Primary defect	Absolute insulin deficiency	Relative insulin deficiency
Incidence	Common	Uncommon
Patients affected	Type 1 DM > type 2 DM, young > elderly	Usually type 2, elderly > young, common in obese
Onset	Acute (Hours to 1–2 days)	Chronic (Days to week)
Neurological symptoms	Later and less	Early and severe
Dehydration	Moderate to severe	Severe to profound
Water deficit	100 mL/kg or 6 liter	100 to 200 mL/kg or 9 liter
Hyperglycemia	Present	Very severe
Blood sugar	>250 mg/dL	>600 mg/dL
Ketoacidosis	Large	Absent or minimal
Arterial pH	<7.3	>7.3
Serum bicarbonate	<15 mEq/L	>15 mEq/L
Anion gap	High	Normal (<14 mEq/L)
Serum osmolality	Variable, <320 mOsm/L	High >320 mOsm/L
Serum sodium	Usually low or normal	Usually high
Serum potassium	Normal or elevated	Normal or elevated
Mortality	Low, <1%	High, 5–20%

presentation, and diagnostic features between HHS and DKA [1, 52].

DIAGNOSIS

Major features of HHS are [1, 52, 53]:

1. Severe dehydration with predominant neurological symptoms.

2. Hyperglycemia, blood sugar >600 mg/dL (>33.3 mmol/L).

3. Effective serum osmolality >320 mOsm/kg.

4. Absent to small ketonemia and ketonuria.

5. Arterial pH >7.30; venous pH >7.25; and serum bicarbonate >15 mEq/L.

TREATMENT

The therapy for HHS is similar to that of DKA since it involves correcting fluid and electrolyte deficits, hyperglycemia, and hyperosmolarity. As hyperosmolality and hypernatremia in HHS develop gradually over several days, it is recommended to carefully correct osmolality at a rate of 3.0–8.0 mOsm/kg/h, gently lower sodium at a rate of 0.5 mEq/L, and reduce blood glucose levels by 180–270 mg/dL (10–15 mmol/L) within the first 24 hours to prevent complications such as osmotic demyelination, cerebral edema, and volume overload [1, 52].

A. Fluid therapy

The primary goal of the initial fluid therapy in HHS is to expand both the intravascular and extravascular volume, increase circulatory volume, improve tissue perfusion, and restore normal kidney perfusion [1, 52]. In HHS, due to a larger fluid deficit (100 to 200 mL/kg or 9 liter), a more vigorous and faster fluid replacement is required than recommended for DKA. The goal of treatment is to replenish around 50% of

the estimated fluid loss within the initial 12 hours [52].

Hypotensive patients: It is appropriate to use the normal saline solution as the principal fluid for restoring circulating volume, correcting hypotension, and reversing dehydration in HHS [52]. Additionally, because of its high sodium concentration (154 mEq/L), normal saline helps avoid a harmful rapid reduction in osmolality in hypernatremic HHS patients. Therefore, an initial bolus of 20 mL/kg of normal saline is recommended for immediate resuscitation in hypotensive patients. Careful monitoring of serum osmolality and adjustment of fluid replacement rate is essential in achieving positive fluid balance and controlled decline in osmolality during initial fluid replacement in HHS.

Subsequent fluid replacement: After achieving hemodynamic stability and correcting hypotension, switch to a 0.45% sodium chloride solution (half-normal saline) to meet maintenance fluid requirements, correct fluid deficits, and replace urinary losses [25].

When treating HHS, it's essential to include the volume of fluid lost through urine in the replacement fluid, unlike in DKA treatment [1]. Hypotonic half-normal saline effectively corrects hypernatremia and hyperosmolality by providing free water.

Once hyperglycemia is controlled and blood glucose levels reach 250 mg/dL [14 mmol/L], it is advisable to start administering 5% dextrose to correct intracellular dehydration and provide free water [52].

B. Insulin treatment

HHS is characterized by severe hyperglycemia. But urgent administration of insulin bolus or infusion to reduce blood sugar rapidly can be dangerous and should be strictly avoided. Instead, the first step of treatment for both HHS and DKA is rapid and adequate fluid replacement.

Administering insulin as an initial management strategy for HHS is contraindicated due to the risk of neurological complications, cardiovascular collapse, and severe hypokalemia. Insulin-induced rapid correction of hyperglycemia and hyperosmolality can cause a fluid shift from the ECF to the ICF compartment [52]. This rapid shift can result in neurological complications such as cerebral edema. Additionally, in a dehydrated patient, the resultant reduction in intravascular volume can lead to cardiovascular collapse and shock. Furthermore, in cases of HHS with severe potassium deficits, insulin can cause a rapid shift of potassium into the intracellular space, resulting in severe hypokalemia.

Insulin therapy is initiated when serum glucose concentration ceases to fall with fluid administration alone, and a fixed-rate intravenous insulin infusion is recommended instead of an insulin bolus. The recommended initial insulin dose for HHS is lower at 0.025–0.05 units/kg/hr compared to the 0.1 units/kg/hr generally used for DKA [52].

C. Electrolyte management

The method and need for administering electrolytes and bicarbonates are similar to DKA.

D. Supportive treatment

Other additional supportive measures to be kept in mind are:

- Nasogastric tube in the unconscious patient.

- Hemodynamic and cardiac monitoring in unstable patients with severe DKA. It is essential to avoid fluid overload.

- If low oxygen, evaluate by ABG, chest x-ray, and provide oxygen.

- Low-dose heparin in comatose obese patients to prevent deep vein thrombosis.

- Recognition and treatment of precipitating factors, i.e., drugs (steroids, mannitol, diuretics, and phenytoin), infections, or cerebrovascular accident.

- Antibiotics, if the infection is detected or suspected.

- Electrocardiogram (ECG): Cardiac monitoring as a guide to potassium therapy.

- Bladder catheterization if sensorium is altered.

- Frequent monitoring of pulse, BP, respiration, and level of consciousness.

MONITORING

In HHS, blood sugar should be monitored half or one hourly and electrolytes frequently. Details of therapy, vital data, urine output, and laboratory parameters are recorded in a continuous flow sheet.

REFERENCES

1. Glaser N, Fritsch M, Priyambada L, et al: ISPAD Clinical practice consensus guidelines 2022: diabetic ketoacidosis and hyperglycemic hyperosmolar state. Pediatr Diabetes. 2022;23(7):835–56.

2. JBDS. JBDS-IP Joint British Diabetes Societies Inpatient Care Group. The Management of Diabetic Ketoacidosis in Adults, March 2023 Update: JBDS Guidelines [Internet]. London: ABCD; 2023 Mar. Available from: https://abcd.care/sites/abcd.care/files/site_uploads/JBDS_Guidelines_Current/JBDS_02_DKA_Guideline_with_QR_code_March_2023.pdf.

3. Tremblay ES, Millington K, Monteaux MC, et al. Plasma β-Hydroxybutyrate for the Diagnosis of Diabetic Ketoacidosis in the Emergency Department. Pediatr Emerg Care. 2021;37(12):e1345–e1350.

4. Dhatariya K. Blood Ketones: Measurement, Interpretation, Limitations, and Utility in the

Management of Diabetic Ketoacidosis. Rev Diabet Stud. 2016;13(4):217–225.

5. Rawla P, Vellipuram AR, Bandaru SS, et al. Euglycemic diabetic ketoacidosis: a diagnostic and therapeutic dilemma. Endocrinol Diabetes Metab Case Rep. 2017;2017:17–0081.

6. Nasa P, Chaudhary S, Shrivastava PK, et al. Euglycemic diabetic ketoacidosis: A missed diagnosis. World J Diabetes. 2021;12(5):514–523.

7. Kitabchi AE, Umpierrez GE, Miles JM, et al. Hyperglycemic crises in adult patients with diabetes. Diabetes Care. 2009;32(7):1335–1343.

8. Kitabchi AE, Umpierrez GE, Murphy MB, et al. Hyperglycemic crises in adult patients with diabetes: a consensus statement from the American Diabetes Association. Diabetes Care. 2006;29(12):2739–48.

9. English P, Williams G. Hyperglycaemic crises and lactic acidosis in diabetes mellitus. Postgrad Med J. 2004;80(943):253–261.

10. DeFronzo RA, Hompesch M, Kasichayanula SK, et al. Characterization of renal glucose reabsorption in response to dapagliflozin in healthy subjects and subjects with type 2 diabetes. Diabetes Care 2013;36(10):3169–3176.

11. Arora S, Cheng D, Wyler B, et al. Prevalence of hypokalemia in ED patients with diabetic ketoacidosis. Am J Emerg Med 2012;30(3):481–4.

12. Adrogué HJ, Lederer ED, Suki WN, et al. Determinants of plasma potassium levels in diabetic ketoacidosis. Medicine (Baltimore) 1986;65(3):163–172.

13. Conte G, Dal Canton A, Imperatore P, et al. Acute increase in plasma osmolality as a cause of hyperkalemia in patients with renal failure. Kidney Int. 1990;38(2):301–7.

14. Umpierrez GE, Murphy MB, Kitabchi AE. Diabetic Ketoacidosis and Hyperglycemic Hyperosmolar Syndrome. Diabetes Spectrum 2002;15(1):28–36.

15. Dhatariya KK, Nunney I, Higgins K, et al. A national survey of the management of diabetic ketoacidosis in the UK in 2014. Diabet Med. 2016;33(2):252–260.

16. Pasquel FJ, Lansang MC, Dhatariya K, et al. Management of diabetes and hyperglycaemia in the hospital. Lancet Diabetes Endocrinol. 2021;9(3):174–188.

17. Mein SA, Schwartzstein RM, Richards JB. Sugar, Sodium, and Water: A Recipe for Disaster. Ann Am Thorac Soc. 2020;17(8):1016–1020.

18. 18. van der Vaart A, Waanders F, van Beek AP, et al. Incidence and determinants of hypophosphatemia in diabetic ketoacidosis: an observational study. BMJ Open Diabetes Res Care. 2021;9(1):e002018.

19. Choi HS, Kwon A, Chae HW, et al. Respiratory failure in a diabetic ketoacidosis patient with severe hypophosphatemia. Ann Pediatr Endocrinol Metab. 2018;23(2):103–106.

20. Kuppermann N, Ghetti S, Schunk JE, et al. Clinical trial of fluid infusion rates for pediatric diabetic ketoacidosis. New England Journal of Medicine 2018;378(24):2275–2287.

21. University Hospitals of Leicester. Management of Diabetic Ketoacidosis (DKA) in Adults Guideline (V4 approved by Policy and Guideline Committee on 27 February 2023 Trust ref: B66/2011) [Guidelines]. NHS; 2023. Available from: https://secure.library.leicestershospitals.nhs.uk/PAGL/Shared%20Documents/Diabetic%20Ketoacidosis%20(DKA)%20in%20Adults%20UHL%20Guideline.pdf.

22. Fluid and insulin therapy in children and young people with diabetic ketoacidosis: An update to the NICE NG18 guideline. Journal of Diabetes Nursing 2021;25:JDN171. Available from: https://www.nice.org.uk/guidance/ng18/chapter/Recommendations#fluid-and-insulin-therapy.

23. Diabetes (type 1 and type 2) in children and young people: diagnosis and management. London: National Institute for Health and Care Excellence (NICE); 2022 Jun 29. (NICE Guideline, No. 18.) Available from: https://www.ncbi.nlm.nih.gov/books/NBK555102/.

24. South Australia (SA) Health. Clinical practice guideline on diabetic ketoacidosis (DKA) in children. Adelaide: SA Health; 2019. Available from: https://www.sahealth.sa.gov.au/wps/wcm/connect/04ac0b-8040d0430e975ebf40b897efc8/Diabetic+Ketoacidosis+%28DKA%29+in+Children+and+Adolescents_Paed_v2_1.pdf?MOD=AJPERES&CACHEID=-ROOTWORKSPACE-04ac0b8040d0430e975ebf-40b897efc8-obYYWor.

25. Diabetes Canada Clinical Practice Guidelines Expert Committee; Goguen J, Gilbert J. Hyperglycemic Emergencies in Adults. Can J Diabetes. 2018;42(1):S109–S114.

26. Myburgh JA, Mythen MG. Resuscitation fluids. N Engl J Med. 2013;369(13):1243–51.

27. Oliver WD, Willis GC, Hines MC, et al. Comparison of PlasmaLyte A and sodium chloride 0.9% for fluid resuscitation of patients with diabetic ketoacidosis. Hosp Pharm 2018;53(5):326–330.

28. Yung M, Letton G, Keeley S. Controlled trial of Hartmann's solution versus 0.9% saline for diabetic ketoacidosis. J Paediatr Child Health. 2017;53(1):12–17.

29. Mahler S, Conrad S, Wang H, et al. Resuscitation with balanced electrolyte solution prevents hyperchloremic metabolic acidosis in patients with diabetic ketoacidosis. Am J Emerg Med. 2011;29(6):670–674.

30. Ramanan M, Attokaran A, Murray L. SCOPE-DKA Collaborators and Queensland Critical Care Research Network (QCCRN). Sodium chloride or PlasmaLyte-148 evaluation in severe diabetic ketoacidosis (SCOPE-DKA): a cluster, crossover, randomized, controlled trial. Intensive Care Med. 2021;47(11):1248–1257.

31. Self W, Evans C, Jenkins C, et al. Clinical Effects of Balanced Crystalloids vs Saline in Adults With Diabetic Ketoacidosis. JAMA Netw Open. 2020;3:(11):e2024596.

32. Van Zyl D, Rheeder P, Delport E. Fluid management in diabetic-acidosis Ringer's lactate versus normal saline: a randomized controlled trial. QJM. 2012;105(4):337–343.

33. Chua HR, Schneider A, Bellomo R. Bicarbonate in diabetic ketoacidosis – a systematic review. Ann Intensive Care 2011;1(1):23.

34. Bergmann KR, Abuzzahab MJ, Nowak J, et al. Resuscitation with Ringer's lactate compared with normal saline for pediatric diabetic ketoacidosis. Pediatr Emerg Care 2021;37(5):e236–e242.

35. Jahangir A, Jahangir A, Siddiqui FS, et al. Normal Saline Versus Low Chloride Solutions in Treatment of Diabetic Ketoacidosis: A Systematic Review of Clinical Trials. Cureus. 2022;14(1):e21324.

36. Catahay JA, Polintan ET, Casimiro M, et al. Balanced electrolyte solutions versus isotonic saline in adult patients with diabetic ketoacidosis: A systematic review and meta-analysis. Heart Lung. 2022;54:74–79.

37. Alghamdi NA, Major P, Chaudhuri D, et al. Saline Compared to Balanced Crystalloid in Patients With Diabetic Ketoacidosis: A Systematic Review and Meta-Analysis of Randomized Controlled Trials. Crit Care Explor. 2022;4(1):e0613.

38. Zardoost P, Khan Z, Wehrum HL, et al. Hypernatremia in Diabetic Ketoacidosis: A Rare Metabolic Derangement Requiring a Cautionary Approach in Fluid Resuscitation. Cureus 2023;15(3):e36689.

39. Dressler DD. Normal Saline vs. Balanced Crystalloid for Diabetic Ketoacidosis. NEJM JOURNAL Watch. 2022 Jul 26. Visit: https://www.jwatch.org/na55108/2022/07/26/normal-saline-vs-balanced-crystalloid-diabetic.

40. Aldhaeefi M, Aldardeer NF, Alkhani N, et al. Updates in the Management of Hyperglycemic Crisis. Front Clin Diabetes Healthc. 2022;2:820728.

41. Effects of Balanced Crystalloids vs. Saline in Adults with Diabetic Ketoacidosis [Internet]. Anaesthesia News. 2021. Available from: https://anaesthesianews.wordpress.com/2021/12/12/effects-of-balanced-crystalloids-vs-saline-in-adults-with-diabetic-ketoacidosis/.

42. Farkas J. Diabetic Ketoacidosis (DKA). emcrit.org. 2021. Available from: https://emcrit.org/ibcc/dka/.

43. Gripp K, Trottier ED, Thakore S, et al. Current recommendations for management of paediatric diabetic ketoacidosis. Canadian Paediatric Society 2022.

44. BSPED Guideline for the Management of Children and Young People under the age of 18 years with Diabetic Ketoacidosis - 2021 [Internet]. British Society for Paediatric Endocrinology and Diabetes; 2021. Available from: https://www.bsped.org.uk/clinical-resources/bsped-dka-guidelines/.

45. Forestell B, Battaglia F, Sharif S, et al. Insulin Infusion Dosing in Pediatric Diabetic Ketoacidosis: A Systematic Review and Meta-Analysis of Randomized Controlled Trials. Crit Care Explor. 2023;5(2):e0857.

46. Kilpatrick ES, Butler AE, Ostlundh L, et al. Controversies Around the Measurement of Blood Ketones to Diagnose and Manage Diabetic Ketoacidosis. Diabetes Care. 2022;45(2):267–272.

47. Ma OJ, Rush MD, Godfrey MM, et al. Arterial blood gas results rarely influence emergency physician management of patients with suspected diabetic ketoacidosis. Acad Emerg Med. 2003;10(8):836–41.

48. Menchine M, Probst MA, Agy C, et al. Diagnostic accuracy of venous blood gas electrolytes for identifying diabetic ketoacidosis in the emergency department. Acad Emerg Med. 2011;18(10):1105–1108.

49. Byrne AL, Bennett M, Chatterji R, et al. Peripheral venous and arterial blood gas analysis in adults: are they comparable? A systematic review and meta-analysis. Respirology. 2014;19(2):168–175.

50. Prasad H, Vempalli N, Agrawal N, et al. Correlation and agreement between arterial and venous blood gas analysis in patients with hypotension-an emergency department-based cross-sectional study. Int J Emerg Med. 2023;16(1):18.

51. Milanesi A, Weinreb JE. Hyperglycemic Hyperosmolar State. [Updated 2018 Aug 1]. In: Feingold KR, Anawalt B, Blackman MR, et al, editors. Endotext [Internet]. South Dartmouth (MA): MDText.com, Inc.; 2000. Available from: https://www.ncbi.nlm.nih.gov/books/NBK278976/.

52. Mustafa OG, Haq M, Dashora U, et al. Management of Hyperosmolar Hyperglycaemic State (HHS) in Adults: An updated guideline from the Joint British Diabetes Societies (JBDS) for Inpatient Care Group. Diabet Med. 2023;40(3):e15005.

53. Zeitler P, Haqq A, Rosenbloom A, et al. Hyperglycemic hyperosmolar syndrome in children: pathophysiological considerations and suggested guidelines for treatment. Rev J Pediatr. 2011;158(1):9–14.

41 | Neurological Disorders

IMPORTANCE OF FLUID REPLACEMENT

Fluid replacement is of utmost importance in patients with traumatic brain injury (TBI) or those undergoing neurosurgery. These patients require the administration of intravenous solutions to achieve three important goals: (1) Achieve hemodynamic stability, (2) Improve cerebral perfusion and ensure adequate cerebral oxygenation to prevent brain damage, and (3) Prevent cerebral edema [1–3].

Aneurysmal subarachnoid hemorrhage (aSAH) patients are prone to volume contraction due to cerebral salt wasting, resulting in increased urine output. Therefore, they require fluid replacement. Furthermore, the combined effect of volume depletion and cerebral vasospasm resulting from aSAH increases the risk of cerebral ischemia and life-threatening ischemic strokes, leading to significant morbidity and mortality [4].

So, patients with aSAH require large volumes of sodium-rich IV fluids to correct hypovolemia, maintain euvolemia and normonatremia [5], and prevent the associated poor outcomes [6, 7].

SELECTION OF FLUIDS

To choose the ideal intravenous solution for neurological disorders, it is essential to understand the benefits and harmful effects associated with the solution's composition, tonicity, and type of buffer [3]. The 2018 ESICM consensus and clinical practice recommendations suggest using crystalloids as first-line resuscitation and preferred maintenance fluids and advise against using colloids in neurointensive care patients [8].

A. Normal saline: Preferred fluid

Isotonic solution normal saline (0.9% sodium chloride) is the most commonly used and preferred crystalloid for neurological patients [9, 10].

As the osmolarity of normal saline is 308 mOsm/L (compared to normal plasma osmolality of about 285 mOsm/kg), its use for resuscitation in neurological patients is without the risk of cerebral edema. Furthermore, as the sodium content of normal saline is 154 mEq/L, it effectively corrects cerebral salt wasting-induced hypovolemia and hyponatremia in patients with aSAH [5].

B. Balanced crystalloid solutions: Not preferred

Compared to saline, the electrolyte composition of balanced crystalloids like Ringer's lactate (RL) and PlasmaLyte is closer to that of plasma, which reduces the risk of acute kidney injury and death among critically ill adults [11–13]. In addition, balanced crystalloids are more beneficial than normal saline because normal saline can cause harmful effects such as significantly lower postoperative pH and hyperchloremia [14]. Administering a large volume of chloride-rich normal saline is likely to cause hyperchloremia, which can lead to poor patient outcomes [15, 16].

But general guidelines for fluid administration do not apply to neurological patients due to their unique physiological and clinical characteristics.

1. **Avoid Ringer's lactate:** As RL is a hypotonic fluid with low plasma osmolarity (i.e., at 273 mOsm/L), it can cause or worsen cerebral edema and, therefore, should be avoided in aSAH, TBI, and those undergoing neurosurgery [1, 2, 17]. Ringer's lactate may increase mortality compared with saline in patients with TBI [18].

2. **PlasmaLyte not preferred:** PlasmaLyte is an isotonic balanced crystalloid with an osmolality of 294 mOsm/L that closely resembles plasma in composition, with a sodium concentration of 140 mEq and a pH of 7.4 [19]. A systematic review and meta-analysis compared several balanced crystalloid solutions and found that, compared to other balanced crystalloids, PlasmaLyte resulted in lower serum concentrations of chloride and lactate and higher base excess [20].

Compared to normal saline, the composition of balanced crystalloids, like PlasmaLyte, is closer to that of plasma, and therefore, their use reduces the risk of acute kidney injury and death among critically ill adults [12, 13, 21. Due to these beneficial effects, the trend of using isotonic balanced solutions, such as PlasmaLyte, is currently growing in critically ill patients [22–25].

However, it's crucial to note that the growing preference for PlasmaLyte in critically ill patients does not extend to those with neurological issues, as its use is not recommended in neurological patients. A secondary analysis of the SMART and BaSICS randomized trial and a systematic review revealed that the use of balanced crystalloids in patients with aSAH and TBI led to adverse outcomes, including increased mortality, emphasizing the importance of avoiding balanced crystalloids including PlasmaLyte in these patients [26–28].

C. Avoid hypotonic fluid and hypoosmolality

Hypoosmolality can induce or aggravate cerebral edema, so avoid infusion of hypotonic fluid such as 5% dextrose and 0.45% saline as resuscitation fluids in neurointensive care patients [8]. Normal plasma osmolality is about 285 mOsm/

kg, while the osmolality of 5% dextrose and 0.45% saline (half-normal saline) is 278 and 154 mOsm/kg, respectively, which can lower plasma osmolality below the normal level. In addition to hypoosmolality, another reason to avoid 5% dextrose is its ability to cause hyperglycemia, especially in stroke patients [9].

D. Albumin: Not beneficial

Human albumin solution (HAS) is a natural colloid commonly available in 5% and 20%. Patients with severe TBI commonly have hypoalbuminemia, and the use of HAS for fluid resuscitation not only corrects hypotension but also reduces fluid volume requirements and avoids changes in osmolality. Nevertheless, patients who received albumin 25% at a dose of 2 gm/kg had a higher risk of developing pulmonary edema and intracerebral hemorrhage [29]. In the SAFE Study (2007), albumin was associated with higher mortality rates in patients with traumatic brain injury [30]. Furthermore, the price of HAS is 100 times greater than that of crystalloid.

Therefore, the use of HAS in neurointensive care patients remains controversial and is not recommended by most current guidelines and literature [2, 8, 31, 32].

E. Hydroxyethyl starch (HES): Harmful

Patients undergoing neurosurgery should not be given HES due to its potential to cause harmful effects like acute kidney injury and coagulopathy and the lack of evidence demonstrating its superiority to crystalloids [8]. Therefore, caution must be exercised when considering using HES in this patient population [2].

MAINTAIN EUVOLEMIA

Current literature recommends that clinicians avoid dehydration and hypervolemia, both of which can be detrimental to the brain, and instead focus on achieving normovolemia through precise fluid management in patients with stroke and TBI [8, 9, 14, 33, 34].

In the past, fluid restriction was encouraged to achieve moderate to severe dehydration and prevent an increase in brain water content and cerebral edema. However, dehydration causes hemoconcentration, increases blood viscosity, and reduces blood pressure. Hypotension can cause inadequate cerebral perfusion, impaired tissue oxygenation in the injured central nervous system, and causing secondary brain injury in TBI [35]. Furthermore, dehydration has been shown to lead to poor outcomes in patients with stroke and TBI [35–37].

As a result, the recent ESICM consensus (2018) and the European guideline on trauma (2023) recommends against using restrictive fluid strategies and permissive hypotension in TBI and neurointensive care patients [8, 21]. The current guidelines of the Brain Trauma Foundation (2017) recommend that patients between the ages of 50 and 69 should maintain a systolic blood pressure (SBP) ≥100 mmHg, whereas patients aged 15 to 49 or over 70 should maintain a SBP ≥110 mmHg [38].

Nevertheless, it is crucial to avoid even hypervolemia because it can be detrimental to the brain. Furthermore, the positive daily fluid balance has been linked to high ICU mortality and worse functional outcomes [33, 34]. Therefore, achieving neutral fluid balances in fluid management is essential for optimal patient outcomes.

AVOID HYPERGLYCEMIA

Hyperglycemia occurs in more than 50% of patients with acute ischemic stroke, either due to acute stress reaction secondary to neuro-endocrine dysfunction or underlying diabetes [39].

It is important to avoid the administration of dextrose solutions in acute neurological settings because hyperglycemia increases the production of free radicals in salvageable areas of the injured brain leading to worsened overall functional outcomes, prolonged hospital stay and even mortality rate [40, 41] In neurocritical patients, hyperglycemia can lead to harmful effects such as increased cerebral edema in patients with cerebral ischemia and an increased risk of hemorrhagic transformation of the infarct [42, 43].

The current guidelines recommend avoiding and treating hyperglycemia and maintaining blood glucose levels between 140 mg/dL (7.8 mmol/dL) and 180 mg/dL (10 mmol/dL) in acute ischemic stroke [9, 44].

However, it is important to avoid hypoglycemia as well [9, 44]. It is worth noting that intensive treatment of hyperglycemia to achieve tight glycemic control (glucose <110 mg/dL) is not beneficial compared to standard treatment and, therefore, should be avoided [45–47].

OSMOTHERAPY

Cerebral edema and acutely increased intracranial pressure (ICP) are the most important modifiable life-threatening threats in patients with neurological injuries such as TBI, spontaneous ICH, and aSAH. Swelling of brain cells due to cerebral edema within the rigid cranial vault causes the brain tissue to compress, increasing intracranial pressure and subsequent neurological symptoms and even acute brain herniation.

The main goal of osmotherapy is to reduce intracranial pressure, maintain cerebral perfusion pressure, preserve or restore the physiology and minimize secondary brain damage. Hyperosmolar therapy, such as mannitol or hypertonic saline, is the primary medical management to control increased intracranial pressure rapidly in patients with signs of intracranial hypertension/brain herniation [48, 49].

A. Mannitol

Mannitol has been the 'gold standard' osmotic agent for almost a century to treat intracranial hypertension. 20% mannitol, with a calculated osmolality of 1,098 mOsm/kg, is the most common formulation of mannitol used for the treatment of elevated ICP. Because of high osmolarity and impermeability to the blood-brain barrier, 20% mannitol creates a significant osmotic gradient between the brain and the serum, reduces brain water content, and decreases cerebral edema and intracranial hypertension.

The usual dosage of mannitol for treating cerebral edema and intracranial hypertension ranges from 0.25 gm/kg to 2 gm/kg and is administered intravenously over a 30–60 minute period every 6 to 8 hours [50]. The osmotic effect of mannitol starts within 15–20 minutes after administration and reaches its maximum effect in the brain after 30 minutes. Its osmotic effect lasts variably for about 90 minutes to 6 hours.

Drawbacks of the utilization of mannitol are:

• Dehydration, hypotension, and hypernatremia: As mannitol is freely filtered at the glomerulus and poorly reabsorbed, it acts as an osmotic diuretic and can cause intravascular dehydration and hypotension [51].

- Acute kidney injury: Mannitol can cause acute kidney injury due to three main factors: (1) Renal vasoconstriction caused by high doses or concentrations of mannitol; (2) Dehydration resulting from profound diuresis; and (3) Hyperosmolarity [52]. When mannitol is administered early, there is a high risk of developing acute kidney injury [53].

- Pulmonary edema and electrolyte abnormalities: The administration of high doses of mannitol or its use in the presence of underlying kidney failure can cause volume expansion, hyponatremia, and hyperkalemia due to the mannitol-induced osmotic shift of water and potassium out of the cells.

- Rebound intracranial hypertension: Mannitol that has crossed the altered blood-brain barrier accumulates in the brain and reverses the osmotic gradient, which can worsen cerebral edema and cause rebound intracranial hypertension.

Due to its potential adverse effects, mannitol is avoided in patients with hypovolemia, hypotension, hypervolemia, hyponatremia, hyperkalemia, and preexisting renal failure. To prevent renal dysfunction during mannitol therapy, monitor serum osmolality, and an objective is to maintain osmolality <320 mOsm/kg. The osmolar gap is a more dependable indicator of serum mannitol levels, where a normal osmolar gap implies adequate mannitol clearance [54], while an osmolar gap exceeding 15–20 mOsm/kg indicates incomplete drug clearance [55].

Mannitol is indicated for patients with signs of transtentorial herniation or progressive neurological deterioration [38] and patients with TBI who cannot receive hypertonic saline [48].

B. Hypertonic saline

Hypertonic saline (HTS) is currently the most popular and preferred osmotherapy agent to reduce cerebral edema and intracranial pressure in TBI, neurosurgical patients, and patients with aSAH and stroke [48]. In addition, it is used as a first-line osmotherapy, as an alternative to mannitol therapy failure, and as adjunctive therapy with mannitol in refractory intracranial hypertension [48, 56].

Two characteristic features of hypertonic saline are high sodium concentration and hyperosmolarity. 3% hypertonic saline contains a high concentration of sodium (513 mEq/L compared to normal serum sodium of 140 mEq/L) and high osmolarity (1026 mOsm/L compared to normal serum osmolarity of 285 mOsm/kg). As hypertonic saline cannot cross the blood-brain barrier, it creates a significant osmotic gradient due to its high sodium concentration and hyperosmolarity. As a result, it drives free water out of the brain, reduces cerebral edema, and decreases intracranial pressure. Furthermore, hypertonic saline has been shown to increase cerebral blood flow, improving oxygenation and reducing the risk of further brain injury.

The most commonly used formulation of hypertonic saline is lower concentrations, such as 3% saline [57], which is safe and provides a greater reduction in intracranial pressure than higher concentrations of hypertonic saline [58]. Two methods for administering hypertonic saline are continuous infusion and intermittent boluses; both effectively reduce increased intracranial pressure [59, 60].

The recommended therapeutic doses of hypertonic saline range from 1.4 to 2.5 mL/kg, and it is administered either as boluses every 4 to 6 hours or through continuous infusion throughout the entire duration of therapy [57].

The benefits of hypertonic saline are:

- Faster resolution of increased ICP [61, 62].

- More effective than mannitol in reducing ICP and therefore preferred for refractory ICP [63–65].

- Reduced incidence of treatment failure for ICP than mannitol [66, 67].

- In hypovolemia, the preferred agent over mannitol due to its potential advantages, such as intravascular volume expansion without a diuretic effect, which helps maintain better hemodynamic stability [68, 69].

- Favorable cerebral hemodynamics resulting in higher cerebral perfusion [66, 70, 71].

- The potential advantage of rapid weaning when treatment is no longer required, while mannitol must be gradually tapered to prevent rebound cerebral edema and increased ICP [72].

Adverse effects: Prolonged and continuous use of hypertonic saline in large volumes carries a risk of developing volume overload, acute pulmonary edema, hyperchloremic metabolic acidosis, and acute kidney injury. To minimize the risk of acute kidney injury during hypertonic saline therapy, it is recommended to maintain an upper serum sodium range of 155–160 mEq/L and a serum chloride range of 110–115 mEq/L [48].

C. Comparison of sugar (mannitol) versus salt (hypertonic saline) solutions

Mannitol and hypertonic saline are both effective and widely used globally in treating cerebral edema and increased ICP. When comparing the effectiveness of mannitol and hypertonic saline, several studies [73–78], as well as systematic reviews and meta-analyses [79, 80], have demonstrated their similar effectiveness. However, there is a growing trend favoring the use of hypertonic saline over mannitol due to the benefits discussed above, as well as recent studies [65, 81–83], systematic reviews, and meta-analyses that strongly support its use.

Even recent guidelines recommend using hypertonic saline over mannitol to manage cerebral edema and increase intracranial pressure in patients with TBI [48].

Nevertheless, the literature does not demonstrate significant superiority in mortality rates between hypertonic saline and mannitol.

REFERENCES

1. Tommasino C, Picozzi V. Volume and electrolyte management. Best Pract Res Clin Anaesthesiol. 2007;21(4):497–516.

2. Ryu T. Fluid management in patients undergoing neurosurgery. Anesth Pain Med (Seoul). 2021;16(3):215–224.

3. Dąbrowski W, Woodcock T, Rzecki Z, et al. The use of crystalloids in traumatic brain injury. Anaesthesiol Intensive Ther 2018;50(2):150-159.

4. Mistry AM, Mistry EA, Ganesh Kumar N, et al. Corticosteroids in the management of hyponatremia, hypovolemia, and vasospasm in subarachnoid hemorrhage: a meta-analysis. Cerebrovasc Dis. 2016;42(3–4):263–271.

5. Connolly ES Jr, Rabinstein AA, Carhuapoma JR, et al. Guidelines for the management of aneurysmal subarachnoid hemorrhage: a guideline for healthcare professionals from the american heart association/american stroke association. Stroke. 2012;43(6):1711–1737.

6. Mapa B, Taylor BE, Appelboom G, et al. Impact of hyponatremia on morbidity, mortality, and complica-

tions after aneurysmal subarachnoid hemorrhage: a systematic review. World Neurosurg. 2016;85:305–314.

7. Zheng B, Qiu Y, Jin H, et al. A predictive value of hyponatremia for poor outcome and cerebral infarction in highgrade aneurysmal subarachnoid haemorrhage patients. J Neurol Neurosurg Psychiatry. 2011;82(2):213–217.

8. Oddo M, Poole D, Helbok R, et al. Fluid therapy in neurointensive care patients: ESICM consensus and clinical practice recommendations. Intensive Care Med. 2018;44(4):449–463.

9. Wijdicks EF, Sheth KN, Carter BS, et al. Recommendations for the management of cerebral and cerebellar infarction with swelling: a statement for healthcare professionals from the American Heart Association/American Stroke Association. Stroke. 2014;45(4):1222–1238.

10. Jauch EC, Saver JL, Adams HP Jr, et al. Guidelines for the early management of patients with acute ischemic stroke: a guideline for healthcare professionals from the American Heart Association/American Stroke Association. Stroke. 2013;44(3):870–947.

11. Sen A, Keener CM, Sileanu FE, et al. Chloride content of fluids used for large-volume resuscitation is associated with reduced survival. Crit Care Med. 2017;45(2):e146–e153.

12. Shaw AD, Bagshaw SM, Goldstein SL, et al. Major complications, mortality, and resource utilization after open abdominal surgery: 0.9% saline compared to plasma-lyte. Ann Surg. 2012;255(5):821–829.

13. Zhou F, Peng ZY, Bishop JV, et al. Effects of fluid resuscitation with 0.9% saline versus a balanced electrolyte solution on acute kidney injury in a rat model of sepsis. Crit Care Med. 2014;42(4):e270–e278.

14. Huang L, Zhou X, Yu H. Balanced crystalloids vs 0.9% saline for adult patients undergoing non-renal surgery: A meta-analysis. Int J Surg 2018;51:1–9.

15. Neyra JA, Canepa-Escaro F, Li X, et al. Association of hyperchloremia with hospital mortality in critically ill septic patients. Crit Care Med 2015;43(9):1938–44.

16. Barlow B, Bastin T, Shadler A, et al. Association of chloride-rich fluids and medication diluents on the incidence of hyperchloremia and clinical consequences in aneurysmal subarachnoid hemorrhage. J Neurocrit Care 2022;15(2):113–121.

17. Rossaint R, Afshari A, Bouillon B, et al. The European guideline on management of major bleeding and coagulopathy following trauma: sixth edition. Crit Care. 2023;27(1):80.

18. Rowell SE, Fair KA, Barbosa RR, et al. The impact of pre-hospital administration of lactated Ringer's solution versus normal saline in patients with traumatic brain injury. J Neurotrauma. 2016;33(11):1054–9.

19. Weinberg L, Collins N, Van Mourik K, et al. Plasma-Lyte 148: A clinical review. World J Crit Care Med 2016;5(4):235–250.

20. Curran JD, Major P, Tang K, et al. Comparison of Balanced Crystalloid Solutions: A Systematic Review and Meta-Analysis of Randomized Controlled Trials. Crit Care Explor. 2021;3(5):e0398.

21. Shaw AD, Schermer CR, Lobo DN, et al. Impact of intravenous fluid composition on outcomes in patients with systemic inflammatory response syndrome. Crit Care. 2015;19(1):334.

22. Semler MW, Self WH, Wanderer JP, et al. Balanced Crystalloids versus Saline in Critically Ill Adults. N Engl J Med. 2018;378(9):829–839.

23. Beran A, Altorok N, Srour O, et al. Balanced Crystalloids versus Normal Saline in Adults with Sepsis: A Comprehensive Systematic Review and Meta-Analysis. J Clin Med. 2022;11(7):1971.

24. Hammond NE, Zampieri FG, Di Tanna GL, et al. Balanced Crystalloids versus Saline in Critically Ill Adults — A Systematic Review with Meta-Analysis. NEJM Evid 2022;1(2).

25. Prabhakar A, Bhargava V. Balanced Salt Solutions: Are We Crystal Clear or Still Murky? ASN Kidney News 2022;14(12):25–26.

26. Mistry AM, Magarik JA, Feldman MJ, et al. Saline versus Balanced Crystalloids for Adults with Aneurysmal Subarachnoid Hemorrhage: A Subgroup Analysis of the SMART Trial. Stroke Vasc Interv Neurol. 2022;2(4):e000128.

27. Zampieri FG, Damiani LP, Biondi RS, et al. Effects of balanced solution on short-term outcomes in traumatic brain injury patients: a secondary analysis of the BaSICS randomized trial. Rev Bras Ter Intensiva. 2022;34(4):410–417.

28. Dong WH, Yan WQ, Song X, et al. Fluid resuscitation with balanced crystalloids versus normal saline in critically ill patients: a systematic review and meta-analysis. Scand J Trauma Resusc Emerg Med. 2022;30(1):28.

29. Martin RH, Yeatts SD, Hill MD, et al. ALIAS (albumin in acute ischemic stroke) trials: analysis of the combined data from parts 1 and 2. Stroke. 2016;47(9):2355–9.

30. SAFE Study Investigators, Australian and New Zealand Intensive Care Society Clinical Trials Group, Australian Red Cross Blood Service, et al. Saline or albumin for fluid resuscitation in patients with traumatic brain injury. N Engl J Med 2007;357(9):874–884.

31. Ma HK, Bebawy JF. Albumin Use in Brain-injured and Neurosurgical Patients: Concepts, Indications, and Controversies. J Neurosurg Anesthesiol. 2021;33(4):293–299.

32. Wiedermann CJ. Use of Hyperoncotic Human Albumin Solution in Severe Traumatic Brain Injury Revisited—A Narrative Review and Meta-Analysis. Journal of Clinical Medicine. 2022;11(9):2662.

33. Wiegers EJA, Lingsma HF, Huijben JA, et al. Fluid balance and outcome in critically ill patients with traumatic brain injury (CENTER-TBI and OzENTER-TBI): a prospective, multicentre, comparative effectiveness study. Lancet Neurol. 2021;20(8):627–638.

34. Kochanek PM, Jha RM. Fluid therapy after brain injury: the pendulum swings again. Lancet Neurol. 2021;20(8):587–589.

35. Rauch S, Marzolo M, Cappello TD, et al. Severe traumatic brain injury and hypotension is a frequent and lethal combination in multiple trauma patients in mountain areas - an analysis of the prospective

international Alpine Trauma Registry. Scand J Trauma Resusc Emerg Med. 2021;29(1):61.

36. Rowat A, Graham C, Dennis M. Dehydration in hospital-admitted stroke patients: detection, frequency, and association. Stroke. 2012;43(3):857–9.

37. Lehmann F, Schenk LM, Bernstock JD, et al. Admission Dehydration Status Portends Adverse Short-Term Mortality in Patients with Spontaneous Intracerebral Hemorrhage. J Clin Med. 2021;10(24):5939.

38. Carney N, Totten AM, O'Reilly C, et al. Guidelines for the Management of Severe Traumatic Brain Injury, Fourth Edition. Neurosurgery. 2017;80(1):6–15.

39. Anadani M, Nelson A, Bruno A. Hyperglycemia Management. Practical Neurology. Cover Focus | January 2022. Available from: https://practicalneurology.com/articles/2022-jan/hyperglycemia-management. Accessed April 25, 2023.

40. Rostami E. Glucose and the injured brain-monitored in the neurointensive care unit. Front Neurol. 2014;5:91.

41. Peng TJ, Andersen LW, Saindon BZ, et al. The administration of dextrose during in-hospital cardiac arrest is associated with increased mortality and neurologic morbidity. Crit Care. 2015;19(1):160.

42. Zhang J, Yang Y, Sun H, et al. Hemorrhagic transformation after cerebral infarction: current concepts and challenges. Ann Transl Med. 2014;2(8):81.

43. Spronk E, Sykes G, Falcione S, et al. Hemorrhagic Transformation in Ischemic Stroke and the Role of Inflammation. Front Neurol. 2021;12:661955.

44. Powers WJ, Rabinstein AA, Ackerson T, et al. Guidelines for the early management of patients with acute ischemic stroke: 2019 update to the 2018 guidelines for the early management of acute ischemic stroke: a guideline for healthcare professionals from the American Heart Association/American Stroke Association. Stroke. 2019;50(12):e344–e418.

45. Hermanides J, Plummer MP, Finnis M, et al. Glycaemic control targets after traumatic brain injury: a systematic review and meta-analysis. Crit Care 2018;22(1):11.

46. Fuentes B, Ntaios G, Putaala J, et al. European Stroke Organisation (ESO) guidelines on glycaemia management in acute stroke. Eur Stroke J. 2018;3(1):5–21.

47. Johnston KC, Bruno A, Pauls Q, et al. Intensive vs Standard Treatment of Hyperglycemia and Functional Outcome in Patients With Acute Ischemic Stroke: The SHINE Randomized Clinical Trial. JAMA. 2019;322(4):326–335.

48. Cook AM, Morgan Jones G, Hawryluk GWJ, et al. Guidelines for the Acute Treatment of Cerebral Edema in Neurocritical Care Patients. Neurocrit Care. 2020;32(3):647–666.

49. Picetti E, Catena F, Abu-Zidan F, et al. Early management of isolated severe traumatic brain injury patients in a hospital without neurosurgical capabilities: a consensus and clinical recommendations of the World Society of Emergency Surgery (WSES). World J Emerg Surg. 2023;18(1):5.

50. Tenny S, Patel R, Thorell W. Mannitol. [Updated 2022 Nov 14]. In: StatPearls [Internet]. Treasure Island (FL): StatPearls Publishing; 2023 Jan-. Available from: https://www.ncbi.nlm.nih.gov/books/NBK470392/.

51. Shah S, Kimberly WT. Today's Approach to Treating Brain Swelling in the Neuro Intensive Care Unit. Semin Neurol. 2016;36(6):502–507.

52. Lin SY, Tang SC, Tsai LK, et al. Incidence and Risk Factors for Acute Kidney Injury Following Mannitol Infusion in Patients With Acute Stroke: A Retrospective Cohort Study. Medicine (Baltimore). 2015;94(47):e2032.

53. Skrifvars MB, Bailey M, Moore E, et al. A post hoc analysis of osmotherapy use in the erythropoietin in traumatic brain injury study-associations with acute kidney injury and mortality. Crit Care Med. 2021;49(4):e394–403.

54. García-Morales EJ, Cariappa R, Parvin CA, et al. Osmole gap in neurologic-neurosurgical intensive care unit: Its normal value, calculation, and relationship with mannitol serum concentrations. Crit Care Med. 2004;32(4):986–91.

55. Human T, Tesoro E, Peacock S. Pharmacotherapy Pearls for Emergency Neurological Life Support. Neurocrit Care 2019.

56. Reina-Rivero R, Gaitán-Herrera G, García-García AE, et al. Osmotherapy in patients with severe brain trauma: which agents should we take into account? Romanian Neurosurgery 2022;36(1):92–97.

57. Susanto M, Riantri I. Optimal Dose and Concentration of Hypertonic Saline in Traumatic Brain Injury: A Systematic Review. Medeni Med J. 2022;37(2):203–211.

58. Mekonnen M, Ong V, Florence TJ, et al. Hypertonic Saline Treatment in Traumatic Brain Injury: A Systematic Review. World Neurosurg. 2022;162:98–110.

59. Roquilly A, Moyer JD, Huet O, et al. Effect of Continuous Infusion of Hypertonic Saline vs Standard Care on 6-Month Neurological Outcomes in Patients With Traumatic Brain Injury: The COBI Randomized Clinical Trial. JAMA. 2021;325(20):2056–2066.

60. Wahdan AS, Al-Madawi AA, El-Shafey KA, et al. Comparison of intermittent versus continuous infusion of 3% hypertonic saline on intracranial pressure in traumatic brain injury using ultrasound assessment of optic nerve sheath. Egyptian Journal of Anaesthesia 2022;38(1):291–299.

61. Lazaridis C, Neyens R, Bodle J, et al. High-Osmolarity Saline in Neurocritical Care: Systematic Review and Meta-Analysis. Crit Care Med. 2013;41(8):1353–61.

62. Rossong H, Hasen M, Ahmed B, et al. Hypertonic Saline for Moderate Traumatic Brain Injury: A Scoping Review of Impact on Neurological Deterioration. Neurotrauma Rep. 2020;1(1):253–260.

63. Kerwin AJ, Schinco MA, Tepas JJ 3rd, et al. The use of 23.4% hypertonic saline for the management of elevated intracranial pressure in patients with severe traumatic brain injury: a pilot study. J Trauma. 2009;67(2):277–82.

64. Kamel H, Navi BB, Nakagawa K, et al. Hypertonic saline versus mannitol for the treatment of elevated intracranial pressure: a meta-analysis of randomized clinical trials. Crit Care Med. 2011;39(3):554–559.

65. Cheng F, Xu M, Liu H, et al. A retrospective study of intracranial pressure in head-injured patients undergoing decompressive craniectomy: a comparison of hypertonic saline and mannitol. Front Neurol. 2018;9:631.

66. Han C, Yang F, Guo S, et al. Hypertonic Saline Compared to Mannitol for the Management of Elevated Intracranial Pressure in Traumatic Brain Injury: A Meta-Analysis. Front Surg. 2022;8:765784.

67. Burgess S, Abu-Laban RB, Slavik RS, et al. A systematic review of randomized controlled trials comparing hypertonic sodium solutions and mannitol for traumatic brain injury: implications for emergency department management. Ann Pharmacother 2016;50(4):291–300.

68. Hawryluk GWJ, Aguilera S, Buki A, et al. A management algorithm for patients with intracranial pressure monitoring: the Seattle International Severe Traumatic Brain Injury Consensus Conference (SIBICC). Intensive Care Med. 2019;45(12):1783–94.

69. Singla A, Mathew PJ, Jangra K, et al. A Comparison of Hypertonic Saline and Mannitol on Intraoperative Brain Relaxation in Patients with Raised Intracranial Pressure during Supratentorial Tumors Resection: A Randomized Control Trial. Neurol India. 2020;68(1):141–145.

70. Shi J, Tan L, Ye J, et al. Hypertonic saline and mannitol in patients with traumatic brain injury: A systematic and meta-analysis. Medicine (Baltimore). 2020;99(35):e21655.

71. Schwimmbeck F, Voellger B, Chappell D, et al. Hypertonic saline vs. mannitol for traumatic brain injury: a systematic review and meta-analysis with trial sequential analysis. J Neurosurg Anesthesiol. 2021;33(1):10–20.

72. El-Swaify ST, Kamel M, Ali SH, et al. Initial neurocritical care of severe traumatic brain injury: New paradigms and old challenges. Surg Neurol Int. 2022;13:431.

73. Francony G, Fauvage B, Falcon D, et al. Equimolar doses of mannitol and hypertonic saline in the treatment of increased intracranial pressure. Crit Care Med. 2008;36(3):795–800.

74. Huang X, Yang L. [Comparison of 20% mannitol and 15% hypertonic saline in doses of similar osmotic burden for treatment of severe traumatic brain injury with intracranial hypertension]. Nan Fang Yi Ke Da Xue Xue Bao. 2014;34(5):723–6. Chinese.

75. Jagannatha AT, Sriganesh K, Devi BI, et al. An equiosmolar study on early intracranial physiology and long term outcome in severe traumatic brain injury comparing mannitol and hypertonic saline. J Clin Neurosci. 2016;27:68–73.

76. Kumar SA, Devi BI, Reddy M, et al. Comparison of equiosmolar dose of hyperosmolar agents in reducing intracranial pressure-a randomized control study in pediatric traumatic brain injury. Childs Nerv Syst. 2019;35(6):999–1005.

77. Huang X, Yang L, Ye J, et al. Equimolar doses of hypertonic agents (saline or mannitol) in the treatment of intracranial hypertension after severe traumatic brain injury. Medicine (Baltimore). 2020;99(38):e22004.

78. Tatro HA, McMillen JC, Hamilton LA, et al. 23.4% Sodium Chloride Versus Mannitol for the Reduction of Intracranial Pressure in Patients With Traumatic Brain Injury: A Single-Center Retrospective Cohort Study. Ann Pharmacother. 2021;55(8):988–94.

79. Chen H, Song Z, Dennis JA. Hypertonic saline versus other intracranial pressure-lowering agents for people with acute traumatic brain injury. Cochrane Database Syst Rev. 2020;1(1):CD010904.

80. Gharizadeh N, Ghojazadeh M, Naseri A, et al. Hypertonic saline for traumatic brain injury: a systematic review and meta-analysis. Eur J Med Res. 2022;27(1):254.

81. Patil H, Gupta R. A Comparative Study of Bolus Dose of Hypertonic Saline, Mannitol, and Mannitol Plus Glycerol Combination in Patients with Severe Traumatic Brain Injury. World Neurosurg. 2019;125:e221–e228.

82. Bhatnagar N, Bhateja S, Jeenger L, et al. Effects of two different doses of 3% hypertonic saline with mannitol during decompressive craniectomy following traumatic brain injury: A prospective, controlled study. J Anaesthesiol Clin Pharmacol. 2021;37(4):523–528.

83. Kochanek PM, Adelson PD, Rosario BL, et al. Comparison of Intracranial Pressure Measurements Before and After Hypertonic Saline or Mannitol Treatment in Children With Severe Traumatic Brain Injury. JAMA Netw Open. 2022;5(3):e220891.

Part 9

Fluid Therapy in Surgical Disorders

42 | Preoperative Fluid Therapy

INTRODUCTION

Fluid therapy in surgical patients is a critical part of perioperative care that involves the administration of fluids to maintain the patient's hemodynamic stability, organ perfusion, and hydration status during and after surgery.

Timely administered intravenous fluid is vital and can be lifesaving in surgical patients. The type and amount of fluids administered depend on various factors, such as the patient's preoperative status, the extent of surgical trauma, the duration of surgery, and associated illnesses and comorbid conditions. Proper fluid management can help reduce complications after major surgery, decrease stay in the hospital, and improve patient outcomes [1].

Understanding the possible fluid and electrolyte imbalances in surgical patients and their proper management is important to achieve optimal outcomes after surgery.

Special considerations for fluid therapy in surgical patients

In surgical patients, several factors can modify the normal physiology of fluid and electrolyte balance in the body, which requires special consideration. Some important factors that need to be considered are:

- In surgical patients, the secretion of ACTH increases due to acute stress. This increased adrenocorticotropic hormone (ACTH) level stimulates the adrenal glands to secrete two hormones: a large amount of cortisol to fight acute stress and aldosterone, which results in sodium retention and urinary loss of potassium. Hypovolemia during major surgery also leads to increased aldosterone secretion. The increased aldosterone secretion for the first 2-3 postoperative days leads to increased sodium and water reabsorption.

- Postoperative pain and stress can cause an increase in antidiuretic hormone (ADH) secretion from the posterior pituitary gland during the first 2-3 postoperative days. By reducing urine output and increasing water reabsorption, ADH helps in the correction of hypotension in postoperative patients. It is important to remember that the amount of maintenance fluid required on the first postoperative day is lower due to the increased ADH secretion.

- Fluid deficit resulting from preoperative oral fluid restriction (nothing by mouth-NPO) must be taken into account and replenished prior to or during the surgery to maintain proper hydration.

- Abnormal blood and fluid loss before, during, and after different surgeries need careful consideration and calculation to determine the suitable type, volume, and infusion rate of fluids required.

- Patients with hypovolemia due to blood or fluid loss before surgery are at a higher risk of developing significant hypotension during surgery and anesthesia. Hence, it is essential to detect and manage hypovolemia before surgery to reduce the risk of adverse outcomes.

- When damage occurs to organs due to surgical problems or direct physical injury, it can impair the functions of organs such as the kidney, brain, lung, skin, or gastrointestinal (GI) tract, which are essential for maintaining normal fluid, electrolyte, and acid-base balance. Hence, detecting and managing hypovolemia before surgery is essential to reduce the risk of adverse outcomes.

- Hypotension during surgery and anesthesia can occur due to several causes, such as hypovolemia from blood or fluid loss, decreased cardiac output, vasodilation, and adverse drug reactions.

- Patients requiring GI surgery are more prone to fluid and electrolyte disturbances due to a combination of factors, such as:
  a. Inability to take fluids orally.
  b. Excess loss of electrolytes and hydrogen-rich gastric secretion due to vomiting, nasogastric suction, or obstruction can cause hypokalemic, hypochloremic metabolic alkalosis with hyponatremia [2].
  c. Paralytic ileus may be a presentation of severe hypokalemia [3], and prolonged postoperative ileus can cause hyponatremia and hypochloremia [4].
  d. Loss of a large amount of diarrheal stool can cause hypokalemia and metabolic acidosis [5].
  e. Loss of fluid and electrolytes occurs due to pancreatic, biliary, or intestinal drainage.
  f. Enemas, laxatives, or mechanical bowel preparation can lead to fluid and electrolyte imbalance.

The goals of fluid therapy in surgical patients are:

- To correct life-threatening imbalances (hypovolemic shock and hyperkalemia) and maintain adequate and effective intravascular volume as a top priority.

- To replace the electrolyte, and water deficits.

- To provide water, electrolytes and nutrients for maintaining the patient's daily needs.

- To avoid creating new disturbances as a result of improper therapy.

- To select proper IV fluid with the correct composition and to determine the appropriate infusion rate.

Fluid therapy in surgical patients can be discussed under three headings: (A) Preoperative, (B) Intraoperative, and (C) Postoperative management.

PREOPERATIVE FLUID THERAPY

Preoperative evaluation and correction of existing fluid and electrolytes disorder are crucial for better surgical patient outcomes. However, in emergency conditions, complete correction is not possible. But it is always better to correct fluid deficit partly by rapid fluid replacement and to correct life-threatening disorders than none at all.

Preoperative fluid therapy can be discussed under four headings:

1. Correction of hypovolemia
2. Correction of anemia
3. Correction of other disorders
4. Preoperative fasting

1. Correction of hypovolemia

Ensuring adequate correction of hypovolemia by choosing the right fluid and the appropriate rate of infusion before surgery is crucial.

Importance of correcting hypovolemia prior to surgery

Correcting hypovolemia before surgery is crucial for several reasons.

Firstly, hypovolemia can cause a decrease in tissue perfusion and oxygen delivery, leading to organ dysfunction and injury. Therefore, it is crucial to promptly and effectively correct hypovolemia before surgery.

Secondly, it increases the risk of intraoperative hypotension, which is associated with higher morbidity and mortality rates. Before surgery, normal baroreceptor reflexes compensate for uncorrected hypovolemia by raising vascular resistance and heart rate. However, during anesthesia induction, these reflexes are disrupted, and compensation is lost, increasing the likelihood of severe hypotension or even acute kidney injury. If the fluid deficit isn't corrected before surgery, the risk of hypotension during and after the procedure is greater. Thus, preoperative correction of the fluid deficit is crucial.

Thirdly, it adversely affects postoperative recovery and increases the risk of postoperative complications, such as acute kidney injury. Lastly, it can increase the risk of adverse reactions to anesthetics [6].

Common causes of hypovolemia in surgical patients: Vomiting, nasogastric suction, blood loss, third space losses, fever, hyperventilation, diuretic therapy, diarrhea, or preoperative bowel preparation are important causes of hypovolemia in surgical patients.

Third space loss and underlying causes in surgical patients: Third space loss refers to the internal redistribution of fluids from the intravascular to the interstitial space, resulting in hypovolemia due to the unavailability of fluid to perfuse vital organs. In addition, the sequestration of a large fluid volume can decrease circulating blood volume, which may cause hypotension or even shock. Crush injuries, acute intestinal obstruction, acute gastric dilatation, acute peritonitis, acute pancreatitis, severe acute cellulitis, massive ascites, and postoperative bowel wall and mesentery swelling are common causes of third space losses.

Determining the preoperative fluid deficit volume: The volume of the preoperative fluid deficit is difficult to determine precisely, but it can be estimated based on the patient's medical history, physical examination, and laboratory values. Physical examination plays a significant role in volume assessment and includes evaluating vital signs, postural blood pressure changes, jugular venous pressure, peripheral edema, and lung sounds.

If available, hemodynamic monitoring is a valuable tool for volume assessment in hemodynamically unstable patients. Dynamic parameters, such as stroke volume variation, pulse pressure variation, and passive leg raising, are more reliable for volume assessment than static parameters, such as central venous pressure.

Selection of fluid for correcting preoperative fluid deficit: The choice of the proper fluid for replacement depends on the nature of loss, hemo-dynamic status, and concentration or compositional abnormality. Ringer's lactate, normal saline (0.9% NaCl), colloids, and whole blood are the most widely used. Crystalloids are preferred over colloids, and a balanced crystalloid like Ringer's lactate is the preferred initial fluid for correcting hypovolemia in surgical patients [7, 8]. Normal saline is preferred for patients with vomiting, hyponatremic hypovolemia, traumatic brain injury, metabolic alkalosis, and hypochloremia [9].

A detailed discussion about the selection of IV solutions is included in the "Selecting Appropriate Type of Fluid" part of Chapter 43 on "Intraoperative Fluid Therapy."

Optimal infusion rate for correcting hypovolemia with IV fluids: The rate of infusion for IV fluids to correct hypovolemia depends on the severity of hypovolemia, the patient's hemodynamic status, the presence of continuing losses, and cardiac status.

Generally, a rate of 500–1000 mL/hour is recommended for mild to moderate hypovolemia, while severe hypovolemia may require an initial rapid infusion of 20–30 mL/kg over 5–15 minutes, followed by adjusted rates of fluid administration based on patient response.

Close monitoring is important to avoid complications such as fluid overload or pulmonary edema. Elderly patients require slower and more careful correction with appropriate monitoring.

2. Correction of anemia

Correction of anemia is a potentially lifesaving and essential aspect of perioperative care, but careful administration is necessary as inappropriate blood transfusion can lead to harm.

Up to 40% of presurgical patients may have anemia, and even mild anemia is independently associated with increased morbidity and mortality rates [10].

Importance of correcting anemia in surgical patients

Correction of anemia is essential:

- To establish hemodynamic stability in surgical patients with acute severe blood loss or anemia.
- To improve tissue oxygenation in the intraoperative and postoperative periods.
- To cope with the possibility of operative blood loss.
- To reduce the risk of perioperative complications such as myocardial ischemia, wound infection, and impaired wound healing.
- To promote postoperative recovery and healing.

Treatment approaches for anemia in preoperative patients: If urgent surgery is not required, it is crucial to investigate the underlying cause of anemia and provide targeted treatment to increase hemoglobin levels, thereby minimizing or avoiding unnecessary blood transfusions and associated harm. Commonly used strategies to improve preoperative hemoglobin levels include specific treatments based on the underlying cause, intravenous (IV) iron therapy to correct iron deficiency, and the selective use of erythropoiesis-stimulating agents (ESAs) in patients with anemia of chronic disease or anemia of inflammation [11–18].

Guidelines for red blood cell transfusions in preoperative patients: Current guidelines suggest restrictive red blood cells (RBC) transfusion as the preferred strategy over liberal transfusion strategies and recommend specific indications for administering red blood cell transfusions in preoperative patients are [11, 13, 17–23]:

Stable non-cardiac patients: It is recommended to avoid administering red blood cell transfusions if their hemoglobin level is >7.0 gm/dL.

Stable specific patient populations: In patients with pre-existing cardiovascular disease, acute coronary syndrome, or those undergoing cardiac surgery, red blood cell transfusions are indicated if their hemoglobin level is 8 gm/dL or less.

The goal for stable patients requiring transfusion is to raise their hemoglobin concentration to 7.0–9.0 gm/dL after transfusion.

Clinical indications: In the case of preoperative patients with persistent active bleeding or hemodynamically unstable or symptomatic anemia due to major hemorrhage, transfusion is necessary even with a higher concentration of hemoglobin.

Benefits of correcting anemia with RBC transfusion 48–72 hours before elective surgery: Among different blood products, red blood cell transfusion is recommended to correct anemia in surgical patients. It is advisable to transfuse blood for anemia correction 48 to 72 hours before elective surgery. This timing is essential because blood stored in an ACD bag/bottle has low levels of 2,3-diphosphoglycerate (2,3

DPG). It takes approximately 48 hours for the body to restore adequate 2,3 DPG levels, which are crucial for oxygen dissociation from hemoglobin and its availability to the tissues. Administering blood transfusion during the early preoperative period ensures maximum oxygen availability during and after surgery [24, 25].

3. Correction of other disorders

Other important disorders that require careful consideration in preoperative patients include fluid overload, hypokalemia, and hyperkalemia.

Fluid overload: Fluid overload is not commonly observed in surgical patients, although it can occur in hospitalized individuals. Excessive fluid administration or the redistribution of fluid from the third space back into the extracellular fluid compartment during the recovery phase of an underlying condition are major contributors to overhydration.

Fluid overload is commonly seen in patients with congestive heart failure, renal failure, or liver cirrhosis. To correct fluid overload before surgery, administering diuretics, restricting salt intake, and limiting fluid intake are essential. In severe cases of renal failure, dialysis may be required.

Hypokalemia: Surgical patients may develop hypokalemia due to several factors, including gastrointestinal losses (e.g., vomiting, nasogastric aspiration, and ureteroenterostomies), potassium-free intravenous fluids or parenteral nutrition administration, excessive renal excretion from diuretics or mannitol use, continuous obligatory renal potassium loss (exceeding 20 mEq per day), metabolic alkalosis (e.g., vomiting), and intracellular potassium shifts due to various causes.

Patients with hypokalemia are at risk of developing intraoperative cardiac arrhythmias, respiratory difficulties after extubation, and postoperative paralytic ileus. Therefore, it is essential to correct hypokalemia.

Hyperkalemia: Hyperkalemia is a less frequent but more severe serious disorder observed in surgical patients. Important causes of hyperkalemia include the release of significant quantities of intracellular potassium into the extracellular space in response to severe injury (such as crush syndrome) or surgical stress, acidosis, and the catabolic state, or the infusion of potassium-rich fluids, especially in oliguric or anuric renal failure. If renal function is normal, dangerous hyperkalemia (serum potassium >6 mEq/L) is rarely seen.

Failure to identify and treat hyperkalemia before surgery can result in potentially life-threatening bradyarrhythmias or cardiac arrest, leading to death.

4. Preoperative fasting

Preoperative fasting is routinely instructed before undergoing anesthesia to allow for gastric emptying, reduce the volume and acidity of gastric contents, and minimize the risks of pulmonary regurgitation and aspiration.

Physiological basis: The gastric emptying time of clear fluids, including up to 5 mL/kg of water, sugared water, tea, and gastric secretions, is typically short, taking about 30 to 60 minutes [26, 27]. In contrast, non-clear fluids such as milk or high-protein clear fluids take much longer to empty from the stomach, usually requiring about 3 to 3.5 hours [28]. Solid food's gastric emptying time can vary due to factors like food type and quantity, but generally, it takes 2 to 6 hours for the food to empty from the stomach.

Fasting guidelines for adults: To prepare for elective surgery, it is recommended that both adults and children avoid consuming solid food for 6 hours preoperatively while encouraging the consumption of clear fluids up to 2 hours before the procedure. Commonly used clear fluids preoperatively include water, lime water, fruit juices without pulp, carbohydrate-rich clear drinks, carbonated beverages, clear tea, and black coffee. This recommendation is strongly supported by various guidelines [8, 29, 30], including the European Society of Anaesthesiology (2011) and the American Society of Anesthesiologists (2023) guidelines [31, 32], as well as numerous current literature sources [33–35].

Harm due to prolonged fasting: Despite the benefits of short periods of preoperative fasting, many centers continue to practice prolonged NPO (nothing by mouth) or overnight fasting protocols to prevent pulmonary aspiration of gastric contents during anesthesia induction, often due to busy hospital practices, staff shortages, fear of legal consequences, and unintentional noncompliance [34, 36–38].

However, the current practice of prolonged preoperative fasting is not only unnecessary but also outdated and harmful. It can lead to adverse consequences such as thirst, hunger, discomfort, fatigue, dehydration, hypotension, hypoglycemia, postoperative nausea and vomiting (PONV), and increased insulin resistance [39–41]. Additionally, young children are at risk of ketone body accumulation [40, 42].

Safety of liberal guidelines: Consuming clear liquids up to two hours before surgery is considered safe as it reduces the acidity of stomach fluids and has been shown to improve patient outcomes [33, 43–45], while not increasing gastric volumes or the risk of reflux and aspiration. Based on this evidence [46], clinicians should benefit their patients by avoiding the practice of prolonged fasting.

Benefits of carbohydrate-containing clear liquids: Carbohydrate-containing clear liquids are recommended for nondiabetic adults up until 2 hours before surgery as per recent guidelines [8, 31, 32], and are preferred over complete fasting or noncaloric clear liquids due to their numerous benefits. These benefits include reducing hunger and thirst [32], decreasing preoperative discomfort [47], lowering the incidence of postoperative nausea and vomiting [48, 49], shortening hospital stays [50–52], decreasing postoperative insulin resistance and insulin requirements [50, 51, 53–57], without increasing the risk of aspiration or other pulmonary complications [45, 50, 58, 59]. Based on this new evidence, clinicians should encourage patients to consume carbohydrate-containing clear liquids up to 2 hours before surgery.

Protein-containing clear liquids: There is currently insufficient evidence to support the consumption of protein-containing clear liquids, which also contain carbohydrates, over clear liquids containing only carbohydrates or noncaloric clear liquids [32].

Chewing gum: Chewing gum is neither beneficial nor harmful. Chewing gum does not warrant delaying elective surgery in adult patients, but it is crucial to remove it before administering any sedative or anesthetic [32].

FASTING GUIDELINES FOR CHILDREN

In children, recommended preoperative fasting is 6 hours for solid food and formula milk, and 4 hours for breast milk [60]. The concept of preoperative fasting time for clear fluids is changing rapidly, and significantly affects the outcome.

In children, longer than recommended preoperative fasting is a common practice [61], and it can have detrimental effects such as ketosis, hypotension, and patient discomfort [40, 42]. The risk of pulmonary aspiration is very low in children (3 in 10,000) [62], and a study has shown that shortening the clear fluid fasting time from 2 hours to 1 hour did not have any impact on the occurrence of regurgitation or pulmonary aspiration [63].

So, various guidelines, including recent European (2022) and Canadian (2019) guidelines, recommend a shorter preoperative fasting time of only 1 hour for clear fluids and 3 hours for breast milk [30, 35, 60, 64–66].

However, the recent ASA guideline (2023) found the evidence of benefits and harms of 1-hour versus 2-hour clear liquid fasting recommendations to be insufficient [32].

Indications of prolonged preoperative fasting: Patients with uncontrolled esophageal reflux, hiatal hernia, esophageal stricture, gastroparesis, diabetes mellitus, gastrointestinal obstruction, or acute abdomen are recommended to have a prolonged preoperative fasting time due to delayed gastric emptying and increased risk for aspiration [32, 67].

REFERENCE

1. Makaryus R, Miller TE, Gan TJ. Current concepts of fluid management in enhanced recovery pathways. Br J Anaesth. 2018;120(2):376–383.

2. National Clinical Guideline Centre (UK). Intravenous Fluid Therapy: Intravenous Fluid Therapy in Adults in Hospital [Internet]. London: Royal College of Physicians (UK); 2013 Dec.

3. Brigode WM, Jones C, Vazquez DE, et al. Scrutinizing the evidence linking hypokalemia and ileus: A commentary on fact and dogma. Int J Acad Med 2015;1(1):21–26.

4. Penfold JA, Wells CI, Du P, et al. Relationships between serum electrolyte concentrations and ileus: A joint clinical and mathematical modeling study. Physiol Rep. 2021;9(3):e14735.

5. Gopchade A. Electrolyte Disturbances in Children Presenting with Acute Diarrhea: A Prospective Cohort Study. JMSCR 2019;7(9):777.

6. Noel-Morgan J, Muir WW. Anesthesia-Associated Relative Hypovolemia: Mechanisms, Monitoring, and Treatment Considerations. Front Vet Sci. 2018;5:53.

7. Malbrain MLNG, Langer T, Annane D, et al. Intravenous fluid therapy in the perioperative and critical care setting: Executive summary of the International Fluid Academy (IFA). Ann Intensive Care. 2020;10(1):64.

8. Irani JL, Hedrick TL, Miller TE, et al. Clinical practice guidelines for enhanced recovery after colon and rectal surgery from the American Society of Colon and Rectal Surgeons and the Society of American Gastrointestinal and Endoscopic Surgeons. Surg Endosc. 2023;37(1):5–30.

9. Semler MW, Kellum JA. Balanced Crystalloid Solutions. Am J Respir Crit Care Med. 2019;199(8):952–960.

10. Musallam KM, Tamim HM, Richards T, et al. Preoperative anaemia and postoperative outcomes in non-cardiac surgery: a retrospective cohort study. Lancet. 2011;378(9800):1396–407.

11. American Society of Anesthesiologists Task Force on Perioperative Blood Management. Practice guidelines for perioperative blood management: an updated report by the American Society of Anesthesiologists Task Force on Perioperative Blood Management*. Anesthesiology. 2015;122(2):241–75.

12. Pagano D, Milojevic M, Meesters MI, et al. 2017 EACTS/EACTA Guidelines on patient blood management for adult cardiac surgery. Eur J Cardiothorac Surg 2018;53(1):79–111.

13. Raphael J, Mazer CD, Subramani S, et al. Society of Cardiovascular Anesthesiologists Clinical Practice Improvement Advisory for Management of Perioperative Bleeding and Hemostasis in Cardiac Surgery Patients. Anesth Analg 2019;129(5):1209–1221.

14. Cho BC, Serini J, Zorrilla-Vaca A, et al. Impact of Preoperative Erythropoietin on Allogeneic Blood Transfusions in Surgical Patients: Results From a Systematic Review and Meta-analysis. Anesth Analg 2019;128(5):981–992.

15. Kaufner L, von Heymann C, Henkelmann A, et al. Erythropoietin plus iron versus control treatment including placebo or iron for preoperative anaemic adults undergoing non-cardiac surgery. Cochrane Database Syst Rev 2020;8(8):CD012451.

16. Guinn NR, Schwartz J, Arora RC, et al. Perioperative Quality Initiative and Enhanced Recovery After Surgery-Cardiac Society Consensus Statement on the Management of Preoperative Anemia and Iron Deficiency in Adult Cardiac Surgery Patients. Anesth Analg 2022;135(3):532–544.

17. Shander A, Corwin HL, Meier J, et al. Recommendations From the International Consensus Conference on Anemia Management in Surgical Patients (ICCAMS). Ann Surg. 2023;277(4):581–590.

18. Kloeser R, Buser A, Bolliger D. Treatment Strategies in Anemic Patients Before Cardiac Surgery. J Cardiothorac Vasc Anesth. 2023;37(2):266–275.

19. Carson JL, Grossman BJ, Kleinman S, et al. Clinical Transfusion Medicine Committee of the AABB. Red blood cell transfusion: a clinical practice guideline from the AABB*. Ann Intern Med. 2012;157(1):49–58.

20. NICE Guideline. Blood Transfusion. (2015). https://www.nice.org.uk/guidance/ng24/chapter/recommendations#red-blood-cells-2. Accessed 8 May 2023.

21. Switzerland SMCW. The Swiss Society of General Internal Medicine Recommends this Top-5 Interventions to be Avoided in Hospital Care 2016 [Internet]. 2016 [cited 8 May 2023]. Available from: https://www.smartermedicine.ch/fileadmin/user_upload/Adaptionen/smartermedicine/Dokumente/Listen_Flyer_neu/SmarterMedicine_Flyer_ENG_web300.pdf.

22. Carson JL, Guyatt G, Heddle NM, et al. Clinical Practice Guidelines From the AABB: Red Blood Cell Transfusion Thresholds and Storage. JAMA. 2016;316(19):2025–2035.

23. Baker L, Park L, Gilbert R, et al. Intraoperative red blood cell transfusion decision-making: A systematic review of guidelines. Ann Surg 2021;274(1):86–96.

24. D'Alessandro A, Liumbruno G, Grazzini G, et al. Red blood cell storage: the story so far. Blood Transfus. 2010;8(2):82–8.

25. Stan A, Zsigmond E. The restoration in vivo of 2,3-diphosphoglycerate (2,3-DPG) in stored red cells, after transfusion. The levels of red cells 2,3-DPG. Rom J Intern Med. 2009;47(2):173–7.

26. Schmitz A, Kellenberger CJ, Liamlahi R, et al. Gastric emptying after overnight fasting and clear fluid intake: a prospective investigation using serial magnetic resonance imaging in healthy children. Br J Anaesth. 2011;107(3):425–9.

27. Beck CE, Chandrakumar T, Sümpelmann R, et al. Ultrasound assessment of gastric emptying time after intake of clear fluids in children scheduled for general anesthesia-A prospective observational study. Paediatr Anaesth. 2020;30(12):1384–1389.

28. Du T, Hill L, Ding L, et al. Gastric emptying for liquids of different compositions in children. Br J Anaesth. 2017;119(5):948–955.

29. Thiele RH, Raghunathan K, Brudney CS, et al. American Society for Enhanced Recovery (ASER) and perioperative quality initiative (POQI) joint consensus statement on perioperative fluid management within an enhanced recovery pathway for colorectal surgery. Perioper Med. 2016;5(1):24.

30. Rosen D, Gamble J, Matava C, et al. Canadian Pediatric Anesthesia Society statement on clear fluid fasting for elective pediatric anesthesia. Canadian journal of anaesthesia 2019;66(8):991–992.

31. Smith I, Kranke P, Murat I, et al. Perioperative fasting in adults and children guidelines from the European Society of Anaesthesiology. Eur J Anaesthesiol 2011;28(8):556–569.

32. Joshi GP, Abdelmalak BB, Weigel WA, et al. 2023 American Society of Anesthesiologists Practice Guidelines for Preoperative Fasting: Carbohydrate-containing Clear Liquids with or without Protein, Chewing Gum, and Pediatric Fasting Duration-A Modular Update of the 2017 American Society of Anesthesiologists Practice Guidelines for Preoperative Fasting. Anesthesiology. 2023;138(2):132–151.

33. Yip A, Hogan S, Carey S. Interventions Aimed at Reducing Fasting Times in Acute Hospital Patients: A Systematic Literature Review. Nutr Clin Pract. 2021;36(1):133–152.

34. Beck CE, Rudolph D, Becke-Jakob K, et al. Real fasting times and incidence of pulmonary aspiration in children: Results of a German prospective multicenter observational study. Paediatr Anesth. 2019;29(10):1040–1045.

35. Disma N, Thomas M, Afshari A, et al. Clear fluids fasting for elective paediatric anaesthesia: the European Society of Anaesthesiology consensus statement. Eur J Anaesthesiol. 2019;36(3):173–174.

36. Salman OS, Asida SM, Ali HS. Current knowledge, practice and attitude of preoperative fasting: A limited survey among Upper Egypt anesthetists. Egyptian Journal of Anaesthesia 2013;29(2):125–130.

37. Panjiar P, Kochhar A, Vajifdar H, et al. A prospective survey on knowledge, attitude and current practices of pre-operative fasting amongst anaesthesiologists: A nationwide survey. Indian J Anaesth. 2019;63(5):350–355.

38. Witt L, Lehmann B, Sümpelmann R, et al. Quality-improvement project to reduce actual fasting times for fluids and solids before induction of anaesthesia. BMC Anesthesiol 2021;21:254.

39. Meisner M, Ernhofer U, Schmidt J. Liberalisation of preoperative fasting guidelines: effects on patient comfort and clinical practicability during elective laparoscopic surgery of the lower abdomen. Zentralbl Chir 2008;133(5):479–85.

40. Dennhardt N, Beck C, Huber D, et al. Optimized preoperative fasting times decrease ketone body concentration and stabilize mean arterial blood pressure during induction of anesthesia in children younger than 36 months: a prospective observational cohort study. Pediatr Anesth 2016;26(8):838–43.

41. Fawcett WJ, Ljungqvist O. Starvation, carbohydrate loading and outcome after major surgery. BJA Education 2017;17(9):312–6.

42. Dennhardt N, Beck C, Huber D, et al. Impact of preoperative fasting times on blood glucose concentration, ketone bodies and acid-base balance in children younger than 36 months: A prospective observational study. Eur J Anaesthesiol 2015;32(12):857–861.

43. Brady MC, Kinn S, Ness V, et al. Preoperative fasting for preventing perioperative complications in children. In: Cochrane database of systematic reviews [Internet]. Wiley; 2009 [cited 2023 May 5]. Available from: http://onlinelibrary.wiley.com/doi/10.1002/14651858.CD005285.pub2/abstract.

44. Brady MC, Kinn S, Stuart P, et al. Preoperative fasting for adults to prevent perioperative complications. In: Cochrane database of systematic reviews [Internet]. Wiley; 2003 [cited 2015 Oct 17]. Available from: http://onlinelibrary.wiley.com/doi/10.1002/14651858.CD004423/abstract.

45. Zhang G, Huang X, Feng J, et al. Oral carbohydrate 2 hours before surgery doesn't increase the risk of reflux and aspiration. A randomized controlled trial in volunteers. Research Square [Internet]. 2023 Jan 11 [cited 2023 May 3];[about 16 p.]. Available from: https://doi.org/10.21203/rs.3.rs-2361859/v1.

46. Sun J, Wei G, Hu L, et al. Perioperative pulmonary aspiration and regurgitation without aspiration in adults: a retrospective observational study of 166,491 anesthesia records. Ann Palliat Med. 2021;10(4):4037–4046.

47. Hausel J, Nygren J, Lagerkranser M, et al. A carbohydrate rich drink reduces preoperative discomfort in elective surgery patients. Anesth Analg 2001;93(5):1344–50.

48. Yilmaz N, Cekmen N, Bilgin F, et al. Preoperative carbohydrate nutrition reduces postoperative nausea and vomiting compared to preoperative fasting. J Res Med Sci 2013;18(10):827–32.

49. Singh BN, Dahiya D, Bagaria D, et al. Effects of preoperative carbohydrates drinks on immediate postoperative outcome after day care laparoscopic cholecystectomy. Surg Endosc 2015;29(11):3267–3272.

50. Awad S, Varadhan KK, Ljungqvist O, et al. A meta-analysis of randomised controlled trials on preoperative oral carbohydrate treatment in elective surgery. Clin Nutr 2013;32:34–44.

51. Smith MD, McCall J, Plank L, et al. Preoperative carbohydrate treatment for enhancing recovery after elective surgery. Cochrane Data-base Syst Rev 2014;(8):CD009161.

52. Amer MA, Smith MD, Herbison GP, et al. Network meta-analysis of the effect of preoperative carbohydrate loading on recovery after elective surgery. Br J Surg. 2017;104(3):187–197.

53. Nygren J, Soop M, Thorell A, et al. Preoperative oral carbohydrate administration reduces postoperative insulin resistance. Clin Nutr 1998;17(2):65–71.

54. Gianotti L, Biffi R, Sandini M, et al. Preoperative oral carbohydrate load versus placebo in major elective abdominal surgery (PROCY): a randomized, placebo-controlled, multicenter, phase III trial. Ann Surg 2018;267(4):623–30.

55. Morrison B, Jones C, Kelliher L, et al. The impact of reduced fasting times and carbohydrate preload on the peri-operative insulin and glucose response in liver resection. Anaesthesia 2018;73:67.

56. Rizvanović N, Nesek Adam V, Čaušević S, Derviševic S, Delibegović S. A randomised controlled study of preoperative oral carbohydrate loading versus fasting in

patients undergoing colorectal surgery. Int J Colorectal Dis. 2019;34(9):1551–1561.

57. Shi M, Hu Z, Yang D, et al. Preoperative oral carbohydrate reduces postoperative insulin resistance by activating AMP-activated protein kinase after colorectal surgery. Dig Surg. 2020;37(5):368–375.

58. Cho EA, Huh J, Lee SH, et al. Gastric Ultrasound Assessing Gastric Emptying of Preoperative Carbohydrate Drinks: A Randomized Controlled Noninferiority Study. Anesth Analg 2021;133(3):690–697.

59. Shin HJ, Koo BW, Lim D, et al. Ultrasound assessment of gastric volume in older adults after drinking carbohydrate-containing fluids: a prospective, nonrandomized, and noninferiority comparative study. Can J Anaesth 2022;69(9):1160–1166.

60. Pre-operative Fasting Guide for Adults and Children. NHS Guidelines. V3 approved by Policyand Guideline Committee on 16 October 2020. Trust Ref: B27/2014. Available from: https://secure.library.leicestershospitals.nhs.uk/PAGL/Shared%20Documents/Pre%20Operative%20Fasting%20for%20Adults%20and%20Children%20UHL%20Guideline.pdf.

61. Aroonpruksakul N, Punchuklang W, Kasikan K, et al. The actual duration of preoperative fasting in pediatric patients, and its effects on hunger and thirst: a prospective observational study. Transl Pediatr. 2023;12(2):146–154.

62. Andersson H, Zarén B, Frykholm P. Low incidence of pulmonary aspiration in children allowed intake of clear fluids until called to the operating suite. Pediatr Ansth. 2015;25(8):770–777.

63. Beck CE, Rudolph D, Mahn C, et al. Impact of clear fluid fasting on pulmonary aspiration in children undergoing general anesthesia: Results of the German prospective multicenter observational (NiKs) study. Paediatr Anaesth. 2020;30(8):892–899.

64. Thomas M, Morrison C, Newton R, et al. Consensus statement on clear fluids fasting for elective pediatric general anesthesia. Paediatr Anesth. 2018;28(5):411–414.

65. Linscott D. SPANZA endorses 1-hour clear fluid fasting consensus statement. Paediatr Anesth. 2019;29(3):292.

66. Frykholm P, Disma N, Andersson H, et al. Pre-operative fasting in children: A guideline from the European Society of Anaesthesiology and Intensive Care. Eur J Anaesthiol. 2022;39(1):4–25.

67. Warner MA, Meyerhoff KL, Warner ME, et al. Pulmonary aspiration of gastric contents: A closed claims analysis. Anesthesiology 2021;135(2):284–91.

43 | Intraoperative Fluid Therapy

Intraoperative hypovolemia and hypotension are common in high-risk prolonged surgeries, such as major abdominal or cardiac procedures, among vulnerable populations, including elderly patients and those with preexisting medical conditions, and are associated with high morbidity, risk of postoperative mortality, and adverse postoperative outcomes [1, 2].

Proper fluid therapy is an essential and critical component of intraoperative management. Its goal is to prevent and correct hypovolemia and hypotension while avoiding fluid overload. Fluid overload is harmful as it carries the risk of impaired tissue oxygenation, pulmonary edema, impaired wound healing, acute kidney injury (AKI), prolonged bowel dysfunction, and longer hospital stay in surgical patients [3, 4]. Adequate fluid therapy ensures proper tissue perfusion and oxygenation, which are crucial for maintaining optimal surgical outcomes.

CAUSES OF INTRAVASCULAR VOLUME DISTURBANCES

Hypovolemia: To avoid hypovolemia and hypotension, along with appropriate fluid replacement, it is essential to diagnose and treat the underlying causes. Causes of intraoperative hypovolemia and hypotension include [5, 6]:

1. Surgical blood loss: This is a major cause of hypovolemia, and the volume of blood loss depends on several factors, including the type and duration of the surgery, as well as any preexisting or acquired defects in hemostasis. Trauma surgery is the most common cause of severe blood loss. Concurrently, the use of anticoagulant therapies like warfarin,

and antiplatelet agents such as clopidogrel, can further elevate the risk of bleeding during surgery.

2. Fluid depletion: This can result from prolonged preoperative fasting, preexisting preoperative fluid deficits, intraoperative fluid loss, and maintenance fluid requirements during the long surgery.

3. Third space losses: These can occur due to the accumulation of fluids in the bowels in intestinal obstruction. In addition, severe acute pancreatitis can cause fluid accumulation in the retroperitoneal space and peritoneal cavity.

4. Insensible losses: These can result from evaporative losses from the mucosal surface of viscera, exposed body cavities, or wounds during prolonged surgery.

5. Anesthesia-related hypotension: This occurs during induction of general anesthesia or spinal or epidural anesthesia due to reduced peripheral vascular resistance and vasodilation.

6. Decreased venous return: This can occur due to high intra-thoracic pressure resulting from mechanical ventilation or abdominal insufflation during laparoscopy.

7. Sepsis: Hypotension during the intraoperative period due to sepsis is caused by a systemic inflammatory response that leads to decreased vascular tone and hypovolemia.

SELECTING THE APPROPRIATE TYPE OF FLUID

During the intraoperative period, hypotension can occur due to multiple causes in addition to blood loss; therefore, selecting an appropriate type of fluid for administration is critical.

Crystalloids, colloids, and blood transfusions are three categories of fluids commonly administered intravenously during intraoperative periods. Crystalloids are the first-line solutions [7] that are used either alone or frequently in combination with colloids or blood transfusion to correct hypovolemia and hypotension during major surgeries with substantial blood loss.

The selection of IV fluid during surgery is critical to avoid harm and may affect outcomes based on factors such as the type and rate of fluid loss, electrolyte and acid-base balance, availability, hemoglobin status, cost, and hospital policy [8].

Crystalloids

Isotonic crystalloids, such as balanced crystalloids like Ringer's lactate or PlasmaLyte, and normal saline, are commonly recommended fluids for maintenance and resuscitation during the intraoperative period [7, 9]. It is important to note that isotonic crystalloids are primarily used as maintenance fluids in surgical patients, while moderately hypotonic dextrose-containing solutions are usually the fluid of choice for the majority of non-surgical adult patients.

A. Balanced crystalloids

Ringer's lactate and PlasmaLyte are balanced salt solutions with a lower chloride content which are recommended as the first choice for crystalloid resuscitation or replacement intraoperatively, compared to normal saline [10–16].

Because the sodium, potassium, and chloride content in balanced crystalloids are similar to that of extracellular fluid, they have fewer adverse effects on electrolytes and acid-base balance when administered intravenously, even in large volumes [13, 17, 18]. Because of low chloride and the presence of buffer, which provides bicarbonate, balanced crystalloids decrease the risk of hyperchloremic metabolic acidosis [19–23].

PlasmaLyte: Ringer's lactate is the most widely recommended and commonly used balanced crystalloid intraoperatively. However, PlasmaLyte is recommended in selected patients due to benefits such as [24, 25]:

- It mimics human plasma more closely (sodium 140 mEq/L, osmolality 295 mOsm/L, and pH 7.4).

- It has acetate as a bicarbonate precursor compared to lactate in RL, so it is effective even in patients with severe shock or liver dysfunction (acetate in PlasmaLyte is metabolized in several organs and not limited to the liver like lactate).

- It contains magnesium instead of calcium in RL and can be safely infused concurrently with blood components.

Because of these benefits, Plasma-Lyte is used intraoperatively in selected patients with liver dysfunction, patients undergoing major liver surgery, and renal transplantation [24, 26].

For further details regarding different aspects of balanced crystalloid solutions, please refer to Chapter 4 on "Balanced and Multi-electrolyte Solutions" and Chapter 8 on "Resuscitation Fluids."

B. Normal saline

Normal saline (0.9% NaCl) is not preferred as an intraoperative fluid due to its supraphysiological concentrations of chloride (154 mEq/L) compared to the normal serum chloride level (100 mEq/L), which increases the risk of hyperchloremic metabolic acidosis and

acute kidney injury [10, 27–29]. In contrast, normal saline is commonly used as an alternative to Ringer's lactate or PlasmaLyte in selected patients with traumatic brain injury, neurosurgical patients, or contraindications to these fluids during intraoperative fluid management [30]. Besides multiple evidence favoring balanced crystalloids over saline, robust evidence to support one fluid over the other in surgical patients is lacking [31, 32].

Colloids

Colloids, such as human albumin, hydroxyethyl starch (HES), and gelatins, are commonly used intraoperatively as replacement solutions to expand the circulating blood volume and correct hypovolemia and hypotension caused by blood loss rather than for maintenance of fluid balance [33].

The benefits of using colloids over crystalloids include better hemodynamic stability due to their greater volume-expanding effect, and the ability to improve hemodynamics with smaller volumes, potentially reducing fluid overload and the risk of edema [30, 34]. Furthermore, colloids have a longer-lasting volume expansion effect providing sustained intravascular volume expansion. Therefore, colloids are generally used as a supplement to crystalloids as the second-line therapy rather than as a substitute for crystalloids as the first-line choice for intraoperative fluid management.

The selection of the formulation of colloids for intraoperative administration is based on weighing the advantages and disadvantages of various available agents.

A. Albumin

Human serum albumin is a colloid of choice for intraoperative fluid management in selected patients because of its effectiveness, the relatively long half-life, which allows for sustained volume expansion, a low risk of causing anaphylactic reactions and is less likely to cause tissue edema compared to other colloid solutions.

Albumin is used selectively intraoperative in patients with sepsis, subarachnoid hemorrhage due to its neuroprotective effect, cardiac surgery, major pediatric surgery, and major abdominal surgery with hypoalbuminemia [30, 35–38].

However, the cost of using albumin for intraoperative fluid management is a major limitation as it is usually 20 to 100 times higher than that of crystalloids [39]. Moreover, the superiority of albumin over other solutions for intraoperative fluid management has not been conclusively demonstrated, and therefore it is used sparingly [40].

It is important to note that administering albumin to patients with traumatic brain injury (TBI) is not recommended as it has been found to be harmful [41–45].

B. Hydroxyethyl starch

For decades, intravenous hydroxyethyl starch solutions were used to correct hypotension in surgical patients, but their use in the perioperative period is highly controversial [46].

HES is effective: Previously, HES was widely used due to its ability to rapidly expand blood volume, resulting in faster hemodynamic stabilization with less volume needed compared to crystalloids, as well as its easy availability, storage, and administration, and lower cost compared to albumin.

HES is harmful: The use of HES in correcting intraoperative hypotension has been called into question due to

harmful effects and adverse outcomes observed in several studies, systematic reviews, and meta-analyses conducted between 2008 and 2018 [47].

In surgical, severe sepsis, trauma, and critically ill patients, HES is found to have the following adverse impacts:

- It carries an increased risk of acute kidney injury and a high risk of renal replacement therapy [34, 48–56].
- It is associated with postoperative excess bleeding and an increased need for blood transfusion [34, 56–59].
- It is linked to an increased risk of mortality and poor outcomes [50, 52, 60, 61].

Advise against the use of HES: Due to significant harmful effects, concerns have been raised regarding the safety of HES. As a result, the European Medicines Agency (EMA) recommended restricted use of HES in 2013 [62], and more stringent recommendations were issued in July 2018 [63]. However, on 24 June 2022, the EMA suspended the use of HES [64]. This decision was made due to non-adherence to the advised suggestions and using HES outside the recommendations outlined in the product information.

To ban or use HES: Despite decades of research, it remains uncertain whether using HES solutions for volume replacement during the perioperative period is safe or linked to organ dysfunction [65]. Therefore, careful consideration is suggested for the use of HES in current literature, rather than banning it, based on the following evidence:

- Several publications have analyzed the risks and benefits of HES, leading to debates and protests against a complete ban [65–69]. Instead, they propose various preventive measures, such as changes in labeling, strict control over the delivery of HES exclusively to hospital pharmacies for surgical and emergency procedures, and discouraging its use in intensive care units, rather than completely withdrawing it from the market.

- When the newer balanced hydroxyethyl starch was used in noncritically ill patients undergoing major surgery with adequate indications, its safety profile was comparable, and several recent RCTs, systematic reviews, and meta-analyses conducted between 2016 and 2022 demonstrated no higher incidence of acute kidney injury, renal replacement therapy or negative effects on survival [61, 70–80].

- In July 2021, the US FDA opted not to ban HES but instead issued a strict notice to revise the Boxed Warning, emphasizing the risks of mortality, kidney injury, and excess bleeding associated with its use [81]. In addition, the FDA strongly emphasized that HES products should only be used when adequate alternative treatments are unavailable.

- The WHO Pharmaceuticals Newsletter No.2 of May 2023 included recommendations from the MHLW and Japan Pharmaceutical and Medical Device Agency (PMDA) (Jan 2023). These recommendations support continuing HES marketing but strictly implementing revised product information.

How to use HES safely?

To avoid adverse effects of HES, the following suggestions are made [62]:

- Use HES solutions sparingly and not routinely to replace plasma volume

in acute blood loss cases when an adequate crystalloid dose is ineffective and alternative treatments are unavailable. Avoid using HES solutions as maintenance fluids.

- HES solutions are contraindicated in patients with sepsis, critically ill patients, burns, renal impairment, or those undergoing renal replacement therapy. Additionally, their use should be avoided in patients with severe coagulopathy, dehydration, volume overload, congestive heart failure, hepatic impairment, and electrolyte disturbances such as hyperkalemia, hypernatremia, and hyperchloremia.

- Restrict the dose of HES solutions to less than 30 mL/kg and the duration to less than 24 hours. Limit the use of HES solutions to the initial phase of volume resuscitation and discontinue their use as soon as hemodynamic goals are achieved. Continuous hemodynamic monitoring aids in assessing the adequacy of fluid replacement.

- Avoid using older generations of HES with large molecular sizes and molar substitution, as they pose a higher risk of adverse effects on kidney function and coagulation [52, 82]. In comparison, a newer balanced 6% HES 130/0.4 is found to be safer for volume replacement therapy in surgical patients, as indicated in several recent publications [70, 72–80].

- Monitor renal function and blood coagulation parameters closely after administering HES.

C. Gelatine

The use of gelatins varies between countries, with gelatins not being available in the USA [83, 84]. However, in the U.K. and European countries, gelatins are commonly used as colloids during the perioperative period when crystalloids alone are ineffective [85], and their usage has increased in the last decade due to safety concerns and restrictions on HES by EMA [86, 87, 88].

Recent studies have shown that the administration of newer balanced gelatins in moderate doses during the perioperative period has no potential for harm (with nonsignificant lower mortality) and has been associated with beneficial effects [89–93]. In addition, a recent Cochrane Review in 2018 comparing gelatins and crystalloids for fluid resuscitation found no significant difference in mortality and similar rates of allergic reactions between the two groups [34]. However, gelatin should be administered with caution during surgery due to the higher risk of anaphylactic shock [94, 95] and the significantly increased risk of fluid overload [96].

In conclusion, due to limited safety studies, gelatin should be used selectively and cautiously in the perioperative setting, taking into consideration its potential benefits and risks, including anaphylaxis and acute kidney injury [86, 97–99].

Chapter 5 on "Colloids Solutions" provides a comprehensive discussion on various aspects of gelatin, including its composition, adverse effects, and precautions.

Blood products

Timely and appropriate intraoperative blood transfusion can be lifesaving but should be used judiciously, as reducing or limiting red blood cells (RBC) transfusion can have beneficial outcomes. One unit of RBC transfusion will increase the hemoglobin level of an average-sized adult by 1 gm/dL.

Keep blood ready: Crossmatch and have red blood cells units readily available for intraoperative blood transfusion in elective major surgeries with a risk of significant blood loss or emergency surgeries with a potential need for blood transfusion. Anticipating the need and placing early orders for crossmatching is a prudent approach, considering that blood may not be immediately accessible and requires time for crossmatching before it can be provided.

When should blood transfusion be given intraoperatively?

The decision to transfuse blood intraoperatively should not be determined solely on hemoglobin levels but should be based on multiple factors, such as: (1) The patient's hemoglobin concentration, (2) The severity of blood loss, (3) Clinical signs of blood loss, and (4) The presence of coagulation disorders.

1. Hemoglobin status: In patients without significant ongoing bleeding, the majority of guidelines recommend a restrictive red blood cell transfusion threshold, suggesting transfusion in stable non-cardiac patients with a hemoglobin level of ≤7.0 gm/dL and in stable patients with preexisting cardiovascular disease with a hemoglobin level of ≤7.5–8.0 gm/dL, aiming for a post-transfusion hemoglobin concentration target of 7.0–9.0 gm/dL [100–108]. However, it is important to note that the recent transfusion guidelines generally advise against transfusing red blood cells when the hemoglobin level is ≥10 gm/dL [109].

2. Severity of blood loss: The decision to transfuse blood intraoperatively should be based on the assessment of the severity of blood loss since the stabilization of hemoglobin concentration after blood loss is a slow process, and therefore, the hemoglobin status in actively bleeding patients may not accurately reflect the extent of blood loss. The estimation of ongoing blood loss, which includes a visual assessment of the surgical field, measurement of blood volume in scaled suction canisters, and evaluation of blood-soaked surgical sponges and drapes, guides the determination of the required number of RBC units to be transfused.

Notably, minor intraoperative blood loss does not necessitate RBC transfusion; however, in cases of major blood loss where a rapid reduction of 30-40% of the blood volume occurs, RBC transfusion becomes essential [110].

3. Clinical signs of blood loss: The correlation between blood loss and clinical signs is often poor [111]. However, the presence of certain indicators such as pallor, tachycardia, systolic hypotension, and a shock index (heart rate divided by systolic blood pressure) >0.85 suggests significant blood loss, which indicates the potential requirement for intraoperative RBC transfusion [111, 112].

It is important to note that in mildly hypovolemic or anemic patients, avoiding intraoperative single-unit RBC transfusion is advisable due to the adverse effects associated with such transfusions [113].

4. Presence of coagulation disorders: Intraoperative blood product transfusion is indicated to correct severe coagulation disorders.

QUANTITY AND STRATEGY FOR FLUID ADMINISTRATION

Providing the optimal quantity of fluid intraoperatively is essential because it ensures adequate tissue perfusion, prevents hypoxia, minimizes the risk of end-organ damage, and influences postoperative outcomes. Intraoperatively, excessive IV fluid administration leads to pulmonary complications and poor wound healing, and fluid restriction posing the risk of hypotension and decreased perfusion are harmful. The volume of IV fluid to be administered intraoperatively should be individualized as it varies in each patient based on hydration status, type of surgery, expected blood loss, age, weight, and coexisting comorbidities.

Minimal or moderate trauma surgery

Patients undergoing such less invasive surgery usually do not have significant fluid shifts or blood loss and commonly receive 1 to 2 liters of infusion of a balanced electrolyte solution to prevent hypovolemia [114]. This fluid is administered slowly over 30 minutes to two hours to replenish the losses caused by preoperative fasting and minor operative losses in patients undergoing such minor surgery.

Major invasive surgery

Different strategies used to determine the volume of IV fluid to be infused intraoperatively in major surgery include:
- The traditional approach
- Restrictive versus liberal fluid therapy
- Goal-directed fluid therapy

A. The traditional approach

In adult patients with no preexisting fluid deficit, the traditional or previously practiced method to calculate the amount of intraoperative fluid volume using standardized formulas (mL/kg/h) is as follows:

1. Correction of fluid deficit due to preoperative starvation

Volume to be replaced for starvation fluid deficit is calculated by multiplying the duration of nothing by mouth-NPO (hours) by the hourly volume based on weight (mL/kg body weight). To determine the duration of NPO, calculate the fasting hours prior to the start of anesthesia.

The volume of fluid to be infused every hour for maintenance requirements is estimated by the 4/2/1 rule: 4 mL/kg/hr for the first 10 kg, 2 mL/kg/hr for the second 10 kg, and 1 mL/kg/hr for every subsequent kg above 20.

The preoperative deficit due to fasting may be replaced by giving half of the calculated volume in the first hour and the other half over the next two hours, in addition to the intraoperative fluid replacement.

2. Maintenance requirement for the period of surgery

Maintenance volume for the intraoperative period = Duration of surgery (hours) multiplied by the volume per hour calculated by the 4/2/1 rule.

3. Correction of ongoing intraoperative losses

The amount of fluid required to correct intraoperative fluid loss due to tissue dissection or hemorrhage depends on the type of surgery. For surgeries with the least trauma (i.e., ophthalmic surgery, cystoscopy, etc.), the fluid requirement is zero, while minimal trauma surgeries (i.e., plastic surgery, herniorrhaphy, etc.) require 2–4 mL/kg body weight, moderate trauma surgeries (i.e., appendicectomy, cholecystectomy, etc.) require 4–6 mL/kg body weight, and severe trauma surgeries (i.e., bowel resection for intestinal obstruction) require 6-8 mL/kg body weight.

4. Replacement for loss of blood

The traditional recommendation was to infuse a crystalloid volume three times the amount of blood lost [115].

Traditional method not recommended: Traditional methods of intraoperative volume management, which rely on fixed formulas and estimations, are criticized for their lack of individualization and failure to consider specific surgical needs. Furthermore, these approaches often result in the administration of excessive crystalloid fluids, leading to increased postoperative body weight due to fluid overload, which can cause tissue edema and adverse outcomes [116]. Additionally, current literature suggests replacing blood loss with crystalloid in a ratio of 1.5:1.0, as opposed to the previous recommendation of a 3:1 ratio [114]. Therefore, traditional approaches are outdated and should be avoided.

B. Restrictive versus liberal fluid therapy

The concepts regarding whether to use a restrictive or liberal fluid strategy for determining the volume of fluid to be administered intraoperatively in major surgery are constantly evolving.

1. Concept of administering liberal and aggressive fluid therapy harmful and outdated

Intraoperatively, hypovolemia and resulting hypotension reduce peripheral tissue perfusion, leading to tissue hypoxia and the risk of end-organ damage. The conventional concept of traditional, liberal, and aggressive intraoperative fluid therapy, which has been practiced for decades, aims to maintain higher cardiac output and increase tissue perfusion and oxygenation. However, the misconception of replacing aggressive IV fluids has been challenged and changed due to the understanding that it leads to fluid overload, which, in turn, causes numerous harmful effects, increases major morbidity, and prolongs the length of hospital stay [117–120].

2. **Restrictive fluid therapy beneficial**

    Intraoperative restrictive fluid therapy is not a fluid restriction. Instead, restrictive zero-balance fluid therapy aims to provide the least amount of fluid that avoids hypovolemia and complications of fluid overload, such as tissue edema. Several studies conducted between 2006 and 2018 have demonstrated the safety, cost-effectiveness, and reduction of major complications and morbidity associated with restrictive fluid therapy [119, 121–126].

3. **Individualize fluid therapy, prefer a moderately liberal fluid regimen and avoid strict restrictive fluid therapy**

    The recent large RELIEF (Restrictive versus Liberal Fluid Therapy for Major Abdominal Surgery) trial (NEJM 2018) compared restrictive versus liberal fluid therapy in 3000 patients. The restrictive group received the most restrictive fluid regimen (median of 3.7 liters of fluids compared to 6.1 liters in the liberal fluid group) and had a higher rate of AKI. Due to the increased rate of acute kidney injury in the restrictive fluid group and the absence of a better rate of disability-free survival, the RELIEF trial concluded that administering a modestly liberal fluid regimen is safer than a restrictive regimen [127].

A systematic review and meta-analysis of randomized controlled trials in major abdominal elective surgery conducted by Messina A et al. (2021) demonstrated a similar higher occurrence of renal major events [128]. Possible explanations of the increased risk of AKI are the gradually decreased volume of fluid given with restrictive fluid, the more rigid restriction termed "zero balance," and the failure to detect hypovolemia clinically during the 'restrictive regimen' [3].

Several studies, including Chappell et al. (2008), Shin et al. (2018), and Miller et al. (2021), have endorsed the findings that both restrictive and liberal fluid therapy can be harmful due to the risks associated with the infusion of excessively high or low fluid volumes, leading to increased morbidity, mortality, cost, and length of stay [117, 129, 130].

Currently, the more highly ranked and effective option available to individualize fluid therapy, compared to restrictive or liberal fluid therapy in major surgery, is goal-directed fluid therapy [131, 132], or the use of hemodynamic monitoring to determine the needs of each individual patient [133].

C. Goal-directed fluid therapy

Perioperative goal-directed therapy (GDT) is an individualized approach aiming to customize optimal fluid management to benefit surgical patients while avoiding both under-correction and overcorrection, thereby mitigating the associated intraoperative harmful effects [128, 134, 135].

Indication: GDT is recommended in invasive, complex, or high-risk major surgery with anticipated significant blood loss [7].

Goals: The primary goals of intraoperative GDT in major or high-risk abdominal surgery are to optimize fluid balance, provide individualized fluid management, prevent complications, and enhance postoperative recovery [135]. GDT achieves these goals by monitoring cardiac output and other basic hemodynamic parameters, which helps increase cardiac output, avoid excessive fluid administration, decrease the risk of tissue edema, and ensure adequate tissue perfusion and oxygen delivery [136]. Additionally, GDT aids in assessing a patient's fluid responsiveness by measuring various hemodynamic parameters, enabling the identification and treatment of volume depletion while avoiding harmful fluid overload [137].

Monitoring techniques: Currently, noninvasive or minimally invasive techniques for GDT, such as esophageal doppler or pulse contour analysis, are increasingly being utilized to monitor cardiac output in high-risk patients [138–140]. Parameters such as pulse pressure variation (PPV) and stroke volume variation (SVV) are commonly used to assess cardiac output and fluid responsiveness. A variation of PPV and SVV greater than 10 to 15% indicates fluid responsiveness in the patient [141]. In such fluid-responsive patients, 250 ml repeated fluid boluses are usually administered. Conversely, when the values of PPV and SVV are less than 10%, fluid administration is discontinued to prevent hypervolemia.

Advantages: GDT is demonstrated to be superior to either renal function test (RFT) or liver function test (LFT) and reduces perioperative complications [132, 142]. The evidence supporting improved outcomes of wound infections and anastomotic leaks due to GDT is strong and reliable [142]. GDT may also reduce several postoperative complications, including postoperative pneumonia and pulmonary edema, while aiding in faster recovery of gastrointestinal function, promoting rapid recovery, shortening hospital stay, and reducing mortality [132, 135, 138, 142–145].

Limitations: Although evidence favors the benefits of intraoperative GDT in major surgery, its implementation into clinical practice remains slow and incomplete [140, 146]. The major drawbacks and limitations of using GDT are its unavailability, high cost, and lack of knowledge among clinicians [139, 140]. Furthermore, there is no clear consensus on the most suitable monitoring device and the most effective goals to be used [147]. Some techniques are too invasive or complex, and clinicians may be unfamiliar with GDT, leading to the potential for inappropriate patient care [148].

MONITORING

For optimal fluid replacement, proper monitoring is essential, and commonly used intraoperative techniques include:

Standard methods: Blood pressure, heart rate, temperature, electrocardiogram (ECG) monitoring, pulse oximetry, central venous pressure, and urine output are routinely monitored during surgery. While these traditional parameters provide valuable information, they may be less sensitive in assessing volume status and determining the appropriate quantity of fluid to be administered intraoperatively.

Dynamic parameters: Various GDT techniques, such as transesophageal doppler ultrasound, echocardiography, and point-of-care ultrasound, are selectively used intraoperatively to assess fluid responsiveness in patients undergoing high-risk surgeries with expected significant blood loss or fluid shifts.

Laboratory parameters: Blood tests such as hemoglobin, hematocrit, serum lactate levels, and arterial blood gas (ABG), if necessary, are intermittently measured during surgery based on the individual's specific needs.

REFERENCES

1. Wesselink EM, Kappen TH, Torn HM, et al. Intraoperative hypotension and the risk of postoperative adverse outcomes: a systematic review. Br J Anaesth. 2018;121(4):706–721.

2. Saugel B, Sessler DI. Perioperative Blood Pressure Management. Anesthesiology 2021;134(2):250–261.

3. Miller TE, Myles PS. Perioperative fluid therapy for major surgery. Anesthesiology. 2019;130(5):825–832.

4. Malbrain MLNG, Langer T, Annane D, et al. Intravenous fluid therapy in the perioperative and critical care setting: Executive summary of the International Fluid Academy (IFA). Ann Intensive Care. 2020;10(1):64.

5. Kouz K, Hoppe P, Briesenick L, et al. Intraoperative hypotension: Pathophysiology, clinical relevance, and therapeutic approaches. Indian J Anaesth. 2020;64(2):90–96.

6. Guarracino F, Bertini P. Perioperative hypotension: causes and remedies. J Anesth Analg Crit Care 2022;2:17.

7. National Institute for Health and Care Excellence (NICE). Perioperative care in adults: Evidence review for intravenous fluid management strategy. NICE guideline [NG180]. Published: 19 August 2020. Available at: https://www.nice.org.uk/guidance/ng180/chapter/Recommendations#intraoperative-care.

8. Langer T, Santini A, Scotti E, et al. Intravenous balanced solutions: from physiology to clinical evidence. Anaesthesiol Intensive Ther. 2015;47:s78–88.

9. Nasa P, Wise R, Elbers PWG, et al. Intravenous fluid therapy in perioperative and critical care setting-Knowledge test and practice: An international cross-sectional survey. J Crit Care. 2022;71:154122.

10. Yunos NM, Bellomo R, Hegarty C, et al. Association between a chloride-liberal vs chloride-restrictive intravenous fluid administration strategy and kidney injury in critically ill adults. JAMA. 2012;308(15):1566–72.

11. Shaw AD, Raghunathan K, Peyerl FW, et al. Association between intravenous chloride load during resuscitation and in-hospital mortality among patients with SIRS. Intensive Care Med. 2014;40(3):342–53.

12. Navarro LH, Bloomstone JA, Auler JO Jr, et al. Perioperative fluid therapy: a statement from the international Fluid Optimization Group. Perioper Med 2015;4:3.

13. Semler MW, Kellum JA. Balanced crystalloid solutions. Am J Respir Crit Care Med. 2021;203(5):520–30.

14. British Association for Parenteral and Enteral Nutrition. GIFTASUP: British Consensus Guidelines on Intravenous Fluid Therapy for Adult Surgical Patients. http://www.bapen.org.uk/resources-and-education/education-and-guidance/bapen-principles-of-good-nu-tritional-practice/giftasup?showall=1&limitstart=. Published February 13, 2018. Accessed [accessed on 12 May 2023].

15. Heming N, Moine P, Coscas R, et al. Perioperative fluid management for major elective surgery. Br J Surg. 2020;107(2):e56–e62.

16. Irani JL, Hedrick TL, Miller TE, et al. Clinical practice guidelines for enhanced recovery after colon and rectal surgery from the American Society of Colon and Rectal Surgeons and the Society of American Gastrointestinal and Endoscopic Surgeons. Surg Endosc. 2023;37(1):5–30.

17. Guidet B, Soni N, Della Rocca G, et al. A balanced view of balanced solutions. Crit Care 2010;14(5):325.

18. Hoorn JE. Intravenous fluids: balancing solutions. J Nephrol 2017;30(4):485–492.

19. Chowdhury AH, Cox EF, Francis ST, et al. A randomized, controlled, double-blind crossover study on the effects of 2-L infusions of 0.9% saline and PlasmaLyte® 148 on renal blood flow velocity and renal cortical tissue perfusion in healthy volunteers. Ann Surg. 2012;256(1):18–24.

20. Burdett E, Dushianthan A, Bennett-Guerrero E, et al. Perioperative buffered versus non-buffered fluid administration for surgery in adults. Cochrane Database Syst Rev. 2012;12:CD004089.

21. Krajewski ML, Raghunathan K, Paluszkiewicz SM, et al. Meta-analysis of high-versus low-chloride content in perioperative and critical care fluid resuscitation. Br J Surg 2015;102(1):24–36.

22. Kilic O, Gultekin Y, Yazici S. The Impact of Intravenous Fluid Therapy on Acid-Base Status of Critically Ill Adults: A Stewart Approach-Based Perspective. Int J Nephrol Renovasc Dis. 2020;13:219–230.

23. Astapenko D, Navratil P, Pouska J, et al. Clinical physiology aspects of chloremia in fluid therapy: a systematic review. Perioper Med 2020;9(1):40.

24. Weinberg L, Collins N, Van Mourik K, et al. PlasmaLyte 148: a clinical review. World J Crit Care Med 2016;5(4):235–250.

25. Ellekjaer KL, Perner A, Jensen MM, et al. Lactate versus acetate buffered intravenous crystalloid solutions: a scoping review. Br J Anaesth. 2020;125(5):693–703.

26. Chatrath V, Ranjana, Kaur J, et al. A comparison of PlasmaLyte a vs 0.9% saline for intraoperative fluid replacement in abdominal surgeries. International Journal of Contemporary Medical Research 2016;3(12):3579–3583.

27. Shaw AD, Bagshaw SM, Goldstein SL, et al. Major complications, mortality, and resource utilization after open abdominal surgery: 0.9% saline compared to PlasmaLyte. Ann Surg. 2012;255(6):821–829.

28. Li H, Sun SR, Yap JQ, et al. 0.9% saline is neither normal nor physiological. J Zhejiang Univ Sci B. 2016;17(3):181–7.

29. Semler MW, Wanderer JP, Ehrenfeld JM, et al. Balanced Crystalloids versus Saline in Critically Ill Adults. N Engl J Med. 2018;378(9):829–839.

30. Boer C, Bossers SM, Koning NJ. Choice of fluid type: physiological concepts and perioperative indications. Br J Anaesth. 2018;120(2):384–396.

31. Maheshwari K, Turan A, Makarova N, et al. Saline versus lactated Ringer's solution: the saline or Lactated Ringer's (SOLAR) Trial. Anesthesiology 2020;132(4):614–624.

32. Bampoe S, Odor PM, Dushianthan A, et al. Perioperative administration of buffered versus nonbuffered crystalloid intravenous fluid to improve outcomes following adult surgical procedures. Cochrane Database Syst Rev 2017;9(9):CD004089.

33. de Keijzer IN, Kaufmann T, Scheeren TWL. Which type of fluid to use perioperatively? J Emerg Crit Care Med. 2019;3:51.

34. Lewis SR, Pritchard MW, Evans DJ, et al. Colloids versus crystalloids for fluid resuscitation in critically ill people. Cochrane Database Syst Rev. 2018;8(8):CD000567.

35. Farag E, Ebrahim ZY. The Perioperative Use of Albumin. Perioperative Fluid Management. 2016:215–34.

36. Wiedermann CJ. Phases of fluid management and the roles of human albumin solution in perioperative and critically ill patients. Curr Med Res Opin. 2020;36(12):1961–1973.

37. Yu YT, Liu J, Hu B, et al. Expert consensus on the use of human serum albumin in critically ill patients. Chin Med J (Engl). 2021;134(14):1639–1654.

38. Xiang F, Huang F, Huang J, et al. Expert Consensus on the Use of Human Serum Albumin in Adult Cardiac Surgery. Chin Med J (Engl). 2023;136(10):1135–1143.

39. Jiang L, Jiang S, Zhang M, et al. Albumin versus other fluids for fluid resuscitation in patients with sepsis: a meta-analysis. PLoS One. 2014;9(12):e114666.

40. Sweeney RM, McKendry RA, Bedi A. Perioperative intravenous fluid therapy for adults. Ulster Med J. 2013;82(3):171–8.

41. Myburgh J, Cooper DJ, Finfer S, et al. Saline or albumin for fluid resuscitation in patients with traumatic brain injury. N Engl J Med. 2007;357(9):874–84.

42. Oddo M, Poole D, Helbok R, et al. Fluid therapy in neurointensive care patients: ESICM consensus and clinical practice recommendations. Intensive Care Med. 2018;44(4):449–463.

43. Ryu T. Fluid management in patients undergoing neurosurgery. Anesth Pain Med (Seoul). 2021;16(3):215–224.

44. Ma HK, Bebawy JF. Albumin Use in Brain-injured and Neurosurgical Patients: Concepts, Indications, and Controversies. J Neurosurg Anesthesiol. 2021;33(4):293–299.

45. Rossaint R, Afshari A, Bouillon B, et al. The European guideline on management of major bleeding and coagulopathy following trauma: sixth edition. Crit Care. 2023;27(1):80.

46. Weiss R, Wenk M, Van Aken H, et al. HES or How to End Science. Anesth Analg. 2018;127(6):1440–1444.

47. Green RS, Butler MB, Hicks SD, et al. Effect of Hydroxyethyl Starch on Outcomes in High-Risk Vascular Surgery Patients: A Retrospective Analysis. J Cardiothorac Vasc Anesth. 2016;30(4):967–72.

48. Brunkhorst FM, Engel C, Bloos F, et al. German Competence Network Sepsis (SepNet). Intensive insulin therapy and pentastarch resuscitation in severe sepsis. N Engl J Med. 2008;358(2):125–139.

49. Mutter TC, Ruth CA, Dart AB. Hydroxyethyl starch (HES) versus other fluid therapies: effects on kidney function. Cochrane Database Syst Rev 2013;(7):CD007594.

50. Perner A, Haase N, Guttormsen AB. Hydroxyethyl starch 130/0.42 versus Ringer's acetate in severe sepsis. N Engl J Med. 2012;367(2):124–34.

51. Myburgh JA, Finfer S, Bellomo R, et al. CHEST Investigators; Australian and New Zealand Intensive Care Society Clinical Trials Group. Hydroxyethyl starch or saline for fluid resuscitation in intensive care. N Engl J Med. 2012;367(20):1901–1911.

52. Zarychanski R, Abou-Setta AM, Turgeon AF, et al. Association of hydroxyethyl starch administration with mortality and acute kidney injury in critically ill patients requiring volume resuscitation: a systematic review and meta-analysis. JAMA. 2013;309(7):678–88.

53. Bayer O, Schwarzkopf D, Doenst T, et al. Perioperative fluid therapy with tetrastarch and gelatin in cardiac surgery–A prospective sequential analysis. Crit Care Med 2013;41(11):2532–42.

54. Wilkes MM, Navickis RJ. Postoperative renal replacement therapy after hydroxyethyl starch infusion: A meta-analysis of randomized trials. Neth J Crit Care 2014;18(4):4–9.

55. Kashy BK, Podolyak A, Makarova N, et al. Effect of hydroxyethyl starch on postoperative kidney function in patients having noncardiac surgery. Anesthesiology 2014;121(4):730–739.

56. Lagny MG, Roediger L, Koch JN, et al. Hydroxyethyl Starch 130/0.4 and the Risk of Acute Kidney Injury After Cardiopulmonary Bypass: A Single-Center Retrospective Study. J Cardiothorac Vasc Anesth 2016;30(4):869–875.

57. Navickis RJ, Haynes GR, Wilkes MM. Effect of hydroxyethyl starch on bleeding after cardiopulmonary bypass: a meta-analysis of randomized trials. J Thorac Cardiovasc Surg 2012;144(1):223–30.

58. Rasmussen KC, Johansson PI, Højskov M, et al. Hydroxyethyl starch reduces coagulation competence and increases blood loss during major surgery: results from a randomized controlled trial. Ann Surg. 2014;259(2):249–54.

59. Tobey R, Cheng H, Gao M, et al. Postoperative Acute Kidney Injury and Blood Product Transfusion After Synthetic Colloid Use During Cardiac Surgery. J Cardiothorac Vasc Anesth 2017;31(3):853–862.

60. Allen CJ, Valle EJ, Jouria JM, et al. Differences between blunt and penetrating trauma after resuscitation with hydroxyethyl starch. J Trauma Acute Care Surg 2014;77(6):859–64.

61. Raiman M, Mitchell CG, Biccard BM, et al. Comparison of hydroxyethyl starch colloids with crystalloids for surgical patients: a systematic review and meta-analysis. Eur J Anaesthesiol. 2016;33(1):42–8.

62. EMA. PRAC confirms that hydroxyethyl-starch solutions (HES) should no longer be used in patients with sepsis or burn injuries or in critically ill patients. 11 October 2018. https://www.ema.europa.eu/en/news/

prac-confirms-hydroxyethyl-starch-solutions-hes-should-no-longer-be-used-patients-sepsis-burn.

63. EMA. Hydroxyethyl starch solutions: CMDh introduces new measures to protect patients. 17 July 2018. Available at: https://www.ema.europa.eu/en/documents/referral/hydroxyethyl-starch-article-107i-referral-hydroxyethyl-starch-solutions-cmdh-introduces-new-measures_en-0.pdf.

64. Hydroxyethyl starch: CMDh Scientific Conclusion and Condition for Lifting suspension of the marketing authorisations. 24 June 2022 Available at: https://www.ema.europa.eu/en/documents/psusa/hydroxyethyl-starch-cmdh-scientific-conclusions-conditions-lifting-suspension-marketing/h/n/psr/j/0031_en.pdf.

65. Zarbock A, Buhre W. Hydroxyethyl Starch in the Perioperative Period: Friend, Foe, or Still an Unsolved Issue? Anesth Analg 2022;134(4):683–685.

66. Vincent JL, Kellum JA, Shaw A, et al. Should hydroxyethyl starch solutions be totally banned? Crit Care. 2013;17(5):193.

67. Wittenstein J, Pelosi P, de Abreu MG. The European Medicines Agency and the Authorization for Hydroxyethyl starch Containing Solutions-Killing the Cow to Get Rid of Ticks? Turk J Anaesthesiol Reanim. 2018;46(3):168–169.

68. Annane D, Fuchs-Buder T, Zoellner C, et al. EMA recommendation to suspend HES is hazardous. Lancet 2018;391(10122):736–738.

69. Priebe HJ. Should hydroxyethyl starch be banned? Lancet. 2018;392(10142):117–118.

70. Ertmer C, Zwissler B, Van Aken H, et al. Fluid therapy and outcome: a prospective observational study in 65 German intensive care units between 2010 and 2011. Ann Intensive Care. 2018;8(1):27.

71. Joosten A, Delaporte A, Ickx B, et al. Crystalloid versus colloid for intraoperative goaldirected fluid therapy using a closed-loop system: a randomized, double-blinded, controlled trial in major abdominal surgery. Anesthesiology. 2018;128(1):55–66.

72. Kammerer T, Brettner F, Hilferink S, et al. No Differences in Renal Function between Balanced 6% Hydroxyethyl Starch (130/0.4) and 5% Albumin for Volume Replacement Therapy in Patients Undergoing Cystectomy: A Randomized Controlled Trial. Anesthesiology 2018;128(1):67–78.

73. Oh HW, Lee JH, Kim HC, et al. The effect of 6% hydroxyethyl starch (130/0·4) on acute kidney injury in paediatric cardiac surgery: a prospective, randomised trial. Anaesthesia 2018;73(2):205–15.

74. Degoul S, Chazard E, Lamer A, et al. Intraoperative administration of 6% hydroxyethyl starch 130/0.4 is not associated with acute kidney injury in elective non-cardiac surgery: A sequential and propensity-matched analysis. Anaesth Crit Care Pain Med. 2020;39(2):199–206.

75. Futier E, Garot M, Godet T, et al. Effect of hydroxyethyl starch vs saline for volume replacement therapy on death or postoperative complications among high-risk patients undergoing major abdominal surgery: the FLASH randomized clinical trial. JAMA. 2020;323(3):225–36.

76. Chappell D, van der Linden P, Ripollés-Melchor J, et al. Safety and efficacy of tetrastarches in surgery and trauma: a systematic review and meta-analysis of randomised controlled trials. Br J Anaesth. 2021;127(4):556–568.

77. Lee MJ, Tannenbaum C, Mao G, et al. Effect of 6% Hydroxyethyl Starch 130/0.4 on Inflammatory Response and Pulmonary Function in Patients Having Cardiac Surgery: A Randomized Clinical Trial. Anesth Analg 2021;133(4):906–914.

78. Wei L, Li D, Sun L. The comparison of albumin and 6% hydroxyethyl starches (130/0.4) in cardiac surgery: a meta-analysis of randomized controlled clinical trials. BMC Surg 2021;21:342.

79. Xu Y, Wang S, He L, et al. Hydroxyethyl starch 130/0.4 for volume replacement therapy in surgical patients: a systematic review and meta-analysis of randomized controlled trials. Perioper Med (Lond). 2021;10(1):16.

80. Pensier J, Deffontis L, Rollé A, et al. Hydroxyethyl Starch for Fluid Management in Patients Undergoing Major Abdominal Surgery: A Systematic Review With Meta-analysis and Trial Sequential Analysis. Anesth Analg. 2022;134(4):686–695.

81. FDA calls for new warning labels on hydroxyethyl starch products. https://www.raps.org/news-and-articles/news-articles/2021/7/fda-calls-for-new-warning-labels-on-hydroxyethyl-s (Accessed on May 18, 2022).

82. Treib J, Haass A, Pindur G, et al. Influence of intravascular molecular weight of hydroxyethyl starch on platelets. Eur J Haematol. 1996;56(3):168–72.

83. Food and Drug Administration. List of Drug Products That Have Been Withdrawn or Removed From the Market for Reasons of Safety or Effectiveness. 63 FR 54082. (1998). Available online at: https://www.gpo.gov/fdsys/pkg/FR-1998-10-08/pdf/98-26923.pdf.

84. Vincent JL. Fluid management in the critically ill. Kidney International 2019;96(1):52–57.

85. Finger S, Liu B, Taylor C, et al. Resuscitation fluid use in critically ill adults: an international cross-sectional study in 391 intensive care units. Crit. Care 2010;14(5):R185.

86. Moeller C, Fleischmann C, Thomas-Rueddel D, et al. How safe is gelatin? A systematic review and meta-analysis of gelatin-containing plasma expanders vs crystalloids and albumin. J Crit Care. 2016;35:75–83.

87. Sümpelmann R, Becke K, Brenner S, et al. Perioperative intravenous fluid therapy in children: guidelines from the Association of the Scientific Medical Societies in Germany. Paediatr Anesth. 2017;27(1):10–18.

88. Protsyk V, Rasmussen BS, Guarracino F, et al. Fluid Management in Cardiac Surgery: Results of a Survey in European Cardiac Anesthesia Departments. J Cardiothorac Vasc Anesth. 2017;31(5):1624–1629.

89. Annane D, Siami S, Jaber S, et al. Effects of fluid resuscitation with colloids vs crystalloids on mortality in critically ill patients presenting with hypovolemic shock: the CRISTAL randomized trial. JAMA. 2013;310(17):1809–17.

90. Marx G, Meybohm P, Schuerholz T, et al. Impact of a new balanced gelatine on electrolytes and pH in the perioperative care. PLoS One. 2019;14(4):e0213057.

91. Mohanan M, Rajan S, Kesavan R, et al. Evaluation of Renal Function with Administration of 6% Hydroxyethyl Starch and 4% Gelatin in Major Abdominal Surgeries: A Pilot Study. Anesth Essays Res. 2019;13(2):219–224.

92. Tseng C, Chen T, Wu M, et al. Resuscitation fluid types in sepsis, surgical, and trauma patients: a systematic review and sequential network meta-analyses. Crit Care. 2020;24(1):693.

93. Sümpelmann R, Camporesi A, Gálvez I, et al. Modified fluid gelatin 4% for perioperative volume replacement in pediatric patients (GPS): Results of a European prospective noninterventional multicenter study. Paediatr Anaesth. 2022;32(7):825–833.

94. Farooque S, Kenny M, Marshall SD. Anaphylaxis to intravenous gelatin-based solutions: a case series examining clinical features and severity. Anaesth. 2019;74(2):174–9.

95. Ring J, Messmer K. Incidence and severity of anaphylactoid reactions to colloid volume substitutes. Lancet. 1977;1(8009):466–9.

96. Katona H, Dobronte L, Soltesz A, et al. Perioperative Gelatin Use Is Associated With Increased Complication Rates and Does Not Prevent Postoperative Fluid Overload in Patients Undergoing Elective Cardiac Surgery. J Cardiothorac Vasc Anesth. 2023;37(3):399–406.

97. Charlesworth M, Shelton CL. Should intravenous gelatins have a role in contemporary peri-operative and critical care? Anaesthesia. 2020;75(2):266–269.

98. Saw MM, Chandler B, Ho KM. Benefits and risks of using gelatin solution as a plasma expander for perioperative and critically ill patients: a meta-analysis. Anaesth Intensive Care 2012;40(1):17–32.

99. Thomas-Rueddel DO, Vlasakov V, Reinhart K, et al. Safety of Gelatin for volume resuscitation – a systematic review and meta-analysis. Intensive Care Medicine 2012;38(7):1134–42.

100. Carson JL, Grossman BJ, Kleinman S, et al. Clinical Transfusion Medicine Committee of the AABB. Red blood cell transfusion: a clinical practice guideline from the AABB*. Ann Intern Med. 2012;157(1):49–58.

101. American Society of Anesthesiologists Task Force on Perioperative Blood Management. Practice guidelines for perioperative blood management: an updated report by the American Society of Anesthesiologists Task Force on Perioperative Blood Management*. Anesthesiology. 2015;122(2):241–75.

102. NICE Guideline. Blood Transfusion. (2015). https://www.nice.org.uk/guidance/ng24/chapter/recommendations#red-blood-cells-2. Accessed 8 May 2023.

103. Carson JL, Guyatt G, Heddle NM, et al. Clinical Practice Guidelines From the AABB: Red Blood Cell Transfusion Thresholds and Storage. JAMA. 2016;316(19):2025–2035.

104. Raphael J, Mazer CD, Subramani S, et al. Society of Cardiovascular Anesthesiologists Clinical Practice Improvement Advisory for Management of Perioperative Bleeding and Hemostasis in Cardiac Surgery Patients. Anesth Analg. 2019;129(5):1209–1221.

105. Mueller MM, Van Remoortel H, Meybohm P, et al. Patient Blood Management: Recommendations From the 2018 Frankfurt Consensus Conference. JAMA. 2019;321(10):983–997.

106. Baker L, Park L, Gilbert R, et al. Intraoperative red blood cell transfusion decision-making: A systematic review of guidelines. Ann Surg 2021;274(1):86–96.

107. Shander A, Corwin HL, Meier J, et al. Recommendations From the International Consensus Conference on Anemia Management in Surgical Patients (ICCAMS). Ann Surg. 2023;277(4):581–590.

108. Kloeser R, Buser A, Bolliger D. Treatment Strategies in Anemic Patients Before Cardiac Surgery. J Cardiothorac Vasc Anesth. 2023;37(2):266–275.

109. Tomic Mahecic T, Dünser M, Meier J. RBC Transfusion Triggers: Is There Anything New? Transfus Med Hemother. 2020;47(5):361–368.

110. Stainsby D, MacLennan S, Hamilton PJ. Management of massive blood loss: a template guideline. Br J Anaesth. 2000;85(3):487–91.

111. Pacagnella RC, Souza JP, Durocher J, et al. A systematic review of the relationship between blood loss and clinical signs. PLoS One. 2013;8(3):e57594.

112. Campos-Serra A, Montmany-Vioque S, Rebasa-Cladera P, et al. The use of the Shock Index as a predictor of active bleeding in trauma patients. Cir Esp (Engl Ed). 2018;96(8):494–500.

113. Ferraris VA, Davenport DL, Saha SP, et al. Surgical outcomes and transfusion of minimal amounts of blood in the operating room. Arch Surg. 2012;147(1):49–55.

114. Joshi GP, O'Connor MF, Nussmeier NA. Intraoperative fluid management. In: UpToDate [Internet]. Post, TW (Ed), UpToDate, Waltham (MA) 2023 [cited May 23, 2023].

115. Kaye AD, Riopelle JM. Intravascular fluid and electrolyte physiology. In: Miller RD, Eriksson LI, Fleisher LA, eds. Miller's Anesthesia. 7th ed. New York: Churchill Livingstone; 2009:1705–173.

116. Brandstrup B, Svendsen PE, Rasmussen M, et al. Which goal for fluid therapy during colorectal surgery is followed by the best outcome: near-maximal stroke volume or zero fluid balance? Br J Anaesth 2012;109(2):191–9.

117. Chappell D, Jacob M, Hofmann-Kiefer K, et al. A rational approach to perioperative fluid management. Anesthesiology 2008;109(4):723–40.

118. Doherty M, Buggy DJ. Intraoperative fluids: how much is too much? Br J Anaesth. 2012;109(1):69–79.

119. Boland MR, Reynolds I, McCawley N, et al. Liberal perioperative fluid administration is an independent risk factor for morbidity and is associated with longer hospital stay after rectal cancer surgery. Ann R Coll Surg Engl. 2017;99(2):113–116.

120. Al-Ghamdi AA. Intraoperative fluid management: Past and future, where is the evidence? Saudi J Anaesth. 2018;12(2):311–317.

121. Brandstrup B. Fluid therapy for the surgical patient. Best Pract Res Clin Anaesthesiol. 2006;20(2): 265–283.

122. Holte K, Foss NB, Andersen J, et al. Liberal or restrictive fluid administration in fast-track colonic surgery:

a randomized, double-blind study. Br J Anaesth. 2007;99(4):500–8.

123. Rahbari NN, Zimmermann JB, Schmidt T, et al. Meta-analysis of standard, restrictive and supplemental fluid administration in colorectal surgery. Br J Surg 2009;96(4):331–41.

124. Lobo SM, Ronchi LS, Oliveira NE, et al. Restrictive strategy of intraoperative fluid maintenance during optimization of oxygen delivery decreases major complications after high-risk surgery. Crit Care 2011;15(5):R226.

125. Wrzosek A, Jakowicka-Wordliczek J, Zajaczkowska R, et al. Perioperative restrictive versus goal-directed fluid therapy for adults undergoing major non-cardiac surgery. Cochrane Database Syst Rev. 2019;12(12):CD012767.

126. Belavić M, Sotošek Tokmadžić V, Brozović Krijan A, et al. A restrictive dose of crystalloids in patients during laparoscopic cholecystectomy is safe and cost-effective: prospective, two-arm parallel, randomized controlled trial. Ther Clin Risk Manag. 2018,14:741–751.

127. Myles PS, Bellomo R, Corcoran T, et al. Restrictive versus Liberal Fluid Therapy for Major Abdominal Surgery. N Engl J Med 2018;378(24):2263–2274.

128. Messina A, Robba C, Calabrò L, et al. Perioperative liberal versus restrictive fluid strategies and postoperative outcomes: a systematic review and metanalysis on randomised-controlled trials in major abdominal elective surgery. Crit Care. 2021;25(1):205.

129. Shin CH, Long DR, McLean D, et al. Effects of Intraoperative Fluid Management on Postoperative Outcomes: A Hospital Registry Study. Ann Surg 2018;267(6):1084–1092.

130. Miller TE, Mythen M, Shaw AD, et al. Association between perioperative fluid management and patient outcomes: a multicentre retrospective study. Br J Anaesth. 2021;126(3):720–729.

131. Zhao X, Tian L, Brackett A, et al. Classification and differential effectiveness of goal-directed hemodynamic therapies in surgical patients: A network meta-analysis of randomized controlled trials. J Crit Care. 2021;61:152–61.

132. Yang T, Tan AY, Leung WH, et al. Restricted Versus Liberal Versus Goal-Directed Fluid Therapy for Non-vascular Abdominal Surgery: A Network Meta-Analysis and Systematic Review. Cureus 2023;15(4):e38238.

133. Temel H, Karslı B, Kayacan N, et al. Evaluation of Intraoperative Fluid Management. Akd Med J 2022;8(1):33–41.

134. Miller TE, Roche AM, Mythen M. Fluid management and goal-directed therapy as an adjunct to Enhanced Recovery After Surgery (ERAS). Can J Anaesth 2015;62(2):158–68.

135. Jessen MK, Vallentin MF, Holmberg MJ, et al. Goal-directed haemodynamic therapy during general anaesthesia for noncardiac surgery: a systematic review and meta-analysis. Br J Anaesth 2022;128(3):416–433.

136. Giglio M, Biancofiore G, Corriero A, et al. Perioperative goal-directed therapy and postoperative complications in different kind of surgical procedures: an updated meta-analysis. J Anesth Analg Crit Care 2021;1:2.

137. Kendrick JB, Kaye AD, Tong Y, et al. Goal-directed fluid therapy in the perioperative setting. J Anaesthesiol Clin Pharmacol 2019;35(Suppl 1):S29–S34.

138. Calvo-Vecino JM, Ripollés-Melchor J, Mythen MG, et al. Effect of goal-directed haemodynamic therapy on postoperative complications in low moderate risk surgical patients: a multicentre randomised controlled trial (FEDORA trial). Br J Anaesth. 2018;120(4):734–744.

139. Fellahi JL, Futier E, Vaisse C, et al. Perioperative hemodynamic optimization: from guidelines to implementation-an experts' opinion paper. Ann Intensive Care. 2021;11(1):58.

140. Flick M, Joosten A, Scheeren Thomas WL, et al. Haemodynamic monitoring and management in patients having noncardiac surgery: A survey among members of the European Society of Anaesthesiology and Intensive Care. European Journal of Anaesthesiology and Intensive Care 2023;2(1):e0017.

141. Michard F. Changes in arterial pressure during mechanical ventilation. Anesthesiology. 2005;103(2):419–28.

142. Peltoniemi P, Pere P, Mustonen H, et al. Optimal Perioperative Fluid Therapy Associates with Fewer Complications After Pancreaticoduodenectomy. J Gastrointest Surg. 2023;27(1):67–77.

143. Pearse RM, Harrison DA, MacDonald N, et al. Effect of a perioperative, cardiac output-guided hemodynamic therapy algorithm on outcomes following major gastrointestinal surgery: a randomized clinical trial and systematic review. JAMA. 2014;311(21):2181–90.

144. Dushianthan A, Knight M, Russell P, et al. Goal-directed haemodynamic therapy (GDHT) in surgical patients: systematic review and meta-analysis of the impact of GDHT on post-operative pulmonary complications. Perioper Med (Lond). 2020;9:30.

145. Virág M, Rottler M, Gede N, et al. Goal-Directed Fluid Therapy Enhances Gastrointestinal Recovery after Laparoscopic Surgery: A Systematic Review and Meta-Analysis. J Pers Med. 2022;12(5):734.

146. Kaufmann T, Saugel B, Scheeren TWL. Perioperative goal-directed therapy - What is the evidence? Best Pract Res Clin Anaesthesiol 2019;33(2):179–187.

147. Chong MA, Wang Y, Berbenetz NM, et al. Does goal-directed haemodynamic and fluid therapy improve peri-operative outcomes?: A systematic review and meta-analysis. Eur J Anaesthesiol 2018;35(7):469–483.

148. Joshi GP, Kehlet H. CON: Perioperative Goal-Directed Fluid Therapy Is an Essential Element of an Enhanced Recovery Protocol? Anesth Analg 2016;122(5):1261–3.

44 | Postoperative Fluid Therapy

Postoperative fluid therapy is crucial for managing patients' fluid needs, ensuring their physiological stability, maintaining hydration and tissue perfusion, restoring fluid balance, and supporting recovery during the postoperative period. The administration of fluid and electrolytes during the postoperative period depends on a thorough patient evaluation, and no single postoperative fluid regimen suits everyone [1].

THE GOAL OF FLUID THERAPY

The aim of postoperative fluid therapy is to keep the patient normovolemic, maintain an adequate circulating blood volume, optimize organ perfusion, promote wound healing, provide adequate calories to prevent catabolism and prevent complications such as hypovolemia, fluid overload, electrolyte imbalances, and acid-base disturbances. In postoperative patients, the major principles of management of fluid balance are:

- To replace ongoing losses (hemorrhage, drainage, third space losses, and insensible losses)
- To provide maintenance requirements
- To correct preexisting deficits (preoperative and intraoperative losses)

CAUSES OF HYPOVOLEMIA

Hypovolemia and hypotension are common postoperative complications, and their important causes include:

- Bleeding: Intraoperative and postoperative blood loss.
- Fluid deficit: Inadequate correction of the preoperative starvation (nothing

by mouth-NPO) deficit, utilization of "zero-balance" or "restrictive fluid strategy" to replace intraoperative losses, failure to adequately replace maintenance fluid requirements during prolonged surgeries, and ongoing fluid losses from the gastrointestinal tract (such as vomiting and diarrhea).

- Drainage: Fluid loss from nasogastric aspirations, drains, and fistulas.

- Third-spacing: Sequestration of several liters of fluid into the soft tissues' interstitial space, peritoneal or pleural cavities, and bowel lumen.

- Insensible losses: Excessive loss due to hyperventilation or pyrexia, prolonged exposure from an open abdominal cavity during laparotomy, and delays in operation due to a long operating theater (OT) list, especially in summer.

INDICATIONS AND DURATION OF IV FLUID ADMINISTRATION

The continuation of postoperative IV fluids should not be a routine practice for all patients. Instead, the fluid management strategy should be personalized according to individual needs, prescribing IV fluids only when necessary and for the shortest duration possible [2].

The need for postoperative IV fluids and the duration of their administration depend on several factors, including the type (minor or major) and nature of the surgery (e.g., limb surgery, abdominal surgery), as well as the patient's volume and hemodynamic status. Patients undergoing minor uncomplicated surgery may not require postoperative IV fluids or only need them temporarily until they can resume oral fluid intake. On the other hand, patients undergoing prolonged major surgeries, such as

emergency laparotomies and intestinal resection with anastomosis, which are performed under general anesthesia and require rest for the intestinal viscera, usually necessitate postoperative fluid administration for a longer duration [1].

It is important to discontinue intravenous fluids and encourage patients to transition to oral fluids as early as possible, provided they are euvolemic, hemodynamically stable, and do not experience active nausea or vomiting symptoms [3–7]. This early transition to oral intake helps preserve gastrointestinal motility, facilitate early mobility, enhance healing and recovery in the postoperative period, and enable earlier discharge [4, 8–10].

DETERMINING THE APPROPRIATE VOLUME OF FLUID INFUSION

It is important to provide the optimum volume of IV fluids to maintain proper hydration while avoiding fluid overload, as it can provide benefits such as improved pulmonary function, gastrointestinal motility, and wound healing [10]. Tailor the volume of IV fluids to individual needs based on the preexisting fluid deficit, ongoing fluid and blood losses, and maintenance fluid requirements [11].

For minor surgeries where expected blood loss is minimal, a small volume replacement of IV fluids (<30 mL/kg) is sufficient. When there is a moderate to severe loss of fluid and blood, accurately estimating the fluid deficit and volume of IV fluid to be infused becomes challenging. In such patients, apart from considering maintenance requirements, the volume of fluid to be infused is determined based on restoring normal perfusion rather than relying on calculations using specific formulas.

The recommended maintenance fluid requirement in adults is 25–30 mL/kg/day according to NICE guidelines, 1.5–2.5 liters of water based on the Adult Surgical Patients by British Consensus Guidelines (GIFTASUP), and 0.5 mL/kg/hr with fluid boluses for resuscitation as stated in the York teaching hospitals NHS foundation trust summary sheet [3, 12, 13].

Parameters suggesting the administration of an adequate volume of IV fluids and the restoration of normal perfusion include hemodynamic stability, clear mental status, adequate urine output (>0.5 mL/kg/hour), and the absence of lactic acidosis. In patients with critical illness, hemodynamic instability, or sepsis following complex major surgery, especially in high-risk patients, goal-directed therapy is an effective modality for optimizing the replacement of IV fluids during the postoperative period [14, 15].

Close monitoring, continuous individualized assessment and reassessment, and appropriate adjustments in fluid administration throughout the postoperative period help optimize patient outcomes and promote a smooth recovery process.

Immediate postoperative IV fluid selection

When IV fluids are indicated postoperatively, their selection needs to be individualized based on the time of administration and their specific indication, whether it is for resuscitation, replacement of ongoing losses, or maintenance purposes.

SELECTION OF IV FLUIDS IMMEDIATELY AFTER SURGERY

Postoperatively, factors such as pain, nausea, stress, hypovolemia, the administration of pain management narcotics, and inhaled anesthetics can stimulate the secretion of antidiuretic hormone (ADH), resulting in water retention [16].

Avoid hypotonic fluids: It is important to note that administering hypotonic solutions combined with ADH-induced electrolyte-free water retention postoperatively can increase the risk of hyponatremia [17–20]. Therefore, in the immediate postoperative period, it is advisable to avoid administering hypotonic IV fluids such as 5% dextrose and fluids containing 0.45% or lower sodium concentration, especially in hemodynamically unstable patients and children [21].

Prefer isotonic fluids: It is recommended to administer an isotonic solution with a higher sodium concentration at a reduced volume during the initial postoperative period to reduce the risk of hyponatremia [22, 23]. Sodium-rich isotonic IV fluids, such as Ringer's lactate with a sodium concentration of 130 mEq/L, normal saline with a sodium concentration of 154 mEq/L, and PlasmaLyte with a sodium concentration of 140 mEq/L, are frequently administered on the first postoperative day.

Before initiating IV fluids, measuring CBC, hematocrit, electrolyte levels, calcium, and glucose is essential. Repeat these parameters at least every 24 hours if IV fluids are continued to ensure the appropriate modifications of IV fluid in the postoperative period.

The selection of IV fluids according to the requirements of different patients is summarized below.

Ringer's lactate

Balanced crystalloid like Ringer's lactate (RL) is widely used and preferred for fluid replacement in most postoperative patients [13]. The benefits of using RL over normal saline include its safety even in large volumes due to its balanced composition [24, 25] and effectiveness as a resuscitation fluid [26–30].

RL contains lactate, which provides bicarbonate and a small amount of potassium, making it suitable for conditions such as duodenal, small bowel, and pancreatic fistulas, as well as diarrhea that causes bicarbonate and potassium loss.

However, it is important to avoid the use of RL in patients with traumatic brain injury, as it is a hypotonic fluid with low plasma osmolarity (273 mOsm/L), which can lead to or worsen cerebral edema [31–33]. Additionally, RL should not be infused concurrently with blood transfusion due to its calcium content [34].

Normal saline

Normal saline is a sodium-rich solution that contains 154 mEq/L of sodium. Normal saline is often termed "abnormal saline" as its chloride concentration is supraphysiological (154 mEq/L of sodium, 50% higher compared to plasma) [35, 36].

Normal saline is recommended as a second-line fluid due to the potential risk of hyperchloremic acidosis and acute kidney injury following the administration of large volumes [37–40]. However, the recent SOLAR study (2020) failed to show any significant differences between using Ringer's lactate and normal saline in causing postoperative complications in elective orthopedic surgery [41].

Nevertheless, normal saline remains the fluid of choice postoperatively for patients with prolonged vomiting or nasogastric suction, those with head injury or undergoing neurosurgical operations, individuals with hyponatremia or metabolic alkalosis, and patients receiving diuretics [3, 15, 32, 42]. It can also be safely infused alongside blood transfusion.

PlasmaLyte

PlasmaLyte, with a more balanced composition, has been found to be a safer fluid than saline in the postoperative period [43]. Both PlasmaLyte and RL are balanced crystalloids, with PlasmaLyte containing acetate as a buffer and RL containing lactate as a buffer. The metabolism of lactate occurs in the liver, while acetate is effectively metabolized regardless of liver failure or severe shock [44, 45]. Consequently, in postoperative patients with liver failure or severe shock, PlasmaLyte may be the preferred balanced solution over RL [46]. An additional advantage of PlasmaLyte is that it does not contain calcium, making it compatible with all blood products. However, the higher cost of PlasmaLyte is a limiting factor in its use.

Human albumin

Because of its high cost (about 100 times greater than crystalloids) and increasing evidence showing limited benefits, it is used in selected postoperative patients with septic shock, severe malnutrition, or liver insufficiency [11, 47].

Other colloids

Colloids like hydroxyethyl starch, gelatins, and dextrans are frequently used intraoperatively for resuscitation but are rarely utilized postoperatively due to their adverse effects on coagulation.

Blood transfusion

The American Association of Blood Banks recommends transfusion in postoperative surgical patients when the hemoglobin concentration is 8 gm/dL or less or when symptoms such as chest pain, orthostatic hypotension, or tachycardia unresponsive to fluid resuscitation, or congestive heart failure are present [48].

POTASSIUM SUPPLEMENTATION

Hypokalemia (serum potassium <3.5 mEq/L) is a common and harmful condition that can occur postoperatively.

Importance

It is important to pay careful attention to potassium supplementation postoperatively because:

- Risk of hypokalemia in postoperative patients due to gastric suction, abdominal drains, high aldosterone levels from surgical stress, potassium shifting into cells, and infusion of potassium free intravenous fluids.

- An audit of fluid prescriptions revealed that inadequate potassium supplementation postoperatively is a common practice [49, 50].

- Hypokalemia carries the risk of cardiac arrhythmias, slower return of gut function, urine retention, and respiratory difficulties after extubation postoperatively [50–52].

- Postoperative maintenance of normal blood potassium levels not only reduces mortality but also enhances postoperative recovery [53].

- Fear of supplementing potassium intravenously and the misconception that potassium-containing balanced crystalloids provide sufficient potassium are common reasons for inadequate postoperative potassium supplementation [50].

- The potassium concentration of Ringer's lactate and PlasmaLyte is only 4 mEq/L and 5 mEq/L, respectively, which is insufficient to meet the recommended daily potassium requirement of 1 mEq/kg.

Timing of potassium supplementation

Postoperatively, when to administer potassium is an important issue that requires careful attention.

A. Traditional practice to supplement potassium late

In the immediate postoperative period, until urine output is established and normal renal status is ensured, patients may not require potassium supplementation in the first 24 hours for the following reasons:

1. Oliguria or azotemia, which indicates reduced kidney function, may necessitate potassium level monitoring before supplementation.

2. Postoperative tissue trauma and metabolic acidosis can lead to the redistribution of potassium from the intracellular compartment to the extracellular compartment, potentially maintaining adequate potassium levels.

3. Intraoperative or postoperative transfusion of stored or hemolyzed blood can introduce a substantial amount of potassium, contributing to the overall potassium balance and potentially obviating the need for immediate supplementation.

So, the routine practice is adding potassium from days 2 to 3 [54].

B. Need for early administration of potassium

To address preexisting potassium deficits, replace ongoing potassium losses, and correct hypokalemia, many patients may require potassium supplementation in the early postoperative period (from day 1), with consideration of their serum potassium levels, urine output, and renal status.

Early administration of intravenous potassium supplementation in patients with appropriate indications, starting immediately after surgery in the operating theater, is both safe and beneficial for promoting the recovery of gastrointestinal function after abdominal surgery [51, 55].

Strategy to provide potassium

It is crucial to remember that the commonly used IV solutions during the first 24 hours postoperatively, such as normal saline, are free of potassium, while balanced crystalloids like Ringer's lactate and PlasmaLyte contain very small amounts of potassium.

As per standard practice, a solution is prepared by adding 20–40 mEq of potassium chloride (KCl) per liter, which is administered with close monitoring. In cases of severe hypokalemia, the preferred method for administering potassium is through an infusion pump when a central line is available.

The total potassium requirement varies from patient to patient, but 60–100 mEq of potassium chloride per day is usually needed to meet daily needs and address mild deficits.

The goal of potassium supplementation is to achieve blood potassium concentrations within the high normal range (i.e., ≥4.00 mEq/L), as studies have shown that this improves postoperative recovery of gastrointestinal motility [56, 57].

CALORIC SUPPLEMENTATION

To provide calories and prevent catabolism, it is essential to administer approximately 100 gm of glucose per day.

Notably, the commonly used IV solutions in the initial 24 hours postoperatively, such as normal saline, Ringer's lactate, and PlasmaLyte, do not contain glucose. Administering a dextrose saline solution (5% dextrose with 0.9% NaCl) [16, 22] or providing 100 gm of glucose per day separately with balanced crystalloids are common options for delivering calories during the initial postoperative period.

SELECTION OF IV FLUIDS DURING THE SUBSEQUENT POSTOPERATIVE PERIOD

Maintenance fluids are administered when a postoperative patient is hemodynamically stable and requires intravenous fluid due to restricted or insufficient oral intake. Furthermore, ongoing fluid losses are replenished by administering an equivalent volume of suitable intravenous fluids.

Maintenance fluids

The goal of postoperative maintenance fluid therapy is to provide sufficient fluid, electrolytes, and some calories to prevent catabolism:

1. Selection of fluid: To counteract the positive sodium and fluid balance resulting from increased secretion of ADH and aldosterone due to postoperative pain and stress, it is advisable to administer maintenance fluids with low-volume and relatively low sodium content [3, 58]. Commonly recommended hypotonic IV solutions for postoperative maintenance fluid therapy include 5% dextrose in half-normal saline (0.45% NaCl with 5% dextrose solution) with 20 mEq per liter of potassium, as well as 0.18% sodium/4% dextrose solution with potassium [3, 59].

2. Volume of IV fluids: The recommended maintenance fluid requirement in adults is 25–30mL/kg/day according to NICE guidelines, 1.5–2.5 liters of water based on the Adult Surgical Patients by British Consensus Guidelines (GIFTASUP), and 0.5 mL/kg/hr with fluid boluses for resuscitation as stated in the York teaching hospitals NHS foundation trust summary sheet [3, 12, 13].

Administration: The volume of maintenance fluid to be administered should be closely monitored and tailored to avoid fluid overload. The infusion rate of postoperative maintenance fluid should be less than 2 mL/kg/hour in patients with normal renal function.

MONITORING

- **Clinical:** Monitoring postoperative patients involves regular assessment of vital signs, such as heart rate, blood pressure, respiratory rate, and oxygen saturation levels.

- **Charting:** It is also important to measure daily weight and maintain strict input and output charts, including tracking drain and nasogastric losses.

- **Laboratory tests:** Daily laboratory assessment, including blood tests for complete blood count, serum biochemistry, and glucose monitoring, is essential for monitoring the patient's overall status and detecting any abnormalities or imbalances. Close monitoring of clinical and laboratory parameters and timely adjustments in fluid prescription based on these findings are crucial for ensuring patient safety and early detection of adverse events.

- **Cumulative fluid balance chart:** Maintain cumulative fluid balance chart: Accurately tracking and recording daily fluid intake and output, noting the daily positive or negative fluid volume, and maintaining a net cumulative fluid balance chart on subsequent days are crucial.

This chart provides clear information about the total postoperative fluid balance, allowing for precise detection of net fluid gain or loss throughout the hospital stay. This practice of monitoring the exact volume of total fluid balance is crucial in preventing potential complications associated with the inappropriate volume of IV fluids administered [60].

REFERENCES

1. Kayilioglu SI, Dinc T, Sozen I, et al. Postoperative fluid management. World J Crit Care Med. 2015;4(3):192–201.

2. Sweeney RM, McKendry RA, Bedi A. Perioperative intravenous fluid therapy for adults. Ulster Med J. 2013;82(3):171–8.

3. Powell-Tuck J, Gosling P, Lobo DN, et al. GIFTASUP: British Consensus Guidelines on Intravenous Fluid Therapy for Adult Surgical Patients. Revised 7 March 2011. Available at: https://www.bapen.org.uk/pdfs/bapen_pubs/giftasup.pdf [accessed on 3 June 2023].

4. Thiele RH, Raghunathan K, Brudney CS, et al. American Society for Enhanced Recovery (ASER) and Perioperative Quality Initiative (POQI) joint consensus statement on perioperative fluid management within an enhanced recovery pathway for colorectal surgery. Perioper Med (Lond) 2016;5:24.

5. Feldheiser A, Aziz O, Baldini G, et al. Enhanced Recovery After Surgery (ERAS) for gastrointestinal surgery, part 2: consensus statement for anaesthesia practice. Acta Anaesthesiol Scand. 2016;60(3):289–334.

6. Miller TE, Myles PS. Perioperative fluid therapy for major surgery. Anesthesiology. 2019;130(5):825–832.

7. O'Rourke K, Morrison B, Sen S, et al. Fluid management for enhanced recovery surgery. 2019;2:37.

8. Lewis SJ, Egger M, Sylvester PA, et al. Early enteral feeding versus "nil by mouth" after gastrointestinal surgery: systematic review and meta-analysis of controlled trials. BMJ. 2001;323(7316):773–6.

9. Malhotra N, Khanna S, Pasrija S, et al. Early oral hydration and its impact on bowel activity after elective caesarean section: Our experience. Eur J Obstet Gynecol Reprod Biol 2005;120(1):53–6.

10. Makaryus R, Miller TE, Gan TJ. Current concepts of fluid management in enhanced recovery pathways. Br J Anaesth. 2018;120(2):376–383.

11. Moemen ME. Fluid therapy: Too much or too little. Egyptian Journal of Anaesthesia 2010;26(4):313–318.

12. National, Clinical Guideline Centre UK. "Intravenous Fluid Therapy: Intravenous Fluid Therapy in Adults in Hospital." (2013).

13. Li W. Fluid Therapy in Post-operative care. Perioperative Care. York teaching hospitals NHS foundation trust Version 1.0 (08/09/2017) [Internet]. Available from: https://www.yorkperioperativemedicine.nhs.uk/health-professionals/preoperative-care/post-operative-care/fluid-therapy/. Accessed June 3, 2023.

14. Parker T, Brealey D, Dyson A, et al. Optimising organ perfusion in the high-risk surgical and critical care patient: a narrative review. Br J Anaesth. 2019;123(2):170–176.

15. Malbrain MLNG, Langer T, Annane D, et al. Intravenous fluid therapy in the perioperative and critical care setting: Executive summary of the International Fluid Academy (IFA). Ann Intensive Care. 2020;10(1):64.

16. Moritz ML, Ayus JC. Maintenance intravenous fluids in acutely ill patients. N Engl J Med. 2015;373(14):1350–60.

17. Chung HM, Kluge R, Schrier RW, et al. Postoperative hyponatremia: a prospective study. Arch Intern Med 1986;146(2):333–6.

18. Steele A, Gowrishankar M, Abrahamson S, et al. Postoperative hyponatremia despite near-isotonic saline infusion: a phenomenon of desalination. Ann Intern Med 1997;126(1):20–5.

19. Plain D5W or hypotonic saline solutions post-op could result in acute hyponatremia and death in healthy children. ISMP Medication Safety Alert 2009;7:1–4.

20. Winata AS, Jen WY, Teng ML, et al. Intravenous maintenance fluid tonicity and hyponatremia after major surgery- a cohort study. Int J Surg. 2019;67:1–7.

21. Moritz ML, Ayus JC. Prevention of hospital-acquired hyponatremia: a case for using isotonic saline. Pediatrics 2003;111(2):227–30.

22. Moritz ML, Ayus JC. Water water everywhere: standardizing postoperative fluid therapy with 0.9% normal saline. Anesth Analg. 2010;110(2):293–5.

23. Oh GJ, Sutherland SM. Perioperative fluid management and postoperative hyponatremia in children. Pediatr Nephrol. 2016;31(1):53–60.

24. Burdett E, Dushianthan A, Bennett-Guerrero E, et al. Perioperative buffered versus non-buffered fluid administration for surgery in adults. Cochrane Database Syst Rev. 2012;12:CD004089.

25. Lehr AR, Rached-d'Astous S, Parker M, et al. Impact of balanced versus unbalanced fluid resuscitation on clinical outcomes in critically ill children: protocol for a systematic review and meta-analysis.Syst Rev. 2019;8(1):195.

26. Miller TE, Bunke M, Nisbet P, et al. Fluid resuscitation practice patterns in intensive care units of the USA: a cross-sectional survey of critical care physicians. Perioper Med (Lond) 2016;5:15.

27. Jonsson AB, Perner A. Changes from 2012 to 2015 in intravenous fluid solutions issued to hospital departments. Acta Anaesthesiol Scand. 2017;61(5):532–538.

28. Semler MW, Self WH, Wanderer JP, et al. Balanced crystalloids versus saline in critically ill adults. New Engl J Med 2018;378(9):829–839.

29. Semler MW, Kellum JA. Balanced crystalloid solutions. Am J Respir Crit Care Med. 2019;199(8):952–960.

30. Gladden LB. Lactate metabolism: A new paradigm for the third millennium. J. Physiol. 2004;558(Pt 1):5–30.

31. Tommasino C, Picozzi V. Volume and electrolyte management. Best Pract Res Clin Anaesthesiol. 2007;21(4):497–516.

32. Myburgh JA, Mythen MG. Resuscitation fluids. N Engl J Med. 2013;369(13):1243–51.

33. Reddy S, Weinberg L, Young P. Crystalloid fluid therapy. Crit Care. 2016;20:59.

34. Ryden SE, Oberman HA. Compatibility of common intravenous solutions with CPD blood. transfusion. 1975;15(3):250–5.

35. Wakim KG. "Normal" 0.9 per cent salt solution is neither "normal" nor physiological. JAMA 1970;214(9):1710.

36. Kellum JA. Abnormal saline and the history of intravenous fluids. Nat. Rev. Nephrol. 2018;14(6):358–360.

37. Reid F, Lobo DN, Williams RN, et al. (Ab)normal saline and physiological Hartmann's solution: a randomized double-blind crossover study. Clin Sci (Lond). 2003;104(1):17–24.

38. Lobo DN, Awad S. Should chloride-rich crystalloids remain the mainstay of fluid resuscitation to prevent "pre-renal" acute kidney injury? con. Kidney International. 2014;86(6):1096–1105.

39. Yunos NM, Bellomo R, Glassford N, et al. Chloride-liberal vs. Chloride-restrictive intravenous fluid administration and acute kidney injury: an extended analysis. Intensive Care Med 2015;41(2):257–64.

40. Heng Li, Sun SR, Yap JQ, et al. 0.9% saline is neither normal nor physiological. J Zhejiang Univ Sci B. 2016;17(3):181–187.

41. Maheshwari K, Turan A, Makarova N, et al. Saline versus lactated ringer's solution: The saline or Lactated Ringer's (SOLAR) trial. Anesthesiology. 2020;132(4):614–24.

42. Mythen MG, Swart M, Acheson N, et al. Perioperative fluid management: Consensus statement from the enhanced recovery partnership. Perioper Med (Lond) 2012;1:2.

43. Shaw AD, Bagshaw SM, Goldstein SL, et al. Major complications, mortality, and resource utilization after open abdominal surgery: 0.9% saline compared to Plasma Lyte. Ann Surg 2012;255(5):821–829.

44. Rizoli S. PlasmaLyte. J Trauma 2011;70(5 Suppl):S17–8.

45. Ergin B, Kapucu A, Guerci P, et al. The role of bicarbonate precursors in balanced fluids during haemorrhagic shock with and without compromised liver function. British Journal of Anaesthesia 2016;117(4):521–8.

46. Weinberg L, Collins N, Van Mourik K, et al. PlasmaLyte 148: A clinical review. World J Crit Care Med. 2016;5(4):235–250.

47. Wiedermann CJ. Phases of fluid management and the roles of human albumin solution in perioperative and critically ill patients. Curr Med Res Opin. 2020;36(12):1961–1973.

48. Carson JL, Grossman BJ, Kleinman S, et al. Red blood cell transfusion: A clinical practice guideline from the AABB. Ann Intern Med. 2012;157(1):49–58.

49. Walsh SR, Walsh CJ. Intravenous fluid-associated morbidity in postoperative patients. Ann R Coll Surg Engl. 2005;87(2):126–30.

50. Harris B, Schopflin C, Khaghani C, et al. Perioperative intravenous fluid prescribing: a multi-centre audit. Perioper Med (Lond). 2015;4:15.

51. Lu G, Yan Q, Huang Y, et al. Prevention and control system of hypokalemia in fast recovery after abdominal surgery. Curr Ther Res Clin Exp. 2013;74:68–73.

52. Muhammad Ali S, Shaikh N, Shahid F, et al. Hypokalemia Leading to Postoperative Critical Arrhythmias: Case Reports and Literature Review. Cureus. 2020;12(5):e8149.

53. Zhu Q, Li X, Tan F, et al. Prevalence and risk factors for hypokalemia in patients scheduled for laparoscopic colorectal resection and its association with post-operative recovery. BMC Gastroenterol. 2018;18(1):152.

54. Prescribing Intravenous Fluids for Adults. Fluid and Electrolyte Guideline Working Party. Queensland Health 2016. Available at: https://www.health.qld.gov.au/__data/assets/pdf_file/0024/700089/ivfluid-glines-adult.pdf (Accessed on 4 June 2023).

55. Rassam SS, Counsell DJ. Perioperative fluid therapy. Contin Educ Anaesth Crit Care and Pain 2005;5(5):161–165.

56. Lu G, Xu L, Zhong Y, et al. Significance of serum potassium level monitoring during the course of post-operative rehabilitation in patients with hypokalemia. World Journal of Surgery. 2014;38(4):790–794.

57. Yang Y, Yang J, Yao X, et al. Association between Blood Potassium Level and Recovery of Postoperative Gastrointestinal Motility during Continuous Renal Replacement Therapy in Patient Undergoing Open Abdominal Surgery. Biomed Res Int. 2019;2019:6392751.

58. Miller TE, Roche AM, Mythen M. Fluid management and goal-directed therapy as an adjunct to enhanced recovery after surgery (ERAS). Can J Anesth/J Can Anesth. 2014;62(2):158–68.

59. Padhi S, Bullock I, Li L, et al. Intravenous fluid therapy for adults in hospital: summary of NICE guidance. BMJ 2013;347:f7073.

60. Balakumar V, Murugan R, Sileanu FE, et al. Both Positive and Negative Fluid Balance May Be Associated With Reduced Long-Term Survival in the Critically Ill. Crit Care Med. 2017;45(8):e749–e757.

45 | TURP Syndrome

Transurethral resection of prostrate (TURP) is the second most common surgical procedure (after cataract extraction) done in men over the age of 65 years. Transurethral resection of prostrate syndrome is rare but potentially dreaded complication of urological endoscopic surgery [1].

DEFINITION

TURP syndrome is a distinct clinical entity characterized by a constellation of sign-symptoms secondary to neurological, cardiovascular and electrolyte imbalance resulting from the absorption of the irrigation fluid through prostatic venous sinusoids or breaches in the prostatic capsule during TURP.

INCIDENCE

The prevalence of TURP syndrome, previously reported to be as high as 2% to 12% in earlier literature, [2, 3], has significantly decreased to 1% or less with the adoption of safer techniques, as demonstrated in recent literature [4, 5].

RISK FACTORS

Following patient and technique-related factors carry a high likelihood of developing TURP syndrome [1, 6–8]:

- Patient-related factors contributing to the development of TURP syndrome include age over 80 years, prostate weight exceeding 75 gm, and resected prostate weight over 45 gm.

- Technique-related factors contributing to fluid absorption during TURP and the development of TURP syndrome include resection time over 90 minutes using Monopolar electrosurgery technique, the use of hypotonic irrigation fluid, irrigation volume greater than 30 liters, high irrigation pressure (height >70 cm), inadequate effluent through the resectoscope, intermittent drainage of fluid, the use of a monopolar instead of a bipolar diathermy system, and an inexperienced surgeon.

ROLE OF IRRIGATION FLUID

The type of irrigation fluid used during TURP surgery can influence the risk of TURP syndrome, with hypotonic irrigation fluids specifically posing an increased risk for its development. Commonly used solutions in TURP include both non-electrolyte solutions like distilled water, 1.5% glycine, 5% dextrose, sorbitol, and mannitol solutions, as well as electrolyte solutions such as normal saline and Ringer's lactate.

A. Distilled sterile water

Due to its affordability, easy availability, and superior visualization compared to 1.5% glycine and normal saline, distilled water is frequently utilized as a substitute for glycine in TURP in resource-limited settings of low-income countries [9, 10]. Due to its extreme hypotonicity compared to glycine and other irrigation fluids, distilled water carries a higher risk of TURP syndrome, including risks of haemolysis, dilutional hyponatremia, shock, and renal failure [11]. Due to high risk of severe adverse effects, currently most of centers do not use distilled water for TURP.

B. Glycine

Irrigation fluid, specifically glycine 1.5% with an osmolality of 200 mOsm/L, is widely utilized for the traditional therapeutic endoscopic urologic procedure TURP. It is preferred due to its favorable characteristics, such as low electrical conductivity and a refractive index similar to water, ensuring clear vision during the procedure. Despite its hypotonic osmolality, glycine is nonhemolytic as it effectively penetrates red blood cells, maintaining their structural integrity and preventing cell swelling or rupture. However, it is crucial to note that the osmolality of 1.5% glycine at 200 mOsm/L can cause serum electrolyte dilution and result in hyponatremia due to its large volume absorption. It is important to be aware that the rapid absorption of glycine can be toxic, leading to increased plasma ammonia levels and potential adverse effects such as cardiodepressant effects and renal toxicity [12]. Due to potential risk of metabolic and electrolyte disturbances, and the availability of safer options, trend to use glycine as preferred irrigation fluid for TURP is declining [13, 14].

C. Normal saline

An isotonic irrigation fluid, normal saline, is commonly used as the preferred and safer choice for TURP but can only be utilized when employing the bipolar electrosurgery technique [15, 16]. The risk of hyponatremia and TURP syndrome is very low when saline is used as an irrigation fluid for TURP, due to its slightly higher sodium concentration and osmolality compared to plasma (154 mEq/L vs. 140 mEq/L and 308 mOsm/L vs. 290 mOsm/L, respectively) [13, 17, 18]. However, it is important to note that the absorption of a large volume of normal saline can lead to adverse effects such as volume overload, heart failure, and hyperchloremic metabolic acidosis [15, 19, 20].

Caution: Do not use normal saline while using monopolar electrosurgery for TURP because saline conducts electricity and diffuses the current, making conventional monopolar cautery ineffective for cutting or coagulating.

Irrigation fluids like 5% dextrose, sorbitol and mannitol are used less frequently.

PATHOPHYSIOLOGY

During a TURP procedure, irrigation fluid can be absorbed through the prostatic venous sinuses or directly into the systemic circulation via disrupted venous channels, resulting in systemic effects due to rapid changes in osmolality and circulating volume [21]. The severity of TURP syndrome is closely related to the rate, volume, and composition of the systemically absorbed irrigation fluid. Various factors influence these factors, including electrolyte concentrations, osmolality, solute content, irrigation fluid delivery pressures, surgery duration, and surgical skill.

Major disturbances due to TURP syndrome are summarized below:

A. Circulatory overload

The average rate of irrigation fluid absorption through the venous network of the prostatic bed during TURP is reported to be 10–30 ml/min of operating time [22]. Typically, approximately 1 liter of fluid is absorbed within one hour. However, when a larger volume of fluid is absorbed, it can result in increased blood volume, leading to circulatory overload. This, in turn, can cause elevated systolic and diastolic blood pressure and potentially lead to heart failure, resulting in pulmonary edema.

B. Dilution and hyponatremia

The excessive absorption of hypotonic irrigating fluids, such as distilled water, 1.5% glycine, or sorbitol, during TURP can lead to the dilution of serum electrolytes, resulting in hyponatremia. This dilution, caused by the hypotonic fluid, increases the water content within the brain, which can potentially cause neurological symptoms.

C. Hemolysis due to hypotonic fluid

When a hypotonic irrigation fluid, such as sterile water, is absorbed in a large volume, its hypotonicity can result in the movement of water into red blood cells, leading to their swelling and potential rupture, which can cause hemolysis. The release of hemoglobin from ruptured cells can contribute to complications such as renal dysfunction and coagulopathy.

SIGNS AND SYMPTOMS

TURP syndrome can manifest with variable clinical presentations, ranging from mild cases that may go unnoticed to severe and life-threatening situations. The severity of symptoms depends on the extent of the abrupt reduction in serum osmolarity, which leads to hyponatremia, as well as the severity of volume overload and intravascular hemolysis.

The earliest common clinical presentation of TURP syndrome includes headaches, anxiety, nausea, bradycardia, irritability, confusion, and visual disturbances, such as flashing lights [23, 24]. Development of intraoperative hypertension is indicative of hypervolemia.

In severe cases of TURP syndrome, the clinical presentation can be life-threatening and may include profound hyponatremia, leading to neurological symptoms such as altered mental status, stupor, seizure, and even coma. Patients may experience severe cardiovascular instability, causing dyspnea, chest pain, hypoxia, and pulmonary edema. If not treated promptly, the patient may develop cyanosis, hypotension, and even cardiac arrest. Additionally, the presence of hemolysis may manifest as hematuria, jaundice, and acute kidney injury, while hypothermia can occur due to the rapid absorption of large volumes of irrigation fluid.

Diagnosis of TURP syndrome is difficult and often delayed when TURP is done under general anesthesia. Unexplained hypertension and refractory bradycardia are the very important warning signs of TURP syndrome. Therefore, all patients undergoing TURP should be closely monitored with electrocardiogram (ECG) and frequent blood pressure monitoring.

Patients with TURP syndrome can experience symptoms related to the toxicity of solute contents in irrigation fluid, such as glycine-induced visual abnormalities and sorbitol-induced gastrointestinal disturbances.

PREVENTION

Measures used to minimize the risk of complication TURP Syndrome include [1, 5, 25–27]:

1. Patient selection: Identify individuals at higher risk of TURP syndrome and correct possible modifiable factors. Patients with preexisting hyponatremia are at greater risk of developing TURP syndrome, so patients on a salt-restricted diet or diuretic therapy need correction before surgery.

2. Selecting an appropriate irrigation fluid: Isotonic solutions, such as normal saline, are preferred to minimize the risk of hyponatremia [28]. To prevent TURP Syndrome, it is advisable to restrict volume or avoid using hypotonic fluids like glycine and sterile or distilled water.

3. Fluid limitation: Careful monitoring and limiting the volume of irrigation

fluid used during TURP procedure can help prevent excessive fluid absorption. Sparingly use intravenous fluids, if needed and avoid the use of hypotonic IV fluids to minimize the risk of TURP syndrome.

4. Bipolar TURP: The new system, bipolar TURP, is preferred over the monopolar TURP system because it uses normal saline for irrigation, maintaining the balance of electrolytes and preventing TURP syndrome [29, 30]. The bipolar TURP procedure allows the use of isotonic electrolyte solutions like normal saline for irrigation, unlike the monopolar TURP technique, where non-electrolyte hypotonic irrigation fluids are used, carrying a high risk of TURP syndrome [5].

5. Operative modifications: Various intraoperative measures that can help prevent TURP syndrome include keeping the patient horizontal and avoiding the Trendelenburg position, limiting resection time to one hour, considering staged procedures for resecting large prostates to avoid prolonged operative times, and preserving the prostatic capsule by avoiding aggressive resection near it.

6. Fluid bag height: The rate of fluid absorption during TURP is influenced by the hydrostatic pressure of the irrigation fluid at the prostatic bed. To prevent excessive absorption, it is important to deliver the irrigation fluid at the lowest required pressure and avoid setting the fluid bag height greater than 60 cm above the patient.

7. Avoid increased bladder pressure: Ensuring smooth bladder drainage is the most crucial factor in minimizing fluid absorption during TURP and preventing TURP syndrome, which

can be achieved by implementing the following methods: suprapubic continuous drainage using Reiter's cannula or trocar cystostomy, utilizing a continuous flow irrigation system, and using a large diameter catheter to maintain low bladder pressure.

8. Experienced surgeons: Having TURP procedures performed by experienced surgeons can reduce complications, shorten surgical times, and improve outcomes.

9. Using regional anesthesia: Performing a TURP under spinal or epidural anesthesia is preferred because the awake and alert state allows for early diagnosis of TURP syndrome, whereas general anesthesia may mask its symptoms [23, 24].

10. Monitoring during TURP: Continuous monitoring of the patient's vital signs can help detect early signs of TURP syndrome. Measure the quantity of fluid absorbed and stop the procedure at predetermined absorption thresholds.

11. Early intervention: Prompt recognition of TURP syndrome symptoms and immediate intervention including use of diuretics, can prevent the progression to severe or life-threatening complications.

MANAGEMENT

Early and prompt treatment of TURP syndrome will prevent its serious central nervous system and cardiac complications. The treatment is planned according to the severity of the symptoms, and in asymptomatic patients with mild hyponatremia, specific therapy is not necessary. The treatment of symptomatic patients is summarized below [21, 23].

1. **Termination of surgery:** When TURP syndrome is diagnosed, the surgical procedure is terminated as early as possible.

2. **Diuretics and fluid restriction:** Discontinue IV fluids and administer furosemide at 1 mg/kg to increase renal water excretion, leading to an increased urine output, which helps eliminate large volumes of absorbed irrigation fluid and reduces circulatory overload.

3. **Hypertonic saline:** To correct severe hyponatremia in symptomatic patients with severe neurological symptoms, such as severe headaches, confusion, altered sensorium, convulsions, and coma, administer 100 ml of 3% hypertonic saline rapidly (to be given over 20 minutes) along with IV furosemide. In cases of acute severe hyponatremia, the administration of 3% NaCl as a rapid intermittent bolus (RIB) is preferred over slow continuous infusion, as recommended for the treatment of acute hyponatremia in recent guidelines. [31–33]. To guide further administration of 3% saline, measure serum sodium and its rate of correction by frequent estimation, and closely monitor the neurological status. Continue 3% saline until neurological symptoms improve.

4. **Hemodialysis:** Hemodialysis is indicated in a few severe cases of TURP syndrome characterized by marked hyponatremia, volume overload, and acute kidney injury. In such cases, diuretics may be less effective, and hemodialysis effectively corrects hyponatremia, removes excess fluid, and eliminates toxic metabolites of irrigation fluids such as glycine, sorbitol, or mannitol.

5. Supportive measures: This involves administering oxygen to treat pulmonary edema and hypoxia, managing seizures with medications such as diazepam, barbiturates, or dilantin, using inotropes to treat hypotension, correcting hypocalcemia, and cautiously transfusing blood with packed red cells to manage anemia.

MONITORING

Monitoring of the management of TURP syndrome includes:

- Continuous monitoring of vital signs, such as blood pressure, heart rate, and oxygen levels, to assess the patient's overall condition.

- Assessing neurological status for any improvement or deterioration in symptoms.

- Meticulous volume assessment, maintaining strict intake-output charting and daily weight to assess the correction of volume overload, plan fluid intake, and adjust diuretic dosages.

- Closely monitoring laboratory tests, including serum electrolytes (especially sodium), osmolality, renal function tests, complete blood count (CBC), and coagulation profile.

REFERENCES

1. Hawary A, Mukhtar K, Sinclair A, et al. Transurethral resection of the prostate syndrome: almost gone but not forgotten. J Endourol. 2009;23(12):2013–20.

2. Koshiba K, Egawa S, Ohori M, et al. Dose transurethral resection of the prostate pose a risk to life? 22-year outcome. J Urol. 1995;153(5):1506–1509.

3. Okamura K, Terai A, Nojiri Y, et al. Evolution of common clinical path for transurethral resection of prostate (TURP). Nihon Hinyokika Gakkai Zasshi Jpn J Urol. 2007;98(1):3–8.

4. The PLASMA system for transurethral resection and haemostasis of the prostate. Medical technologies guidance. January 6, 2021. Available from: www.nice.org.uk/guidance/mtg53.

5. Zeng XT, Jin YH, Liu TZ, et al. Clinical practice guideline for transurethral plasmakinetic resection

of prostate for benign prostatic hyperplasia (2021 Edition). Mil Med Res. 2022;9(1):14.

6. Mebust WK, Holtgrewe HL, Cockett ATK, et al. Transurethral prostatectomy: Immediate and postoperative complications. A cooperative study of 13 participating institutions evaluating 3,885 patients. 1989. J Urol. 2002;167(2 Pt 2):999–1003.

7. Fujiwara A, Nakahira J, Sawai T, et al. Prediction of clinical manifestations of transurethral resection syndrome by preoperative ultrasonographic estimation of prostate weight. BMC Urol. 2014;14:67.

8. Nakahira J, Sawai T, Fujiwara A, et al. Transurethral resection syndrome in elderly patients: a retrospective observational study. BMC Anesthesiol. 2014;14:30.

9. Watcharaporn T, Choonraklai V. Sterile water give better visualization than 0.9%NaCl and 1.5% Glycine irrigation in Transurethral resection of prostate gland. The Thai Journal of UROLOGY. 2008;29(1):26–30.

10. Meena R, Maranna H, Bains L, et al. Biochemical Changes Using Sterile Water and 1.5% Glycine in TURP: A Randomized Study. MAMC J Med Sci 2020;6(2):81–9.

11. Chen SS, Lin AT, Chen KK, et al. Hemolysis in transurethral resection of the prostate using distilled water as the irrigant. J Chin Med Assoc. 2006;69(6):270–5.

12. Park HP. Irrigation fluids used for transurethral resection of the prostate: a double-edged sword. Korean J Anesthesiol. 2019;72(2):87–88.

13. Yousef AA, Suliman GA, Elashry OM, et al. A randomized comparison between three types of irrigating fluids during transurethral resection in benign prostatic hyperplasia. BMC Anesthesiol. 2010;10:7.

14. Hahn RG. Glycine 1.5% for Irrigation Should Be Abandoned. Urol Int 2013;91(3):249–255.

15. Michielsen DPJ, Debacker T, De Boe V, et al. Bipolar transurethral resection in saline-an alternative surgical treatment for bladder outlet obstruction? J Urol. 2007;178(5):2035–9.

16. Cheung GY, Tempany S, Man Chu MH. Complications Associated With Intraoperative Use of Irrigation Fluid for Endoscopic Procedures. Update in Anaesthesia. World Federation of Societies of Anaesthesiologists Published 17 September 2019.

17. Zeltser I, Pearle MS, Bagley DH. Saline is our friend. Urology 2009;74(1):28–9.

18. Michielsen DPJ, Coomans D, Braeckman JG, et al. Bipolar transurethral resection in saline: the solution to avoid hyponatraemia and transurethral resection syndrome. Scand J Urol Nephrol 2010;44(4):228–35.

19. Johansson J, Lindahl M, Gyllencreutz E, et al. Symptomatic absorption of isotonic saline during transcervical endometrial resection. Acta Anaesthesiol Scand 2017;61(1):121–124.

20. Okuma N, Hino H, Kuroki M, et al. Symptomatic absorption of normal saline during transurethral resection of the prostate: a case report. JA Clin Rep. 2022;8(1):43.

21. O'Donnell AM, TH Foo I. Anaesthesia for transurethral resection of the prostate. Continuing Education in Anaesthesia Critical Care & Pain 2009;9(3):92–96.

22. Gravenstein D. Transurethral resection of the prostate (TURP) syndrome: a review of the pathophysiology and management. Anesth Analg 1997;84(2):438–46.

23. Demirel I, Ozer AB, Bayar MK, et al. TURP syndrome and severe hyponatremia under general anaesthesia. BMJ Case Rep. 2012;2012:bcr-2012–006899.

24. McGowan-Smyth S, Vasdev N, Gowrie-Mohan S. Spinal Anesthesia Facilitates the Early Recognition of TUR Syndrome. Curr Urol. 2016;9(2):57–61.

25. Rassweiler J, Teber D, Kuntz R, et al. Complications of transurethral resection of the prostate (TURP)–incidence, management, and prevention. Eur Urol 2006;50(5):969–79.

26. Aziz W, Ather MH. Frequency of electrolyte derangement after transurethral resection of prostate: need for postoperative electrolyte monitoring. Adv Urol. 2015;2015:415735.

27. Gamit B, Thakkar NB. Role of preoperative assessment of serum sodium in transurethral resection of prostate to avoid transurethral resection of prostate syndrome: a comparative study. Int Surg J. 2020;7(8):2630–5.

28. Virkar ND, Nerurkar AA, Patkar GA, et al. Effect of Saline Irrigation for Transurethral Resection of Prostate on Acid Base and Electrolyte StatusA Prospective Cohort Study. Journal of Clinical and Diagnostic Research. 2022;16(1):UC01-UC04.

29. Issa MM. Technological advances in transurethral resection of the prostate: bipolar versus monopolar TURP. J Endourol 2008;22(8):1587–95.

30. Cleves A, Dimmock P, Hewitt N, et al. The TURis System for Transurethral Resection of the Prostate: A NICE Medical Technology Guidance. Appl Health Econ Health Policy. 2016;14(3):267–79.

31. Hoorn EJ, Zietse R. Diagnosis and treatment of hyponatremia: compilation of the guidelines. J Am Soc Nephrol. 2017;28(5):1340–1349.

32. Garrahy A, Dineen R, Hannon AM, et al. Continuous Versus Bolus Infusion of Hypertonic Saline in the Treatment of Symptomatic Hyponatremia Caused by SIAD. J Clin Endocrinol Metab 2019;104(9):3595–3602.

33. Baek SH, Jo YH, Ahn S, et al. Risk of Overcorrection in Rapid Intermittent Bolus vs Slow Continuous Infusion Therapies of Hypertonic Saline for Patients With Symptomatic Hyponatremia: The SALSA Randomized Clinical Trial. JAMA Intern Med. 2021;181(1):81–92.

46 | Burns

INTRODUCTION

Fluid management in burns is a crucial aspect of burn care as it significantly impacts patient outcomes, particularly in severe cases where larger volumes of IV fluids must be administered within the first hours, exceeding the needs of other trauma patients [1].

However, it is a complex and controversial topic, as no one-size-fits-all approach can be universally applied to every clinical scenario. Therefore, it is essential to have a comprehensive understanding of fluid therapy in order to make proper decisions regarding the selection, volume, and administration of fluids from the array of available fluid regimens.

IMPORTANCE OF FLUID MANAGEMENT

Effective, optimal, and timely fluid management is crucial for resuscitation in burn patients because:

- Severe hypovolemia and hypotension in severe burns can lead to life-threatening shock or shock-induced renal failure [2].
- Delayed or insufficient fluid resuscitation is associated with higher mortality [3].
- Severe hypotension and suboptimal fluid resuscitation cause rapid conversion of viable but ischemic deep-dermal burn to non-viable full-thickness burn, leading to greater mortality [4].

- Acute loss of protein (especially in the first 24 hours) due to leaky capillaries in the burned tissue causes hypoproteinemia, which accentuates edema formation in the burn as well as non-burn areas. Proper fluid therapy is essential for its prevention.
- Over-aggressive fluid therapy is harmful as it can lead to fluid creep and other complications [3, 5].

CAUSES OF HYPOTENSION

Causes of hypovolemia and hypotension in burns are multifactorial, including extensive loss of plasma from damaged blood vessels, increased capillary permeability, fluid shifts into the interstitial space, and loss of albumin and other proteins [6]. Additionally, the release of inflammatory mediators can lead to vasodilation and reduced systemic vascular resistance [7]Decreased cardiac output, which occurs in the early postinjury phase, also contributes to hypotension [8]. The combination of these factors can result in inadequate circulating blood volume and impaired tissue perfusion in burn patients.

GOALS

Providing timely and effective fluid resuscitation in burns is vital because a delay of more than 2 hours post-burn injury is associated with higher complications and mortality [4]. The objectives of proper fluid therapy in burns are:

- To restore and maintain adequate intravascular volume, optimize tissue perfusion, and improve oxygenation.
- To replace lost fluids, prevent complications such as hypovolemic shock and organ dysfunction, and correct electrolyte imbalances.

- To preserve heat-injured but viable soft tissue.
- To avoid the detrimental effects of over-resuscitation and associated complications like fluid creep.

INDICATIONS OF IV FLUIDS ADMINISTRATION

Common indications of intravenous fluid administration in burns are [9, 10]:

- Adults with more than 15–20% nonsuperficial burns.
- Children with more than 10% burns.
- Electric burns with hemochromogens in the urine.
- Patients at the extremes of age or elderly patients with preexisting cardiac or pulmonary disease, where the compensatory response to even minor hypovolemia is reduced.

Estimation of burn area: The "Rule of Nines" in burns is the most popular and quick method to estimate the percentage of total body surface area (TBSA) affected by burns: Head and neck (9%), each upper limb (front and back) (9% each, total 18%), anterior trunk (18%), posterior trunk (18%), each lower limb (front and back) (18% each, total 36%), and perineum (1%). The "Rule of Nines" provides a rough estimation but may not be precise for irregularly distributed burns or specific areas like the hands, feet, or face.

PLANNING FLUID THERAPY ON DIFFERENT POST-BURN DAYS

During the different stages of burns, the body undergoes varying degrees of fluid loss, resulting in the need for different volumes of fluids. Understanding the distinct pathophysiology during each stage is crucial for designing appropriate treatment strategies on different post-burn days.

For a basic understanding, fluid therapy in burns is broadly categorized into three phases:

A. Initial 24 hours

B. During the first 24–48 hours

C. Fluid therapy after 48 hours

A. INITIAL FLUID RESUSCITATION

During this period, the inflammatory response triggered by a burn injury results in increased capillary permeability and damaged blood vessels, leading to significant fluid loss from the blood vessels into the surrounding tissues. The leakage of fluid rich in sodium and proteins from the intravascular compartment into the interstitial spaces of the burn area contributes to the formation of edema. Hence, it is crucial to promptly and cautiously initiate IV fluid resuscitation during the initial phase to replace lost fluid, maintain blood pressure, and minimize edema formation.

Fluid therapy in burns is tailored based on factors such as the extent and degree of burn injury, hemodynamic status, coexisting morbid conditions, body weight, age, preexisting medical conditions, burn location, and time since the burn injury. To ensure adequate and effective fluid resuscitation during the initial phase of burns, it is crucial to establish appropriate vascular access, select the suitable replacement fluid, accurately determine the required fluid volume through proper calculations, and decide on the optimal rate of fluid administration.

Vascular access

Establishing vascular access is crucial for the timely and effective administration of large amounts of IV fluids, but it can be challenging in burn patients due to technical issues such as edema [11]. Commonly employed options for IV fluid administration include the reliable insertion of large bore IV in peripheral veins, with the utilization of vessels underlying burned skin if necessary. In cases where peripheral intravenous access is unavailable, alternatives such as tunneled central venous catheterization, central line placement, or the use of intraosseous access in emergent situations can be considered.

Choice of replacement fluid

The mainstays for initial fluid resuscitation in burns include the use of crystalloids like Ringer's lactate, normal saline, and PlasmaLyte, and colloids like albumin and hydroxyethyl starch. The selection of these fluids is individualized based on factors such as the severity of the burn, hemodynamic status, and response to therapy.

1. Crystalloid resuscitation

For initial fluid resuscitation in burns, the primary options are crystalloids such as Ringer's lactate, normal saline, and PlasmaLyte.

a. Ringer's lactate: Crystalloid solution Ringer's lactate (RL) is the recommended first-line intravenous fluid for initial fluid resuscitation in burns [9, 10, 12]. The preference for RL over normal saline is based on several reasons, which are as follows:

- RL is a balanced crystalloid solution that closely resembles plasma electrolyte composition, enabling the administration of large volumes without causing electrolyte imbalances.

- With a high sodium concentration of 130 mEq/L, RL effectively replaces the significant amount of sodium and water lost from the intravascular space into the interstitial spaces of the burn area, correcting hypotension.

- RL is free of glucose, so it does not carry the risk of hyperglycemia and associated problems even when rapidly infused in large volumes.

- RL's conversion of lactate into bicarbonate helps correct metabolic acidosis commonly seen in burn patients.

- Using RL instead of normal saline for initial fluid resuscitation in burns prevents the risk of hyperchloremic acidosis associated with large volumes of normal saline.

b. Normal saline: Normal saline is an isotonic crystalloid solution that is widely available, inexpensive, and compatible with most medications. However, due to its 50% higher chloride concentration than plasma (154 mEq/L vs. 100 mEq/L), administering normal saline in large volumes can result in dilutional hyperchloremic acidosis, which makes it less favorable for initial fluid resuscitation in burns [3, 13]. Furthermore, normal saline lacks electrolytes such as potassium or calcium.

c. PlasmaLyte: PlasmaLyte, a newer balanced crystalloid solution similar to RL, is gaining popularity for its use in critically ill patients, including those with burn injuries [14]. Its utilization as the primary crystalloid solution for large burns is increasing due to its favorable characteristics, including a composition closer to plasma than RL and lactate as a bicarbonate precursor that can be metabolized even in patients with shock [15, 16]. However, the limited use of this fluid in burns is attributed to its high cost and the lack of evidence demonstrating its superiority over other fluids in burn management [17].

2. Colloid resuscitation

Colloids like albumin and fresh frozen plasma are commonly used, while hydroxyethyl starch and gelatins are avoided. The role of colloids in the initial resuscitation of burns is controversial, as their use is typically considered an adjunct to crystalloids rather than a primary choice of fluid. The limited utilization of colloids is primarily attributed to their higher cost and the absence of survival benefits [3, 18].

Capillary leakage is maximum within the initial 8 hours after the burn and persists for subsequent 24–48 hours [19]. Consequently, the use of colloids for resuscitation is generally avoided during the initial 8–12 hours, as it has minimal effect on intravascular retention due to the significantly high protein leakage [12, 20]. Furthermore, the use of colloids within 12 hours of a burn injury may have detrimental effects, as it can potentially worsen alveolar exudative inflammation [21].

However, judicious administration of colloids after 12–18 hours provides advantages, such as a reduction in the overall fluid volume requirement, a significant decrease in fluid load, and a minimized risk of "fluid creep" and edema formation [5, 18, 22].

a. Human albumin: Human albumin, the most widely used colloid, is recommended as an adjunct to crystalloid resuscitation in patients with severe burns and shock, particularly after the initial 12 to 18 hours [21]. Its major benefit lies in reducing the total volume requirement of crystalloid in burn patients during the early period, thereby reducing the risk of fluid overload and fluid creep [1, 23–28]. The use of albumin is suggested in patients with severe burns who have serum albumin concentrations below 30 gm/L [21] and a projected fluid volume requirement exceeding 6 mL/kg/%TBSA in 24 hours [29]. Notably, albumin administration decreases the occurrence of compartment syndrome, improves outcomes, and reduces mortality rates in patients undergoing burn shock resuscitation [25, 30].

b. Fresh frozen plasma (FFP): Natural colloids like human albumin and fresh frozen plasma are widely prescribed [31] and advocated in major burns [1, 19]. The use of FFP in burn resuscitation remains controversial, but recent literature suggests a growing trend of using FFP as a potential adjunct to crystalloids and as an alternative to albumin in severe burns because [32–35]:

- FFP effectively reduces the large amounts of crystalloid fluids required during burn resuscitation [18, 32, 36].

- Its composition is more consistent with the lost body fluid [21].

- FFP improves clotting factors and hemostasis and has a longer shelf life compared to albumin [37].

- FFP exerts a protective effect on the endothelium in burns by preventing the disruption of the endothelial glycocalyx, thus reducing the microvascular leak commonly associated with large burns [33, 38, 39].

- In the first study comparing FFP and albumin recently conducted, patients treated with FFP had significantly lower mortality [40]. However, further studies with larger sample sizes are needed to confirm these findings.

- FFP is preferred over albumin in certain guidelines [21].

- The risk of transfusion-transmitted infections is low due to recent advancements in screening techniques and more rigorous testing [41].

- In many resource-limited countries like India, FFP is preferred due to the limited availability and comparatively high cost of albumin [42]. However, the cost comparison between the two varies across different countries.

c. Hydroxyethyl starch: When hydroxyethyl starch (HES) was added to RL in severe burn injury, studies did not find a volume-sparing effect [43], and due to the lack of benefits and the increased risk of mortality, acute kidney injury and coagulopathy associated with HES [44, 45], recommendations strongly advise against its use in burns [46].

d. Gelatin: Gelatins are not recommended in burns as they have not shown superiority over crystalloids, and the evidence does not support their safety [1].

3. Hypertonic resuscitation fluid

Physiological considerations: Due to the distribution of sodium in the extracellular fluid (ECF), the sodium concentration of an IV fluid determines its ability to expand the ECF, including the intravascular volume, which plays a crucial role in maintaining hemodynamic stability. Due to its higher sodium concentration of 513 mEq/L, a smaller volume of 3% hypertonic saline is required for initial resuscitation compared to Ringer's lactate, which has a sodium concentration of 130 mEq/L. The osmolality of 3% hypertonic saline solution, which is significantly higher at 1027 mOsm/kg compared to the normal serum osmolality of around 285 mOsm/kg, creates an osmotic gradient.

Clinical considerations: Hypertonic fluid resuscitation is considered an attractive choice as it increases plasma osmolality, shifts water into the intravascular space, reduces intracellular water volume, limits the development of cellular edema, and also reduces the requirements of total resuscitation fluid volume and prevents fluid creep [9, 18]. However, its use should be approached cautiously due to the potential risks of hypernatremia, hyperchloremia, renal failure, and increased mortality rate [9, 47]. Based on current data, the use of hypertonic saline as a safe and viable adjunct to burn resuscitation is not supported [34].

Formulas used to calculate fluid volume

Numerous formulas have been proposed to calculate the appropriate resuscitative volume, but it is important to remember that these formulas serve as rough guides for predicting initial fluid resuscitation [48]. Subsequent infusion rates should be adjusted hourly based on individual responses rather than blindly following a set regimen.

The Parkland and modified Brooke formulas are the two most widely used and popular formulas for calculation in adults. It is important to note that the 24 hours for resuscitation is calculated from the time of the burn accident and not from the time of admission or initiation of treatment. It is also important to note that this formula provides an initial estimate and may require adjustments based on hourly urine output, the patient's clinical condition, and ongoing assessment of their fluid status.

1. Parkland formula: The Parkland formula, also known as the Baxter Formula, was developed in 1968 by Baxter and Shires, and it remains the most frequently used formula for calculating the volume required for burn resuscitation. The estimated requirement of Ringer's lactate for patients with burns in the first 24 hours can be calculated using the widely used Parkland formula as follows [49]:

The Volume Required (ml) =
   $4 \times$ %TBSA of Burns $\times$
      Body Weight (kg)

For example, if a patient weighs 70 kilograms and has a burn affecting 30% of their TBSA, the fluid requirement in the first 24 hours would be:

Fluid Volume =
   4 mL $\times$ 30% $\times$ 70 kg
      = 8,400 mL or 8.4 Liters

Out of the total fluid requirement for the first 24 hours, half is administered within the first 8 hours following the burn injury, while the remaining half is given over the next 16 hours. This initial 50% volume administration within the first 8 hours is necessary to compensate for the maximum capillary leakage and the loss of protein and sodium-rich fluids that occur during this time. As the rate of fluid loss decreases after the initial 8 hours, a smaller volume is needed to meet the ongoing needs.

The calculated fluid should be administered as a continuous infusion at a constant flow rate, as administering a large amount of intravenous fluid in bolus form can result in increased edema, while slower infusion rates can lead to hemodynamic instability [50].

2. Modified Brooke formula: The modified Brooke formula provides a lower total volume for fluid resuscitation, aiming to prevent "fluid creep" or excessive fluid administration. The formula is as follows:

The Volume Required (ml) =
2 × %TBSA of Burns ×
Body Weight (kg)

3. American Burn Association guideline: According to the American Burn Association (2008) recommendation, the initial rate of crystalloid fluid resuscitation in the first 24 hours post-burn is estimated to be 2–4 mL/kg/% TBSA [9]. This guideline is derived from the modified Brooke and Parkland formulas, which are widely used and accepted for burn resuscitation.

4. WHO formula for mass burn casualties: In 2021, the World Health Organization Technical Working Group on Burns (WHO TWGB) recommended an initial fluid rate of 100 mL/kg/24 h, either orally or intravenously, as a resuscitation formula for burns beyond 20% TBSA (total body surface area), which is suitable for resource-limited situations [51]. This formula offers the advantages of simplicity, usability, and safety for primary management, including transfers, while reducing the risk of early complications, particularly in situations such as mass burn casualties when immediate expertise is not readily available [52].

Altered fluid requirement in patients with burns: Patients who typically require a large resuscitation fluid volume include those with full-thickness burns, high voltage electric injury, inhalation injury, and those who need escharotomy, whereas obese burn patients generally have lower requirements for resuscitation fluid volumes.

Volume overload and fluid creep

Several reports have documented a high incidence of receiving more resuscitation fluid than predicted, leading to volume overload when utilizing the Parkland formula for calculating fluid requirements [48, 53–55].

Fluid creep in burns refers to the inadvertent accumulation of excessive fluid in the body due to overly aggressive fluid resuscitation, which can result in complications such as tissue edema, compartment syndromes, infections, pneumonia, acute respiratory distress syndrome (ARDS), respiratory failure, acute kidney injury (AKI), increased need for renal replacement therapy (RRT), multiorgan failure, and even death [5, 55–58].

Several factors contribute to the development of fluid creep, including the overestimation of burn size, errors in judgment due to a lack of experience, overly enthusiastic or inattentive resuscitation practices, failure to recognize the need for colloids to conserve crystalloid administration in large volumes, inadequate monitoring of urine output, and inability to adjust fluid administration based on individual patient response [59].

To prevent fluid creep, several measures can be employed, including:

- Following an early fluid restriction regimen [29, 57, 60].

- Administering colloids such as albumin or fresh frozen plasma alongside crystalloids in cases with high fluid requirements, aiming to reduce overall fluid needs and minimize the risk of fluid creep [5, 18, 22, 26, 61].

- Avoid routine use of fluid boluses to correct hypotension.

- Implementing permissive hypoperfusion, a safe and well-tolerated strategy in studies involving adults and children [60, 62].

- Close clinical monitoring, including hourly urine volume assessment and making timely fluid volume adjustments as necessary.

Blood transfusion

Patients with severe thermal burns may uncommonly require a blood transfusion to correct anemia, which can result from associated traumatic injury, blood loss during surgical procedures, decreased red blood cell production, increased red blood cell destruction, and iatrogenic blood testing [63, 64]. Implementing a restrictive transfusion strategy with a red blood cell transfusion threshold of 7 gm/dL is well tolerated, markedly reduces transfusion volume, and helps prevent numerous complications associated with aggressive transfusion [64–66]. Patients should receive blood transfusions one unit at a time unless they are hemodynamically unstable or actively bleeding, and before administering a second unit, reassessment of the patient is necessary [63].

B. SUBSEQUENT FLUID THERAPY
(During the first 24–48 Hours)

During the first 24–48 hours following burns, it is common for the patient's body weight to increase by 5–15% of their pre-injury level due to fluid retention [67]. The goal of fluid management during this stage is to ensure sufficient fluid administration to maintain hemodynamic stability while restricting the total volume of administered fluids to achieve euvolemia and avoid fluid overload and fluid creep.

During this stage, although increased capillary permeability persists, it is relatively less pronounced compared to the first 24 hours, potentially leading to a lower volume of fluid loss. Consequently, the total fluid requirements for the second 24 hours are reduced, usually by nearly half compared to the

requirements of the first 24 hours, for resuscitation fluid [68]. The volume is adjusted based on the patient's response to resuscitation, closely monitoring parameters such as hourly urine volume and other indicators.

If adequate urine output is maintained for more than 2 hours during the first 24–48 hours, it suggests adequate fluid resuscitation and the patient is gradually switched to maintenance fluid [69]. While calculating the maintenance fluid volume in burns, consider normal maintenance fluid plus evaporative loss from the burned skin. Maintenance fluid can be administered either intravenously, using D5/0.45 NaCl + 20 mEq potassium chloride per liter, or through enteral feeds.

The use of colloids for resuscitation is beneficial at this stage due to the decreased capillary permeability. This decrease in permeability results in reduced loss of colloids from the intravascular compartment into the interstitial spaces, providing two advantages. Firstly, it allows greater intravascular retention, ensuring effective hemodynamic stability. Secondly, it reduces the risk of tissue edema by decreasing protein leakage. Colloids, such as albumin or fresh frozen plasma, can be administered as 20–60% of the calculated plasma volume, which helps reduce fluid requirements and minimize the risk of fluid overload.

C. FLUID THERAPY AFTER 48 HOURS

During this early post-resuscitation phase (48–72 hours), capillary permeability decreases, resulting in decreased fluid loss. The primary focus shifts from aggressive fluid resuscitation to maintaining a balanced crystalloid status. The volume of fluid required is typically reduced compared to the initial

48 hours, emphasizing the importance of adjusting fluid administration to prevent fluid overload while ensuring proper hydration and electrolyte balance.

After the initial 48 hours of resuscitation, the fluid requirement consists of the sum of normal maintenance requirements, replacement of abnormal evaporative water loss, and continuous loss of plasma.

Fluid therapy is initiated based on the calculated maintenance requirements (100 mL/kg for the first 10 kg, + 50 mL/kg for 10–20 kg, and + 20 mL/kg for >20 kg) and is closely monitored. To calculate the required volume of IV fluid, subtract any orally consumed or NGT-administered fluid from the estimated fluid requirements.The fluid regimen is adjusted according to the patient's response to resuscitation, ongoing fluid losses, and clinical parameters.

MONITORING

Monitoring the burn patient is an essential component of fluid resuscitation, as no resuscitation formula should be considered a "license" to put the patient on autopilot. Careful and precise monitoring, along with necessary adjustments in the regimen, is vital for achieving adequate fluid resuscitation tailored to each patient's needs. Modalities used to monitor patients with burns can be categorized into clinical monitoring, laboratory tests, noninvasive monitoring, and invasive monitoring.

A. Clinical monitoring

The American Burn Association recommends monitoring pulse, blood pressure, urine output, mental status, and oxygen saturation in patients with burns [9].

Heart rate: The pulse rate holds limited usefulness but surpasses blood pressure measurement in sensitivity when monitoring fluid therapy [3]. Typically, a pulse rate below 110 to 120 beats per minute in a young adult suggests adequate resuscitation. However, if the heart rate exceeds 140 beats per minute, persistent severe tachycardia may indicate hypovolemia, although it can also arise from untreated pain or agitation [12]. Weak pulses may be attributed to inadequate fluid resuscitation, peripheral edema, or pressure on blood vessels caused by elevated compartment pressures.

Blood pressure: Manual blood pressure measurements can be challenging, inaccurate, and potentially misleading in edematous or charred extremities due to the progressive attenuation of auditory blood pressure signals as edema develops beneath the burn wound.

Sensorium: Anxiety and restlessness can be early signs of hypovolemia and hypoxia, indicating the need for attention and correction.

Urine volume: Accurate measurement and monitoring of urine output are crucial, requiring a urinary catheter in all patients with burns ≥20% TBSA [12]. Hourly measurement of urine output serves as the primary indicator for assessing adequate fluid resuscitation, evaluating tissue perfusion, and guiding timely adjustments in volume administration [70, 71].

Measure the hourly volume of urine, calculate the urine output as mL/kg, and adjust the rate of fluid administration in response to the patient's urine output as follows [72]:

- If the urine output is <0.5 mL/kg/hour, increase the rate of infusion based on the hourly urine volume. Additionally, considering a fluid challenge with 250 ml of Ringer's lactate in addition to the ongoing fluid may be considered.

- If the urine output is between 0.5 to 1 mL/kg/hour, it suggests adequate fluid replacement. Therefore, the fluid infusion should be continued at the same ongoing rate, and reassessment should be done hourly.

- If the urine output is between 1–2 mL/kg/hour, the fluid infusion rate should be reduced by 10%, and reassessment should be done hourly.

- If the urine output is >2 mL/kg/hour, the fluid infusion rate should be reduced by 20%, and reassessment should be done hourly.

It's important to note that increased urine output can occur in patients undergoing diuretic therapy or with conditions like glycosuria, hypertonic saline infusion, or dextran infusion attributed to the clearance of an osmotic load. However, this elevated urine output does not accurately indicate the patient's volume status and may potentially worsen severely depleted intravascular volume.

B. Laboratory tests

The laboratory tests performed for monitoring burns depend on the severity and extent of the burns and typically include complete blood count, electrolyte levels, blood urea nitrogen, creatinine, serum lactate and glucose levels, creatine phosphokinase, and mixed venous blood gas analysis.

Serum lactate level is a commonly used and valuable monitoring tool for hemodynamic resuscitation in patients with burns, as it helps assess tissue perfusion and metabolic status [73]. Estimating serum lactate levels early, upon hospital admission and periodically thereafter, is helpful in assessing the adequacy of tissue perfusion. An

increase in serum lactate levels suggests inadequate end-organ perfusion, while a reduction in serum lactate levels after fluid infusion indicates adequate fluid resuscitation in burns [74].

Mixed venous oxygen saturation (SvO_2) plays a crucial role in evaluating the patient's respiratory function, and a decrease in SvO_2 suggests inadequate end-organ perfusion.

C. Noninvasive monitoring

Noninvasive monitoring methods, such as noninvasive blood pressure (NIBP), pulse oximetry, continuous electrocardiogram (ECG) monitoring, ultrasonography, Transthoracic echocardiography, pulse-contour analysis, and transpulmonary thermodilution can be utilized effectively in burns for comprehensive and noninvasive assessment, if available [75–77].

D. Invasive monitoring

Invasive monitoring is beneficial for selected high-risk patients with large burns and complex comorbidities, and various techniques used for monitoring include central venous pressure, transesophageal echocardiography, transpulmonary thermodilution, arterial blood pressure, and pulmonary artery catheterization to optimize their management. However, evidence supporting patient outcomes benefits after major burn trauma due to invasive monitoring to guide fluid resuscitation is lacking [78].

ENDPOINTS OF BURN SHOCK RESUSCITATION

The clinical interpretation of hemodynamic status can be challenging, and there are no single parameters that definitively determine the endpoints of resuscitation in burns. Therefore, simultaneous consideration of various parameters is essential, which may suggest hemodynamic improvement and guide in optimizing fluid administration.

The primary indicators of the adequacy of resuscitation include improvement in mental status (normalization of sensorium), urine output of 0.5 to 1 mL/kg/hour without osmotic diuresis, normalization of heart rate and blood pressure (mean arterial blood pressure >70 mm Hg), and a reduction in lactate concentration and base deficit values [79, 80]. Base excess, lactate levels, and their correction rates reliably predict mortality [79].

Patients who are hemodynamically unstable, with coexisting comorbidities such as renal, hepatic, or cardiovascular disease, or elderly persons may need advanced hemodynamic monitoring for better monitoring if available.

COMPLICATIONS OF FLUID RESUSCITATION

Volume overload and fluid creep are common problems in burns, as discussed. In addition, large-volume resuscitation can lead to uncommon yet severe complications, which are described below:

- Abdominal compartment syndrome (ACS) is characterized by sustained intra-abdominal pressure (>20 mmHg) and new onset multiorgan dysfunction, including oliguria and decreased pulmonary compliance.

- Extremity compartment syndromes occur when there is an increase in pressure within a closed muscle compartment due to blood accumulation or soft tissue edema, resulting in impaired capillary flow to the enclosed muscle. These

syndromes are characterized by clinical signs such as swelling, tightness, muscle pain, pallor, coolness of the distal extremity, and, in severe cases, late loss of pulses.

- Pulmonary complications in burns can manifest as pleural effusions, pulmonary edema, respiratory failure, and prolonged intubation, contributing to significant respiratory challenges.

- Orbital compartment syndrome, a rare yet devastating complication of over-resuscitation, occurs due to a rapid increase in intraocular pressure. It is a surgical emergency characterized by orbital pain, double vision, acute-onset vision loss, and features such as a fixed dilated pupil and ophthalmoplegia.

NUTRITION ROUTE AND TIMING

Paying attention to nutrition is crucial in burns because it is a hypermetabolic state characterized by increased catabolism leading to increased caloric and protein requirements, significant loss of protein and micronutrients caused by the compromised skin barrier, and the need for increased energy expenditure to compensate for heat loss through the exposed surface [81]. Timely and adequate nutritional support in burns provides essential nutrients for tissue healing, supports immune function, reduces the risk of infection, minimizes protein catabolism and maintains lean body mass, and promotes wound healing and overall recovery [82]. So, early nutrition should be initiated proactively rather than waiting to address it later.

Route: Oral feed, enteral nutrition (EN), and parenteral nutrition (PN) are all viable options for providing nutritional supplementation in burns.

Enteral nutrition is recommended as first-line nutrition support in hemodynamically stable burns patients if oral feeding is not possible or if patients cannot meet the increased nutritional requirements through oral feeding alone. EN is preferred, and PN is not recommended routinely in burns because of adverse effects like overfeeding, impaired immunity, liver failure, and higher mortality [82].

The preferred method for enteral nutrition is nasogastric (NG) tubes, but feeding by nasoduodenal and nasojejunal tubes is indicated in a few patients with delayed gastric emptying.

PN is administered in burn patients only when EN is not feasible, not tolerated (e.g., abdominal distention, high residuals, diarrhea), or is inadequate to meet desired total nutrient requirements [83].

Timing of nutrition support: In burn patients, early EN (within 24 hours) is as safe as late EN (after 24 hours) [84], and it is recommended to initiate early EN, preferably within the first 24 hours after a burn injury [83, 85].

The advantages of early enteral nutrition in burns are [85, 86]:

- Protection of the gastrointestinal tract, preventing increased bacterial translocation and reducing the risk of sepsis.

- Enhanced nutrient adequacy, preventing the development of malnutrition and nutrient depletion.

- Reduced rates of complications and infections, shorter hospital stays, lower costs, and decreased morbidity and mortality.

For comprehensive information on nutritional considerations in burns, including energy, protein, carbohydrate, and lipid requirements, as well as the role of glutamine and micronutrients, please refer to the Chapter 56 on "Parenteral Nutrition in Specific Disease."

OLIGURIA IN BURNS

Oliguria during the resuscitation period (first 48 hours post burns) is commonly due to inadequate resuscitation and is almost never an indicator of acute kidney injury. It should be treated with increased fluid administration, not by fluid restriction or administration of diuretics.

Patients with high voltage electric injuries, deep burns involving muscle, and associated crush injuries are prone to developing rhabdomyolysis and myoglobinuric acute kidney injury, which can lead to oliguria. Weakness, muscular pain, oliguria with dark red to brown urine, and significantly elevated creatine phosphokinase (CPK) levels suggest myoglobinuric acute kidney injury, which may need diuretics.

Urinary output is no longer a reliable indicator to monitor fluid resuscitation once a diuretic has been administered [12]. Diuretics are also required in patients with extensive burns who remain oliguric despite receiving fluid volume far over estimated needs.

FLUID IN HIGH VOLTAGE ELECTRIC INJURIES

Management of high voltage electric injury is more complex and challenging than standard burn resuscitation due to the potential presence of significant and extensive deep muscle injury that may be hidden beneath normal-looking skin, making it difficult to estimate the severity and extent of burns accurately [87]. Additionally, severe electric injuries can cause damage to deep tissues and muscles, leading to acute kidney injury through rhabdomyolysis-induced precipitation of urinary hemochromogens in the renal tubules.

In such cases, administration of additional fluid is necessary to achieve a high urine flow (0–1.5 ml per kg per hour or 75–100 ml/hour in adults) in order to facilitate the rapid clearance of heme pigments, thus eliminating the need for diuretics and preventing acute kidney injury [12]. As various formulas tend to underestimate the fluid requirements for resuscitation significantly, optimal fluid administration is more accurately guided by monitoring urine output and other clinical, laboratory, and hemodynamic parameters to determine appropriate resuscitation endpoints [87].

If oliguria persists despite adequate hydration, additional measures for diuresis can be employed, such as the use of osmotic diuretics (such as mannitol), loop diuretics (like furosemide), or urine alkalization through sodium bicarbonate titration.

REFERENCES

1. Guilabert P, Usúa G, Martín N, et al. Fluid resuscitation management in patients with burns: update. Br J Anaesth. 2016;117(3):284–96.

2. Schaefer TJ, Nunez Lopez O. Burn Resuscitation and Management. [Updated 2023 Jan 23]. In: StatPearls [Internet]. Treasure Island (FL): StatPearls Publishing; 2023 Jan-. Available from: https://www.ncbi.nlm.nih.gov/books/NBK430795/.

3. Sánchez-Sánchez M, García-de-Lorenzo A, Asensio MJ. First resuscitation of critical burn patients: progresses and problems. Med Intensiva. 2016;40(2):118–24.

4. Barrow RE, Jeschke MG, Herndon DN. Early fluid resuscitation improves outcomes in severely burned children. Resuscitation 2000;45(2):91–96.

5. Saffle JR. Fluid Creep and Over-resuscitation. Crit Care Clin. 2016;32(4):587–98.

6. Snell JA, Loh NH, Mahambrey T, et al. Clinical review: the critical care management of the burn patient. Crit Care. 2013;17(5):241.

7. Nielson CB, Duethman NC, Howard JM, et al. Burns: Pathophysiology of Systemic Complications and Current Management. J Burn Care Res. 2017;38(1):e469–e481.

8. Williams FN, Herndon DN, Suman OE, et al. Changes in cardiac physiology after severe burn injury. J Burn Care Res. 2011;32(2):269–74.

9. Pham TN, Cancio LC, Gibran NS. American Burn Association practice guidelines burn shock resuscitation. J Burn Care Res. 2008;29(1):257–66.

10. ISBI Practice Guidelines Committee; Steering Subcommittee; Advisory Subcommittee. ISBI Practice Guidelines for Burn Care. Burns. 2016;42(5):953–1021.

11. Bittner EA, Shank E, Woodson L, et al. Acute and perioperative care of the burn-injured patient. Anesthesiology. 2015;122(2):448–64.

12. American Burn Association. Advanced Burn Life Support Course Provider Manual. American Burn Association; 2018. Chapter 4, Shock and Fluid Resuscitation. Available from: https://ameriburn.org/wp-content/uploads/2019/08/2018-abls-providermanual.pdf (accessed on 11 June 2023).

13. Orbegozo Cortes D, Rayo Bonor A, Vincent JL. Isotonic crystalloid solutions: A structured review of the literature. Br J Anaesth. 2014;112(6):968–81.

14. Cappuyns L, Tridente A, Stubbington Y, et al. Review of Burn Resuscitation: Is PlasmaLyte® a Comparable Alternative to Ringer's Lactate? J Burn Care Res. 2023;44(1):81–86.

15. Rizoli S. PlasmaLyte. J Trauma. 2011 May;70(5 Suppl):S17–8.

16. Weinberg L, Collins N, Van Mourik K, et al. PlasmaLyte 148: a clinical review. World J Crit Care Med 2016;5(4):235–250.

17. Chaussard M, Dépret F, Saint-Aubin O, et al. Physiological response to fluid resuscitation with Ringer lactate versus PlasmaLyte in critically ill burn patients. J Appl Physiol (1985). 2020;128(3):709–714.

18. Kao Y, Loh EW, Hsu CC, et al. Fluid Resuscitation in Patients With Severe Burns: A Meta-analysis of Randomized Controlled Trials. Acad Emerg Med 2018;25(3):320–329.

19. Cartotto R, Greenhalgh D. Colloids in acute burn resuscitation. Crit Care Clin. 2016;32(4):507–23.

20. Haberal M, Sakallioglu Abali AE, et al. Fluid management in major burn injuries. Indian J Plast Surg. 2010;43(Suppl):S29–36.

21. Yu YT, Liu J, Hu B, et al. Expert consensus on the use of human serum albumin in critically ill patients. Chin Med J (Engl). 2021;134(14):1639–1654.

22. Lawrence A, Faraklas I, Watkins H, et al. Colloid administration normalizes resuscitation ratio and ameliorates "fluid creep". J Burn Care Res. 2010;31(1):40–7.

23. Hunter JE, Drew PJ, Potokar TS, et al. Albumin resuscitation in burns: a hybrid regime to mitigate fluid creep. Scars Burn Heal 2016;2:2059513116642083.

24. Müller Dittrich MH, Brunow de Carvalho W, Lopes Lavado E. Evaluation of the "Early" Use of Albumin in Children with Extensive Burns: A Randomized Controlled Trial. Pediatr Crit Care Med 2016;17(6):e280–e286.

25. Navickis RJ, Greenhalgh DG, Wilkes MM. Albumin in Burn Shock Resuscitation: A Meta-Analysis

of Controlled Clinical Studies. J Burn Care Res. 2016;37(3):e268–78.

26. Eljaiek R, Heylbroeck C, Dubois MJ. Albumin administration for fluid resuscitation in burn patients: A systematic review and meta-analysis. Burns 2017;43(1):17–24.

27. Blanco-Schweizer P, Sánchez-Ballesteros J, Bendito B, et al. Resuscitation with albumin using BET formula keeps at bay fluid administration in burned patients. An observational study. Burns 2020;46(4):860–867.

28. Comish P, Walsh M, Castillo-Angeles M, et al. Adoption of rescue colloid during burn resuscitation decreases fluid administered and restores end-organ perfusion. Burns. 2021;47(8):1844–1850.

29. Chung KK, Wolf SE, Cancio LC, et al. Resuscitation of severely burned military casualties: fluid begets more fluid. J Trauma. 2009;67(2):231–237.

30. Cochran A, Morris SE, Edelman LS, et al. Burn patient characteristics and outcomes following resuscitation with albumin. Burns. 2007;33(1):25–30.

31. Greenhalgh DG. Burn resuscitation: the results of the ISBI/ABA survey. Burns. 2010;36(2):176–82.

32. Hoelscher VS, Harvin JA, Cotton BA, et al. Impact of Fresh Frozen Plasma Infusions during Resuscitation in Thermally-Injured Patients, J Burn Care Res 2018;39(1):S76.

33. Gurney JM, Kozar RA, Cancio LC. Plasma for burn shock resuscitation: is it time to go back to the future? Transfusion. 2019;59(S2):1578–1586.

34. Satahoo SS, Palmieri TL. Fluid Resuscitation in Burns: 2 cc, 3 cc, or 4 cc?. Curr Trauma Rep 2019;5:99–105.

35. Cartotto R, Callum J. A Review on the Use of Plasma During Acute Burn Resuscitation. J Burn Care Res. 2020;41(2):433–440.

36. O'Mara MS, Slater H, Goldfarb IW, et al. A prospective, randomized evaluation of intra-abdominal pressures with crystalloid and colloid resuscitation in burn patients. J Trauma. 2005;58(5):1011–8.

37. Rijnhout TWH, Noorman F, De Kort B, et al. Prolonged (post-thaw) shelf life of -80°C frozen AB apheresis plasma. Transfusion. 2020;60(8):1846–1855.

38. Schött U, Solomon C, Fries D, et al. The endothelial glycocalyx and its disruption, protection and regeneration: a narrative review. Scand J Trauma Resusc Emerg Med. 2016;24:48.

39. Cruz MV, Carney BC, Luker JN, et al. Plasma Ameliorates Endothelial Dysfunction in Burn Injury. J Surg Res. 2019;233:459–466.

40. Vural S, Yasti CA, Dolapçi M. Comparison of Albumin and Fresh Frozen Plasma as Colloid Therapy in Patients With Major Burns. Cureus. 2023;15(1):e33485.

41. Busch MP, Bloch EM, Kleinman S. Prevention of transfusion-transmitted infections. Blood. 2019;133(17):1854–1864.

42. Ravishankar J, Jagannathan SY, Arumugam P, et al. Evaluating the appropriateness of blood component utilization in burns patients. International Journal of Research in Medical Sciences 2016;4(12):5364–5371.

43. Béchir M, Puhan MA, Fasshauer M, et al. Early fluid resuscitation with hydroxyethyl starch 130/0.4 (6%) in severe burn injury: a randomized, controlled, double-blind clinical trial. Crit Care. 2013;17(6):R299.

44. Myburgh JA, Finfer S, Bellomo R, et al. Hydroxyethyl starch or saline for fluid resuscitation in intensive care. N Engl J Med. 2012;367(20):1901–11.

45. Perner A, Haase N, Guttormsen AB, et al. Hydroxyethyl starch 130/0.42 versus Ringer's acetate in severe sepsis. N Engl J Med. 2012;367(2):124–34.

46. EMA. PRAC confirms that hydroxyethyl-starch solutions (HES) should no longer be used in patients with sepsis or burn injuries or in critically ill patients. 11 October 2018. https://www.ema.europa.eu/en/news/prac-confirms-hydroxyethyl-starch-solutions-hes-should-no-longer-be-used-patients-sepsis-burn.

47. Huang PP, Stucky FS, Dimick AR, et al. Hypertonic sodium resuscitation is associated with renal failure and death. Ann Surg. 1995;221(5):543–54.

48. Blumetti J, Hunt JL, Arnoldo BD, et al. The Parkland formula under fire: is the criticism justified? J Burn Care Res. 2008;29(1):180–6.

49. Baxter CR, Shires T. Physiological response to crystalloid resuscitation of severe burns. Ann N Y Acad Sci. 1968;150(3):874–94.

50. Gueugniaud PY, Carsin H, Bertin-Maghit M, et al. Current advances in the initial management of major thermal burns. Intensive Care Med 2000;26(7):848–56.

51. Leclerc T, Potokar T, Hughes A, et al. A simplified fluid resuscitation formula for burns in mass casualty scenarios: Analysis of the consensus recommendation from the WHO Emergency Medical Teams Technical Working Group on Burns. Burns. 2021;47(8):1730–1738.

52. Bhat S, Humphries YM, Gulati S. The problems of burn resuscitation formulas: A need for a simplified guideline. J Burns Wounds 2004;3(7).

53. Cartotto RC, Innes M, Musgrave MA, et al. How well does the Parkland formula estimate actual fluid resuscitation volumes? J Burn Care Rehabil. 2002;23(4):258–65.

54. Sullivan SR, Friedrich JB, Engrav LH, et al. "Opioid creep" is real and may be the cause of "fluid creep" Burns. 2004;30(6):583–90.

55. Lindahl L, Oksanen T, Lindford A, et al. Initial fluid resuscitation guided by the Parkland formula leads to high fluid volumes in the first 72 h, increasing mortality and the risk for kidney injury. Burns Open 2023;7(3):51–58.

56. Pruitt BA Jr. Protection from excessive resuscitation: "pushing the pendulum back." J Trauma. 2000;49(3):567–8.

57. Saffle JR. The Phenomenon of "Fluid Creep" in Acute Burn Resuscitation. J Burn Care Res 2007;28(3):382–95.

58. Daniels M, Fuchs PC, Lefering R, et al. Is the Parkland formula still the best method for determining the fluid resuscitation volume in adults for the first 24 hours after injury? - A retrospective analysis of burn patients in Germany. Burns. 2021;47(4):914–921.

59. Atiyeh BS, Dibo SA, Ibrahim AE, et al. Acute burn resuscitation and fluid creep: it is time for

colloid rehabilitation. Ann Burns Fire Disasters. 2012;25(2):59–65.

60. Walker TL, Rodriguez DU, Coy K, et al. Impact of reduced resuscitation fluid on outcomes of children with 10-20% body surface area scalds. Burns. 2014;40(8):1581–6.

61. Chung KK, Blackbourne LH, Wolf SE, et al. Evolution of burn resuscitation in operation Iraqi freedom. J Burn Care Res. 2006;27:606–11.

62. Arlati S, Storti E, Pradella V, et al. Decreased fluid volume to reduce organ damage: a new approach to burn shock resuscitation? A preliminary study. Resuscitation. 2007;72(3):371–8.

63. ISBI Practice Guidelines Committee; Advisory Subcommittee; Steering Subcommittee. ISBI Practice Guidelines for Burn Care, Part 2. Burns. 2018;44(7):1617–1706.

64. Palmieri TL, Holmes JH 4th, Arnoldo B, et al. Transfusion Requirement in Burn Care Evaluation (TRIBE): A Multicenter Randomized Prospective Trial of Blood Transfusion in Major Burn Injury. Ann Surg. 2017;266(4):595–602.

65. Higgins S, Fowler R, Callum J, et al. Transfusion-related acute lung injury in patients with burns. J Burn Care Res. 2007;28(1):56–64.

66. Palmieri TL. Burn injury and blood transfusion. Curr Opin Anaesthesiol. 2019;32(2):247–251.

67. Tang Y, Chen I, Yen J, et al. Fluid Restriction for Treatment of "Fluid Creep" after Acute Burn Resuscitation. Hong Kong j. emerg. med. 2014;21:222–229.

68. "Practical Handbook of Burns Management" by the National Programme for Prevention, Management, and Rehabilitation of Burn Injuries (NPPMRBI) under the Ministry of Health and Family Welfare, Government of India.

69. Gupta AK, Asirvatham E, Reddy KA, et al. Fluid resuscitation in adult burns. Curr Med Issues 2021;19:103–9.

70. Paratz JD, Stockton K, Paratz ED, et al. Burn resuscitation–hourly urine output versus alternative endpoints: a systematic review. Shock 2014;42(4):295–306.

71. Cancio LC, Salinas J, Kramer GC. Protocolized resuscitation of burn patients. Crit Care Clin 2016;32(4):599–610.

72. Care of Burns in Scotland. National Managed Clinical Network. Fluid Resuscitation Protocol in Burns-Specific ICU Fluid Guidance. NSD610-006.07 V1. Oct 2020 [Internet]. Available from: https://www.cobis.scot.nhs.uk/wp-content/uploads/2021/07/NSD610-006.07.pdf.

73. Mokline A, Abdenneji A, Rahmani I, et al. Lactate: prognostic biomarker in severely burned patients. Ann Burns Fire Disasters. 2017;30(1):35–38.

74. D'souza NT, Kujur AR, Rajeswari D. Understanding the role of serum lactate as an end point in burn resuscitation. Indian J Burns 2020;28(1):7–12.

75. Coşkun F, Akıncı E, Ceyhan MA, et al. Our new stethoscope in the emergency department: handheld ultrasound. Ulus Travma Acil Cerrahi Derg 2011;17(6):488–92.

76. Jafarian AA, Farhoodi A, Jafarian Z, et al. Investigating the possibility of using noninvasive basic monitoring in patients with acute burns undergoing general anesthesia. Arch Trauma Res 2020;9(4):173–175.

77. Burmeister DM, Smith SL, Muthumalaiappan K, et al. An Assessment of Research Priorities to Dampen the Pendulum Swing of Burn Resuscitation. J Burn Care Res. 2021;42(2):113–125.

78. Davenport LM, Dobson GP, Letson HL. The role of invasive monitoring in the resuscitation of major burns: a systematic review and meta-analysis. Int J Burns Trauma. 2019;9(2):28–40.

79. Causbie JM, Sattler LA, Basel AP, et al. State of the Art: An Update on Adult Burn Resuscitation. European Burn Journal. 2021;2(3):152–167.

80. Belaunzaran M, Raslan S, Ali A, et al. Utilization and Efficacy of Resuscitation Endpoints in Trauma and Burn Patients: A Review Article. Am Surg. 2022;88(1):10–19.

81. Clark A, Imran J, Madni T, et al. Nutrition and metabolism in burn patients. Burns Trauma. 2017;5:11.

82. Williams FN, Branski LK, Jeschke MG, et al. What, how, and how much should patients with burns be fed? Surg Clin North Am. 2011;91(3):609–29.

83. McClave SA, Taylor BE, Martindale RG, et al. Guidelines for the Provision and Assessment of Nutrition Support Therapy in the Adult Critically Ill Patient: Society of Critical Care Medicine (SCCM) and American Society for Parenteral and Enteral Nutrition (A.S.P.E.N.). JPEN J Parenter Enteral Nutr 2016;40(2):159–211.

84. Wasiak J, Cleland H, Jeffery R. Early versus delayed enteral nutrition support for burn injuries. Cochrane Database Syst Rev 2006;(3):CD005489.

85. Rousseau AF, Losser MR, Ichai C, et al. ESPEN endorsed recommendations: Nutritional therapy in major burns. Clin Nutr. 2013;32(4):497–502.

86. Chourdakis M, Bouras E, Shields BA, et al. Nutritional therapy among burn injured patients in the critical care setting: An international multicenter observational study on "best achievable" practices. Clin Nutr. 2020;39(12):3813–3820.

87. Culnan DM, Farner K, Bitz GH, et al. Volume Resuscitation in Patients with High-Voltage Electrical Injuries. Ann Plast Surg. 2018;80(3 Suppl 2):S113–S118.

47 | Urinary Diversion

Urinary diversion is a surgical procedure that creates a new route to reroute urine flow from the normal pathway to an alternate path for elimination from the body.

INDICATIONS

Urinary diversion becomes necessary when the bladder can no longer safely store urine due to various conditions, such as:

- Bladder carcinoma: Surgical removal of the bladder for carcinoma.

- Traumatic injuries: Extensive damage to the bladder, urethra, or pelvis.

- Medical conditions: Malfunctioning bladder due to neurologic bladder dysfunction.

- Congenital defect: Bladder exstrophy is a congenital condition in which the bladder is located outside the body.

- Miscellaneous causes: Severe radiation injury to the bladder, intractable urinary incontinence, or vesicovaginal fistulae.

METHODS OF URINARY DIVERSION

There are several types of urinary diversion procedures, and the choice of procedure depends on the specific medical condition, extent of urinary tract involvement, and personal preference [1].

Urinary diversions are classified into two types [2]:

1. Incontinent diversions, where urine is redirected into an intestinal segment and continuously drained into an external collection bag (e.g., ileal conduit).

2. Continent diversions, where urine is collected and stored within the body, requiring either self-catheterization (e.g., catheterizable ileal pouch) or voluntary voiding to empty the reservoir (e.g., orthotopic neobladder).

Four common methods of urinary diversion includes:

A. Ileal conduit urinary diversion

The most commonly performed and simplest type of incontinent urinary diversion with the fewest surgical complications involves attaching the ureters to a segment of the ileum, creating a stoma on the abdomen for continuous urine drainage into an external collecting bag. The drawbacks of ileal conduit urinary diversion include the need for an external collecting bag for continuous urine drainage, potential changes in body image, and the possibility of leakage or odors.

B. Ileal pouch urinary reservoir

In this continent cutaneous diversion method, a pouch is created from portions of the ileum to store urine within the abdomen. The ureters are redirected to drain into this pouch, and intermittent self-catheterization is required several times a day to empty the urine from the pouch. The advantages of the ileal pouch reservoir surgery include not requiring an external bag for urine collection and eliminating the issue of odor associated with external urine drainage.

C. Orthotopic neobladder

This is a form of continent urinary diversion in which a surgically created reservoir is made from a segment of the intestine and placed in the same anatomical position as the original bladder, connected to the urethra. The neobladder closely resembles the storage function of a urinary bladder, allowing patients to void normally by increasing intra-abdominal pressure and significantly improving their quality of life and self-image after radical cystectomy. If voiding is not adequate despite the aforementioned efforts, patients may need to perform self CIC (clean intermittent catheterization).

D. Ureterosigmoidostomy

This urinary diversion procedure involves connecting the ureters to the sigmoid colon, allowing urine to be diverted into the colon and eliminated with bowel movements.

Ureterosigmoidostomy, which was once a common urinary diversion procedure, is now rarely used and considered a last resort option due to potential risks, such as electrolyte imbalances, urinary tract infections, worsening of kidney function, and the risk of colon malignancy. Safer and more advanced methods of urinary diversion have largely replaced it. However, due to advantages such as providing urinary continence without the need for a stoma and external appliances, simplicity, and the relatively quick performance of the procedure, ureterosigmoidostomy is still performed in some complex pediatric cases in resource-limited settings [3].

PATHOPHYSIOLOGY OF METABOLIC AND ELECTROLYTE DISTURBANCES

The factors that determine metabolic derangements and electrolyte imbalances in urinary diversion include the type of bowel segment used for the anastomosis, the length and surface area of the bowel segment exposed to urine, and the duration of contact time between urine and the bowel [4].

Urinary diversions involve using a part of the bowel that is not physiologically designed to handle and withstand urine's fluid composition [5]. Metabolic and electrolyte imbalances are more common in traditional ureterosigmoidostomy compared to other newer methods of urinary diversion. In ureterosigmoidostomy, urine containing chloride, sodium, and ammonium is diverted to the sigmoid colon, which acts as a reservoir. Due to the sigmoid colon serving as a large-sized reservoir and the prolonged transit time of urine in the colonic segment, which leads to a longer contact period in the colon, there is a significant exchange of urinary electrolytes with plasma through the colonic mucosa, resulting in fluid and electrolyte disturbances.

Common abnormalities encountered in ureterosigmoidostomy include metabolic acidosis, hypokalemia, hyperammonemia, diarrhea, urolithiasis, and metabolic bone diseases.

A. Metabolic acidosis

Metabolic acidosis commonly occurs in urinary diversions when urine comes into contact with the bowel wall, leading to the reabsorption of urinary ammonia, hydrogen, and chloride in exchange for the excretion of sodium and bicarbonate ions, which contributes to its development [4].

The absorption of chloride-rich urine by the luminal anion exchange pump of the colonic mucosa leads to the secretion of HCO_3 in exchange, causing bicarbonate loss in the bowel and resulting in hyperchloremia and metabolic acidosis.

An additional mechanism contributing to the development of hyperchloremic acidosis in urinary diversion is the absorption of ammonium [4]. When urine comes into contact with the colonic mucosa, fecal bacteria convert urinary ammonia into a large amount of ammonium ions. This leads to excessive intestinal absorption of urinary ionized ammonium, along with chloride as ammonium chloride, causing a loss of bicarbonate and a gain of chloride, resulting in hyperchloremic metabolic acidosis [6]. Loss of bicarbonate due to diarrhea (due to colon irritation by urine) also contributes to hyperchloremic metabolic acidosis.

B. Hypokalemia

Hypokalemia is more common in sigmoid diversions compared to ileal diversions, possibly because the colon has a lower capacity for potassium absorption than the ileum. In ureterosigmoidostomy, hypokalemia develops due to both loss of potassium in the colonic mucosa (secretion) and renal wasting [7]. Renal potassium wasting plays a relatively major role in potassium depletion, and it occurs due to acidosis, volume depletion, and activation of the renin-angiotensin-aldosterone system [8]. Diarrhea due to colon irritation by urine leads to direct loss of potassium and contributes to hypokalemia.

C. Metabolic bone diseases

In patients with urinary diversion, the long-term risk of metabolic bone diseases is a concern, and the factors contributing to these conditions include [4, 5, 7, 9]:

- Demineralization of bone due to chronic metabolic acidosis.

- Metabolic acidosis impairs the renal activation of vitamin D, which is essential for proper bone mineralization.

- Hypomagnesemia in ureterosigmoidostomy, resulting from urinary loss of magnesium, can lead to hypoparathyroidism by reducing parathyroid hormone (PTH) release and causing PTH insensitivity, adversely affecting bone formation.

- Impaired intestinal absorption of both calcium and vitamin D occurs when intestinal segments are used during diversion, leading to fat-soluble vitamin D deficiency, further aggravating bone demineralization.

- The associated presence of CKD contributes to metabolic bone diseases.

Metabolic bone diseases are late complications that can lead to osteomalacia and osteoporosis, increasing the risk of fractures [2].

D. Urolithiasis

The risk of renal stone formation is high (3% and 43%) in patients with ureterosigmoidostomy [10], and the mechanisms of its development are as follows [4, 5, 7, 11, 12]:

- Chronic metabolic acidosis leads to the release of bone calcium through the process of demineralization, resulting in hypercalciuria.

- Metabolic acidosis reduces urine citrate levels, and since citrate inhibits stone formation, a low concentration of citrate in the urine predisposes to the development of calcium-containing kidney stones.

- The increased intestinal absorption of bivalent anions, particularly sulfates, leads to elevated serum sulfate concentrations. The excretion of elevated urinary sulfate is coupled with the associated loss of urinary divalent cations, which can cause hypercalciuria and hypermagnesuria and raise the risk of stone formation.

- Dehydration due to diarrhea can lead to concentrated urine, which favors stone formation in the presence of the above predisposing factors.

- Anatomical changes that increase bacterial colonization, urinary stasis, mucus reflux into the upper tract, and exposure to surgical material such as sutures and staples may act as a nidus.

E. Hyperammonemia

In patients with ureterosigmoidostomy, urinary tract infections with urea-splitting organisms and urinary tract obstruction increase ammonia's production and subsequent colonic absorption significantly [13]. In patients with chronic liver disease or acute hepatic dysfunction, the liver cannot metabolize the increased ammonia load efficiently, leading to hyperammonemia and encephalopathy [4].

URINARY DIVERSION METHOD SELECTION

Selecting the appropriate urinary diversion method is crucial to prevent metabolic and electrolyte disturbances. In ureterosigmoidostomy, fluid and electrolyte disturbances are more common due to the larger capacity of the sigmoid colon and longer urinary contact time. To decrease these complications, the ileal conduit method for urinary diversion is effective because the ilial loop serves as a conduit and not as a reservoir. Urine is continuously drained into an external collecting bag, which reduces the contact time between urine and intestinal mucosa, thus minimizing the risk of metabolic and electrolyte disturbances. The incidence of stone formation is significantly lower with the ileal conduit diversion method, ranging from 9% to 11%, compared to 17% to 27% with the Kock pouch diversion [14].

The risk of metabolic and electrolyte disturbances is also reduced when methods like the ileal pouch urinary reservoir and orthotopic neobladder are used for urinary diversion, as they have smaller capacities, resulting in a smaller bowel surface area exposed to urine.

TREATMENT

Treating metabolic derangements and electrolyte imbalances in urinary diversion involves various approaches, depending on the specific imbalance present. Long-term planning with oral agents is desirable, as fluid and electrolyte abnormalities are usually chronic and persistent. In a few patients with severe dehydration, acidosis, and hypokalemia, vigorous hydration, alkalinization, and potassium repletion are needed [15].

A. Metabolic acidosis

Metabolic consequences and disturbances are frequently observed in patients following urinary diversion. Metabolic acidosis can lead to harmful effects in these patients, such as bone loss, increased protein catabolism, and decreased albumin synthesis, resulting in the loss of muscle mass and strength, making them frail and more susceptible to falls and fractures [2]. Initiating prophylactic treatment of metabolic acidosis early, at the stage of subclinical acidosis, and effectively restoring normal acid-base balance is crucial in preventing such metabolic complications [16].

The treatment for hyperchloremic metabolic acidosis requires administering alkalizing agents or blockers of chloride transport [8]. Alkalinizing therapy is commonly initiated with oral sodium bicarbonate (1–2 gm three times a day), but in some patients, it may cause significant gastrointestinal symptoms, such as excessive flatulence. Sodium citrate and citric acid (Shohl's solution) are used together as an effective alternative. Potassium citrate may also be used if excessive sodium administration is a problem (as in cardiac diseases) and potassium supplementation is desirable.

In patients with persistent hyperchloremic metabolic acidosis, where sodium loads are undesirable due to fluid retention/pulmonary edema and hypertension, chlorpromazine or nicotinic acid may be used to reduce the severity of acidosis. These agents impair chloride transport, limit the development of acidosis, and reduce the requirements for alkalizing agents rather than directly correcting the acidosis [8]. Chlorpromazine is usually given at a dose of 25 mg three times a day, whereas nicotinic acid is administered at a dose of 400 mg three to four times a day [17, 18].

Patients with ureterosigmoidostomy are advised to consume a low-sodium chloride diet to minimize their chloride intake and prevent acidosis [10].

B. Hypokalemia

Hypokalemia and total body potassium depletion are common in patients with ureterosigmoidostomies and are usually associated with hyperchloremic metabolic acidosis. Therefore, the treatment must involve simultaneous and cautious correction of both hypokalemia and metabolic acidosis.

In cases of severe potassium deficits, it is crucial to replace potassium before addressing the acidosis to avoid life-threatening hypokalemia. Conversely, correcting hypokalemia without treating metabolic acidosis can lead to hyperkalemia.

For prolonged oral correction, supplementing potassium citrate 15 mEq (approximately 1.6 gm b.i.d. to q.i.d.) helps in correcting both hypokalemia and acidosis in urinary diversion [19].

C. Metabolic bone diseases

Early and adequate correction of metabolic acidosis is crucial for preventing metabolic bone diseases and improving bone health; if the improvement is not achieved, oral calcium and vitamin D3 supplementation may be considered [9].

D. Hyperammonemia

Hyperammonemia can be managed through a low-protein diet and the administration of medications like oral neomycin and/or lactulose while simultaneously addressing disorders that can increase ammonia production, such as acute or chronic liver disease, urinary tract obstruction, and urinary tract infection [19].

REFERENCE

1. Moon A, Vasdev N, Thorpe AC. Continent urinary diversion. Indian J Urol. 2013;29(4):303–9.

2. Gupta A, Atoria CL, Ehdaie B, et al. Risk of fracture after radical cystectomy and urinary diversion for bladder cancer. J Clin Oncol. 2014;32(29):3291–8.

3. Przydacz M, Corcos J. Revisiting Ureterosigmoid-ostomy, a Useful Technique of Urinary Diversion in Functional Urology. Urology. 2018;115:14–20.

4. Vasdev N, Moon A, Thorpe AC. Metabolic complications of urinary intestinal diversion. Indian J Urol. 2013;29(4):310–5.

5. Sperling CD, Lee DJ, Aggarwal S. Urinary Diversion: Core Curriculum 2021. Am J Kidney Dis 2021;78(2):293–304.

6. McDougal WS, Stampfer DS, Kirley S, et al. Intestinal ammonium transport by ammonium and hydrogen exchange. J Am Coll Surg 1995;181(3):241–8.

7. Van der Aa F, Joniau S, Van Den Branden M, et al. Metabolic changes after urinary diversion. Adv Urol. 2011;2011:764325.

8. Wintner A, Dahl DM. Use of Intestinal Segments in Urinary Diversion. In: Partin AW, Dmochowski RR, Kavoussi LR, Peters CA, editors. Campbell-Walsh Urology 12th Ed. Elsevier; 2021.p.3200–3201.

9. Cano Megías M, Muñoz Delgado EG. Bone and metabolic complications of urinary diversions. Endocrinol Nutr. 2015;62(2):100–5.

10. Pedrazaa IA, Pérez de la Cruz SM, López de Aldaa A. Percutaneous nephrolithotomy in a patient with a ureterosigmoidostomy diversion. Uro-Technology Journal 2022;6(4):17–20.

11. Terai A, Ueda T, Kakehi Y, et al. Urinary calculi as a late complication of the Indiana continent urinary diversion: Comparison with the kock pouch procedure. J Urol 1996;155(1):66–8.

12. Okhunov Z, Duty B, Smith AD, et al. Management of urolithiasis in patients after urinary diversions. BJU Int. 2011;108(3):330–336.

13. Albersen M, Joniau S, Van Poppel H, et al. Urea-splitting urinary tract infection contributing to hyperammonemic encephalopathy. Nat Clin Pract Urol 2007;4(8):455–58.

14. Zhong W, Yang B, He F, et al. Surgical management of urolithiasis in patients after urinary diversion. PLoS One. 2014;9(10):e111371.

15. Tollefson MK, Elliott DS, Zincke H, et al. Long-term outcome of ureterosigmoidostomy: an analysis of patients with >10 years of follow-up. BJU Int. 2010;105(6):860–3.

16. Stein R, Rubenwolf P. Metabolic consequences after urinary diversion. Front Pediatr. 2014;2:15.

17. Koch MO, McDougal SW. Chlorpromazine: Adjuvant therapy for the metabolic derangements created by urinary diversion through intestinal segments. J Urol 1985;134(1):165–9.

18. Koch MO, McDougal SW. Nicotinic acid: Treatment for the hyperchloremic acidosis following urinary diversion through intestinal segments. J Urol 1985;134(1):162–4.

19. Van der Aa F, De Ridder D, Van Poppel H. Nutrition issues in gastroenterology, SERIES #73. When the Bowel becomes the bladder: Changes in Metabolism After Urinary Diversion. Practical Gastroenterology. 2012;36(37):15–28.

Part 10

Fluid Therapy in Pediatrics

Fluid therapy in children is an essential aspect of managing critically ill individuals, and appropriate fluid therapy can be lifesaving. The primary goal of resuscitation fluids is to establish hemodynamic stability, ensuring adequate intravascular volume and tissue perfusion. Maintenance fluids, on the other hand, are administered to achieve proper hydration and maintain electrolyte balance.

INDICATIONS OF IV FLUID THERAPY

Oral fluid replacement is always a safe and preferred mode. The indications of IV fluid therapy include correcting or maintaining fluid and electrolyte balance in conditions such as shock, severe dehydration, uncontrolled vomiting or diarrhea, inability to drink, paralytic ileus leading to abdominal distension, impaired sensorium, and other serious complications.

Goals: IV fluid replacement aims can be broadly categorized into three groups: Resuscitation, maintenance, and replacement [1]. Distinguishing these reasons is crucial because the choice of fluids, their composition, volume, and administration rates vary depending on the patient's clinical status and specific indications. It's essential to select the appropriate IV fluids tailored to each situation.

- **Fluid resuscitation:** The primary role of fluid resuscitation is to rapidly correct hypovolemia, raise blood pressure, ensure adequate blood flow to vital organs, and improve organ perfusion.

- **Maintenance fluids:** The goal of maintenance IV fluid is to provide an adequate amount of water and electrolytes to replace the ongoing daily physiologic losses in children and infants who are euvolemic and hemodynamically stable but unable to take adequate fluid orally or via the enteral route to meet their requirements.

- **Replacement fluids:** The aim of replacement IV fluids is to replace preexisting deficits and correct ongoing losses, such as gastrointestinal losses from vomiting and diarrhea, by providing appropriate fluid and correcting fluid, electrolytes, and acid-base disorders.

SPECIAL CONSIDERATIONS FOR FLUID THERAPY IN CHILDREN AND INFANTS

Fluid therapy in children needs special consideration and care because fluid balance is more delicately balanced in young infants and children due to the following reasons:

A. **Greater insensible losses:** Due to their higher basal metabolic rate and larger surface area compared to total body weight, young infants experience greater fluid loss, increasing the risk of dehydration.

B. **Greater urinary loss:** Neonates have a reduced renal ability to concentrate urine compared to adults (600 vs. 1,200 mOsm/kg), making them more vulnerable to fluid loss in the form of urine, even in a fluid deficit state.

C. **Thirst mechanism:** The thirst mechanism is the primary and the most effective way older children and adults can correct negative fluid balance. However, young infants cannot express their need for fluids during fluid loss, which increases their vulnerability to dehydration.

D. **Larger turnover:** Infants require special consideration due to their larger turnover; an infant exchanges about half of their total extracellular fluid (ECF) volume per day, compared to one-seventh in an adult.

E. **Fluid overload:** Fluid overload can easily occur in young children due to their relatively small circulatory volume (80 mL/kg), which is notably less compared to their daily IV fluid requirement (100 mL/kg).

Example: For a 5 kg child,
fluid need = 500 ml,
circulatory volume = 400 ml

For a 50 kg adult, fluid need = 2500 ml, circulatory volume = 5000 ml

F. **Meticulous calculation for smaller total fluid required:** As the total volume of fluid needed in children is smaller (a requirement in ml) compared to adults (a requirement in liters), meticulous calculation is required to avoid under or overhydration, especially in preterm babies, sick neonates and children with renal failure.

G. **Volume and distribution of body water:** Neonates have relatively larger water content. The water content is around 80% of body weight compared to 60% in adolescents and adults. The ECF volume is half of the intracellular fluid volume in adults. In contrast, ECF and ICF volumes are almost equal in neonates.

RESUSCITATIONS IV FLUIDS IN CHILDREN

In hypovolemic, hypotensive children, appropriate aggressive administration of fluids is essential and life-saving, as it restores circulating intravascular volume and ensures adequate tissue perfusion.

A. Selection of resuscitation fluids

The choice of resuscitation fluids for initial administration is determined by the clinical status, underlying etiology, and coexisting electrolyte and acid-base disorders.

1. Crystalloids vs. colloids debate

Colloids, as resuscitation fluids, offer benefits such as a more potent effect, longer intravascular persistence, and the potential to reduce fluid volume requirements compared to crystalloids. However, colloids are more expensive than crystalloids, and evidence supporting significant benefits of colloids over crystalloids, such as mortality benefits, reduction in the risk of acute kidney injury (AKI), need for blood transfusion, or the need for renal replacement therapy, is lacking [2].

Additionally, crystalloids are readily available and low-cost; therefore, crystalloids are preferred over colloids. Current guidelines, The Surviving Sepsis Campaign Guidelines in Children (2020) and European Resuscitation Council (ERC) guidelines (2021), recommend crystalloids over colloids [3, 4], and colloids are not included in the Pediatric Advanced Life Support Guidelines (2021) [5].

Use of albumin: The administration of albumin is generally safe and effective, but its limitations include being 30 to 100 times more costly than crystalloids, limited availability, and an increased risk of mortality in patients with traumatic brain injury [6–9].

Recent European Resuscitation Council (ERC) guidelines (2021) recommend using albumin as a second-line fluid choice in children who need large volumes of crystalloids [4]. The use of albumin as a resuscitation fluid may be beneficial in selected patients such as dengue, cerebral malaria [4], nephrotic syndrome with shock, and sepsis with septic shock [10–13].

Use of hydroxyethyl starch (HES): Due to harmful effects like increased risk of mortality, coagulopathy, and AKI [2, 14–16], current guidelines like EMA Guidelines (2018), NICE guidelines (2020), and Surviving Sepsis Campaign Guidelines (2020) recommend against using starches for the acute resuscitation of children [3, 17, 18].

Use of gelatin: The Surviving Sepsis Campaign Guidelines (2020) [3] recommend against using gelatin for the acute resuscitation of children due to the lack of benefits [19, 20] and potentially harmful effects, such as the risk of coagulopathy [21] and anaphylactic shock [22].

Due to this evidence, the use of hydroxyethyl starch and gelatin is not preferred for resuscitation in children.

2. Normal saline vs. balanced crystalloids debate

All guidelines and consensus recommend using effective, inexpensive, and readily available dextrose-free crystalloids such as normal saline or balanced crystalloids like Ringer's lactate or PlasmaLyte for resuscitation [2–4, 18, 23, 24]. However, controversies persist regarding the best choice of crystalloid.

Physiological basis: To understand the superiority of one crystalloid over another, it is essential to comprehend the composition of each fluid and the benefits and potentially harmful effects associated with its composition (Table 48.1).

Normal saline: Isotonic crystalloid normal saline contains 154 mEq/L of sodium and chloride but lacks buffers and electrolytes normally present in plasma, such as potassium, calcium, and magnesium. Compared to plasma, the higher sodium content of normal saline (154 mEq/L vs. 140 mEq/L) effectively expands the intravascular compartment in hemodynamically unstable patients. However, the supraphysiological concentration of chloride in normal saline (154 mEq/L compared to the normal serum chloride concentration of 100 mEq/L, a 50% greater concentration) can lead to harmful hyperchloremia [25]. In children with severe metabolic alkalosis and hypochloremia (e.g., profound vomiting), normal saline is the preferred IV fluid, and balanced crystalloids like Ringer's lactate (RL) or PlasmaLyte are avoided because lactate or acetate could worsen the alkalosis.

Ringer's lactate (RL): This balanced physiological solution contains 130 mEq/L sodium, 109 mEq/L chloride, 4 mEq/L potassium, 3 mEq/L calcium, and 28 mEq/L buffer lactate. This sodium-rich fluid effectively expands extracellular fluid (ECF) and corrects hypovolemia and hypotension. With a chloride concentration of 109 mEq/L, which is closer to the normal serum chloride level, RL eliminates the risk of hyperchloremia and acidosis associated with saline. Moreover, the presence of 28 mEq/L of lactate in RL allows for its metabolism and conversion into bicarbonate, providing a valuable buffering effect. However, due to its sodium concentration of 130 mEq/L, RL is a hyponatremic solution, and administering it in large volumes could potentially lead to hyponatremia [26].

PlasmaLyte: PlasmaLyte is a newer balanced crystalloid solution that more closely mimics human plasma compared to RL in its electrolyte content, thereby offering all the benefits of RL. PlasmaLyte contains 140 mEq/L sodium, as opposed to 130 mEq/L sodium in RL, and

Table 48.1 Composition of common resuscitation fluids

	Sodium mEq/L	Potassium mEq/L	Chloride mEq/L	Calcium mEq/L	Magnesium mEq/L	Buffers mEq/L	Osmolality mOsm/L
Plasma	135–140	3.5–5.5	98–106	4.5–5.5	1.5–3.0	HCO_3 22–26	290
Saline	154	0	154	0	0	0	308
Ringer's lactate	130	4.0	109	3.0	0	Lactate 28	273
PlasmaLyte	140	5.0	98	0	3.0	Acetate 27 Gluconate 23	295

therefore has no risk of hyponatremia even with large-volume resuscitation. Additionally, PlasmaLyte includes acetate and gluconate as bicarbonate precursors, providing better buffering action than lactate in RL. Unlike lactate in RL, acetate in PlasmaLyte has extrahepatic metabolism, thus maintaining its superior buffering action even in the presence of liver dysfunction [27, 28].

Evidence-based selection: The use of normal saline is known to induce hyperchloremia [29], which can, in turn, lead to acute kidney injury, organ dysfunction, and a higher mortality rate, particularly in cases of septic shock [30–33]. On the contrary, various recent studies have demonstrated lower length of stay, AKI, and mortality rates when using balanced crystalloids in children and adults with sepsis [34–36].

A recent systematic review demonstrated improvement in blood pH and bicarbonate values with fluid bolus therapy using balanced crystalloids compared to normal saline among critically ill children [37]. Furthermore, in a recent randomized trial conducted by Sankar et al. (2023) involving over 700 children treated for septic shock in India, the use of fluid boluses with a balanced crystalloid solution (PlasmaLyte A) demonstrated a decreased incidence of new or progressive acute kidney injury, when compared to the use of fluid boluses with normal saline [38]. Given these advantages, the recent Surviving Sepsis Guidelines (2020), ERCs guidelines (2021), the advanced life support guidelines (2021), and the Latin American Consensus (2022) all advocate for the preference of balanced crystalloids over normal saline when resuscitating children with sepsis [3–5].

Avoid hypotonic fluids: Hypotonic IV fluids like half normal saline and multi-electrolyte solutions (such as Isolyte-P, Isolyte-G, and Isolyte-M) can lead to hyponatremia, resulting in life-threatening cerebral edema and seizures, and are therefore avoided.

Avoid dextrose-containing fluids: Avoiding rapid administration of dextrose-containing fluids, such as dextrose saline, for resuscitation is essential due to the risk of hyperglycemia, osmotic diuresis, and potential worsening of dehydration. Additionally, in cases of traumatic brain injury, these fluids pose a risk of neurologic injury.

It is advisable to refrain from using dextrose-based salt-poor fluids like half-normal saline or salt-free fluids like 5% or 10% dextrose solution for rapid infusion during fluid resuscitation, as the rapid infusion of these dextrose-based solutions during the initial phase can result in hyperglycemia and the previously mentioned adverse effects. However, it's important to note that as the dextrose from these solutions is metabolized in subsequent periods, the remaining salt-poor or salt-free fluid becomes hypotonic, posing a potential risk of harmful hyponatremia [5].

However, it remains crucial to conduct bedside blood glucose testing to promptly detect hypoglycemia and administer timely treatment using a 10% dextrose solution.

Avoid potassium-containing fluids: Dehydration may be associated with acute kidney injury and hyperkalemia, and therefore, the rapid administration of potassium-containing fluids for resuscitation carries the potential risk of hyperkalemia and is hence avoided. Potassium is usually included in IV fluids in the presence of significant hypokalemia or once the patient voids and normal renal function is documented.

3. Role of blood transfusion

In cases of severe trauma causing hemorrhagic shock, the recent guidelines recommend the early introduction of blood as the preferred resuscitation fluid while minimizing the utilization of crystalloid solutions [4, 5].

B. Administration of resuscitation fluids

For the safe, optimal, and effective administration of resuscitation fluid, it is crucial to carefully consider its timing, method, volume, and duration.

1. Timing

Administering resuscitation fluid early and appropriately improves outcomes and lowers mortality rates in the pediatric population [3, 39]. Therefore, the initial management within the crucial first hours, often called the "golden hours," becomes imperative [40].

2. Bolus vs. continuous infusion administration

The administration of resuscitation fluids as a bolus therapy is essential as it helps restore blood pressure, improves cardiac output, enhances oxygen delivery, and optimizes organ perfusion [41], making it a recommended approach in all guidelines for the resuscitation of children with severe dehydration and shock [3–5, 18]. However, the Surviving Sepsis Campaign Guidelines (2020) and Latin American Consensus (2022) do not recommend administration of fluid as a bolus in centers without intensive care facilities and to children without hypotension [3, 42].

3. The volume of fluid bolus

The administration of the optimum volume of a fluid bolus is critical because it helps provide adequate fluid, correct hypotension, and maintain sufficient tissue perfusion while avoiding fluid overload:

- The Fluid Expansion as Supportive Therapy (FEAST) trial in 2011 showed that large fluid boluses (20 to 40 mL/kg) led to poor outcomes, including increased mortality [43]. This finding has influenced some clinical guidelines to recommend smaller fluid boluses [44].

- In 2016, the World Health Organization (WHO) updated its guidelines, recommending the administration of fluid boluses at a rate of 10 to 20 mL/kg over 30 to 60 minutes [45].

- The Surviving Sepsis Campaign International Guidelines 2020 recommend administering 10–20mL/kg per bolus over the first hour in children [3].

- More recent UK Resus Council Guidelines (2021), European Resuscitation Councils Guidelines (2021), Advanced Paediatric Life Support (APLS 2021), and the Latin American Consensus (2022) have shifted their recommendation to administering smaller volumes of resuscitation boluses (e.g., 10 mL/kg instead of 20 mL/kg) for the initial management of shock in children [4, 5, 42].

- However, the decision to use smaller fluid bolus volumes in these guidelines is based on concerns about the potential detrimental effects of fluid overload from larger bolus volumes rather than strong evidence supporting the safety of using 10 mL/kg instead of 20 mL/kg fluid boluses for resuscitation in children [44].

- If hypotension persists after the initial bolus, fluid boluses should be repeated up to 40–60 mL/kg in intensive care and 40 mL/kg when intensive care is unavailable, with close monitoring [3].

4. Avoiding volume overload

Once clinical improvement, such as a decrease in heart rate, normalization of blood pressure, improvement in alertness, and urine output, occurs with the initial resuscitation, it's crucial to restrict fluid and avoid excessive fluid replacement to prevent fluid overload [46]. The benefits of avoiding fluid overload in critically ill patients include more ventilator-free days, shorter ICU stays, reduced risk of acute kidney injury, and decreased in-hospital mortality [47, 48].

5. Additional measures

It is essential to search and treat underlying etiology, hypoxemia, electrolyte abnormalities, and metabolic acidosis during the resuscitation.

MAINTENANCE FLUIDS FOR CHILDREN

Intravenous maintenance fluids are crucial for supportive care in critically ill children. These fluids are used when children cannot receive hydration reliably through oral or enteral routes or when conditions such as respiratory issues, neurological impairments, gastrointestinal problems, perioperative states, or severe acute or chronic illnesses make enteral hydration unsuitable [49].

However, the oral or enteral route should always be the first choice when possible, as it can reduce the length of hospital stays for term neonates and also cut costs [50]. Given the potential pros and cons of maintenance intravenous fluids, they should be administered only when clinically necessary.

A. Goals

Before administering maintenance IV fluids, first rehydrate dehydrated patients; then start the maintenance IV fluids and discontinue them as soon as adequate oral or enteral fluid intake becomes possible.

The primary objective of maintenance IV fluid is to compensate for daily physiological losses such as urine, feces, and sweat. Maintenance IV fluids help in maintaining the normal water and electrolyte balance and provide sufficient calories to prevent starvation, ketosis, and protein degradation. Importantly, these fluids are not intended to correct existing fluid deficits or electrolyte imbalances but to prevent them in euvolemic children requiring intravenous hydration. Concurrently, some children might also need additional fluid replacement to address continuous losses from sources like diarrhea, vomiting, and other related issues.

B. Maintenance requirements of IV fluids

Maintenance IV fluids contain water, dextrose, sodium, potassium, and chloride and occasionally include bicarbonate, acetate, and lactate. Although these fluids don't provide adequate calories and lack protein, fat, minerals, and vitamins, this isn't usually a concern for children since the fluids are meant to be given for a short time.

1. Fluid volume calculation

It is crucial to calculate children's maintenance fluid requirements to meet

Table 48.2 Calculating maintenance fluid volume and rate based on weight

Body weight	Fluid volume per day (100/50/20 rule)	Fluid volume per hour (4/2/1 rule)
0–10 kg	100 mL/kg/day	4 mL/kg/hr
11–20 kg	1000 + 50 mL/kg/day >10 kg	40 mL/kg/hr + 2 mL/kg/hr >10 kg
Over 20 kg	1500 + 20 mL/kg/day >20 kg	60 mL/kg/hr + 1 mL/kg/hr >20 kg
Usually, the maximum volume is 2500 ml/day, and the rate is 100 ml/hour		

Table 48.3 Water requirements in children

Causes of increased water requirements	Causes of decreased water requirements
Preterm infants, Fever, burns, gastrointestinal-GI losses (vomiting, diarrhea), hyperventilation, loss in third space, adrenal insufficiency, polyuria, hyperosmolar state like diabetic ketoacidosis, and sweating due to increased physical activity	Oligo-anuria, SIADH as in postoperative stress, acute neurological or respiratory infections (e.g., meningitis, encephalitis, pneumonia, and bronchiolitis), persistent nausea, head injury and coma, hypothermia, ventilator use with fully humidified air and high humidity atmosphere

their physiological needs and preventing imbalances.

The Holliday-Segar method, commonly used even today for its simplicity, is a standard formula for calculating maintenance water requirements in healthy children and young people, as summarized in Table 48.2.

To determine a child's daily and hourly fluid requirements, calculate the amount of fluid volume based on the child's weight. Using the formula outlined in Table 48.2, the calculation for a child weighing 25 kg is as follows:

For the daily fluid requirement for a 25 kg child: (10 kg × 100 mL) + (10 kg × 50 mL) + (5 kg × 10 mL) = 1,000 mL + 500 mL + 50 mL = 1,550 mL/day.

For the hourly fluid requirement for a 25 kg child: (10 kg × 4 mL) + (10 kg × 2 mL) + (5 kg × 1 mL) = 40 mL + 20 mL + 5 mL = 65 mL/hour.

2. Electrolyte calculation

Traditionally, the Holliday-Segar method calculated electrolyte concentration in children based on human and cow milk composition, suggesting 2-3 mEq/kg of sodium and 2 mEq/kg of potassium. For a child weighing 10 kg, this would mean the maintenance IV fluid should contain 25 mEq/L sodium and 20 mEq/L potassium, implying the use of hypotonic IV fluid for maintenance therapy.

However, recent American (2018), Canadian (2018), NICE (2020), and European clinical guidelines no longer recommend determining the electrolyte content of maintenance IV fluids in children based solely on weight [18, 49–51]. Instead, they emphasize the selection based on the appropriate tonicity of the maintenance IV fluid. As a result, the traditional weight-based method of calculating the electrolyte content of the maintenance IV fluid in children is now viewed as harmful and is discouraged.

3. Modifying factors for water requirements

Water requirements in children can vary widely depending on several factors, as summarized in Table 48.3.

C. Prescribing maintenance IV fluid

Several factors, such as the composition of the fluid (tonicity, dextrose, and potassium content), volume, and infusion rate, need to be considered when prescribing maintenance intravenous fluids. It's crucial to assess a child's hydration status and to check serum electrolytes, glucose, and kidney function before initiating IV fluid treatment. Monitoring these parameters during therapy is also essential.

1. Use of hypotonic maintenance fluids is outdated and harmful

For over six decades, hypotonic solution was used as a standard maintenance IV fluid for hospitalized children worldwide [52]. The selection of hypotonic multi-electrolyte solutions such as Isolyte-P was based on the fluid and electrolyte requirement in healthy children at rest [53].

Moritz and Ayus, in their 2003 review, highlighted the risks of administering hypotonic fluids to children [54]. Consequently, the use of such fluids for maintenance therapy has come under scrutiny. Over the last two decades, numerous studies and literature have clearly shown a potential risk of severe hyponatremia and associated fatal complications, leading to significant morbidity and mortality in children receiving hypotonic maintenance fluids, especially among postoperative children [51, 55–68].

The harmful effects of hypotonic maintenance fluids prompted a patient safety alert from the National Health Service, advocating the removal of 0.18% saline from general-use areas for children, like emergency departments and pediatric wards [69].

The current recommendations advise against using hypotonic maintenance fluids as IV solutions for hospitalized children, as corroborated by various literature [70–72] and recent guidelines [18, 49–51].

Based on this evidence, the routine use of hypotonic fluids for intravenous maintenance fluid therapy in hospitalized children should be avoided, and the use of such low sodium-containing fluids should be limited to specific scenarios, such as hypernatremia with the free-water deficit or a renal-concentrating defect with ongoing urinary free-water losses, where extra free water is needed [73, 74].

2. Physiological basis of shift from hypotonic to isotonic maintenance fluids

While using hypotonic maintenance fluid may be appropriate for healthy children, it's often not suitable for hospitalized ones.

Two primary causes for the development of hyponatremia in hospitalized children are the administration of hypotonic fluid, which contains electrolyte-free water, and water retention resulting from elevated antidiuretic hormone (ADH) levels.

Hospitalized children are more prone to nonosmotic stimuli for ADH production because of factors like pain, nausea, anxiety, stress, postoperative conditions, and hypovolemia. Administering hypotonic maintenance fluid to hospitalized children with elevated ADH activity can impair the excretion of electrolyte-free water, leading to water retention, iatrogenic hyponatremia, and related neurological complications [70, 75, 76]. Based on this physiological understanding, combined with the above evidence of the harmful effects of hypotonic maintenance fluids, current recommendations have shifted from using hypotonic solutions to favoring isotonic solutions as the preferred maintenance fluid.

3. Current guidelines recommends isotonic maintenance fluids

Isotonic maintenance fluids such as normal saline, Ringer's lactate, or PlasmaLyte are associated with a lower risk of hyponatremia in hospitalized children compared to hypotonic fluids, as demonstrated in several studies [64, 77–80] and systematic reviews and meta-analyses [57, 63, 67, 72, 81–84]. While concerns and fears exist about potential hypernatremia, congestive heart failure, or pulmonary edema when using isotonic fluids as maintenance IV fluids [85–87], these risks seem to be largely theoretical unless the child has an impaired ability to excrete sodium [51, 72]. According to the recent AAP practice guideline (2018) as well as systematic reviews and meta-analyses by Hasim et al. (2021) and Amer et al. (2023), there is no identified risk of hypernatremia associated with the use of isotonic maintenance fluids in children [49, 67, 84].

Since isotonic fluids are demonstrated to be beneficial and safe [74], they are recommended by all guidelines as the preferred maintenance IV fluid for hospitalized children [18, 24, 49–51, 88].

4. Commercial vs. custom-made solutions

While custom-made solutions offer the flexibility to tailor the fluid composition to an individual child's specific medical needs, they may require more time and expertise to prepare; therefore, readily available and cost-effective commercial solutions are usually preferred. Other benefits of ready-to-use solutions include

a lower risk of reconstitution errors, stability problems, and microbiological contaminations [50].

5. Choosing appropriate isotonic maintenance fluids

The American guidelines (2018) [49], Canadian guidelines (2018) [51], and NICE guidelines (2020) [18], all recommend isotonic crystalloids as maintenance IV fluids for hospitalized children, but none of these guidelines specify whether to choose normal saline or balanced crystalloids. Recent European guidelines (ESPNIC 2022) recommend the use of isotonic balanced solutions for maintenance fluid therapy in acutely and critically ill children, as these solutions have shown a slight reduction in hospital stay length [50]. The latest systematic review by Amer et al. (2023) also proposes the utilization of balanced isotonic fluid for maintenance fluid therapy, given its lower association with acute kidney injury risk compared to 0.9% saline [84]. The potential disadvantage of using normal saline is the risk of hyperchloremic metabolic acidosis due to excess chloride, which might decrease renal perfusion and induce acute kidney injury. Conversely, the advantage of using balanced solutions as maintenance fluids is their inclusion of buffers that deliver bicarbonate, helping in preventing acidosis. Nonetheless, avoiding solutions with lactate buffers, like Ringer's lactate, is suggested in children suffering from severe liver dysfunction [50].

6. Dextrose content in maintenance IV fluids

Isotonic fluids like normal saline, Ringer's lactate, or PlasmaLyte are the preferred maintenance intravenous fluids in children, but they lack dextrose. Therefore, including 5–10% dextrose in the IV maintenance fluid prescription is crucial to meet daily energy needs and prevent conditions such as hypoglycemia, starvation, ketoacidosis, and protein degradation in children with limited glycogen stores [18, 49, 50].

Typically, older children are given a 5% dextrose concentration, while neonates, who have higher relative glucose requirements and are at greater risk of becoming hypoglycemic, often receive a 10% dextrose solution. The practice of providing a blanket prescription of 5% or 10% dextrose can lead to hyperglycemia in some cases [18]. The usual practice is to initially use dextrose 5% and increase it to 10% for children who develop hypoglycemia or for those requiring additional calories during extended IV therapy.

Blood glucose levels should be monitored initially upon starting IV fluid therapy, at least daily thereafter, and more frequently if there's an increased risk of hypoglycemia or hyperglycemia. The aim is to supply a sufficient amount of dextrose to prevent hypoglycemia while avoiding excess glucose that may cause hyperglycemia in critically ill children [50].

Although dextrose does impact the osmolarity of IV fluids, it is metabolized quickly when administered intravenously, so the dextrose component does not influence the tonicity of the intravenous fluids [49].

7. Potassium content in maintenance IV fluids

Traditionally, the Holliday-Segar formula recommends hypotonic intravenous maintenance fluid therapy containing 20 mEq/L of potassium.

Recent American guidelines (2018) and European guidelines (2022) recommend adding an appropriate amount of potassium to isotonic maintenance fluids and regularly monitoring potassium levels to avoid hypokalemia [49, 50]. However, current guidelines do not specify the amount of potassium supplement needed in maintenance fluids [18, 49–51].

In a recent randomized clinical trial by Lehtiranta et al. (2020), the incidence of hypokalemia was 19% among children receiving isotonic fluid therapy [89]. Consequently, the study recommends routinely adding potassium to commercially available isotonic maintenance fluids in acutely ill children, even in the absence of hypokalemia at admission.

For children with normal serum potassium levels and renal function, 10–20 mEq/L potassium should be added to isotonic maintenance fluids based on the child's clinical status. The standard concentration for most commercially available fluids is 20 mmol/L of potassium chloride.

Routine magnesium, calcium, and phosphate addition in intravenous maintenance fluid is not recommended for acutely and critically ill children [50].

8. Exceptions to standard recommendations

American guidelines exclude children with conditions such as neurosurgical disorders, congenital or acquired cardiac disease, hepatic disease, cancer, renal dysfunction, diabetes insipidus, severe watery diarrhea, or severe burns from the standard recommendations for maintenance fluids [49].

D. Rate of maintenance fluids - controversy

Current guidelines do not recommend an optimal rate of maintenance fluid therapy in children [18, 49, 50]. The rate of maintenance IV fluids should be individualized based on the child's specific needs, hydration status, and ongoing frequent assessments.

Careful monitoring of weight, urine output, and electrolyte levels is essential for identifying overhydration, underhydration, hyponatremia, or hypernatremia, allowing timely and proper adjustments to the fluid infusion rate. In hypovolemic children, the rate of fluid therapy needs to be increased, while in cases of volume overload, the rate should be decreased.

E. Avoid fluid overload

Fluid administered as a maintenance fluid is an important cause of volume overload, which is a modifiable contributor of non-resuscitation fluid [90–94]. Fluid creep, defined as the unintended excess administration of intravenous fluids to keep venous access lines open and fluids given with medications and IV flushes, also significantly contributes to volume overload [95].

It is important to pay attention to fluid overload because it is common and is associated with poor clinical outcomes such as prolonged need for mechanical ventilation [96, 97], acute kidney injury [98], and higher mortality rates [48, 94, 99].

Fluid-restrictive strategies focusing on preventing fluid overload due to maintenance fluids include:

- The most recent ESPNIC guideline from 2022 advises the use of a restrictive intravenous fluid volume approach, in contrast to the traditional Holliday-Segar method, which tends to overestimate fluid needs in acutely ill children [50].

In critically ill children likely to secrete excess ADH, reducing the maintenance fluid volume to 65–80% or two-thirds of the amount suggested by the Holliday and Segar formula can help avoid water overload and hyponatremia [50, 100].

Postoperative children with acute central nervous system conditions like head injuries, meningitis, or pulmonary issues such as pneumonia and who are on mechanical ventilation are particularly susceptible to increased endogenous ADH secretion [100].

- Consider all sources of fluid, including IV medications, line flushes, maintaining vein patency, administering blood products, and enteral intake, when calculating daily fluid requirements and preparing a fluid prescription [50]. This meticulous calculation will prevent fluid creep, limit fluid intake, and ensures an accurate fluid prescription which avoids fluid overload.

- In edematous children, due to conditions such as heart failure, renal failure, or hepatic failure, consider limiting the volume of maintenance fluid therapy to 50–60% of the amount recommended by the Holliday and Segar formula to minimize the risk of volume overload [18, 50].

- It's crucial to recognize that once children reach adult size, the upper limit for daily maintenance fluid is 2500 ml per day for males and 2000 ml per day for females [18].

MAINTENANCE FLUID FOR NEONATES

The fluid and electrolyte requirements of neonates are unique, and it's important to individualize them based on factors such as birth weight, gestational age, and corrected age when planning their fluid therapy. The goal of maintenance fluid therapy is to keep an infant in a neutral water balance while also providing the water necessary for growth and maintaining electrolyte balance.

A. Physiological considerations

Managing fluids in preterm neonates is particularly challenging due to physiological factors such as increased insensible water loss, reduced renal function, and low weight at birth. The principles of maintenance fluid therapy differ between neonates and older children due to various factors such as:

1. **Excess of total body water:** The distribution of total body water (TBW) changes with the fetus's gestational age, constituting 90% of body weight in extremely preterm neonates and decreasing to 75% in term neonates. After birth, this extra water must be mobilized and excreted, which explains why fluid requirements are lower on the first day of life and increase incrementally on subsequent days.

2. **Increased insensible water loss:** Due to their higher body-surface-area-to-body-weight ratio, small-sized neonates with a relatively large surface area experience greater insensible water loss. The maturity of a neonate's skin is an important factor influencing insensible water loss; preterm babies experience a greater loss due to their immature epithelial layer, which results in thinner and more permeable skin. Additionally, insensible water loss in neonates increases due to extra-renal factors such as elevated body and environmental temperatures, particularly when they are placed under open radiant warmers instead of incubators or are undergoing phototherapy.

3. **Functional immaturity of the neonatal kidney:** As renal function matures with increasing gestational age, the neonatal kidney's impaired capacity at birth makes it less efficient at excreting acute sodium or water loads compared to the kidneys of infants or older children. In neonates, urine output is low on day 1, characterized by oliguria. On days 2 to 3, postnatal diuresis occurs, leading to an increase in urine output accompanied by sodium loss. On days 4 to 5, urine output varies depending on fluid intake.

B. Prescribing maintenance fluids

When planning fluid prescriptions in neonates, it's important to pay attention to the rate of infusion, tonicity, as well as the content of dextrose, potassium, and calcium.

1. Rate of infusion: Administering maintenance fluid at appropriate rates is crucial for ensuring adequate hydration while preventing fluid overload, which can result in significant morbidity [101]. To avoid harmful fluid overload, it is important to administer maintenance fluid in neonates carefully, based on a proper understanding of the complexity of their fluid dynamics [102]. It's important to note that fluid requirements are lower on the first day of life and increase incrementally on each subsequent day.

According to updated NICE guidelines (2020), the recommended IV fluid maintenance rates for term neonates are as follows [18]:

• **First 24 hours of life:** During the initial period when urine output is low on day 1, a conservative IV fluid rate of 50 to 60 mL/kg/day is recommended to accommodate the neonate's limited physiological capacity for handling larger fluid volumes, to facilitate the mobilization and excretion of extra water after birth, and to achieve gradual expected physiologic weight loss.

- **Day 2 to 4:** Fluid rates increase by approximately 20 mL/kg/day after day 1. On day 2, the rate rises to 70 to 80 mL/kg/day. By day 3, the rate further escalates to 80 to 100 mL/kg/day, and on day 4, it reaches 100 to 120 mL/kg/day.

- **Day 5:** The fluid requirement stabilizes during this period, and a rate of 120 to 150 mL/kg/day is recommended.

The rate of administration for maintenance fluids in neonates should be closely monitored and adjusted based on the patient's response to therapy, taking into account clinical parameters such as changes in body weight and urine output, as well as laboratory parameters like serum sodium concentration [103]. In a neonate, if there is a weight loss of >5% or a serum sodium level exceeding 150 mEq/L, even without isotonic fluid administration, it is necessary to increase the fluid infusion rate. The use of 500 ml or smaller volume bags is recommended for administering IV fluids to neonates.

2. Tonicity of fluid: It's crucial to understand the basic principles of selecting the appropriate tonicity for IV maintenance fluid therapy in neonates and to modify the initial prescription at different stages based on physiological considerations.

3. Selection of solution based on tonicity: Although isotonic fluids are preferred and recommended over hypotonic fluids for maintenance therapy in children, recent guidelines from America (2018), Canada (2018), and Europe (2022) either exclude neonates or do not provide specific recommendations for them [49–51]. No guidelines recommend a particular sodium concentration for maintenance fluids from the second to the seventh day of life for neonates.

The use of isotonic fluids for maintenance therapy in neonates significantly increases the risk of hypernatremia, as demonstrated by recent randomized clinical trials [104, 105] and the latest systematic review and meta-analysis [84]. The NICE guidelines suggest that a sodium content of 131 to 154 mEq/L for maintenance therapy might be too high for term neonates in their initial days of life. Consequently, the 2020 revised NICE guidelines recommendations emphasize the use of professional judgment to minimize the incorrect use of isotonic crystalloids in very young neonates, especially during the first 7 days [18]. Additionally, hypotonic fluids are found to be unsafe due to the risk of hyponatremia [104, 106].

Given the adverse effects of both isotonic and hypotonic fluids, it is wise to closely monitor serum sodium levels and adjust the sodium concentration in maintenance fluid prescriptions for individual neonates instead of adhering to a one-size-fits-all approach.

4. Planning sodium concentration of initial prescription

- **Day 1:** For term neonates, it is advisable to administer no or minimal sodium on day 1. This accommodates the newborn's limited physiological capacity to excrete sodium and aims to prevent hypernatremia during the crucial postnatal adaptation phase until postnatal diuresis and weight loss occur [18].

- **Day 2 to 7:** Alongside 10% dextrose, sodium should be added in an appropriate concentration to maintain sodium levels within the normal range. A reasonable approach may be to provide 0.45% or 0.225% saline with 10% dextrose initially, and the sodium concentration in the prescription should be adjusted subsequently based on serum sodium levels.

- **After day 7:** For term neonates who are 8 days old or older and require maintenance IV fluids, initiation should begin with isotonic crystalloids containing sodium levels ranging from 131–154 mEq/L and 5–10% dextrose [18].

In addition to these general guidelines, close monitoring of serum sodium levels throughout all stages is essential, and the sodium concentration in maintenance fluid should be adjusted as needed.

5. Dextrose content of fluids: Dextrose 10%, with or without additional sodium chloride, is commonly used as a maintenance fluid in neonates, as opposed to the dextrose 5% typically used in older children. This higher concentration is preferred for neonates due to their higher requirements, limited glycogen stores, and increased risk of hypoglycemia. The recommended rate for dextrose infusion in neonates is about 4–6 mg/kg/min.

6. Potassium content of fluids: Neonates usually require no potassium supplementation for the first two days of maintenance fluid therapy. Subsequently, the addition of 2–3 mEq/kg/day of potassium chloride to the infusate should be considered, provided there is good urine output and normal renal function.

Hypocalcemia is common in newborns, and neonates may require calcium gluconate supplementation if their total serum calcium level falls below 6.5 mg/dL or if their ionized calcium level is less than 0.8–0.9 mmol/L.

PRESCRIPTION SUMMARY OF MAINTENANCE FLUID THERAPY

- The commonly used method for calculating maintenance water requirements in children is the Holliday-Segar formula, which uses either the 100/50/20 rule for daily fluid volume or the 4/2/1 rule for hourly fluid volume. In critically ill children, it's advised to limit the fluid volume to two-thirds of the amount suggested by the Holliday-Segar formula to prevent water overload and hyponatremia.

- For hospitalized children, current recommendations advocate the use of isotonic solutions like normal saline, Ringer's lactate, or PlasmaLyte; the traditional use of hypotonic fluids for maintenance IV fluid is now considered harmful and obsolete, and such fluids should be removed from general-use areas for children. Since isotonic solutions are dextrose-free, it's important to include 5% dextrose in maintenance IV fluids for older children to provide calories and prevent starvation ketoacidosis. An appropriate amount of potassium chloride should be added to isotonic maintenance fluids to avoid hypokalemia.

- Most guidelines do not specify a preference between normal saline and balanced crystalloids. However, current European guidelines recommend using isotonic balanced solutions for maintenance fluid therapy in acutely and critically ill children.

- In children with hypernatremia (serum sodium >145 mEq/L), D5W with 0.45% NaCl and close monitoring of serum sodium levels are recommended.

- In neonates, fluid requirements are initially lower on the first day of life and increase in the subsequent days. Maintenance fluid therapy typically begins with dextrose 10%, with sodium being added after 24-48 hours. The use of isotonic fluids for maintenance is not recommended in the first days of life due to the significant risk of hypernatremia in neonates.

The effective monitoring of resuscitation and maintenance fluid administration is crucial in pediatric care, involving adjustments according to clinical status, urine volume, and laboratory parameters.

REFERENCES

1. National Clinical Guideline Centre. IV Fluids in Children: Intravenous Fluid Therapy in Children and Young People in Hospital. Quality standard. London: National Institute for Health and Care Excellence (UK); 2016 Sep 21. Accessed 2023 Aug 22. Available from: https://www.nice.org.uk/guidance/qs131.

2. Lewis SR, Pritchard MW, Evans DJ, et al. Colloids versus crystalloids for fluid resuscitation in critically ill people. Cochrane Database Syst Rev. 2018;8(8):CD000567.

3. Weiss SL, Peters MJ, Alhazzani W, et al. Executive Summary: Surviving Sepsis Campaign International Guidelines for the Management of Septic Shock and Sepsis-Associated Organ Dysfunction in Children. Pediatr Crit Care Med 2020;21(2):e52–e106.

4. Van de Voorde P, Turner NM, Djakow J, et al. European Resuscitation Councils Guidelines 2021: Paediatric Life Support. Resuscitation. 2021;161:327–387.

5. Skellett S, Maconochie I, Bingham B, et al. Paediatric advanced life support Guidelines. Resuscitation Council UK. Published May 2021. Visit: https://www.resus.org.uk/library/2021-resuscitation-guidelines/paediatric-advanced-life-support-guidelines.

6. Myburgh J, Cooper DJ, Finfer S, et al. Saline or albumin for fluid resuscitation in patients with traumatic brain injury. NEJM 2007;357(9):874–884.

7. Brackney C, Diaz L, Milbrandt E, et al. Is albumin use SAFE in patients with traumatic brain injury? Crit Care 2010;14(2):307.

8. Cooper DJ, Myburgh J, Heritier S, et al. Albumin resuscitation for traumatic brain injury: is intracranial hypertension the cause of increased mortality? J Neurotrauma 2013;30(7):512–518.

9. Rossi S, Picetti E, Zoerle T, et al. Fluid management in acute brain injury. Curr Neurol Neurosci Rep 2018;18(11):74.

10. SAFE Study Investigators, Finfer S, McEvoy S, et al. Impact of albumin compared to saline on organ function and mortality of patients with severe sepsis. Intensive Care Med. 2011;37(1):86–96.

11. Caironi P, Tognoni G, Masson S, et al. Albumin replacement in patients with severe sepsis or septic shock. N Engl J Med. 2014;370(15):1412–1421.

12. Charpentier J, Mira JP. Efficacy and tolerance of hyperoncotic albumin administration in septic shock patients: the EARSS study. Intensive Care Med. 2011;37(Suppl 1):S115–S0438.

13. Xu JY, Chen QH, Xie JF, et al. Comparison of the effects of albumin and crystalloid on mortality in adult patients with severe sepsis and septic shock: A meta-analysis of randomized clinical trials. Crit. Care 2014;18(6):702.

14. Perner A, Haase N, Guttormsen AB, et al. Hydroxyethyl starch 130/0.42 versus ringer's acetate in severe sepsis. N Engl J Med 2012;367(2):124–134.

15. Myburgh JA, Finfer S, Bellomo R, et al. Hydroxyethyl starch or saline for fluid resuscitation in intensive care. N Engl J Med 2012;367(20):1901–1911.

16. Zarychanski R, Abou-Setta AM, Turgeon AF, et al. Association of hydroxyethyl starch administration with mortality and acute kidney injury in critically ill patients requiring volume resuscitation: a systematic review and meta-analysis. JAMA. 2013;309(7):678–88.

17. EMA. PRAC confirms that hydroxyethyl-starch solutions (HES) should no longer be used in patients with sepsis or burn injuries or in critically ill patients. 11 October 2018. https://www.ema.europa.eu/en/news/prac-confirms-hydroxyethyl-starch-solutions-hes-should-no-longer-be-used-patients-sepsis-burn.

18. National Institute for Health and Care Excellence. Intravenous fluid therapy in children and young people in hospital. NICE guideline. Published: December 9, 2015. Last updated: June 11, 2020. Available from: www.nice.org.uk/guidance/ng29.

19. Upadhyay M, Singhi S, Murlidharan J, et al. Randomized evaluation of fluid resuscitation with crystalloid (saline) and colloid (polymer from degraded gelatin in saline) in pediatric septic shock. Indian Pediatr 2005;42(3):223–231.

20. Thomas-Rueddel DO, Vlasakov V, Reinhart K, et al. Safety of gelatin for volume resuscitation–a systematic review and meta-analysis. Intensive Care Med. 2012;38(7):1134–42.

21. Moeller C, Fleischmann C, Thomas-Rueddel D, et al. How safe is gelatin? A systematic review and meta-analysis of gelatin-containing plasma expanders vs crystalloids and albumin. J Crit Care 2016;35:75–83.

22. Farooque S, Kenny M, Marshall SD. Anaphylaxis to intravenous gelatin based solutions: a case series examining clinical features and severity. Anaesth. 2019;74(2):174–9.

23. World Health Organization. Pocket book of hospital care for children. 2nd ed. Guidelines for the management of common childhood illnesses. WHO, 2013.

24. Leung LCK, So LY, Ng YK, et al. Initial intravenous fluid prescription in general paediatric in-patients aged >28 days and <18 years: consensus statements. Hong Kong Med J. 2021;27(4):276–286.

25. Yunos NM, Bellomo R, Story D, et al. Bench-to-bedside review: chloride in critical illness. Crit Care. 2010;14(4):226.

26. Moritz ML, Ayus JC. 0.9% saline and balance crystalloids in acute ill patients: Trading one problem for another. Journal of Critical Care 2021;63:254–256.

27. Shin WJ, Kim YK, Bang JY, et al. Lactate and liver function tests after living donor right hepatectomy: a comparison of solutions with and without lactate. Acta Anaesthesiol Scand. 2011;55(5):558–64.

28. Weinberg L, Collins N, Van Mourik K, et al. PlasmaLyte 148: a clinical review. World J Crit Care Med 2016;5(4):235–250.

29. Anantasit N, Thasanthiah S, Lertbunrian R. Balanced salt solution versus normal saline solution as initial fluid re- suscitation in pediatric septic shock: A randomized, double-blind controlled trial. Crit Care Shock 2020;23(4):158–168.

30. Hoorn EJ. Intravenous fluids: balancing solutions. J Nephrol 2017;30(4):485–492.

31. Barhight MF, Lusk J, Brinton J, et al. Hyperchloremia is independently associated with mortality in critically ill children who ultimately require continuous renal replacement therapy. Pediatr Nephrol 2018;33(6):1079–1085.

32. Stenson EK, Cvijanovich NZ, Anas N, et al. Hyperchloremia Is Associated With Complicated Course and Mortality in Pediatric Patients With Septic Shock. Pediatr Crit Care Med 2018;19(2):155–160.

33. Ginter D, Gilfoyle E, Wade A, et al. Hyperchloremia and association with acute kidney injury in critically ill children. Pediatr Nephrol. 2023;38(7):2233–2242.

34. Emrath ET, Fortenberry JD, Travers C, et al. Resuscitation With Balanced Fluids Is Associated With Improved Survival in Pediatric Severe Sepsis. Crit Care Med 2017;45(7):1177–1183.

35. Semler MW, Self WH, Wanderer JP, et al. Balanced crystalloids versus saline in critically ill adults. N Engl J Med 2018;378(9):829–839.

36. Self WH, Semler MW, Wanderer JP, et al. Balanced crystalloids versus saline in noncritically ill adults. N Engl J Med 2018;378:819–828.

37. Lehr AR, Rached-d'Astous S, Barrowman N, et al. Balanced Versus Unbalanced Fluid in Critically Ill Children: Systematic Review and Meta-Analysis. Pediatr Crit Care Med 2022;23(3):181–191.

38. Sankar J, Muralidharan J, Lalitha AV, et al. Multiple Electrolytes Solution Versus Saline as Bolus Fluid for Resuscitation in Pediatric Septic Shock: A Multicenter Randomized Clinical Trial. Crit Care Med 2023.

39. Kight BP, Waseem M. Pediatric Fluid Management. [Updated 2023 Jan 16]. In: StatPearls [Internet]. Treasure Island (FL): StatPearls Publishing; 2023 Jan.

Available from: https://www.ncbi.nlm.nih.gov/books/NBK560540/.

40. Chong SL, Ong GY, Venkataraman A, et al. The golden hours in paediatric septic shock--current updates and recommendations. Ann Acad Med Singap. 2014;43(5):267–74.

41. San Geroteo J, Levy M, Gotchac J, et al. Fluid bolus therapy in pediatric sepsis: a narrative review. Eur J Med Res. 2022;27(1):246.

42. Fernández-Sarmiento J, De Souza DC, Martinez A, et al. Latin American Consensus on the Management of Sepsis in Children: Sociedad Latinoamericana de Cuidados Intensivos Pediátricos [Latin American Pediatric Intensive Care Society] (SLACIP) Task Force: Executive Summary. J Intensive Care Med. 2022;37(6):753–763.

43. Maitland K, Kiguli S, Opoka RO, et al. Mortality after fluid bolus in African children with severe infection. N Engl J Med. 2011;364(26):2483–95.

44. 2022 exceptional surveillance on intravenous fluid therapy in children and young people (NICE guidelines NG29, NG51, NG143, CG84, CG102 and NG18). Surveillance report Published: 21 October 2022 www.nice.org.uk.

45. World Health Organization. Updated guideline: paediatic emergency triage, assessment and treatment. Geneva: WHO 2016.

46. Russotto V. Conservative fluid management: Turn off the tap after use? European Society of Intensive Care Medicine (ESICM) [Internet]. April 25, 2017. Available from: https://www.esicm.org/article-review-conservative-fluid-management-april-2017/.

47. Sinitsky L, Walls D, Nadel S, et al. Fluid overload at 48 hours is associated with respiratory morbidity but not mortality in a general PICU: retrospective cohort study. Pediatr Crit Care Med. 2015;16(3):205–209.

48. Alobaidi R, Morgan C, Basu RK, et al. Association between fluid balance and outcomes in critically ill children: a systematic review and meta-analysis. JAMA Pediatr. 2018;172(3):257–268.

49. Feld LG, Neuspiel DR, Foster BA, et al. Clinical practice guideline: maintenance intravenous fluids in children. Pediatrics 2018;142(6):e20183083.

50. Brossier DW, Tume LN, Briant AR, et al. ESPNIC clinical practice guidelines: intravenous maintenance fluid therapy in acute and critically ill children- a systematic review and meta-analysis. Intensive Care Med. 2022;48(12):1691–1708.

51. Friedman JN. Risk of acute hyponatremia in hospitalized children and youth receiving maintenance intravenous fluids. Canadian Paediatric Society. Posted: 2018 Dec 18. Last updated: May 5, 2021. [Accessed 2023 Aug 28]. Available from: https://cps.ca/en/documents/position/acute-hyponatremia-in-hospitalized-children-and-youth.

52. Saba TG, Fairbairn J, Houghton F, et al. A randomized controlled trial of isotonic versus hypotonic maintenance intravenous fluids in hospitalized children. BMC Pediatrics. 2011;11:82.

53. Holliday MA, Segar WE. The maintenance need for water in parenteral fluid therapy. Pediatrics 1957;19(5):823–32.

54. Moritz ML, Ayus JC. Prevention of hospital-acquired hyponatremia: A case for using isotonic saline. Pediatrics 2003;111(2):227–230.

55. Hoorn EJ, Geary D, Robb M, et al. Acute hyponatremia related to intravenous fluid administration in hospitalized children: An observational study. Pediatrics 2004;113(5):1279–84.

56. Moritz Ml, Ayus JC. Preventing neurological complications from dysnatremias in children. Pediatr Nephrol. 2005;20(12):1687–700.

57. Choong K, Kho ME, Menon K, et al. Hypotonic versus isotonic saline in hospitalised children: a systematic review. Arch Dis Child. 2006;91(10):828–35.

58. Beck CE. Hypotonic versus isotonic maintenance intravenous fluid therapy in hospitalized children: a systematic review. Clin Pediatr (Phila). 2007;46(9):764–70.

59. Koczmara C, Hyland S, Greenall J. Hospital-acquired acute hyponatremia and parenteral fluid administration in children. Can J Hosp Pharm. 2009;62(6):512–5.

60. Choong K, Arora S, Cheng J, et al. Hypotonic versus isotonic maintenance fluids after surgery for children: a randomized controlled trial. Pediatrics. 2011;128(5):857–66.

61. Rey C, Los-Arcos M, Hernández A, et al. Hypotonic versus isotonic maintenance fluids in critically ill children: a multicenter prospective randomized study. Acta Paediatr. 2011;100(8):1138–43.

62. Grissinger M. Hyponatremia and death in Healthy children From plain dextrose and Hypotonic Saline Solutions after Surgery. P T. 2013;38(7):364–88.

63. Foster BA, Tom D, Hill V. Hypotonic versus isotonic fluids in hospitalized children: a systematic review and meta-analysis. J Pediatr 2014;165(1):163–169.

64. Flores Robles CM, Cuello García CA. A prospective trial comparing isotonic with hypotonic maintenance fluids for prevention of hospital-acquired hyponatraemia. Paediatr Int Child Health. 2016;36(3):168–74.

65. McNab S. Intravenous maintenance fluid therapy in children. J Paediatr Child Health. 2016;52(2):137–40.

66. Torres SF, Iolster T, Schnitzler EJ, et al. Hypotonic and isotonic intravenous maintenance fluids in hospitalised paediatric patients: a randomised controlled trial. BMJ Paediatr Open. 2019;3(1):e000385.

67. Hasim N, Bakar MAA, Islam MA. Efficacy and Safety of Isotonic and Hypotonic Intravenous Maintenance Fluids in Hospitalised Children: A Systematic Review and Meta-Analysis of Randomised Controlled Trials. Children. 2021;8(9):785.

68. Ratnjeet K, Pallavi P, Jhamb U, et al. 0.45% Versus 0.9% Saline in 5% Dextrose as Maintenance Fluids in Children Admitted With Acute Illness: A Randomized Control Trial. Pediatr Emerg Care. 2022;38(9):436–441.

69. National Patient Safety Agency. Patient Safety Alert 22. Reducing the risk of hyponatraemia when administering intravenous infusions to children. 2007. https://www.sps.nhs.uk/wp-content/uploads/2018/02/2007-NRLS-0409-Hyponatraemia-cen-PSA-2007-03-28-v1.pdf.

70. Moritz ML, Ayus JC. Maintenance intravenous fluids in acutely ill patients. N Engl J Med. 2015;373(14):1350–1360.

71. Duke T. Maintenance intravenous fluids for children: enough evidence, now for translation and action. Paediatr Int Child Health 2016;36(3):165–7.

72. Padua AP, Macaraya JR, Dans LF, et al. Isotonic versus hypotonic saline solution for maintenance intravenous fluid therapy in children: a systematic review. PediatrNephrol 2015;30(7):1163–72.

73. Narsaria P, Lodha R. Isn't it time to stop using 0.18% saline in dextrose solutions for intravenous maintenance fluid therapy in children? Indian Pediatr. 2014;51(12):964–6.

74. Hall AM, Ayus JC, Moritz ML. Things We Do For No Reason: The Default Use of Hypotonic Maintenance Intravenous Fluids in Pediatrics. J Hosp Med. 2018;13(9):637–640.

75. Steele A, Gowrishankar M, Abrahamson S, et al. Postoperative hyponatremia despite near-isotonic saline infusion: A phenomenon of desalination. Ann. Intern. Med. 1997;126(1):20–25.

76. Skippen P, Adderley R, Bennett M, et al. Iatrogenic hyponatremia in hospitalized children: can it be avoided? Paediatr Child Health. 2008;13(6):502–506.

77. Kannan L, Lodha R, Vivekanandhan S, et al. Intravenous fluid regimen and hyponatraemia among children: a randomized controlled trial. Pediatr Nephrol 2010;25(11):2303–2309.

78. Neville KA, Sandeman DJ, Rubinstein A, et al. Prevention of Hyponatremia during Maintenance Intravenous Fluid Administration: A Prospective Randomized Study of Fluid Type versus Fluid Rate. J Pediatr 2010;156(2):313–319.e1–2.

79. McNab S, Duke T, South M, et al. 140 mmol/L of sodium versus 77 mmol/L of sodium in maintenance intravenous fluid therapy for children in hospital (PIMS): a randomised controlled double-blind trial. Lancet 2015;385(9974):1190–7.

80. Friedman JN, Beck CE, DeGroot J, et al. Comparison of isotonic and hypotonic intravenous maintenance fluids: A randomized clinical trial. JAMA Pediatr 2015;169(5):445–51.

81. McNab S, Ware RS, Neville KA, et al. Isotonic versus hypotonic solutions for maintenance intravenous fluid administration in children. Cochrane Database Syst Rev 2014;12:CD009457.

82. Wang J, Xu E, Xiao Y. Isotonic versus hypotonic maintenance IV fluids in hospitalized children: a meta-analysis. Pediatrics 2014;133(1):105–13.

83. Yang G, Jiang W, Wang X, et al. The efficacy of isotonic and hypotonic intravenous maintenance fluid for pediatric patients: A meta-analysis of randomized controlled trials. Pediatr Emerg Care 2015;31(2):122–6.

84. Amer BE, Abdelwahab OA, Abdelaziz A, et al. Efficacy and safety of isotonic versus hypotonic intravenous maintenance fluids in hospitalized children: an updated systematic review and meta-analysis of randomized controlled trials. Pediatr Nephrol. 2023.

85. Holliday MA. Isotonic saline expands extracellular fluid and is inappropriate for maintenance therapy. Pediatrics. 2005;115(1):193–194.

86. Holliday MA, Ray PE, Friedman AL. Fluid therapy for children: facts, fashions and questions. Arch Dis Child. 2007;92(6):546–550.

87. Kannan L, Lodha R. Appropriate fluid for intravenous maintenance therapy in hospitalized children--current status. Indian J Pediatr. 2011;78(3):357–9.

88. World Health Organization. Hospital Care for Children: Guidelines for the Management of Common Illnesses with Limited Resources, 2nd edn. Geneva:WHO. Available from: http://www.who.int/maternal_child_adolescent/documents/child_hospital_care/en/2013.

89. Lehtiranta S, Honkila M, Kallio M, et al. Risk of Electrolyte Disorders in Acutely Ill Children Receiving Commercially Available Plasmalike Isotonic Fluids: A Randomized Clinical Trial. JAMA Pediatr 2021;175(1):28–35.

90. Van Regenmortel N, Verbrugghe W, Roelant E, et al. Maintenance fluid therapy and fluid creep impose more significant fluid, sodium, and chloride burdens than resuscitation fluids in critically ill patients: a retrospective study in a tertiary mixed ICU population. Intensive Care Med. 2018;44(4):409–417.

91. Lindén-Søndersø A, Jungner M, Spångfors M, et al. Survey of non-resuscitation fluids administered during septic shock: a multicenter prospective observational study. Ann Intensive Care. 2019;9(1):132.

92. Maes T, Meuwissen A, Diltoer M, et al. Impact of maintenance, resuscitation and unintended fluid therapy on global fluid load after elective coronary artery bypass surgery. J Crit Care. 2019;49:129–135.

93. Al-Lawati ZH, Sur M, Kennedy CE, et al. Profile of Fluid Exposure and Recognition of Fluid Overload in Critically Ill Children. Pediatr Crit Care Med. 2020;21(8):760–766.

94. Barhight MF, Nelson D, Chong G, et al. Non-resuscitation fluid in excess of hydration requirements is associated with higher mortality in critically ill children. Pediatr Res. 2022;91(1):235–240.

95. Bulfon AF, Alomani HL, Anton N, et al. Intravenous Fluid Prescription Practices in Critically Ill Children: A Shift in Focus from Natremia to Chloremia? J Pediatr Intensive Care. 2019;8(4):218–225.

96. Ingelse SA, Wiegers HM, Calis JC, et al. Early Fluid Overload Prolongs Mechanical Ventilation in Children With Viral-Lower Respiratory Tract Disease. Pediatr Crit Care Med. 2017;18(3):e106–e111.

97. Kong X, Zhu Y, Zhu X. Association between early fluid overload and mortality in critically-ill mechanically ventilated children: a single-center retrospective cohort study. BMC Pediatr. 2021;21(1):474.

98. Naveda Romero OE, Naveda Meléndez AF. Fluid overload and kidney failure in children with severe sepsis and septic shock: A cohort study. Arch Argent Pediatr. 2017;115(2):118–124.

99. Raina R, Sethi SK, Wadhwani N, et al. Fluid Overload in Critically Ill Children. Front Pediatr. 2018;6:306.

100. The Royal Children's Hospital Melbourne. IV fluids - for children beyond the newborn period. Clinical Practice Guidelines. Updated October 2020. Accessed September 1, 2023. Available from: https://www.rch.org.au/clinicalguide/guideline_index/intravenous_fluids/.

101. Segar JL. A physiological approach to fluid and electrolyte management of the preterm infant: Review. J Neonatal Perinatal Med. 2020;13(1):11–19.

102. Rutledge A, Murphy HJ, Harer MW, et al. Fluid Balance in the Critically Ill Child Section: "How Bad Is Fluid in Neonates?" Front Pediatr. 2021;9:651458.

103. Lindower JB. Water balance in the fetus and neonate. Semin Fetal Neonatal Med 2017;22(2):71–75.

104. Balasubramanian K, Kumar P, Saini SS, et al. Isotonic versus hypotonic fluid supplementation in term neonates with severe hyperbilirubinemia - a double-blind, randomized, controlled trial. Acta Paediatr. 2012;101(3):236–41.

105. Dathan K, Sundaram M. Comparison of isotonic versus hypotonic intravenous fluid for maintenance fluid therapy in neonates more than or equal to 34 weeks of gestational age - a randomized clinical trial. J Matern Fetal Neonatal Med. 2022;35(25):6338–6345.

106. Tuzun F, Akcura Y, Duman N, et al. Comparison of isotonic and hypotonic intravenous fluids in term newborns: is it time to quit hypotonic fluids. J Matern Fetal Neonatal Med. 2022;35(2):356–361.

Replacement Fluid Therapy and its Monitoring in Children

INTRODUCTION

Replacement fluid therapy represents the third crucial pillar in comprehensive fluid management for children, complementing fluid resuscitation and maintenance strategies. IV fluids replacement aims to replenish preexisting deficits (fluids lost before treatment) and address ongoing losses, such as gastrointestinal issues due to vomiting and diarrhea, by administering the appropriate solutions to correct fluid, electrolyte, and acid-base disorders.

The five crucial steps to planning optimal and effective replacement fluid therapy in children are as follows:

1. Severity assessment: Assess the severity of dehydration, which can be categorized as mild, moderate, or severe.

2. Laboratory assessment: Utilize laboratory tests to evaluate dehydration in children.

3. Establish the type of dehydration: Determine the type of dehydration based on sodium concentration, specifically identifying if it is hyponatremic, isonatremic, or hypernatremic. Plan treatment based on this differentiation.

4. Identifying the underlying cause: Identify the etiology of fluid loss, such as diarrhea, vomiting, diabetic ketoacidosis, etc., and individualize treatment based on it.

5. Monitoring: Close clinical assessments, periodic laboratory tests, strict measurement of urine volume, and maintaining a daily weight chart help to assess the child's

Table 49.1 Assessment of dehydration		
Ask	**Look**	**Feel**
Stool frequency/ consistency Vomiting frequency Thirst level Urine output	Sunken eyes Dry mouth and tongue Level of alertness Signs of lethargy or irritability Abnormal respiratory patterns	Anterior fontanelle and skin turgor Pulse, heart rate, temperature, and blood pressure Postural changes in blood pressure Peripheral perfusion, and capillary refill time

response to therapy, facilitating necessary adjustments based on their condition.

ASSESSMENT OF THE SEVERITY OF DEHYDRATION

The first step in replacement fluid management is to assess the severity of dehydration, which helps to decide both the urgency of intervention and the volume of fluid necessary for effective rehydration.

Determining the extent of dehydration involves three assessment steps: Asking specific questions, looking at visible signs, and physical examinations, as summarized in Table 49.1.

In the evaluation of dehydration, obtaining a detailed history is critical and immensely helpful as it provides information about the etiology of fluid loss, the severity and volume of fluid depletion, fluid intake, alertness to thirst in the child, and a decline in urine output. Ten standard criteria suggested for clinical assessment of dehydration include:

- General observation (general appearance, respiratory pattern).
- Vital signs (heart rate and radial pulse).
- Detailed physical examinations (examining eyes, tears, mucous membranes, skin elasticity, and capillary refill time).

Table 49.2 Degree of fluid deficit and clinical signs in dehydration				
Severity of dehydration	**Age**	**Weight loss**	**Fluid deficit**	**Clinical signs**
Mild dehydration	Older child	<3%	30 mL/kg	Thirst, mild oliguria, normal or slightly increased pulse, and no other detectable signs
	Infant	<5%	50 mL/kg	
Moderate dehydration	Older child	3–6%	60 mL/kg	Increased thirst, oliguria, irritability, restlessness, weakness, slightly sunken eyes and anterior fontanelle, reduced tear production, cool and pale skin, tachycardia, mild decrease in skin turgor, and delayed capillary refill (>1.5 seconds)
	Infant	6–10%	100 mL/ kg	
Severe dehydration	Older child	>6%	90 mL/kg	Marked tachycardia, low blood pressure, significantly sunken eyes and anterior fontanelle, loss of skin turgor, absence of tears, severe oliguria or anuria, restlessness coupled with apathy, pallor, cold and clammy skin, very delayed capillary refill (>3 seconds), weak or non-palpable radial pulse, circulatory collapse, drowsiness, coma, hyperpyrexia, and cyanosis
	Infant	>10%	150 mL/ kg	

- Charting urine output [1].

Based on the clinical severity assessment, dehydration is categorized into mild, moderate, and severe degrees, which provide clinicians with reasonable estimates of the percentage and volume of fluid deficit, as summarized in Table 49.2.

Caution: Identifying the misleading signs during children's dehydration assessment is crucial. These signs include:

- Obese infants may be significantly dehydrated, yet the only noticeable sign might be tachycardia.

- The degree of dehydration in marasmic infants is often overestimated.

- With hypernatremic dehydration, skin, and circulatory changes might be deceptively inconspicuous, with predominant neurological signs.

- A raised blood urea level can indicate more severe dehydration than what is apparent from physical signs or may provide a clue to an underlying renal disease.

LABORATORY ASSESSMENT

Blood tests should not be performed routinely in assessing dehydration in children, especially for those who are stable with mild to moderate dehydration and when the etiology is apparent [2]. However, laboratory evaluations are recommended for children with severe dehydration who require intravenous therapy, exhibit signs of shock, are suspected of having electrolyte disturbances such as hyponatremia or hypernatremia, or have preexisting medical conditions predisposing them to electrolyte abnormalities.

If laboratory evaluations are necessary, the commonly performed laboratory tests include the following:

Serum blood urea nitrogen (BUN) and creatinine concentrations: A disproportionate increase in the BUN, with little or no change in the creatinine concentration, indicates moderate dehydration. However, a BUN may also be disproportionately increased in a child with a gastrointestinal bleed or receiving glucocorticoids. High values of both BUN and creatinine suggest renal insufficiency.

Serum electrolytes: Measuring levels of sodium, potassium, and chloride is useful for the establishment of diagnoses of electrolyte disorders, which assists in planning specific treatment regimens. The measurement of serum sodium is essential in detecting hyponatremia (<130 mEq/L) and hypernatremia (>150 mEq/L), which are common in dehydration. Evaluating serum potassium levels is crucial in identifying hypokalemia, the most common electrolyte abnormality in children, frequently caused by diarrheal losses and vomiting [3].

Serum bicarbonate, pH, and anion gap: Evaluating serum bicarbonate levels is crucial in determining the severity of dehydration. These levels directly correlate with the extent of dehydration, with lower venous bicarbonate levels indicating a greater degree of dehydration [4].

Metabolic acidosis, evidenced by low bicarbonate levels, may arise from diarrhea, secondary renal insufficiency, or lactic acidosis from shock. Calculating the anion gap assists in narrowing down the diagnosis of various causes of metabolic acidosis. Conversely, metabolic alkalosis, marked by high bicarbonate levels, can result from losing gastric fluid through vomiting or nasogastric aspiration.

Blood glucose: This is not a specific investigation for dehydration, but it can be low due to poor intake or extremely high in cases of diabetic ketoacidosis.

Hemoglobin and hematocrit levels: Elevated levels can be a sign of hemoconcentration, which occurs in dehydration. However, in anemic children, acute dehydration can temporarily elevate the hemoglobin concentration to normal levels, which may be misleading.

Urine specific gravity: A high urine specific gravity can indicate concentrated urine, a common sign of dehydration.

Amongst all these tests, the pH and HCO_3, creatinine, and urine density demonstrate a significant relationship with the actual degree of dehydration [5].

THE TYPE OF DEHYDRATION AND TREATMENT BASED ON IT

Depending on the proportion of salt and water loss, and the resultant sodium concentration, dehydration can be classified into three types: hyponatremic, isonatremic, or hypernatremic dehydration. In children with dehydration, isonatremic dehydration is the most

Table 49.3 Types of dehydration			
Dehydration	**Isonatremic**	**Hyponatremic**	**Hypernatremic**
Incidence [3]	58–61%	31–35%	7%
Serum sodium level	135–145 mEq/L	<135 mEq/L	>145 mEq/L
Plasma osmolality	Normal	Low	High
Types of fluid loss	Proportional loss of water and sodium	Excess sodium loss compared to water, combined with hypotonic fluid intake	Greater loss of water compared to sodium
Mechanism of sodium fluctuation	N/A	Sodium dilution due to excessive intake of hypotonic fluids	Fluid depletion due to insufficient intake
ECF volume	Moderately decreased	Severely decreased	Decreased
ICF volume	Maintained	Normal or increased	Decreased
Common etiologies	Diarrhea or vomiting	Diarrhea, vomiting, or excessive perspiration with hypotonic fluid intake	Excessive salt or solute intake coupled with inadequate water consumption
History of thirst	Normal	Normal	Excessive
Skin temperature	Cold	Cold	Cold or hot
Skin turgor	Poor	Extremely poor	Unaffected
Skin feel	Dry	Clammy	Doughy
Mucous membrane	Dry	Slightly moist	Parched
CNS status	Lethargic	Drowsy or comatose	Hyperirritability
Pulse rate	Rapid, weak	Very rapid and thready	Moderately rapid
Blood pressure level	Low	Very low or shock	Moderately low
Initial selection of IV fluids	0.9% NaCl or Ringer's lactate	0.9% NaCl or hypertonic NaCl	Hypotonic fluid. If shock, 0.9% NaCl or RL

common (58–61%), followed by hyponatremic dehydration (31–35%), with a small group presenting with hypernatremic dehydration (7%) [3, 6, 7]. The clinical presentations differ significantly among these three types of dehydration, and the amount and type of fluid to be replaced vary accordingly. Table 49.3 provides a differential diagnosis of dehydration.

Clinically, patients with hyponatremic dehydration are hemodynamically most unstable, while those with hypernatremic dehydration are least unstable. To administer the appropriate sodium concentration to children with dehydration with varying serum sodium levels, it is essential to remember the sodium concentration (measured in mEq/L) present in IV fluids, as outlined in Table 49.4.

Treatment plans according to types of dehydration

1. Isonatremic or isotonic dehydration
2. Hyponatremic or hypotonic dehydration
3. Hypernatremic or hypertonic dehydration

A child with severe dehydration, irrespective of sodium concentration, necessitates the administration of IV fluids, which is divided into three essential steps: resuscitation, addressing maintenance needs, and correcting both preexisting deficits and ongoing losses.

1. **Fluid resuscitation:** The first step in managing hemodynamically unstable or hypotensive children with dehydration is the prompt and adequate replenishment of fluids using a dextrose-free isotonic solution for resuscitation. This approach remains unchanged, regardless of the child's sodium status.

2. **Maintenance fluids:** This step aims to ensure that children receive adequate water and electrolytes through IV dextrose-containing isotonic solution, thereby compensating for the daily physiological losses.

The previous chapter comprehensively discusses strategies for resuscitation and maintenance fluid therapy in children.

3. **Replacement fluids:** After the initial fluid replacement for resuscitation, the subsequent step involves administering replacement fluids to correct preexisting deficits and address ongoing losses. The serum sodium concentration and the underlying cause of the fluid loss should guide the planning and design of the replacement fluid regimen.

Isonatremic or isotonic dehydration

Isonatremic or isotonic dehydration is characterized by a serum sodium concentration within the normal range of 135–145 mEq/L, maintaining the body fluids' normal tonicity at 275–290 mOsm/kg.

Pathophysiology: In this type of dehydration, the sodium concentration remains unaltered due to an equal

Table 49.4 Sodium concentration of IV fluids								
Type of fluid	0.9% NaCl	PlasmaLyte	RL	0.45% NaCl	0.33% NaCl	Isolyte P	3% NaCl	7.5% NaHCO₃
Sodium concentration	154 mEq/L	140 mEq/L	130 mEq/L	77 mEq/L	57 mEq/L	25 mEq/L	51 mEq/dL	22.5 mEq/ 25 ml amp.

proportionate loss of sodium and water, with the fluid deficit primarily occurring from extracellular space. There is no fluid shift between the intracellular fluid and the extracellular fluid or vice versa due to the normal serum osmolality.

Causes: Isonatremic dehydration is the most common type of dehydration in children, commonly resulting from gastrointestinal losses like vomiting, diarrhea, and diabetic ketoacidosis.

Treatment: For effective fluid replacement in isonatremic or isotonic dehydration, it is vital to consider the appropriate route, rate, type, and volume of the fluid to be administered.

Oral vs. IV fluid replacement: Oral fluid intake is the preferred method for fluid replacement and should be encouraged. Oral fluid replacement is usually adequate for mild to moderate hypovolemia or during the later stages of severe hypovolemia once the patient has stabilized. IV fluid replacement is necessary when rapid restoration of fluid is indicated, when the child cannot consume oral fluids, or if oral intake is contraindicated or insufficient to correct dehydration.

Selection of replacement fluid: The goal of fluid replacement is to correct dehydration and replace electrolytes without causing iatrogenic complications. The preferred fluids for rehydration therapy in isonatremic dehydration are isotonic solutions such as Ringer's lactate and normal saline.

Potassium is usually added to the IV fluids once the patient voids and normal renal function is documented unless there is a presence of significant hypokalemia.

While selecting the appropriate fluid for treatment, it is essential to consider the pH status. When isonatremic dehydration is accompanied by metabolic acidosis due to an underlying cause such as diarrhea, administering a balanced crystalloid like Ringer's lactate or PlasmaLyte is beneficial and effective, as it supplies a buffer and corrects acidosis. Conversely, when dehydration coexists with alkalosis due to an underlying cause such as vomiting, administering normal saline offers the advantage of correcting metabolic alkalosis.

Volume of replacement fluid: The volume of the replacement fluid to be administered for correcting dehydration is calculated based on the degree of dehydration. The fluid deficit for mild, moderate, and severe dehydration is about 3%, 6%, and 9% in children and less than 5%, 6–10%, and more than 10% in infants, respectively. To convert these percentages to a volume of fluid deficit, the approximate amounts are 30 mL/kg, 60 mL/kg, and 90 mL/kg for mild, moderate, and severe dehydration in children, and 50 mL/kg, 100 mL/kg, and 150 mL/kg for infants, respectively.

The calculated total fluid volume is divided into two portions: the initial volume administered for resuscitation until the patient stabilizes hemodynamically and the remaining volume scheduled for administration within the next 24 hours. The volume for subsequent administration is determined by subtracting the volume of fluid used during acute resuscitation from the total deficit fluid volume.

Rate of fluid replacement: The rate of fluid replacement to correct dehydration differs in the initial and subsequent phases. In children with hypovolemic shock, initial fluid therapy for resuscitation is administering frequent small-volume boluses of dextrose-free isotonic fluid at a rate of 10 mL/kg over less than 10 minutes to rapidly correct hypotension and ensure adequate hydration [8–10]. If hypotension persists after the initial bolus, fluid boluses should be repeated up to 40–60 mL/kg in ICU and 40 mL/kg in wards, with close monitoring [11].

Subsequent fluid to correct dehydration is administered at a calculated rate to ensure the total volume of the fluid deficit is infused within the first 24 hours [12]. The practice of replacing 50% of the deficit fluids over the first 8 hours, followed by the remaining 50% over the next 16 hours, can be clinically impractical and may carry the risk of too-rapid replacement if adjustments are not made on time [12].

Designing a fluid prescription: In children with isonatremic or hyponatremic dehydration, the complete fluid deficit is usually corrected over 24 hours; conversely, a slower correction is recommended for managing hypernatremic dehydration. The planning of fluid prescription, which considers the volume of resuscitation fluid, maintenance needs, existing fluid deficits, and ongoing losses, is summarized in Table 49.5.

Hyponatremic or hypotonic dehydration

Hyponatremic dehydration characterized by serum sodium <135 mEq/L occurs in about 31–35% of children with dehydration due to diarrhea [3, 6, 7]. This condition is less common than isonatremic dehydration but more common than hypernatremic dehydration.

Pathophysiology: Hyponatremic dehydration in children can occur due to a relatively greater loss of sodium compared to water or when fluid losses are replaced with hypotonic fluids. Hypovolemia due to fluid depletion stimulates the secretion of the antidiuretic hormone, which prevents the excretion of water by the kidney and thereby delays the correction of hyponatremia.

Causes: An excessive loss of sodium in watery stool, which is especially common in cases of cholera, can lead to hyponatremic dehydration. On average,

---

Table 49.5 Designing a fluid prescription in children
Step 1: Calculate total fluid requirements in 24 hours (maintenance + deficit + ongoing losses)
• Maintenance requirements: Determine the fluid volume based on body weight using the 100/50/20 rule. In critically ill children with high ADH, utilize 2/3 of the maintenance volume.
• Calculate the volume of fluid deficit: Depending on the degree of dehydration, loss of fluid volume is 30 mL/kg for mild, 60 mL/kg for moderate, and 90 mL/kg for severe dehydration, respectively.
Step 2: Determine the volume of deficit fluid to be administered after resuscitation.
• The initial volume for resuscitation is dictated by clinical response.
• Calculate the subsequent volume to be administered by subtracting the resuscitation volume from the sum of the maintenance and deficit volumes.
• Administer the calculated subsequent volume over 24 hours using 5% dextrose and isotonic balanced crystalloids or saline with 10–20 mEq/L potassium chloride to correct the remaining fluid deficit after resuscitation.
Step 3: Every 4 hours, assess and calculate ongoing fluid losses through careful history and evaluation, then administer additional fluids based on the losses noted in the previous 4-hour period. Assess, calculate and replace fluid more frequently if ongoing fluid losses are very rapid.
Step 4: Close monitoring and modifying fluid prescription as per need.

the sodium concentration in diarrhea is about 50 mEq/L, but in choleric stool, it can be very high, ranging from 90 to 140 mEq/L. Diuretic use is an additional cause of hyponatremic dehydration due to excessive loss of sodium.

Furthermore, using low-sodium hypotonic fluids, such as plain water, fruit juice, 5% dextrose, 0.22% saline, or Isolyte-P, to compensate for the combined loss of sodium and water can precipitate hyponatremia. This type of dehydration can also occur due to excessive perspiration or through diuresis accompanied by abnormally high renal sodium loss.

Fluid loss comes mainly from the extracellular fluid (ECF) [intravascular + interstitial] compartment rather than intracellular fluid (ICF). Due to severe ECF depletion, patients with hyponatremic dehydration are more hemodynamically unstable, with a higher chance of circulatory collapse.

Clinical features: Symptoms related to low serum sodium can vary depending on its severity and the duration of its onset. These may range from headaches, nausea, malaise, and lethargy when the serum sodium level is below 125 mEq/L to more severe and life-threatening symptoms such as drowsiness, seizures, brain stem herniation, respiratory arrest, and coma, which occur rarely and mainly when the level falls below 120 mEq/L.

Management: The management of hyponatremic dehydration is almost similar to that of isonatremic dehydration, except in very few patients with significant neurological symptoms due to severe hyponatremia. The most widely used fluid in the treatment of hyponatremic dehydration is normal saline, which contains 154 mEq/L of sodium, effectively raising serum sodium levels. Hypertonic saline is selectively used in a few children with severe symptomatic hyponatremia.

Moreover, the addition of potassium should be considered based on the serum potassium levels. It's less commonly known but vital to recognize and understand that potassium supplementation in cases of hyponatremic dehydration with hypokalemia can also correct hyponatremia. This correction occurs because the administered potassium enters cells and shifts sodium from the intracellular to the extracellular fluid in exchange for potassium. Concurrently, the increase in intracellular osmolality, brought about by the influx of potassium into cells, promotes water movement into the cells. This dual action of sodium moving into the extracellular fluid and water migrating into the intracellular fluid helps in correcting hyponatremia.

Important considerations in management

(Also refer Chapter 20 on "Hyponatremia")

1. Avoid rapid correction of hyponatremia (>12 mEq/L in first 24 hr).

2. Hypertonic saline should be used judiciously and is required in very few children with severe hyponatremia (serum Na$^+$ <120 mEq/L) or when severe neurological symptoms are present. The goal of administering hypertonic saline is to aggressively correct symptomatic hyponatremia during the initial three to four hours to reduce cerebral edema. In order to rapidly raise the serum sodium level and control severe neurological symptoms, the calculated volume of hypertonic saline should be infused as a bolus instead of a slow infusion [13]. Administer boluses of hypertonic saline with caution due to the potential risk of volume overload.

3. Avoid consumption of clear water or infusion of hypotonic solutions,

as there is a high risk of inducing symptomatic hyponatremia.

4. It is essential to closely monitor serum sodium levels and adjust the sodium concentration of the infused fluid as required.

Hypernatremic or hypertonic dehydration

Hypernatremic dehydration characterized by serum sodium >145 mEq/L is the least common cause of dehydration, which occurs in about 7% of children with dehydration due to diarrhea [3, 6, 7].

Causes: Hypernatremic dehydration occurs when there is a greater loss of water compared to sodium. Common causes of hypernatremic dehydration include excessive salt or solute intake from consuming incorrectly prepared, highly concentrated oral rehydration solutions or high-solute beverages during diarrhea and increased insensible losses due to fever or sweating. A free water deficit due to poor water intake is a common cause of hypernatremic dehydration, which can occur due to inadequate water access, a poor thirst mechanism (due to neurologic impairment), severe vomiting, or anorexia. Thirst is a potent physiological response that prevents a free water deficit. Hypernatremic dehydration can also occur due to additional free water loss due to urinary concentrating defects in children with conditions such as diabetes insipidus, renal tubular disorders, or post-obstructive diuresis.

Pathophysiology: In hypernatremic dehydration, due to water deficit, there is a decrease in both extracellular and intracellular fluid volumes. A decrease in ECF volume due to water deficit increases the serum sodium concentration, leading to hypernatremia. Hypernatremia creates an osmotic imbalance, leading to water movement from brain cells into the hypertonic extracellular fluid, causing shrinkage of brain cells, altered neuronal function, and neurological symptoms. Severe brain shrinkage in acute hypernatremia can lead to vascular rupture, resulting in life-threatening complications such as cerebral bleeding, subarachnoid hemorrhage, or even death.

Clinical features: Hypernatremic dehydration is a dangerous type of dehydration due to the complications associated with both hypernatremia and its treatment. Symptoms of hypernatremic dehydration are variable and includes:

- Children are hemodynamically more stable because fluid loss occurs proportionately from both ICF and ECF compartments, and therefore, the reduction in intravascular volume is less significant.

- Characteristic symptoms include an intense thirst that seems disproportionate to the apparent degree of dehydration, a shrill cry or mewing sound, muscle weakness, fever, and tachycardia. Reduced skin turgor, a doughy skin texture, and warm extremities are characteristic features.

- Neurological symptoms observed include lethargy, hyperirritability, confusion, muscle twitching, and, in severe cases, seizures.

- Rapid correction of hypernatremia can lead to brain edema and cause neurological symptoms like headache, altered mental status, and convulsions.

Management: Since hypernatremic dehydration is frequently iatrogenic, prevention is always preferable. A water deficit is the cause in many children, so cautious replacement with hypotonic fluid is usually necessary.

Recommended rate of correction: A more gradual correction, extending over a period of 48 hours or more, is considered safer. The recommended sodium reduction rate in hypernatremic dehydration cases is <0.5 mEq/L per hour and/or <12 mEq/L over a 24-hour period. Avoid allowing IV infusions to run rapidly, as this can lead to a rapid correction of hypernatremia, potentially causing cerebral edema and associated complications such as convulsions.

Fluid management during shock: A few children with hypernatremic dehydration, presenting with hypotension or shock, may require initial resuscitation with IV normal saline, even in the presence of hypernatremia. Avoid using Ringer's lactate instead of normal saline for the initial resuscitation in cases of hypernatremic dehydration, as its lower sodium content (130 mEq/L compared to 154 mEq/L in normal saline) carries a higher risk of a rapid reduction in serum sodium levels.

Subsequent fluid management: Once volume expansion occurs and the child becomes hemodynamically stable, the IV fluid should be switched to a hypotonic solution compared to the patient's plasma to provide free water and correct hypernatremia. Since there are no specific recommendations for the selection of fluids or the rate of administration during the correction of hypernatremic dehydration, the treatment plan should be adjusted based on close clinical monitoring and serial sodium estimations every 2–4 hours.

Selection of replacement fluids: At this stage, to facilitate the gradual reduction of high serum sodium levels, a prudent approach would be the cautious administration of solutions such as 0.9%

normal saline with dextrose (D5NS) or 0.45% normal saline with dextrose (D5-1/2NS), rather than using 5% dextrose or 0.22% saline.

It's critical to select the appropriate sodium concentration of the IV fluid and adjust the type of fluid based on the serum sodium reduction rate to prevent rapid correction of hypernatremia. If the rate of serum sodium reduction is slow, less than 0.5 mEq/L/h, administering a more hypotonic solution like D5-1/2NS to provide additional free water is advised. On the other hand, switching to an IV fluid with a higher sodium concentration, such as D5NS, would be wise if the serum sodium level decreases rapidly.

Volume of replacement fluid: As water deficit is a common cause of hypernatremic dehydration in children, they are often administered maintenance fluids at a higher rate, i.e., 1.25–1.5 times the normal rate. When hypotonic fluid compared to the patient's plasma is administered to treat hypernatremic dehydration, the rate of fluid delivery is a critical factor in determining the decrease in serum sodium levels. If the rate of reduction of serum sodium is slower than desired, infusing a larger volume of fluid to deliver more free water can be achieved by increasing the rate of fluid administration. Conversely, if the reduction rate of serum sodium is too rapid, it is advisable to reduce the rate of fluid administration.

Hypernatremia with volume overload: In cases of hypernatremia induced by salt poisoning, signs of overhydration and volume expansion should be apparent. Enhancing sodium excretion can be achieved by using a loop diuretic to increase urinary sodium losses and replacing urine output with free water.

If the serum sodium concentration exceeds 180 mEq/L, or if the patient exhibits renal or cardiac compromise due to the electrolyte imbalance, dialysis might be necessary to correct the abnormalities. Under such circumstances, peritoneal dialysis may be favored over hemodialysis, as the correction process is relatively slow.

(Also refer to the Chapter 21 on "Hypernatremia" for further details.)

IDENTIFY THE CAUSE AND TREATMENT BASED ON IT

Diarrhea, vomiting, and diabetic ketoacidosis are the common causes of dehydration in children, and it is essential to thoroughly understand the different fluid management strategies for each disorder.

Diarrhea

Diarrhea in children, characterized by frequent loose or watery stools, is the most common cause of dehydration in young individuals. Severe cases can lead to electrolyte and acid-base disorders. Therefore, proper assessment is vital for effectively and appropriately managing these cases. The Chapter 34 on "Gastrointestinal Losses and Upper GI Bleeding" provides a detailed discussion on the etiology and pathophysiology of volume, fluid, electrolytes, and acid-base disorders related to diarrhea, as well as its management.

A. Electrolytes and acid-base disorders in diarrhea: Several electrolytes and acid-base disorders commonly encountered in diarrhea are briefly summarized below. The Chapter 34 on "Gastrointestinal Losses and Upper GI Bleeding" provides detailed information on the pathophysiology of electrolytes and acid-base disorders in diarrhea.

1. Hypokalemia: In diarrhea, hypokalemia is a common electrolyte disorder that occurs due to the loss of diarrheal fluid, which is rich in potassium. Increased aldosterone production due to severe hypovolemia stimulates the renal reabsorption of sodium and increases urinary and intestine secretion of potassium, which also contributes to the development of hypokalemia.

2. Metabolic acidosis: Diarrheal fluid is rich in bicarbonate. Such fluid loss often results in a normal anion gap (AG) metabolic acidosis. Severe volume depletion can lead to hypoperfusion, causing concurrent lactic acidosis and further aggravating metabolic acidosis.

3. Sodium disturbances: In most cases of diarrhea, water loss, and sodium loss occur in the same proportion, so serum sodium concentration remains unaltered. However, children with severe diarrhea may develop hyponatremia if they drink large quantities of low-salt fluids like water or formula, receive hypotonic IV fluids, or have diarrhea with high sodium content, such as cholera. A small proportion of children with significant loss of electrolyte-poor diarrheal fluid can develop hypernatremia due to a net loss of water exceeding the loss of sodium.

B. The assessment of dehydration: Several clinical diagnostic criteria for assessing the severity of dehydration in cases of diarrhea have been proposed, with the three most commonly used being the WHO scale for dehydration (developed by the WHO) [14], the Gorelick scale (GS) developed by the Philadelphia Children's Hospital (Gorelick et al., 1997) [1], and the Clinical Dehydration Scale (CDS) developed by the Toronto Children's Hospital (Friedman et al., 2004) [15]. In recent studies, the diagnostic accuracy of the "WHO" scale for dehydration and the Gorelick scale was found to be more accurate in determining the degree of dehydration in children compared to the Clinical Dehydration Scale [5, 16].

According to WHO criteria, children having dehydration are categorized into three distinct groups:

- Group A signifies severe dehydration, identified by the presence of at least two of the following signs: Sunken eyes, a poor ability to drink or an inability to drink, and a skin pinch that retracts very slowly (taking 2 seconds or more), or the child is lethargic or unconscious.

- Group B indicates some dehydration, marked by two or more of the following signs: Sunken eyes and a strong desire to drink, characterized by noticeable thirst, restlessness, and irritability.

- Group C, on the other hand, represents no dehydration, characterized by an insufficient number of signs to qualify as either some or severe dehydration.

C. Management: In cases of no dehydration or some dehydration (or mild to moderate dehydration), the optimal approach for replacing ongoing fluid and electrolyte losses is supplementation with oral rehydration solutions (ORS) or homemade solutions, while children with severe dehydration need IV supplementation of fluids. Avoid fluids with high sugar content, such as cola, apple juice, and sports drinks, which have low sodium ($\leq$20 mEq/L) and high osmolality (ranging from 350–750 mOsm/L).

1. No dehydration: In children with no dehydration (plan A) who have less than a 5% fluid deficit, the volume of ORS or homemade solutions provided is 10 mL/kg/per purge, and they are encouraged to continue breastfeeding.

2. Some dehydration: In children with some dehydration (plan B), characterized by a 5–10% fluid deficit, 75 mL/kg of ORS is administered over 4 hours in sips (5 mL or one teaspoon every 2 minutes), with the continuation of breastfeeding. After 4 hours, reassess the child's hydration, classify the degree of dehydration, and select the appropriate plan to determine the necessary amounts of ORS.

3. Severe dehydration: In children with severe dehydration having >10% fluid deficit (plan C) or those unable to consume fluids via the oral or nasogastric (NG) route, administration of intravenous rehydration fluids is necessary.

In older children (>1 year) with severe dehydration, the recommended rate of IV fluid administration is 30 mL/kg in the first 30 minutes, followed by 70 mL/kg over the next 2.5 hours; thus, a total of 100 mL/kg of fluid is delivered in 3 hours. For infants, the recommended rate of IV fluid administration is 30 mL/kg during the first hour and an additional 70 mL/kg over the subsequent five hours, thus providing a total 100 mL/kg in a six-hour period.

In children who are able to drink, administer ORS orally while setting up the IV drip. If IV access is unavailable, ORS can be administered via a nasogastric tube at a rate of 20 mL/kg/h.

4. Selection of IV fluids: For the treatment of severe dehydration due to diarrhea, the selection of appropriate IV fluids is categorized as follows:

- Preferred solution: Ringer's lactate or PlasmaLyte.

- Acceptable solutions: Normal saline, 0.45% NaCl (half-strength saline).

- Unacceptable and harmful solutions: Sodium-free or poor solutions such as 5% dextrose, 0.22% saline, or multi-electrolyte solutions like Isolyte-P.

Balanced crystalloids vs. normal saline: In acute severe diarrheal dehydration cases, there has been a persistent debate over whether to opt for balanced crystalloids like Ringer's lactate or the conventionally favored normal saline for resuscitation. Previous studies indicated no significant differences in clinical improvement or biochemical resolution between Ringer's lactate and normal saline, thereby preferring the latter as the preferred option due to its comparable efficacy, lower cost, and greater availability [17, 18].

However, by recommending Ringer's lactate as the preferred IV fluid to correct dehydration due to severe diarrhea, the World Health Organization (WHO) challenged this popular practice [14]. A recent analysis by the Cochrane Database Systematic Review (2023) favored the use of balanced crystalloid such as Ringer's lactate over normal saline, highlighting their potential to reduce the duration of hospital stays and the risk of hypokalemia following intravenous correction without increasing the risk of hyponatremia [19]. Furthermore, the review demonstrated that metabolic acidosis, a common complication of dehydration, can induce vomiting and hinder food intake in recovering children, potentially prolonging their hospital stay, and if untreated, its severe form can adversely affect the body's metabolic functions.

Balanced crystalloid Ringer's lactate (RL), which provides 28 mEq/L of bicarbonate through hepatic conversion of lactate, facilitates quicker resolution of metabolic acidosis, supporting the preference for balanced crystalloids [20].

The review raised concerns about the potassium-free composition of normal saline, warning that it could increase the risk of hypokalemia, thereby inducing detrimental effects like muscular weakness and diminished gastrointestinal motility, which consequently interfere with children's capacity to accept oral fluids and feedings [19].

Considering this evidence, the Cochrane Review suggested that balanced solutions, having a range of electrolytes and additional cations similar to those found in human plasma, stand as a potentially superior choice for rehydration compared to the traditional 0.9% saline solution that contains only sodium and chloride [19].

5. Management of dehydration in severe acute malnutrition (SAM): An important aspect to note is that the approach to managing dehydration in children with SAM differs significantly from that in children without malnutrition, as outlined below [21]:

- As children with SAM have low glucose reserves and high total body sodium, so always correct dehydration slowly and provide adequate carbohydrates with close monitoring in children with SAM.

- The preferred route is oral, and NG tube administration is utilized for children who have difficulty drinking adequately. IV fluids carry a risk of overhydration and heart failure; thus, their use should be reserved for treating shock.

- The recommended rate of administering oral fluid is 5–10 mL/kg/h for a maximum duration of 12 hours.

- For dehydrated children with severe acute malnutrition, the WHO guidelines advise the usage of ReSoMal, an oral rehydration solution that has a lower sodium content

(45 mEq/L) and higher potassium content (40 mEq/L), as opposed to the older WHO ORS formulation which contains a higher level of sodium (90 mEq/L) and a lower level of potassium (20 mEq/L).

- However, ReSoMal should be cautiously administered due to the potential risk of severe hyponatremia, and it is not advised for children with suspected cholera or profuse watery diarrhea [22].

- **Preparing ReSoMal solution:** If ReSoMal is unavailable, a comparable solution can be prepared using the standard WHO reduced osmolarity ORS, which contains 75 mEq/L of sodium, 20 mEq/L of potassium, and 13.5 gm/L glucose, by following these steps:

  a. Dissolve the WHO reduced osmolarity ORS in 2L of clean water. This increases the volume to 2L instead of the standard 1L.

  b. Add 45 mL of potassium chloride solution. As every 15 mL of USP solution contains 20 mEq of potassium, adding 45 mL will supply an additional 60 mEq of potassium.

  c. Add 50 gm of sucrose to the solution.

  d. The final composition will consist of 37.5 mEq/L sodium, 40 mEq/L potassium, and about 32 gm/L of glucose/sucrose.

Vomiting

Loss of gastric fluid, either due to vomiting or NG suction, is an important cause of dehydration. Hypokalemic, hypochloremic metabolic alkalosis can occur due to the loss of gastric fluid in severe persistent vomiting. Infants with pyloric stenosis are at high risk of developing such disorders [23]. Volume depletion resulting from dehydration increases plasma aldosterone, promoting renal excretion of potassium and renal reabsorption of sodium to maintain circulatory volume. As the potassium concentration in gastric fluid is very low (10 mEq/L), urinary potassium loss is the primary cause of hypokalemia in cases of vomiting or NG suction. As gastric fluid contains hydrochloric acid, the loss of about 60–80 mEq/L hydrogen ions leads to metabolic alkalosis, and the loss of about 90 mEq/L of chloride leads to hypochloremia. The Chapter 34 on "Gastrointestinal Losses and Upper GI Bleeding" provides detailed information about electrolyte disorders due to the loss of gastric fluid and its management.

Management: The strategy for managing vomiting depends on its severity. Often, vomiting will stop without any specific medical treatment. The severity of vomiting can be classified using a scale with three levels: Mild (1–2 times per day), moderate (3–7 times per day), and severe (vomiting nearly everything or experiencing 8 or more episodes per day) [24].

Oral rehydration: In cases of mild to moderate vomiting, oral replacement may be adequate; important considerations to provide optimal oral fluids include:

- Oral fluid replacement can effectively maintain hydration in children who are vomiting if they can tolerate the oral intake.

- After vomiting, wait for about 20–30 minutes and then initiate oral rehydration therapy (ORT).

- For initial rehydration, the most effective method is to frequently administer small volumes (about 5 mL/dose) of glucose-electrolyte solution every 1–2 minutes until the child begins to rehydrate and can tolerate higher dosages [25, 26]. It is vital to avoid the common mistake of giving too much liquid too quickly, as this can exacerbate vomiting.

- Once there is no vomiting for 3–4 hours, gradually increase the amount of liquids.

- Oral rehydration therapy is recommended to correct electrolyte disturbances, restore hydration, and assist in recovering a child having vomiting [25].

- Low-osmolarity ORS solution (240–250 mOsm/l) is preferred for oral rehydration therapy [2].

- If ORS is unavailable, other fluids that can be used for initial rehydration include clear fluids such as ice chips or sips of water, sugar water, lemon-lime soda, clear broths weak herbal teas, Popsicles, or gelatin desserts. However, avoiding sports drinks, sodas, and fruit juices is advisable due to their high carbohydrate content.

- Solid foods should be avoided for about 24 hours after an episode of vomiting because they can stimulate further vomiting.

- If the oral rehydration therapy (ORT) regimen is carefully followed at home, it can help avoid emergency department visits and hospitalizations [27].

- If children fail to show improvement following ORT, hospital admission for intravenous fluid administration may be necessary.

Antiemetics: To control persistent vomiting effectively, administer ondansetron 15 to 30 minutes before initiating or resuming oral rehydration therapy [28]. This intervention reduces the failure rate of ORT and, by facilitating the consumption of ORT, it decreases the need for IV fluids [29].

Intravenous therapy: In children requiring the administration of IV fluid, the preferred solution is normal saline with the addition of 10 mEq/L of potassium chloride. This potassium-containing normal saline will effectively correct plasma electrolyte imbalances and acid-base disturbances in cases of hypokalemic hypochloremic alkalosis due to gastric losses [30].

To determine the appropriate volume of IV fluid to administer, it is recommended to measure the urine output every 1–6 hours and plan a volume-to-volume replacement.

In severe vomiting with associated known or probable metabolic alkalosis, the use of balanced crystalloids like RL and PlasmaLyte should be avoided as they can exacerbate the alkalosis by providing buffers.

Diabetic ketoacidosis

Diabetic ketoacidosis (DKA) is a serious and potentially life-threatening metabolic complication of diabetes mellitus commonly encountered in clinical settings. It is characterized by a triad of hyperglycemia, metabolic acidosis, and either ketonemia or ketonuria, usually accompanied by disorders such as dehydration, hypokalemia, and hyponatremia in a few children.

To plan effective strategies for managing DKA, it is essential to understand the pathophysiology of hyperglycemia, ketoacidosis, and the associated fluid and electrolyte disorders. A detailed exploration of these disorders and relevant therapeutic strategies can be found in the Chapter 40 on "Diabetic Ketoacidosis and Hyperosmolar Hyperglycemic State".

Fluid management is a crucial aspect of treating DKA, and based on recent evidence, the concepts and trends regarding the prescription of IV fluids are changing, as summarized below:

- During DKA treatment, the risk of developing cerebral edema is highlighted, and in the past, slow rehydration has been recommended to avoid this risk [31]. A recent study, however, has shown that neither the rate of infusion nor the sodium chloride concentration significantly influences the risk of cerebral injury [32].

- Normal saline has traditionally been the fluid of choice, and current guidelines and textbooks still recommend its use for both volume resuscitation and deficit replacement in DKA [33].

- However, normal saline isn't truly "normal" or "physiological because it lacks bicarbonate and has a chloride concentration 50% higher than that of serum chloride [34, 35]. When large volumes of this chloride-rich (154 mEq/L) saline are administered, there's a potential for hyperchloremia. This can cause hyperchloremic acidosis, lead to acute kidney injury (AKI), prolong the time to DKA resolution, and result in a longer hospital stay [36–38].

- Recent literature suggests that using balanced crystalloids, like PlasmaLyte, in children with DKA provides multiple benefits: faster pH correction, reduced risk of hyperchloremic metabolic acidosis, cost savings, and decreased likelihood of cerebral edema [39–43].

- Several adult DKA studies indicate that balanced crystalloids like PlasmaLyte lead to a quicker resolution of metabolic acidosis and lesser hyperchloremia compared to normal saline, suggesting that balanced crystalloids may be a better acute management option for adults with DKA [37, 44–47].

- Recently updated guidelines for children, including the Surviving Sepsis Guidelines (2020), ERC guidelines (2021), advanced life support guidelines (2021), and the Latin American Consensus (2022), favor balanced crystalloids over normal saline, even outside the context of DKA [8, 9, 11]. The rationale for choosing balanced crystalloids (e.g., Ringer's lactate, PlasmaLyte) over saline is their associated benefits, such as improved blood pH and bicarbonate values in critically ill children, as well as a reduced risk of AKI [48, 49].

- With growing evidence supporting balanced crystalloids for DKA in both children and adults, as well as for critically ill children and those with sepsis, the prevailing trend is a preference for balanced crystalloids over saline; its use is included in recent guidelines for treating DKA [42, 50, 51].

- A recent literature review by Othman et al. (2023) found that treating DKA with PlasmaLyte instead of normal saline resulted in beneficial effects such as rise in bicarbonate levels and blood pressure, decreased chloride and potassium levels, and an earlier resolution of DKA without exacerbating ketosis [33]. Notably, using PlasmaLyte could shorten ICU and hospital stays without increasing the incidence of AKI or mortality rates.

- Although current recommendations generally favor the use of balanced crystalloids over saline, they are

Table 49.6 Monitoring fluid therapy
Physical examination: Assess hydration status and look for dehydration or volume overload
Vital signs: To assess hemodynamic status
Fluid balance and weight chart: Measure fluid intake, urine volume and watch for change in body weight
Laboratory parameters: Serial measurements of serum sodium and potassium. Additional test considering clinical status

based on evidence of only mild to moderate certainty [38, 40]. While some pediatric studies demonstrate comparable effects between the two fluids [52], ongoing trials like the BRISK-ED study will further clarify the best fluid choice for DKA [53].

MONITORING

A child receiving IV fluids should be closely monitored, especially with significant ongoing fluid loss. This monitoring includes frequent physical examinations, maintaining a fluid balance chart, daily weight tracking, and laboratory tests, as summarized in Table 49.6. Planning of initial fluid administration is based on the severity of dehydration, and meticulous subsequent monitoring is crucial in facilitating necessary adjustments and optimizing the volume and type of IV fluids, minimizing complications from inappropriate administration.

Physical examination and vital signs

Meticulous clinical examinations conducted frequently are crucial for evaluating hydration status and monitoring the response to fluid repletion. Skin turgor, thirst and urine output are the most commonly used monitoring parameters to assess dehydration (see Tables 49.1 and 49.2 for a comprehensive list of parameters) [54]. If the examination points to dehydration, continued rehydration is warranted. On the other hand, symptoms like puffy eyes, swelling of the lower limbs, and pulmonary congestion suggest fluid overload and necessitate fluid restriction.

Monitoring the patient's vital signs is essential to gauge intravascular volume status. A child having hypotension and tachycardia may require a fluid bolus for swift correction.

Fluid balance and weight chart

It is essential to monitor a child's total fluid intake, as it's often in excess of the prescribed volumes. Fluid intake includes not only the IV fluids ordered but also any additional fluids used as diluents for medication.

Strict measurement of urine volume is a valuable indicator of hydration status. A good urine output (≥1 mL/kg/hour) suggests successful rehydration therapy, while oliguria suggests inadequate fluid replacement in a child with normal kidney function.

Accurate daily weight measurements are crucial to determine total fluid balance and assess therapeutic response to fluid therapy. For accurate daily weight measurements, use the same scales and ensure the child is in similar lightweight clothing. A decrease in weight may indicate dehydration, insufficient fluid replacement, or ongoing fluid loss that exceeds the volume of fluid administered. On the other hand, a sudden weight increase can suggest successful hydration, but excessive gain points to potential fluid overload.

To assess hydration status in children with profuse ongoing fluid loss, calculate the fluid balance and measure weight every 4–6 hours or more frequently.

Laboratory tests

In children receiving IV fluids, it's important to monitor serial laboratory tests, including CBC and hematocrit, serum sodium and potassium, pH and bicarbonate, renal functions, and blood glucose. Which test to order and the frequency of testing is unclear [55], and it depends on the individual patient's clinical presentation and the severity of their underlying etiology.

In a child receiving resuscitation and maintenance intravenous fluids, serum sodium is checked daily for stable patients, but in those with severe dehydration and large ongoing volume losses, it may require serial estimations every four to six hours. Serum sodium concentration indicates the body's free water content: hyponatremia typically reflects an excess of water, while hypernatremia usually indicates a water deficit.

Commonly used isotonic fluids in children, such as normal saline, are potassium-free, while balanced crystalloids like Ringer's lactate and PlasmaLyte contain only 4 mEq/L and 5 mEq/L of potassium, respectively. The most common cases of fluid loss in children are diarrhea and vomiting, and both disorders are associated with hypokalemia. Given these factors, it is essential to measure serum potassium in such children and to add potassium chloride to the IV fluid to correct any potassium deficit.

Since metabolic acidosis and alkalosis can result from diarrhea and vomiting, it's important to diagnose these conditions and tailor fluid replacement accordingly. Based on this information fluid chosen are balanced crystalloids like Ringer's lactate and PlasmaLyte to treat metabolic acidosis, and normal saline is the preferred fluid for treating metabolic alkalosis.

REFERENCES

1. Gorelick MH, Shaw KN, Murphy KO. Validity and reliability of clinical signs in the diagnosis of dehydration in children. Pediatrics. 1997;99(5):E6.

2. National Collaborating Centre for Women's and Children's Health (UK). Diarrhoea and Vomiting Caused by Gastroenteritis: Diagnosis, Assessment and Management in Children Younger than 5 Years. London: RCOG Press; 2009 Apr. (NICE Clinical Guidelines, No. 84.) 5, Fluid management. Available from: https://www.ncbi.nlm.nih.gov/books/NBK63837/.

3. Chakravarthi GK, Kumar P. Study on incidences of electrolyte disorders among children with dehydration. Int J Pediatr Res. 2019;6(7):352–358.

4. Hoxha TF, Azemi M, Avdiu M, et al. The usefulness of clinical and laboratory parameters for predicting severity of dehydration in children with acute gastroenteritis. Med Arch 2014;68(5):304–7.

5. Can YY, Taşar MA, Gökçeoğlu AU. Are the Clinical Evaluation Scales and Laboratory Tests Adequate in Determining Dehydration Degree in Acute Diarrhea? J Pediatr Emerg Intensive Care Med 2022;9:85–93.

6. Shankar P, Mahamud S, Aara A. Study of electrolyte disturbances and renal parameters in acute gastroenteritis under 5 years of age in a tertiary care hospital of Bengaluru, India. Int J Contemp Pediatr. 2020;7(9):1910–1917.

7. Rashid N, Sadia G, Noor F. Frequency and Outcome of Sodium Imbalance in Dehydrated Children Presenting with Acute Watery Diarrhea PJMHS 202;14(1):341–343.

8. Skellett S, Maconochie I, Bingham B, et al. Paediatric advanced life support Guidelines. Resuscitation Council UK. Published May 2021. Visit: https://www.resus.org.uk/library/2021-resuscitation-guidelines/paediatric-advanced-life-support-guidelines.

9. Van de Voorde P, Turner NM, Djakow J, et al. European resuscitation council guidelines 2021: paediatric life support. Resuscitation. 2021;161:327–387.

10. Fernández-Sarmiento J, De Souza DC, Martinez A, et al. Latin American Consensus on the Management of Sepsis in Children: Sociedad Latinoamericana de Cuidados Intensivos Pediátricos [Latin American Pediatric Intensive Care Society] (SLACIP) Task Force: Executive Summary. J Intensive Care Med. 2022;37(6):753–763.

11. Weiss SL, Peters MJ, Alhazzani W, et al. Executive Summary: Surviving Sepsis Campaign International Guidelines for the Management of Septic Shock and Sepsis-Associated Organ Dysfunction in Children. Pediatr Crit Care Med 2020;21(2):e52–e106.

12. Powers KS. Dehydration: Isonatremic, Hyponatremic, and Hypernatremic Recognition and Management. Pediatr Rev. 2015;36(7):274–85.

13. Baek SH, Jo YH, Ahn S, et al. Risk of Overcorrection in Rapid Intermittent Bolus vs Slow Continuous Infusion Therapies of Hypertonic Saline for Patients With Symptomatic Hyponatremia: The SALSA Randomized Clinical Trial. JAMA Intern Med. 2021;181(1):81–92.

14. World Health Organization. The treatment of diarrhoea: a manual for physicians and other senior health workers, 4th rev. World Health Organization. 2005. https://apps.who.int/iris/handle/10665/43209.

15. Friedman JN, Goldman RD, Srivastava R, et al. Development of a clinical dehydration scale for use in children between 1 and 36 months of age. J Pediatr. 2004;145(2):201–7.

16. Hoxha T, Xhelili L, Azemi M, et al. Comparing the Accuracy of the Three Dehydration Scales in Children with Acute Diarrhea in a Developing Country of Kosovo. Mater Sociomed. 2015;27(3):140–3.

17. Mahajan V, Sajan SS, Sharma A, et al. Ringers lactate vs normal saline for children with acute diarrhea and severe dehydration- A double blind randomized controlled trial. Indian Pediatr 2012;49(12):963–968.

18. Kartha GB, Rameshkumar R, Mahadevan S. Randomized double-blind trial of Ringer Lactate versus normal saline in pediatric acute severe diarrheal dehydration. J Pediatr Gastroenterol Nutr 2017;65(6):621–626.

19. Florez ID, Sierra J, Pérez-Gaxiola G. Balanced crystalloid solutions versus 0.9% saline for treating acute diarrhoea and severe dehydration in children. Cochrane Database Syst Rev 2023;5(5):CD013640.

20. Naseem M, Dubey AP, Mishra TK, et al. Effect of Rehydration with Normal Saline versus Ringer Lactate on Serum Sodium Level of Children with Acute Diarrhea and Severe Dehydration: A Randomized Controlled Trial. Indian Pediatr. 2020;57(6):519–522.

21. Cherukuri N, Wadhwa SP. Acute Watery Diarrhea. In: Standard Treatment Guidelines. Indian Academy of Pediatrics (IAP); 2022. Available from: https://iapindia.org/pdf/Ch-020-STG-Acute-Watery-Diarrhea.pdf.

22. Houston KA, Gibb JG, Maitland K. Oral rehydration of malnourished children with diarrhoea and dehydration: A systematic review. Wellcome Open Res. 2017;2:66.

23. Breaux CW Jr, Hood JS, Georgeson KE. The significance of alkalosis and hypochloremia in hypertrophic pyloric stenosis. J Pediatr Surg. 1989;24(12):1250–2.

24. Schmitt Pediatric Guidelines LLC. Vomiting without diarrhea. Seattle Children's. Reviewed September 8, 2023. Available from: https://www.seattlechildrens.org/conditions/a-z/vomiting-without-diarrhea/.

25. American Academy of Pediatrics, Provisional Committee on Quality Improvement, Subcommittee on Acute Gastroenteritis. Practice parameter: the management of acute gastroenteritis in young children. Pediatrics. 1996;97(3):424–435.

26. King CK, Glass R, Bresee JS, et al. Managing acute gastroenteritis among children: oral rehydration, maintenance, and nutritional therapy. MMWR Recomm Rep. 2003;52(RR-16):1–16.

27. Tieder JS, Robertson A, Garrison MM. Pediatric hospital adherence to the standard of care for acute gastroenteritis. Pediatrics. 2009;124(6):e1081–e1087.

28. Cheng A. Emergency department use of oral ondansetron for acute gastroenteritis-related vomiting in infants and children. Paediatr Child Health. 2011;16(3):177–182.

29. Freedman SB, Adler M, Seshadri R, et al. Oral ondansetron for gastroenteritis in a pediatric emergency department. N Engl J Med. 2006;354(16):1698–1705.

30. Hayes W. Ab-normal saline in abnormal kidney function: risks and alternatives. Pediatr Nephrol. 2019;34(7):1191–1199.

31. Duck SC, Wyatt DT. Factors associated with brain herniation in the treatment of diabetic ketoacidosis. J Pediatr. 1988;113(1 Pt 1):10–4.

32. Kuppermann N, Ghetti S, Schunk JE, et al. PECARN DKA FLUID Study Group. Clinical Trial of Fluid Infusion Rates for Pediatric Diabetic Ketoacidosis. N Engl J Med. 2018;378(24):2275–2287.

33. Othman MI, Nashwan AJ, Alfayoumi M, et al. PlasmaLyte-148 Versus Normal Saline 0.9% in Diabetic Ketoacidosis Management: A Review. Cureus. 2023;15(6):e41079.

34. Li H, Sun SR, Yap JQ, et al. 0.9% saline is neither normal nor physiological. J Zhejiang Univ Sci B. 2016;17(3):181–7.

35. Reddy S, Weinberg L, Young P. Crystalloid fluid therapy. Crit Care. 2016;20:59.

36. Goad NT, Bakhru RN, Pirkle JL, et al: Association of hyperchloremia with unfavorable clinical outcomes in adults with diabetic ketoacidosis. J Intensive Care Med 2019;35(11):1307–1313.

37. Oliver WD, Willis GC, Hines MC, et al. Comparison of PlasmaLyte A and Sodium Chloride 0.9% for Fluid Resuscitation of Patients With Diabetic Ketoacidosis. Hosp Pharm 2018;53(5):326–330.

38. Alghamdi NA, Major P, Chaudhuri D, et al. Saline Compared to Balanced Crystalloid in Patients With Diabetic Ketoacidosis: A Systematic Review and Meta-Analysis of Randomized Controlled Trials. Crit Care Explor. 2022;4(1):e0613.

39. Bergmann KR, Abuzzahab MJ, Nowak J, et al. Resuscitation with Ringer's lactate compared with normal saline for pediatric diabetic ketoacidosis. Pediatr Emerg Care 2021;37(5):e236–e242.

40. Catahay JA, Polintan ET, Casimiro M, et al. Balanced electrolyte solutions versus isotonic saline in adult patients with diabetic ketoacidosis: A systematic review and meta-analysis. Heart Lung. 2022;54:74–79.

41. Jahangir A, Jahangir A, Siddiqui FS, et al. Normal Saline Versus Low Chloride Solutions in Treatment of Diabetic Ketoacidosis: A Systematic Review of Clinical Trials. Cureus. 2022;14(1):e21324.

42. Gripp KE, Trottier ED, Thakore S, et al. Current recommendations for management of paediatric diabetic ketoacidosis. Paediatr Child Health. 2023;28(2):128–138.

43. Tamzil R, Yaacob N, Noor NM, et al. Comparing the clinical effects of balanced electrolyte solutions versus normal saline in managing diabetic ketoacidosis: A

systematic review and meta-analyses. Turk J Emerg Med 2023;23(3):131–138.

44. Chua HR, Venkatesh B, Stachowski E, et al. PlasmaLyte 148 vs 0.9% saline for fluid resuscitation in diabetic ketoacidosis. J Crit Care 2012;27(2):138–45.

45. Van Zyl D, Rheeder P, Delport E. Fluid management in diabetic-acidosis Ringer's lactate versus normal saline: a randomized controlled trial. QJM. 2012;105(4):337–343.

46. Self WH, Semler MW, Wanderer JP, et al. Balanced Crystalloids versus Saline in Noncritically Ill Adults. N Engl J Med 2018;378(9):819–828.

47. Ramanan M, Attokaran A, Murray L. et al. Sodium chloride or PlasmaLyte-148 evaluation in severe diabetic ketoacidosis (SCOPE-DKA): a cluster, crossover, randomized, controlled trial. Intensive Care Med. 2021;47(11):1248–1257.

48. Lehr AR, Rached-d'Astous S, Barrowman N, et al. Balanced Versus Unbalanced Fluid in Critically Ill Children: Systematic Review and Meta-Analysis. Pediatr Crit Care Med 2022;23(3):181–191.

49. Sankar J, Muralidharan J, Lalitha AV, et al. Multiple Electrolytes Solution Versus Saline as Bolus Fluid for Resuscitation in Pediatric Septic Shock: A Multicenter Randomized Clinical Trial. Crit Care Med 2023.

50. JBDS. JBDS-IP Joint British Diabetes Societies Inpatient Care Group. The Management of Diabetic Ketoacidosis in Adults, March 2023 Update: JBDS Guidelines [Internet]. London: ABCD; 2023 Mar. Available from: https://abcd.care/sites/abcd.care/files/site_uploads/JBDS_Guidelines_Current/JBDS_02_DKA_Guideline_with_QR_code_March_2023.pdf.

51. BSPED Guideline for the Management of Children and Young People under the age of 18 years with Diabetic Ketoacidosis - 2021 [Internet]. British Society for Paediatric Endocrinology and Diabetes; 2021. Available from: https://www.bsped.org.uk/clinical-resources/bsped-dka-guidelines/.

52. Williams V, Jayashree M, Nallasamy K, et al. 0.9% saline versus PlasmaLyte as initial fluid in children with diabetic ketoacidosis (SPinK trial): a double-blind randomized controlled trial. Crit Care 2020;24(1):1.

53. Yan JW, Slim A, Van Aarsen K, et al. Balanced crystalloids (RInger's lactate) versus normal Saline in adults with diabetic Ketoacidosis in the Emergency Department (BRISK-ED): a protocol for a pilot randomized controlled trial. Pilot Feasibility Stud. 2023;9(1):121.

54. Meyers RS. Pediatric fluid and electrolyte therapy. J Pediatr Pharmacol Ther. 2009;14(4):204–11.

55. Feld LG, Neuspiel DR, Foster BA, et al. Clinical practice guideline: maintenance intravenous fluids in children. Pediatrics 2018;142(6):e20183083.

50 | Oral Rehydration Therapy

INTRODUCTION AND ADVANTAGES

Oral rehydration therapy (ORT) is a remarkable innovation that changed the outcome of millions of children suffering from diarrhea globally [1, 2]. ORT is a wonderful discovery that has saved more lives than any other treatment modality over the past century [3]. ORT is a cost-effective, noninvasive alternative to intravenous fluids, offering the benefits of being less expensive and having a lower complication rate.

ORT eliminates the need for IV fluid infusion, which requires a skilled professional to establish a venous line, especially in infants, and also avoids the risks of pulmonary edema or electrolyte imbalance associated with IV fluid therapy. The efficacy of ORT is often underestimated due to its low cost, leading to a lack of trust and subsequent underuse [4].

ORAL REHYDRATION SOLUTIONS VS. ORAL REHYDRATION THERAPY

The terms "oral rehydration therapy" and "oral rehydration solutions" are often used interchangeably. Oral rehydration therapy refers to the broader practice of using a variety of solutions, including oral rehydration solution (ORS), for rehydration, typically containing a mixture of salt, sugar, and water. On the other hand, ORS represents specific formulations, such as the WHO-recommended mixture of glucose and electrolytes, which are scientifically designed to treat dehydration effectively. Thus, ORS stands out as the most scientifically advanced and effective method for treating dehydration among all ORT options.

A variety of ORT comprises different salt and sugar solutions used for correcting dehydration. These include:

- **Oral rehydration solutions (ORS):** It is a simple, inexpensive, and effective glucose and electrolyte solution, specially engineered and promoted extensively by the World Health Organization (WHO) for treating dehydration [5, 6]. ORS is a safe, widely available, and easy-to-use method for correcting dehydration that doesn't require skilled medical personnel, making it a highly practical solution, especially in settings with limited healthcare access.

  ORS can successfully treat up to 90% of dehydration cases resulting from diarrhea [7], reducing diarrhea-related deaths by 93% [8] making it the preferred treatment for rehydration unless contraindicated. Since ORS is effective and beneficial and shows no clinical difference in results compared to intravenous rehydration in cases of mild-to-moderate dehydration [9, 10], it is considered an important first-line therapy by WHO, the Center for Disease Control, and the European Society [5, 11–13].

  ORS include the WHO Standard (or Old) ORS (1978) with an osmolality

of 311 mOsm/L and a sodium concentration of 90 mmol/L, the WHO low osmolarity ORS (2002) with an osmolality of 245 mOsm/L and a sodium concentration of 75 mmol/L, ReSoMal (Rehydration Solution for Malnutrition) with an osmolality of 300 mOsm/L and a sodium concentration of 45 mmol/L.

- **Modified ORS:** These are solutions based on rice powder, those containing amino acids or zinc, offering alternative options for rehydration.

- **Homemade electrolyte solution:** In the absence of availability of commercial ORS, a homemade solution can be prepared by dissolving approximately 30 gm (6 teaspoons) of sugar and 2.5 gm (0.5 teaspoons) of salt in a liter of clean water.

- **Readily available home fluids:** When ORS is not available, options like salt and sugar-containing lemon water, salted and sugared buttermilk, green coconut water, thin rice kanji, dal water, and vegetable soup can be used as alternatives.

INDICATIONS

ORT is recommended to prevent dehydration in patients with inadequate oral intake or increased fluid losses and treat existing dehydration. ORT should be utilized for most children with mild to moderate dehydration, and it is important to remember that vomiting is not a contraindication for its use.

CONTRAINDICATIONS

Clinical settings in which ORT is not advised or is contraindicated are summarized below:

- Severe continuous, intractable, or uncontrolled vomiting.

- Severe dehydration accompanied by shock or hemodynamic instability. However, after shock correction, patients can still receive ORS safely even while continuing IV fluid therapy, meaning severe dehydration is not an absolute contraindication to ORT.

- The presence of an acute surgical abdomen, severe abdominal distention, or paralytic ileus.

- Altered mental status, convulsions, or a stuporous or comatose condition make oral intake unsafe due to the risk of aspiration. However, if a nasogastric tube can be passed, these patients could still receive ORT through this method.

PHARMACOLOGICAL BASIS

ORS is a specially formulated oral solution consisting of a balanced mix of electrolytes, including sodium and potassium, and glucose, which stimulates intestinal fluid absorption. This composition ensures rapid uptake of fluids and electrolytes into the bloodstream, effectively correcting dehydration resulting from diarrhea or similar conditions. It is important to remember that ORS provides water, replaces sodium and potassium deficits, and corrects acidosis in diarrhea, but per se does not reduce the frequency, severity, volume, or duration of stool output [14]. ORS effectively corrects dehydration caused by diarrhea, regardless of the underlying cause or the patient's age [1].

The pharmacological basis of the absorption of ORS depends on the body's physiological response to the electrolytes and glucose contained in the solution, as explained below [15–19].

Effect of salt-containing water without glucose

Oral intake of salt-containing water for correcting dehydration due to diarrhea is ineffective. This ineffectiveness arises because the intestinal absorption of sodium, which occurs in healthy individuals, is impaired during diarrhea, so neither sodium nor water will be absorbed. In contrast, oral intake of excess sodium-containing water can lead to increased secretion of water into the intestinal lumen, worsening diarrhea [20].

Adding glucose to salt-containing water - a key discovery of the century

In diarrhea, every sodium absorption mechanism, excluding the coupled sodium and chloride absorption, remains intact [17]. Adding glucose to a saline solution activates a new intestinal absorption mechanism for ORS [18, 20].

The absorption of glucose molecules is unaffected by the diarrhoeal disease state. The glucose molecules are absorbed, and through the action of the sodium/glucose co-transport cotransporter (SGLT1), located on the apical membrane of intestinal epithelial cells, sodium is concurrently absorbed with glucose [20].

Since each glucose molecule co-transports one sodium ion (Na^+), the optimal glucose-to-sodium ratio in rehydration fluids for effective ORS absorption is approximately one to one. The glucose-to-sodium ratio in rehydration fluids should not exceed 2:1 to ensure effective fluid repletion, as a higher glucose concentration can worsen diarrhea and increase sodium loss.

This oral rehydration formula, based on a glucose/salt solution, effectively counteracts dehydration even during persistent diarrhea. Consequently, ORS has revolutionized the management of dehydration associated with diarrhea, offering a highly effective solution.

RECOMMENDED COMPOSITION OF ORS

The composition of the rehydration solution is crucial for optimal absorption. The desired characteristics of electrolytes and glucose in the prepared ORS, as recommended by WHO and UNICEF, are summarized in Table 50.1 [21].

The effectiveness of ORS in gastrointestinal reabsorption depends on three main factors: The optimal concentrations of sodium and glucose and the appropriate osmolality of the solution. Furthermore, including potassium to counterbalance potassium deficits and citrate as a buffer in correcting acidosis establishes ORS as a comprehensive remedy for diarrheal dehydration. The Importance and optimal concentrations of each ORS component are summarized below.

Table 50.1 WHO and UNICEF's criteria for acceptable ORS	
Glucose	At least equal that of sodium but should not exceed **111** mmol/L
Sodium	Within the range of **60–90** mmol/L
Glucose sodium ratio	At least 1:1 and should not exceed 2:1
Potassium	Within the range of **15–25** mmol/L
Citrate	Within the range of **8–12** mmol/L
Chloride	Within the range of **50–80** mmol/L
Total osmolarity	Within the range of **200–310** mOsm/L (including that contributed by glucose)

Glucose content

The addition of glucose is the most critical part of ORS. It is important to remember that adding glucose is essential for sodium absorption during a diarrheal state, and a glucose-free salt solution will not be absorbed in patients with diarrhea.

When 2 gm/dL (20 gm/L) of glucose is added to water as per the recommendation of WHO/UNICEF, the resultant 2% solution provides 111 mmol of glucose per liter, facilitating optimal sodium and water absorption in the ORS solution.

A higher glucose concentration (>3%) solution is not recommended for ORS due to its dual detrimental impacts [20]. It not only exacerbates diarrhea, intensifying water loss through osmotic effects but also increases the risk of electrolyte imbalances, notably hypernatremia.

Replacing glucose with a complex carbohydrate, like rice or wheat, can offer a more effective and superior option for optimal ORS formulation compared to traditional glucose-based ORS [22]. Complex carbohydrates are metabolized in the intestine and slowly release glucose, which helps in sodium absorption [23].

Avoid adding sweeteners to ORS or using glucose-rich or fizzy drinks, such as sweet teas, sweet coffee, soft drinks, undiluted fruit juices, and sports drinks, as an ORT. Altering the glucose-to-sodium ratio impairs the effective absorption of salt and water and can induce osmotic diarrhea.

Sodium content

Sodium losses in diarrhea can be substantial, ranging from 50–60 mEq/L in non-cholera diarrhea to more than 100 mEq/L in cases like cholera, requiring due attention [20]. To compensate for this sodium loss, the sodium component of ORS is vital. Its effective intestinal absorption plays a crucial role in rectifying hypovolemia in cases of dehydration. The recommended sodium concentration in ORS should be between 60–90 mmol/L.

For efficient sodium absorption, it's essential to have both the addition of glucose and a maintained 1:1 ratio of sodium to glucose within the solution. The combined concentration of sodium and glucose in the ORS mixture determines the osmolality of ORS. The previous standard WHO ORS, which contained 90 mEq/L of sodium, had an osmolality of 311 mOsm/L, while the currently recommended low osmolarity WHO ORS, with 75 mEq/L of sodium, has an osmolality of 245 mOsm/L.

Osmolarity

The concentration of glucose and electrolytes in ORS is meticulously balanced to ensure an optimal osmolarity. The previous standard WHO ORS contained 90 mEq/L of sodium and 111 mmol/L of glucose, resulting in an osmolality of 311 mOsm/L. In contrast, the current WHO and UNICEF recommended low osmolarity ORS includes 75 mEq/L of sodium and 75 mmol/L of glucose, leading to an osmolality of 245 mOsm/L

The advantages of reduction of osmolarity in the ORS solution due to the significant reduction of glucose content are:

- Avoids the impairment of fluid absorption caused by hyperosmolarity and enhances intestinal water absorption due to its lower osmolality [17].

- Improves fluid absorption, providing significant benefits, such as a 33% reduction in IV fluid requirements compared to the standard WHO-ORS solution [24].

- Effectively reduces both stool volume and the duration of diarrhea [25, 26], and ensures better hydration compared to the standard WHO ORS [22].

Potassium content

As diarrheal fluid is rich in potassium, hypokalemia is common in diarrheal dehydration, requiring potassium supplementation. In ORS, the recommended range of potassium is 15–25 mmol/L, and both the standard WHO and lower osmolarity WHO ORS achieve this by containing 1.5 gms of potassium chloride, which provides 20 mmol/L of potassium.

Citrate content to correct acidosis

Diarrheal fluid is rich in HCO_3, so metabolic acidosis can occur in diarrheal dehydration, requiring attention and correction.

In ORS, citrate is added to correct metabolic acidosis, with the recommended concentration being between 8–12 mmol/L. Both the standard and lower osmolarity WHO ORS fulfill this by containing 2.9 gms of trisodium citrate dihydrate, which provides 10 mmol/L of citrate. This citrate is metabolized to bicarbonate in the body, offering an effect similar to directly adding 10 mEq/L of bicarbonate.

Although both sodium bicarbonate and trisodium citrate can effectively correct the metabolic acidosis resulting from diarrhea [27], the WHO recommends the use of trisodium citrate in ORS. This preference is attributed to its prolonged shelf life, increased stability, non-soiling nature of the sachet, superior taste, and its being more cost-effective.

TYPES OF ORAL REHYDRATION SOLUTIONS

The most commonly used oral rehydration solutions include WHO Standard (Old) ORS (1978), current WHO low osmolarity ORS (2002), ReSoMal (REhydration SOlution for MALnutrition), and Rice-based ORS. The compositions and content of these commonly used ORS are summarized in Table 50.2 and Table 50.3.

WHO Standard ORS

WHO Standard ORS was first introduced in the late sixties when cholera-induced diarrhea was highly prevalent. This simple but incredible discovery has contributed substantially to the dramatic reduction in global mortality from diarrheal diseases during that period.

As diarrhea induced by cholera is profuse and characterized by a high mean stool sodium concentration of about 90 mmol/L, the sodium content in the original WHO Standard ORS was intentionally set high at 90 mEq/L to compensate for this significant sodium

Table 50.2 Compositions of commonly used oral rehydration solutions (ORS)				
	WHO Standard ORS (1978)	WHO low osmolarity ORS (2002)	ReSoMal	Rice-based ORS
Osmolality (mOsm/L)	311	245	300	200
Glucose (mmol/L)	111	75	125	75
Sodium (mEq/L)	90	75	45	75
Potassium (mEq/L)	20	20	40	20
Chloride (mEq/L)	80	65	70	65
Citrate (mEq/L)	10	10	7.0	10
ResoMal, REhydration SOlution for MALnutrition				

Table 50.3 Content of commonly used oral rehydration solutions (ORS)				
	WHO Standard ORS (1978)	WHO low osmolarity ORS (2002)	ReSoMal	Rice-based ORS
Osmolality mOm/L	311	245	300	200
Glucose	20.0 gm/L	13.5 gm/L	10.0 gm/L	-
Sucrose	-	-	25.0 gm/L	-
Processed rice oowder	-	-	-	50.0 gm/L
Sodium chloride	3.5 gm/L	2.6 gm/L	1.75 gm/L	2.6 gm/L
Tri-Sodium citrate dihydrate	2.9 gm/L	2.9 gm/L	1.45 gm/L	2.9 gm/L
Potassium chloride	1.5 gm/L	1.5 gm/L	2.54 gm/L	1.5 gm/L
Potassium citrate	-	-	0.65 gm/L	-
ResoMal, REhydration SOlution for MALnutrition				

loss. This formula, which WHO and UNICEF have recommended for over 25 years, contains 90 mEq/L of sodium, 20 mEq/L of potassium, and 10 mEq/L of citrate, ensures adequate rehydration, provides electrolytes, and also corrects metabolic acidosis.

However, this ORS's "hyperosmolar" nature had its downsides, notably increasing the risk of hypernatremia and exacerbating stool output due to osmotic effects, especially in infants and young children [20].

These limitations, compounded by the formula's inability to reduce the volume of stool and duration of diarrhea and its unsuitability for well-nourished children with non-cholera diarrhea due to its high sodium content, prompted the search for improved ORS compositions [28].

WHO low osmolarity ORS

In 2002, WHO introduced a revised ORS formula with 75 mEq/L of sodium and an osmolality of 245 mOsm/L, offering a reduction in both sodium content and osmolality compared to the conventional WHO ORS formula.

Reasons and benefits of shifting to revised low osmolarity WHO ORS (2002) [29–31]:

1. **Adaptation to changing pattern of diarrheal diseases:** The evolution of diarrheal diseases, marked by a decline in cholera due to enhanced water and sanitation and a rise in rotavirus infections, prompted a reassessment of ORS formulations. The original ORS formulation, containing 90 mEq/L of sodium, was specifically designed to replace the significant sodium losses associated with cholera, having a mean stool sodium concentration of 88.9 mmol/L. In contrast, the mean stool sodium concentration in rotavirus infections is only 37.2 mmol/L, making the revised ORS with 75 mEq/L sodium a safer and more effective option.

2. **Improved patient tolerance:** The old WHO ORS often led to gastrointestinal discomfort, exacerbated diarrhea, and failed to reduce vomiting and stool volume, mainly due to its high osmolality [32, 33]. The revised formula addresses these issues, improving patient tolerance and acceptance.

3. **Enhanced efficacy and comfort:** The revised WHO ORS formula, with its lower osmolarity (245 mOsm/L) compared to plasma (290 mmol/L), facilitates faster intestinal absorption of sodium and water, resulting in several benefits [26, 34]:
   - Lower stool volumes: A 25% reduction in stool output or volume compared to the original WHO ORS formula.
   - Less vomiting: A reduction in vomiting by approximately 30%, minimizing further fluid loss.
   - Reduced need for IV fluids: Over a 30% reduction in the requirements for IV therapy requiring less hospitalization.
   - Shortened diarrhea duration: The diarrhea length is reduced by 24–48 hours.

4. **Safety even in cholera:** Proven safe and effective not only in managing dehydration caused by rotavirus diarrhea but also in cholera cases, without leading to significant symptomatic hyponatremia [35].

In light of these substantial benefits, the revised hypo-osmolar ORS has been endorsed as the standard by the

WHO and is supported by American and European medical authorities, largely replacing the old WHO ORS high sodium formulation [12, 36, 37].

ReSoMal

Introduced in 2002, ReSoMal (REhydration SOlution for MALnutrition) is a specially designed ORS formula that offers optimal rehydration and electrolytes supplementation and addresses micronutrient deficiencies in malnourished children with diarrhea [38].

ReSoMal, strongly recommended by WHO for rehydration in severe acute malnutrition (SAM), has a different composition compared to the old WHO ORS, such as [29]:

- **Lower sodium** content (45 mEq/L) to prevent the risk of hypernatremia, fluid overload, and cardiac failure.
- **Higher potassium** content (40 mEq/L) to address the potassium deficiency commonly found in malnourished children.
- **Higher glucose** content (30 gm/L glucose/sucrose) to provide optimal calories.
- **Contains microminerals** such as magnesium, zinc, and copper concentrations to correct micronutrient deficiencies.

Due to its lower sodium concentration of 45 mEq/L, ReSoMal carries a risk of hyponatremia. It should be used cautiously and is unsuitable for treating cholera, a condition that results in very high sodium losses.

Rice-based ORS

Rice-based ORS uses processed rice powder as a substitute for the glucose or sucrose found in WHO ORS, and its electrolyte content, including sodium, potassium, chloride, and citrate, is similar to that of the Low Osmolarity WHO ORS. Benefits of Rice-based ORS include:

Increased efficacy: With an osmolality of 200 mOsm/L, rice-based ORS is significantly less osmolar than both the Standard WHO ORS at 311 mOsm/L and the low osmolarity WHO ORS at 245 mOsm/L.

The reduced osmolality of rice-based ORS significantly lessens both stool output and diarrhea duration in adults and children suffering from cholera [22, 39–41]. However, these advantages are not observed in infants and children with non-cholera diarrhea, and rice-based ORS doesn't prove to be superior to the standard glucose-based ORS [40].

Better taste: Rice-based ORS tends to be more accepted and popular, especially in regions where rice is a staple food.

Superior nutritional profile: This formula offers protein alongside calories, contributing to enhanced nutrition that helps in recovery during the acute stage of illness [42].

Gastrointestinal comfort: Patients often experience better gastrointestinal comfort due to the complex carbohydrates present in rice powder.

ZINC IN ORS

Administering zinc supplementation has reduced the duration and severity of diarrhea and has also been shown to prevent subsequent episodes [43–45]. In children with diarrhea, WHO recommends providing 20 mg per day of zinc for 10–14 days (10 mg per day for infants under six months) [45]. Because of its lifesaving properties, safety, and cost-effectiveness, zinc sulfate is a promising addition to ORS for enhanced diarrhea treatment [43].

TREATMENT PLAN BASED ON SEVERITY OF DEHYDRATION

Oral rehydration treatment is tailored according to the patient's degree of dehydration. There are three distinct plans - A, B, and C, each designed to address specific levels of dehydration based on the child's clinical condition.

Plan A: Home treatment – for <5% fluid loss – no dehydration

• Administer 50–100 ml of ORS after each loose stool for children under 2 years of age, and increase the amount for those over 2 years of age.

• Avoid offering high osmolality fluids like undiluted juices, and instead, provide low sodium maintenance oral rehydration solution "ad libitum."

Plan B: Clinic-based ORT – for 5–10% fluid loss – some signs of dehydration

• Administer ORS at the clinic and reassess the patient to determine whether admission or home discharge is appropriate.

• Administer 75 mL/kg body weight ORS within 4 hours (or 10 mL/kg/ hour ORS for 4 hours).

• Reassessment at 4-hour intervals. Increase the amount and rate if diarrhea continues or rehydration is inadequate.

• Allow early breastfeeding 'ad libitum' in infants. In children provide home made foods such as rice and dal water, vegetable soup, yogurt drink with salt (salted Lassi), sugar and salt containing lemon water, and coconut water.

• If diarrhea persists, provide extra ORS or maintenance solution (i.e., 5–10 mL/kg or an amount equal to the volume of diarrhea) after each stool.

Plan C: Admission and IV fluid therapy – for >10% fluid loss – severe signs of dehydration

• Admit the patient for intravenous fluid therapy.

METHOD OF ADMINISTRATION

Practical considerations for effectively administering ORS are summarized below:

• Encourage early administration of ORS for rehydration and replacement of ongoing losses.

• After a vomiting episode, wait for about 20–30 minutes before administering ORS. Once the vomiting has subsided, start by giving frequent small volumes of ORS (about 5 mL per dose) and gradually increasing the amount as tolerated.

• In patients with severe persistent vomiting, administering ondansetron 15 to 30 minutes prior to initiating or resuming ORS can effectively control vomiting, reduce the ORT failure rate, and decrease the need for IV fluids.

• Do not add salt or glucose to the prepared ORS solution. It will make the fluid hyperosmolar and will aggravate the diarrhea and dehydration.

• ORS should be given in small amounts (by small spoon, small cup, dropper, or syringe) at short intervals (every one or two minutes). Large fluid volume can stimulate the gastrocolic reflex, resulting in a quick passage of stool or vomiting.

• A child should never be kept on ORS fluid alone for more than 24 hours. Fasting has been shown to prolong diarrhea. Encourage early breastfeeding after the initial 4-hour rehydration period with ORS, even if the child continues to have diarrhea or vomiting.

- A nasogastric (NG) tube is used for children who have difficulty drinking adequately or who refuse to drink. For patients with persistent vomiting, it allows the continuous, steady administration of ORS at a slow rate.

- To prepare the ORS solution, pour the entire contents of the sachet into a clean container containing precisely 1 liter of clean water, then mix well until it's fully dissolved. It's crucial to measure the volume of water accurately when diluting the ORS sachet, as the effectiveness of the solution is dependent on achieving a precise concentration. Any error in the preparation process could change the solution's composition, either diminishing its effectiveness or causing potential adverse effects.

- ORS solution should be consumed within 12 hours if stored at room temperature or within 24 hours if kept refrigerated; otherwise, it should be discarded.

MONITORING ORS THERAPY

Monitoring of ORS therapy is essential to assess hydration status and analyze the patient's response to treatment to ensure optimal rehydration and recovery. Here are the key components:

Clinical assessment: Evaluating the patient's hydration levels before and after treatment by regularly checking for signs of dehydration like sunken eyes, poor skin turgor, and dry mouth, along with monitoring vital signs such as pulse rate, blood pressure, and temperature,

assists in assessing the effectiveness of the ORS therapy.

Laboratory assessment: Routine serum electrolyte testing before starting ORS in diarrhea patients is unnecessary. However, laboratory evaluation is essential for selected patients undergoing ORS therapy, especially those with severe dehydration, suspected sepsis, persistent vomiting, an existing medical condition, or a lack of response to initial rehydration measures.

Progress evaluation: Mothers should be instructed to record and maintain a simple chart noting the prescribed and actual amounts of ORS administered, the number of vomiting and diarrhea episodes, and the frequency, volume, and color of urine; this information is crucial for adjusting the treatment to optimize its effectiveness [46].

Emergency reporting: The mother should be instructed to contact the doctor during ORS therapy if the child exhibits signs of increased dehydration, persistent vomiting, reduced urine output, fever, unresponsiveness, or if there is no improvement in the child's condition.

REFERENCES

1. Hirschhorn N. The treatment of acute diarrhea in children. An historical and physiological perspective. Am J Clin Nutr. 1980;33(3):637–63.

2. Hartman S, Brown E, Loomis E, et al. Gastroenteritis in Children. Am Fam Physician. 2019;99(3):159–165.

3. Guandalini S. Treatment of acute diarrhea in the new millennium. J Pediatr Gastroenterol Nutr 2000;30(5):486–489.

4. Satheesh G, Unnikrishnan MK. The alarming need for universalising Oral Rehydration Therapy: How many more children must die? Journal of Global Health Economics and Policy. 2022;2:e2022007.

5. World Health Organization. Oral rehydration salts: production of the new ORS. World Health Organization 2006.

6. Ofei SY, Fuchs GJ 3rd. Principles and practice of Oral rehydration. Curr Gastroenterol Rep. 2019;21(12):67.

7. Lenters LM, Das JK, Bhutta ZA. Systematic review of strategies to increase use of oral rehydration

solution at the household level. BMC Public Health. 2013;13(3):S28.

8. Munos MK, Walker CL, Black RE. The effect of oral rehydration solution and recommended home fluids on diarrhoea mortality. Int J Epidemiol. 2010;39 Suppl 1(Suppl 1):i75–87.

9. Spandorfer PR, Alessandrini EA, Joffe MD, et al. Oral versus intravenous rehydration of moderately dehydrated children: a randomized, controlled trial. Pediatrics. 2005;115(2):295–301.

10. Hartling L, Bellemare S, Wiebe N, et al. Oral versus intravenous rehydration for treating dehydration due to gastroenteritis in children. Cochrane Database Syst Rev. 2006;2006(3):CD004390.

11. Centers for Disease Control and Prevention. Guidelines for the Management of Acute Diarrhea after a Disaster. 2014. Available from: https://www.cdc.gov/disasters/disease/diarrheaguidelines.html.

12. Guarino A, Ashkenazi S, Gendrel D, et al. European Society for Pediatric Gastroenterology, Hepatology, and Nutrition/European Society for Pediatric Infectious Diseases evidence-based guidelines for the management of acute gastroenteritis in children in Europe: update 2014. J Pediatr Gastroenterol Nutr. 2014;59(1):132–52.

13. Powers KS. Dehydration: isonatremic, hyponatremic, and hypernatremic recognition and management. Pediatr Rev 2015;36(7):274–85.

14. Mahalanabis D, Sack RB, Jacobs B, et al. Use of an oral glucose-electrolyte solution in the treatment of paediatric cholera--a controlled study. J Trop Pediatr Environ Child Health. 1974;20(2):82–7.

15. Loo DD, Zeuthen T, Chandy G, et al. Cotransport of water by the Na+/glucose cotransporter. Proc Natl Acad Sci U S A. 1996;93(23):13367–70.

16. Chen L, Tuo B, Dong H. Regulation of intestinal glucose absorption by ion channels and transporters. Nutrients. 2016;8(1):43.

17. Sarangi G, Mohanty N, Kadam N. The Prospects of ORS And Miles Ahead; New Indian Journal of Pediatrics, 2019;8(3):39–54.

18. Goodall RM. Oral Rehydration Therapy: How it Works. Rehydration Project: Focus on Diarrhea, Dehydration and Rehydration. Updated 2019 Jul 18. Available from: https://rehydrate.org/ors/ort-how-it-works.htm.

19. Buccigrossi V, Lo Vecchio A, Bruzzese E, et al. Potency of oral rehydration solution in inducing fluid absorption is related to glucose concentration. Sci Rep 2020;10(1):7803.

20. WHO. Oral rehydration salts (ORS) a new reduced osmolarity formulation. updated: 23 August, 2019. [ONLINE] Available via http://www.rehydrate.org/ors/expert-consultation.html (Accessed 27 September 2023).

21. World Health Organization. 2002. "New Formula Oral Rehydration Solution." In WHO Drug Information. Vol. 16, No. Geneva: WHO. Available at http://apps.who.int/medicinedocs/en/d/Js4950e/2.4.html.

22. Gregorio GV, Gonzales ML, Dans LF, et al. Polymer-based oral rehydration solution for treating acute watery diarrhoea. Cochrane Database Syst Rev. 2016;12(12):CD006519.

23. Aghsaeifard Z, Heidari G, Alizadeh R. Understanding the use of oral rehydration therapy: A narrative review from clinical practice to main recommendations. Health Sci Rep. 2022;5(5):e827.

24. CHOICE study group. Multicenter, Randomized, double-blind clinical trial to evaluate the efficacy and safety of a reduced Osmolarity Oral Rehydration salts solution in children with acute watery diarrhea. Pediatrics. 2001;107(4):613–8.

25. Hahn S, Kim Y, Garner P. Reduced osmolarity oral rehydration solution for treating dehydration due to diarrhoea in children: systematic review. BMJ 2001;323(7304):81–5.

26. Hahn S, Kim S, Garner P. Reduced osmolarity oral rehydration solution for treating dehydration caused by acute diarrhoea in children. Cochrane Database Syst Rev 2002;(1):CD002847.

27. Islam M, Samadi AR, Ahmed SM, et al. Oral rehydration therapy: Efficacy of sodium citrate equals to sodium bicarbonate for correction of acidosis in diarrhoea. Gut 1984;25(8):900–4.

28. Suh JS, Hahn WH, Cho BS. Recent Advances of Oral Rehydration Therapy (ORT). Electrolyte Blood Press. 2010;8(2):82–6.

29. Houston KA, Gibb JG, Maitland K. Oral rehydration of malnourished children with diarrhoea and dehydration: a systematic review. Wellcome Open Res. 2017;2:66.

30. Mohanty N, Thapa BR, Mathai J, et al. Low Osmolarity Oral Rehydration Salt Solution (LORS) in Management of Dehydration in Children. Indian Pediatr. 2021;58(3):266–272.

31. Bawankar B. Use of Low Osmolarity Oral Rehydration Salt solution (LORS) in the treatment of dehydration in children. Asian J Biomed Pharmaceut Sci. 2022;12(92):137.

32. Hirschhorn N, Nalin DR, Cash RA, Greenough WB 3rd. Formulation of oral rehydration solution. Lancet. 2002;360(9329):340–341.

33. Duggan C, Fontaine O, Pierce NF, et al. Scientific rationale for a change in the composition of oral rehydration solution. JAMA. 2004;291(21):2628–31.

34. World Health Organisation (WHO), United Nations Children Fund (UNICEF) Joint Statement: Clinical management of acute diarrhea. WHO 2004. Available from: https://www.who.int/publications/i/item/WHO_FCH_CAH_04.7 Accessed October 2, 2023.

35. Alam NH, Yunus M, Abu S, et al. Symptomatic hyponatremia during treatment of dehydrating diarrheal disease with reduced osmolarity oral rehydration solution. JAMA. 2006;296(5):567–73.

36. Pocket book of hospital care for children 2nd edition. Guidelines for the management of common childhood illnesses.In: Geneva: World Health Ogantization;2013.

37. USAID Global Health Supply Chain Program. Manual for Procurement & Supply of Quality-Assured MNCH Commodities. MODULE 3, ORAL REHYDRATION, ORS-1. [Internet]. [cited 2023 October 3]. Available from: https://www.ghsupplychain.org/sites/default/files/2019-02/MNCH%20Commodities-OralRehydration.pdf.

38. Ashworth A, Khanum S, Jackson A, et al. Guidelines for the inpatient treatment of severely malnourished children. In: Geneva: World Health Organization;2003;51.

39. Gore SM, Fontaine O, Pierce NF. Impact of rice based oral rehydration solution on stool output and duration of diarrhoea: meta-analysis of 13 clinical trials. British Medical Journal, 1992;304(6822):287–91.

40. Fontaine O, Gore SM, Pierce NF. WITHDRAWN: Rice-based oral rehydration solution for treating diarrhoea. Cochrane Database Syst Rev. 2007;1998(4):CD001264.

41. Sundari TA, Soetjiningsih I, Yati Soenarto SS, et al. Efficacy of reduced osmolarity oral rehydration solution, rice-based oral rehydration solution, and standard WHO oral rehydration solution in children with acute diarrhea – a randomized open trial. Paediatr Indones 2009;49(3):169–176.

42. Molla AM, Ahmed SM, Greenough WB 3rd. Rice-based oral rehydration solution decreases the stool volume in acute diarrhoea. Bull World Health Organ. 1985;63(4):751–6.

43. Walker CL, Black RE. Zinc for the treatment of diarrhoea: effect on diarrhoea morbidity, mortality and incidence of future episodes. Int J Epidemiol. 2010;39(Suppl 1):i63–9.

44. Lazzerini M, Wanzira H. Oral zinc for treating diarrhoea in children. Cochrane Database Syst Rev 2016;12(12):CD005436.

45. World Health Organization. Intervention. Zinc supplementation in the management of diarrhoea. WHO; updated 2023 Aug 9. Available from: https://www.who.int/tools/elena/interventions/zinc-diarrhoea.

46. Kailemia M, Kariuki N, Laving A, et al. Caregiver oral rehydration solution fluid monitoring charts versus standard care for the management of some dehydration among Kenyan children: a randomized controlled trial. Int Health. 2018;10(6):442–450.

Part 11

Fluid Therapy in Obstetrics

51 | Maternal Changes and Fluid Management during Pregnancy

During pregnancy, delivery, and in the postpartum period, administration of IV fluids may be required. It is essential to provide appropriate and timely fluid management whenever needed. This chapter aims to provide a basic understanding of the physiological changes that occur in the mother during pregnancy, as well as guidelines for fluid management in the cases of hyperemesis gravidarum and normal delivery.

MATERNAL PHYSIOLOGICAL CHANGES DURING PREGNANCY

Many physiological hemodynamic changes occur during pregnancy, starting just after conception and resolving within six weeks of delivery. An increase in weight gain during pregnancy is attributable to an increased size of the gravid uterus and breasts and an increase in blood volume and extravascular extracellular fluid [1]. Pregnancy-induced hemodynamic and cardiovascular changes ensure optimal growth and development of the fetus, and it also helps in the prevention of blood loss during delivery.

It is essential to understand changes in the circulatory system during pregnancy, such as an increase in cardiac output, retention of sodium and water leading to an expansion of blood volume, and a reduction in systemic vascular resistance and blood pressure. These physiological changes can significantly impact fluid management in pregnant patients, so understanding these changes can help in planning for fluid management in pregnant patients more efficiently.

BLOOD VOLUME CHANGES

Maternal plasma volume and red blood cell increase as early as the fourth week of pregnancy and peak at 28 to 34 weeks of gestation. During pregnancy, there is a retention of 900 to 1000 mEq of sodium and 6 to 8 liters of total body water, causing the expansion of total body volume [2–4].

The increased blood volume during pregnancy helps the body to meet the increased circulatory needs of the fetoplacental unit, which are necessary to sustain the pregnancy. This increased blood volume also allows most women to tolerate significant blood loss during childbirth.

The maternal plasma volume increases by 40% to 50% during pregnancy. In comparison, the red cell volume only increases by 15% to 20%, resulting in hemodilution and a condition known as physiological anemia of pregnancy or relative anemia [5, 6].

CARDIOVASCULAR SYSTEM CHANGES

During pregnancy, cardiac output increases by 30% to 40%. The maximum increase usually occurs around 28–30 weeks of gestation [7]. This increase is due to both increased stroke volume and heart rate.

BLOOD PRESSURE CHANGES

Reduced systemic vascular resistance leads to a fall in blood pressure (BP) during pregnancy. The BP typically falls early in gestation and is usually 10 mmHg below baseline in the second trimester [2]. However, in the third trimester of pregnancy, systemic vascular resistance gradually increases, leading to a slow increase in blood pressure reaching nonpregnant levels by the end of the pregnancy [8].

CHANGES DURING LABOR AND DELIVERY

During labor and delivery, significant hemodynamic changes occur due to anxiety, exertion, pain, uterine contractions, uterine involution, and bleeding. During the first stage of labor, each uterine contraction displaces about 300 to 500 ml of blood into the general circulation and increases central blood volume by as much as 500 ml. As blood volume increases, the stroke volume of the heart also increases, leading to a 50% increase in cardiac output with each contraction.

In addition, maternal pushing efforts in the second stage of labor can further increase cardiac output. Immediately postpartum, cardiac output increases to 80 percent above pre-labor values due to significant autotransfusion associated with uterine involution.

Thus, the cardiac output can increase to 75% above its baseline level during labor and delivery. An increase in blood volume and cardiac output protects the mother from average blood loss of delivery (300–400 ml for a vaginal delivery and 500–800 ml for a cesarean section).

FLUID THERAPY IN HYPEREMESIS GRAVIDARUM

INTRODUCTION

Nausea and vomiting of pregnancy (NVP) is the most frequent problem in the first trimester of pregnancy, which affects 50%–90% of all pregnant women [9,

10]. These symptoms are worse in the morning (but often persist throughout the day) and are usually limited to the first trimester of pregnancy.

Hyperemesis gravidarum (HG) is a severe form of nausea and vomiting that affects a small percentage of pregnant women, ranging from 0.3% to 3%. It can lead to significant weight loss, dehydration, ketoacidosis, hypokalemic metabolic alkalosis from the loss of gastric hydrochloric acid, and nutritional deficiencies [11–15].

Two serious nutritional deficiencies reported with hyperemesis in pregnancy are vitamin B1 (thiamine) deficiency (which can cause Wernicke's encephalopathy) and vitamin K^+ deficiency (which can cause maternal coagulopathy and fetal intracranial hemorrhage) [16].

Hyperemesis gravidarum is the major reason for hospitalization during the first half of pregnancy and remains the second leading cause of hospitalization throughout pregnancy [17, 18].

MANAGEMENT

Management of hyperemesis gravidarum includes adequate hydration, antiemetic medications, electrolyte replacement, vitamin supplementation, and dietary management [19, 20]. Intravenous hydration is an essential intervention aimed at fluid resuscitation and correcting fluid deficit, ketones, electrolytes deficit (primarily hypokalemia), and acid-base balance [21]. In addition, as pregnant women are in a catabolic condition, sufficient caloric requirements must be administered [22].

A. lindications of IV fluids

Common indications of IV fluid administration in hyperemesis gravidarum are [23, 24]:

- Persistent vomiting (three or more times per 24 hours) despite antiemetic medical therapy.
- 5% or more weight loss of prepregnancy weight.
- Severe dehydration with the presence of signs and symptoms due to significant fluid loss such as fatigue, dizziness, decreased skin turgor, postural changes in blood pressure and pulse, ketonuria, electrolyte imbalance, acid-base abnormality like hypochloremic metabolic alkalosis, increased hematocrit, increased BUN to creatinine ratio and abnormal urine specific gravity.

B. Outpatient vs. inpatient IV hydration

Ambulatory (outpatient) intravenous hydration is the recommended first-line treatment for patients with severe or persistent nausea and vomiting. Multiple studies have found this treatment option to be as effective as inpatient care [25, 26].

Hospitalization is recommended if vomiting persists even after rehydration and outpatient management fails [27].

C. Selection of IV fluids

Normal saline (NS) and Ringer's lactate are the mainstay of the management of dehydration and are equally effective in treating complications of hyperemesis gravidarum [28, 29]. Usually, Ringer's lactate (RL) is preferred for the initial aggressive rehydration, and normal saline is used for the subsequent slower rehydration [30].

Why is Ringer's lactate preferred for the initial aggressive rehydration and in patients of HG with severe hyponatremia?

The speed at which one rehydrates depends on the severity of their dehydration. In patients of hyperemesis gravidarum with severe dehydration, 2 liters of Ringer's lactate is infused rapidly initially (first 1 liter RL over 2 hours followed by second 1-liter RL over 4 hours). In severe hyponatremia, avoid rapid administration of a large volume of high sodium containing normal saline (sodium 154 mEq/L), as it can lead to rapid correction of sodium levels and may cause central pontine myelinolysis [30]. Therefore in symptomatic and severe hyponatremia (serum sodium <120 mEq/L), choose low sodium containing Ringer's lactate (130 mEq/L sodium) which carries lower risk of rapid correction of hyponatremia.

Why is normal saline preferred for the subsequently slow rehydration in and in patients of HG with less severe hyponatremia associated with hypochloremia?

For hospitalized women with hyperemesis gravidarum who are hypovolemic with minimal symptoms of hyponatremia and have serum sodium levels >120 mEq/L (low risk of rapid correction) and hypochloremia, normal saline is an appropriate choice for rehydration. Normal saline containing 154 mEq/L sodium and chloride is a preferred fluid in HG for hydration because it corrects vomiting-induced hypochloremia, hyponatremia, hypokalemia, and metabolic alkalosis effectively [31].

If hypokalemic, the woman may require potassium supplementation [12, 32]. Usually, 20 mEq/L of potassium chloride is added to either normal saline or half-normal saline (depending on the serum sodium status) and infused slowly (over 6 to 8 hours) to correct hypokalemia.

In severe hypokalemia, consider potassium replacement using one liter of normal saline with 40 mEq potassium chloride to be infused over 4–6 hours. 10 mEq of potassium per hour is a safe infusion rate if urine output is adequate.

D. Role of dextrose solutions

Avoid dextrose-containing IV fluids for the initial fluid replacement, but it may be beneficial for the subsequent IV fluid infusion. Two reasons to avoid dextrose containing IV fluids for the initial fluid replacement are [33]:

1. Risk of Wernicke's encephalopathy: As thiamine (vitamin B1) deficiency occurs in about 60% of hyperemesis gravidarum patients [34], dextrose-containing IV fluids can precipitate Wernicke's encephalopathy in such patients [10]. Supplement 100 mg of thiamine intravenously with the initial IV fluid on the first day and another 100 mg daily for the next two or three days to prevent Wernicke's encephalopathy [25, 33, 35].

2. Risk of worsening of hypokalemia: Hypokalemia is a common electrolyte abnormality in hyperemesis gravidarum [16]. It is recommended to avoid using dextrose-containing solutions for initial fluid replacement, as dextrose administration stimulates insulin release, which can cause extracellular potassium to be shifted into cells and worsen hypokalemia.

After thiamine supplementation and supplementing potassium, maintain hydration with the dextrose-based solution as it fulfills the caloric requirement and helps in faster improvement of nausea [36]. In addition, evidence suggests better improvement with dextrose saline than normal saline in moderate-severe cases [37]. Finally, select 10% dextrose to provide nutritional supplementation rather than the low-calorie-containing 5% solution [38].

Continue administering IV hydration until ketosis and vitamin deficiencies are corrected, and the patient is able to tolerate oral fluids. Afterward, check and address any associated magnesium, calcium, and phosphorus deficits.

To effectively address fluid deficit with hyponatremia and hypokalemia, it is crucial to monitor the input-output chart and check the blood urea and serum electrolyte levels daily [25]. This will allow for the accurate selection of the appropriate IV fluids necessary for treatment.

FLUID THERAPY DURING NORMAL LABOR AND VAGINAL DELIVERY

INTRODUCTION

Labor is a period of prolonged and vigorous exercise for pregnant mothers. During labor, effective skeletal and smooth muscle contractions require increased energy demand. Glucose is an essential source of maternal energy, which plays an important part in the improvement of muscle performance and overcoming fatigue. Depletion of glycogen stores and fat metabolism to meet glucose demands may cause ketonemia, hypoglycemia, and acidosis. An adequate resource of glucose is needed to maintain exercise tolerance and muscle efficiency during labor. Dehydration adversely affects exercise performance and may be a factor contributing to a longer duration of labor. Providing adequate dextrose and fluids to pregnant mothers during labor can help to provide the necessary energy and hydration they need and may also lead to a faster labor process, shorter labor duration, and potentially a reduced need for oxytocin and cesarean delivery

[39, 40]. To assess the hydration status, it is important to monitor urinary output and the presence or absence of ketonuria [41].

ORAL LIQUID INTAKE

Previously, the policy during active labor was "nil by mouth," or restriction of oral intake. This policy was based on the concern that a woman may require general anesthesia for an emergency cesarean section and inhale stomach contents during surgery, leading to aspiration pneumonia [42]. However, the risk of aspiration pneumonia is very low [43], and restricting oral intake can cause dehydration and ketosis [44]. Therefore, this policy is not necessary and may cause harm to the woman [44].

Women with low complication risks and at low risk of cesarean section delivery are allowed and encouraged to consume moderate amounts of clear liquids orally during labor [45–47]. However, to avoid aspiration during uncomplicated labor, it is more important to consider how much suspended particulate matter the fluid ingested contains rather than the volume of fluid permitted to be consumed [45].

During labor, it is necessary to restrict oral intake in patients who are at high risk of aspiration (e.g., morbid obesity, diabetes mellitus, and difficult airway) or those who may need a cesarean section [45].

ORAL SOLID FOOD INTAKE

Avoiding particulate-containing fluids and solid food during active labor and delivery is the standard practice and a recommendation by the American College of Obstetricians and Gynecologists (2009) and the American Society of Anesthesiologists Task Force on Obstetric Anesthesia (2016) [45–47]. This recommendation is because gastric emptying time is remarkably prolonged during labor.

However, the incidence of aspiration is low with current obstetric anesthesia techniques in recent literature. Therefore, solid food restriction in women at low risk of requiring general anesthesia is questioned [42, 48, 49].

Cochrane review (2013) found no evidence to support restriction to eating or drinking in women at low risk of requiring anesthesia for Cesarean section [50]. However, a recent systematic review (Ciardulli et al. 2017) of 10 randomized trials in women with a low-risk singleton (one fetus) pregnancies found that less restrictive policies resulted in a slightly shorter duration of labor [51].

PARENTERAL FLUIDS IN NORMAL LABOR

During normal labor, intravenous fluids are usually administered for proper hydration and to prevent prolonged labor. But as per current evidence from the Cochrane database of systematic reviews (2013), the World Health Organization (2014), and the American College of Obstetricians and Gynecologists (2019), continuous IV fluid infusion is not routinely recommended in normal labor [39, 52].

Regardless of solution type, possible harmful effects to mother and newborn due to the administration of intravenous fluids during labor are:

1. Discomfort, stress, and restriction in freedom of movement.

2. Peripheral swelling and increased risk of fluid overload due to excessive IV fluids.

3. Postpartum breast swelling and feeding issues due to the large volume of IV fluids infusion [53].

4. Fetal volume expansion causes a bloated newborn at birth and greater weight loss of the newborn after birth [54, 55].

Moreover, oral food and liquids are more effective than intravenous fluids in providing energy and nutrition for the increased demand during labor [50]. Thus, instead of administering intravenous fluids to all women during labor, they should be given only to selected patients, considering their limitations and drawbacks.

Conclusion: During normal labor, avoid the "nil by mouth" policy and do not administer intravenous fluids routinely to prevent dehydration and ketosis [39, 52].

A. Indications of IV fluids during labor

When oral fluid intake is restricted, administering IV fluids in a moderate amount shortens the course of labor [39]. So the administration of IV fluid is indicated in selected pregnant mothers.

Common indications for intravenous fluid administration during labor include:

• High-risk pregnancies or restricted oral intake because of the possible need for cesarean delivery.

• Women who develop ketosis in labor [39].

• Following epidural or spinal anesthesia for cesarean delivery to prevent or treat hypotension [56].

• Infusion of oxytocin for induction or augmentation of labor.

• Need to administer intravenous fluids for other clinical reasons such as nausea, vomiting, diarrhea, maternal exhaustion, prolonged labor, blood volume loss, and administration of antibiotics or other medications [57].

B. Type and volume of IV fluids

When IV fluids are indicated, the selection of the type, the volume, and the infusion rate of IV fluid differ on the clinical status of individual women and the anticipated duration of labor [39].

For nulliparous women who are not allowed oral intake during labor, the infusion of dextrose solution significantly reduces the total labor length without increasing the complication rate [40, 58–60].

Because of its cost-effectiveness, safety, and advantages, dextrose should be the default solute for IV fluids during labor [59, 61]. Maintenance intravenous fluid usually administered is 5% dextrose in 0.45 percent saline, normal saline, or Ringer's lactate solution [62]. Avoid administering sodium-free 5% dextrose solution because it may cause maternal and neonatal hyponatremia and increase maternal and newborn morbidity [39].

Rate of infusion: IV fluid administration at a rate of 250 ml/hour, rather than 125 ml/hour, is associated with a shorter duration of labor and lesser need for cesarean section delivery. This data support increased hydration among nulliparous women in labor when oral intake is restricted [63].

FLUID MANAGEMENT DURING SURGERY

PREOPERATIVE ORAL INTAKE

Liquid intake: The uncomplicated patient undergoing elective cesarean delivery may have clear liquids up to 2 hours before induction of anesthesia (American Society of Anesthesiologists (ASA) recommendation 2016) [45]. Consuming high-calorie carbohydrate drinks up to two hours before surgery can reduce preoperative thirst, hunger, anxiety, and the risk of dehydration in patients undergoing abdominal surgery [64, 65].

In pregnant women with a higher risk for aspiration during labor (e.g., morbid obesity, diabetes mellitus, and difficult airway), the recommendation is to restrict oral liquid intake for 6 or more hours, determined on a case-by-case basis [45].

Solid food intake: During elective surgery (e.g., planned cesarean delivery or postpartum tubal ligation) recommended fasting period for solid food is 6 to 8 hours [45].

REFERENCES

1. Cunningham FG, Leveno KJ, Bloom SL, et al. William Obstetrics 24th edition 2014.
2. Cheung KL, Lafayette RA. Renal Physiology of Pregnancy. Advances in Chronic Kidney Disease. 2013;20(3):209–14.
3. Theunissen IM, Parer JT. Fluid and Electrolytes in Pregnancy. Clin Obstet Gynecol 1994;37(1):3–15.
4. Lindheimer MD, Katz AI. Sodium and Diuretics in Pregnancy. N Engl J Med 1973;288(17):891–4.
5. Ueland K. Maternal Cardiovascular Hemodynamics. VII. Intrapartum Blood Volume Changes. Am J Obstet Gynecol 1976;126(6):671–7.
6. Taylor DJ, Lind T. Red Cell Mass During and After Normal Pregnancy. British Journal of Obstetrics and Gynaecology 1979;86(5):364–70.
7. Mashini IS, Albazzaz SJ, Fadel HE, et al. Serial noninvasive evaluation of cardiovascular hemodynamics during pregnancy. Am J Obstet Gynecol. 1987;156(5):1208–1213.
8. Wilson M, Morganti AA, Zervodakis I et al. Blood Pressure, the Renin-aldosterone System, and Sex Steroids Throughout Normal Pregnancy. Am J Med 1980;68(1):97–104.
9. Jarnfelt-Samsioe A. Nausea and Vomiting in Pregnancy: A Review. Obstet Gynecol Surv 1987;42(7):422–7.
10. Jarvis S, Nelson-Piercy C. Management of Nausea and Vomiting in Pregnancy. BMJ 2011;342:d3606.
11. Kallen B. Hyperemesis During Pregnancy and Delivery Outcome: A Registry Study. Eur. J. Obstet. Gynecol. Reprod. Biol. 1987;26(4):291–302.
12. Goodwin TM. Hyperemesis Gravidarum. Clin Obstet Gynecol 1998;41(3):597–605.

13. Broussard CN, Richter JE. Nausea and Vomiting of Pregnancy. Gastroenterol Clin North Am 1998;27(1):123–51.

14. American College of Obstetricians and Gynecologists. Practice Bulletin Summary No. 153: Nausea and Vomiting of Pregnancy. Obstet Gynecol. 2015;126(3):687–688.

15. MacGibbon KW, Fejzo MS, Mullin PM. Mortality Secondary to Hyperemesis Gravidarum: A Case Report. Womens Health Gynecol 2015;1(2):011.

16. London V, Grube S, Sherer DM, et al. Hyperemesis Gravidarum: A review of recent literature. Pharmacology 2017;100(3–4):161–171.

17. Gazmararian JA, Petersen R, Jamieson DJ, et al. Hospitalizations During Pregnancy Among Managed Care Enrollees. Obstet. Gynecol. 2002;100(1):94–100.

18. Poursharif B, Korst LM, Fejzo MS, et al. The psychosocial burden of hyperemesis gravidarum. J Perinatol. 2008;28(3):176–181.

19. Bottomley C, Bourne T. Management Strategies for Hyperemesis. Best Pract Res Clin Obstet Gynaecol 2009;23(4):549–64.

20. Tan PC, Omar SZ. Contemporary approaches to hyperemesis during pregnancy. Curr Opin Obstet Gynecol 2011;23(2):87–93.

21. Bustos M, Venkataramanan R, Caritis S. Nausea and vomiting of pregnancy - what's new? Auton Neurosci Basic Clin. 2017;202:62–72.

22. Tamay AG, Kuscu NK. Hyperemesis Gravidarum: Current Aspect. J Obstet Gynaecol 2011;31(8):708–712.

23. Intravenous (IV) Hydration Therapy for Hyperemesis Gravidarum. HMSA 2015.

24. Liu C, Zhao G, Qiao D, et al. Emerging Progress in Nausea and Vomiting of Pregnancy and Hyperemesis Gravidarum: Challenges and Opportunities. Front Med (Lausanne). 2022;8:809270.

25. The Management of Nausea and Vomiting of Pregnancy and Hyperemesis Gravidarum. RCOG Green-top Guideline No. 69. June 2016.

26. Mitchell-Jones N, Farren JA, Tobias A, et al. Ambulatory versus inpatient management of severe nausea and vomiting of pregnancy: a randomised control trial with patient preference Arm BMJ Open 2017;7(12):e017566.

27. Cunningham FG, Leveno KJ, Bloom SL, et al. Chapter 54: Gastrointestinal Disorders, Williams Obstetrics, 25 2018 McGraw-Hill Education.

28. Rao A. Hyperemesis Gravidarum in Pregnancy. Intrapartum NICE Guidelines August 2016.

29. Adibah I, Khursiah D, Ahmad AI, et al. Hartman's solution or normal saline in the treatment of hyperemesis gravidarum among south east asian population: a randomised controlled trial". International Medical Journal 2008;7:2.

30. Deb S. NHS Guidelines on Management of Hyperemesis Gravidarum. 2017.

31. Guideline for Management and Treatment of Hyperemesis Gravidarum. Initiated By: Cwm Taf Morgannwg University Health Board Gynaecology Forum. Date Approved: 28th July 2022. Available from: https://wisdom.nhs.wales/health-board-guidelines/cwm-taf-gynaecology-file/hyperemesisctm-guideline-august-2022pdf/ [Accessed March 23, 2023].

32. Morantz C, Torrey B. Practice Guideline Briefs. Am Fam Physician 2004;70:601–02.

33. Chiossi G, Neri I, Cavazzuti M, et al. Hyperemesis gravidarum complicated by wernicke encephalopathy: background, case report, and review of the literature. Obstet Gynecol Surv 2006;61(4):255–68.

34. Van Stuijvenberg ME, Schabort I, Labadarios D, et al. The nutritional status and treatment of patients with hyperemesis gravidarum. Am J Obstet Gynecol 1995;172(5):1585–91.

35. Giugale LE, Young OM, Streitman DC. Iatrogenic wernicke encephalopathy in a patient with severe hyperemesis gravidarum. Obstet Gynecol 2015;125(5):1150–1152.

36. Tan P, Norazilah MJ, Omar SZ. Dextrose saline compared with normal saline rehydration of hyperemesis gravidarum; a randomized controlled trial Obstet Gynaecol 2013;121(2 Pt 1):291–298.

37. McParlin C, O'Donnell A, Robson SC, et al. Treatments for Hyperemesis Gravidarum and Nausea and Vomiting in Pregnancy: A Systematic Review. JAMA. 2016;316(13):1392–1401.

38. Fejzo MS, Trovik J, Grooten IJ, et al. Nausea and vomiting of pregnancy and hyperemesis gravidarum. Nat Rev Dis Primers. 2019;5(1):62.

39. Dawood F, Dowswell T, Quenby S. intravenous fluids for reducing the duration of labour in low risk nulliparous women. The Cochrane Data Base of Systematic Reviews. 2013(6):CD007715.

40. Movahed F, Pakniat H, Ataee, M, et al. Normal saline and dextrose-saline infusion comparison in the duration of active phase in nulliparous Women. Biotech Health Sci. 2015;2(4):e31666.

41. ACOG Committee Opinion No. 766: Approaches to limit intervention during labor and birth. February 2019;133(2):e164–e173.

42. Sperling JD, Dahlke JD, Sibai BM. Restriction of oral intake during labor: whither are we bound? Am J Obstet Gynecol 2016;214(5):592–6.

43. Robinson M, Davidson A. Aspiration Under Anaesthesia: Risk Assessment and Decision-Making. Cont Educ Anaesth Crit Care Pain. 2014;14(4):171–175.

44. Ozkan SA, Kadioglu M, Rathfisch G. Restricting oral fluid and food intake during labor: a qualitative analysis of women's views. International Journal of Caring Sciences. 2017;10(1):235–242.

45. Practice Guidelines for Obstetric Anesthesia: An updated report by the american society of anesthesiologists task force on obstetric anesthesia and the society for obstetric anesthesia and perinatology. Anesthesiology, 2016;124(2):270–300.

46. ACOG Committee Opinion No. 441: Oral Intake During Labor. American College of Obstetricians and Gynecologists. Obstet Gynecol 2009;114(3):714.

47. O'Sullivan G, Scrutton M. NPO During Labor. Is there any scientific validation? Anesthesiol Clin North America 2003;21(1):87–98.

48. WHO Recommendation on Oral Fluid and Food Intake During Labor, For Women At Low Risk (May 2014). The WHO Reproductive Health Library; Geneva: World Health Organization.

49. Lee L, Dy J, Azzam H. Practice Guidelines for the Society of Obstetricians and Gynaecologists of Canada: Management of Spontaneous Labor at Term in Healthy Women J Obstet Gynaecol Can 2016;38(9):843–865.

50. Singata M, Tranmer J, Gyte GM. Restricting Oral Fluid and Food Intake During Labour. Cochrane Database of Systematic Reviews 2013;2013(8):CD003930.

51. Ciardulli A, Saccone G, Anastasio H, et al. Less-Restrictive Food Intake During Labor in Low-Risk Singleton Pregnancies A Systematic Review and Meta-analysis Obstet Gynecol 2017;129(3):473–80.

52. WHO Recommendation on the Use of Intravenous Fluids with the Aim of Shortening the Duration of Labor (May 2014). The WHO Reproductive Health Library; Geneva: World Health Organization.

53. Kujawa-Myles S, Noel-Weiss J, Dunn S, et al. Maternal intravenous fluids and postpartum breast changes: a pilot observational study. Int Breastfeed J. 2015;10(1):18.

54. Watson J, Hodnett E, Armson BA, et al. A randomized controlled trial of effect of intrapartum intravenous fluid management on breastfed newborn weight loss. J Obstet Gynecol Neonatal Nurs. 2012;41(1):24–32.

55. Noel-Weiss J, Woodend AK, Peterson WE, et al. An observational study of associations among maternal fluids during parturition, neonatal output, and breastfed newborn weight loss. Int Breastfeed J 2011;6:9.

56. Hofmeyr GJ, Cyna A, Middleton P. Prophylactic Intravenous Preloading for Regional Analgesia in Labor. Cochrane Database Syst Rev. 2004;11(4):CD000175.

57. Rebecca Dekker. Evidence on: IV Fluids During Labor. May 31 2017 https://evidencebasedbirth.com/iv-fluids-during-labor/.

58. Swidan KH, Abou-gamrah AA, Abdel Shafy A, et al. Effect of Normal Saline Infusion versus Dextrose 5% Infusion on The Duration of Labor in Nulliparous Women: Randomized Controlled Trial. The Egyptian Journal of Hospital Medicine. 2017;68(3):1452–1461.

59. Paré J, Pasquier JC, Lewin A, et al. Reduction of total labor length through the addition of parenteral dextrose solution in induction of labor in nulliparous: results of DEXTRONS prospective randomized controlled trial. American Journal of Obstetrics and Gynecology. 2017;216(5):508.e1–508.e7.

60. Yulghunlu FA, Shafaie FS, Mirghafourvand M, et al. The effects of intravenous Dextrose 5%, Ringer's Solution, and oral intake on the duration of labor stages in nulliparous women: a double-blind, randomized, controlled trial. The Journal of Maternal-Fetal & Neonatal Medicine. 2020;33(2):289–296.

61. Shrivastava VK, Garite TJ, Jenkins SM, et al. A Randomized, Double-blinded, Controlled Trial Comparing Parenteral Normal Saline with and without Dextrose on the Course of Labor in Nulliparous. Am J Obstet Gynecol 2009;200(4):379.e1–6.

62. Funai EF, Norwitz ER, et al. Management of Normal Labor and Delivery. UptoDate Mar 07, 2019.

63. Ehsanipoor RM, Saccone G, Seligman NS, et al. Intravenous fluid rate for reduction of cesarean delivery rate in nulliparous women: a systematic review and meta-analysis. Acta Obstet Gynecol Scand 2017;96(7):804–811.

64. Hausel J, Nygren J, Lagerkranser M, et al. A carbohydrate-rich drink reduces preoperative discomfort in elective surgery patients. Anesth Analg. 2001;93(5):1344–50.

65. Singh JP. Preoperative oral carbohydrate drink improves surgical outcome. 2018;6(2):72–73.

52 | Fluid Management for Cesarean Delivery

INTRODUCTION

Spinal anesthesia is the most common type of anesthesia used in cesarean sections [1].

Maternal hypotension is the most common complication of spinal anesthesia for cesarean delivery. Maternal hypotension is defined as systolic blood pressure (SBP) <90 mmHg or a reduction in mean arterial blood pressure >30% fall from baseline [2].

The incidence of maternal hypotension during spinal anesthesia for elective cesarean delivery is much higher (70–80%) [3] as compared to the incidence of hypotension caused by spinal anesthesia in nonpregnant women (about 33%) [4].

Mechanism of maternal hypotension: Spinal anesthesia blocks the sympathetic nerve fibers innervating smooth muscles of arteries and veins, which causes reduced peripheral vascular resistance and vasodilatation. Vasodilatation in the lower part of the body is the crucial mechanism of the development of hypotension due to spinal anesthesia in uncomplicated pregnancy [5].

Consequences of maternal hypotension: Maternal hypotension after spinal anesthesia for cesarean section causes both maternal and fetal/neonatal adverse effects [6]. Spinal hypotension can result in maternal nausea, vomiting, and dizziness due to a reduction in cerebral perfusion, which induces transient brainstem ischemia [7]. In addition, treatment of spinal hypotension can cause iatrogenic pulmonary edema or severe maternal hypertension. Severe and sustained hypotension can decrease uteroplacental perfusion, which can cause fetal hypoxia, acidosis, and neonatal depression [8].

MANAGEMENT

The goal of management is to optimize maternal, uterine, and fetal perfusion, which is crucial for the mother's safety and the baby's wellbeing.

Major steps in treating spinal hypotension are fluid loading, vasopressor, and non-pharmacological measures. Combinations of interventions will be more effective than single ones [9].

THE GOAL OF BLOOD PRESSURE

Treatment aims to maintain systolic blood pressure ≥100 mmHg or ≥90% of an accurately measured baseline blood pressure [10, 11].

FLUID LOADING

Before the initiation of spinal anesthesia, it is important for the patient to have large-diameter intravenous access (preferably 16 or 18 gauge) in place. This will allow for the rapid administration of fluids, medications, and blood products if necessary.

The two most important determinants for the optimal and effective treatment of spinal hypotension are: (1) The type of fluid (crystalloid compared with colloid solutions) and, (2) The timing of administration [given before spinal anesthesia (preloading) or given immediately after spinal block placement (co-loading) as rapid infusions.

A. Preloading

Preloading is a method where IV fluid is administered immediately before spinal anesthesia to reduce post-spinal hypotension (PSH).

Crystalloid preloading: Rapid administration of 10–20 mL/kg of intravenous Ringer's lactate just 15–20 minutes before spinal anesthesia was previously a routine practice to minimize hypotension resulting from sympathetic blockade. But fluid preloading with crystalloid is clinically ineffective due to its rapid redistribution and therefore is currently not recommended before spinal anesthesia [9, 12, 13].

Colloid preloading: In contrast to crystalloid preloading, colloid preloading significantly reduces hypotension and improves maternal hemodynamics [9, 14].

As preloading is not superior to co-loading (irrespective of the type of IV solution used), one should not waste significant time in administering a predetermined IV fluid volume and consequently delay spinal anesthesia initiation [15].

B. Co-loading

In co-loading, IV fluids are rapidly administered and started simultaneously with spinal anesthesia to reduce post-spinal hypotension. Using co-loading protocols is less time consuming with better (or at least similar) effects than preloading [16].

Co-loading is a more rational and physiological approach. In fluid co-loading, IV fluid administration coincides precisely with the time of the maximal vasodilatory effect of spinal anesthesia and thereby compensates for the "relative hypovolemia" and prevents post-spinal hypotension [17].

Crystalloid co-loading: A balanced electrolyte solution (e.g., Ringer's lactate solution) is the most commonly used intravenous fluid for bolus administration. Usually, a bolus of about 10–15 ml per kg or 500 to 1000 mL of Ringer's lactate is infused as fast as possible in fluid co-loading.

Use dextrose free IV fluids for crystalloid co-loading because it avoids maternal hyperglycemia. The immediate effect of maternal hyperglycemia is fetal hyperglycemia, but it may cause neonatal hypoglycemia after delivery. When dextrose containing IV fluid is administered to the mother before delivery, glucose crosses the placental barrier and can result in fetal hyperglycemia and and hyperinsulinemia. After delivery, the glucose supply is ceased, but neonatal insulin levels are still elevated, which causes neonatal hypoglycemia [18].

The volume of fluid given during spinal anesthesia may vary depending on the patient's underlying co-morbidities and their current volume status, with a smaller volume typically being given to patients with severe preeclampsia.

Crystalloid co-loading is more effective than crystalloid preloading in preventing hypotension during spinal anesthesia for elective cesarean delivery [19–22]. Additionally, crystalloid co-loading is similar in effectiveness to colloid preloading [23].

Colloid co-loading: For colloid co-loading third generation colloids such as tetrastarch (Hydroxyethyl starch 130/0.4) seem safer than other colloids [24]. Colloid co-loading is not superior to colloid preloading [17].

Both crystalloid and colloid co-loading are equally effective in decreasing the incidence of spinal hypotension in cesarean delivery [21, 25]. However, the volume needed for colloid co-loading is less than that required for crystalloid co-loading [23].

Because of less adverse effects, lesser cost, ready availability, and restricted or second line usage of colloids in most studies [26], current literature recommends the use of crystalloids than colloids co-loading in cesarean delivery [27].

Factors affecting fluid requirements: Total requirement of intravenous fluids (crystalloids) during and after cesarean delivery varies considerably but is usually 2 to 3 liters. The requirement of fluid volume may be higher in patients with sepsis syndrome, vomiting, prolonged labor without adequate fluid intake, and increased blood loss.

In patients with preeclampsia, spinal anesthesia tends to cause less hypotension than it does in normal pregnant women. Therefore, it is recommended to use mild to moderate intravascular volume loading during spinal anesthesia in patients with preeclampsia.

The loading of a large volume of fluid carries the risk of pulmonary edema in preeclampsia [19].

VASOPRESSORS

Vasopressor therapy is a crucial component in minimizing spinal hypotension. Fluid loading protocols alone are not usually sufficient to achieve reasonable control in post-spinal hypotension [16]. Besides crystalloid or colloid co-loading, a significant proportion of patients require vasopressors to control spinal hypotension [28].

Vasopressor treatment aims to restore systemic vascular resistance. Alpha-adrenergic agonist drugs are the most appropriate agents to treat or prevent hypotension following spinal anesthesia [11]. In addition, prophylactic vasopressors are superior in preventing adverse neonatal outcomes compared to reactive treatment [29].

Phenylephrine and ephedrine are the two most widely used and recommended vasoconstrictor agents in treating spinal hypotension [15]. Phenylephrine is a synthetic selective direct alpha-adrenergic agonist. Ephedrine is a synthetic mixed adrenergic agonist. Ephedrine is a stimulant that directly activates alpha and beta-adrenergic receptors and indirectly stimulates the release of endogenously stored norepinephrine. Recently, even norepinephrine (noradrenaline) has been found to be helpful in preventing and treating spinal hypotension during cesarean delivery.

A. Phenylephrine

A combined approach using titrated phenylephrine with crystalloid co-loading is probably the best option for the management of hypotension during spinal anesthesia for cesarean section [6, 21]. Phenylephrine infusions co-administered with crystalloid has shown to eliminate the likelihood of spinal hypotension [30].

Pharmacology: Phenylephrine is a drug that acts selectively on the alpha-1 adrenergic receptors found on the vascular smooth muscle cells in blood vessels, resulting in vasoconstriction. It is a potent agent that increases total peripheral vascular resistance and increases both systolic and diastolic blood pressure. The onset of action is <1 minute, and its duration of effect is short lasting (15 to 20 minutes). At higher doses, phenylephrine can cause bradycardia due to the activation of baroreceptors, which can lead to a reduction in maternal cardiac output [31].

Preparation: Injection phenylephrine, available as a 1 ml ampoule, contains 10 mg of phenylephrine.

Method of administration (bolus vs. infusion)

In the treatment of spinal hypotension, prophylactic phenylephrine infusion is superior to bolus administration because of the lower incidence of intraoperative nausea and vomiting [32, 33]. An international consensus statement for the management of spinal hypotension by AAGBI (2018) recommends prophylactic phenylephrine infusion as the first line of management [11].

Dose: To prepare an infusion, add 1 ml (10 mg) of phenylephrine solution in 100 ml of normal saline. Each ml of this infusion will provide 100 mcg of phenylephrine (100 mcg/ml solution).

1. **IV bolus:** A commonly used dose of a prophylactic bolus of IV phenylephrine is 50 to 100 mcg (0.5 to 1 ml). Repeat the dose every 2 to 5 minutes as required, but do not give more than a total dose of 200 micrograms (mcg).

2. **IV infusion:** Currently recommended dose of phenylephrine infusion is 25–50 mcg/min. (0.25 to 0.5 ml/min) [11, 16] Prophylactic phenylephrine infusion is started with an infusion pump as soon as the spinal anesthesia is given. The dose is titrated according to maternal systolic blood pressure response and pulse rate.

   A higher incidence of post-spinal hypotension occurs with the lower dose (25 mcg/min), and a higher incidence of reactive hypertension and bradycardia occurs with the higher dose (50 mcg/min) [31, 34].

3. **IV bolus followed by infusion:** When phenylephrine is infused after spinal anesthesia, there will be a delay in achieving adequate blood pressure levels. However, an initial phenylephrine bolus immediately after the spinal anesthesia, followed by a phenylephrine infusion, will maintain blood pressure without adverse effects [5].

B. Ephedrine

Ephedrine is a sympathomimetic drug that stimulates both alpha and beta-adrenergic receptors. As a result, it stimulates the heart rate, increases cardiac output, and variably increases peripheral resistance, leading to an increase in blood pressure.

Previously, ephedrine was the first-line treatment for spinal hypotension. But the trend to use ephedrine in the treatment of post-spinal anesthesia hypotension is decreasing because:

- Repeated administration of ephedrine diminishes its vasoconstrictive effect [35].

- Delayed onset of action of ephedrine may result in a longer period of hypotension than phenylephrine.

- The relatively long duration of the effect of ephedrine makes accurate titration of blood pressure difficult [36].

- Ephedrine may increase the risk of fetal acidosis by crossing the placenta to a greater extent [37].

Currently, ephedrine is preferred to treat spinal hypotension in a pregnant patient with bradycardia, as it typically increases heart rate.

The commonly used dose of ephedrine is 5 to 10 mg IV boluses or 1 to 5 mg/min IV infusion.

C. Phenylephrine versus ephedrine

Ephedrine was previously the first-line therapy for parturients with spinal hypotension [38]. But phenylephrine is currently vasopressor of choice in the treatment of spinal hypotension in the absence of maternal bradycardia [39–41]. Reflex bradycardia and decreased cardiac output are the primary concerns associated with phenylephrine.

As compared to ephedrine, phenylephrine is preferred and superior because of its faster onset [42], ease to titrate, better preservation of uterine blood flow, does not cause or worsen maternal tachycardia [43, 44], less reactive hypertension [45], less incidence of fetal acidosis [46], and less maternal nausea and vomiting [47, 48].

However, ephedrine may be more beneficial in patients with bradycardia, compromised cardiac functions, uteroplacental insufficiency, and preeclampsia [16].

Vasopressor selection based on maternal heart rate:

1. Hypotension and tachycardia: This is the usual response to spinal anesthesia, and phenylephrine is a preferred vasoconstrictor agent in treatment.

2. Hypotension and bradycardia: This is the unusual response that resembles a vagal reaction; rather than 'appropriate' tachycardia and vasoconstriction. Ephedrine is a preferred vasoconstrictor agent for spinal hypotension associated with bradycardia [40].

D. Norepinephrine as vasopressor

Norepinephrine (NE, noradrenalin) is recently introduced to prevent and treat spinal hypotension during cesarean delivery [49, 50]. Norepinephrine (NE) is a potent vasopressor having both alpha-adrenergic agonistic activity, and weak beta-adrenergic agonistic activity. NE has minimal cardiac depressant effect [51]. NE has a similar effect to phenylephrine in maintaining blood pressure but may be associated with higher heart rates (closer to baseline), and greater cardiac output [52, 53].

Because of beneficial cardiac effects and potency, NE may be preferred in mothers with low baseline heart rates or poor cardiac function, where phenylephrine is relatively contraindicated [51].

More research is needed to evaluate the safety and efficacy of norepinephrine before its routine use in obstetric patients [51, 54]. Table 52.1 summarizes all vasopressors used in spinal hypotension during cesarean delivery.

NON-PHARMACOLOGICAL MEASURES

In the supine position, the gravid uterus compresses the maternal abdominal aorta and inferior vena cava, which decreases cardiac output [55]. Positioning protocols for the prevention of post-spinal hypotension are targeted to relieve aortocaval compression imparted by the gravid uterus and increase venous return [16]. Left lateral uterine displacement with 15° table tilt reduces inferior vena cava compression and is routinely recommended in addition to other measures [11, 56, 57].

Table 52.1 Vasopressors in spinal hypotension during cesarean delivery			
Vasopressor	**Phenylephrine**	**Ephedrine**	**Norepinephrine (noradrenaline)**
Mechanism of action	Selective direct α 1 receptor agonist	Direct α and β agonist and indirect release of norepinephrine	Direct α 1 and β 1 agonist
Arterial vasoconstriction	Potent	Less potent	Potent
Chronotropic effect	Negative	Positive	Positive
Maternal heart rate	Reflex bradycardia	Tachycardia	Increased
Cardiac output	Decrease	Increase	Modest increase
Onset of action	Faster	Slower	Immediate
Duration of action	Short-acting (15 to 20 minutes)	Relatively long duration (about 60 min), so longer period of hypotension	Very short (1 to 2 minutes)
Advantage	No maternal tachycardia, better titratability	No maternal bradycardia	Less negative effects on heart rate and cardiac output
Selection	Currently preferred vasopressor in post-spinal hypotension. Preferred in maternal tachycardia	Preferred in maternal bradycardia in post-spinal hypotension	Beneficial effects in mothers with bradycardia and compromised cardiac function in recent studies
Strength of injectable solution and dilution	10 mg/mL (1 mL diluted in 100 ml of normal saline equals 100 mcg/mL)	30 mg/mL, 50 mg/mL (1 mL diluted in 10 ml of normal saline equals 3 mg/mL or 5 mg/mL)	1mg/mL (2 mL diluted in 500 ml of D5W or D5NS equals 4 mcg/mL)
Commonly used doses	50 to 100 mcg IV bolus or 25 to 100 mcg/min IV infusion	5 to 10 mg IV boluses or 1 to 5 mg/min IV infusion	Further studies are required before its routine use

POSTOPERATIVE CARE AFTER CESAREAN DELIVERY

Early oral intake

After cesarean delivery, fluids or food is traditionally avoided until bowel functions return (confirmed by bowel sounds or passage of flatus or stools). But in uncomplicated cesarean delivery, evidences to justify the restriction of oral fluids or food is lacking.

Current evidence suggests that early oral intake (within six hours of delivery) may have several benefits for postpartum care. These benefits include promoting the return of bowel function (through the stimulation of the gastrocolic reflex), encouraging early ambulation, reducing the duration of intravenous fluid administration, decreasing the risk of sepsis, shortening the time to breastfeeding, decreasing the length of hospital stay, and reducing the cost of hospitalization [58–61].

Nausea and vomiting after cesarean delivery can delay early oral intake. In the management of postoperative nausea and vomiting (PONV), the combination of anti-emetics is more effective than monotherapy [62].

During cesarean delivery, intraoperative nausea and vomiting (IONV) are common [7]. Measures to reduce IONV during cesarean are the prevention of hypotension with liberal perioperative administration of IV fluids, maintaining normal blood pressure with prophylactic use of vasopressors (i.e., phenylephrine or ephedrine), administration of anti-emetics (metoclopramide and ondansetron) and minimizing visceral manipulation (e.g., uterine exteriorization) [63, 64].

REFERENCES

1. Shibli KU, Russell IF. A survey of anaesthetic techniques used for caesarean section in the UK in 1997. Int J Obstet Anesth 2000;9(3):160–7.

2. Miller RD. Miller's Anaesthesia. 8th ed. Saunders, an Imprint of Elsevier Inc; 2015. Chapter 56:p.1773.

3. Mercier FJ, Augè M, Hoffmann C, et al. Maternal Hypotension during Spinal Anesthesia for Caesarean Delivery. Minerva Anestesiol 2013;79(1):62–73.

4. Montoya BH, Oliveros CI, Moreno DA. Managing Hypotension Induced by Spinal Anesthesia for Caesarean Section. Rev. Col. Anest. Mayo-Julio 2009;37(2):131–140.

5. Kuhn JC, Hauge TH, Rosseland LA, et al. Hemodynamics of Phenylephrine Infusion Versus Lower Extremity Compression during Spinal Anesthesia for Cesarean Delivery: A Randomized, Double-Blind, Placebo-Controlled Study. Anesthesia and Analgesia 2016;122(4):1120–9.

6. Butwick AJ, Columb MO, Carvalho B. Preventing Spinal Hypotension during Caesarean Delivery: What is the latest? Br J Anaesth. 2015;114(2):183–6.

7. Balki M, Carvalho JC. Intraoperative Nausea and Vomiting during Cesarean Section under Regional Anesthesia. Int J Obstet Anesth 2005;14(3):230–41.

8. Mueller MD, Brühwiler H, Schüpfer GK, et al. Higher Rate of Fetal Acidemia after Regional Anesthesia For Elective Cesarean Delivery. Obstet Gynecol 1997;90(1):131–4.

9. Chooi C, Cox JJ, Lumb RS, et al. Techniques for Preventing Hypotension during Spinal Anaesthesia for Caesarean Section. Cochrane Database Syst Rev. 2017;8(8):CD002251.

10. Klöhr S, Roth R, Hofmann T, et al. Definitions of Hypotension after Spinal Anaesthesia for Caesarean Section: Literature Search and Application to Parturients. Acta Anaesthesiol Scand 2010;54(8):909–21.

11. Kinsella SM, Carvalho B, Dyer RA, et al. International Consensus Statement on the Management of Hypotension with Vasopressors during Caesarean Section under Spinal Anaesthesia. Anaesthesia 2018;73(1):71–92.

12. Mercier FJ. Fluid Loading for Cesarean Delivery under Spinal Anesthesia: Have we studied all the Options? Anesth Analg. 2011;113(4):677–80.

13. Kee WDN. Prevention of Maternal Hypotension after Regional Anaesthesia for Caesarean Section. Current Opinion in Anaesthesiology 2010;23(3):304–9.

14. Melchor JR, Espinosa Á, Hurtado EM, et al. Colloids Versus Crystalloids in the Prevention of Hypotension Induced by Spinal Anesthesia in Elective Cesarean Section. A Systematic Review and Meta-Analysis. Minerva Anestesiologica 2015;81(9):1019–30.

15. Apfelbaum JL, Hawkins JL, Agarkar M, et al. Practice Guidelines for Obstetric Anesthesia: An Updated Report by the American Society of Anesthesiologists Task Force on Obstetric Anesthesia and the Society for Obstetric Anesthesia and Perinatology. Anesthesiology 2016;124(2):270–300.

16. Hasanina A, Mokhtar AM, Badawy A, et al. Post-Spinal Anesthesia Hypotension during Cesarean Delivery, a Review Article. Egyptian Journal of Anaesthesia 2017;33(2):189–193.

17. Carvalho B, Mercier FJ, Riley ET, et al. Hetastarch co-loading is as Effective as Preloading for the Prevention of Hypotension Following Spinal Anesthesia for Cesarean Delivery. Int J Obstet Anesth 2009;18(2):150–5.

18. Sumikura H. Neonatal Hypoglycemia after Cesarean Section. J Anesth 2013;27(2):167–168.

19. Loubert C. Fluid and Vasopressor Management for Cesarean Delivery under Spinal Anesthesia: Continuing Professional Development. Can J Anaesth 2012;59(6):604–19.

20. Ni HF, Liu HY, Zhang J, et al. Crystalloid Coload Reduced the Incidence of Hypotension in Spinal Anesthesia for Cesarean Delivery, When Compared to Crystalloid Preload: A Meta-Analysis. Biomed Res Int. 2017;2017:3462529.

21. Ferre F, Martin C, Bosch L, et al. Control of spinal anesthesia-induced hypotension in adults. Local Reg Anesth 2020;13:39–46.

22. Artawan IM, Sarim BY, Sagita S, et al. Comparison the effect of preloading and coloading with crystalloid fluid on the incidence of hypotension after spinal anesthesia in cesarean section. Bali J Anaesthesiol 2020;4(1):3–7.

23. Tawfik MM, Hayes SM, Jacoub FY, et al. Comparison between Colloid Preload and Crystalloid Co-Load in Cesarean Section under Spinal Anesthesia: A Randomized Controlled Trial. International Journal of Obstetric Anesthesia 2014;23(4):317–23.

24. Van Der Linden P, James M, Mythen M, et al. Safety of Modern Starches used During Surgery. Anesth Analg. 2013;116(1):35–48.

25. Wani SA, Pandit BH, Din MU, et al. Comparative Study to Evaluate the Effect of Colloid Coloading Versus Crystalloid Coloading for Prevention of Spinal Anaesthesia Induced Hypotension and Effect on Fetal Apgar score in Patients Undergoing Elective Lower Segment Caesarean Section: A Prospective Observational Study. Int J Reprod Contracept Obstet Gynecol 2018;7(5):1868–1875.

26. Evans L, Rhodes A, Alhazzani W, et al. Surviving sepsis campaign: international guidelines for management of sepsis and septic shock 2021. Intensive Care Med. 2021;47(11):1181–1247.

27. Rijs K, Mercier FJ, Lucas DN, et al. Fluid loading therapy to prevent spinal hypotension in women undergoing elective caesarean section: Network meta-analysis, trial sequential analysis and meta-regression. Eur J Anaesthesiol. 2020;37(12):1126–1142.

28. Jacob JJ, Williams A, Verghese M, et al. Crystalloid preload versus crystalloid coload for parturients undergoing cesarean section under spinal anesthesia. Journal of Obstetric Anesthesia and Critical Care 2012;2(1):10–15.

29. Mercier FJ. Cesarean Delivery Fluid Management. Curr Opin Anaesthesiol. 2012;25(3):286–91.

30. Kee WDN, Khaw KS, Ng FF. Prevention of Hypotension During Spinal Anesthesia for Cesarean Delivery: An Effective Technique using Combination Phenylephrine Infusion and Crystalloid Cohydration. Anesthesiology 2005;103(4):744–50.

31. Stewart A, Fernando R, McDonald S, et al. The Dose-Dependent Effects of Phenylephrine for Elective Cesarean Delivery under Spinal Anesthesia. Anesthesia and Analgesia 2010;111(5):1230–7.

32. Siddik-Sayyid SM, Taha SK, Kanazi GE, et al. A Randomized Controlled Trial of Variable Rate Phenylephrine Infusion with Rescue Phenylephrine Boluses versus Rescue Boluses Alone on Physician Interventions during Spinal Anesthesia for Elective Cesarean Delivery. Anesth Analg. 2014;118(30:611–8.

33. George RB, McKeen DM, Dominguez JE, et al. Randomized Trial of Phenylephrine Infusion Vs. Bolus for Nausea & Vomiting during Cesarean in Obese Women. Can J Anaesth. 2018;65(3):254–262.

34. Allen TK, George RB, White WD, et al. A Double-Blind, Placebo-controlled Trial of Four Fixed Rate Infusion Regimens of Phenylephrine for Hemodynamic Support during Spinal Anesthesia for Cesarean Delivery. Anesth Analg. 2010;111(5):1221–9.

35. Kee WDN, Khaw KS. Vasopressors in obstetrics: What should we be using? Curr Opin Anaesthesiol 2006;19(3):238–43.

36. Kee WDN, Khaw KS, Lee BB, et al. A Randomized Controlled Study of colloid Preload before Spinal Anaesthesia for Caesarean Section. Br J Anaesth. 2001;87(5):772–4.

37. Kee WDN, Khaw KS, Tan PE, et al. Placental transfer and Fetal Metabolic Effects of Phenylephrine and Ephedrine during Spinal Anesthesia for Cesarean Delivery. Anesthesiology 2009;111(3):506–12.

38. Ralston DH, Shnider SM, DeLorimier AA. Effects of Equipotent Ephedrine, Metaraminol, Mephentermine, and Methoxamine on Uterine Blood Flow in the Pregnant Ewe. Anesthesiology. 1974;40(4):354–370.

39. Van De Velde M. Belgian Guidelines for Safe Regional Anesthesia and Obstetric Anesthesia and Analgesia. Acta Anaesthesiol Belg 2013;64(3):95–96.

40. Nag DS, Samaddar DP, Chatterjee A, et al. Vasopressors in Obstetric Anesthesia: A Current Perspective. World J Clin Cases. 2015;3(1):58–64.

41. Heesen M, Stewart A, Fernando R. Vasopressors for the Treatment of Maternal Hypotension Following Spinal Anaesthesia for Elective Caesarean Section: Past, Present and Future. Anaesthesia 2015;70(3):252–7.

42. Dyer RA, Reed AR, Dyk DV, et al. Hemodynamic Effects of Ephedrine, Phenylephrine, and the Coadministration of Phenylephrine with Oxytocin during Spinal Anesthesia for Elective Cesarean Delivery. Anesthesiology 2009;111(4):753–65.

43. Cooper DW, Carpenter M, Mowbray P, et al. Fetal and Maternal Effects of Phenylephrine and Ephedrine during Spinal Anesthesia for Cesarean Delivery. Anesthesiology 2002;97(6):1582–1590.

44. Gunda CP, Malinowski J, Tegginmath A, et al. Vasopressor Choice for Hypotension in Elective Cesarean Section: Ephedrine or Phenylephrine. Arch Med Sci 2010;6(2):257–263.

45. Lee A, NganKee WD, Gin T. A Dose-Response Meta-Analysis of Prophylactic Intravenous Ephedrine for the Prevention of Hypotension during Spinal Anesthesia for Elective Cesarean Delivery. Anesth Analg 2004;98(2):483–439.

46. Veeser M, Hofmann T, Roth R, et al. Vasopressors for the Management of Hypotension after Spinal Anesthesia for Elective Caesarean Section. Systematic Review and Cumulative Meta-Analysis. Acta Anaesthesiol Scand 2012;56(7):810–6.

47. Prakash S, Pramanik V, Chellani H, et al. Maternal and Neonatal Effects of Bolus Administration of Ephedrine and Phenylephrine during Spinal Anaesthesia for Caesarean Delivery: A Randomised Study. Int J Obstet Anesth 2010;19(1):24–30.

48. Habib AS. A Review of the Impact of Phenylephrine Administration on Maternal Hemodynamics and Maternal and Neonatal Outcomes in Women Undergoing Cesarean Delivery under Spinal Anesthesia. Anesth Analg 2012;114(2):377–90.

49. Kee WDN, Lee SW, Ng FF, et al. Randomized Double-Blinded Comparison of Norepinephrine and Phenylephrine for Maintenance of Blood Pressure during Spinal Anesthesia for Cesarean Delivery. Anesthesiology 2015;122(4):736–45.

50. Onwochei DN, Kee WDN, Fung L, et al. Norepinephrine Intermittent Intravenous Boluses to Prevent Hypotension during Spinal Anesthesia for Cesarean Delivery: A Sequential Allocation Dose-Finding Study. Anesth Analg 2017;125(1):212–8.

51. Hasanin AM, Amin SM, Agiza NA, et al. Norepinephrine Infusion for Preventing Postspinal Anesthesia Hypotension during Cesarean Delivery: A Randomized Dose-finding Trial. Anesthesiology 2019;130(1):55–62.

52. Kee WDN. The Use of Vasopressors during Spinal Anaesthesia for Caesarean Section. Curr Opin Anaesthesiol 2017;30(3):319–325.

53. Kee WDN, Lee SWY, Ng FF, et al. Prophylactic Norepinephrine Infusion for Preventing Hypotension during Spinal Anesthesia for Cesarean Delivery. Anesth Analg 2018;126(6):1989–1994.

54. Dong L, Dong Q, Song X, et al. Comparison of Prophylactic Bolus Norepinephrine and Phenylephrine on Hypotension during Spinal Anesthesia for Cesarean Section. Int J Clin Exp Med. 2017;10(8):12315–12321.

55. Lees MM, Scott DB, Kerr MG, et al. The Circulatory Effects of Recumbent Postural Change in Late Pregnancy. Clin Sci 1967;32(3):453–465.

56. Lee SWY, Khaw KS, Kee WDN, et al. Haemodynamic effects from aortocaval compression at different angles of lateral tilt in non-labouring term pregnant women. British Journal of Anaesthesia 2012;109(6):950–6.

57. Kundra P, Velraj J, Amirthalingam U, et al. Effect of positioning from supine and left lateral positions to left lateral tilt on maternal blood flow velocities and waveforms in full-term parturients. Anaesthesia 2012;67(8):889–93.

58. Guo J, Long S, Li H, et al. Early versus Delayed Oral Feeding for Patients after Cesarean. Int J Gynaecol Obstet. 2015;128(2):100–5.

59. Huang H, Wang H, He M. Early Oral Feeding Compared with Delayed Oral Feeding after Cesarean Section: A Meta-Analysis. J Matern Fetal Neonatal Med. 2016;29(3):423–9.

60. Hsu YY, Hung HY, Chang SC, et al. Early Oral Intake and Gastrointestinal Function after Cesarean Delivery: A Systematic Review and Meta-Analysis. Obstet Gynecol. 2013;121(6):1327–34.

61. Ogbadua AO, Agida TE, Akaba GO, et al. Early Versus Delayed Oral Feeding after Uncomplicated Cesarean Section under Spinal Anesthesia: A Randomized Controlled Trial. Niger J Surg. 2018;24(1):6–11.

62. Ituk U, Habib AS. Enhanced Recovery after Cesarean Delivery. F1000Research 2018;7:F1000 Faculty Rev-513.

63. Habib AS, George RB, McKeen DM, et al. Antiemetics Added to Phenylephrine Infusion during Cesarean Delivery: A Randomized Controlled Trial. Obstet Gynecol. 2013;121(3):615–23.

64. Jelting Y, Klein C, Harlander T, et al. Preventing nausea and vomiting in women undergoing regional anesthesia for cesarean section: challenges and solutions. Local Reg Anesth. 2017;10:83–90.

53 | Fluid Management in Preeclampsia and Postpartum Hemorrhage

Preeclampsia and postpartum hemorrhage are two common problems that need meticulous fluid management.

FLUID MANAGEMENT IN PREECLAMPSIA

Preeclampsia (PE) is a condition that is characterized by hypertension and significant proteinuria that occurs after 20 weeks of pregnancy.

One of the common clinical symptoms of preeclampsia is generalized edema. However, it's important to note that peripheral edema can occur in normal pregnancies. Therefore, one should suspect preeclampsia when weight gain is sudden and rapid (> 2.3 kg/week).

Fluid management for the patient with preeclampsia presents a challenge for the obstetrician as there are considerable controversies and data on the ideal fluid strategy are limited and insufficient [1].

In preeclampsia, two paradoxical findings, intravascular volume depletion, and increased extracellular fluid volume, lead to confusion and different opinions regarding optimal fluid management.

Excessive administration of IV fluids and mobilization of fluid sequestered in the extravascular space into the vascular space carries a high risk of pulmonary edema in preeclampsia [2].

Fluid management should be customized to the specific clinical situation and closely monitored to achieve optimal fluid balance. Fluid management aims to maintain circulating volume and preserve kidney function while minimizing the risk of pulmonary edema.

Basic principles of fluid balance in preeclampsia [1, 3, 4]

- As patients with preeclampsia are edematous, it is important to carefully infuse optimal IV fluids with the aim of restricting fluid to avoid pulmonary edema.

- Aggressive fluid therapy carries a risk of pulmonary edema; therefore, fluid management requires frequent clinical assessment and meticulous attention. Record fluid balance carefully.

- For precise infusion of intravenous fluids, use a volumetric infusion pump.
- Replace obvious blood loss during delivery.
- Pulmonary edema carries a higher risk of death compared to oliguric renal failure. Therefore, it is important to avoid the overuse of crystalloid solutions to treat postpartum hemorrhage (PPH) in patients with preeclampsia.
- Avoiding IV fluids preloads before spinal anesthesia.
- To maintain optimal fluid balance, restrict fluid intake to a maximum of 40 ml per hour plus the previous hour's urine output, up to a total of 80 ml per hour or 1 mL/kg/hr. The type of fluids preferred are balanced crystalloids (Hartmann's solution, Ringer's lactate, or PlasmaLyte).
- As oliguria is common with severe preeclampsia, maintain fluid restriction until there is a postpartum diuresis.
- Administer infused drugs in concentrated solutions to avoid excessive fluid volume administration.
- Do not chase an increased urine output that follows delivery, as it carries a risk of volume overload.
- Insert the indwelling catheter and measure urine output hourly with a urometer.
- In preeclampsia, a central line is usually only indicated if there is significant obstetric bleeding or severe heart dysfunction. Before insertion of the central line, always check the coagulation profile and platelet count because

Preeclampsia is often complicated by HELLP syndrome.

- Monitor SpO$_2$ closely. Fluid overload is the most likely cause of a decrease in oxygen saturation. Deterioration of SpO$_2$ below 95% may indicate impending pulmonary edema. Use diuretics only when the diagnosis of pulmonary edema is confirmed.

Antenatal fluid management

Careful fluid balance is essential. In preeclampsia, it is important to restrict intravenous and oral fluid intake in order to prevent fluid overload and pulmonary edema. When the administration of syntocinon (oxytocin) is indicated, it is advisable to use a high-concentration infusion (30 IU in 500 mL) or, for even more concentrated solutions, dilute it in just 50 mL and deliver it using an infusion pump to prevent fluid overload [4].

Women with preeclampsia have an increased risk of requiring a cesarean delivery. Therefore, keeping them on a "nil by mouth" or limiting oral fluid intake to 30 ml per hour or less is recommended to minimize the risk of complications during surgery [3, 5].

In the antepartum period, furosemide is used only to treat patients with severe preeclampsia complicated by pulmonary edema [6].

Fluid management during labor

Intravenous fluid in preeclampsia: to use or not?

Fluid management in preeclampsia is complex, and there is limited and insufficient data on the ideal fluid strategy for women with this condition [1].

Volume restriction

Acute pulmonary edema is a common cause of death in women with preeclampsia and often leads to admission to the intensive care unit [7]. Pulmonary edema kills, but oliguria and renal failure do not, so administer fluid cautiously in preeclampsia.

A fluid restriction regimen is associated with lower rates of pulmonary edema and good maternal outcome [8, 9]. Multiple recent guidelines recommend against plasma volume expansion (NICE, SOGC, SOMANZ) and recommend fluid restriction (NICE, GAIN, CMQCC, SOGC) [9–13]. For women with severe preeclampsia and without any fluid losses, it is recommended to restrict total fluid intake to 80 ml/hour, which includes oral, drug, and intravenous fluids [9, 10].

Volume expansion

Women with preeclampsia have reduced plasma volume and are usually oliguric. Therefore, fluid restriction is generally recommended in preeclampsia but may not be appropriate for all women. Achieving proper fluid balance before delivery is essential [14]. Intravenous fluid administration may be used judiciously as maintenance therapy or for resuscitation [15]. Replacement therapy is administered according to an estimated deficit and is usually transfused rapidly.

Common indications of fluid administration in preeclampsia are the following [15, 16]:

1. As a vehicle to administered IV labetalol or IV hydralazine for the adequate and more reliable control of severe hypertension.

2. To replace ongoing blood and fluid loss.

3. As a vehicle for administering agents for induction/augmentation of labor and anticonvulsant medication.

4. Maintenance therapy. The preeclamptic woman who is fasting may need intravenous fluid to maintain hydration. Maintenance fluid is commonly given intravenously slowly over 24 hours, and its volume should match the urinary output combined with the insensible loss [15].

5. Oliguria due to suspected or confirmed intravascular volume deficit [17].

The choice of intravenous fluids: colloids vs. crystalloids

The theoretical benefits of colloids are that they remain in the vascular compartment longer than crystalloids, and a smaller volume of solution is required for volume expansion. However, most of the previous comparative trials of colloids and crystalloids excluded pregnant women in their studies, so choosing between these two solutions during labor is controversial [18].

There is no evidence in the literature of general critical care to support the use of colloids over crystalloids for fluid resuscitation, and current studies favor the use of crystalloids over colloids [18–20].

Fluid during spinal anesthesia

Spinal or epidural anesthesia is generally considered better and safer for cesarean section in preeclampsia due to improved hemodynamic stability and better outcomes for newborns [21].

Women with preeclampsia develop less hypotension after spinal anesthesia than healthy women [22–24].

General anesthesia carries a higher risk compared to neuraxial anesthesia in preeclampsia. Some of the significant risks associated with general anesthesia include the risk of aspiration [25] and an abrupt, severe increase in hypertension during intubation and extubation [5, 26]. Such sudden, severe hypertension carries a risk of hypertensive crisis and stroke [27].

Additionally, preeclampsia-associated tissue edema can lead to narrowing around the larynx, making endotracheal intubation difficult [28].

A prophylactically or routine fixed intravenous fluid preload bolus should never be administered before initiating neuraxial anesthesia in preeclampsia [4, 5, 9].

Administer crystalloid/colloid carefully for co-loading. As a general rule, 500 mL to 1000 mL is sufficient unless the fluids are being used to replace blood loss [3, 5].

Phenylephrine is the optimal first-line vasopressor to reverse spinal hypotension in preeclampsia. However, prophylactic vasopressor infusion in preeclampsia is not usually required, and the dose of phenylephrine to treat hypotension may be lower than in healthy women.

It is essential to monitor the blood pressure carefully during cesarean section, as the fetus may not tolerate sudden decreases in blood pressure well. If necessary, a low dose of phenylephrine can be administered to treat spinal hypotension [22, 29].

Postpartum fluid management

- Intravascular volume increases in the postpartum period because of the mobilization of extracellular fluid to the intravascular space and "autotransfusion" of blood from the contracted uterus.

- The greatest risk of postpartum eclampsia is in the first 48 hours because of the profound shift of third space fluid to intravascular volume space after delivery, which may worsen hypertension [30].

- After delivery, it is common for patients to experience a short period of oliguria lasting up to 6 hours. To manage postpartum oliguria, it is recommended to restrict fluid intake after delivery and wait for natural diuresis, which typically occurs within 36–48 hours [5]. During this time, the combined of intravenous and oral fluids intake should be kept at 80 mL per hour or less. The intravenous fluids should be gradually reduced and eventually stopped when the patient can take and tolerate more than 80 mL of oral fluids per hour.

- This approach can help to prevent excess fluid overload.

- Replace appropriate blood products in postpartum hemorrhage, as in cases of placental abruption.

Oliguria in preeclampsia

- A short period (up to 6 hours) of oliguria in the immediate postpartum period is common and physiological, so wait and observe [11].

- Avoid administering fluids to treat this physiological oliguria (<15 mL/h urine output during the initial six hours in the postpartum period) [9].

- If oliguria persists after 6 hours, exclude pre-existing renal disease or a rising creatinine, and subsequently try the fluid challenge to rule out a pre-renal failure.

- A fluid bolus of 250–500 ml of normal saline or Ringer's lactate can be tried as a fluid challenge [13].

- Both dopamine and furosemide should be avoided to treat persistent oliguria [11].

- It is unlikely that short-term oliguria caused by severe preeclampsia will result in irreversible kidney damage.

- Postpartum persistent oliguria (beyond 24 hours) and increased plasma creatinine suggest postpartum renal failure [11].

FLUID MANAGEMENT IN POSTPARTUM HEMORRHAGE

Postpartum hemorrhage (PPH) is a major cause of maternal mortality and is estimated to cause around 30% of maternal deaths or 10 deaths every hour [31, 32]. The definition of PPH varies in different guidelines (Table 53.1). But the common definition of postpartum hemorrhage is blood loss of ≥500 ml for a vaginal delivery and ≥1000 ml for a cesarean birth [32, 33]. In addition, PPH is classified into two categories based on the severity of blood loss: minor (500–1000 mL) or major (more than 1000 mL). Major PPH is further divided into moderate PPH (1000–2000 mL) and severe PPH (more than 2000 mL) [34].

Uterine atony is the most common cause of primary postpartum hemorrhage, accounting for 80% of PPH. Other important causes of PPH are placenta previa, uterine rupture, trauma, placental abruption, and retained placenta.

Diagnosis and estimation

It is challenging to estimate blood loss accurately in PPH. But all possible efforts

Table 53.1 Postpartum hemorrhage definitions	
Guidelines	**Definitions**
World Health Organization (WHO) 2012 [35]	Blood loss >500 mL within 24 hours
International Federation of Gynecology and Obstetrics (FIGO) 2012 [36]	Blood loss >500 ml in a vaginal birth and >1000 ml in a cesarean section
Royal College of Obstetricians and Gynaecologists (RCOG) 2016 [34]	Minor PPH: Blood loss 500–1000 ml without clinical shock Major PPH: Blood loss >1000 mL and continuous bleeding or clinical shock
Royal Australian and New Zealand College of Obstetricians and Gynaecologists, (RANZCOG) 2017 [37]	Blood loss >500 ml during the puerperium Severe PPH: Blood loss >1000 mL
American College of Obstetricians and Gynecologists (ACOG) 2017 [38]	Blood loss ≥1000 ml or more, or signs and symptoms of hypovolemia due to blood loss
NHS Obstetric Hemorrhage Clinical Guideline 2018 [39]	Primary minor PPH: Blood loss of 500–1000 ml within 24 hours of the birth of a baby Primary moderate PPH: Blood loss 1000–1500 mL within 24 hours Primary severe PPH: Blood loss ≥1500 mL within 24 hours Massive PPH: Blood loss ≥2000 mL within 24 hours, hemodynamic instability or sign of shock
A NATA consensus statement 2019 [40]	Primary PPH: Blood loss >500 mL within 24 hours Severe PPH: Blood loss >1000 mL within 24 hours with signs/symptoms of hypovolaemia Massive life-threatening PPH: Blood loss >2500 mL or hypovolemic shock

should be made for its assessment because PPH can be a serious and potentially life-threatening condition.

The volume and speed at which blood is lost in PPH are often underestimated because the blood loss may be concealed. In addition, the physiological hemodynamic changes that occur during pregnancy may mask the typical clinical signs of hypovolemia. Hemodynamic changes which may occur after PPH is variable and depend on several factors such as hematocrit before delivery, cardiovascular status, and the rate of blood loss.

So, the correlation between blood loss and clinical signs is not reliable [41].

Clinical and laboratory parameters that can provide clues for early or undetected postpartum hemorrhage are summarized in Table 53.2.

Shock index: This is a simple-to-use parameter helpful to assess the amount of blood loss and the degree of hypovolemia in hemorrhagic shock, including PPH [43, 44]. The calculation of the shock index is simple: divide the heart rate by the systolic blood pressure. The normal value of the shock index is between 0.5 and 0.7, and a higher value

indicates the presence of shock and is associated with hemodynamic instability.

The peak shock index may be a superior parameter for detecting PPH compared to heart rate or systolic blood pressure [45]. However, the shock index alone is not a good screening tool and should be used with other parameters [46].

Other methods: Various methods, such as visual estimation, direct measurement using calibrated drapes, and the gravimetric technique (which involves weighing blood-soaked materials), are used for estimating blood loss after vaginal birth. However, there is insufficient evidence to support the use of one method over another [47].

Due to the variable clinical signs of hemorrhagic shock and the lack of a rapid and reliable method to accurately detect the amount of blood lost early, the delay in diagnosis of postpartum hemorrhage and its severity is common. This can lead to a delay in therapy. Therefore, the initial step in the appropriate management of PPH is maintaining a high index of suspicion, and the onset of symptoms and signs of volume loss warrants aggressive volume replacement.

Table 53.2 Clues for early or undetected postpartum hemorrhage [42]	
Clinical parameters	**Laboratory parameters**
Tachycardia (>100 bpm) in the absence of clinical hypovolemia and with adequate pain control	Hb fall >2 gm/dL before administration of IV fluids
Hypotension (BP ≤85/45 mmHg or blood pressure fall by 20% from the baseline value)	Severe metabolic acidosis (e.g., base excess <-4, pH <7.2)
Oliguria (urine volume <500 ml/day)	Shock index of >0.9
Persistent or recurrent maternal hypotension despite active fluid resuscitation and/or use of vasopressor drugs	High serum lactate level >4.0 mmol/L
Excessive requirement of IV fluids	Presence of coagulopathy
Cool extremities, tachypnea, inappropriate fear, restlessness, or confusion	-

Management

The medical strategy described as damage control resuscitation (DCR) is used to manage severe acute PPH. Its goal is to limit secondary blood loss, stabilize the patient's condition as quickly as possible and prevent further tissue damage [48, 49].

The main measures for damage control resuscitation include:

1. Hypotensive fluid resuscitation.
2. Blood product transfusion.
3. To identify and control the sources of bleeding as quickly as possible by medical and damage control surgery.

Supportive measures such as raising the legs, administering oxygen, and warming the body in patients with PPH can help improve hemodynamic stability.

Fluid resuscitation

Draw blood for baseline measurements, and obtain an intravenous line with wide a bore cannula. Compared to 18 gauge, 14 gauge cannula can infuse almost double the fluid volume.

Until blood is available, start immediate rapid replacement with crystalloids or colloids for resuscitation and to maintain adequate tissue perfusion.

All crystalloids administered during resuscitation should be warmed and, if possible, given using rapid infusion devices to improve effectiveness and speed.

How much crystalloid to infuse?

For resuscitation in PPH, infuse crystalloids initially to maintain blood pressure while waiting for blood products. Two modalities with different approaches used for fluid resuscitation in PPH are the conventional aggressive approach and the currently recommended hypotensive fluid resuscitation approach [48].

Aggressive fluid resuscitation

The conventional aggressive approach is a traditionally used method in which large volume (>2 liters) of crystalloids are administered to rapidly expand the effective circulating blood volume and restore blood pressure and hemodynamic stability [50, 51]. But current recommendations advise against using an aggressive resuscitation strategy due to the potential for adverse effects, such as coagulopathy due to dilution of coagulation factors, third spacing of fluids, and hypothermia, which can occur due to infusion of large volumes of cold crystalloids [52], and resultant adverse maternal outcomes [53].

Hypotensive fluid resuscitation

Permissive hypotension, also known as hypotensive fluid resuscitation, is an alternative method currently recommended as the preferred strategy for treating PPH. This more cautious approach involves restricting the use of crystalloid fluids to maintain the patient's blood pressure lower than normal to limit secondary blood loss until control of bleeding is achieved and to prevent fluid overload [50, 54]. The aim of administering small crystalloid volumes is to provide adequate tissue perfusion and oxygen delivery to the body's tissues but reduce the risk of dilutional coagulopathy and prevent the disruption of pre-formed blood clots [48, 55]. Multiple studies have shown that hypotensive resuscitation can improve survival rates and is considered a safe and effective fluid resuscitation strategy [50, 56–58].

Recent guidelines recommend avoiding using more than 2 liters of crystalloid solutions or 1.5 liters of colloids in the treatment of PPH before resorting to blood transfusion [34, 59]. In treating PPH, it is more important to rapidly replace fluids and warm the solutions than to focus on the specific type of fluid being infused [34].

Goals of fluid therapy

Crystalloids should be followed immediately with packed red cell replacement using packed red blood cells (RBC) to restore oxygen-carrying capacity and maintain hemoglobin greater than 8 gm/dL.

The goal of therapy is to maintain systolic pressure of 80–90 mm of Hg, urine output >0.5 mL/kg/hr, and normal mental status. It is important to remember that, due to the benefits of permissive hypotension in PPH, the goal of therapy is not to maintain blood pressure in the normal range. So rather than following the standard practice of fluid administration, clinicians should adjust fluid infusion to maintain a target systolic blood pressure of 80–90 mm Hg until major bleeding has been controlled [60].

An alternative goal of fluid administration during the bleeding phase of severe postpartum hemorrhage is to achieve a low mean arterial pressure, which has been recommended to be between 50–60 mm Hg [60] and 55–65 mm Hg [40].

Colloids vs. crystalloids

Colloid solutions may be used as an alternative or an adjunct to crystalloids with the assumption of its greater and longer duration of volume expansion effect. But no colloid solution has been demonstrated to be superior to crystalloids. Compared to crystalloids, colloids are more expensive and carry a greater risk of adverse effects [61, 62]. According to guidelines from the World Health Organization (2012), an intravenous fluid replacement for PPH should be with isotonic crystalloids rather than colloids [35]. A Cochrane review (2018) that compared the use of colloids and crystalloids for fluid resuscitation in critically ill patients (excluding pregnant patients who had undergone cesarean section) found that resuscitation with colloids was not associated with an improvement in survival [20].

Based on these findings, for the resuscitation of women with PPH, isotonic crystalloids should be used in preference to colloids. Avoid dextrans in obstetric practice as they may interfere with platelet function and cross-matching and are hazardous [39]. Also, avoid using hydroxyethyl starch for resuscitation in major PPH [34].

Which crystalloid to give?

Ringer's lactate and normal saline are the two most commonly used crystalloid solutions for initial fluid resuscitation. They are routinely used, inexpensive, readily available solutions without significant side effects. Until blood is available, infuse crystalloid at a volume that is approximately three times the estimated volume of blood loss [39, 63].

Normal saline is usually administered in a labor ward because of its easy availability, low cost, and compatibility with blood transfusions and most drugs. But the infusion of large quantities (>2 L) of normal saline can cause hyperchloremic acidosis [63, 64] and acute kidney injury [65]. Ringer's lactate solution, compared to normal saline, has an electrolyte composition that more closely resembles plasma and can also buffer acidosis due to the metabolism of lactate to bicarbonate. Because of these properties, Ringer's lactate is considered more physiological than normal saline and is increasingly recommended as the first-choice resuscitation fluid [66].

Dextrose-containing IV solutions, such as 5% dextrose or dextrose with saline, should not be used in treating PPH because the rapid infusion of these solutions can cause hyperglycemia and resultant diuresis.

Blood replacement

Timely and adequate blood replacement is crucial and lifesaving in the treatment of severe PPH.

Intravenous fluids vs. blood

Because of the potential harms of large-volume crystalloid resuscitation (e.g., dilution coagulopathy, volume overload, and hypothermia) [67, 68], early blood transfusion should be managed after initial fluid administration.

The trend is growing (hemostatic resuscitation) to transfuse blood components early to correct hypovolemia and allow permissive hypotension in severe acute PPH [40, 48, 55, 69]. The rationale of this strategy is to reduce the contribution of crystalloid solutions and thereby prevent side effects associated with the administration of a large volume of crystalloids.

Indications of blood replacement

There are no clear guidelines for determining when a red blood cell transfusion should be infused [70, 71]. Patients with acute hemorrhage can have normal hemoglobin, so it is important to pay close attention to the clinical evaluation [71].

Common indications of red cell transfusion in PPH are [34, 38, 71–75]:

- Women with a hemoglobin value <6 gm/dL, irrespective of symptoms.

- Clinically severe uncontrollable postpartum hemorrhage.
- Blood loss of 1500 ml or more usually requires blood/pack cell transfusion.
- Blood is usually administered to symptomatic women (maternal tachycardia >110 beats per minute, dizziness, syncope) with active bleeding, irrespective of hemoglobin status. Do not wait for laboratory results; the decision to provide a blood transfusion should be based on clinical signs to avoid delay.
- The combination of a higher shock index (>9) and lactate levels (>4.0 mmol/L), with immediate postpartum lower hemoglobin, predicts the requirement for blood transfusion.
- Blood transfusion is usually not required when blood loss due to PPH is small, and the woman is asymptomatic.
- Women with PPH rarely require a blood transfusion if the hemoglobin is more than 10.0 gm/dL.

Selection of blood product

Packed red blood cells (PRBCs) are preferred for resuscitation and to avoid crystalloids-induced dilutional coagulopathy in women with massive hemorrhage. In cases of life-threatening PPH when the patient's blood group is unavailable or there is an anticipated delay in receiving cross-matched blood, consider using O Rh negative blood [34, 76].

Packed red blood cells are the preferred treatment for hypovolemic shock caused by hemorrhage, and each unit can be expected to increase the hemoglobin level by about 1 gm/dL [77].

Transfusion ratios: When a large volume of transfusion is required, recommended proportionate administration of red blood cells, fresh frozen plasma (FFP), and platelets are in a 1:1:1 ratio, which resembles the replacement of whole blood [38, 78]. Blood products transfused in a ratio, mimicking whole blood replacement, are associated with lesser complications and better survival [79].

Post-transfusion goals

The post-transfusion goals in the management of PPH are to maintain the following [80]:

- Hemoglobin level greater than 8 gm/dL.
- Platelet counts greater than 50,000/mm3.
- Fibrinogen level greater than 150–200 mg/dL.
- Prothrombin time is less than 1.5 times the normal value.

Adverse effects

With the changing trend to use early transfusions to achieve faster hemodynamic stability and avoid using the large volume of crystalloids, a higher incidence of transfusion-related complications due to the administration of multiple units has been observed. Complications frequently encountered are hyperkalemia, hypocalcemia, allergic reactions, citrate toxicity, volume overload, and transfusion-related acute lung injury (TRALI).

Hyperkalemia and hypocalcemia (low ionized calcium) are common electrolyte abnormalities seen whenever multiple units of stored PRBCs are transfused rapidly. The risk of hyperkalemia is high following a massive transfusion because older stored PRBCs contain about 5 mEq of potassium per unit (300 mL).

The risk of developing hypocalcemia is high after rapidly transfusing large amounts of blood due to the presence of citrate, an anticoagulant, in the blood. Each unit of packed red blood cells contains about 3 mg of citrate. In very sick patients, the liver's ability to eliminate citrate may be impaired, leading to citrate accumulation in the blood. Accumulated citrate binds to circulating ionized calcium, leading to hypocalcemia and can cause citrate toxicity. Therefore, monitoring for and managing citrate toxicity in patients receiving large amounts of PRBCs or who have compromised liver function is essential Patients receiving large amounts of blood need the administration of calcium injections to prevent or correct hypocalcemia.

Ringer's lactate and blood should not be administered in the same line because the calcium in the RL solution may cause clotting.

REFERENCES

1. Pretorius T, van Rensburg G, Dyer RA, et al. The Influence of Fluid Management on Outcomes in Preeclampsia: A Systematic Review and Meta-Analysis. Int J Obstet Anesth 2018;34:85–95.

2. Dimitriadis E, Rolnik DL, Zhou W, et al. Pre-eclampsia. Nat Rev Dis Primers 2023;9(1):8.

3. Wong S. NHS Hypertension – Management in Pregnancy Guideline (GL952). February 2018 (https://www.royalberkshire.nhs.uk/Downloads/GPs/GP%20protocols%20and%20guidelines/Maternity%20Guidelines%20and%20Policies/Medical%20conditions%20and%20complications/Hypertension_guideline_V3.1_GL952_JUN19.pdf Accessed on 20 Nov 2018).

4. The Diagnosis and Management of Preeclampsia and Eclampsia - Clinical Practice Guideline. Institute of Obstetricians and Gynaecologists, Royal College of Physicians of Ireland. September 2011. (https://rcpi-live-cdn.s3.amazonaws.com/wp-content/uploads/2017/02/Preeclampsia_Approved_120716.pdf Accessed on 27 June 2019).

5. Regional Guideline for the Management of Preeclampsia (July 2015). Maternity, Children and Young People Strategic Clinical Network. Review July 2017 (https://www.nwcscnsenate.nhs.uk/files/6814/7160/2738/Eclampsia_Guidelines_FINAL_Ratified_MCYP_SG_Sept20_15.pdf Accessed on 21/11/2018).

6. Dennis AT, Solnordal CB. Acute Pulmonary Oedema in Pregnant Women. Anaesthesia 2012;67(6):646–59.

7. Dennis AT. Management of Preeclampsia: Issues for Anaesthetists. Anaesthesia 2012;67(9):1009–20.

8. Tuffnell DJ, Jankowicz D, Lindow SW, et al. Outcomes of Severe Preeclampsia/Eclampsia in Yorkshire 1999/2003. BJOG 2005;112(7):875–80.

9. Magee LA, Pels A, Helewa M, et al. Diagnosis, evaluation, and management of the hypertensive disorders of pregnancy: executive summary. J Obstet Gynaecol Can. 2014;36(5):416–41.

10. Hypertension in Pregnancy: Diagnosis and Management. NICE Guideline [NG133]. Published: 25 June 2019 (www.nice.org.uk/guidance/ng133 Accessed on 27 June 2019).

11. Lowe SA, Bowyer L, Lust K, et al. Guideline for the Management of Hypertensive Disorders of Pregnancy 2014. Aust N Z J Obstet Gynaecol. 2015;55(5):e1–29.

12. Guidelines for the Management of Severe Preeclampsia and Eclampsia. GAIN March 2012.

13. Druzin ML, Shields LE, Peterson NL, et al. Improving Health Care Response to Preeclampsia: CMQCC Preeclampsia Toolkit Preeclampsia Care Guidelines CDPH-MCAH Approved: 12/20/13.

14. Hypertensive Disorders in Pregnancy: Executive Summary. New York State Department of Health May 2013 (https://www.health.ny.gov/professionals/protocols_and_guidelines/hypertensive_disorders/2013_hdp_executive_summary.pdf).

15. Anthony J, Schoeman LK. Fluid Management in Preeclampsia. Obstetric Medicine 2013;6(3):100–104.

16. Eclampsia and Severe Preeclampsia - Clinical Guidelines. Royal Cornwall Hospitals NHS Trust. 20 October 2015 (https://doclibrary-rcht.cornwall.nhs.uk/GET/d10140812).

17. Shunker S. Preeclampsia Management in ICU. Liverpool Hospital October 2013 (https://www.aci.health.nsw.gov.au/__data/assets/pdf_file/0004/306472/liverpoolPreeclampsia_Management_in_ICU.pdf Accessed on 28 November 2018).

18. Perel P, Roberts I, Ker K. Colloids versus crystalloids for fluid resuscitation in critically ill patients. Cochrane Database Syst Rev. 2013;(2):CD000567.

19. Rhodes A, Evans LE, Alhazzani W, et al. Surviving Sepsis Campaign: International Guidelines for Management of Sepsis and Septic Shock: 2016. Crit Care Med. 2017;45(3):486–552.

20. Levis SR, Pritchard MW, Evans DJ, et al. Colloids versus Crystalloids for Fluid Resuscitation in Critically Ill People. Cochrane Database of Systematic Reviews 2018;8(8):CD000567.

21. Sivevski AG, Sholjakova M, Kartalov A, et al. Comparison of Low Dose Spinal Anesthesia with General Anesthesia in Pre-Eclamptic Parturients Undergoing Emergency Cesarean Section. Anaesth Pain & Intensive Care 2015;19(1):37–43.

22. Kinsella SM, Carvalho B, Dyer RA, et al. International Consensus Statement on the Management of Hypotension with Vasopressors during Caesarean Section Under Spinal Anaesthesia. Anaesthesia 2018;73(1):71–92.

23. Aya AG, Mangin R, Vialles N, et al. Patients with Severe Preeclampsia Experience Less Hypotension during Spinal Anesthesia for Elective Cesarean Delivery than Healthy Parturients: A Prospective Cohort comparison. Anesth Analg 2003;97(3):867–72.

24. Sivevski AG, Ivanov E, Karadjova D. Spinal-Induced Hypotension in Preeclamptic and Healthy Parturients Undergoing Cesarean Section. Open Access Macedonian Journal of Medical Sciences. 2019;7(6):996–1000.

25. ACOG Practice Bulletin No. 202: Gestational Hypertension and Preeclampsia. Obstetrics & Gynecology January 2019;133(1):1–25.

26. Loughran PG, Moore J, Dundee JW. Maternal Stress Response Associated with Cesarean Delivery Under General and Epidural Anaesthesia. Br J Obstet Gynaecol 1986;93(9):943–9.

27. Huang CJ, Fan YC, Tsai PS. Differential Impacts of Modes of Anaesthesia on the Risk of Stroke Among Preeclamptic Women who Undergo Caesarean Delivery: A Population-based Study. Br J Anaesth 2010;105(6):818–26.

28. Santos AC, Birnbach DJ. Spinal Anesthesia for Cesarean Delivery in Severely Preeclamptic Women: Don't throw Out the Baby with the Bathwater! Anesth Analg 2005;101(3):859–61.

29. Leslie D, Collis RE. Hypertension in Pregnancy. BJA Education 2016;16(1):33–37.

30. Sibai BM. Diagnosis, Prevention, and Management of Eclampsia. Obstet Gynecol. 2005;105(2):402–410.

31. Say L, Chou D, Gemmill A, et al. Global causes of maternal death: a WHO systematic analysis. Lancet Glob Health 2014;2(6):e323–33.

32. Weeks A. "The prevention and treatment of postpartum hemorrhage: what do we know, and where do we go to next?" BJOG: An International Journal of Obstetrics and Gynaecology. 2015;122(2):202–12.

33. Mousa HA, Blum J, Abou El Senoun G, et al. Treatment for primary postpartum hemorrhage. Cochrane Database Syst Rev. 2014;2014(2):CD003249.

34. Mavrides E, Allard S, Chandraharan E, et al. Prevention and management of postpartum haemorrhage. BJOG 2016;124:e106–e149.

35. WHO recommendations for the prevention and treatment of postpartum haemorrhage recommendations on prevention and treatment of postpartum haemorrhage [Internet] 2012.

36. Lalonde A. Prevention and treatment of postpartum hemorrhage in low-resource settings. Int J Gynaecol Obstet 2012;117(2):108–18.

37. Royal Australian and New Zealand College of Obstetricians and Gynaecologists. Management of Postpartum Haemorrhage (PPH). 2017. (Available at: https://ranzcog.edu.au/RANZCOG_SITE/media/RANZCOG-MEDIA/Women%27s%20Health/Statement%20and%20guidelines/Clinical-Obstetrics/Management-of-Postpartum-Haemorrhage-(C-Obs-43)-Review-July-2017.pdf?ext=.pdf).

38. Committee on Practice Bulletins-Obstetrics. Practice Bulletin No. 183: Postpartum Hemorrhage. Obstet Gynecol 2017;130(4):e168–e186.

39. Obstetric Hemorrhage Clinical Guideline V2.3 Royal Cornwall Hospitals NHS Trust, August 2019 (https://

doclibrary-rcht.cornwall.nhs.uk/DocumentsLibrary/RoyalCornwallHospitalsTrust/Clinical/MidwiferyAndObstetrics/ObstetricHaemorrhageClinicalGuideline.pdf Accessed on 6 November 2019).

40. Muñoz M, Stensballe J, Ducloy-Bouthors AS, et al. Patient blood management in obstetrics: prevention and treatment of postpartum haemorrhage. A NATA consensus statement. Blood Transfus. 2019;17(2):112–136.

41. Pacagnella RC, Souza JP, Durocher J, et al. A systematic review of the relationship between blood loss and clinical signs. PLoS One 2013;8(3):e57594.

42. Hofer S, Blaha J, Collins PW, et al. Haemostatic support in postpartum haemorrhage: A review of the literature and expert opinion. Eur J Anaesthesiol. 2023;40(1):29–38.

43. Nathan HL, El Ayadi A, Hezelgrave NL, et al. Shock index: an effective predictor of outcome in postpartum haemorrhage? BJOG 2015;122(2):268–75.

44. Koch E, Lovett S, Nghiem T, et al. Shock index in the emergency department: utility and limitations. Open Access Emerg Med. 2019;11:179–199.

45. Huang L, Gan X, Luo D, et al. The Ability of Shock Index In Detecting Postpartum Haemorrhage: A Retrospective Case-Control Study. Research Square 2022.

46. Makino Y, Okada A, Ikeda Y, et al. Predictive accuracy of the shock index for severe postpartum hemorrhage in high-income countries: A systematic review and meta-analysis J Obstet Gynaecol Res. 2022:48(8):2027–2037.

47. Diaz V, Abalos E, Carroli G. Methods for blood loss estimation after vaginal birth. Cochrane Database Syst Rev 2018;9(9):CD010980.

48. Escobar MF, Nassar AH, Theron G, et al. FIGO recommendations on the management of postpartum hemorrhage 2022. Int J Gynaecol Obstet. 2022;157 Suppl 1(Suppl 1):3–50.

49. Leibner E, Andreae M, Galvagno SM, et al. Damage control resuscitation. Clin Exp Emerg Med. 2020;7(1):5–13.

50. Owattanapanich N, Chittawatanarat K, Benyakorn T, et al. Risks and benefits of hypotensive resuscitation in patients with traumatic hemorrhagic shock: a meta-analysis. Scand J Trauma Resusc Emerg Med. 2018;26:107.

51. Wang H, Chen MB, Zheng XW, et al. Effectiveness and safety of hypotensive resuscitation in traumatic hemorrhagic shock: a protocol for meta-analysis. Medicine. 2019;98(48):e18145.

52. Gillissen A, van den Akker T, Caram-Deelder C, et al. Association between fluid management and dilutional coagulopathy in severe postpartum haemorrhage: a nationwide retrospective cohort study. BMC Preg Childbirth. 2018;18(1):398.

53. Henriquez DDCA, Bloemenkamp KWM, Loeff RM, et al. Fluid resuscitation during persistent postpartum haemorrhage and maternal outcome: A nationwide cohort study. Eur J Obstet Gynecol Reprod Biol. 2019;235:49–56.

54. Carrick MM, Leonard J, Slone DS, et al. Hypotensive resuscitation among trauma patients. Biomed Res Int. 2016;2016:8901938.

55. Carvajal JA, Ramos I, Kusanovic JP, et al. Damage-control resuscitation in obstetrics. J Matern Fetal Neonatal Med. 2022;35(4):785–798.

56. Albreiki M, Voegeli D. Permissive hypotensive resuscitation in adult patients with traumatic haemorrhagic shock: a systematic review. Eur J Trauma Emerg Surg 2018;44(2):191–202.

57. Tran A, Yates J, Lau A, et al. Permissive hypotension versus conventional resuscitation strategies in adult trauma patients with hemorrhagic shock: A systematic review and meta-analysis of randomized controlled trials. J Trauma Acute Care Surg. 2018;84(5):802–808.

58. Safiejko K, Smereka J, Filipiak KJ, et al. Effectiveness and safety of hypotension fluid resuscitation in traumatic hemorrhagic shock: A systematic review and meta-analysis of randomized controlled trials. Cardiol J. 2022;29(3):463–471.

59. Queensland Maternity and Neonatal Clinical Guidelines Program. 2018 Primary postpartum hemorrhage MN18.1-V7-R23.

60. Spahn DR, Bouillon B, Cerny V, et al. The European guideline on management of major bleeding and coagulopathy following trauma. Crit Care. 2019;23(1):98.

61. Mutter TC, Ruth CA, Dart AB. Hydroxyethyl starch (HES) versus other fluid therapies: effects on kidney function. Cochrane Database Syst Rev 2013;7:CD007594.

62. Perner A, Haase N, Guttormsen AB, et al. Hydroxyethyl starch 130/0.42 versus Ringer's acetate in severe sepsis. (6S Trial) N Engl J Med 2012;367(2):124–34.

63. Postpartum hemorrhage - prevention and management. Clinical practice guidelines at the Royal Hospital for Women 21 June 2018.

64. Yunos M, Bellomo R, Story D, et al. Bench-to-bedside review: Chloride in critical illness. Critical Care; 2010;14(4):226.

65. Yunos NM, Bellomo R, Glassford N, et al. Chloride-liberal vs. chloride-restrictive intravenous fluid administration and acute kidney injury: an extended analysis. Intensive Care Med 2015;41(2):257–64.

66. Myburgh JA, Mythen MG. Resuscitation fluids. N Engl J Med 2013;369(13):1243–1251.

67. Cotton BA, Guy JS, Morris Jr JA, et al. The cellular, metabolic, and systemic consequences of aggressive fluid resuscitation strategies. Shock. 2006;26(2):115–21.

68. Ley EJ, Clond MA Srur MK, et al. Emergency department crystalloid resuscitation of 1.5 L or more is associated with increased mortality in elderly and nonelderly trauma patients. J Trauma. 2011;70(2):398–400.

69. Peña PCA, Meza MJM, Martínez BYI. Integral management of reanimation in the patient with critical bleeding: reanimation of damage control. Med Crit. 2021;35(4):200–205.

70. Fuller AJ, Bucklin B. Blood component therapy in obstetrics. Obstet Gynecol Clin North Am 2007;34(3):443–58.

71. Blood Transfusion in Obstetrics. Green-top Guideline No. 47. Royal College of Obstetricians and Gynaecologists May 2015 (https://www.rcog.org.uk/media/sdqcorsf/gtg-47.pdf).

72. American Society of Anesthesiologists Task Force on Perioperative Blood Transfusion and Adjuvant Therapies. Practice guidelines for perioperative blood transfusion and adjuvant therapies: an updated report by the American Society of Anesthesiologists Task Force on Perioperative Blood Transfusion and Adjuvant Therapies. Anesthesiology 2006;105(1):198–208.

73. Lyndon A, Lagrew D, Shields L, et al. Improving Health Care Response to Obstetric Hemorrhage. Version 2.0. A California Quality improvement toolkit. Department of Public Health. 2015.

74. Shields LE, Wiesner S, Fulton J, et al. Comprehensive maternal hemorrhage protocols reduce the use of blood products and improve patient safety. Am J Obstet Gynecol. 2015;212(3):272–80.

75. Attali E, Many A, Kern G, et al. Predicting the need for blood transfusion requirement in postpartum hemorrhage. J Matern Fetal Neonatal Med. 2022;35(25):7911–7916.

76. Bonnet MP, Benhamou D. Management of postpartum haemorrhage. F1000Res. 2016;5:F1000 Faculty Rev-1514.

77. Müller M, Geisen C, Zacharowski K, et al. Transfusion of packed red cells—indications, triggers and adverse events. Dtsch Arztebl Int 2015;112(29–30):507–17.

78. Collins P, Abdul-Kadir R, Thachil J. Management of coagulopathy associated with postpartum hemorrhage: guidance from the SSC of the ISTH. J Thromb Haemost. 2016;14(1):205–10.

79. Holcomb JB, Tilley BC, Baraniuk S, et al. Transfusion of plasma, platelets, and red blood cells in a 1:1:1 vs a 1:1:2 ratio and mortality in patients with severe trauma: the PROPPR randomized clinical trial. JAMA. 2015;313(5):471–482.

80. Hunt BJ, Allard S, Keeling D, et al. A practical guideline for the haematological management of major haemorrhage. Br J Haematol 2015;170(6):788–803.

54 | Hyponatremia during Labor

Labor per se does not cause hyponatremia (defined as serum sodium <130 mEq/L), but during labor, women are at increased risk of developing the same [1]. Hyponatremia following prolonged labor is not uncommon and is potentially hazardous to the mother and neonate [2, 3].

PHYSIOLOGICAL PREDISPOSING FACTORS

Women in labor are at greater risk of developing hyponatremia than non-pregnant women [4] because of:

1. Lower baseline plasma sodium. The normal range of serum sodium concentration is lower (130–140 mEq/L) in pregnancy compared to its value in non-pregnant adults (135–145 mEq/L) [4, 5]. In the late third trimester, about 6 to 8 liter of water is retained, which is responsible for the dilutional hyponatremia and the lower baseline plasma sodium value.

2. An impaired renal ability to excrete water [6, 7]. In healthy women, the normal capacity of kidneys to excrete a water load is 900 ml/h. While in late pregnancy, the maximum renal ability to excrete a water load reduces to 600 mL/h [8]. In the presence of the tendency of kidneys to retain water, hyponatremia is likely to occur if the excess fluid is consumed orally or administered intravenously.

3. Antidiuretic effect of endogenous oxytocin. As the structure of oxytocin is similar to vasopressin, oxytocin causes water retention and results in dilutional hyponatremia in laboring women [9]. Reasons for the higher concentration of oxytocin during labor are the greater release of endogenous secretion of oxytocin and IV administration of synthetic oxytocin to induce or augment labor.

CAUSES

Causes of maternal hyponatremia are:

1. Excessive oral water intake during prolonged labor [10, 11].

2. Hyponatremia is likely in women who choose home delivery but are transferred to the hospital after prolonged labor due to unsuccessful delivery or obstetric complications [3]. The mechanism for developing hyponatremia in such patients is the high endogenous secretion of oxytocin and excessive oral hypotonic fluid intake.

3. Liberal fluid administration causes iatrogenic maternal fluid overload.

4. Increased oral fluid intake and intravenous fluid administration are major causes of hyponatremia. Hyponatremia occurs when the intake of low sodium-containing fluid exceeds a woman's ability to excrete it during labor. Water retention causes a decrease in the concentration of sodium by diluting the blood. As a result, the incidence of hyponatremia at delivery among women is 1% for those with a total fluid intake (oral + IV) of up to 1 liter during labor and 5% for those with a total fluid intake between 1 to 2.5 liters [2]. The risk of hyponatremia increases to as high as 26% for those with a total fluid intake above 2.5 liters.

5. Administration of a large volume of oxytocin in hypotonic solutions (i.e., 5% dextrose) for a prolonged period for induction and augmentation of labor can cause hyponatremia [2].

6. Other causes: Hyperemesis gravidarum, psychiatric disorders, and maternal medications like diuretics, antidepressants like selective serotonin reuptake inhibitors [SSRIs], and synthetic recreational drugs like ecstasy.

HARMFUL EFFECTS

Hyponatremia during labor can produce deleterious consequences for both the mother and the neonate. In addition to the usual symptoms of hyponatremia (e.g., nausea, lethargy, headache, agitation, confusion, drowsiness, seizures, etc.), maternal hyponatremia is associated with the prolongation of the second stage of labor, instrumental birth, and emergency cesarean birth for failure to progress [2].

As water diffuses freely across the placenta, maternal hyponatremia can lead to neonatal hyponatremia [12, 13]. Significant hyponatremia in newborns may cause irritability, lethargy, and feeding difficulties in mild cases and seizures, respiratory distress, apnea, hyperbilirubinemia, and coma in severe cases [10, 14–16].

PREVENTION

Measures which help to prevent hyponatremia are [1]:

1. Strict fluid balance chart and early recognition: Record oral/intravenous fluid intake and urine output every four hours for close monitoring. When an electrolyte imbalance is suspected, it is important to measure the serum electrolytes. If a woman's fluid balance exceeds positive 1500 ml, her risk of developing hyponatremia is high, and her blood sodium level should be checked.

2. Neutral fluid balance: Maternal dilutional hyponatremia can be prevented during labor by maintaining a neutral fluid balance. Therefore, excessive fluid intake during labor should not be encouraged for women.

3. Avoid the administration of hypotonic IV fluids like 5% dextrose during labor.

4. When oxytocin is to be administered in a high dose for a prolonged period, use a higher concentration of oxytocin to reduce the total volume of infused fluid, use electrolyte-containing solutions such as normal saline or Ringer's lactate as a diluent, and avoid electrolyte free solution like 5% dextrose as a diluent.

5. During labor, it is important to monitor serum sodium levels in women who require oxytocin infusion, have a

positive fluid balance exceeding 1500 ml, develop symptoms of hyponatremia, or have a serum sodium level less than 130 mEq/L.

TREATMENT

Treatment depends on the underlying cause. The basic principle of treating dilutional maternal hyponatremia is a fluid restriction (oral and intravenous), discontinuation of oxytocin infusion, and co-administration of furosemide if there is any evidence of fluid overload [1]. Administration of hypertonic saline is necessary for patients with severe clinical symptoms due to hyponatremia (such as seizures or loss of consciousness) with close monitoring of sodium levels.

Hypovolemic depletion hyponatremia is less common during labor and may need IV fluid administration. Normal saline is a preferred solution in such women. For detailed information about the treatment of hyponatremia, please refer to Chapter 20 on "Hyponatremia".

REFERENCES

1. GAIN Guideline for the prevention, diagnosis and management of hyponatraemia in labour and the immediate postpartum period march 2017.
2. Moen V, Burdin L, Rundgren M, et al. Hyponatremia complicating labour—rare or unrecognised? A prospective observational study. BJOG 2009;116(4):552-61.
3. Lassey SC, Napoe GS, Carusi D, et al. Hyponatremia among parturients transferred to the hospital after prolonged labor during an attempted home birth. Obstet Gynecol. 2019;134(1):106–108.
4. Costantine MM. Physiologic and pharmacokinetic changes in pregnancy. Front Pharmacol. 2014;5:65.
5. Narelle H. Biochemical Changes in Pregnancy-What Should A Clinician Know? J Gynecol Women's Health. 2017;4(1):555626.
6. Schrier RW. Body water homeostasis: clinical disorders of urinary dilution and concentration. J Am Soc Nephrol 2006;17(7):1820–1832.
7. Cheung KL, Lafayette RA. Renal physiology of pregnancy. Adv Chronic Kidney Dis. 2013;20(3):209–14.
8. Hytten FE, Klopper AI. Response to a water load in pregnancy. J Obstet Gynaecol Br Commonw 1963;70:811–6.
9. Chunling Li, Weidong W, Sandra NS, et al. Molecular Mechanisms of Antidiuretic Effect of Oxytocin. J Am Soc Nephrol. 2008;19(2):225–32.
10. Johansson S, Lindow S, Kapadia H, et al. Perinatal water intoxication due to excessive oral intake during labour. Acta Paediatr. 2002;91(7):811–4.
11. Solomon N, Many A, Orbach R, et al. Maternal and neonatal hyponatremia during labor: a case series. J Matern Fetal Neonatal Med. 2019;32(16):2711–2715.
12. West CR, Harding JE. Maternal water intoxication as a cause of neonatal seizures. J. Paediatric Child health. 2004;40(12):709–710.
13. Walter KN, Montgomery J, Amess P, et al. Hyponatraemia and brain oedema in newborns following oral water intoxication during prolonged labour. Klinische Paädiatrie. 2012;224(4):266–267.
14. Chapman TH, Hamilton M. Water intoxication presenting as maternal and neonatal seizures: a case report. Journal of medical Case Reports. 2008;2:366.
15. Ophir E, Solt I, Odeh M, et al. Water intoxication - a dangerous condition in labor and delivery rooms. Obstet Gynecol Surv 2007;62(11):731–8.
16. Valerio E, Fantinato M, Giovannini IA, et al. Severe asymptomatic maternal antepartum hyponatremia leading to neonatal seizures: prevention is better than cure. Matern Health Neonatol Perinatol. 2015;1:25.

Part 12

Parenteral Nutrition

55 | Parenteral Nutrition: Principles and Requirements

INTRODUCTION

Parenteral nutrition (PN) is currently one of the most sophisticated forms of intravenous therapy. Appropriate use of parenteral nutrition is lifesaving when there is no other option for nutrition.

DEFINITION

Parenteral nutrition is a method of intravenous administration of nutrients, vitamins, electrolytes, and medications to patients who cannot take or tolerate enteral nutrition or have a non-functional gastrointestinal tract.

PN is an effective means of sustaining life and promoting recovery in critically ill patients incapable of ingesting, absorbing, or assimilating nutrients. Similarly, PN is a life-supporting therapy even for non-critically ill patients with pre-existing malnutrition and for non-stressed but hospitalized patients who cannot take oral intake for 5 to 7 or more days.

BASIC PRINCIPLES OF NUTRITION

1. Avoid malnutrition as it is harmful [1].

2. If the intestines are functioning properly, utilize them. When possible, it is recommended to use enteral nutrition instead of parenteral nutrition. However, ensuring the safe and sufficient delivery of nutrition is of higher priority than the route of delivery.

3. Avoid overfeeding, as it can cause significant complications. Excess carbohydrates can cause hyperglycemia, hepatic steatosis, and increased CO_2 production; excess protein can cause azotemia and metabolic acidosis, and excess fat can cause hyperlipidemia [2, 3].

4. While planning PN, more critical factors are the method of delivery, timing, and the type of formula rather than the specific amounts of nutrients provided.

5. During acute stress, the body mobilizes endogenous amino acids and energy stores. It is not possible to make catabolic patients anabolic entirely. The goal of nutritional support is to prevent the wasting of protein and to provide essential and conditionally essential nutrients.

Importance of avoiding malnutrition

Malnutrition should be prevented due to its harmful consequences, including:

1. Malnutrition leads to increased morbidity and mortality and should be avoided. In addition, it leads to increased susceptibility to infection, poor wound healing, pulmonary complications (weakness of respiratory muscles leading to the decreased ventilatory drive, reduction of vital capacity, and depressed lung defense due to reduces cough pressure and removal of secretions), electrolyte disturbances, and postoperative complications.

2. Malnutrition leads to a prolonged recovery period and a longer duration of hospitalization.

3. It can negatively impact the quality of life and is associated with higher morbidity and mortality.

Goals of parenteral nutrition

The role of PN is supportive. The principal goals of nutritional support are:

1. To sustain or improve nutrition by administering all necessary nutrients such as proteins, carbohydrates, lipids, electrolytes, minerals, trace elements, and vitamins.

2. To decrease the negative impacts of catabolism, it is essential to maximize protein synthesis, limit the breakdown of body protein, and slow down the rate of weight loss.

3. To boost the immune function and to improve wound healing.

4. Restoring glycogen storage increases the strength of cardiac and diaphragmatic muscles and improves cardiopulmonary function.

5. To maintain or correct acid-base and electrolyte disturbances.

Table 55.1 Planning of parenteral nutritional support
1. Selection of patient: Determine if PN is truly indicated. PN is recommended only when potential benefits (improvement in prognosis and quality of life) exceed the risks.
2. Select and establish an appropriate route of administration on the basis of long-term vs. short-term requirements.
3. Calculations of nutritional requirements: Calculate the requirements of fluid, energy, glucose, lipids, proteins, minerals, and vitamins for individual patients (along with disease-specific modifications).
4. Prescribe parenteral nutrition: Convert nutritional requirements to prescription. Prepare or select an optimal formula to deliver nutrients.
5. Administration, monitoring, and avoiding complications of PN support.

6. To accelerate recovery and improve the quality of life.

Planning parenteral nutrition

Planning of parenteral nutritional therapy is summarized in Table 55.1.

ENTERAL NUTRITION VS. PARENTERAL NUTRITION

Preference of EN over PN

Enteral nutrition (EN) is preferred when the gastrointestinal tract is functional and accessible. The potential benefits of enteral feeding are:

1. Maintains mucosal integrity: Provides nutrients that are needed in the intestinal lumen to maintain the structural and functional integrity of the gastrointestinal (GI) tract. Enteral feeding prevents the atrophy of intestinal mucosa and maintains mucosal functions of the gut. Intact mucus membrane preserves the barrier functions of the bowel and prevents bacterial translocation, and therefore prevents the possible risk of sepsis.

2. Unlike standard PN, EN provides gut-preferred fuels such as glutamate and short-chain fatty acids.

3. More physiological as the liver is not bypassed. The complete volume of nutrient-rich venous blood from all parts of the gastrointestinal tract passes from the liver before it returns to the heart. So hepatic take-up, process, and storing of various nutrients from the venous blood and subsequent release on neural or hormonal command is maintained with EN.

4. Prevents cholelithiasis by stimulating gall bladder motility.

5. Fewer serious complications and avoids known and potential complications of PN.

6. Less costly and easier to maintain than PN. Because of the potential advantages of EN, the provision of even "token" enteral supplementation is recommended to patients receiving total PN support whenever possible.

Contraindications EN

Major contraindications of enteral nutrition are:

1. Gastrointestinal causes: Active severe gastrointestinal bleeding, small or large bowel obstruction, perforation, generalized peritonitis, severe paralytic ileus, high output external fistula, and intractable vomiting or diarrhea refractory to medical management.

2. Cardiac causes: Active shock or severe hemodynamic instability

with poor end-organ perfusion and hypotensive patients on a high dose of inotropes/vasopressors. Avoid EN in patients who are hemodynamically unstable and not fully resuscitated [4, 5], but due to multiple benefits of EN [6, 7], initiate EN after adequately fluid resuscitation once the patient is stable and/or doses of vasopressors are declining [8, 9].

3. Lack of access: Unobtainable safe access to the gastrointestinal tract.

4. Complications of enteral feeding: Patients with enteral feeding complications (i.e., pulmonary aspiration, severe diarrhea, and intestinal ischemia or infarct precipitated by enteral feeding in patients with ischemic bowel syndrome) should not be fed by the enteral route.

Advantages of PN over EN

Potential advantages of parenteral nutrition over enteral nutrition are:

1. Ensured desired volume delivery of nutrients without the concerns of gastrointestinal intolerance or compliance with transnasal feeding tubes.

2. Improved metabolic, electrolyte, and micronutrient management.

3. Better acid-base manipulation.

4. Drug delivery capabilities (histamine H2 blockers, metoclopramide, insulin, heparin, etc.).

So, PN not only delivers nutrition but also regulates fluid, electrolyte, and acid-base homeostasis.

Factors considered while selecting parenteral nutritional support

The decision to use parenteral nutrition should take into account several important factors, including:

1. Age and premorbid state (healthy or otherwise).

2. Nutritional status, including endogenous fuel (fat) and protein (muscle) stores, weight loss, and serum albumin value.

3. Duration of starvation and degree of the anticipated insult.

4. Underlying disease, its severity, and concomitant medical therapy.

5. Gastrointestinal function and the possibility of resuming normal intake soon.

INDICATIONS OF PARENTERAL NUTRITION

Parenteral nutrition is required in patients who cannot, should not, or will not eat enough to maintain adequate nutrition and are at risk of developing malnutrition. PN prevents the adverse effects of malnutrition and prevents or corrects specific nutrient deficiencies when the gastrointestinal tract cannot be used efficiently or safely for a prolonged period. Additionally, using PN can reduce total hospitalization costs due to faster recovery and reduced complications of the underlying condition.

However, PN is expensive and has the potential for serious complications. So benefits of PN should be weighed against the potential risks before initiating PN. Important indications of PN are summarized in Table 55.2 [10–12].

ADVANTAGES AND DISADVANTAGES OF PN

Major advantages and disadvantages of the parenteral nutrition are as follows:

Major advantages

1. Lifesaving when the GI tract cannot be used.

2. Ensured desired volume delivery of nutrients when:

<table>
<tr><td colspan="1" align="center">**Table 55.2 Indications of parenteral nutrition**</td></tr>
</table>

A. General indications

1. Critical illness with inadequate oral or enteral nutrition for >5–7 days

2. In critically ill patients with severe malnutrition or high nutrition risk, initiate PN as soon as feasible if oral or enteral nutrition is not possible or inadequate

B. Anticipated or actual inadequate oral or enteral intake

1. Conditions that impair the absorption of nutrients

    a. GI fistula

    b. Short bowel syndrome

    c. Small bowel obstruction

    d. Effects of radiation or chemotherapy

2. Need for bowel rest

    a. Severe acute necrotizing pancreatitis

    b. Inflammatory bowel disease

    c. Mesenteric ischemia

    d. Peritonitis

    e. Perioperative (bowel resection, major gastrointestinal surgery)

3. Motility disorders

    a. Prolonged ileus

4. Inability to achieve or maintain enteral access

    a. Haemodynamic instability

    b. Massive gastrointestinal bleeding

    c. Unacceptable aspiration risk

    d. Hyperemesis gravidarum, eating disorders

C. Significant multiorgan system disease

- Significant renal, hepatic, and pulmonary diseases or critical illness (multi organ failure, severe head injury, burns, etc.), which prevents adequate oral or EN

- GI intolerance prevents oral or EN.
- Less than 2 to 3 feet of the small intestine.

3. Easier correction of fluid and electrolyte disturbances.

Major disadvantages

1. High cost.

2. Catheter-associated infections and complications.

3. Fluid overload and electrolyte abnormalities.

4. More risk of metabolic problems like hyperglycemia, hypercholesterolemia, hepatic dysfunction, and refeeding syndrome.

5. Leads to intestinal mucosal atrophy, causing damage to the gut barrier. Loss of this first line of defense predisposes patients on PN to risk bacteremia and infection.

6. Daily PN is cumbersome.

CONTRAINDICATIONS OF PN

Contraindications of PN are broadly discussed in two groups:

General contraindications

1. If enteral or oral nutrition meets the patient's nutritional requirements.

2. Patients are well-nourished, stable, non-catabolic, and within the short

term (five to seven days), oral or enteral nutrition is likely to be initiated. For Most patients who require short-term support, the risks of PN outweigh the benefits.

3. Severe liver failure, cardiac failure, cardiogenic shock, and blood dyscrasias.

4. Cautious use in hemodynamic instability, volume overload, azotemia (BUN >100 mg/dL), severe hyperglycemia (glucose >300 mg/dL), or electrolyte disturbances (Na^+ >150 mEq/L, K^+ <3 mEq/L, Cl^- <85 mEq/L and phosphorus <2 mg/dL), where administration of PN carries high risk.

5. Undue high risk in the insertion of catheter solely for PN.

6. To prolong life in terminally ill patients with a poor expected outcome when there is little prospect of good quality of life.

Disease-specific contraindications

1. Excess use of carbohydrates results in the production of a large amount of carbon dioxide and therefore should be avoided in patients with compromised pulmonary function and with ventilator support during the weaning period.

2. Use lipid administration with caution if the triglyceride level is consistently more than 350 mg/dL or in patients with severe sepsis, a moderate degree of jaundice, low platelet count (<50,000 to 60,000/mm), and ARDS or severe respiratory disease.

3. Avoid the use of excess PN volume in patients with heart or kidney failure.

4. In patients with hepatic encephalopathy and severe renal failure, modified amino acids are preferred over standard amino acids.

It is important to remember that parenteral nutrition must not be undertaken lightly. It is potentially harmful and dangerous if not administered with due precautions.

Timing of parenteral nutrition initiation

Even in critical patients, the decision to start PN is never an emergency. Before starting PN, if the patient is hemodynamically stable and there are no electrolyte or blood glucose abnormalities, the risks of adverse effects of PN are low. At times adequate initial therapy of critical illness may sufficiently improve clinical status to permit oral or EN, and the patient may not require PN. Early PN benefits severely malnourished, critically ill patients, patients with severe necrotizing acute pancreatitis, and high output fistula with large nutrient losses.

NUTRITIONAL REQUIREMENTS

Basic nutritional requirements include a balanced amount of fluid, macronutrients (carbohydrates, lipids, proteins), and micronutrients (electrolytes, minerals, trace elements, and vitamins).

Fluid requirements

The total fluid requirement in an adult patient can be calculated by adding abnormal losses to normal daily fluid requirements. In adult patients of average-sized, the fluid requirements are about 25–30 mL/kg/d. Correct volume deficit before initiating PN. Search and replace fluid additionally to replace abnormal fluid losses caused by diuretic therapy, diarrhea, vomiting, nasogastric tube drainage, wound output, perspiration, etc. Patients with fluid overload due to cardiac, pulmonary, hepatic, or renal failure need fluid restriction. The volume of fluid delivered by the enteral route should be subtracted from the estimated total fluid requirement. Significant minerals are lost with enteric fluid loss, so an extra amount of these nutrients and fluid must be added to the parenteral solution.

Energy requirements

PN should provide adequate energy to patients. Four components of daily energy requirements/total energy expenditure (TEE) are resting energy expenditure-REE (normally two-thirds of TEE), activity energy expenditure (activity factor-AF, normally one-fourth to one-third of TEE), the thermal effect of food (Thermal factor-TF, normally 10% of TEE) and associated illness (disease factor-DF). Adult patients' appropriate total energy requirement is 20–30 kcal/kg/d [13].

Total energy expenditure can be estimated by any of three methods (Table 55.3):

1. By using a simple calculation based on calories per kilogram of body weight.

2. By using Harris-Benedict (HB) equation to calculate resting energy expenditure, plus additional calories for activity and illness or,

3. By calculating energy expenditure with indirect calorimetry.

1. Simple body weight-based calculation

Energy requirements can be calculated roughly by multiplying actual body weight in kilogram by 25–30 kcal, which needs modifications considering physical activity and associated illness (Table 55.4). In obese patients, use ideal body weight for calculation. Severely malnourished critically ill patients are at high risk for refeeding syndrome, and therefore while initiating PN,

Table 55.3 Methods for estimating total energy expenditure (kcal)
1. Simple body weight based calculation: • REE (kcal/day) = 30 × weight in kg
2. Harris-Benedict equation: • REE (Man) = 66 + (13.7 × W) + (5.0 × H) - (6.7 × A)   • REE (Women) = 655 + (9.6 × W) + (1.8 × H) - (4.7 × A)
3. Indirect calorimetry: • REE (Man) = (3.9 × VO2) + (1.1 × VCO2) - 61
A: Age in years; H: Height in cm; W: Weight in kg; REE: Resting energy expenditure

Table 55.4 Guidelines for adjustment in energy requirements		
AF = Activity factor	**DF = Disease factor**	**TF = Thermal factor**
1.2 bed rest	1.10 on ventilator	1.1 38°C
1.3 out of bed	1.25 general surgery	1.2 39°C
1.4 active	1.3 sepsis	1.3 40°C
-	1.6 multiorgan failure	1.4 41°C
-	1.7 30–50% burns	-
-	1.8 50–70% burns	-
-	2.0 70–90% burns	-

administer hypocaloric PN (energy intake less than 20 kcal/kg/d) with adequate protein intake.

2. **Harris-Benedict equation**

   While calculating REE by the Harris-Benedict equation, undernourished patients use actual body weight, and obese persons use ideal body weight.

   To calculate TEE from REE, it is necessary to correct for physical activity (activity factor-AF), associated illness (disease factor-DF), and temperature (TF) as per Table 55.4.

   So, TEE = REE × AF × DF × TF

3. **Indirect calorimetry**

   Above both methods fails to provide accurate calculations of the actual energy used, especially for patients who are significantly underweight, overweight, or critically ill. Therefore, indirect calorimetry using the multicomponent metabolic carts [14] is considered the gold standard method to evaluate energy expenditure in clinical practice. As this accurate and non-invasive technique helps in planning the prescription of nutrition and prevents both under and over-feeding in patients by spontaneously breathing and ventilation, its routine use to optimize nutrition care should be encouraged [15, 16].

   Calculation based on body weight and the HB equation is simple but often overestimates energy expenditure.

Because of the complications of overfeeding, it is wiser to administer lesser calories rather than too many calories.

Providing energy requirements in parenteral nutrition

The approximate proportion of various macronutrients, including carbohydrates, lipids, and proteins, in the parenteral solution for energy supplementation is summarized in Table 55.5. Generally, the energy content of parenteral nutrition predominantly consists of carbohydrates and lipids (non-protein calories), as proteins are primarily directed towards anabolic processes rather than serving as an energy source. In clinical practice, a common approach is to provide approximately 60–70% of calories from glucose and 30–40% from lipids. This combination of fuel sources in critically ill patients significantly reduces carbon dioxide (CO_2) production, improving patient outcomes

In clinical practice, glucose and lipids are usually given roughly 60–70% glucose and 30–40% lipids.

This mixed fuel nutrient in stressed patients significantly reduces CO_2 production and, therefore, reduces the respiratory work of breathing.

Avoidance of overfeeding in parenteral nutrition

Overfeeding is associated with several significant complications that must be carefully managed to optimize patient outcomes. These complications include:

Table 55.5. Macronutrient composition in parenteral nutrition solutions

Macronutrient	% Contribution	Calories per gm
Carbohydrates	50–60%	1 gm dextrose = 3.4 kcal
Lipids	20–30%	1 gm lipid = 9 kcal
Proteins	15–20%	1 gm protein = 4 kcal

1. Severe hyperglycemia: Overfeeding can lead to severe hyperglycemia, resulting in glycosuria, osmotic diuresis, and dehydration.
2. Increased risk of infections: Hyperglycemia caused by overfeeding can elevate the risk of nosocomial infections.
3. Increased oxygen consumption: Excessive calorie administration can lead to increased oxygen consumption and carbon dioxide production. This heightened metabolic rate may necessitate increased respiratory effort, potentially causing problems in patients with compromised lung function.
4. Hepatic steatosis: Overfeeding and excess calorie intake can contribute to the accumulation of fat in the liver, leading to hepatic steatosis. This condition can result in long-term hepatic dysfunction [17].

Carbohydrates

Dextrose is the least expensive and most commonly used - a primary source of calories in parenteral nutrition.

A. Caloric value, preparations, and requirements

Each gm of hydrated dextrose monohydrate used to prepare parenteral nutrition supplies 3.4 kcal (The caloric contribution of dietary carbohydrate is 4 kcal/gm). Commercially made formulas are available in a concentration ranging from 5% to 70% (Table 55.6).

Most central parenteral nutrition (CPN) formulations use dextrose in concentrations ranging from 50–70%, which is then diluted to 15–30% when mixed with other macronutrients. Usually, 50–70% of the total energy requirement is provided in the form of dextrose. Dextrose requirements are about 4–5 mg/kg/min in stable patients and less than 4 mg/kg/min in critically ill, trauma, and sepsis patients and should not exceed 5 mg/kg/min [13, 18]. The minimal requirement of carbohydrates for PN is about 2 gm/kg/d of glucose [19].

Start with no more than 150 to 200 gm of dextrose on the first day of PN. In patients with diabetes or patients at risk for refeeding syndrome, start with a lower dose (100 to 150 gm) of dextrose.

B. Functions and advantages

1. Low cost: Dextrose is the least expensive macronutrient and hence, most commonly used.
2. Supplies calories: Parenteral carbohydrate in the form of dextrose in PN is the primary source of calories. Many tissues, such as erythrocytes, white blood cells, and renal medulla, rely primarily on glucose as an energy source and cannot easily use alternative fuels. Brain tissues, red blood cells, immune cells, and renal medulla preferentially use glucose as fuel [19]. So, it is safer to provide a minimum of 100–150 gm (about 2 gm/kg body weight) of dextrose per day to meet these demands [18].

Table 55.6 Characteristics of dextrose solutions						
Solution concentration	5%	10%	20%	25%	50%	70%
Dextrose content (gm/L)	50	100	200	250	500	700
Supply of calories (kcal/L)	170	340	680	850	1,700	2,380
Osmolarity (mOsm/L)	253	505	1,010	1,330	2,525	3,535

3. Nitrogen-sparing effect: Adequate carbohydrate supplementation has an important nitrogen-sparing effect, especially in patients with metabolic stress. When calories are provided as glucose, it stimulates insulin secretion, reduces muscle protein breakdown, and reduces the release of glucose from the liver. Thus, dextrose prevents protein catabolism by inhibiting the release of amino acid precursors from skeletal muscle for gluconeogenesis. In addition, glucose oxidation is also stimulated, thus sparing the oxidation of amino acids.

C. Disadvantages

1. Low-calorie supply: Dextrose is a poor source of calories (3.4 kcal/gm of dextrose vs. 9.0 kcal/gm of fat). So to meet the total calorie requirements, the patient either needs a larger fluid volume (if we use diluted dextrose solution) or a highly concentrated dextrose solution (which can cause thrombophlebitis).

2. Hyperglycemia: The development of hyperglycemia is the most common drawback of dextrose in PN. The risk and severity of hyperglycemia are greater with IV dextrose than with the same amount of oral or enteral administration because IV dextrose bypasses the entero-insular axis. Hyperglycemia due to a larger amount of dextrose limits the increment in the dose of dextrose in PN.

3. Increased CO_2 production (high respiratory quotient): Carbohydrates produce more carbon dioxide compared to lipids, which increases the work of respiratory muscles to eliminate carbon dioxide. Therefore, carbohydrate is not preferred as an only source of calorie in respiratory compromised patients and patients weaning from ventilator support.

4. Thrombophlebitis: Concentrated dextrose solution (above 10%) has high osmolarity as compared to plasma osmolarity (280 mOsm/L), so it can cause thrombophlebitis, requiring a central line for administration.

D. Administration of dextrose infusion and monitoring

The infusion rate of dextrose should not exceed the body's glucose oxidative capacity. The maximum rate of dextrose oxidation is approximately 4–5 mg/kg/min (5.8–7.2 gm/kg/day). Providing an excess amount of dextrose increases the risk of complications such as hyperglycemia, fatty liver, respiratory problems due to excess CO_2 production, and increased infectious-related mortality. Therefore, in patients at high risk of developing hyperglycemia (pre-existing diabetes, sepsis, obesity, steroid therapy, etc.), initiate carbohydrate infusion at a low rate (i.e., 1–2 gm/kg body weight/day). Monitor dextrose infusion closely and maintain blood sugar levels between 140–180 mg/dL [20]. Administer regular insulin only if necessary. Insulin therapy is usually initiated in diabetic patients when blood sugar is more than 140 mg/dL and in non-diabetic patients when blood sugar is more than 180 mg/dL [21].

To control hyperglycemia, insulin can be administered using different regimens, but the continuous infusion of insulin and adding insulin to the nutrition bag are common and efficient methods [21–23].

E. Example of calculation of carbohydrate/dextrose requirements

Example: For a 60 kg male with 25 kcal/kg/d energy requirements, how much 50% dextrose solution is needed (considering 60% of daily total energy requirement in the form of carbohydrates) in a day?

Calculation:

1. Total caloric requirements will be 60×25=1500 kcal/day, and carbohydrate requirement will be 900 (60% of 1500) kcal/day as dextrose.

2. Divide caloric requirements from carbohydrates by 3.4 (there is 3.4 kcal/gm of dextrose) to determine the gm of dextrose required. 900 divided by 3.4 = 264.7 gm of dextrose/day.

3. D50% has 50 gm of dextrose per 100 ml. So to provide 264.7 gm of dextrose/day required volume of D50 will be about 529 ml/day (22 ml per hour).

Protein

Protein supplementation is an essential component of parenteral nutrition. The primary source of protein supplementation in parenteral nutrition is free amino acids. Amino acids given in PN are not provided as an energy substrate. But the rationale for its supplementation is that they are essential for synthesizing protein, replacing nitrogen losses, and preventing further skeletal muscle breakdown.

A. Calorie value and preparations

When an amino acid is oxidized for energy, it provides 4 calories per gm. 6.25 gm of protein contains 1 gm of nitrogen. The standard amino acid solution contains approximately 40–50% essential amino acids (N=9) and the rest 50–60% nonessential amino acids (N=10) plus semi-essential (N=4) amino acids. Crystalline amino acid solutions used in PN are of high biological quality.

Standard commercially made crystalline amino acid formulations are available in 3 to 15% concentrations. 10% solution of amino acids contains 100 gm of protein per liter.

B. Requirements

Approximately 15 to 20% of total energy requirements should come from protein. Protein and energy requirements are closely related. To minimize protein catabolism, a sufficient amount of non-protein calories, such as carbohydrates and fats, must be administered simultaneously. A calorie to nitrogen ratio of 100–150:1 will be satisfactory for normal patients. The protein requirement for an average stable adult is about 0.8–1.5 gm/kg/day. When patients receive protein without adequate calories, the requirement for protein increases because, in addition to its use for protein synthesis, the protein supplied is also utilized for energy production. Amino acid administration is essential to prevent protein-energy malnutrition (PEM). PEM may lead to immunosuppression and infection in critically ill patients.

Table 55.7 Recommended daily protein intake	
Clinical condition	**Protein requirements** (gm/kg ideal body wt/day)
Stable	0.8–1.5
Critically ill, trauma, sepsis	1.2–2.5
Acute kidney injury (undialysed)	0.8–2.0
Renal replacement therapy	Additional 0.2 gm/kg/d, up to 2.5 gm/kg/d
Burns	1.5–2.0
Hepatic failure	1.2–2.0
Traumatic brain injury	1.5–2.5

Protein requirement is higher (1.5–2.5 gm/kg/day) in massive burns, severe trauma, hypoproteinemia, protein-losing enteropathy or nephropathy, or in patients receiving dialysis treatment. In critically ill patients with sepsis, a large amount of nitrogen loss results from abnormal metabolism. General guidelines for protein requirement in hospitalized patients are summarized in Table 55.7 [13].

For critically ill patients, optimal protein intake is approximately 1.5 gm/kg/day. This amount of protein intake can decrease the degree of nitrogen loss in catabolic patients, mostly by enhancing visceral protein synthesis and, to a lesser extent, by diminishing peripheral protein catabolism. Delivering an additional amount of protein does not further reverse this trend and does not yield a positive nitrogen balance. On the contrary, if excess protein (>1.7 gm/kg/day) is provided, it results in excess ureagenesis rather than contributing to protein anabolism.

C. Functions and advantages

1. Protein synthesis: The main function of protein is the growth and maintenance of cells and tissues in a steady stage.

2. Reduces the rate of protein catabolism: In critically ill patients, protein catabolism exceeds protein synthesis and leads to net protein loss. Administration of an adequate amount of protein along with calories decreases body protein loss but does not prevent the loss completely.

3. Calorie supplementation: 1 gm of protein provides 4 kcal energy. Patients receiving inadequate calories from carbohydrates and lipids will utilize protein for energy production. Thus, excess protein is needed for nitrogen balance when energy intake is low.

D. Contraindications and adverse effects

1. Hepatic insufficiency: In patients with hepatic insufficiency, infusion of standard amino acids may cause metabolic alkalosis, increased levels of ammonia, stupor, or coma.

2. Renal failure: A patient with impaired renal function may develop a marked rise in BUN.

3. Metabolic or respiratory alkalosis may be exacerbated by the excess acetate ions present in amino acid solutions.

4. Rapid administration may cause nausea, vomiting, headache, chills, or fever.

5. Administration of excess protein or insufficient calorie supplementation results in the production of an increased amount of urea. Renal loss of excess nitrogen leads to water loss and may cause hypertonic dehydration (especially in young children) unless extra water is provided.

E. Monitoring

In stable patients receiving an amino acid infusion, the adequacy of protein support can be assessed by analyzing nitrogen balance.

Nitrogen Balance =
Nitrogen Intake – Nitrogen Loss

Nitrogen Intake =
Protein Intake [gm] / 6.25

Nitrogen Loss = 24-Hour UUN + 4

Where 24-hour UUN represents the gm of nitrogen excreted in the urine over 24 hours, and the addition of + 4 accounts for 4 gm of nitrogen lost each day as insensible losses via the skin and gastrointestinal tract.

Positive nitrogen balance suggests anabolism or nitrogen retention. Nitrogen loss greater than nitrogen intake (negative nitrogen balance) suggests net nitrogen loss. If the blood urea nitrogen (BUN) level exceeds 100 mg/dL or a patient with hepatic encephalopathy shows clinical worsening with a rising ammonia level while infusing amino acids, the dose of standard amino acids needs to be reduced or discontinued [24].

F. Example of calculation of protein/ amino acid solution requirements

Example: For a 60 kg male with 1.0 gm per kg per day protein requirements, considering basic requirements and adding stress factors, how much amino acid solution is needed for PN in a day?

1. Total daily protein requirements will be 60 kg × 1.0 gm/kg = 60 gm per day.
2. 100 ml solution of 5% and 10% of amino acid preparation provides 5 gm and 10 gm of amino acid, respectively. So, to provide 60 gm of amino acid/day required volume

of 5% and 10% of amino acid preparations will be 1200 and 600 ml/day, respectively.

Lipids

Lipid injectable emulsions (ILEs, formerly known as Intravenous Fat Emulsion) are an essential component of PN formulations that have two main functions: to provide an energy-dense source of calories that help in reducing the dextrose load needed to meet energy goals and supply essential fatty acids (EFAs) such as linoleic and linolenic acids which prevent or correct essential fatty acid deficiency.

A. Contents of lipid emulsion

Different lipid emulsions contain varying amounts and proportions of omega-3, omega-6, and omega-9 fatty acids. Lipid emulsions containing soybean oil are the mainstay and the first-generation lipids for parenteral nutrition and have been used extensively with fair success for decades [25, 26]. This formulation for PN also contains three other components: egg yolk phospholipids as an emulsifying

Table 55.8 Classification, composition, and benefits of lipid injectable emulsions

Generation of ILEs	Composition of ILEs	The ratio of ω-6:ω-3 FAs	Rationale and benefits	Selected ILEs products
First	100% soy oil	7:1	Used to supply EFA and energy	Intralipid, nutrilipid
Second	50% soy oil, 50% MCT	7:1	MCT is added to reduce the soy content and the amount of ω-6 FA	Lipofundin MCT/ LCT
Third	20% soy oil, 80% olive oil	9:1/NA	Reduce the soy content. Less prone to inflammatory processes and immune suppression	ClinOleic/ clinolipid
Fourth	30% soy oil, 30% MCT, 25% olive oil, 15% fish oil	2.5:1	Reduce the soy content, ω-6 to ω-3 FA ratio, infectious complications, and hospital stay. Preferred in critically ill and surgical patients	SMOFlipid

EFA: Essential fatty acid; FA: Fatty acid; ω-3, Omega 3; ω-6, Omega 6; ILE: Lipid injectable emulsion; LCT: Long chain triglycerides; MCT: Medium-chain triglyceride; MUFA: Monounsaturated fatty acid; Soy: Soybean agent to mix two immiscible liquid phases, fine droplets of oil suspended in water; glycerin to make the formulation isotonicity with plasma; and sodium hydroxide, which adjusts the final pH around 8.0 [27, 28].

First-generation soybean oil containing lipid emulsions are composed mainly of omega-6 FA-rich linoleic acid with low content (about 10%) of omega-3 FA containing α-linolenic acid (ALA), and therefore has a high (7:1) omega-6/omega-3 FAs ratio. The high content of omega-6 FA in soybean-based lipid emulsions has pro-inflammatory and immunosuppressive harmful effects and therefore is associated with adverse outcomes in critically ill patients [25, 29, 30].

Alternative lipid emulsions, such as generation 2 (combining soybean oil with medium-chain triglycerides), generation 3 (using olive oil), and generation 4 (using fish oil) lipid emulsions, have been developed to decrease the harmful effects of the omega-6-rich linoleic acid content and to lower the ratio of omega-6 to omega-3 fatty acids as summarized in Table 55.8 [26, 31–33].

B. Caloric values, preparations, and requirements

Lipid is the richest source of calories; 1 gm of lipid provides 9 kcal (vs. dextrose provides 3.4 kcal/gm and protein provides 4.0 kcal/gm). The lipid emulsions are available as 10% (1.1 kcal/ml), 20% (2.0 kcal/ml), and 30% (3.0 kcal/ml) solution and have low osmolarity (260 mOsm/L). The use of 30% lipid emulsion is approved for preparing a total nutrient admixture or "3 in 1" delivery system in a pharmacy admixture program. Still, it is not recommended for direct intravenous administration.

In PN, lipids should be infused to provide about 25–40% of non-protein calories [34]. ILE requirements are 1 gm/kg/d in stable patients and less than 1 gm/kg/d in critically ill, trauma, and sepsis patients (ASPEN 2019) [13]. Lipid emulsions should be started usually at a dose of 0.7 gm/kg/day, the upper recommended dose is 1 gm/kg/day, and it should not exceed 1.5 gm/kg/day (ESPEN 2019) [18]. In obese patients, underfeeding help in the mobilization of the endogenous fat store and, as a result, improves insulin sensitivity and glycemic control [35].

C. Functions and advantages

1. Dense calorie supplementation: IV lipid emulsion is a concentrated calorie source (9 kcal/gm), so it is the other major calorie-rich fuel that provides energy effectively. Providing more energy in a given volume (compared to IV dextrose fluids) is an essential advantage of lipid emulsion in critically ill, volume overloaded patients.

2. Avoids hyperglycemia: Lipid emulsion provides a portion of the total calorie requirement, thereby allowing a lower rate of dextrose infusion and reducing the potential adverse effects of infusing excess glucose for calories.

3. Protein sparing effect: IV lipid emulsion is more effective than IV dextrose in providing energy. In PN, adequate supplementation of calories by curtailing protein oxidation prevents protein catabolism and exerts a protein-sparing effect.

4. Less CO_2 production (lower respiratory quotient): Compared to carbohydrates, lipids produce less CO_2 and, therefore, are preferred in respiratory compromised patients.

Lipids' respiratory quotient (RQ) is the least (RQ of lipids 0.7 vs. 0.8 for proteins and 1.0 for carbohydrates). The respiratory quotient is the ratio of CO_2 production to O_2 consumption. So, IV lipid emulsion has the advantages of better glucose tolerance, less hyperinsulinemia, less fatty infiltration of the liver, and less production of CO_2. Because of these benefits, lipid emulsion is widely utilized in patients with hyperglycemia, diabetes, liver disease, and respiratory failure.

5. Prevention of essential fatty acid deficiency: Lipid emulsion assists in wound healing, the production of red blood cells (RBC), and prostaglandin synthesis. PN administration without lipid supplementation for more than 2 weeks should be avoided because it can lead to essential fatty acid deficiency, causing dry, scaly skin rash, hair loss, thrombocytopenia, anemia, poor wound healing, and increased susceptibility to infection. To prevent essential fatty acid deficiency, supplement about 2% to 4% of total caloric intake as linoleic acid and 0.25% to 0.5% as alpha-linolenic acid beyond 2 weeks of administering PN.

6. Reduced risk of thrombophlebitis due to lower osmolality: Hypertonic solutions are irritant to veins, thus increasing the risk of thrombophlebitis. Unlike the hypertonic dextrose solutions, the osmolarity of lipid emulsion is low (260 mOsm/L), almost the same as that of plasma. So the addition of lipid emulsion reduces the osmolarity and, therefore, reduces the risk of thrombophlebitis due to PN. Besides, lipid emulsion exerts a protective effect on vascular endothelium. For the same reason, lipid emulsion is an important component of solutions for peripheral parenteral nutrition (PPN).

The advantages of including lipid emulsion in PN are summarized in Table 55.9.

D. Adverse effects and disadvantages

The adverse effects of lipid administration are:

1. Increased triglyceride levels: Infusion of lipid emulsion causes an increase in plasma triglycerides, cholesterol, phospholipids, and concentration of lipoproteins. When lipid emulsion is infused rapidly and/or in high doses, the rate of infusion of triglyceride exceeds the rate of hydrolysis of triglyceride by endothelial enzyme lipoprotein lipase and, therefore, can cause hypertriglyceridemia [36].

2. Sepsis: Lipid emulsion carries a risk of infection when administered separately over a prolonged time.

3. Fat embolism: Lipid is less stable when infused with amino acids and

---

Table 55.9 Advantages of lipid emulsion in PN solutions

- Large amount of calories in a small volume.
- Improve glucose tolerance and reduce insulin levels.
- Reduces the risk of refeeding syndrome.
- Lower osmolarity. Reduces the risk of thrombophlebitis. Safe for PPN.
- Supply of essential fatty acid.
- Less CO_2 production than glucose oxidation, which is beneficial in respiratory compromised patients weaning from ventilator support.

glucose as a combined "three-in-one solution". Destabilized particles of fat coalesce into larger droplets and subsequently form fat emboli. For the same reason, a three-in-one solution has a shorter storage life, and improperly mixed or delayed in the use of solution carries the risk of fat embolism.

4. Less frequent complications: Immediate or early adverse reactions include dyspnea, cyanosis, nausea or vomiting, headache, allergic reactions, chest and back pain, or thrombocytopenia. Delayed complications with prolonged administration include hepatic dysfunction, fat overload syndrome, pancreatitis, and delayed gastric emptying.

Most adverse effects are instead due to hypertriglyceridemia than due to lipids per se. Hypertriglyceridemia occurs due to the infusion of lipids at a rate faster than lipid clearance. Thus, if lipids are infused at proper infusion rates and serum triglycerides are monitored regularly, most adverse effects of lipids are avoided.

E. Indications

Lipid administration is indicated in all patients needing a home or prolonged PN. Lipid administration is also indicated in patients who need PPN, high caloric supplementation but fail to tolerate carbohydrates, critically ill patients, and patients with hyperglycemia, diabetes mellitus, and respiratory failure.

F. Contraindications

Avoid lipid emulsion in patients with severe hypertriglyceridemia (reduce dose if serum triglycerides >400 mg/dL and do not use if serum triglycerides >1000 mg/dL), in patients who are at risk of developing fat embolism, hypersensitivity to lipid emulsion, severe metabolic acidosis, in patients with acute shock, anemia, severe coagulopathy, and evidence of intravascular coagulation [34]. In addition, lipid emulsions should be used cautiously in obese patients because of the greater risk of hyperglycemia and hypertriglyceridemia.

G. Administration and monitoring

IV lipid emulsion used to prevent essential fatty acid deficiency is given 3 to 4 days a week; while used as a calorie source, it is provided daily. The lipid can be administered IV either separately by piggyback infusion with the 2-in-1 system (containing dextrose and amino acids) or as 3 in 1 admixture (all-in-one infusion) of dextrose, protein, and lipids in a single bag. Lipid emulsions may also provide rich media for the growth of bacteria and fungi. Therefore, scrupulous handwashing before handling lipids is mandatory to reduce the risk of touch contamination. As exposure of the lipids to light causes the formation of potentially toxic peroxides, avoid it by wrapping it in aluminum foil or carbon paper.

Since most complications are associated with rapid IV lipid infusion (greater than 1.0 kcal/kg/hr or 0.11 gm/kg/hr), the rate should not exceed 0.7 kcal/kg/hr. Usually, lipid emulsions should be administered slowly over 12 hours. However, avoid a prolonged infusion of lipids and discard bottles and tubing hung alone after 12 hours. PN solution bag may hang for a maximum of 24 hours and discard any remaining solution and tubing after 24 hours [37].

In patients with lipid infusion, triglyceride levels should be monitored at least weekly. Lipid infusion should be reduced or discontinued if the triglyceride level exceeds 400 mg/dL to decrease the risk of pancreatitis or decreased diffusion capacity in patients with severe chronic obstructive lung disease.

H. Selection of lipid emulsions (ILE)

The most commonly used soybean based first-generation lipid emulsions are usually recommended for short-term use (<2 weeks) in stable critical patients with normal LFTs [33].

Newer lipid emulsions for PN are developed which has a lower content of harmful omega-6 FA and contains omega-3 FA in a higher amount [31]. In contrast to omega-6 FA, omega-3 FA-enriched newer lipid emulsions (i.e., fish oil containing ILE) has beneficial anti-inflammatory and immunomodulatory effects, which reduces the risk of infection and sepsis and shorten ICU and hospital stay and therefore preferred in high-risk patients requiring PN such as sepsis, critically ill and surgical patients [33, 38–40]. Lipid emulsion preparation containing a mixture of soybean oil, medium-chain triglycerides (MCTs), olive oil and fish oils, such as SMOF lipid is available commercially [41].

I. Example of calculation of lipids/ lipid emulsion requirements

Example: For a 60 kg male with 25 kcal/kg/d energy requirements, how much lipid emulsion is needed (considering 30% of total energy requirement in the form of lipid) in a day?

1. Total caloric requirements will be 60 × 25 = 1500 kcal/day, and lipid requirement will be 450 (30% of 1500) kcal/day.

2. 10% and 20% of lipid emulsions provide 1.1 kcal/cc and 2.0 kcal/cc, respectively. So, to provide 600 kcal/day required volume of 10% and 20% of lipid emulsion will be about 409 ml (450 ÷ 1.1) and 225 ml (450 ÷ 2.0) respectively.

Diseases-specific amino acids

Modified specialized solutions with adjusted amino acid contents are available for the specific disease state.

A. For hepatic encephalopathy

Specific "hepatic formula" for parenteral nutrition is a modified amino acid solution rich in branched-chain amino acids (BCAAs) (valine, leucine, and isoleucine) and has a low content of aromatic amino acids (AAA) (phenylalanine, tryptophan, and tyrosine), and sulfur-containing amino acids like methionine [42].

Potential mechanisms by which branched-chain amino acids benefits are:

- Compared with non-branched chain amino acids (Non-BCAAs), which are metabolized by the liver, BCAAs are uniquely oxidized chiefly in skeletal muscle and adipose tissues (and not in the liver). BCAAs enhances detoxification and removal of ammonia in skeletal muscles, reduces plasma ammonia concentration, and may reduce hepatic encephalopathy [43].

- In hepatic insufficiency due to liver cirrhosis, high aromatic amino acids (AAA) and low BCAAs/AAA ratio play an important role in developing hepatic encephalopathy [44]. BCAAs and aromatic amino acids are transported into the brain via the same carrier [45]. So, BCAAs compete with aromatic amino acids, potentially decreasing the passage of aromatic amino acids across the blood-brain barrier, reducing the release of neurotransmitters, notably serotonin, and thereby having beneficial effects on brain function [46, 47].

A high concentration of BCAAs (35–45%) in "hepatic formula" corrects the amino acid imbalance and is recommended in selected patients of liver cirrhosis with hepatic encephalopathy grades III–IV refractory to standard management [42].

BCAAs-enriched formulations show highly significant improvement in mental recovery [48, 49], but no evidence suggests improvement in the patient's outcome [4, 49].

Because of increased cost and controversial efficiency, BCAAs should not be used as the first-line treatment for hepatic encephalopathy [4].

In patients with liver diseases, use standard amino acid (and reduce the cost of therapy) in the absence of encephalopathy, grades I or II hepatic encephalopathies, once the encephalopathy resolves, and for preoperative nutrition after liver transplantation [50].

B. For acute kidney injury (AKI)

Supplementation of protein leads to accumulation of end products such as urea with worsening of uremia. Therefore, protein restriction was previously practiced to reduce uremic symptoms and avoid or delay initiating dialysis therapy. But as per current recommendations, protein restriction should be avoided in patients with renal insufficiency [4, 51].

Recommended doses of protein in non-dialysis AKI patients are 0.8–1.0 gm/kg/day in non-catabolic AKI [51], and in AKI patients on renal replacement therapy (RRT) are 1.0–1.5 gm/kg/d as per KDIGO guidelines (2012) [51], or additional protein 0.2 gm/kg/day, up to 2.5 gm/kg/day as per ASPEN guidelines (2016) [4].

The role of specially designed amino acid-containing solutions ("nephro-solutions") is controversial but may benefit patients who do not require dialysis [52].

Immunomodulators

Immunonutrients are specific nutrients that have the potential to modify inflammatory or immune responses with beneficial effects on mucosal barrier function, cellular defense, and local or systemic inflammation [53]. The use of immune-modulating nutrients such as glutamine, arginine, and omega-3 fatty acids are common. However, a recent Cochrane Database Systematic Review (2019) found the effect of these immunonutrition supplements on the duration of ventilator days, ICU length of stay, or oxygenation in patients with acute respiratory distress syndrome to be uncertain [54].

A. Glutamine

Glutamine is the body's most abundant amino acid, which is primarily synthesized by skeletal muscles. glutamine is the primary energy source for rapidly dividing cells such as intestinal epithelial cells, vascular epithelial cells, and proliferating immune cells. Glutamine is vital for maintaining the gut barrier function and is considered a "fuel for the immune system," which exerts antioxidant and cytoprotective effects, helps defend the body against pathogens, and decreases infectious complications [55].

Studies in septic and critically ill patients have shown that administering glutamine does not improve outcomes such as mortality, organ failure, infectious complications, or length of stay [56–58]. Some studies have even shown harmful effects [58–60], leading to the recommendation against administering glutamine in septic critically ill patients [61]. In recent guidelines, parenteral glutamine is not recommended in critically ill, unstable, and complex ICU patients and with multiorgan failure, especially with liver and renal failure (Canadian guidelines 2015, ASPEN guidelines 2016, ESPEN guideline 2019) [4, 18, 62].

As clinical benefits of parenteral glutamine are documented in various studies [63–67], IV glutamine may be used in selected patients on PN who are stable, together with adequate parenteral energy and protein after excluding hemodynamic instability, hepatic or renal failure [68].

Parenteral glutamine supplementation is preferred over enteral for patients in the intensive care unit [69]. When IV glutamine supplementation is indicated in PN, the recommended dose of glutamine is 0.2–0.4 gm/kg/day (0.3–0.6 gm/kg/day of alanyl-glutamine dipeptide) [70].

B. Omega 3 fatty acids

Omega-3 fatty acids have anti-inflammatory and immunomodulatory effects and have been shown to improve clinical outcomes in surgical, trauma, cancer, and critically ill patients, as well as during long-term parenteral nutrition due to their inflammation-resolving effects [29, 30, 71].

Administration of injectable lipid emulsion containing omega-3 fatty acids provides significant benefits such as the reduction in risk of infection, sepsis, and length of stay in both ICU as well as hospital, and therefore is preferred over standard lipid emulsions (without omega-3 fatty acids) in hospitalized adult patients requiring PN [30, 40, 71].

Omega-3 fatty acids are abundant in fish oil. Newly designed **SMOFlipid** solution is a **S**oybean oil (30%), **M**edium-chain triglycerides (30%), **O**live oil (25%), and **F**ish oil (15%)

containing **lipid** emulsion, which is used to provide omega-3 fatty acids enriched PN [26]. The higher cost of omega-3 fatty acids enriched lipid emulsions is a concern. But improved clinical outcomes (reduced infectious complications and shorter hospital and ICU stays) offset the overall costs [72, 73].

C. Arginine

Arginine is a nutrient that boosts the immune system and is considered a nonessential amino acid under normal circumstances. However, during times of catabolism, it becomes a conditionally essential nutrient. Arginine plays an essential role in protein synthesis, nitric oxide generation, and immunomodulation, thereby playing a major role in cellular defense and wound healing. In addition, arginine supplementation reduces the rate of infectious complications and the duration of hospitalization postoperatively [74].

Intravenous or enteral arginine supplementation as a standalone treatment is not recommended for critically ill patients or those with severe sepsis [4, 75, 76]. For patients requiring enteral nutrition therapy, an immune-modulating formula containing both arginine and fish oils should be used in the perioperative or postoperative period, including in malnourished patients undergoing major cancer surgery and in severe trauma cases in the SICU [4, 76].

Micronutrients

Electrolytes, trace elements, and vitamins come under micronutrients. Requirements of micronutrients for PN in the normal adult are summarized in Table 55.10. The minerals and vitamins required in parenteral nutrition are much lesser than in enteral nutrition because of better bioavailability with direct

Nutrient	Requirements	Nutrient	Requirements
Table 55.10 Recommended daily parenteral requirements of micronutrients			
Electrolytes		**Fat soluble vitamin**	
Sodium	1.0–2.0 mEq/kg	Vitamin A	990 mcg (3300 IU)
Potassium	1.0–2.0 mEq/kg	Vitamin D	5.0 mcg (200 IU)
Magnesium	8.0–20 mEq	Vitamin E	10 mg (10 IU)
Phosphate	20–40 mmol	Vitamin K	150 mcg
Calcium	10–15 mEq	-	-
Trace minerals		**Water soluble vitamins**	
Chromium	≤10 mcg	Thiamine (B1)	6.0 mg
Copper	0.3–0.5 mg	Riboflavin (B2)	3.6 mg
Manganese	55 mcg	Niacin (B3)	40 mg
Selenium	60–100 mcg	Pantothenic acid (B5)	15 mg
Zinc	3.0–5.0 mg	Pyridoxine (B6)	6.0 mg
-	-	Folic acid (B9)	600 mcg
-	-	Cobalamin B12	5.0 mcg
-	-	Ascorbic acid (Vit C)	200 mg
-	-	Biotin	60 mcg

intravenous infusion. These value needs to be modified considering the clinical situations.

Electrolytes

As electrolytes are essential to perform critical metabolic activities, it is a must in all PN formulas. As sodium influences intravascular volume status, it is restricted in patients at risk of volume overload (e.g., cardiac, liver, and renal failure) and given liberally when volume expansion is desired (those with GI losses). Potassium requirement increases in patients with increased renal loss of potassium, in those who receive amphotericin B therapy, and in severely malnourished patients while initiating PN.

After meeting phosphate requirements, sodium and potassium cations are usually added to parenteral nutrition solutions in the form of chloride or acetate salts. The choice of the salt form

has an impact on acid-base balance. The liver metabolizes acetate into bicarbonate, which acts as an alkaline buffer. Therefore, acetate is a preferred salt in patients with metabolic acidosis. Loss of a large amount of chloride (such as nasogastric aspiration) can cause metabolic alkalosis. Sodium and potassium are provided in such patients, preferably as chloride salt for PN.

The use of sodium bicarbonate in PN is incompatible as it forms insoluble coprecipitates, mainly with calcium and magnesium. Thus, bicarbonate salts should never be infused through a common intravenous line with PN.

Trace elements

Trace elements, in small amounts, are crucial for efficient substrate utilization and other supporting functions and therefore are an essential component of PN. A deficiency of trace elements develops quickly in stressed patients or patients with increased GI losses.

On the other hand, stable patients do not develop evidence of deficiency, even though trace elements are not supplemented for about two months. Commercial preparations are available as injections in various combinations, providing required trace elements.

Most trace element PN formulations contain zinc, copper, chromium, manganese, and selenium but do not have iron and iodine [13]. Selenium supplementation is recommended for patients receiving long-term PN because of the risk of muscle weakness and fatal cardiomyopathy caused by selenium deficiency.

The daily requirement of iodine is 70–150 mcg and 1 mg of elemental iron, but most PN formulations do not contain these trace elements. In most patients receiving PN, iron is not supplemented because of adequate body storage. Note that iron is not generally part of commercially available standard additives and not added to PN solutions because it can cause lipid emulsions to destabilize and therefore is incompatible with lipid-containing PN formulas like "3 in 1" solutions. In addition, iron is not given routinely to patients who are critically ill because free iron may promote bacterial growth and increase susceptibility to infection [77].

The requirements for many trace elements in PN are lower than for oral or enteral nutrition. This is because the gut absorbs only a portion of the supplemented nutrient, sometimes less than 10% (e.g., chromium).

However, it is important to remember that some trace elements' parenteral requirements are higher than actual body requirements. These increased requirements result from increased urinary losses, as they are delivered via systemic rather than portal circulation (and therefore not captured by the liver).

Vitamins

Vitamins are essential for normal metabolism and are an important part of PN. Requirements of trace elements for PN are generally lower than in EN, but the reverse is true for vitamins.

Parenteral requirements of vitamins are higher than those required through oral or enteral administration due to the following reasons.

1. Vitamins supplemented orally are generally absorbed much more than most trace elements.

2. Vitamins get degraded during preparations and storage. For example, vitamin A, riboflavin, and vitamin K are degraded by light, and thiamine is degraded by sulfite ions used as a preservative for amino acid solutions.

3. Vitamins are lost partially due to adherence to tubing and delivery bags.

The recommended dose for water-soluble vitamins is four to five times the usual and minimum daily requirements for fat-soluble vitamins. Commercially available aqueous multivitamin preparations will provide normal daily requirements for most vitamins except for vitamin K.

Commercially available aqueous multivitamin preparations will provide normal daily requirements. Vitamin K is beneficial to most patients on PN and is administered as multivitamin preparation or added separately to lipid emulsions, but it may be detrimental to patients receiving oral anticoagulants [78, 79]. It is important to remember that vitamins and trace elements are added to PN shortly before use because of the concern about stability.

REFERENCES

1. Saunders J, Smith T. Malnutrition: causes and consequences. Clin Med (Lond). 2010;10(6):624–627.
2. Griffiths RD. Too much of a good thing: the curse of overfeeding. Crit Care. 2007;11(6):176.
3. Preiser JC, van Zanten AR, Berger MM, et al. Metabolic and nutritional support of critically ill patients: consensus and controversies. Crit Care. 2015;19(1):35.
4. McClave SA, Taylor BE, Martindale RG, et al. Guidelines for the provision and assessment of nutrition support therapy in the adult critically ill patient: Society of Critical Care Medicine (SCCM) and American Society for Parenteral and Enteral Nutrition (A.S.P.E.N.). JPEN J Parenter Enteral Nutr 2016;40(2):159–211.
5. Reignier J, Boisramé-Helms J, Brisard L, et al. Enteral versus parenteral early nutrition in ventilated adults with shock: a randomised, controlled, multicentre, open-label, parallel-group study (NUTRIREA-2). Lancet 2018;391(10116):133–143.
6. Windsor AC, Kanwar S, Li AG, et al. Compared with parenteral nutrition, enteral feeding attenuates the acute phase response and improves disease severity in acute pancreatitis. Gut. 1998;42(3):431–435.
7. Khalid I, Doshi P, DiGiovine B. Early enteral nutrition and outcomes of critically ill patients treated with vasopressors and mechanical ventilation. Am J Crit Care 2010;19:261–268.
8. Merchan C, Altshuler D, Aberle C, et al. Tolerability of enteral nutrition in mechanically ventilated patients with septic shock who require vasopressors. J Intensive Care Med. 2017;32(9):540–546.
9. Simo Es Covello LH, Gava-Brandolis MG, Castro MG, et al. Vasopressors and nutrition therapy: safe dose for the outset of enteral nutrition? Crit Care Res Pract. 2020;2020:1095693.
10. ASPEN Board of Directors and the Clinical Guidelines Task Force. Guidelines for the use of parenteral and enteral nutrition in adult and pediatric patients [erratum in JPEN J Parenter Enteral Nutr. 2002;26(2):144.
11. Wilkinson RE, Dickerson RN. "New" Indications for Parenteral Nutrition. Hosp Pharm. 2016;51(10):795–797.
12. Worthington P, Balint J, Bechtold M, et.al. When is parenteral nutrition appropriate? JPEN J Parenter Enteral Nutr. 2017;41(3):324–377.
13. Appropriate Dosing for Parenteral Nutrition: ASPEN Recommendations. American Society Parenteral and Enteral Nutrition 2019. http://www.nutritioncare.org/uploadedFiles/Documents/Guidelines_and_Clinical_Resources/PN%20Dosing%201-Sheet-FINAL.pdf.
14. Gupta RD, Ramachandran R, Venkatesan P, et al. Indirect calorimetry: from bench to bedside. Indian J Endocrinol Metab. 2017;21(4):594–599.
15. Delsoglio M, Achamrah N, Berger MM, et al. Indirect calorimetry in clinical practice. J Clin Med. 2019;8(9):1387.
16. Achamrah N, Delsoglio M, De Waele E, et al. Indirect calorimetry: the 6 main issues. Clin Nutr 2020.
17. Nowak K. Parenteral nutrition-associated liver disease. Clin Liver Dis (Hoboken). 2020;15(2):59–62.
18. Singer P, Blaser AR, Berger MM, et al. ESPEN guideline on clinical nutrition in the intensive care unit. Clin Nutr. 2019;38(1):48–79.
19. Singer P, Berger MM, Van den Berghe G, et al. ESPEN guidelines on Parenteral Nutrition: intensive care. Clin Nutr 2009;33:246e51.
20. American Diabetes Association. 15. Diabetes care in the hospital: Standards of Medical Care in Diabetesd2020. Diabetes Care 2020;43(Suppl. 1):S193–S202.
21. Gosmanov AR, Umpierrez GE. Management of hyperglycemia during enteral and parenteral nutrition therapy. Curr Diab Rep. 2013;13(1):155–162.
22. Li F, Zhang W, Liu B, et al. Management of glycemic variation in diabetic patients receiving parenteral nutrition by continuous subcutaneous insulin infusion (CSII) therapy. Sci Rep 2018;8:5888.
23. McCulloch A, Bansiya V, Woodward JM. Addition of insulin to parenteral nutrition for control of hyperglycemia. JPEN J Parenter Enteral Nutr. 2018;42(5):846–854.
24. Cerra FB, Benitez MR, Blackburn GL, et al. Applied nutrition in ICU patients. A consensus statement of the American College of Chest Physicians. Chest. 1997;111(3):769–78.
25. Raman M, Almutairdi A, Mulesa L, et al. Parenteral nutrition and lipids. Nutrients. 2017;9(4):388.
26. Mundi MS, Salonen BR, Bonnes SL, et al. Parenteral nutrition lipid emulsions and potential complications. Practical Gastroenterology 2017;41(8):32–37.
27. Hippalgaonkar K, Majumdar S, Kansara V. Injectable lipid emulsions- advancements, opportunities and challenges. AAPS PharmSciTech. 2010;11(4):1526–1540.
28. Fell GL, Nandivada P, Gura KM, et al. Intravenous lipid emulsions in parenteral nutrition. Adv Nutr. 2015;6(5):600–610.
29. Klek S. Omega-3 fatty acids in modern parenteral nutrition: a review of the current evidence. J Clin Med. 2016;5(3):34.
30. Calder PC, Adolph M, Deutz NE, et al. Lipids in the intensive care unit: recommendations from the ESPEN Expert Group. Clin Nutr. 2018;37(1):1–18.
31. Sadu Singh BK, Narayanan SS, Khor BH, et al. Composition and functionality of lipid emulsions in parenteral nutrition: examining evidence in clinical applications. Front Pharmacol. 2020;11:506.
32. Calder PC, Waitzberg DL, Klek S, et al. Lipids in parenteral nutrition: biological aspects. JPEN J Parenter Enteral Nutr. 2020;44(1):S21–S27.
33. Mirtallo JM, Ayers P, Boullata J, et al. ASPEN lipid injectable emulsion safety recommendations, part 1: background and adult considerations. Nutr Clin Pract. 2020;35(5):769–782.

34. Adolph M, Heller AR, Koch T, et al. Lipid emulsions - Guidelines on Parenteral Nutrition, Chapter 6. Ger Med Sci. 2009;7:Doc22.

35. Koretz RL, Lipman TO, Klein S. American Gastroenterological Association. AGA technical review on parenteral nutrition. Gastroenterology. 2001;121(4):970–1001.

36. Anez-Bustillos L, Dao DT, Baker MA, et al. Intravenous fat emulsion formulations for the adult and pediatric patient: understanding the differences. Nutr Clin Pract. 2016;31(5):596–609.

37. Infection Control Manual. UNC Health Care. February 2018. https://spice.unc.edu/wp-content/uploads/2018/05/Intravascular-Catheter-Related-Infections-IC0032.pdf.

38. Mayer K, Klek S, Martindale RG, et al. Lipid use in hospitalized adults requiring parenteral nutrition. JPEN J Parenter Enteral Nutr. 2020;44(Suppl 1):S28–S38.

39. Martindale RG, Berlana D, Boullata JI, et al. Summary of proceedings and expert consensus statements from the international summit "Lipids in Parenteral Nutrition". JPEN J Parenter Enteral Nutr. 2020;44(Suppl 1):S7–S20.

40. Pradelli L, Mayer K, Klek S, et al. ω-3 Fatty-Acid enriched parenteral nutrition in hospitalized patients: systematic review with meta-analysis and trial sequential analysis. JPEN J Parenter Enteral Nutr 2020;44(1):44–57.

41. Goulet O, Antébi H, Wolf C, et al. A new intravenous fat emulsion containing soybean oil, medium-chain triglycerides, olive oil, and fish oil: a single-center, double-blind randomized study on efficacy and safety in pediatric patients receiving home parenteral nutrition. JPEN J Parenter Enteral Nutr. 2010;34(5):485–95.

42. Plauth M, Schuetz T, Working group for developing the guidelines for parenteral nutrition of The German Association for Nutritional Medicine. Hepatology - Guidelines on Parenteral Nutrition, Chapter 16. Ger Med Sci. 2009;7:12.

43. Dam G, Aamann L, Vistrup H, et al. The role of Branched Chain Amino Acids in the treatment of hepatic Encephalopathy. J Clin Exp Hepatol. 2018;8(4):448–451.

44. Dejong CH, van de Poll MC, Soeters PB, et al. Aromatic amino acid metabolism during liver failure. J Nutr. 2007;137(6 Suppl 1):1579S–1585S.

45. Holeček M. Branched-chain amino acids in health and disease: metabolism, alterations in blood plasma, and as supplements. Nutr Metab (Lond). 2018;15:33.

46. Fernstrom JD. Branched-chain amino acids and brain function. J Nutr. 2005;135(6 Suppl):1539S–46S.

47. Varshney P, Saini P. Role of Branched Chain Amino Acids supplementation on quality of life in liver cirrhosis patients. Research J. Pharm. and Tech. 2020;13(7):3516–3519.

48. Naylor CD, O'Rourke K, Detsky AS, et al. Parenteral nutrition with branched-chain amino acids in hepatic encephalopathy. A meta-analysis. Gastroenterology 1989;97:1033.

49. Gluud LL, Dam G, Les I, et al. Branched-chain amino acids for people with hepatic encephalopathy. Cochrane Database Syst Rev 2017;5:CD001939.

50. EASL Clinical Practice Guidelines on nutrition in chronic liver disease. J Hepatol. 2019;70(1):172–193.

51. Kellum JA, Lameire N, Aspelin P, et al. KDIGO clinical practice guideline for acute kidney injury. Kidney Int Suppl. 2012;2(1):1–138.

52. Stein J, Boehles HJ, Blumenstein I, et al. Amino acids – Guidelines on Parenteral Nutrition, Chapter 4. GMS Ger Med Sci 2009;7:24.

53. Calder PC. Immunonutrition. BMJ. 2003;327(7407):117–118.

54. Dushianthan A, Cusack R, Burgess VA, et al. Immunonutrition for acute respiratory distress syndrome (ARDS) in adults. Cochrane Database Syst Rev. 2019;1(1):CD012041.

55. Cruzat V, Macedo Rogero M, Keane KN, et al. Glutamine: metabolism and immune function, supplementation and clinical translation. Nutrients. 2018;10(11):1564.

56. Andrews PJ, Avenell A, Noble DW, et al. Randomised trial of glutamine, selenium, or both, to supplement parenteral nutrition for critically ill patients. BMJ 2011;342:d1542.

57. Wernerman J, Kirketeig T, Andersson B, et al. Scandinavian glutamine trial: A pragmatic multi-centre randomised clinical trial of intensive care unit patients. Acta Anaesth. Scand. 2011;55:812–818.

58. Heyland D, Muscedere J, Wischmeyer PE, et al. Canadian Critical Care Trials Group. A randomized trial of glutamine and antioxidants in critically ill patients. N Engl J Med. 2013;368(16):1489–97.

59. Heyland DK, Elke G, Cook D, et al. Canadian Critical Care Trials Group. Glutamine and antioxidants in the critically ill patient. JPEN Parenter. Enter. 2015;39(4):401–9.

60. van Zanten AR, Sztark F, Kaisers UX, et al. High-protein enteral nutrition enriched with immune-modulating nutrients vs standard high-protein enteral nutrition and nosocomial infections in the ICU: A randomized clinical trial. JAMA. 2014;312(5):514–24.

61. De Waele E, Malbrain MLNG, Spapen H. Nutrition in Sepsis: A Bench-to-Bedside Review. Nutrients. 2020;12(2):395.

62. Canadian clinical practice guidelines for nutrition support in the mechanically ventilated, critically ill adult, 9.4a composition of PN: Glutamine (CCCN) 2015 https://www.criticalcarenutrition.com/docs/CPGs%202015/4.1c%202015.pdf.

63. Novak F, Heyland DK, Avenell A, et al. Glutamine supplementation in serious illness: a systematic review of the evidence. Crit Care Med 2002;30:2022–9.

64. Manzanares W, Dhaliwal R, Jiang X, et al. Antioxidants micronutrients in the critically ill: a systematic review and meta-analysis. Crit Care 2012;16:R66.

65. Pradelli L, Iannazzo S, Zaniolo O, et al. Effectiveness and cost-effectiveness of supplemental glutamine dipeptide in total parenteral nutrition therapy for critically ill patients: a discrete event simulation model based on Italian data. Int J Technol Assess Health Care. 2012;28(1):22–8.

66. Wischmeyer PE, Dhaliwal R, McCall M, et al. Parenteral glutamine supplementation in critical illness: a systematic review. Crit Care. 2014;18(2):R76.

67. Stehle P, Ellger B, Kojic D, et al. Glutamine dipeptide-supplemented parenteral nutrition improves the clinical outcomes of critically ill patients: a systematic evaluation of randomised controlled trials. Clin Nutr ESPEN 2017;17:75–85.

68. Stehle P, Kuhn KS. Glutamine: an obligatory parenteral nutrition substrate in critical care therapy. BioMed Res Int. 2015:ID545467.

69. Wernerman J. Glutamine supplementation. Ann Intensive Care. 2011;1(1):25.

70. Singer P, Berger MM, Van den Berghe G, et al. ESPEN guidelines on parenteral nutrition: intensive care. Clin Nutr. 2009;28(4):387–400.

71. Mayer K, Klek S, García-de-Lorenzo A, et al. Lipid use in hospitalized adults requiring parenteral nutrition. JPEN J Parenter Enteral Nutr. 2020;44(1):S28–S38.

72. Wu GH, Gao J, Ji CY, et al. Cost and effectiveness of omega-3 fatty acid supplementation in Chinese ICU patients receiving parenteral nutrition. Clinicoecon Outcomes Res. 2015;7:369–375.

73. Pradelli L, Muscaritoli M, Klek S, et al. Pharmacoeconomics of parenteral nutrition with ω-3 fatty acids in hospitalized adults. JPEN J Parenter Enteral Nutr. 2020;44(S1):S68–S73.

74. Casaer MP, Van den Berghe G. Nutrition in the acute phase of critical illness. N Engl J Med. 2014;370(13):1227–36.

75. Canadian Clinical Practice Guidelines for Composition of Enteral Nutrition. 4.1a EN composition: Diets supplemented with arginine and select other nutrients. (CCCN) 2015 https://www.criticalcarenutrition.com/docs/systematic_reviews_2018/4.1a%20%20Arginine_2018.pdf.

76. Weimann A, Braga M, Carli F, et al. P. ESPEN guideline: Clinical nutrition in surgery. Clin Nutr. 2017;36(3):623–650.

77. Lapointe M. Iron supplementation in the intensive care unit: when, how much, and by what route? Crit Care. 2004;8 Suppl 2(Suppl 2):S37–S41.

78. Singh H, Duerksen DR. Vitamin K and nutrition support. Nutr Clin Pract. 2003;18:359–365.

79. Shearer MJ. Vitamin K in Parenteral Nutrition. Gastroenterology2009;137:S105–S118.

56 | Parenteral Nutrition in Specific Diseases

In specific diseases, individuals have nutritional needs that differ from the usual guidelines, necessitating a personalized nutritional strategy. These conditions require a tailored nutritional approach to meet their distinct requirements. This chapter will discuss the unique nutritional considerations, goals, indications, timing for initiating parenteral nutrition, nutritional requirements, and management of several common disorders.

ACUTE KIDNEY INJURY (AKI)

Nutritional considerations

In acute kidney injury, the rapid decline in kidney function not only leads to water, electrolyte, and acid-base disturbances but also affects carbohydrate, protein, and lipid metabolism and significantly affects nutrition. In AKI, excessive protein catabolism and inadequate intake of nutrition lead to protein-energy wasting (PEW) and malnutrition.

Malnutrition is common in hospitalized patients with AKI, is a poor prognostic marker, and is a significant predictor of morbidity and mortality in AKI [1–4]. In addition, patients with AKI given low calories and amino acids are associated with higher hospital mortality [5]. So, do not restrict protein intake in AKI patients to avoid or delay the initiation of dialysis [6, 7].

Goal, indications, and timing for initiation of parenteral nutrition (PN)

The general goals of nutrition support are to prevent malnutrition, maintain nutritional status, and limit the complications of AKI by providing adequate amounts of energy, protein, and nutrients.

AKI patients with mild catabolism can be fed orally. Moderate to severely catabolic patients with AKI need nutritional support, and enteral nutrition is the preferred route in such patients. However, total or supplementary PN has indicated if enteral nutrition is inadequate or cannot be given in patients with significant gastrointestinal (GI) dysfunction [8].

When to initiate PN in patients with AKI is an important question to be answered. Early PN may delay recovery in AKI and prolong the duration of renal replacement therapy due to substantial catabolism of the extra amino acids leading to higher levels of plasma urea and, therefore, should be avoided [9].

Compared with early initiation, late initiation of PN is associated with rapid recovery and lesser complications in critically ill adults [10]. Recent ESPEN guidelines (2019) recommended starting PN within three to seven days and providing half of the predicted or measured energy need in the beginning [11].

Nutritional requirements and management

Nutritional requirements of AKI depend on various factors such as underlying disease, associated comorbidities, the need for renal replacement therapy (RRT), including its type and frequency, and pre-existing nutritional status, as summarized in Table 56.1.

A. AKI treated conservatively (non-dialytic therapy)

1. **Energy requirements:** It varies as per the clinical status of patients with AKI.

   Energy required for uncomplicated AKI is in any stage is 20–30 kcal/kg/day, which is similar to that required by a normal adult individual [7, 12].

   Energy requirement increases (about 25 to 35 kcal/kg/day) in critically ill patients with AKI (e.g., severe sepsis, respiratory failure, burns, and multi-organ failure) [13, 14] and during continuous renal replacement therapy (CRRT) [15].

   Providing higher calories does not improve patients' outcomes in AKI [16]. In AKI patients, indirect calorimetry is the standard and clinically recommended method to calculate energy requirements which helps to avoid overfeeding.

Table 56.1 Guidelines for nutritional requirements in acute kidney injury			
Nutritional requirements	ESPEN 2006	KDIGO 2012	ASPEN 2016
Energy	20–30 kcal/kg/d	20–30 kcal/kg/d	25–30 kcal/kg/d
Protein			
Noncatabolic AKI without dialysis	0.6–0.8 gm/kg, max. 1.0 gm/kg	0.8–1.0 gm/kg	1.2–2 gm/kg
RRT, in hypercatabolism	1.0–1.5 gm/kg	1.0–1.5 gm/kg for RRT, up to 1.7 gm/kg for CRRT	Additional 0.2 gm/ kg up to 2.5 gm/kg
Carbohydrates	3–5 gm/kg (max. 7 gm/kg)	-	-
Lipid	0.8–1.2 gm/kg (max. 1.5 gm/kg)	-	-

2. **Protein requirements:** Protein requirements in AKI needs due attention as it is variable based on the condition of the individual patient (Table 56.1). Protein requirements recommended for patients of AKI, not on dialysis is 0.8–1.0 gm/kg/day for stable, non-catabolic patients (KDIGO 2012) and 1.2–2 gm/kg for critical ICU patients (ASPEN 2016) [6, 7]. Avoid supplementation of the greater amount of protein in AKI because retention of nitrogenous waste will aggravate uremic complications and can also contribute to acidosis [7].

3. **Non-protein caloric supplements:** In AKI receiving PN, carbohydrates, and lipids represent about 65–70% (3 to 5 gm/kg/d) and 30–35% (0.8 to 1.0 gm/kg/d) of the calorie intake of total non-protein energy supply respectively [7, 17].

4. **Fluid and electrolytes requirements:** Adjust/restrict fluid intake as per the urine output to avoid volume overload in oliguric patients. Most of oliguric patients also need sodium restriction. Maximally concentrated PN solutions are infused through a central line in oliguric patients. Avoid hyperkalemia, hypermagnesemia, and hyperphosphatemia by restricting potassium, magnesium, and phosphorus in PN.

B. AKI treated with renal replacement therapy

A large amount of amino acids is lost into the effluent fluid during RRT, and its variable depending on the type of modality (i.e., the approximate amount of amino acid lost is about 3–6 gm during conventional hemodialysis, 7–10 gm during sustained low-efficiency dialysis (SLED), and 14–22 gm per session during continuous venovenous hemofiltration (CVVH) respectively [18]. To compensate for the protein loss, protein replacement KDIGO recommended are 1.0–1.5 gm/kg/d for AKI on intermittent RRT and up to 1.7 gm/kg/d in patients on continuous renal replacement therapy (CRRT) [7]. To replace a significant loss of amino acid in CRRT, it is recommended to increase protein intake to a range of 1.5–2.5 gm/kg/day [6, 14, 19].

BURNS

Nutritional considerations

Malnutrition in patients with burns carries a high risk of complications such as infection and delayed wound healing and therefore is very important in managing moderate-to-severe burn injury.

Important causes of malnutrition in burns are:

1. Loss of protein and micronutrients as the skin barrier is lost.

2. Increased energy expenditure to overcome heat loss through the exposed surface and to maintain body temperature.

3. Persistent and prolonged post-burn hypermetabolic state and increased catabolism.

Feeding route: In burn patients, enteral nutrition (EN) is recommended over PN because of the advantages of early EN, such as protection of the gastrointestinal tract, improved nutrient adequacy, reduction in rates of complications, infection, length of hospital stay, cost, morbidity, and mortality [20, 21]. EN is preferred, and PN is not recommended routinely in burns because of adverse effects like overfeeding, impaired immunity, liver failure, and higher mortality [22]. PN is administered in burn patients only when EN is not feasible, not tolerated, or inadequate to meet with desired total nutrient requirements [6].

Nutritional requirements and management

Energy requirements: In patients with burns, nutritional support is provided to meet increased energy requirements due to the hypermetabolic state without causing overfeeding [23]. Indirect calorimetry is the standard and preferred method to determine energy requirements in burns [6]. However, different equations used to determine energy requirements in burns are less reliable because they overestimate or underestimate caloric requirements [24]. When indirect calorimetry is not available or

feasible, alternatively Toronto equation is recommended in adults [20].

Protein requirement: Protein requirement is significantly higher in burns because of the need for protein for wound healing, immune function, to replace ongoing losses, and to reduce protein catabolism [23]. ESPEN (2013) and ASPEN (2016) guidelines recommend 1.5 to 2 gm protein/kg/day in adults [6, 20].

Carbohydrate requirement and glycaemic control: Administer carbohydrates to provide up to 60% of total energy intake from nutrition and non-nutritional sources [20]. However, carbohydrate administration carries the risk of hyperglycemia, and poor glucose control adversely affects outcomes in burns [25]. So, while infusing carbohydrates, monitor blood glucose levels closely, and keep glucose levels under 144 mg/dL (and over 81 mg/dL), preferably by continuous intravenous insulin infusion to achieve tight glycemic control.

Lipid requirement: Administer lipids to provide <35% of total energy intake from fat and monitor total fat delivery [20].

As metabolic demands are high in patients with severe burns, administration of PN via central venous access is preferred.

Glutamine and micronutrients requirement: Supplementation of 0.3 gm/kg/day glutamine is beneficial. Patients with major burns have increased micronutrient requirements due to hypermetabolism, wound healing requirements, and cutaneous exudative losses and need an early supplementation with supra-nutritional amounts of zinc, copper, selenium, and vitamin B1, C, D, and E to prevent deficiency-related complications [20].

CANCER

Cancer-related malnutrition (CRM), weight loss, and cachexia occur in 30 to 80 percent of cancer patients, which contribute to excess morbidity and mortality [26, 27].

Malnutrition reduces the benefit of cancer therapy, increases chemotherapy-related toxicity, leads to poor quality of life, and reduces patient survival.

Why malnutrition occurs in cancer patients?

Malignancy per se or treatment of the malignancy (such as chemotherapy, radiotherapy, or surgical treatment) can lead to loss of test, decreased appetite, nausea, vomiting or diarrhea, oral lesions, severe mucositis, and GI complications such as dysphagia, ileus, intestinal obstruction, malabsorption, short bowel syndrome, and fistulae, which can lead to malnutrition [28].

Nutritional support reduces symptoms, improves the quality of life, reduces weight loss, prevents catabolism, and improves outcomes in cancer patients.

Indications of PN [27, 29, 30]

- PN is not recommended routinely in well-nourished cancer patients because of the lack of advantages and associated harmful effects.

- Access to the digestive tract is not possible for a prolonged period due to GI complications such as perforation, intestinal obstruction, high-output entero-cutaneous fistulas, or chylothorax.

- Chemotherapy or radiotherapy-induced GI toxicity limiting oral/enteral intake for more than 1–2 weeks in cancer patients.

- As anticancer therapy is ineffective in rapidly progressive malignant diseases and terminal stages of malignancy, PN is unlikely to benefit such patients.

- In patients receiving hematopoietic stem cell transplantation, PN is recommended if oral/EN is limited due to severe mucositis, ileus, or intractable vomiting.

Nutritional requirements

The total daily energy expenditure is about 20–25 kcal/kg/day for bedridden cancer patients and 25–30 kcal/kg/day for ambulatory cancer patients [27, 29]. Recommended protein intake is >1 gm/kg/day and, preferably up to 1.5 gm/kg/day [27].

The proportion of carbohydrates and lipids is roughly 40–50% or less and up to 50% of non-protein energy requirements, respectively [31]. The requirement of lipids is about 0.5–1.5 gm/kg/day (up to a maximum of 2 gm/kg/d).

Higher fat to carbohydrate ratio to provide non-protein energy is recommended in weight-losing, cachectic cancer patients with insulin resistance because of the advantages of lipids, such as increased energy density and ability to reduce the glycemic load [27].

CARDIAC DISEASE

Patients with chronic heart failure (CHF) carry the risk of malnutrition due to decreased energy intake, increased energy expenditure and impaired anabolism, and high mortality in patients with CHF with cardiac cachexia [32]. Reduced bowel perfusion due to decreased cardiac function can cause edema of the bowel wall leading to malabsorption [32].

In cardiac patients, oral supplementation and enteral nutrition are preferred, and PN is needed in very few patients who cannot take adequate oral or enteral nutrition.

Because of the potential risk of volume overload and hyponatremia, PN should be used cautiously, preferably using concentrated PN solutions. Lipid emulsion can provide greater calories (9 kcal/gm) with a smaller volume.

CRITICAL ILLNESS

Critical illness refers to seriously ill medical or surgical conditions that need intensive care and is associated with a greater risk of infection, longer ICU stays, and higher mortality. Malnutrition is quite common in critical illness (occurs in about 38% to 78% of patients) and increases morbidity, mortality, and hospital-related cost [33]. Malnutrition in critical illness usually occurs due to multiple causes, such as increased energy expenditure, marked catabolism, decreased food intake for a prolonged period due to anorexia, and different medical or surgical gastrointestinal disorders.

In critical illness, adequate nutrition is important because malnutrition is associated with impaired clinical outcome, starvation or underfeeding leads to increased morbidity and mortality, and timely optimum nutrition decrease hospital stay and morbidity [34–36].

Metabolic changes: Depending on the duration of critical illness, it is divided into three stages: acute early phase, acute late phase, and post-acute late phase [11]. Different metabolic changes according to these stages help in planning the appropriate nutritional therapy considering varying needs. In the acute early phase, catabolism-induced increased endogenous generation of energy helps to meet the demand of the body in critically ill patients, and therefore, early use of PN with the provision of standard energy requirements is likely to cause overfeeding [37]. Characteristics of metabolism at the different time frames in critical illness as summarized in Table 56.2 [11].

Enteral nutrition vs. parenteral nutrition

In critically ill patients, EN is preferred and recommended over PN because of its safety and various advantages by all recent international guidelines [6, 11, 38]. In the CALORIES trial, PN is found to be as safe as EN in a critically ill patient when the dose of PN is hypocaloric, which is equivalent to EN dose [39]. So, the advantages of EN may be due to differences in the intake of calories rather than the route; therefore, using PN in an appropriate dose is as safe as EN [40].

Table 56.2 Metabolic characteristic of critical illness

Stage	ICU days	Metabolism	Characteristic
Acute phase early period	1–2	Catabolism	Metabolic instability and severe increase in catabolism
Acute phase late period	3–7	Catabolism	Significant muscle wasting and stabilization of the metabolic disturbances
Post-acute late phase	After day 7	Anabolism	Improvement and rehabilitation
		Catabolism	Chronicity with persistent inflammatory/catabolic state and prolonged hospitalization.

When to provide nutrition in critical illness?

The timing of the initiation of PN is important and controversial critically ill patients. No benefit or harm was documented with early nutrition in the recent TARGET Trial (2018) [41, 42]. In the largest nutrition EPaNIC trial (2011), the potential harm with early PN and benefits such as enhanced recovery, fewer complications, and reduced healthcare costs were demonstrated with the late initiation PN [10]. So, in adequately nourished critically ill patients with low nutrition risk, if PN is indicated, it should be administered late because of the harmful effects of early PN and the benefits of the late initiation PN. Recent European guidelines recommend initiation of PN between ICU days 3 and 7 (ESPEN 2019), while American guidelines recommend initiation of PN after 7 days (ASPEN/SCCM 2016) [6, 11].

Indications of PN

Adequate nutrition is beneficial during and after the ICU stay in critical illness. Therefore, in critically ill patients, exclusive or supplemental PN is indicated when oral/EN is contraindicated or fails to achieve nutritional targets, which prevents underfeeding associated risks and poor outcomes:

- Critically ill patients who are well-nourished and have a low risk for malnutrition generally do not need exclusive PN in the first seven days of an ICU stay [6, 43].
- In critical patients with high nutrition risk or severe malnutrition, initiate exclusive PN at the earliest following ICU admission if EN is not feasible [6].
- Supplemental PN: If oral/EN fails to meet >60% of energy and protein requirements after seven to ten days, the use of supplemental PN is recommended in patients with a low or high nutritional risk [6]. Supplemental PN is a step-up approach that helps to provide timely and optimal nutrition support during critical illness.

Nutritional requirements and management

How to initiate PN in critical illness?

Current literature is against the traditional practice of aggressive nutrition in the early stages of critical illness [44]. Both European and American guidelines recommend a strategy to provide hypocaloric PN (≤20 kcal/kg/d or 70–80% of estimated energy requirements) with an adequate protein supplementation (≥1.2 gm protein/kg/d) in the first week of hospitalization in the ICU to avoid overfeeding [6, 11]. The strategy to provide hypocaloric PN reduces peripheral insulin resistance and risk of hyperglycemia and improves glycemic control with resultant increases in the safety of PN. After the patient stabilizes, the dose of PN may be increased gradually to achieve 100% of the estimated energy requirements [6].

The nutritional requirements of critical and stable patients are summarized in Table 56.3 [6, 11, 12].

Energy expenditure: Indirect calorimetry is the preferred method to calculate caloric needs [6, 11]. The approximate total energy expenditure in critically ill patients is about 20 to 30 kcal/kg/day [12]. Initial administration of 70–80% of the measured energy expenditure is beneficial, whereas higher or lower energy intakes are both harmful [45–47]. Critical patients with low serum phosphorus levels (less than 0.65 mmol/L or 2 mg/dL) are prone to develop refeeding

Table 56.3 Nutritional requirements in critical and stable patients		
	Critically ill patients	**Stable patients**
Total calories	20 to 30 kcal/kg/d	20 to 30 kcal/kg/d
Protein	1.3 (1.2–2.0) gm/kg/d	0.8 to 1.5 gm/kg/d
Carbohydrate	Not >5 mg/kg/min	4–5 mg/kg/min
Lipid	Less than 1.5 gm/kg/d (100 gm/wk)	1 gm/kg/d
Fluid	Minimum needed to deliver adequate macronutrients	30 to 40 mL/kg/d

syndrome. So in such patients, restrict calorie intake to 50% of the calculated energy needs for 2 to 3 days to prevent the refeeding syndrome [48].

Protein requirements: In the acute phase of critical illness, increased catabolism causes loss of protein and muscle wasting [49, 50], and therefore requirements of protein increase considerably with illness severity. Inadequate protein supplementation may be harmful, and supplementation of protein intake may be beneficial and found to reduce the mortality in critically ill patients in recent literature [45, 51–53].

As per current recommendations, a higher amount of protein should be provided to critically ill patients (i.e., up to 1.3 gm/kg/day as per ESPEN guidelines (2019) and 1.2–2.0 gm/kg/day as per ASPEN/SCCM guideline (2016) [6, 11]. Administration of protein in a low dose initially (<0.8 gm/kg/day before day 3) and subsequently gradually increasing its dose (>0.8 gm/kg/d after day 3) is beneficial and reduces mortality [54].

Combining exercise with calorie and protein supplementation is very important because it helps to maintain muscle mass and function, reduces protein catabolism, and improves outcomes [11, 55, 56].

Carbohydrate requirements: Carbohydrate is the preferred source of energy

in the early phase of critically ill patients. The minimum amount of carbohydrate requirement recommended in ICU patients by 2003 ESPEN guidelines was 2 gm/kg of glucose per day [34] and 1–2 gm/kg/day by the German Association for Nutritional Medicine [57]. But in current literature, the lower limit is removed due to a lack of evidence, and 2019 ESPEN guidelines recommend that in ICU patients receiving PN, the amount of glucose should not exceed 5 mg/kg/min [11].

Avoid Hyperglycemia in critically ill patients because it is harmful and is associated with an increased risk of complications and higher mortality. In critically ill patients, the recommended target blood glucose ranges from 140 or 150 to 180 mg/dL [6, 58]. The use of insulin infusion is recommended for achieving normoglycaemia because controlling blood sugar decreases mortality in critically ill patients. Insulin infusion is used when blood glucose is >150 mg/dL to maintain it below 180 mg/dL [59].

Lipid emulsions: For critically ill patients who are hemodynamically stable, lipid emulsion is an essential part of PN, as it provides a dense source of non-protein calories and essential fatty acids [11].

Requirements: Administration of intravenous lipid emulsions can be initiated safely at a rate of 0.7 gm/kg/

day, and the total dose of lipid should not exceed 1.5 gm lipids/kg/day or a maximum of 100 gm/week and should generally provide about 30% of total calories [6, 11, 60, 61].

Selection of lipid emulsions: Lipid emulsions containing soybean oil are the mainstay and the first-generation lipids for parenteral nutrition. Alternative lipid emulsions, such as Generation 2 (combining soybean oil with medium-chain triglycerides), Generation 3 (using olive oil), and Generation 4 (using fish oil) lipid emulsions, have been developed to decrease the harmful effects of the omega-6-rich linoleic acid content and to lower the ratio of omega-6 to omega-3 fatty acids [62]. Because of the potential risks associated with the use of pure soybean oil emulsions in critically ill patients, 2016 SCCM/ASPEN guidelines recommend against its use during the first week of starting PN [6]. On the contrary, omega-3 fatty acid enriched fish oil containing PN is beneficial and reduces the risk of infection and sepsis, and shortens the length of stay in both ICU and hospital [63].

So current literature recommends the use of fish-oil containing lipid emulsions as part of PN in surgical and high-risk critically ill adult patients (e.g., sepsis, acute respiratory distress syndrome (ARDS), persistent inflammation catabolism syndrome [PICS]), although evidence to support its use in non-surgical patients is not sufficient [6, 11, 64, 65]. Because of clinical benefits over the standard lipid emulsions, provide 0.1–0.2 gm/kg/day fish oil containing lipid emulsions [rich in EPA (eicosapentaenoic acid) + DHA (docosahexaenoic acid)] in patients receiving PN [11].

Monitoring: While administering lipid emulsions, measure serum triglyceride concentrations at baseline, monitor it regularly, and adjust the dose of lipid emulsions to maintain triglyceride levels below 400 mg/dL (4.5 mmol/L) [64].

Micronutrients and glutamine

Vitamins and trace elements (micronutrients) are essential components of PN. As commercially available PN formulations do not contain vitamins and trace elements, their separate administration is needed. In addition, a high dose of micronutrients may improve the outcomes of critically ill patients [66].

Parenteral glutamine supplementation is not recommended in critically ill, unstable, and complex ICU patients and patients with multi-organ failure, especially with liver and renal failure in recent guidelines (Canadian guidelines 2015, ASPEN guidelines 2016, ESPEN guideline 2019) [6, 11, 67].

GASTROINTESTINAL FISTULAE

Gastrointestinal (GI) fistulas divert intestinal contents, most commonly to the skin (cutaneous, gastrointestinal fistula). Common causes of GI fistula are crohn's disease, injury to the bowel, bowel surgery, radiation injury, abscess, and foreign body penetration.

High output GI fistulas (loss greater than 500 ml of fluid in 24 hours) might cause massive loss of fluid, electrolytes, proteins, vitamins, and trace minerals resulting in complications like severe dehydration, fluid, electrolytes, acid-base abnormalities, and malnutrition (which occurs in about 55–90% of patients) [68, 69]. In addition to these abnormalities, profound nutrient depletion and sepsis are leading causes of death in patients with high-output GI fistulas [70].

Nutritional support

The provision of optimum nutrition is necessary because it significantly improves clinical outcomes by accelerating the spontaneous healing rate, enhancing the closer of the fistula, and reducing the mortality rate in patients with high-output GI fistulas [71, 72]. Therefore, PN is started in patients with high output fistula after initial fluids and electrolytes resuscitation and control of sepsis.

Indication: PN has a supportive role, and its indications in patients with GI fistula are [71, 73, 74]:

- High-output fistula (e.g., >500 mL/ day), presence of distal intestinal obstruction, or length of intestinal before the fistula less than 75 cm because these patients cannot tolerate oral or EN.

- When oral or EN fails to provide adequate nutrition beyond 7 days.

- Supplemental PN is provided when EN alone cannot achieve the nutritional goal to meet their metabolic needs.

PN improves nutritional status by providing adequate nutrition, allows time to correct sepsis and thereby prepare them for reconstructive surgery, and helps to postpone extremely hazardous emergency surgical intervention in severely ill patients with GI fistulas.

Nutritional requirements and management: Patients with high-output fistula requires 25 to 35 kcal/kg per day of total caloric intake and 1.5–2.0 gm/kg/d of protein [75]. As protein loss in the effluent of high output fistula can be as high as 75 gm/day, ASPEN-FELANPE clinical guidelines recommend more protein (up to 2.5 gm/kg/d) supplementation in adult patients with high output fistula [73].

Lipids are usually given roughly 20–30% of calories. The use of lipid emulsion containing omega-3 fatty acid-enriched fish oil in PN is beneficial because it is a calorically dense nutrient and has an immune-enhancing effect that reduces the risk of sepsis and shortens the duration of hospitalization [63].

Vitamins and trace elements deficiency is common in malnourished patients, and its supplementation is recommended. The recommended vitamin C and zinc dose is about ten times the daily allowance, while the dose of other vitamins is two times normal [76].

INFLAMMATORY BOWEL DISEASE (IBD)

Inflammatory bowel diseases are chronic, relapsing, and debilitating inflammatory disorders of the gastrointestinal tract, and their most common causes are crohn's disease (CD) and ulcerative colitis (UC).

Malnutrition occurs in about 6% to 16% of patients with IBD [77, 78].

The etiology of malnutrition in IBD is multifactorial, results from decreased food intake, poor digestion, malabsorption, increased losses of nutrients, increased energy requirements, a short length of the intestine due to resection, and drug or surgery-related factors [79, 80].

Adequate correction of malnutrition is essential in patients with IBD because it worsens the prognosis and adversely affects the quality of life by increasing complication rates and mortality [81, 82].

PN does not increase the remission rate or decrease the need for surgery in patients with IBD. Therefore, PN and bowel rest should not be used routinely as primary therapies for IBD. PN is less effective than steroid therapy in the treatment of CD. Correction of dehydration and replacement of various micronutrients are more critical than bowel rest alone.

Indications of PN

- EN is preferred over the PN, and PN is indicated only in selected patients with IBD [81–84].

- If oral or EN is insufficient to deliver nutrition targets (cannot supply >60% of energy needs) in patients with crohn's disease due to GI tract dysfunction or short bowel.

- If oral or EN is not possible due to severe vomiting or diarrhea and absence of access.

- If oral or EN is contraindicated due to paralytic ileus, an obstructed bowel, intestinal ischemia, or severe shock.

- If the patient develops complications such as an anastomotic leak or a high output intestinal fistula.

- In the perioperative period, provide PN if oral or EN cannot be initiated within 7 days.

- In the postoperative period, provide PN if oral or EN cannot be initiated within 7 days.

LIVER DISEASE

The liver is labeled a "workhorse" because it performs multiple complex tasks such as metabolism, alteration, synthesis, storage of various nutrients, and detoxifying different toxic substances.

Malnutrition is commonly seen in patients with liver disease, and its prevalence is about 20% in compensated cirrhosis and as high as 50%–90% in advanced cirrhosis [85, 86].

Important causes of malnutrition are excessive use of alcohol, decreased food intake, impaired gastric emptying, impaired digestion, malabsorption, altered metabolism, increased resting energy expenditure, insufficient nutrient storage and synthesis, and abnormal nutrient losses [86, 87].

Early detection of malnutrition in liver disease is important because it adversely affects outcomes by causing loss of muscle mass (sarcopenia), increased rate of complications (encephalopathy, variceal bleeding, and infection), a longer stay in the hospital, and higher mortality [88–91]. Early diagnosis and proper treatment of malnutrition, ascites, and hyponatremia can reduce morbidity and mortality in patients with liver disease.

Indications of PN

Selective use of PN is beneficial in patients with hepatic failure as it reduces complication rates, duration of mechanical ventilation, and stay in ICU [92].

Common indications of PN are [92–95]:

- When oral or EN are inadequate or contraindicated, PN is used as second-line treatment according to the current recommendation for non-cirrhotic patients.

- PN is beneficial in patients with poor oral intake for a prolonged period and problems like hepatic encephalopathy, gastrointestinal bleeding, and impaired gut motility or ileus.

- In patients with moderate or severe malnutrition, prompt administration of PN is recommended, as in other critically ill patients.

- To provide early postoperative nutrition after liver transplantation and surgery when oral nutrition or EN is not feasible. Postoperative PN helps to reduce rates of complication, length of mechanical ventilation, and ICU stay.

- Considered PN in the presence of problems like unprotected airways, compromised cough and swallow reflexes, and hepatic encephalopathy.

Nutritional requirements and management

Nutritional requirements in patients with liver diseases vary depending upon the type of liver disease, the severity of illness, malnutrition, and associated complications.

Energy requirements

Energy expenditure usually increases in patients with acute liver failure, alcoholic steatohepatitis, and cirrhosis, but it is normal in non-alcoholic fatty liver disease (NAFLD). The basal metabolic rate should be calculated using the actual body weight for patients with cirrhosis of the liver without ascites, but for patients with cirrhosis of the liver with ascites, use the ideal body weight for the calculation [6, 94].

Energy requirements increase in cirrhotic patients with acute complications, refractory ascites, malnutrition, or hepatic encephalopathy, but not for overweight or obese patients (as summarized in Table 56.4) [6, 92, 94, 96, 97].

In cirrhotic patients, carbohydrates should provide 50–60%, and lipids should provide about 40–50% of non-protein energy requirements [93].

Protein requirements

PROVIDING optimum protein supplementation to the cirrhotic patient is the most important and challenging part of nutri-tion. Protein restriction to prevent the development of hepatic encephalopathy (HE) is one of the most common misconceptions. Restriction of protein should be avoided because it increases protein catabolism, and on the contrary, high protein supplement actually improves mental status and does not precipitate or worsen HE [98–100].

The requirement for protein increases in malnourished and/or sarcopenic cirrhotic patients, patients requiring frequent or large-volume paracentesis, and obese cirrhotic patients for preserving lean body mass, as summarized in Table 56.5 [6, 92, 94].

Vitamins and micronutrients

Vitamins and micronutrient deficiencies are frequently seen in patients with liver diseases, especially those with alcoholic cirrhosis. Such patients require the supplementation of vitamins (both fat and water-soluble) and micronutrients. In addition, increased prothrombin time (PT) is frequently encountered in patients with liver diseases, and vitamin K is routinely supplemented to correct PT; however, evidence regarding its efficacy is limited [101, 102].

Zinc deficit is common in patients with cirrhosis of the liver, and evidence of the benefits of zinc supplementation in hepatic encephalopathy is growing [103–107].

Table 56.4 Energy requirements in liver diseases	
Requirements	**Clinical conditions**
25–30 kcal/kg/d	Compensated liver cirrhosis
30–35 kcal/kg/d	Acute liver failure, alcoholic hepatitis, decompensated cirrhosis (in nonobese individuals), cirrhotic with malnutrition, hepatic encephalopathy, preoperatively and postoperative cirrhotic patients
25 kcal/kg/d	Obese cirrhotic patient
35–40 kcal/kg/d	Critically ill cirrhotic patients

Table 56.5 Protein requirements in liver diseases	
Requirements	**Clinical conditions**
1.2 gm/kg/d	Non-malnourished compensated liver cirrhosis
1.5 gm/kg/d	Decompensated cirrhosis (in nonobese individuals), malnourished and/or sarcopenic cirrhotic patients
1.2–1.5 gm/kg/d	Preoperatively and postoperative cirrhotic patients, hepatic encephalopathy
1.5–2 gm/kg/d	High volume recurrent ascites with sarcopenia
2.0–2.5 gm/kg/d	Obese cirrhotic patient
>1.2 gm/kg/d	Critically ill cirrhotic patients

Fluid and salt requirements

Cirrhosis affects the patient's ability to handle salt and water and may cause ascites and dilutional hyponatremia. Ascites is the common complication of cirrhosis of the liver, and in patients with severe anasarca and ascites, salt and water restriction may be necessary. Hyponatremia is prevalent in patients with ascites due to cirrhosis and is associated with higher morbidity and mortality [108].

Salt restriction: Dietary sodium restriction is the first-line therapy in ascites, and recent guidelines recommend intake of about 80–113 mEq sodium or 5–6.5 gm of salt per day [92, 109]. While prescribing a low-salt, unpalatable diet, it is essential to consider the trade-off between reducing caloric intake, which can lead to a risk of malnutrition from decreased food intake, and its moderate advantage in reducing ascites [94, 110]. Therefore, salt restriction is not recommended in patients with cirrhosis in the absence of ascites.

Fluid restriction: Restriction of fluid to 1 to 1.5 L per day should be considered only in patients with clinical hypervolemia with severe hyponatremia (serum sodium <125 mmol/L) [109]. Fluid restriction is not recommended in

hypovolemic hyponatremia and mild to moderate hyponatremia.

PANCREATITIS

Nutritional considerations

Acute pancreatitis (AP) is severe in about 20% of patients, and severe acute pancreatitis increases the mortality rate by 19–30% [111]. Severe acute pancreatitis is a hypercatabolism state leading to sustained protein catabolism and increased energy requirements with resultant nutritional risk [112]. Timely adequate nutrition plays a key role in the management of severe acute pancreatitis.

The concept of "Pancreatic Rest" is changing: Formerly, in the early stages of severe acute pancreatitis, patients were kept nil by mouth and given PN to provide rest to the pancreas. The previously popular concept of "Pancreatic Rest" was based on the presumption that oral or enteral feeding could stimulate pancreatic enzyme secretion, causing autodigestion of the pancreas and surrounding tissues and worsening pancreatitis.

The rationale for discarding "Pancreatic Rest" and changing to EN in the early phases of severe acute pancreatitis are:

1. The lack of oral or enteral nutrition leads to a loss of intestinal mucosal

barrier function and increased bacterial translocation, resulting in an increased risk of complications such as pancreatic infection and necrosis [113].

2. During acute pancreatitis, the secretion of pancreatic enzymes decreases significantly, with the most severe cases having the lowest secretion. As a result, even if EN is taken, it does not increase secretion because it is already reduced, making EN not harmful in severe acute pancreatitis [114, 115].

3. The beneficial effects of oral/EN are improvement in nutritional status, stimulation of intestinal motility, increase in splanchnic blood flow, and maintenance of gut integrity which inhibits bacterial translocation, reduction of pancreatic infection, decrease in local and systemic inflammation risk, and reduced mortality [116–118].

4. Use of parenteral nutrition for bowel rest has a potential risk for hyperglycemia, electrolyte imbalances, catheter-related infections, and sepsis, and is more expensive than EN [119, 120].

To conclude, the concept of "Pancreatic Rest" is outdated, detrimental, and should be abandoned [117, 121–123].

Enteral vs. parenteral nutrition

In the early phases of severe acute pancreatitis, EN is safer, more effective, and is preferred compared with parenteral nutrition according to different studies [124–128], current reviews [113, 116–118], and recent guidelines [6, 112, 123, 129–133].

Compared to PN, oral or EN has demonstrated multiple benefits such as decreased infectious complications, risk of complications, mean length of hospital stay, rate of multiple organ failure, and mortality rate in patients of severe acute pancreatitis in several studies [124–128, 134, 135].

Timing of initiation of EN: The early EN (i.e., initiated within 72 hours [112, 132, 136], 48 hours [6, 125, 130, 135, 137–141], or 24 hours [123, 142, 143] had significant benefits over the delayed EN such as decrease complication rate, organ failure, mortality, length of stay in the hospital, and cost-effectiveness.

It is very important to start EN early in moderate to severe acute pancreatitis because the inability to provide EN for >72–96 hours carries the risk of the rapid deterioration of nutrition status and resultant complications such as increased mortality, frequency of infected necrosis, and length of stay in hospital [6, 138].

Route of nutritional support: The most effective route of nutritional support in acute pancreatitis is determined based on the severity of diseases, associated local and systemic complications, and nutritional status at the time of admission.

Oral feeding: Patients with mild acute pancreatitis should consume normal food intake as tolerated, and the use of EN or PN is not recommended [6]. Recent guidelines [AGA (2018), NICE (2018), and ESPEN (2020)] recommend early initiation of oral feeding in patients with mild acute pancreatitis instead of traditional 'nil-by-mouth' or delayed oral feeding (initiation after reduction of serum amylase and lipase levels, resolution of abdominal pain and bowel sounds become normal) [112, 123, 132].

Early oral feeding (within 24 hours) is safe, and well-tolerated, with no differences in adverse events compared to standard oral refeeding or EN, may shorten the length of hospital stay as well as costs, and help in rapid clinical improvement [144–147]. Oral feeding is usually started when abdominal pain, nausea, and vomiting decreases, the patient feels hungry and intestinal obstruction or ileus are excluded (it is not necessary to wait until abdominal pain resolves completely or serum lipase concentrations decline) [112, 122, 129, 148, 149]. If the patient is unable to take oral intake within 72 hours, EN should be initiated on day 4 [145].

Enteral nutrition (EN): EN is a cheaper, safer, and the most preferred modality for nutritional support in severe acute pancreatitis, where feeding is provided directly into the stomach via a nasogastric tube (NG) or post-pyloric region by a nasojejunal tube (NJ) [128]. If a patient with acute pancreatitis is unable to eat, providing nutrition by enteral feeding is beneficial and preferred over parenteral nutrition.

It is important to remember that enteral feeding can be administered safely and successfully even in the presence of complications such as pseudocysts, ascites, and/or fistulas [150, 151].

In severe acute pancreatitis with high intraabdominal pressure (IAP) and abdominal compartment syndrome having abdominal distension, paralytic ileus, and high gastric residual volume, EN may be initiated cautiously by using nasojejunal as a preferred route [112, 131]. Monitor the intraabdominal pressure and the clinical condition continuously and closely in such patients. EN is initiated gently at a 10–20 mL/h rate via the nasojejunal route when intraabdominal pressure (IAP) is <15 mmHg, but IAP >15 mmHg may need temporary reduction or discontinuation of EN due to higher rates of feeding intolerance [112, 131, 152].

Because of physiological benefits, at least a small amount of EN may be administered supplementary to PN in patients with severe AP and open abdomen, if feasible [112].

Gastric vs. jejunal nutrition

Nasogastric feeding is a preferred route for EN because it is simpler, cheaper, easier to insert, requires less time to start nutrition, can provide adequate nutrition effectively, is safe in patients with low risk of aspiration, and as compared to the nasojejunal route of feeding carries a similar risk of exacerbation of pain, tolerance to EN, infectious complications, mortality, and length of hospital stay [112, 129, 153–161].

Nasojejunal feeding is preferred for EN in patients with a high risk of aspiration, who cannot tolerate gastric feeding, severe gastroparesis, partial gastric outlet obstruction due to pancreatic edema or pseudocysts, and in patients who have undergone minimally invasive necrosectomy [112, 117, 136, 162].

Mild acute pancreatitis: About 80% of acute pancreatitis patients experience a mild form of the disease that resolves on its own, allowing them to consume solid food without requiring nutritional support, such as EN or PN [6, 112]. In mild acute pancreatitis, starting with a soft low-fat solid diet is safe, effective (as it does not worsen abdominal pain, provides more calories than a clear liquid diet, and results in shorter hospital stays), and well-tolerated [146, 163–167]. Therefore, the traditional practice of initially providing a liquid diet and advancing to a solid oral diet is not recommended in mild acute pancreatitis.

Indications of PN

Routine use of PN is unnecessary, as PN is now known to be more expensive, riskier, and no more effective than EN in patients with acute pancreatitis. PN should not be initiated until all attempts are made with EN for at least 2–3 days. In acute pancreatitis, PN is indicated in selected patients [6, 112, 129, 133, 168, 169]:

1. If EN is not possible or contraindications (e.g., prolonged paralytic ileus, duodenal obstruction from pancreatic edema or pseudocyst, complex pancreatic fistulae, hemodynamic instability, and the need for inotrope support).

2. Unable to achieve targeted nutritional demand through EN.

3. When enteral access cannot be maintained, or the patient cannot tolerate a nasal tube due to nasal irritation.

4. If enteral feeding leads to exacerbation of abdominal pain and therefore, patients are unable to tolerate EN.

5. In abdominal compartment syndrome with IAP >20 mmHg, patients cannot tolerate EN, and PN is indicated.

When tolerance to EN increases with recovery, the volume of PN should be decreased gradually, and PN should be transitioned to EN as soon as possible.

Nutritional requirements and management

Severe acute pancreatitis is characterized by substantial protein catabolism, so protein requirements are higher than in healthy individuals. Therefore, when PN is administered, a mixed source of energy from carbohydrates, fat, and protein should be preferred, and particular attention should be given to avoiding overfeeding and hyperglycemia. Rough guidelines for nutritional requirements in severe acute pancreatitis are:

1. Energy: 25–30 kcal/kg/day

2. Protein: 1.2 to 1.5 gm/kg/day

3. Carbohydrate: 4–6 gm/kg/day

4. Lipid: up to 2 gm/kg/day

Carbohydrate supplementation: Hyperglycemia frequently occurs in patients with acute pancreatitis due to pancreatic endocrine dysfunction. Blood sugar should be monitored closely, and insulin treatment is recommended to treat hyperglycemia with a goal of keeping blood sugar less than 180 mg/dL (10 mmol/L).

Lipid infusion: As hypertriglyceridemia is an important cause of acute pancreatitis; lipids should be infused with proper monitoring of triglyceride levels. In the absence of severe hypertriglyceridemia (>350 mg/dL) or thrombocytopenia, IV lipids appear safe and effective, especially if glucose intolerance is present. The triglyceride level should be checked before initiating PN, monitored regularly, and kept below 400 mg/dL. When the triglyceride level exceeds 400 mg/dL (4.5 mmol/L), lipid infusion should be discontinued temporarily. To prevent hypertriglyceridemia, IV lipids should be administered gradually over a period of 10–12 hours.

Glutamine supplementation: The use of glutamine supplementation is beneficial and recommended in patients with severe acute pancreatitis receiving parenteral nutrition [112]. The advantages of glutamine are limited only to patients receiving parenteral nutrition, so do not supplement glutamine to patients of severe acute pancreatitis receiving enteral nutrition. The recommended dose of L-glutamine is 0.20 gm/kg per day, and glutamine supplementation in PN is found to reduce infectious complications and mortality [170, 171].

PERIOPERATIVE NUTRITION

Malnutrition in hospitalized patients is very common, with about 20% and 40% incidence [172]. Many major surgical diseases (e.g., malignancy, inflammation, gastrointestinal dysfunction, and burns) result in malnutrition, causing catabolic effects leading to inflammatory responses, protein catabolism, and nitrogen losses. Gastrointestinal surgery-related causes of malnutrition are pre-existing chronic disease, anorexia, prolonged ileus, pre and postoperative fasting, malabsorption syndrome, intestinal obstruction, and previous surgical bowel resection [173]. Compared with well-nourished patients, malnutrition in surgical patients is associated with detrimental effects like longer hospital stays, increased hospital costs, and increased postoperative morbidity and mortality (increased susceptibility to infection, poor wound healing, and risk for death after surgery) [174–176].

The decision to use PN in surgical patients depends on the state of health before surgery, the severity of malnutrition, whether the surgery is emergency or elective, the type of surgical procedure, the expected duration for return of normal gastrointestinal function, and how much energy and nutrient requirements patient can tolerate by oral or EN route postoperatively. PN is lifesaving in patients with prolonged gastrointestinal failure. Perioperative nutritional support aims to provide adequate macronutrients and micronutrients to minimize the catabolism and aggravation of malnutrition, promote muscle, immune, and cognitive functions, and decreases infectious and non-infectious postoperative complication rates with resultant fast postoperative recovery [177, 178].

Preoperative parenteral nutrition

Preoperative PN is indicated in severely malnourished patients (weight loss >10–15%, serum albumin <3.0 gm/dL, body mass index (BMI) <18.5 or nutrition risk index (NRI) score <83.5) who cannot achieve adequate nutrition orally or enterally [179, 180]. Preoperative PN aims to provide adequate energy, protein, micronutrients and restore glycogen stores [181].

Preoperative PN for 7–10 days in severely malnourished patients reduces the rate of postoperative complications and improves outcome, provided the operation can be safely postponed [180, 181, 182]. Restoration of the nutritional and metabolic status usually takes about 7 to 14 days, and PN is continued in the postoperative period. In patients with mild to moderate malnutrition, surgery need not be delayed for preoperative PN or EN, and avoid preoperative PN in such patients.

Postoperative parenteral nutrition

Postoperative parenteral nutrition should not be used routinely because of the increased risk of postoperative complications [182, 183].

Indications of postoperative nutritional support

Postoperative PN is indicated in the following conditions [6, 179, 180, 184–186]:

1. Previously well-nourished patients are unlikely to resume oral and enteral feeds within 10 days due to postoperative complications impairing gastrointestinal function and preventing normal oral feeding, such as intestinal obstruction. But in well-nourished patients with a delayed return of gut function likely to resume oral intake or EN within 7 days, PN is not indicated.

2. Previously malnourished patients in whom oral intake or EN is not feasible or not tolerated within 5–7 days.

3. In previously severely malnourished patients undergoing emergency surgery, initiate PN as soon as possible.

4. Supplemental PN: Combining EN and PN should be considered for patients who require nutritional support but cannot meet at least 50% of their energy and nutrient needs via oral or enteral intake for more than seven days.

Timing of initiating PN in postoperative patients

The optimal timing of initiation of PN is determined based on the patient's clinical condition and preoperative nutritional status [6, 179, 180, 185].

1. Immediate postoperative PN support (started on PO day 1) may be appropriate in patients as a continuation of preoperative nutritional support for severe malnutrition.

2. Initiate PN as soon as possible in patients with severe malnutrition if oral intake or EN is unlikely.

3. For patients who are nutritionally at risk and oral intake or EN is not possible, initiating PN within 3 to 5 days may be appropriate.

4. In the absence of preoperative malnutrition, PN should be delayed for around 5 days after surgery as early PN does not provide any benefit in most non-critically ill patients [39, 187].

5. Initiate supplemental PN after 7 days if oral and enteral intake alone cannot achieve 50% or more of estimated energy and nutrient requirements in well-nourished, stable adult patients.

Common disorders for which postoperative PN is indicated include gastrointestinal anastomotic failure, gastrointestinal fistulas, postoperative mechanical bowel obstruction, diffuse peritonitis, paralytic ileus, severe acute pancreatitis, bowel ischemia, short bowel syndrome, etc.

In patients receiving PN postoperatively, supplement vitamins and trace elements with PN [177].

PULMONARY DISEASES

Nutritional considerations

There is a strong association between malnutrition and lung function. In chronic obstructive pulmonary disease (COPD), malnutrition is common (occurs in about 10% to 60% of patients) [188, 189] and is associated with higher morbidity, mortality rate, and healthcare costs [190–193].

The important causes of malnutrition in patients with COPD are decreased food intake, increased energy expenditure, depression, social isolation, aging, inflammation, and the use of medication such as corticosteroids [194].

1. Effect of malnutrition on lung function: When calorie intake is inadequate in critically ill patients with pulmonary disorders, protein is catabolized to provide energy. When

protein is used as a source of calories, it leads to catabolic muscle wasting. So, malnutrition can lead to reduced muscle strength and impairment of respiratory muscle function, which can decrease ventilatory drive and decreased response to hypoxia due to progressive diaphragmatic weakness with resultant precipitation or aggravation of respiratory failure [193, 195, 196]. Malnutrition-induced muscle weakness also adversely affects weaning from mechanical ventilators [197]. Moreover, malnutrition also alters pulmonary defense mechanisms and increases susceptibility to infection [198].

2. Effect of pulmonary diseases on nutritional status: In advanced pulmonary diseases, a combination of, (a) Higher energy requirements due to increased work of breathing and systemic inflammation, and (b) Poor food intake lead to catabolism and resultant malnutrition and weight loss [199]. Underweight patients with the chronic pulmonary disease have a significantly increased risk of all-cause mortality [200].

3. Effect of nutritional support on lung function: Nutritional support in COPD patients has shown modest improvement in various parameters such as respiratory (inspiratory and expiratory muscle strength) and non-respiratory (handgrip and quadriceps) muscle strength, respiratory muscle function, exercise tolerance, and quality of life and these benefits are greater in malnourished patients [201–205].

Nutritional requirements

Administration of nutrition by oral or enteral route is preferred. But

if the gastrointestinal function is Administration of nutrition by oral or enteral route is preferred. But if the gastrointestinal function is impaired for a prolonged period, and adequate oral or EN is not feasible, PN is indicated. Patients with ARDS, COPD, respiratory failure and patients on mechanical ventilators need special consideration for their nutritional requirements. The nutritional needs of COPD patients vary and are determined by their clinical state (stable or exacerbation) and disease severity (ranging from mild to very severe) [206]:

1. In COPD, requirements of Energy and protein are higher in moderately or severely malnourished patients, acutely unwell patients with infection, and patients who exercise to increase muscle mass [193].

2. The recommended energy intake for patients with COPD is about 30 kcal/kg/day for weight maintenance [207] and may be as high as 45 kcal/kg/day for patients aiming to achieve weight gain [208]. In malnourished patients, energy requirements may be as high as 1.7 of resting energy expenditure (REE) [209].

3. The recommended daily protein requirement varies based on clinical status, as summarized in Table 56.6 [193].

4. Avoid overfeeding: Excess supplementation of dextrose and lipids is harmful. Administration of total energy that exceeds energy requirements increases CO_2 production and the work of breathing, which may be detrimental in patients vulnerable to the retention of CO_2.

5. Lipids in stable patients: In respiratory disorders, the use of lipids is suggested because it provides more

energy with less production of CO_2 and therefore reduces the work of breathing. So in spontaneously ventilated patients with COPD, the use of a higher amount of lipids (up to about 50%) and lesser carbohydrates (about 30%) is preferred [210]. While administering lipid emulsion as a part of PN, selecting lipid preparation containing omega-3 fatty acids-rich fish-oil is beneficial due to its anti-inflammatory action in high-risk, critical patients with ARDS [64, 211].

6. Lipids in patients on a ventilator: It is recommended to use a low carbohydrate formula, which contains more lipids and less carbohydrates, for patients on a ventilator as it may shorten the duration of mechanical ventilation [212–214]. However, several studies failed to demonstrate the reduction in the duration of ventilatory support [215, 216], and recent ASPEN-SCCM Clinical Guidelines (2016) recommend against the use of high-fat/low-carbohydrate formulations to manipulate the respiratory quotient and reduce CO_2 production in acute respiratory failure patients in ICU [6].

7. As patients with acute respiratory failure are susceptible to fluid accumulation, a concentrated nutritional formula that restricts fluid volume is recommended [6].

8. Avoid hypokalemia, hypophosphatemia, hypocalcemia, and hypomagnesemia because they can adversely affect the strength of respiratory muscles. To avoid these abnormalities caused by refeeding syndrome, it is important to gradually initiate PN in severely malnourished patients with respiratory disorders.

9. Vitamin D deficiency is common in patients with COPD [217–219]. The low value of vitamin D carries the risk of recurrent pulmonary infections [220], worsening lung function [221], and faster decline in lung function [222].

Vitamin D supplementation substantially reduced the risk of respiratory tract infections [223] as well as the exacerbation rates of COPD [224, 225].

So, GOLD guidelines 2020 recommends screening all COPD patients hospitalized for exacerbations to detect vitamin D deficiency and supplement vitamin D if necessary [206].

SHORT BOWEL SYNDROME

Short bowel syndrome (SBS), also known as a small gut syndrome, is a relatively uncommon condition characterized by malabsorption which occurs most commonly due to extensive surgical resection of the small intestine.

Because of the short length of the remaining intestine, the area available

Table 56.6 Protein requirement in COPD patients		
Requirements	**Clinical state**
0.8–1.5 gm/kg/d	Stable, non-malnourished COPD patients without nutritional risk
Up to 1.5 gm/kg/d	In acutely unwell (exacerbating) COPD patients, for daily requirements and avoid further protein losses
	For pulmonary rehabilitation, with exercise to gain or retain lean muscle mass
	Malnourished outpatients to achieve weight gain

for absorption reduces with the resultant malabsorption of macronutrients and/or water and electrolytes, causing diarrhea, dehydration, electrolyte imbalances, and malnutrition. These symptoms are severe if: (1) More than 75% of the small bowel is resected, (2) The terminal ileum and ileocaecal valve are removed, or (3) The remaining bowel is diseased with impaired absorption [226]. After massive intestinal resection, an intact colon, if in continuity, is vital in supporting the remaining small intestine in digestion and thereby reduces the dependency on PN [227–229].

The common causes of short bowel syndrome in adults are re-surgery performed for complications, mesenteric infarction, malignancy and radiation, surgical resection for crohn's disease, intestinal trauma, mesenteric vascular occlusion, and volvulus [230, 231].

Pathophysiology and presentations

1. Severe diarrhea, electrolyte disturbances, and malnutrition: Loss of intestinal absorptive surface area, rapid transit time, and/or dysfunction of the remaining bowel reduces intestinal absorption leading to:

   • Large volume diarrhea, hypovolemia, metabolic acidosis, hypokalemia, hypomagnesemia, and hypocalcemia.

   • Malnutrition, weight loss, and deficit of water and fat-soluble vitamins.

2. Gastric acid hypersecretion: Production of gastric acid secretion inhibitory hormones (normally secreted in the jejunum and distal ileum) reduces after the massive intestinal loss. Due to the loss of inhibitory hormones, gastrin levels increase, stimulating gastric acid secretion [232, 233].

3. D-lactic acidosis: Bacterial fermentation of malabsorbed carbohydrates in the colon produces a substantial amount of D-lactic acid, which can lead to high anion gap metabolic acidosis [234].

4. Nephrolithiasis: Due to multiple factors, the risk of calcium oxalate nephrolithiasis is high in patients with SBS [235, 236]. Normally oxalate in the diet combines with intraluminal calcium and is excreted in stool as insoluble calcium oxalate. In patients with SBS, large amounts of unabsorbed fat are available, and calcium preferentially binds with the same in the intact colon due to malabsorption. The resultant increased unbound oxalate is absorbed freely and rapidly by the intact colon leading to hyperoxaluria, which predisposes patients to a higher risk of oxalate stone formation [237]. In patients with SBS, chronic dehydration, hypocitraturia, hypomagnesuria, low urine volume, and low pH increases the risk of developing kidney stones [235, 236]. In addition, in patients with SBS, multiple factors like chronic dehydration, hypocitraturia, hypomagnesuria, low urine volume, and low pH increases the risk of developing kidney stones [235, 238].

Nutritional management

Before the advent of PN, survival in acute SBS was very poor. The selection of nutritional treatment is based upon the severity of SBS and frequently needs home parenteral nutrition in severe cases. The need for nutrition requirement is variable in SBS, and it ranges from temporary support in the postoperative period to long-term supplementation depending on how much of the gastrointestinal tract is left, the site of resection, and the presence of the colon in continuity with the small bowel. Patients with SBS generally need PN when the length of the remaining functional small bowel is <50–70 cm with the presence of a colon in continuity or the length of the small bowel is <100–150 cm when the colon is absent [228, 239]. The metabolic and nutrient therapy of SBS is divided into 3 clinical stages:

A. First acute stage: The initial acute phase following resection usually lasts for three to four weeks and is characterized by large-volume diarrhea causing significant losses of fluid and electrolytes:

- In the initial acute phase of illness, patients need prompt administration of electrolytes containing intravenous fluids in large volumes to replace huge losses and correct fluid and electrolyte disturbances. The selection of IV fluid is based on existing electrolyte and acid-base disturbance, but supplementing balanced crystalloids or half normal saline with potassium is usually adequate.

- In critically ill unstable patients, patients should be kept NPO (nothing by mouth). Oral intake is not adequate in the majority of such patients at this stage and may carry the risk of aspiration and, therefore, can be harmful.

- PN is indicated if EN is not possible within one week in patients with severe SBS. PN is initiated only after correcting fluid and electrolyte disturbances and achieving hemodynamic stability. PN is the primary source of nutrition in the initial phase, but progression to EN is attempted when the bowel begins to adapt.

- Supplemental oral or EN helps to prevent mucosal atrophy and is essential to promote gut adaptation but administer combined feeding cautiously to avoid overfeeding [231]. EN in bolus form may cause diarrhea, so slow continuous overnight tube feeding is recommended in the initial acute phase, and it significantly increases the net absorption of lipids, proteins, and energy [240].

B. Second adaptive stage: Structural adaptation (hyperplasia with the resultant increase in absorptive surface area) and functional adaptation (slowed transit time to allow increased nutrient absorption) of the bowel may last for up to 2 years [231]:

- As enteral feeding is necessary for bowel adaptation in SBS, it should be started as soon as the volume of fecal loss decreases. The PN is reduced gradually, and oral or enteral intake is increased with caution to avoid excessive diarrhea and aim to provide adequate nutrition.

- In patients requiring PN, administration of a minimal 1 gm/kg/week of intravenous lipid emulsion is recommended to prevent essential fatty acid (EFA) deficiency [230].

- Overfeeding and the use of soybean-based lipid emulsions in patients receiving long-term PN increases the risk of intestinal failure-associated liver disease (IFALD) [241]. On the other hand, IV fish oil-containing lipid emulsions reduce the risk of IFALD in these patients [242–244].

- Administration of glutamine in either PN or EN is not recommended in SBS patients [230].

- As patients with SBS are at risk for fat-soluble vitamin deficiency, supplementation of vitamins A, D, E, and K is necessary [226].

- If the terminal ileum is resected or resection is greater than 100 cm of ileum, an injection of vitamin B12 should be given monthly [245].

- Hypomagnesemia is common because of the malabsorption of magnesium due to loss of the distal ileum, and its management consists of supplementation of magnesium and correction of sodium depletion [226, 246].

C. Third maintenance stage: In about 50% of adult patients, intestinal adaptation occurs significantly, and intestinal failure reverses completely within the first two years. No further improvement or adaptive changes occur in this stable phase, so long-term treatment is planned:

- The selection of treatment is based on the severity of SBS. Most patients with a severe type of SBS need home-based parenteral nutrition (HPN) for months to years or lifelong. Patients with adequate adaptation and absorption may not need PN.

- In patients with home-based PN, continuous PN infusion is avoided, and overnight cycle PN is recommended because it reduces the risk of intestinal failure associated liver disease (IFALD) [230], provides freedom from the infusion pump during the day, and maximizes the convenience of patients [247].

- Oral diet or EN is started using small volume and should be advanced slowly to small frequent meals [248].

- Patients with D-lactic acidosis need appropriate hydration, restriction of carbohydrate containing diet and administration of non-absorbable antibiotics against D-lactate forming bacteria, and thiamine supplementation.

REFERENCES

1. Fiaccadori E, Lombardi M, Leonardi S, et al. Prevalence and clinical outcome associated with preexisting malnutrition in acute renal failure: a prospective cohort study. J Am Soc Nephrol. 1999;10(3):581–93.

2. Cano NJ, Aparicio M, Brunori G, et al. ESPEN guidelines on parenteral nutrition: adult renal failure. Clin Nutr. 2009;28(4):401–14.

3. Li C, Xu L, Guan C, et al. Malnutrition screening and acute kidney injury in hospitalised patients: a retrospective study over a 5-year period from China. Br J Nutr. 2020;123(3):337–346.

4. Meyer D, Mohan A, Subev E, et al. Acute kidney injury incidence in hospitalized patients and implications for nutrition support. Nutr Clin Pract. 2020;35(6):987–1000.

5. Bufarah MNB, Costa NA, Losilla MPRP, et al. Low caloric and protein intake is associated with mortality in patients with acute kidney injury. Clin Nutr ESPEN. 2018;24:66–70.

6. McClave SA, Taylor BE, Martindale RG, et al. Guidelines for the provision and assessment of nutrition support therapy in the adult critically ill patient: Society of Critical Care Medicine (SCCM) and American Society for Parenteral and Enteral Nutrition (A.S.P.E.N.). JPEN J Parenter Enteral Nutr 2016;40(2):159–211.

7. Kellum JA, Lameire N, Aspelin P, et al. KDIGO clinical practice guideline for acute kidney injury. Kidney Int Suppl. 2012;2(1):1–138.

8. Blumenkrantz MJ, Kopple JD, Koffler A, et al. Total parenteral nutrition in the management of acute renal failure. Am J Clin Nutr. 1978;31(10):1831–40.

9. Gunst J, Vanhorebeek I, Casaer MP, et al. Impact of early parenteral nutrition on metabolism and kidney injury. J Am Soc Nephrol. 2013;24(6):995–1005.

10. Casaer MP, Mesotten D, Hermans G, et al. Early versus late parenteral nutrition in critically ill adults. N Engl J Med. 2011;365(6):506–17.

11. Singer P, Blaser AR, Berger MM, et al. ESPEN guideline on clinical nutrition in the intensive care unit. Clin Nutr. 2019;38(1):48–79.

12. Appropriate Dosing for Parenteral Nutrition: ASPEN Recommendations. American Society Parenteral and Enteral Nutrition 2019. http://www.nutritioncare.org/uploadedFiles/Documents/Guidelines_and_Clinical_Resources/PN%20Dosing%201-Sheet-FINAL.pdf.

13. Druml W, Kierdorf HP, Working group for developing the guidelines for parenteral nutrition of The German Association for Nutritional M. Parenteral nutrition in patients with renal failure – Guidelines on Parenteral Nutrition, Chapter 17. Ger Med Sci 2009;7:Doc11.

14. Gervasio JM, Garmon WP, Holowatyj M. Nutrition support in acute kidney injury. Nutr Clin Pract. 2011;26(4):374–81.

15. Honoré PM, De Waele E, Jacobs R, et al. Nutritional and metabolic alterations during continuous renal replacement therapy. Blood Purif. 2013;35(4):279–84.

16. Bellomo R, Cass A, Cole L, et al. Calorie intake and patient outcomes in severe acute kidney injury:

findings from The Randomized Evaluation of Normal vs. Augmented Level of Replacement Therapy (RENAL) study trial. Crit Care. 2014;18(2):R45.

17. Sabatino A, Fiaccadori E. Critically ill patient on renal replacement therapy: nutritional support by enteral and parenteral routes. In: Rajendram R, Preedy VR, Patel VB, eds. Diet and Nutrition in Critical Care. Springer-Verlag New York; 2015:671–683.

18. Oh WC, Mafrici B, Rigby M, et al. Micronutrient and amino acid losses during renal replacement therapy for acute kidney injury. Kidney Int Rep 2019;4(8):1094–1108.

19. Patel JJ, McClain CJ, Sarav M, et al. Protein Requirements for critically ill patients with renal and liver failure. Nutr Clin Pract. 2017;32(1_suppl):101S–111S.

20. Rousseau AF, Losser MR, Ichai C, et al. ESPEN endorsed recommendations: Nutritional therapy in major burns. Clin Nutr. 2013;32(4):497–502.

21. Chourdakis M, Bouras E, Shields BA, et al. Nutritional therapy among burn injured patients in the critical care setting: An international multicenter observational study on "best achievable" practices. Clin Nutr. 2020;39(12):3813–3820.

22. Williams FN, Branski LK, Jeschke MG, et al. What, how, and how much should patients with burns be fed? Surg Clin North Am. 2011;91(3):609–29.

23. Clark A, Imran J, Madni T, et al. Nutrition and metabolism in burn patients. Burns Trauma. 2017;5:11.

24. Wise AK, Hromatka KA, Miller KR. Energy Expenditure and protein requirements following burn injury. Nutr Clin Pract. 2019;34(5):673–680.

25. Jeschke, MG. Clinical review: Glucose control in severely burned patients - current best practice. Crit Care 2013;17(4):232.

26. Hébuterne X, Lemarié E, Michallet M, et al. Prevalence of malnutrition and current use of nutrition support in patients with cancer. JPEN J Parenter Enteral Nutr. 2014;38(2):196–204.

27. Arends J, Baracos V, Bertz H, et al. ESPEN expert group recommendations for action against cancer-related malnutrition. Clin Nutr. 2017;36(5):1187–1196.

28. Mattox TW. Cancer cachexia: cause, diagnosis, and treatment. Nutr Clin Pract. 2017;32(5):599–606.

29. Bozzetti F, Arends J, Lundholm K, et al. ESPEN guidelines on parenteral nutrition: non-surgical oncology. Clin Nutr. 2009;28(4):445–54.

30. Virizuela JA, Camblor-Álvarez M, Luengo-Pérez LM, et al. Nutritional support and parenteral nutrition in cancer patients: an expert consensus report. Clin Transl Oncol. 2018;20(5):619–629.

31. Yalcin S, Gumus M, Oksuzoglu B, et al. Turkey Medical Oncology Active Nutrition Platform. Nutritional aspect of cancer care in medical oncology patients. Clin Ther. 2019;41(11):2382–2396.

32. Anker SD, Laviano A, Filippatos G, et al. ESPEN Guidelines on parenteral nutrition: on cardiology and pneumology. Clin Nutr. 2009;28(4):455–60.

33. Lew CCH, Yandell R, Fraser RJL, et al. Association between malnutrition and clinical outcomes in the intensive care unit: a systematic review. JPEN J Parenter Enteral Nutr 2017;41(5):744–58.

34. Singer P, Berger MM, Van den Berghe G, et al. ESPEN guidelines on parenteral nutrition: intensive care clinical nutrition 2009;28(4):387–400.

35. Tappenden KA, Quatrara B, Parkhurst ML, et al. Critical role of nutrition in improving quality of care: an interdisciplinary call to action to address adult hospital malnutrition. JPEN J Parenter Enteral Nutr. 2013;37(4):482–97.

36. Singer P. Preserving the quality of life: nutrition in the ICU. Crit Care 2019;23:139.

37. van Zanten ARH, De Waele E, Wischmeyer PE. Nutrition therapy and critical illness: practical guidance for the ICU, post-ICU, and long-term convalescence phases. Crit Care 2019;23:368.

38. Canadian Critical Care Society (CCCS) and Canadian Critical Care Trials Group (CCTG). (2015) Canadian Clinical Practice Guidelines: Summary of Revisions to the Recommendations, [Online], Available at: https://www.criticalcarenutrition.com/docs/CPGs%202015/Summary%20CPGs%202015%20vs%202013.pdf.

39. Harvey SE, Parrott F, Harrison DA, et al; CALORIES Trial Investigators. Trial of the route of early nutritional support in critically ill adults. N Engl J Med. 2014;371(18):1673–1684.

40. Elke G, van Zanten AR, Lemieux M, et al. Enteral versus parenteral nutrition in critically ill patients: an updated systematic review and meta-analysis of randomized controlled trials. Crit Care. 2016;20(1):117.

41. TARGET Investigators, for the ANZICS Clinical Trials Group, Chapman M, Peake SL, et al. Energy-dense versus routine enteral nutrition in the critically ill. N Engl J Med. 2018;379(19):1823–34.

42. Rice TW, Wheeler AP, Thompson BT, et al. Initial trophic vs full enteral feeding in patients with acute lung injury: the EDEN randomized trial. JAMA. 2012;307(8):795–803.

43. The magnificent seven. Evidence based quality principles agreed by all critical care units in the east of England. https://drive.google.com/file/d/0BwwIbl4F418eGpuaFg4Z1RGZlE/view.

44. Lambell KJ, Tatucu-Babet OA, Chapple LA, et al. Nutrition therapy in critical illness: a review of the literature for clinicians. Crit Care. 2020;24(1):35.

45. Weijs PJ, Looijaard WG, Beishuizen A, et al. Early high protein intake is associated with low mortality and energy overfeeding with high mortality in non-septic mechanically ventilated critically ill patients. Crit Care. 2014;18(6):701.

46. Tian F, Wang X, Gao X, et al. Effect of initial calorie intake via enteral nutrition in critical illness: a meta-analysis of randomised controlled trials. Crit Care. 2015;19(1):180.

47. Zusman O, Theilla M, Cohen J, et al. Resting energy expenditure, calorie and protein consumption in critically ill patients: a retrospective cohort study. Crit Care. 2016;20(1):367.

48. Doig GS, Simpson F, Heighes PT, et al. Restricted versus continued standard caloric intake during the management of refeeding syndrome in critically ill

adults: a randomised, parallel-group, multicentre, single-blind controlled trial. Lancet Respir Med. 2015;3(12):943–52.

49. Puthucheary ZA, Rawal J, McPhail M, et al. Acute skeletal muscle wasting in critical illness. JAMA. 2013;310(15):1591–600.

50. van Gassel RJJ, Baggerman MR, van de Poll MCG. Metabolic aspects of muscle wasting during critical illness. Curr Opin Clin Nutr Metab Care. 2020;23(2):96–101.

51. Nicolo M, Heyland DK, Chittams J, et al. Clinical outcomes related to protein delivery in a critically ill population: a multicenter, multinational observation study. JPEN J. Parenter. Enter. Nutr. 2016;40(1):45–51.

52. Weijs PJM, Mogensen KM, Rawn JD, et al. Protein intake, nutritional status and outcomes in ICU survivors: a single center cohort study. J Clin Med. 2019;8(1):43.

53. Suzuki G, Ichibayashi R, Yamamoto S, et al. Effect of high-protein nutrition in critically ill patients: A retrospective cohort study. Clin Nutr ESPEN. 2020;38:111–117.

54. Koekkoek WACK, van Setten CHC, Olthof LE, et al. Timing of PROTein INtake and clinical outcomes of adult critically ill patients on prolonged mechanical VENTilation: The PROTINVENT retrospective study. Clin Nutr. 2019;38(2):883–890.

55. Burtin C, Clerckx B, Robbeets C, et al. Early exercise in critically ill patients enhances short-term functional recovery. Crit Care Med. 2009;37(9):2499–505.

56. Schaller SJ, Anstey M, Blobner M, et al. International Early SOMS-guided Mobilization Research Initiative. Early, goal-directed mobilisation in the surgical intensive care unit: a randomised controlled trial. Lancet. 2016;388(10052):1377–1388.

57. Bolder U, Ebener C, Hauner H, et al. Working group for developing the guidelines for parenteral nutrition of The German Association for Nutritional Medicine. Carbohydrates - guidelines on parenteral nutrition, chapter 5. Ger Med Sci 2009;7:Doc23.

58. Silva-Perez LJ, Benitez-Lopez MA, Varon J, et al. Management of critically ill patients with diabetes. World J Diabetes. 2017;8(3):89–96.

59. Jacobi J, Bircher N, Krinsley J, et al. Review guidelines for the use of an insulin infusion for the management of hyperglycemia in critically ill patients. Crit Care Med. 2012;40(12):3251–76.

60. Singer P, Berger MM, Van den Berghe G, et al. ESPEN guidelines on parenteral nutrition: intensive care. Clin Nutr 2009;33:246–251.

61. Calder PC, Jensen GL, Koletzko BV, et al. Lipid emulsions in parenteral nutrition of intensive care patients: current thinking and future directions. Intensive Care Med. 2010;36(5):735–49.

62. Mundi MS, Salonen BR, Bonnes SL, et al. Parenteral nutrition lipid emulsions and potential complications. Practical Gastroenterology 2017;41(8):32–37.

63. Pradelli L, Mayer K, Klek S, et al. ω-3 Fatty-acid enriched parenteral nutrition in hospitalized patients: systematic review with meta-analysis and trial sequential analysis. JPEN J Parenter Enteral Nutr 2020;44(1):44–57.

64. Martindale RG, Berlana D, Boullata JI, et al. Summary of proceedings and expert consensus statements from the international summit "Lipids in Parenteral Nutrition". JPEN J Parenter Enteral Nutr. 2020;44(Suppl 1):S7–S20.

65. Calder PC, Adolph M, Deutz NEP, et al. Lipids in the intensive care unit: report from the ESPEN Expert group. ClinNutr 2018;37:1–18.

66. Manzanares W, Dhaliwal R, Jiang X, et al. Antioxidant micronutrients in the critically ill: a systematic review and meta-analysis. Crit Care. 2012;16(2):R66.

67. Canadian Clinical Practice Guidelines for Nutrition Support in the Mechanically Ventilated, Critically Ill Adult, 9.4a Composition of PN: Glutamine (CCCN) 2015 https://www.criticalcarenutrition.com/docs/CPGs%202015/4.1c%202015.pdf.

68. Szczygie B, Pertkiewicz M, Naber T, et al. Basics in clinical nutrition: Nutrition support in GI fistulas. the European e-Journal of Clinical Nutrition and Metabolism 2009;4:e313–e314.

69. Williams LJ, Zolfaghari S, Boushey RP. Complications of enterocutaneous fistulas and their management. Clin Colon Rectal Surg. 2010;23(3):209–220.

70. Kumar P, Maroju NK, Kate V. Enterocutaneous fistulae: etiology, treatment, and outcome-a study from South India. Saudi J Gastroenterol. 2011;17:391–5.

71. Polk TM, Schwab CW. Metabolic and nutritional support of the enterocutaneous fistula patient: a three-phase approach. World J Surg 2012;36:524–533.

72. Tang QQ, Hong ZW, Ren HJ, et al. Nutritional management of patients with enterocutaneous fistulas: practice and progression. Front Nutr. 2020;7:564379.

73. Kumpf VJ, de Aguilar-Nascimento JE, Diaz-Pizarro Graf JI, et al. FELANPE; American Society for Parenteral and Enteral Nutrition. ASPEN-FELANPE Clinical Guidelines: Nutrition Support of Adult Patients with Enterocutaneous Fistula. JPEN J Parenter Enteral Nutr. 2017;41(1):104–112.

74. Grainger JT, Maeda Y, Donnelly SC, et al. Assessment and management of patients with intestinal failure: a multidisciplinary approach. Clin Exp Gastroenterol. 2018;11:233–241.

75. Gribovskaja-Rupp I, Melton GB. Enterocutaneous fistula: proven strategies and updates. Clin Colon Rectal Surg 2016; 29:130.

76. Evenson AR, Fischer JE. Current management of enterocutaneous fistula. Journal of gastrointestinal surgery: official journal of the Society for Surgery of the Alimentary Tract. 2006;10:455–64.

77. Casanova MJ, Chaparro M, Molina B, et al. Prevalence of malnutrition and nutritional characteristics of patients with inflammatory bowel disease. J Crohn's Colitis. 2017;11(12):1430–9.

78. Nguyen GC, Munsell M, Harris ML. Nationwide prevalence and prognostic significance of clinically diagnosable protein-caloric malnutrition in hospitalized inflammatory bowel disease patients. Inflamm Bowel Dis. 2008;14(8):1105–11.

79. Pulley J, Todd A, Flatley C, et al. Malnutrition and quality of life among adult inflammatory bowel disease patients. JGH Open. 2019;4(3):454–460.

80. Balestrieri P, Ribolsi M, Guarino MPL, et al. Nutritional aspects in inflammatory bowel diseases. Nutrients. 2020;12(2):372.

81. Forbes A, Escher J, Hebuterne X, et al. ESPEN guideline: Clinical nutrition in inflammatory bowel disease. Clin Nutr. 2017;36:321–47.

82. Bischoff SC, Escher J, Hebuterne X, et al. ESPEN practical guideline: clinical nutrition in inflammatory bowel disease. Clin Nutr. 2020;39:632–53.

83. Lamb CA, Kennedy NA, Raine T, et al. British Society of Gastroenterology consensus guidelines on the management of inflammatory bowel disease in adults. Gut. 2019:68(Suppl 3):s1–s106.

84. Sood A, Ahuja V, Kedia S, et al. Diet and inflammatory bowel disease: The Asian Working Group guidelines. Indian J Gastroenterol. 2019;38(3):220–246.

85. Nutritional status in cirrhosis. Italian multicentre cooperative project on nutrition in liver cirrhosis. J Hepatol 1994;21:317–25.

86. Cheung K, Lee SS, Raman M. Prevalence and mechanisms of malnutrition in patients with advanced liver disease, and nutrition management strategies. Clin Gastroenterol Hepatol 2012;10(2):117–25.

87. Saunders J, Brian A, Wright M, et al. Malnutrition and nutrition support in patients with liver disease. Frontline Gastroenterol. 2010;1(2):105–111.

88. Dasarathy S. Consilience in sarcopenia of cirrhosis. J Cachexia Sarcopenia Muscle 2012;3:225–237.

89. Huisman EJ, Trip EJ, Siersema PD, et al. Protein energy malnutrition predicts complications in liver cirrhosis. Eur J Gastroenterol Hepatol 2011;23:982–989.

90. Alberino F, Gatta A, Amodio P, et al. Nutrition and survival in patients with liver cirrhosis. Nutrition 2001;17(6):445–450.

91. Sam J, Nguyen GC. Protein-calorie malnutrition as a prognostic indicator of mortality among patients hospitalized with cirrhosis and portal hypertension. Liver Int 2009;29(9):1396–402.

92. European Association for the Study of the Liver. Electronic address: easloffice@easloffice.eu, European Association for the Study of the Liver. EASL Clinical Practice Guidelines on nutrition in chronic liver disease. J Hepatol 2019;70(1):172–193.

93. Plauth M, Schuetz T, Working group for developing the guidelines for parenteral nutrition of The German Association for Nutritional Medicine. Hepatology - Guidelines on Parenteral Nutrition, Chapter 16. Ger Med Sci. 2009;7:Doc12.

94. Plauth M, Bernal W, Dasarathy S, et al. ESPEN guideline on clinical nutrition in liver disease. Clin Nutr 2019;38(2):485–521.

95. Bischoff SC, Bernal W, Dasarathy S, et al. ESPEN practical guideline: Clinical nutrition in liver disease. Clin Nutr. 2020;39(12):3533–3562.

96. Maharshi S, Sharma BC, Sachdeva S, et al. Efficacy of nutritional therapy for patients with cirrhosis and minimal hepatic encephalopathy in a randomized trial. Clin Gastroenterol Hepatol. 2016;14(3):454–460.e453.

97. Kato A, Tanaka H, Kawaguchi T, et al. Nutritional management contributes to improvement in minimal hepatic encephalopathy and quality of life in patients with liver cirrhosis: a preliminary, prospective, open-label study. Hepatol Res. 2013;43(5):452–458.

98. Amodio P, Bemeur C, Butterworth R, et al. The nutritional management of hepatic encephalopathy in patients with cirrhosis: International Society for Hepatic Encephalopathy and Nitrogen Metabolism Consensus. Hepatology. 2013;58(1):325–336.

99. Gheorghe L, Iacob R, Vădan R, et al. Improvement of hepatic encephalopathy using a modified high-calorie high-protein diet. Rom J Gastroenterol.2005;14(3):231–8.

100. Cordoba J, Lopez-Hellin J, Planas M, et al. Normal protein diet for episodic hepatic encephalopathy: results of a randomized study. Journal of hepatology. 2004;41(1):38–43.

101. Saja MF, Abdo AA, Sanai FM, et al. The coagulopathy of liver disease: does vitamin K help? Blood Coagul Fibrinolysis. 2013;24(1):10–7.

102. Aldrich SM, Regal RE. Routine Use of Vitamin K in the treatment of cirrhosis-related coagulopathy: Is it A-O-K? Maybe not, we say. P T. 2019;44(3):131–136.

103. Takuma Y, Nouso K, Makino Y, et al. Clinical trial: oral zinc in hepatic encephalopathy. Aliment Pharmacol Ther. 2010;32(9):1080–90.

104. Katayama K, Saito M, Kawaguchi T, et al. Effect of zinc on liver cirrhosis with hyperammonemia: a preliminary randomized, placebo-controlled double-blind trial. Nutrition 2014;30(11–12):1409–1414.

105. Mousa N, Abdel-Razik A, Zaher A, et al. The role of antioxidants and zinc in minimal hepatic encephalopathy: a randomized trial. Therap Adv Gastroenterol. 2016;9(5):684–91.

106. Shen YC, Chang YH, Fang CJ, et al. Zinc supplementation in patients with cirrhosis and hepatic encephalopathy: a systematic review and meta-analysis. Nutr J. 2019;18(1):34.

107. Al-Alfy M, Amin Hegazy A, Soliman Hammad K, et al. Zinc replacement in hepatic encephalopathy among the Egyptian patients. Al-Azhar Medical Journal 2020;49(2):839–848.

108. John S, Thuluvath PJ. Hyponatremia in cirrhosis: pathophysiology and management. World J Gastroenterol. 2015;21(11):3197–3205.

109. Aithal GP, Palaniyappan N, China L, et al. Guidelines on the management of ascites in cirrhosis Gut 2021;70(1):9–29.

110. Haberl J, Zollner G, Fickert P, et al. To salt or not to salt?-That is the question in cirrhosis. Liver Int. 2018;38(7):1148–1159.

111. Baron TH, Morgan DE. Acute necrotizing pancreatitis. N Engl J Med. 1999;340(18):1412–7.

112. Arvanitakis M, Ockenga J, Bezmarevic M, et al. ESPEN guideline on clinical nutrition in acute and chronic pancreatitis. Clin Nutr. 2020;39(3):612–631.

113. Zheng Z, Ding Y, Qu Y, et al. A narrative review of acute pancreatitis and its diagnosis, pathogenetic mechanism, and management. Ann Transl Med 2021;9(1):69.

114. Niederau C, Niederau M, Lüthen R, et al. Pancreatic exocrine secretion in acute experimental pancreatitis. Gastroenterology 1990;99(4):1120–1127.

115. Borcham B, Ammori BJ. A prospective evaluation of pancreatic exocrine function in patients with acute pancreatitis: correlation with extent of necrosis and pancreatic endocrine insufficiency. Pancreatology 2003;3(4):303–308.

116. Boxhoorn L, Voermans RP, Bouwense SA, et al. Acute pancreatitis. Lancet 2020;396(10252):726–34.

117. Lakananurak N, Gramlich L. Nutrition management in acute pancreatitis: Clinical practice consideration. World J Clin Cases. 2020;8(9):1561–1573.

118. Mederos MA, Reber HA, Girgis MD. Acute pancreatitis: a review. JAMA. 2021;325(4):382–390.

119. Ioannidis O, Lavrenticva A, Botsios D. Nutrition support in acute pancreatitis. JOP. 2008;9(4):375–90.

120. Mutch KL, Heidal KB, Gross KH, et al. Cost-analysis of nutrition support in patients with severe acute pancreatitis. Int J Health Care Qual Assur. 2011;24(7):540–547.

121. Uomo G. Pancreatic rest or not? The debate on the nutrition in acute pancreatitis continues JOP. 2013;14(2):216–7.

122. Rinninella E, Annetta MG, Serricchio M, et al. Nutritional support in acute pancreatitis: from physiopathology to practice: an evidence-based approach. Eur Rev Med Pharmacol Sci 2017;21(2):421–432.

123. Crockett SD, Wani S, Gardner TB, et al. American Gastroenterological Association Institute Clinical Guidelines Committee. American Gastroenterological Association Institute Guideline on Initial Management of Acute Pancreatitis. Gastroenterology. 2018;154(4):1096–1101.

124. Al-Omran M, Albalawi ZH, Tashkandi MF, et al. Enteral versus parenteral nutrition for acute pancreatitis. Cochrane Database Syst Rev. 2010;(1):CD002837.

125. Vaughn VM, Shuster D, Rogers MAM, et al. Early versus delayed feeding in patients with acute pancreatitis: a systematic review. Ann Intern Med. 2017;166(12):883–892.

126. Li W, Liu J, Zhao S, et al. Safety and efficacy of total parenteral nutrition versus total enteral nutrition for patients with severe acute pancreatitis: a meta-analysis. J Int Med Res 2018;46(9):3948–58.

127. Wu P, Li L, Sun W. Efficacy comparisons of enteral nutrition and parenteral nutrition in patients with severe acute pancreatitis: a meta-analysis from randomized controlled trials. Biosci Rep 2018;38(6):BSR20181515.

128. Yao H, He C, Deng L, et al. Enteral versus parenteral nutrition in critically ill patients with severe pancreatitis: a meta-analysis. Eur J Clin Nutr 2018;72(1):66–68.

129. Tenner S, Baillie J, DeWitt J, et al. American College of Gastroenterology guideline: management of acute pancreatitis. Am J Gastroenterol 2013;108(9):1400–1415.

130. Greenberg JA, Hsu J, Bawazeer M, et al. Clinical practice guideline: management of acute pancreatitis. Can J Surg. 2016;59(2):128–140.

131. Reintam Blaser A, Starkopf J, Alhazzani W, et al. Early enteral nutrition in critically ill patients: ESICM clinical practice guidelines. Intensive Care Med 2017;43(3):380–98.

132. National Institute for Health and Care Excellence. Pancreatitis (NICE guideline NG104). 2018. www.nice.org.uk/guidance/ng104.

133. Leppäniemi A, Tolonen M, Tarasconi A, et al. 2019 WSES guidelines for the management of severe acute pancreatitis. World J Emerg Surg 2019;14:27.

134. Petrov MS, Kukosh MV, Emelyanov NV. A randomized controlled trial of enteral versus parenteral feeding in patients with predicted severe acute pancreatitis shows a significant reduction in mortality and in infected pancreatic complications with total enteral nutrition. Dig Surg 2006;23(5–6):336–344.

135. Petrov MS, Pylypchuk RD, Uchugina AF. A systematic review on the timing of artificial nutrition in acute pancreatitis. Br J Nutr 2009;101(6):787–93.

136. Ramanathan M, Aadam AA. Nutrition management in acute pancreatitis. Nutr Clin Pract 2019;34(S1):S7–S12.

137. Li JY, Yu T, Chen GC, et al. Enteral nutrition within 48 hours of admission improves clinical outcomes of acute pancreatitis by reducing complications: a meta-analysis. PLoS One 2013;8(6):e64926.

138. Wereszczynska-Siemiatkowska U, Swidnicka-Siergiejko A, Siemiatkowski A, et al. Early enteral nutrition is superior to delayed enteral nutrition for the prevention of infected necrosis and mortality in acute pancreatitis. Pancreas. 2013;42(4):640–646.

139. Wu XM, Liao YW, Wang HY, et al. When to initialize enteral nutrition in patients with severe acute pancreatitis? A retrospective review in a single institution experience (2003–2013). Pancreas 2015;44(3):507–11.

140. Feng P, He C, Liao G, et al. Early enteral nutrition versus delayed enteral nutrition in acute pancreatitis A PRISMA-compliant systematic review and meta-analysis. Medicine. 2017;96(96):e8648.

141. Song J, Zhong Y, Lu X, et al. Enteral nutrition provided within 48 hours after admission in severe acute pancreatitis: a systematic review and meta-analysis. Medicine (Baltimore) 2018;97(34):e11871.

142. Bakker OJ, van Brunschot S, Farre A, et al. Timing of enteral nutrition in acute pancreatitis: meta-analysis of individuals using a single-arm of randomised trials. Pancreatology 2014;14(5):340–6.

143. Qi D, Yu B, Huang J, et al. Meta-analysis of early enteral nutrition provided within 24 hours of admission on clinical outcomes in acute pancreatitis. JPEN J Parenter Enteral 2018;42(7):1139–47.

144. Eckerwall GE, Tingstedt BB, Bergenzaun PE, et al. Immediate oral feeding in patients with mild acute pancreatitis is safe and may accelerate recovery–a randomized clinical study. Clin Nutr 2007;26(6):758–63.

145. Bakker OJ, van Brunschot S, van Santvoort HC, et al. Early versus on-demand nasoenteric tube feeding in acute pancreatitis. N Engl J Med. 2014;371(21):1983–1993.

146. Horibe M, Nishizawa T, Suzuki H, et al. Timing of oral refeeding in acute pancreatitis: A systematic review and meta-analysis. United European Gastroenterol J. 2016;4(6):725–732.

147. Lozada-Hernández EE, Barrón-González O, Vázquez-Romero S, et al. Non-inferiority comparative clinical trial between early oral REFEEDING and usual oral REFEEDING in predicted mild acute biliary pancreatitis. BMC Gastroenterol. 2020;20(1):228.

148. Spanier BWM, Bruno MJ, Mathus-Vliegen EM. Enteral nutrition and acute pancreatitis: a review. Gastroenterol Res Pract. 2011;2011:857949.

149. Working Group IAP/APA Acute Pancreatitis Guidelines. IAP/APA evidence-based guidelines for the management of acute pancreatitis. Pancreatology. 2013;13(4 suppl 2):e1–15.

150. Meier R, Ockenga J, Pertkiewicz J, et al. ESPEN guidelines on enteral nutrition: Pancreas. Clin Nutr. 2006;25(2):275–284.

151. Olah A, Romics Jr. L. Enteral nutrition in acute pancreatitis: A review of the current evidence. World J Gastroenterol. 2014;20(43):16123–16131.

152. Sun JK, Li WQ, Ke L, et al. Early enteral nutrition prevents intra-abdominal hypertension and reduces the severity of severe acute pancreatitis compared with delayed enteral nutrition: a prospective pilot study. World J Surg. 2013;37(9):2053–2060.

153. Eatock FC, Chong P, Menezes N, et al. A randomized study of early nasogastric versus nasojejunal feeding in severe acute pancreatitis. Am J Gastroenterol 2005;100:432–9.

154. Kumar A, Singh N, Prakash S, et al. Early enteral nutrition in severe acute pancreatitis: A prospective randomized controlled trial comparing nasojejunal and nasogastric routes. J Clin Gastroenterol. 2006;40(5):431–434.

155. Petrov MS, Correia MI, Windsor JA. Nasogastric tube feeding in predicted severe acute pancreatitis. A systematic review of the literature to determine safety and tolerance. JOP 2008;9(4):440–8.

156. Singh N, Sharma B, Sharma M, et al. Evaluation of early enteral feeding through nasogastric and nasojejunal tube in severe acute pancreatitis: a noninferiority randomized controlled trial. Pancreas 2012;41(1):153–9.

157. Chang YS, Fu HQ, Xiao YM, et al. Nasogastric or nasojejunal feeding in predicted severe acute pancreatitis: a meta-analysis. Crit Care 2013;17(3):R118.

158. Nally DM, Kelly EG, Clarke M, et al. Nasogastric nutrition is efficacious in severe acute pancreatitis: a systematic review and meta-analysis. Br J Nutr 2014;112(11):1769–78.

159. Guo YJ, Jing X, Tian ZB. Comparison of nasogastric feeding versus nasojejunal feeding for severe acute pancreatitis: a systematic review and meta-analysis. Int J Clin Exp Med 2016;9(11):22814–22823.

160. Zhu Y, Yin H, Zhang R, et al. Nasogastric nutrition versus nasojejunal nutrition in patients with severe acute pancreatitis: a meta-analysis of randomized controlled trials. Gastroenterol Res Pract 2016;2016:6430632.

161. Dutta AK, Goel A, Kirubakaran R, et al. Nasogastric versus nasojejunal tube feeding for severe acute pancreatitis. Cochrane Database Syst Rev. 2020;3(3):CD010582.

162. Lee PJ, Papachristou GI. Management of Severe Acute Pancreatitis. Curr Treat Options Gastroenterol. 2020:1–12.

163. Jacobson BC, Vander Vliet MB, Hughes MD, et al. A prospective, randomized trial of clear liquids versus low-fat solid diet as the initial meal in mild acute pancreatitis. Clin Gastroenterol Hepatol 2007;5(8):946–951.

164. Moraes JM, Felga GE, Chebli LA, et al. A full solid diet as the initial meal in mild acute pancreatitis is safe and result in a shorter length of hospitalization: results from a prospective, randomized, controlled, double-blind clinical trial. J Clin Gastroenterol 2010;44(7):517–522.

165. Meng WB, Li X, Li YM, et al. Three initial diets for management of mild acute pancreatitis: A meta-analysis. World J Gastroenterol 2011;17(37):4235–4241.

166. Rajkumar N, Karthikeyan VS, Ali SM, et al. Clear liquid diet vs soft diet as the initial meal in patients with mild acute pancreatitis: a randomized interventional trial. Nutr Clin Pract. 2013;28(3):365–70.

167. Lariño-Noia J, Lindkvist B, Iglesias-García J, et al. Early and/or immediately full caloric diet versus standard refeeding in mild acute pancreatitis: a randomized open-label trial. Pancreatology 2014;14(3):167–173.

168. Gianotti L, Meier R, Lobo DN, et al. ESPEN Guidelines on parenteral nutrition: pancreas. Clin Nutr 2009;28(4):428–435.

169. Baron TH, DiMaio CJ, Wang AY, et al. American Gastroenterological Association Clinical Practice Update: Management of pancreatic necrosis. Gastroenterology. 2020;158(1):67–75.

170. Asrani V, Chang WK, Dong Z, et al. Glutamine supplementation in acute pancreatitis: a meta-analysis of randomized controlled trials. Pancreatology 2013;13(5):468–474.

171. Zhong X, Liang CP, Gong S. Intravenous glutamine for severe acute pancreatitis: A meta-analysis. World J Crit Care Med. 2013;2(1):4–8.

172. Barker LA, Gout BS, Crowe TC. Hospital malnutrition: prevalence, identification and impact on patients and the healthcare system. Int J Environ Res Public Health. 2011;8(2):514–527.

173. Cerantola Y, Grass F, Cristaudi A, et al. Perioperative nutrition in abdominal surgery: recommendations and reality. Gastroenterol Res Pract. 2011;2011:739347.

174. Culebras JM. Malnutrition in the twenty-first century: an epidemic affecting surgical outcome. Surg Infect (Larchmt). 2013;14(3):237–243.

175. Leandro-Merhi VA, de Aquino JL. Determinants of malnutrition and post-operative complications in hospitalized surgical patients. J Health Popul Nutr. 2014;32(3):400–410.

176. Inciong JFB, Chaudhary A, Hsu HS, et al. Hospital malnutrition in northeast and southeast Asia: A systematic literature review. Clin Nutr ESPEN. 2020;39:30–45.

177. Braga M, Ljungqvist O, Soeters P, et al. ESPEN guidelines on parenteral nutrition: surgery. Clin Nutr. 2009;28(4):378–86.

178. Abunnaja S, Cuviello A, Sanchez JA. Enteral and parenteral nutrition in the perioperative period: state of the art. Nutrients. 2013;5(2):608–623.

179. Weimann A, Braga M, Carli F, et al. ESPEN guideline: Clinical nutrition in surgery. Clin Nutr. 2017;36(3):623–650.

180. Worthington P, Balint J, Bechtold M, et al. When is parenteral nutrition appropriate? JPEN J Parenter Enteral Nutr. 2017;41(3):324–377.

181. Lakananurak N, Gramlich L. The role of preoperative parenteral nutrition. Nutrients. 2020 6;12(5):1320.

182. Ward N. Nutrition support to patients undergoing gastrointestinal surgery. Nutr. J. 2003;2:18.

183. Klein S, Kinney J, Jeejeebhoy K, et al. Nutrition support in clinical practice: review of published data and recommendations for future research directions. Clin Nutr 1997;16:193.

184. de-Aguilar-Nascimento JE, Salomão AB, Waitzberg DL, et al. ACERTO guidelines of perioperative nutritional interventions in elective general surgery. Rev. Col. Bras. Cir. [online]. 2017;44(6):633–648.

185. Wischmeyer PE, Carli F, Evans DC, et al. Perioperative Quality Initiative (POQI) 2 Workgroup. American society for enhanced recovery and perioperative quality initiative joint consensus statement on nutrition screening and therapy within a surgical enhanced recovery pathway. Anesth Analg. 2018;126(6):1883–1895.

186. Lobo DN, Gianotti L, Adiamah A, et al. Perioperative nutrition: Recommendations from the ESPEN expert group. Clin Nutr. 2020;39(11):3211–3227.

187. Doig GS, Simpson F, Sweetman EA, et al. Early PN Investigators of the ANZICS Clinical Trials Group. Early parenteral nutrition in critically ill patients with short-term relative contraindications to early enteral nutrition: a randomized controlled trial. JAMA. 2013;309(20):2130–8.

188. Mete B, Pehlivan E, Gülbaş G, et al. Prevalence of malnutrition in COPD and its relationship with the parameters related to disease severity. Int J Chron Obstruct Pulmon Dis. 2018;13:3307–3312.

189. Ting HYT, Chan SHY, Luk EKH, et al. Prevalence of malnutrition in COPD inpatients and its relationship with nutritional intakes and clinical outcomes. J Aging Sci. 2020;8(1):219.

190. Steer J, Norman E, Gibson G, et al. P117 Comparison of indices of nutritional status in prediction of in-hospital mortality and early readmission of patients with acute exacerbations of COPD. Thorax. 2010;65(4):A127.

191. Hoong JM, Ferguson M, Hukins C, et al. Economic and operational burden associated with malnutrition in COPD. Clinical Nutrition. 2017;36(4):1105–1109.

192. Elia M. The cost of malnutrition in England and potential cost savings from nutritional interventions (full report). BAPEN. 2015.

193. Holdoway A, Anderson L, Banner J et al. Managing malnutrition in COPD. 2nd ed. 2020. Available at: www.malnutritionpathway.co.uk/copd.

194. Schols AM. Nutrition in chronic obstructive pulmonary disease. Curr Opin Pulm Med. 2000;6(2):110–5.

195. Dias CM, Pássaro CP, Cagido VR, et al. Effects of undernutrition on respiratory mechanics and lung parenchyma remodeling. J Appl Physiol (1985). 2004;97(5):1888–96.

196. Gea J, Sancho-Muñoz A, Chalela R. Nutritional status and muscle dysfunction in chronic respiratory diseases: stable phase versus acute exacerbations. J Thorac Dis. 2018;10(12):S1332–S1354.

197. Wilson DO, Rogers RM. The role of nutrition in weaning from mechanical ventilation. Journal of Intensive Care Medicine. 1989;4(3):124–133.

198. Rodríguez L, Cervantes E, Ortiz R. Malnutrition and gastrointestinal and respiratory infections in children: a public health problem. Int J Environ Res Public Health. 2011;8(4):1174–1205.

199. Nguyen HT, Collins PF, Pavey TG, et al. Nutritional status, dietary intake, and health-related quality of life in outpatients with COPD. Int J Chron Obstruct Pulmon Dis. 2019;14:215–226.

200. Guo Y, Zhang T, Wang Z, et al. Body mass index and mortality in chronic obstructive pulmonary disease: A dose-response meta-analysis. Medicine (Baltimore). 2016;95(28):e4225.

201. Ferreira IM, Brooks D, White J, et al. Nutritional supplementation for stable chronic obstructive pulmonary disease. Cochrane Database Syst Rev 2012;12:CD000998.

202. Collins PF, Stratton RJ, Elia M. Nutritional support in chronic obstructive pulmonary disease: a systematic review and meta-analysis. Am J Clin Nutr 2012;95(6):1385–1395.

203. Collins PF, Elia M, Stratton RJ. Nutritional support and functional capacity in chronic obstructive pulmonary disease: a systematic review and meta-analysis. Respirology 2013;18(4):616–629.

204. Naz I, Sahin H. The effect of nutritional support on pulmonary rehabilitation outcomes in COPD patients with low body mass index. Eur Resp J 2018;52.

205. Aldhahir AM, Rajeh AMA, Aldabayan YS, et al. Nutritional supplementation during pulmonary rehabilitation in COPD: A systematic review. Chron Respir Dis. 2020;17:1479973120904953.

206. Global strategy for diagnosis, management and prevention of COPD. The Global Initiative for Chronic Obstructive Lung Diseases (GOLD). 2020 report. Available from: https://goldcopd.org/gold-reports/.

207. Slinde F, Gronberg AM, Svantesson U, et al. Energy expenditure in chronic obstructive pulmonary diseaseevaluation of simple measures. Eur J Clin Nutr 2011;65(12):1309–1313.

208. Ganzoni A, Heilig P, Schonenberger K, et al. High-caloric nutrition in chronic obstructive lung disease. Schweiz Rundsch Med Prax 1994;83(1):13–6.

209. Baarends EM, Schols AM, Pannemans DL, et al. Total free living energy expenditure in patients with severe chronic obstructive pulmonary disease. Am J Respir Crit Care Med. 1997;155(2):549–54.

210. Rondanelli M, Faliva MA, Peroni G, et al. Food pyramid for subjects with chronic obstructive pulmonary diseases. Int J Chron Obstruct Pulmon Dis. 2020;15:1435–1448.

211. de Batlle J, Sauleda J, Balcells E, et al. Association between Omega3 and Omega6 fatty acid intakes and serum inflammatory markers in COPD. J Nutr Biochem. 2012;23(7):817–21.

212. al-Saady NM, Blackmore CM, Bennett ED. High fat, low carbohydrate, enteral feeding lowers PaCO2 and reduces the period of ventilation in artifcially ventilated patients. Intensive Care Med. 1989;15(5):290–295.

213. Faramawy MA, Abd Allah A, El Batrawy S, et al. Impact of high fat low carbohydrate enteral feeding on weaning from mechanical ventilation. Egypt J Chest Dis Tuberc 2014;63(4):931–8.

214. Yartsev A. Nutritional manipulation of carbon dioxide production. Deranged Physiology February 27, 2016 https://derangedphysiology.com/main/required-reading/endocrinology-metabolism-and-nutrition/Chapter%205.1.4/nutritional-manipulation-carbon-dioxide-production.

215. Van den Berg B, Bogaard WCJ. High fat, low carbohydrate, enteral feeding in patients weaning from the ventilator. Intensive Care Med. 1994;20(7):479–475.

216. El Koofy NM, Rady HI, Abdallah SM, et al. The effect of high fat dietary modification and nutritional status on the outcome of critically ill ventilated children: single-center study. Korean J Pediatr. 2019;62(9):344–352.

217. Persson LJ, Aanerud M, Hiemstra PS, et al. Chronic obstructive pulmonary disease is associated with low levels of vitamin D. PLoS One. 2012;7(6):e38934.

218. Fernández-Lahera J, Romera D, Gómez Mendieta A, et al. Prevalence of vitamin D deficiency in patients with chronic obstructive pulmonary disease. Eur. Respir. J. 2015;46:PA3977.

219. Horadagoda C, Dinihan T, Roberts M, et al. Body composition and micronutrient deficiencies in patients with an acute exacerbation of chronic obstructive pulmonary disease. Intern Med J. 2017;47(9):1057–1063.

220. Ginde AA, Mansbach JM, Camargo CA Jr. Association between serum 25-hydroxyvitamin D level and upper respiratory tract infection in the Third National Health and Nutrition Examination Survey. Arch Intern Med. 2009;169(4):384–390.

221. Black PN, Scragg R. Relationship between serum 25-hydroxyvitamin D and pulmonary function in the third national health and nutrition examination survey. Chest. 2005;128(6):3792–3798.

222. Afzal S, Lange P, Bojesen SE, et al. Plasma 25-hydroxyvitamin D, lung function and risk of chronic obstructive pulmonary disease. Thorax. 2014;69(1):24–31.

223. Martineau AR, Jolliffe DA, Hooper RL, et al. Vitamin D supplementation to prevent acute respiratory tract infections: systematic review and meta-analysis of individual participant data. BMJ 2017;356:i6583.

224. Zendedel A, Gholami M, Anbari K, et al. Effects of vitamin D intake on FEV1 and COPD exacerbation: A randomized clinical trial study. Glob J Health Sci 2015;7(4):243–248.

225. Jolliffe DA, Greenberg L, Hooper RL, et al. Vitamin D to prevent exacerbations of COPD: systematic review and meta-analysis of individual participant data from randomised controlled trials. Thorax. 2019;74(4):337–345.

226. Nightingale J, Woodward JM. Guidelines for management of patients with a short bowel. Gut 2006;55(4):iv1–12.

227. Nguyen BT, Blatchford GJ, Thompson JS, et al. Should intestinal continuity be restored after massive intestinal resection? Am J Surg. 1989;158(6):577–579.

228. Messing B, Crenn P, Beau P, et al. Long-term survival and parenteral nutrition dependence in adult patients with the short bowel syndrome. Gastroenterology. 1999;117(5):1043–1050.

229. Marino IR, Lauro A. Surgeon's perspective on short bowel syndrome: Where are we? World J Transplant 2018;8(6):198–202.

230. Pironi L, Arends J, Bozzetti F, et al. Home artificial nutrition & chronic intestinal failure special interest group of ESPEN. ESPEN guidelines on chronic intestinal failure in adults. Clin Nutr. 2016;35(2):247–307.

231. Massironi S, Cavalcoli F, Rausa E, et al. Understanding short bowel syndrome: Current status and future perspectives. Dig Liver Dis. 2020;52(3):253–261.

232. Nightingale JM, Kamm MA, van der Sijp JR, et al. Gastrointestinal hormones in short bowel syndrome. Peptide YY may be the' colonic brake' to gastric emptying. Gut 1996;39(2):267–72.

233. Szczygiel B, Jonkers-Schuitema CF, Naber T. Basics in clinical nutrition: Nutritional support in extensive gut resections (short bowel). e-SPEN, Euro E-J Clinic Nutr Metab. 2010;5(1):e63–e68.

234. Kowlgi NG, Chhabra L. D-lactic acidosis: an underrecognized complication of short bowel syndrome. Gastroenterol Res Pract. 2015;2015:476215.

235. Johnson E, Vu L, Matarese LE. Bacteria, Bones, and Stones: Managing Complications of Short Bowel Syndrome. Nutr Clin Pract. 2018;33(4):454–466.

236. Yang J, Sun H, Wan S, et al. Risk factors for nephrolithiasis in adults with short bowel syndrome. Ann Nutr Metab 2019;75(1):47–54.

237. Hylander E, Jarnum S. Jensen HJ, et al. Enteric hyperoxaluria: dependence on small intestinal resection, colectomy, and steatorrhoea in chronic inflammatory bowel disease. Scand J Gastroenterol. 1978;13(5):577–588.

238. Parks JH, Worcester EM, R. Corey O'Connor RC, et al. Urine stone risk factors in nephrolithiasis patients with and without bowel disease. Kidney Int. 2003;63(1):255–65.

239. Amiot A, Messing B, Corcos O, et al. Determinants of home parenteral nutrition dependence and survival of 268 patients with non-malignant short bowel syndrome. Clin Nutr. 2013;32(3):368–74.

240. Joly F, Dray X, Corcos O, et al. Tube feeding improves intestinal absorption in short bowel syndrome patients. Gastroenterology 2009;136(3):824–31.

241. Pironi L, Sasdelli AS. Intestinal failure-associated liver disease. Clin Liver Dis 2019;23(2):279–91.

242. Lal S, Pironi L, Wanten G, et al. Home Artificial Nutrition & Chronic Intestinal Failure Special Interest Group of the European Society for Clinical Nutrition

and Metabolism (ESPEN). Clinical approach to the management of Intestinal Failure Associated Liver Disease (IFALD) in adults: A position paper from the Home Artificial Nutrition and Chronic Intestinal Failure Special Interest Group of ESPEN. Clin Nutr. 2018;37(6 Pt A):1794–1797.

243. Wang C, Venick RS, Shew SB, et al. Long-term outcomes in children with intestinal failure-associated liver disease treated with 6 months of intravenous fish oil followed by resumption of intravenous soybean oil. JPEN J Parenter Enteral Nutr. 2019;43(6):708–716.

244. Lauro A, Lacaille F. Short bowel syndrome in children

and adults: from rehabilitation to transplantation. Expert Rev Gastroenterol Hepatol. 2019;13(1):55–70.

245. Jeejeebhoy KN. Short bowel syndrome: a nutritional and medical approach. CMAJ. 2002;166(10):1297–1302.

246. Miranda SC, Ribeiro ML, Ferriolli E, et al. Hypomagnesemia in short bowel syndrome patients. Sao Paulo Medical Journal 2000;118(6):169–172.

247. Bielawska B, Allard JP. Parenteral nutrition and intestinal failure. Nutrients. 2017;9(5):466.

248. Olieman J, Kastelijn W. Nutritional feeding strategies in pediatric intestinal failure. Nutrients. 2020;12(1):177.

57 | Parenteral Nutrition: Administration and Complications

INTRODUCTION

Parenteral nutrition (PN) is currently one of the most sophisticated forms of intravenous therapy. Appropriate use of parenteral nutrition provides life-saving treatment for patients who could not otherwise be nourished.

ADMINISTRATION OF PARENTERAL NUTRITION

SELECTION OF MACRONUTRIENTS

Selecting an appropriate macronutrient mixture while administering parenteral nutrition in day-to-day practice is essential. Broad guidelines in the selection of the most suitable macronutrient solutions based on requirements for different patients are:

Indications of only dextrose containing crystalloids; avoid PN

In cases where patients are stable, not malnourished, and unable to consume oral intake for a brief period (less than a week), using PN support is unnecessary [1]. Instead, dextrose infusions (>100 gm/day in adults), electrolytes, and vitamins serve as the primary approach for short-term therapy in such individuals. Providing adequate dextrose (calculated as the daily energy requirement in kcal ÷ 3.4 = gm/day dextrose) fulfills calorie needs and helps conserve nitrogen [2].

Indications of amino acids plus dextrose-containing solutions, withhold lipid emulsion

Parenteral nutrition combining amino acids and dextrose may suffice to address nutritional needs over a short duration (less than one week) in patients who are stable and not malnourished, as long as their total caloric requirements remain relatively low. However, it is advisable to introduce lipid administration within ≤7 days of starting PN to prevent essential fatty acid deficiency [3]. Early lipid administration is also crucial for minimizing the risk of hyperglycemia resulting from high glucose intake.

Indications of PN with all three macronutrients (dextrose + amino acids + lipids)

PN solutions that incorporate all three macronutrients are widely utilized in clinical practice. The addition of lipid emulsion provides additional calories, reduces the osmolarity of the solution, and prevents essential fatty acid deficiency. PN solutions containing all three macronutrients are commonly recommended for patients:

- Those in need of PN support for prolonged period.

- Patients requiring peripheral parenteral nutrition (PPN) with significant calorie supplementation but unable to tolerate carbohydrates.

- Critically ill patients, and those with hyperglycemia, diabetes mellitus, and respiratory failure.

DELIVERING PARENTERAL NUTRITION

For proper supplementation of PN, it is essential to understand different fundamental aspects of delivering PN, as classified below:

1. Routes of nutrient delivery:

   Peripheral parenteral nutrition vs. central parenteral nutrition.

2. Systems of delivering PN:

   Multiple bottle system, multichamber-bag PN, or hospital compounded PN.

3. Duration of delivering PN:

   Continuous infusion of PN vs. cyclic infusion of PN.

1. Routes of nutrient delivery

The two routes used for nutrient delivery are peripheral parenteral nutrition, and central parenteral nutrition (CPN), which is compared in Table 57.1.

a. Peripheral parenteral nutrition

Peripheral parenteral nutrition is the frequently used method to deliver all the required nutrients through peripheral veins [4–6]. PPN aims to provide enough calories and nutrition for a short period (less than 2 weeks). PPN is generally intended when central PN is undesirable or unavailable.

Table 57.1 Comparison of peripheral and central parenteral nutrition		
	PPN	**CPN**
Route of administration	Peripheral veins	Central venous access
Access site	Peripheral veins	Large peripheral veins or central veins
Location of catheter distal tips	Below the level of the axillary vein	Central circulation (usually SVC or uncommonly IVC)
Duration of therapy	less than 2 weeks	>7–14 days
Nutritional needs	Low	High
Daily caloric requirement	1000–1500	2000–3000
Daily volume need (mL)	2000–3000	1000–2000
PN osmolarity (mOsm/L)	Low (600–850)	High (>800–900)
Carbohydrate	30%	55%–60%
Fat emulsion	Major caloric source	Minor caloric source
Prerequisite	Good peripheral veins	Successful cannulation of large peripheral or central veins
Fluid permitted	No fluid restriction	Needs fluid restriction
Advantages	Easy insertion, lower risk of infection/complications	No limit to osmolality, pH, or volume of infusion
Disadvantages	Short life span, only for low osmolality infusion	Complex insertion, higher complication risk, and cost
Common complication	Thrombophlebitis of veins	Catheter sepsis
PICC: Peripherally inserted central catheter; CVCs: Central venous catheters; SVC: Superior vena cava; IVC: Inferior vena cava		

Composition: The osmolarity of formulas for PPN should be less than 900 mOsm/L [7]. Formulas for PPN contain low concentrated dextrose (5–10%) and amino acids along with concentrated, calorie-dense lipids (usually 20% lipid emulsion), which can provide the patient's average basal energy and protein needs [8]. Lipid emulsion is an essential part of PPN. Lipid emulsion reduces the osmolarity of PPN because of its low osmolarity (260 mOsm/L) and therefore decreases the risk of thrombophlebitis of peripheral veins.

Prerequisite: For PPN, the peripheral vein should be readily accessible, and fluid restriction should not be an issue.

Indications [9]

1. Requirements of PN for a short period (less than a week). Postoperative patients requiring PN support are the most suitable candidates for PPN.
2. Nutritional needs <1500–1800 kcals per day.
3. Central venous catheter insertion is not possible, carries a high risk, or is contraindicated (e.g., patients with coagulopathy).
4. Sepsis or bacteremia in patients with CPN to avoid central vein catheterization for a few days.

Contraindications

1. In patients with high nutritional requirements (i.e.,

hypermetabolism, preexisting moderate to severe malnutrition, or high risk of protein depletion), PPN is not suitable, as it cannot provide enough nutrients.

2. Patients who need fluid restriction (oliguric patients and edematous patients due to cardiac, hepatic, or renal failure).

3. Critically ill patients who will not tolerate the high fluid volume of PPN required for providing their increased nutritional needs.

4. If PPN does not allow complete nutritional requirements, PN should be administered centrally.

5. If PN is required for a prolonged period (>2 weeks).

Advantages

1. Easy and safe venous access.

2. It avoids morbidity and risks of CPN and saves the cost of a central catheter.

Disadvantages

1. Larger volume is required to provide even maintenance nutritional requirements.

2. Difficulty in meeting high nutritional requirements (because the volume required to provide the same is prohibitively high in sick patients).

3. The concentration of nutrients in peripheral parenteral nutrition is kept low to prevent thrombophlebitis of peripheral veins. So, a larger volume is required to meet the nutritional needs compared to central parenteral nutrition formulas.

Prevention of thrombophlebitis due to PPN

Various measures, which can prevent or reduce thrombophlebitis, are:

1. Add heparin (1U/ml of total volume) and low-dose hydrocortisone to the PPN formulas [10, 11].

2. Place a glycerine trinitrate transdermal patch on the skin overlying the tip of the IV catheter.

3. Topical NSAID creams and gel may inhibit the local inflammatory response.

4. Limiting the osmolarity of PPN to 600 mOsm/L.

5. Chang peripheral lines every 72–96 hours.

b. Central parenteral nutrition

Central parenteral nutrition is the most effective method to deliver high concentration PN in a smaller volume into large diameter central veins (usually superior vena cava or uncommonly inferior vena cava) in patients who needs PN for >7–14 days. It is important to remember that the location of the distal tip determines central versus peripheral venous access and not the site of catheter insertion. When the distal end is located in the large-diameter central vein, administered hypertonic and acidic PN solutions mix quickly with surrounding turbulent blood flow and therefore avoid complications due to the local irritation of veins such as thrombophlebitis.

Goals and indications: The goal of CPN is to provide nutritional maintenance requirements and correct existing nutritional deficits. CPN is mandatory to provide long term PN support (weeks, months, or years) when volume and concentration of solution preclude peripheral administration (i.e., osmolarity exceeds 800–900 mOsm/L, pH <5 or pH >9, or fluid restriction is necessary), and to provide greater nutritional requirements to moderately to severely stressed patients [12].

Composition: As per patients' requirements, the composition of solutions for CPN varies. Most of the CPN solutions contain a higher concentration of dextrose (50–70%) and amino acids (8.5–10%), which makes these solutions hypertonic (osmolarity of CPN 1000–1900 mOsm/L as compared to plasma osmolarity 280 mOsm/L). These hypertonic CPN solutions are too irritant for a peripheral vein and should be infused only through central venous access. For safe and adequate delivery of CPN, it is essential to establish central vascular access with proper selection of the type of catheter and the site of insertion.

CPN permits the administration of a lower amount of fat emulsion than PPN because a higher concentration of dextrose and amino acids in CPN provides a significant amount of calories.

Selection of catheter for CPN: For CPN, a catheter made up of polyurethane and silicone is used routinely. Catheters made up of polyurethane are selected for short-term and medium-term use [12]. The advantage of polyurethane catheters is decreased catheter breakage but has a greater risk of thrombosis and catheter-related infection [13–15]. Silicon rubber catheter is preferred for long term or life-long PN therapy because of the reduced risk of thrombosis and infection, and is appropriate for using ethanol locks (to prevent bloodstream infections), but has decreased mechanical stability [14, 16]. Antimicrobial impregnated central venous catheters are superior in reducing central venous catheter-related bloodstream infection (CRBSI) [17].

Sites for insertion of a catheter for CPN

Short-term central access: Central venous access through a percutaneous non-tunneled catheter is commonly used and preferred for patients in the acute care setting for short duration therapies (<14 days) [12, 18]. In this method, the catheter is placed via the Seldinger technique into the internal jugular, subclavian, or femoral veins. For CPN, an upper body insertion site is preferred, and femoral vein catheterization is discouraged because of the higher risk of infection and thrombotic complications [19, 20].

This approach has the advantage of easy insertion, lesser cost, and better patient comfort and mobility for the short-term need. However, when the patient needs central venous access for the long-term PN, avoid this modality due to a higher risk of infection.

Percutaneous inserted central catheter (PICC): A 50–60 cm long polyurethane catheter is inserted in a peripheral vein in the antecubital area of the arm (cephalic or basilic vein) and threaded into the subclavian vein in such a way that the catheter tip is placed in the lower portion of superior vena cava or right atrium.

The use of PICCs is preferred in adult patients for short-term and medium-term PN (usually more than 2 weeks or less than six months) [21–24].

The use of PICCs has grown substantially in recent years because they are convenient, carry a low risk of placement-related complications, and are long-lasting and cost-effective.

The use of PICCs has grown substantially in recent years because it is convenient, low risk of placement-related complications, long-lasting and cost-effective [18, 25]. However, PICCs are associated with a higher risk of catheter-related venous thrombosis [18, 24, 26–28]. The PICCs are also associated with a higher risk of catheter-related bloodstream infection [18, 22,

29, 30], but the supporting evidence is insufficient [24, 25, 31–33].

While using PICC, to reduce the risk of infection, use the sutureless device and secure the catheter (to prevent migration of catheter) by subcutaneously anchored stabilization device [24, 34].

Long-term central access: "Tunneled" catheters (such as Hickman, Broviac, Hohn, or Groshong) and implanted subcutaneous ports are more stable, acceptable, and safe for patients who need PN for medium or long-term use (e.g., >3 months-years) [12]. The tunneled device is preferred in patients who require daily or routine access for long term PN [23, 35]. Implanted ports are cosmetically more desirable, have lower rates of infection [36], and are preferred when the need for access is less frequent (e.g., medication like chemotherapy) but rarely used for PN due to the requirement of venous access regularly [35].

"Tunneled" catheters are usually placed in the subclavian or internal jugular vein, with the distal tip positioned in the lower portion of the superior vena cava. After exiting from great veins, the "Tunneled" catheter traverses for about 10 cm under the skin in the subcutaneous tunnel, with the external portion of the catheter lying on the anterior chest wall.

The femoral vein is not preferred and usually avoided for long-term central access for PN due to the high risk of infection at the exit site (at the groin) and an increased risk of venous thrombosis [12]. A subcutaneous tunnel is created, so the catheter exits from the skin several inches away from the venipuncture location.

The tunnel acts as a barrier and reduces the risk of infection substantially. The dacron cuff around the catheter is positioned in the subcutaneous tissue 2 to 3 centimeters from the exit site, stabilizing the catheter and acting as a mechanical barrier limiting bacterial entry and preventing ascending microbial infection [16].

Methods used to confirm the catheter tip position are chest radiography, fluoroscopy, point-of-care transthoracic echocardiography, or continuous electrocardiography [19, 37, 38]. In addition to accurately assessing the position of the tip of the catheter, a post-procedure chest X-ray also detects pneumothorax, malpositions, and kinking [39].

The central line must be handled with a strict aseptic technique for safe use, and the single-lumen catheter is preferred to prevent infection. Use a central line exclusively for administering PN and avoid its usage for administering of IV solutions or medications, blood sampling, and central venous pressure (CVP) monitoring.

2. Systems of delivering parenteral nutrition

Three different systems used for delivering parenteral nutrition are a "multiple bottle" system, commercially available multichamber bags parenteral nutrition (MCB-PN), and hospital compounded parenteral nutrition.

a. Multiple bottle system

In the past, separate bottles were used to infuse individual substrates (carbohydrates, lipids, and amino acids) for PN [40, 41]. The advantages of multiple bottle systems are lower cost, flexibility, and ease of making adjustments in PN composition, particularly in critically ill patients with rapidly changing requirements [42].

Disadvantages of multiple bottle system are [40, 42]:

- Frequent manipulations during administering PN through multiple bottle systems carry a greater risk of nosocomial infections.

- Adjustment of different flow rates for different nutrients, adding different minerals and vitamins, and monitoring hyperglycemia, hypertriglyceridemia, and electrolyte disorders in each patient are cumbersome and are not without frequent mistakes.

- Simultaneous administration of various nutrients without maintaining proper proportion carries the risk of physicochemical incompatibilities.

- When costs of disposables and time spent by the nurse for administration of PN are considered, a multiple bottle system is costlier than commercially available multichambered PN formulations [43].

b. Multichamber-bag PN (MCBPN)

These products are standardized, easy-to-use nutrient mixtures, commercially available as two or three-chamber bags. Two-chamber bag systems ("2CB" or 2 in 1 formulation) contain dextrose and amino acids with or without electrolytes. Three-chamber bag systems (all-in-one admixture (AIO), "Three in One" system, 3 in 1 formulation) contain dextrose, amino acids, and lipid injectable emulsion (ILE), with/without electrolytes.

The advantages of three multichamber-bag PN products are:

- Convenience: The easy, convenient, and most preferred way for the single-line administration of PN. As all nutrients are available in a single container (referred to as premixed, "ready-to-use" commercial bags),

it saves time and reduces the workload [44, 45].

- Less infection: Decrease bloodstream infection rates due to less handling during preparation and delivery (reduced connections and reduced need of changing bags) [46–49].

- Safer: Lesser chances of various calculations and compounding human errors and better stability and sterility as manufactured with high standards [44, 45, 50].

- Recommended standard practice: SCCM-ASPEN guidelines (2016) and other literature recommend using standardized commercially available PN formulations compared to compounded PN admixtures when the formulation meets the patient's metabolic needs [1, 51, 52].

- Lower cost: Cost-saving during preparation, handling, and delivery (requiring fewer bags and tubings and no extra pump for lipid emulsion) [40, 49, 53–55].

- Due to slow continuous infusion, better assimilation, and utilization of nutrients with lesser chances of metabolic complications.

- Storage is more convenient with long shelf life [44].

Disadvantages of Multichamber-bag PN are:

- Lack of flexibility: Changes in composition/proportion of contents are not possible.

- Inappropriate overuse due to easy commercial availability of different formulations with a wide choice.

- Absence of transparent color: Due to the presence of lipids, three in one solution is opaque, which impairs visual inspection of the solution for particulate matter, precipitation, or fungal growth.

C. Hospital compounded PN admixture

This PN formulation containing various nutrients is designed to meet the nutritional needs of specific clinical conditions. Aseptic tailormade compounding of PN admixture in a hospital needs a sophisticated manufacturing system and skilled pharmacists, so its availability is problematic. The use of personalized hospital compounded PN is decreasing because of multiple limitations [56–59] and a greater risk of sepsis [60].

3. Duration and mode of delivering parenteral nutrition

Two methods used for administering PN include continuous infusion of PN and cyclic infusion of PN.

a. Continuous parenteral nutrition

Parenteral nutrition infuses over 24 hours continuously at a constant rate by a pump. Continuous PN is the most common regimen used for acute, critical, and hospitalized patients. Slow continuous infusion of PN by infusion pumps avoids volume overload and side effects secondary to rapid administration of carbohydrates and lipids (such as hyperglycemic and triglyceridemia), allows better utilization of nutrients, and provides nutritional requirements throughout the day. Drawbacks of this modality are poor mobility due to attachment to the pump and increased risk of fatty liver due to continuous high insulin levels.

b. Cyclic/intermittent parenteral nutrition

Cyclic/intermittent PN is the method in which PN is infused at a higher rate over 10 to 14 hours (typically at night when the patient is sleeping) and then stopped [61]. Cyclic PN improves the quality of life, decreases the incidence of hepatobiliary complications, and may limit or reverse PN-associated liver dysfunction [62–64]. In addition, this regimen allows for a 10 to 14 hour break each day from the pump, enabling the person to engage in normal daily activities. Cyclic PN should be attempted cautiously in the presence of glucose intolerance, edema, or fluid tolerance and is not suitable for critically ill patients [52]. However, cyclic PN is effective and safe for stable, chronically ill patients who require long-term nutrient support (e.g., home parenteral nutrition) [65].

DESIGNING PARENTERAL NUTRITION FORMULA

PN is a high-alert medication, and planning appropriate and safe prescriptions for the individual is complex. The parenteral nutrition formula can be designed by following steps:

Step 1: Calculate the daily nutritional requirements and convert them into a prescription.

Table 57.2 Factors determining PN requirements
• Weight of the patient
• Clinical status: stable or critical
• Medical or surgical conditions for which PN is indicated
• Nutritional status/malnutrition, volume status, urine volume
• Coexisting disorders (diabetes, hypertension, congestive heart failure, renal disorders, liver diseases, pulmonary diseases, sepsis, etc.)
• Electrolyte and acid base status

Step 2: Choosing the appropriate commercially available formula for the infusion.

Step 1: Calculate the daily nutritional requirements and convert them into a prescription

The first step in preparing a PN prescription is to calculate the daily nutritional requirements. It is essential to conduct a comprehensive evaluation of the patient and take into account all the factors that influence these requirements (refer to Table 57.2) to determine these requirements.

Sample calculation of the daily requirements of energy, protein dextrose, and lipids with consideration of fluid for a 60 kg patient, who is stable, euvolemic with good urine output and moderate stress is summarized below:

1. Fluid requirement: Approximately 35 mL/kg.

   So, 35 (mL/kg) × 60 (kg) = 2100 ml/day.

2. Caloric requirements: Approximately 25 kcal/kg.

   So, 25 (kcal/kg) × 60 (kg) = 1500 kcal/day.

3. Protein requirements: For stable patients, 1 gm/kg body weight.

   So, 1 (gm/kg) × 60 (kg) = 60 gm/day.

   1 gm of protein provides 4 kcal, so 60 gm of protein will provide 60 × 4 = 240 kcal.

4. Lipids requirements: 30% of total calories.

   So, 30% of 1500 (kcal/day) = 450 kcal.

   1 gm of fat provides 9 kcal, so to provide 450 kcal, 450/9 = 50 gm of fat will be required.

5. Carbohydrate requirement:

   Total caloric requirements minus the sum of protein and fat calories.

   So, 1500 – (240 + 450 kcal) = 1500 – 690 = 810 kcal.

   1 gm of dextrose in solution provides 3.4 kcal. So to provide 810 kcal, 810/3.4 = 238 gm of dextrose will be required.

So, the total daily requirement of the patient is 2100 ml fluid volume, a total calorie requirement of 1500 kcal, 60 gm of amino acids, 50 gm of fat, and 238 gm of dextrose. In addition, electrolytes, trace elements, and vitamins should be added as per requirement.

Step 2: Choosing the appropriate commercially available formula for the infusion

According to the prescription, the PN solution is prepared either in a hospital pharmacy or a commercially available formula that best matches the prescribed nutrients is chosen for administration. Micronutrients are coadministered in the proper dose.

PN solution is prepared in hospital pharmacies only for a limited number of patients due to lack of facilities, higher risk of sepsis, and no advantage in clinical outcomes [1]. Due to these limitations, standardized commercially available PN products are widely used and preferred over tailormade hospital compounded PN solutions.

One or more commercially available readymade PN solutions that closely match the prescription are selected.

The volume of fluid permitted to the patient and the concentration of nutrients in the PN solution are inversely proportionate. Select a PN solution with a greater concentration of various nutrients if the patient needs fluid restriction (e.g., central PN). When the patient needs PN, and a larger fluid volume is permitted, a PN solution with a low concentration of nutrients (e.g., in peripheral PN) is selected.

Various commercially available PN products and their classification based on their composition and routes of administration (peripheral vs. central venous access) are summarized in Table 57.3 and Table 57.4. In addition, the classification of various lipid emulsion products based on their lipid source is summarized in Table 57.5. A summary of commercially available PN products in these tables can assist clinicians in selecting PN solutions quickly and accurately.

INITIATION OF PN

- It is essential to evaluate the patient's nutritional status by careful history, physical examination, and

Table 57.3 Commercially available products for peripheral PN and their composition							
Solution	Manufacturer	Volume (ml)	Calorie (kcal)	Osmolarity mOsm/L	Dextrose (gm)	Amino acids (gm)	Lipids (gm)
Amino acid containing solutions							
Aminosyn-PF 7%	Hospira	500	140	561	-	35	-
Aminoven 5%	Fresenius Kabi	500	100	490	-	25	0
Aminoven infant 10%	Fresenius Kabi	100	4	885	-	10	0
Amino acid and dextrose containing double chamber bag							
Aminomix peripheral	Fresenius Kabi	1000	390	770	63	35	-
Aminosyn II 4.25%/10%	Pfizer/Hospira	1000	483	894	100	42.5	-
Clinimix 4.25/10	Baxter	1000	510	930	100	42.5	-
Nutriflex peri	B Braun	1000	480	900	80	40	-
Lipid emulsions							
Intralipid 10%	Fresenius Kabi	500	550	260	-	-	50
Intralipid 20%	Fresenius Kabi	500	1000	260	-	-	100
Lipofundin MCT/ LCT 20%	B Braun	500	954	380	-	-	100
Clinolipid 20%	Baxter	500	1000	270	-	-	100
Lipoplus	B. Braun	500	955	410	-	-	100
SMOFlipid 20%	Fresenius Kabi	500	1000	270	-	-	100
Amino acid, dextrose and lipid containing triple chamber bag							
Kabiven peri	Fresenius Kabi	1440	1000	750	97	34	51
Nutriflex lipid peri	B Braun	1000	765	840	64	32	40
PeriOlimel N4	Baxter	1000	700	760	75	25.3	30
Smofkabivan peri	Fresenius Kabi	1448	1000	850	103	46	41

Table 57.4 Commercially available products for Central PN and their composition

Solution	Manufacturer	Volume (ml)	Calorie (kcal)	Osmolarity mOsm/L	Dextrose (gm)	Amino acids (gm)	Lipids (gm)
Amino acid containing solutions							
Aminoven 10%	Fresenius Kabi	1000	400	999	-	100	-
Aminosyn 10%	Hospira	1000	400	938	-	100	-
FreAmine 10%	B Braun	1000	388	950	-	97	-
Travasol 10%	Baxter	1000	400	999	-	100	-
Amino acid and dextrose containing double chamber bag							
Aminomix Novum	Fresenius Kabi	1000	1000	1779	200	50	-
Aminosyn II 4.25%/20%	Pfizer	1000	850	1295	200	42.5	-
Clinimix 8/10	Baxter	1000	663	1308	100	80	-
Nutriflex plus	B Braun	1000	792	1400	150	48	-
Amino acid, dextrose and lipid containing triple chamber bag							
Kabiven	Fresenius Kabi	1026	872	1060	100	34	40
Nutriflex lipid plus	B Braun	1250	1265	1540	150	48	50
Olimel N9/ Triomel N9	Baxter	1000	1070	1170	110	56.9	40
Smofkabivan	Fresenius Kabi	986	1100	1500	125	50	38

Table 57.5 Commercially available lipid emulsion products and their composition

Lipid source	Product	Manufacturer	Soybean oil	MCT oil	Olive oil	Fish oil	ω-6: ω-3 Ratio
Soybean oil-based	Intralipid Ivelip Lipofundin N Liposyn III	Fresenius Kabi Baxter B Braun Hospira	100%	-	-	-	7:1
SO/MCT-based	Lipofundin MCT/LCT	B Braun	50%	50%	-	-	7:1
	Structolipid	Fresenius Kabi	64%	36%	-	-	7:1
Olive oil-based	ClinOleic Clinolipid	Baxter Baxter	20%	-	80%	-	9:1
Fish oil containing emulsions	Lipoplus (Lipidem)	B. Braun	40%	50%	-	10%	3:1
	SMOFlipid	Fresenius Kabi	30%	30%	25%	15%	2.5:1
	Omegaven	Fresenius Kabi	-	-	-	100%	1:8

laboratory studies before initiation of PN.

- PN may be initiated in hemodynamically stable patients who can tolerate the fluid volume. Correct electrolyte abnormalities and hyperglycemia before the initiation of PN.

- PN should be initiated slowly (no more than 50% of the calculated requirements on the first day) to avoid adverse effects like hyperglycemia and electrolyte disturbances [66]. PN is increased gradually over 4 to 7 days to achieve the nutrition goal.

- PN may precipitate refeeding syndrome in severely malnourished patients due to rapid fall in potassium, magnesium, and phosphorus levels. So slow initiation and close monitoring of the patient's electrolytes is necessary to avoid adverse effects on cardiac and respiratory function.

Care of PN mixture

- Store reconstituted PN bags in a refrigerator until 30 min before using.

- Always examine the PN solution before administration to exclude particulate matter, cloudiness, or an oily layer in the bag.

- Follow strict aseptic techniques while connecting and administering PN.

- To administer dextrose/amino acids PN formulations, use an infusion set with an in-built air vent and a 0.22-micron filter [52]. For administering lipids containing PN formulations, use a 1.2 micron - larger sized filter to avoid clogging of the filter.

- Do not use a three-way stopcock as it increases the risk of infection.

- Do not insert a needle for air venting in a PN bag.

- Do not add any medication to the PN bag.

- Do not allow the PN solution to hang for more than 24 hours.

- Do not use the PN line to draw blood for the test, administer medications, or measure central venous pressure.

MONITORING OF PN

Every patient receiving PN should be monitored carefully for the prevention or early detection of complications and to judge the effectiveness of therapy. Meticulous monitoring is aimed at monitoring, detecting, or assess:

- Metabolic status, including hyperglycemia and hypoglycemia.

- Risk of refeeding syndrome or clues of overfeeding.

- Micronutrient deficiency and toxicity.

- Fluid and electrolytes status.

- Catheter-related complications, including sepsis.

- Hepatic and other long-term complications.

A clinical data and laboratory study used routinely for monitoring patients receiving PN is summarized in Table 57.6:

- Always obtain a chest X-ray to check catheter placement after insertion.

- Record vital signs at least every 4 hours. Temperature elevation is one of the earliest signs of catheter-related sepsis.

- Patients should be weighed daily at the same time each morning after voiding on the same scale. Weight gain may indicate fluid overload.

- Perform site care and dressing change at least three times weekly or whenever the dressing becomes wet.

Table 57.6 Monitoring the patient on parenteral nutrition

Clinical data monitoring

History: Focused on patient's sense of well-being, strength to perform routine activities, fever, and medical history for signs of fluid overload or glucose and electrolyte imbalance.

Vital signs: Monitor temperature, pulse, blood pressure, and respiratory rate.

Fluid balance: Strict input/output chart, daily weight, and signs of fluid overload or dehydration.

Local care: Inspecting and dressing vascular access site (to rule out infection).

Delivery system: Inspection of solution for contamination and watch for the proper functioning of infusion pump, catheter function, and timely changing of tubing and bags.

Monitoring of laboratory data during PN

Parameter	Baseline and initial period	Stable period	Long term
Blood glucose	6 hourly	1–2 times/ week	Monthly
BUN, creatinine, electrolytes, HCO_3, PO_4, Ca^{2+}, Mg^{2+}	Daily	Weekly	Monthly
CBC, liver function test (LFT), triglycerides, PT	Weekly	Weekly	Monthly
Micronutrient tests, as indicated			

- Patients receiving PN should be monitored carefully to detect early signs of complications such as fluid overload, electrolyte imbalances, nutritional problems, or allergic reactions.

- Monitor serum glucose levels every 6 hours initially, then once a day. Watch for the symptoms of hyperglycemia, such as thirst and polyuria. Maintain blood glucose <180 mg/dL [1, 67].

- Monitor renal function, electrolyte levels, liver function, phosphate, calcium, and magnesium daily in the first week of initiating PN. Once the patient is stable, these tests are performed once or twice a week and less frequently in the long term.

- Monitoring response to nutritional therapy. There is no single criterion that can reliably indicate the effectiveness of PN. Improvement in clinical status and visceral protein concentrations (e.g., albumin, prealbumin, and transferrin) are most commonly used to monitor nutritional status. When interpreting visceral protein values, it is essential always to consider the patient's fluid status, organ function, and presence of infection. If nutritional recovery is inappropriate, a nitrogen balance study may guide changes in amino acid intake. Similarly, if traditional methods of calculating calorie requirements are unsatisfactory, indirect calorimetry is indicated.

- If the patient receiving PN develops fever, chills, or hypotension, its most common cause is a catheter-related bloodstream infection. Therefore, for diagnosis of CRBSI, blood cultures should be drawn immediately before initiating antibiotic therapy.

TERMINATION OF PN

- PN is the temporary method of nutritional supplementation. The ultimate goal is slow and smooth transit from PN to oral/enteral food intake once the gastrointestinal function returns.

- During the transition period, discontinue PN when the patient can tolerate 60–70% of the total nutritional requirements orally or enterally.
- If the patient cannot tolerate oral or enteral supplementation and intake is less than 60% of nutritional requirements, restart PN in 2–3 days.
- Plan a gradual transition from PN to oral or enteral nutrition to avoid overfeeding during the phase of reduction of PN and worsening of nutritional status when PN is discontinued.
- If there is a need for abrupt discontinuation of PN, administer 10% dextrose for a few hours to prevent hypoglycemia.
- After discontinuing PN, monitor blood glucose closely for several hours to detect hypoglycemia.

- During the transition period, closely and carefully monitor clinical status, hydration status, weight, and laboratory tests.

COMPLICATIONS OF PARENTERAL NUTRITION

The primary complications of parenteral nutrition include mechanical, metabolic, and infectious complications. However, most complications are reduced with careful management and supervision by an experienced nutritional support team. Commonly encountered complications are summarized in Table 57.7.

MECHANICAL COMPLICATIONS

Potential mechanical complications related to central venous catheter placement are malposition of the catheter, pneumothorax, hemothorax,

Table 57.7 Complications of PN			
	Mechanical	**Metabolic/GI**	**Infectious**
First 48 hours	Malposition, Haemothorax Pneumothorax Chylothorax Air embolism, Cardiac arrhythmia Injury to the subclavian/carotid artery	Fluid overload Hyperglycemia Hypophosphatemia Hypokalemia Hypomagnesemia Refeeding syndrome	-
First two weeks	Catheter displacement Catheter thrombosis Catheter occlusion Air embolism	Hyperglycemic coma Acid base imbalance Electrolyte imbalance	Catheter induced sepsis Exit site infection
Three months induced onwards infection	Fracture or tear of the catheter Catheter thrombosis Air embolism Blood loss	Essential fatty Acid deficiency Vitamin or trace element Deficiency PN metabolic Bone diseases PN liver diseases	Tunnel infection Catheter Sepsis Exit site

arterial injury, thoracic duct injury, nerve injury, air embolism, cardiac arrhythmia, and cardiac perforation with tamponade. Ultrasound-guided central venous catheter insertion by trained and experienced personnel can reduce mechanical complications significantly [68].

Post subclavian and jugular CVC insertion, chest X-ray in the upright or semi-upright position is helpful to exclude malposition of the catheter, pneumothorax, or hemothorax and confirm the correct tip position (in the inferior third of superior vena cava or at the junction of the superior vena cava and the right atrium, parallel to the vessel wall). Avoid excessive advancement of a catheter because the tip of the CVC in the cardiac chamber carries the risk of cardiac arrhythmia. It is also important to avoid the inadequate length of insertion because the infusion of high osmolarity PN solutions with a catheter tip at a higher level can cause direct damage to the vein (thrombophlebitis) [69].

The osmolarity of PN solutions is three to eight times the normal serum osmolality. PN with high osmolarity in the long term can cause injury to endothelium and vein wall inflammation with resultant upper extremity deep venous thrombosis.

Most patients are asymptomatic, but swelling of the neck or arm with erythema, tenderness, and warmth is the common presentation in a few patients [70].

Catheter-related thrombosis is treated primarily with anticoagulation, and thrombolytic therapy is offered in selected patients having a high risk of thrombosis [71]. Removal of the catheter is recommended in catheter-related thrombosis if the catheter is non-functional or not needed, anticoagulation is contraindicated, inadequate improvement in symptoms with anticoagulation, or the thrombosis is limb or life-threatening [70, 71].

CATHETER-RELATED BLOODSTREAM INFECTION

In patients receiving CPN, catheter-related bloodstream infection (CRBSI) is the most common and serious complication that increases hospital stay and cost and is associated with significantly high morbidity and mortality.

In most cases, it is preventable with proper aseptic techniques and is often related to non-adherence to aseptic techniques, suboptimal catheter care, and inadequate patient education.

The upper body insertion site (internal jugular or subclavian vein) is preferred over the femoral site to reduce the risk of infection [19].

CRBSI is usually caused by the migration of skin organisms at the catheter exit site for short-term catheters and direct contamination of the catheter or catheter hub in long-term CVC [72].

The risk of line infection can be minimized by:

- Strict asepsis when handling (connecting/disconnecting) the line.
- Single-lumen central venous catheters should be dedicated solely to the infusion of parenteral nutrition.
- Use of a dedicated lumen on a multiple lumen CVC or a PICC line for administration of PN.
- Use of antibiotic-coated or antibiotic-impregnated catheters.

Fever in a patient with no other identifiable infection source raises suspicion of catheter-related infection. Staphylococcus and candida are the most frequent pathogens. Whenever catheter-related sepsis is suspected, the following steps should be considered:

1. Evaluate the catheter insertion site and culture any drainage.

2. Obtain blood cultures: For diagnosis of CRBSI, blood cultures should be drawn from each lumen of the catheter and two sets of blood cultures from peripheral veins via separate venipuncture sites before initiating antibiotic therapy [73]. Catheter tip cultures cannot be used as a substitute for blood cultures to confirm catheter-related bloodstream infection [74, 75].

3. Begin empiric antibiotic therapy:

   In uncomplicated patients, it is unnecessary to remove the CVC. Instead, treat CRBSI immediately by administering broad-spectrum antibiotics through the lumen to salvage the catheter.

   It is unnecessary to remove the CVC in uncomplicated patients and treat CRBSI immediately by administering broad-spectrum antibiotics through lumen for catheter salvage.

4. Remove catheter: Indications of catheter removal are [76]:

   • Tunnel and pocket infections.

   • Clinical deterioration, septic shock, or presence of severe complications such as endocarditis, septic thrombosis, or abscess formations.

   • Repeated positive blood culture besides antibiotic therapy.

   • Although guidewire exchange has a lower risk of technical complications, it is not recommended as an alternative approach to removal.

METABOLIC COMPLICATIONS

The most common problems caused by PN are hyperglycemia, fluid overload, electrolyte imbalances, refeeding syndrome, and hepatobiliary complications. Therefore, proper monitoring and adjustments in the composition and rate of PN are essential to reduce the metabolic complications caused by PN.

A. Hyperglycemia

Hyperglycemia occurs in more than half of patients receiving PN [77, 78] and is associated with increased hospital complications and mortality [77, 79].

The risk factors for hyperglycemia are excess and rapid administration of dextrose, obesity (BMI>25 kg/m2), preexisting diabetes mellitus or liver impairment, hyperglycemia before starting PN, surgical indications of PN, corticosteroid use, presence of infection, and critical illness [78, 80, 81]. Hyperglycemia in a previously normoglycemic patient should also raise suspicion of infection.

Hyperglycemia is the greatest danger from PN during the first 24 hours. It may lead to osmotic diuresis and glycosuria, leading to excessive excretion of free water by the kidney, thus causing hyperosmolar nonketotic dehydration, coma, and even death. Therefore, it is best treated by prevention.

As blood glucose values above 180 mg/dL are associated with a higher incidence of complications [77], the current recommendation is to keep glucose concentration 140–180 mg/dL [82–85].

Various insulin regimens used to control hyperglycemia in patients receiving PN are [86]:

1. **Continuous intravenous insulin infusion:** Ideal for unstable and critically ill patients receiving PN requiring maximal flexibility in dose modifications.

2. **Insulin added to PN:** Directly adding insulin to the parenteral nutrition bag is a convenient and physiologically favorable method to treat hyperglycemia, particularly in general wards where separate IV insulin administration may not be feasible. However, this method is inappropriate in unstable patients and increases the risk of infectious complications.

3. **Insulin added to PN and supplemental subcutaneous insulin using a sliding scale:** This regimen is widely used for non-critically ill T2DM patients and provides better glycemic control after PN interruption [87].

4. **Subcutaneous insulin injection:** This regimen is useful in stable patients on PN before discontinuation of IV insulin for transitioning from IV to subcutaneous insulin administration.

Measures to prevent hyperglycemia during PN administration

- Do not overfeed the patient (starting dose less than 20–25 kcal/kg/d).

- Restrict dextrose in PN to 100–150 gm/day initially and administer it slowly (2–3 mg/kg/minute).

- Increase the portion of lipid administration if needed (to supply calories and to limit the required dextrose).

- Consider other sources of IV dextrose such as peritoneal dialysis solution, antibiotic drips, etc.

- Monitor blood glucose closely (every 4–6 hours) and increase insulin doses accordingly.

B. Hypoglycemia

Although the incidence of hypoglycemia is low among hospitalized patients receiving PN, it needs careful attention because of its detrimental consequences [88, 89].

PN associated hypoglycemia may be a consequence of:

- Overtreatment of hyperglycemia with the use of insulin via PN, IV infusion, or subcutaneous injection. The risk of hypoglycemia is higher when insulin is administered by drip.

- "Rebound hypoglycemia" after abrupt discontinuation of PN formulations (e.g., cyclic infusion of parenteral nutrition) [65].

Patients prone to develop hypoglycemia are advanced age, poor nutritional status, previous history of diabetes, renal failure, liver disease, ICU patients, patients on long-term PN, insulin administered by drip, and inadequate monitoring [88].

Measures to prevent hypoglycemia are:

- Slow tapering: Before discontinuing of the PN, tapper down infusion at half the rate for 1–2 h to reduce the risk of rebound hypoglycemia.

- If PN infusion needs to be discontinued abruptly, administer dextrose-containing fluid for about 1 or 2 hours to avoid the risk of hypoglycemia.

- When insulin is added to the PN solution, the risk of hypoglycemia is low on abrupt discontinuation of PN.

- As aggressive treatment of hyperglycemia to achieve tight blood glucose control carries the risk of hypoglycemia, a target blood glucose in the range of 140–180 mg/dL is recommended to reduce the incidence of hypoglycemia [82].

- Close monitoring of blood glucose and meticulous adjustment of insulin dosage (avoid higher insulin to dextrose ratio in PN).

C. Refeeding syndrome

This is a potentially serious but often neglected condition that can occur due to shifts of fluid, electrolytes, metabolic, and vitamin disturbances during re-initiation of nutritional therapy in patients with malnutrition or prolonged fasting. It can cause significant morbidity and even mortality.

Common high-risk factors for refeeding syndrome are [90, 91]:

- Severe malnutrition, BMI less than 18.5 kg/m2, recent weight loss (>10% within the last 3–6 months), poor or no nutritional intake for more than 5 days.

- Alcoholism abuse, anorexia nervosa, depression, bariatric surgery, bowel resections, malabsorption, insulin, chemotherapy, antacids, or diuretics.

- Low baseline levels of phosphate, potassium, or magnesium.

Pathophysiology: Refeeding syndrome is related to the shift from the catabolic to the anabolic metabolic pathways, which occurs with the reintroduction of glucose (refeeding) after a prolonged phase of starvation [92].

During the starvation (catabolic) period, the body adapts to less carbohydrates; fat becomes the primary source of energy requirements, and levels of blood glucose and insulin decline.

Prolonged fasting leads to severe depletion of intracellular phosphate, potassium, and magnesium and deficiencies of various vitamins, including thiamine.

The initiation of carbohydrate-containing nutrition leads to a rise in blood glucose levels, which in turn causes a rapid increase in insulin secretion.

Endogenous insulin surge causes massive shifts of phosphorus, potassium, and magnesium intracellularly, leading to severe hypophosphatemia, hypokalemia, hypomagnesemia, and potentially lethal complications. Hypophosphatemia is the hallmark of the syndrome.

Thiamine requirements increase significantly during the nutritional replenishment, so in the state of thiamine deficiency, re-initiation of feeding can cause metabolic acidosis and neurologic abnormalities (i.e., confusion, Wernicke's encephalopathy or dry beriberi) or cardiovascular complications (i.e., peripheral edema, congestive heart failure, or wet beriberi). In addition, thiamine is an essential coenzyme in carbohydrate metabolism. Therefore, glucose is converted to lactate instead of adenosine triphosphate (ATP) via the Krebs cycle, causing lactic metabolic acidosis when thiamine is lacking.

Clinical features: Symptoms generally appear within the first 2–5 days of initiating nutritional therapy, and it's highly variable, ranging from mild to severe and life-threatening, depending on the severity of malnutrition and comorbidities [92]. The clinical symptoms of the refeeding syndrome are nonspecific and chiefly due to underlying hypophosphatemia, hypokalemia, hypomagnesemia, sodium retention, and thiamine deficiency:

- Cardiovascular: Fluid overload, congestive heart failure, arrhythmias, bradycardia/tachycardia, and hypotension.

- Respiratory: Respiratory failure, pulmonary edema, hypoventilation, and failure to wean from the ventilator.

- Neurological: Paraesthesia, ataxia, delirium, Wernicke's encephalopathy.
- Musculoskeletal: Weakness, fatigue, myalgias, and rhabdomyolysis.
- Miscellaneous: Abdominal pain, constipation, vomiting, anemia, metabolic acidosis.

Measures for the prevention and treatment [91–95]

- Search and recognize high-risk patients for refeeding syndrome.
- Order baseline laboratory tests to assess potassium, magnesium, and phosphorus status before initiating nutrition support.
- Prophylactic administration of adequate electrolytes (even if blood levels are in the low-normal range), vitamin (thiamine, water, and fat-soluble), and micronutrient (Zn, Fe, Se) in "standard" maintenance doses, concurrently with the nutrition support. An approximate daily dose of electrolytes supplementation suggested is 1–1.5 mEq/kg potassium, 0.2–0.4 mEq/kg magnesium, and 0.3–0.6 mmol/kg phosphate. If values of electrolytes are severely low, it is recommended to delay the initiation of nutrition support until the electrolyte imbalances are corrected.
- The recommended dose of thiamine is 100 mg per day, to be administered before initiating dextrose-containing IV fluids and to be given for a period of 5–7 days or longer.
- Start refeeding gradually and cautiously in a stepwise manner to avoid excessive nutritional replenishment and limit the resultant risk of refeeding syndrome. First, start caloric supplementation in low dose (no more than 50% of energy requirements [NICE guidelines] or 100–150 gm of dextrose or 10–20 kcal/kg for the first 24 hours [ASPEN guidelines 2020]) and increase the dose slowly (advance by 33% of a goal every 1 to 2 days).

- Careful administration of sodium and fluids to avoid fluid overload.
- Close clinical and laboratory indices monitoring. Measure vital signs every 4 hours on the first day and maintain daily weight and intake output chart. Monitor serum potassium, magnesium, and phosphorus every 12 hours for the first three days.
- If overt symptoms and abnormal electrolyte values, curtail nutritional supplementation. In patients with refeeding hypophosphatemia, reduce energy intake temporarily or restrict it for 48 hours and gradually increase subsequently. Reduce fluid intake if edema or congestive heart failure and replace electrolytes aggressively according to the serum electrolyte levels.

D. Hepatic abnormalities

In patients receiving parenteral nutrition, liver diseases are common, and their prevalence ranges from 4.3% to 65% [96, 97]. Three major and most frequently encountered hepatobiliary complications are steatosis (accumulation of fat in the liver due to overfeeding), cholestasis (impaired or blocked secretion of bile), and gallbladder sludge/stones (due to gallbladder inactivity and stasis) [98, 99]. The broad spectrum of hepatic manifestations of PN-associated liver disease ranges from a benign and temporary rise in liver function tests to steatosis to fibrosis and, eventually, progress to portal hypertension and end-stage liver failure in a few [100].

Elevated serum conjugated bilirubin >2 mg/dL is the primary marker of PN-associated liver disease, which generally occurs early in therapy (within 2 weeks of initiation of PN). Therefore, when a patient receiving PN develops hepatic complications, it is essential to exclude other causes of liver disease.

Three terms used to describe the spectrum of liver disorders in patients receiving PN are PNAC (Parenteral nutrition-associated cholestasis), PNALD (Parenteral nutrition-associated liver disease), and IFALD (Intestinal failure-associated liver disease) [101]. Parenteral nutrition-associated liver disease is the general term used to describe the different hepatic and serum abnormalities associated with liver injury in adult and pediatric patients receiving long-term PN [102]. As long-term administration of PN can cause cholestasis, the term Parenteral nutrition-associated cholestasis (PNAC) is frequently used in the pediatric literature [103].

The term "Intestinal failure-associated liver disease" (IFALD) is now preferred to "PNALD" or "PNAC" for describing liver disease associated with PN in both pediatric and adult patients, as it more accurately reflects the multifactorial nature of the problem and its relation to intestinal failure [104, 105]. However, both terms, PNALD and IFALD, are used interchangeably in clinical practice to describe hepatic dysfunction secondary to intestinal failure in patients who are on PN.

Major risk factors for the development of PNALD are [98, 99]:

- Excessive energy intake or overfeeding.
- Glucose overload or excessive carbohydrate administration.

- Excess administration of lipid >1 gm/kg/d.
- Administration of soybean oil-based lipid emulsion.
- Continuous infusion of PN.
- Lack of enteral stimulation.
- Carnitine and choline deficiency.

Interventions recommended to prevent or treat hepatic complications are:

- Avoiding excessive calorie administration: Avoid administration of >25 to 30 kcal/kg calories to reduce the risk of steatosis or fat deposition in the liver.
- Avoiding excessive carbohydrate administration: Avoid administration of >5 mg/kg/min/d carbohydrate to prevent PNALD/IFALD [96].
- Appropriate carbohydrates to lipids ratio: PN solution should contain about 70–85% carbohydrates and 15–30% lipids to provide nonprotein energy [106].
- Restrict the dose of soybean-based lipid emulsions (<1 gm/kg body weight/d) to treat children with PNALD [21, 107].
- Change the composition of lipid emulsions: Supplementation (partial or complete) of omega-3-fatty acids enriched fish oil to soybean-based lipid emulsions (with the reduced n6/n3 ratio) is recommended to prevent and treat PNALD [103, 108–110].
- Prefer cyclic PN instead of continuous PN: Cyclic PN (9 for 12 to 16 hours) allows time for the mobilization of fats during the non-administration period of PN [105]. Therefore, a switch to cyclic PN infusion helps stabilize or improve impaired liver function [64, 65, 111].
- Early oral or enteral nutrition: Even small amounts of oral or

enteral nutrition (EN) stimulates enterohepatic circulation of bile acids and reduce the risk for PNALD.

REFERENCES

1. McClave SA, Taylor BE, Martindale RG, et al. Guidelines for the provision and assessment of nutrition support therapy in the adult critically ill patient: Society of Critical Care Medicine (SCCM) and American Society for Parenteral and Enteral Nutrition (A.S.P.E.N.). JPEN J Parenter Enteral Nutr 2016;40(2):159–211.

2. Bolder U, Ebener C, Hauner H, et al. Carbohydrates - Guidelines on Parenteral Nutrition, Chapter 5. Ger Med Sci. 2009;7:Doc23.

3. Adolph M, Heller AR, Koch T, et al. Lipid emulsions - Guidelines on Parenteral Nutrition, Chapter 6. Ger Med Sci. 2009;7:Doc22.

4. Anderson ADG, Palmer D, MacFie J. Peripheral parenteral nutrition. Br J Surg. 2003;90(9):1048–1054.

5. Correia MI, Guimarães J, de Mattos LC, et al. Peripheral parenteral nutrition: an option for patients with an indication for short-term parenteral nutrition. Nutr Hosp. 2004;19(1):14–8.

6. Mirtallo J, Canada T, Johnson D, et al. Task force for the revision of safe practices for parenteral nutrition. Safe practices for parenteral nutrition. JPEN J Parenter Enteral Nutr. 2004;28(6):S39–70.

7. Kuwahara T, Asanami S, Tamura T, et al. Effects of pH and osmolality on phlebitic potential of infusion solutions for peripheral parenteral nutrition. J Toxicol Sci 1998;23(1):77–85.

8. Isaacs JW, Millikan WJ, Stackhouse J, et al. Parenteral nutrition of adults with a 900 milliosmolar solution via peripheral veins. Am J Clin Nutr. 1977;30(4):552–9.

9. Pertkiewicz M, Dudrick SJ. Basics in clinical nutrition: Parenteral nutrition, ways of delivering parenteral nutrition and peripheral parenteral nutrition (PPN). e-SPEN, the European e-Journal of Clinical Nutrition and Metabolism 4 (2009):e125–e127.

10. Alpan G, Eyal F, Springer C, et al. Heparinization of alimentation solutions administered through peripheral veins in premature infants: a randomized, controlled study. Pediatrics. 1984;74(3):375–378.

11. Roongpisuthipong C, Puchaiwatananon O, Songchitsomboon S, et al. Hydrocortisone, heparin, and peripheral intravenous infusion. Nutrition. 1994;10(3):211–3.

12. Pittiruti M, Hamilton H, Biffi R, et al. ESPEN Guidelines on Parenteral Nutrition: Central Venous Catheters (access, care, diagnosis and therapy of complications) Clin Nutr. 2009;28(4):365–77.

13. Cohen AB, Dagli M, Stavropoulos SW Jr, et al. Silicone and polyurethane tunneled infusion catheters: a comparison of durability and breakage rates. J Vasc Interv Radiol. 2011;22(5):638–41.

14. Wildgruber M, Lueg C, Borgmeyer S, et al. Polyurethane versus silicone catheters for central

15. venous port devices implanted at the forearm. Eur J Cancer. 2016;59:113–124.

15. Busch JD, Vens M, Mahler C, et al. Complication rates observed in silicone and polyurethane catheters of totally implanted central venous access devices implanted in the upper arm. J Vasc Interv Radiol. 2017;28(8):1177–1183.

16. Micic D, Semrad C, Chopra V. Choosing the Right central venous catheter for parenteral nutrition. Am J Gastroenterol. 2019;114(1):4–6.

17. Wang H, Tong H, Liu H, et al. Effectiveness of antimicrobial-coated central venous catheters for preventing catheter-related blood-stream infections with the implementation of bundles: a systematic review and network meta-analysis. Ann Intensive Care. 2018;8(1):71.

18. Chopra V, Flanders SA, Saint S, et al. Michigan Appropriateness Guide for Intravenous Catheters (MAGIC) Panel. The Michigan Appropriateness Guide for Intravenous Catheters (MAGIC): results from a multispecialty panel using the RAND/UCLA appropriateness method. Ann Intern Med. 2015.15;163(6 suppl):S1–S40.

19. Practice Guidelines for Central Venous Access 2020: An Updated Report by the American Society of Anesthesiologists Task Force on Central Venous Access. Anesthesiology. 2020;132(1):8–43.

20. Infusion Nurses Society. Infusion therapy standards of practice. J Infus Nurs. 2016;39(1 suppl):S11–S159.

21. Pironi L, Arends J, Bozzetti F, et al. ESPEN guidelines on chronic intestinal failure in adults. Clin Nutr. 2016;35(2):247–307.

22. Christensen LD, Holst M, Bech LF, et al. Comparison of complications associated with peripherally inserted central catheters and Hickman™ catheters in patients with intestinal failure receiving home parenteral nutrition. Six-year follow up study. Clin Nutr. 2016;35(4):912–917.

23. Kovacevich DS, Corrigan M, Ross VM, et al. American society for parenteral and enteral nutrition guidelines for the selection and care of central venous access devices for adult home parenteral nutrition administration. JPEN J Parenter Enteral Nutr. 2019;43(1):15–31.

24. Pironi L, Boeykens K, Bozzetti F, et al. ESPEN guideline on home parenteral nutrition. Clin Nutr. 2020;39(6):1645–1666.

25. Cotogni P, Mussa B, Degiorgis C, et al. Comparative complication rates of 854 central venous access devices for home parenteral nutrition in cancer patients: a prospective study of over 169,000 catheter-days. JPEN J Parenter Enteral Nutr. 2021;45(4):768–776.

26. Chopra V, Anand S, Hickner A, et al. Risk of venous thromboembolism associated with peripherally inserted central catheters: a systematic review and meta-analysis. Lancet. 2013;382(9889):311–325.

27. Johansson E, Hammarskjöld F, Lundberg D, et al. Advantages and disadvantages of peripherally inserted central venous catheters (PICC) compared to other central venous lines: a systematic review of the literature. Acta Oncol. 2013;52(5):886–92.

28. Taxbro K, Hammarskjöld F, Thelin B, et al. Clinical impact of peripherally inserted central catheters vs implanted port catheters in patients with cancer: an open-label, randomised, two-centre trial. Br J Anaesth 2019;122(6):734–741.

29. Advani S, Reich NG, Sengupta A, et al. Central line-associated bloodstream infection in hospitalized children with peripherally inserted central venous catheters: extending risk analyses outside the intensive care unit. Clin Infect Dis. 2011;52(9):1108–1115.

30. Chopra V, Ratz D, Kuhn L, et al. PICC-associated bloodstream infections: prevalence, patterns, and predictors. Am J Med. 2014;127(4):319–328.

31. Touré A, Duchamp A, Peraldi C, et al. comparative study of peripherally-inserted and Broviac catheter complications in home parenteral nutrition patients. Clin Nutr. 2015;34(1):49–52.

32. Hon K, Bihari S, Holt A, et al. Rate of catheter-related bloodstream infections between tunneled central venous catheters versus peripherally inserted central catheters in adult home parenteral nutrition: a meta-analysis. JPEN J Parenter Enteral Nutr. 2019;43(1):41–53.

33. Mateo-Lobo R, Riveiro J, Vega-Piñero B, et al. Infectious complications in home parenteral nutrition: a systematic review and meta-analysis comparing peripherally-inserted central catheters with other central catheters. Nutrients. 2019;11(9):2083.

34. Zerla PA, Canelli A, Cerne L, et al. Evaluating safety, efficacy, and cost-effectiveness of PICC securement by subcutaneously anchored stabilization device. J Vasc Access. 2017;18(3):238–242.

35. Cheung E, Baerlocher MO, Asch M, et al. Venous access: a practical review for 2009. Can Fam Physician. 2009;55(5):494–496.

36. Maki DG, Kluger DM, Crnich CJ. The risk of bloodstream infection in adults with different intravascular devices: a systematic review of 200 published prospective studies. Mayo Clin Proc. 2006;81(9):1159–1171.

37. Saugel B, Scheeren TWL, Teboul JL. Ultrasound-guided central venous catheter placement: a structured review and recommendations for clinical practice. Crit Care. 2017;21(1):225.

38. Hill S, Moureau NL. (2019) Tip Position. In: Moureau N. (eds) Vessel Health and Preservation: The Right Approach for Vascular Access. Springer, Cham.

39. Venugopal AN, Koshy RC, Koshy SM. Role of chest X-ray in citing central venous catheter tip: A few case reports with a brief review of the literature. J Anaesthesiol Clin Pharmacol. 2013;29(3):397–400.

40. Menne R, Adolph M, Brock E, et al. Cost analysis of parenteral nutrition regimens in the intensive care unit: three compartment bag system vs multibottle system. JPEN J Parenter Enteral Nutr. 2008;32(6):606–612.

41. Hellerman Itzhaki M, Singer P. Advances in medical nutrition therapy: parenteral nutrition. Nutrients. 2020;12(3):717.

42. Pertkiewicz M, Dudrick SJ. Basics in clinical nutrition: Systems for parenteral nutrition, different systems for parenteral nutrition (AIO vs. MB). e-SPEN, the European e-Journal of Clinical Nutrition and Metabolism. 2009;4:123–124.

43. Raper S, Milanov S, Park GR. The cost of multicompartment 'big bag' total parenteral nutrition in an ICU. Anaesthesia. 2002;57(1):96–7.

44. Pichard C, Schwarz G, Frei A, et al. Economic investigation of the use of three compartment total parenteral nutrition bag: prospective randomized unblinded controlled study. Clin Nutr. 2000;19(4):245–251.

45. Berlana D, Almendral MA, Abad MR, et al. Cost, time, error assessment during preparation of parenteral nutrition: multichamber bags versus hospital-compound bags. JPEN J Parenter Enteral Nutr. 2019;43(4):557–565.

46. Turpin RS, Canada T, Rosenthal V, et al. Bloodstream infections associated with parenteral nutrition preparation methods in the United States: a retrospective, large database analysis. JPEN J Parenter Enteral Nutr. 2012;36(2):169–176.

47. Pontes-Arruda A, Zaloga G, Wischmeyer P, et al. Is there a difference in bloodstream infections in critically ill patients associated with ready-to use versus compounded parenteral nutrition? Clin Nutr. 2012;31(5):728–734.

48. Turpin RS, Solem C, Pontes-Arruda A, et al. The impact of parenteral nutrition preparation on bloodstream infection risk and costs. Eur J Clin Nutr. 2014;68(8):953–958.

49. Alfonso JE, Berlana D, Ukleja A, et al. Clinical, ergonomic, and economic outcomes with multichamber bags compared with (hospital) pharmacy compounded bags and multibottle systems: a systematic literature review. JPEN J Parenter Enteral Nutr. 2017;41(7):1162–1177.

50. Gervasio J. Compounding vs standardized commercial parenteral nutrition product: pros and cons. JPEN J Parenter Enteral Nutr. 2012;36(2 Suppl):40S–41S.

51. Slattery E, Rumore MM, Douglas JS, et al. 3-in-1 vs 2-in-1 parenteral nutrition in adults: a review. Nutr Clin Pract. 2014;29(5):631–5.

52. Ayers P, Adams S, Boullata J, et al. A.S.P.E.N. parenteral nutrition safety consensus recommendations. JPEN J Parenter Enteral Nutr. 2014;38(3):296–333.

53. Turpin RS, Canada T, Liu FX, et al. Nutrition therapy cost analysis in the US: pre-mixed multi-chamber bag vs compounded parenteral nutrition. Appl Health Econ Health Policy. 2011;9(5):281–292.

54. Berlana D, Sabin P, Gimeno-Ballester V, et al. Cost analysis of adult parenteral nutrition systems: three-compartment bag versus customized. Nutr Hosp. 2013;28(6):2135–2141.

55. Berlana D, Barraquer A, Sabin P, et al. Impact of parenteral nutrition standardization on costs and quality in adult patients. Nutr Hosp. 2014;30(2):351–358.

56. Driscoll DF. Compounding TPN admixtures: then and now. JPEN J Parenter Enteral Nutr. 2003;27(6):433–8.

57. Beattie C, Allard J, Raman M. Comparison between premixed and compounded parenteral nutrition solutions in hospitalized patients requiring parenteral nutrition. Nutr Clin Pract. 2016;31(2):229–234.

58. Baras Z, Theilla M, Singer P. From compound to "ready to use" parenteral nutrition bags use in a tertiary

medical center: An observational study. Clin. Nutr. 2019;38:S270–S271.

59. Yu J, Wu G, Tang Y, et al. Efficacy, safety, and preparation of standardized parenteral nutrition regimens: three-chamber bags vs compounded monobags-a prospective, multicenter, randomized, single-blind clinical trial. Nutr Clin Pract. 2017;32(4):545–551

60. Gupta N, Hocevar SN, Moulton-Meissner HA, et al. Outbreak of Serratia marcescens bloodstream infections in patients receiving parenteral nutrition prepared by a compounding pharmacy. Clin Infect Dis. 2014;59(1):1–8.

61. Stout MS, Cober MP. Cyclic parenteral nutrition infusion: considerations for the clinician. Practical gastroenterology series #97. Published 2011.

62. Gonzaleza KW, Weaver KL, Biondo DJ, et al. Cycling parenteral nutrition in a neonatal surgical patient: An argument for increased utilization. Journal of Pediatric Surgery Case Reports 2017;16:C1–4.

63. Gabe SM, Culkin A. Abnormal liver function tests in the parenteral nutrition fed patient. Frontline Gastroenterol. 2010;1(2):98–104.

64. Arenas Villafranca JJ, Nieto Guindo M, Álvaro Sanz E, et al. Effects of cyclic parenteral nutrition on parenteral-associated liver dysfunction parameters. Nutr J. 2017;16(1):66.

65. Stout SM, Cober MP. Metabolic effects of cyclic parenteral nutrition infusion in adults and children. Nutr Clin Pract. 2010;25(3):277–281.

66. Mehanna H, Nankivell PC, Moledina J, et al. Refeeding syndrome--awareness, prevention and management. Head Neck Oncol. 2009;1:4.

67. American Diabetes Association. 15. Diabetes Care in the Hospital: Standards of Medical Care in Diabetes-2019. Diabetes Care. 2019;42(1):S173–S181.

68. Ozakin E, Can R, Acar N, et al. An evaluation of complications in ultrasound-guided central venous catheter insertion in the emergency department. Turk J Emerg Med. 2016;14(2):53–58.

69. Roldan CJ, Paniagua L. Central venous catheter intravascular malpositioning: causes, prevention, diagnosis, and correction. West J Emerg Med. 2015;16(5):658–664.

70. Wall C, Moore J, Thachil J. Catheter-related thrombosis: A practical approach. J Intensive Care Soc. 2016;17(2):160–167.

71. Kakkos SK, Gohel M, Baekgaard N, et al. Editor's Choice – European Society for Vascular Surgery (ESVS) 2021 Clinical practice guidelines on the management of venous thrombosis. Eur J Vasc Endovasc Surg 2021;61(1):9–82.

72. O'Grady NP, Alexander M, Burns LA, et al. Guidelines for the prevention of intravascular catheter-related infections. Clin Infect Dis. 2011;52(9):162–193.

73. Mermel LA, Allon M, Bouza E, et al. Clinical practice guidelines for the diagnosis and management of intravascular catheter-related infection: 2009 Update by the Infectious Diseases Society of America [published correction appears in Clin Infect Dis. 2010;50(7):1079.

74. Peterson LR, Smith BA. Nonutility of catheter tip cultures for the diagnosis of central line-associated bloodstream infection. Clin Infect Dis 2015;60(3):492–3.

75. Bloodstream Infection Event (Central Line-Associated Bloodstream Infection and Non-central Line Associated Bloodstream Infection). National Healthcare Safety Network 2021.

76. Böll B, Schalk E, Buchheidt D, et al. Central venous catheter-related infections in hematology and oncology: 2020 updated guidelines on diagnosis, management, and prevention by the Infectious Diseases Working Party (AGIHO) of the German Society of Hematology and Medical Oncology (DGHO). Ann Hematol. 2021;100(1):239–259.

77. Olveira G, Tapia MJ, Ocón J, et al. Study Group of Hyperglycemia in Parenteral Nutrition: Nutrition Area of the Spanish Society of Endocrinology and Nutrition (SEEN). Parenteral nutrition-associated hyperglycemia in non-critically ill inpatients increases the risk of in-hospital mortality (multicenter study). Diabetes Care. 2013;36(5):1061–6.

78. Elizabeth PC, Ramón PR, Alberto MM. Hyperglycemia associated with parenteral nutrition in noncritical patients. Human Nutrition & Metabolism. 2020;22:200114.

79. Pasquel FJ, Spiegelman R, McCauley M, et al. Hyperglycemia during total parenteral nutrition: an important marker of poor outcome and mortality in hospitalized patients. Diabetes Care 2010;33(4):739–41.

80. Alchaer M, Khasawneh R, Heuberger R, et al. Prevalence and risk factors of total parenteral nutrition induced hyperglycemia at a single institution: retrospective study. Metab Syndr Relat Disord. 2020;18(5):267–273.

81. Sangrador Pelluz C, Pardo Pastor J, Navas Moya E, et al. Predictive factors of hyperglycaemia in patients with parenteral nutrition. Med Clin (Barc). 2020;154(5):157–162.

82. McMahon MM, Nystrom E, Braunschweig C, et al. American Society for Parenteral and Enteral Nutrition (A.S.P.E.N.) Board of Directors; American Society for Parenteral and Enteral Nutrition. A.S.P.E.N. clinical guidelines: nutrition support of adults with hyperglycemia. JPEN J Parenter Enteral Nutr. 2013;37(1):23–36.

83. Yatabe T, Inoue S, Sakaguchi M, et al. The optimal target for acute glycemic control in critically ill patients: a network meta-analysis. Intensive Care Med. 2017;43(1):16–28.

84. Rhodes A, Evans LE, Alhazzani W, et al. Surviving Sepsis Campaign: International guidelines for management of sepsis and septic shock 2016. Intensive Care Med. 2017;43(3):304–77.

85. American Diabetes Association. 15. Diabetes care in the hospital: Standards of Medical Care in Diabetesd2020. Diabetes Care 2020;43(Suppl. 1):S193–S202.

86. Schönenberger KA, Aberer F, Papazafiropoulou AK. Management of Hyperglycemia in Hospitalized Patients Receiving Parenteral Nutrition. Front. Clin. Diabetes Healthc. 2022;3:829412.

87. Olveira G, Abuín J, López R, et al. Regular insulin added to total parenteral nutrition vs subcutaneous glargine in non-critically ill diabetic inpatients, a multicenter randomized clinical trial: INSUPAR trial. Clin Nutr. 2020;39(2):388–394.

88. Kinnare KF, Bacon CA, Chen Y, et al. Risk factors for predicting hypoglycemia in patients receiving concomitant parenteral nutrition and insulin therapy. J Acad Nutr Diet. 2013;113(2):263–8.

89. Olveira G, Tapia MJ, Ocón J, et al. Hypoglycemia in noncritically ill patients receiving total parenteral nutrition: a multicenter study. (Study group on the problem of hyperglycemia in parenteral nutrition; Nutrition area of the Spanish Society of Endocrinology and Nutrition). Nutrition. 2015;31(1):58–63.

90. Nutrition support for adults: oral nutrition support, enteral tube feeding and parenteral nutrition Clinical guideline [CG32] 2006. Last updated: 04 August 2017. Available from: https://www.nice.org.uk/guidance/cg32.

91. da Silva JSV, Seres DS, Sabino K, et al. Parenteral nutrition safety and clinical practice committees, american society for parenteral and enteral nutrition. ASPEN consensus recommendations for refeeding syndrome. Nutr Clin Pract. 2020;35(2):178–195.

92. Ponzo V, Pellegrini M, Cioffi I, et al. The Refeeding Syndrome: a neglected but potentially serious condition for inpatients. A narrative review. Intern Emerg Med. 2021;16(1):49–60.

93. Mehanna HM, Moledina J, Travis J. Refeeding syndrome: what it is, and how to prevent and treat it. BMJ. 2008;336(7659):1495–8.

94. Friedli N, Stanga Z, Culkin A, et al. Management and prevention of refeeding syndrome in medical inpatients: an evidence-based and consensus-supported algorithm. Nutrition 2018;47:13–20.

95. Singer P, Blaser AR, Berger MM, et al. ESPEN guideline on clinical nutrition in the intensive care unit. Clin Nutr. 2019;38(1):48–79.

96. Lakananurak N, Tienchai K. Incidence and risk factors of parenteral nutrition-associated liver disease in hospitalized adults: A prospective cohort study. Clin Nutr ESPEN. 2019;34:81–86.

97. Fousekis FS, Mitselos IV, Christodoulou DK. New insights into intestinal failure–associated liver disease in adults: A comprehensive review of the literature. Saudi J Gastroenterol 2021;27(1):3–12.

98. Kumpf VJ. Parenteral nutrition-associated liver disease in adult and pediatric patients. Nutr Clin Pract. 2006;21(3):279–290.

99. Nowak K. Parenteral nutrition-associated liver disease. Clin Liver Dis (Hoboken). 2020;15(2):59–62.

100. Mitra A, Ahn J. Liver disease in patients on total parenteral nutrition. Clin Liver Dis. 2017;21(4):687–695.

101. Khalaf RT, Sokol RJ. New Insights into Intestinal Failure–Associated Liver Disease in Children. Hepatology. 2020;71(4):1486–1498.

102. Guthrie G, Burrin D. Impact of Parenteral lipid emulsion components on cholestatic liver disease in neonates. Nutrients. 2021;13(2):508.

103. Bischoff SC, Bernal W, Dasarathy S, et al. ESPEN practical guideline: Clinical nutrition in liver disease. Clin Nutr. 2020;39(12):3533–3562.

104. Lacaille F, Gupte G, Colomb V, et al. Intestinal failure-associated liver disease: A position paper of the ESPGHAN Working Group of Intestinal Failure and Intestinal Transplantation. J Pediatr Gastroenterol Nutr 2015;60(2):272–83.

105. Rochling FA. Intravenous Lipid emulsions in the prevention and treatment of liver disease in intestinal failure. Nutrients. 2021;13(3):895.

106. Mirtallo J, Canada T, Johnson D, et al. Safe practices for parenteral nutrition. J Parenter Enteral Nutr 2004;28(6):S39–S70.

107. Wales PW, Allen N, Worthington P, et al. A.S.P.E.N. clinical guidelines: support of pediatric patients with intestinal failure at risk of parenteral nutrition-associated liver disease. J Parenter Enteral Nutr 2014;38(5):538–557.

108. Pironi L, Colecchia A, Guidetti M, et al. Fish oil-based emulsion for the treatment of parenteral nutrition associated liver disease in an adult patient. European e-J Clin Nutr Metabol 2010;5(5):e243–e246.

109. Yan JH, Guan BJ, Gao HY, et al. Omega-3 polyunsaturated fatty acid supplementation and non-alcoholic fatty liver disease: A meta-analysis of randomized controlled trials. Medicine 2018;97(37):e12271.

110. Lal S, Pironi L, Wanten G, et al. Clinical approach to the management of Intestinal Failure Associated Liver Disease (IFALD) in adults: A position paper from the Home Artificial Nutrition and Chronic Intestinal Failure Special Interest Group of ESPEN. Clin Nutr 2018;37(6 Pt A):1794–7.

111. Hwang T, Lue M, Chen L. Early use of cyclic TPN prevents further deterioration if liver functions for the TPN patient with impaired liver function. Hepatogastroenterology 2004;47(35):1347–50.

Index

Abbreviations

ABG	Arterial blood gas		CT Scan	Computerized tomography scan
ADH	Antidiuretic hormone		CVC	Central venous catheter
ADHF	Acute decompensated heart failure		CVP	Central venous pressure
AG	Anion gap		CVVH	Continuous veno venous haemofiltration
AKI	Acute kidney injury		D5W	Dextrose 5%
ANP	Atrial natriuretic peptide		D5NS	Dextrose saline
AP	Acute pancreatitis		DBP	Diastolic blood pressure
ARBs	Angiotensin receptor blockers		DCR	Damage control resuscitation
ARDS	Acute respiratory distress syndrome		DDAVP	Desmopressin
ATN	Acute tubular necrosis		DF	Disease factor
BBB	Blood-brain barrier		DI	Diabetes insipidus
BCAAs	Branched chain amino acids		DKA	Diabetic ketoacidosis
BLS	B-lines score		DM	Diabetes mellitus
BP	Blood pressure		DPG	2-3 Diphosphoglycerate
BUN	Blood urea Nitriogen		ECF	Extracellular fluid
CAD	Coronary artery disease		ECG	Electrocardiogram
CaSR	Calcium sensing receptor		EEO	End-expiratory occlusion
CBC	Complete blood count		EFA	Essential fatty acid
CCB	Calcium channel blocker		EFSA	European food safety authority
CD	Crohn's disease		EN	Enteral nutrition
CHF	Congestive heart failure		ERCP	Endoscopic retrograde cholangiopancreatography
CKD	Chronic kidney disease		ESAs	Erythropoiesis-stimulating agents
CNIs	Calcineurin inhibitors		ESR	Erythrocyte sedimentation rate
CNS	Central nervous system		ESRD	End stage renal disease
CO	Cardiac output		FA	Fatty acid
COPD	Chronic obstructive pulmonary disease		FFA	Free fatty acid
CPK	Creatine phosphokinase		FFP	Fresh frozen plasma
CPN	Central parentral nutrition		GBS	Glasgow blatchford score
CRBSI	Catheter-related bloodstream infection		GDT	Goal-directed therapy
CRRT	Continuous renal replacement therapy		GFR	Glomerular filtration rate
CSW	Cerebral salt wasting			

GI	Gastrointestinal		NPO	Nil per os (nothing by mouth)
HAS	Human albumin solution		NS	Normal saline 0.9% NaCl
HE	Hepatic encephalopathy		NSAIDs	Non-steroidal anti-inflammatory drugs
HES	Hydroxyethyl starch		ORS	Oral rehydration solution
HHNK	Hyperosmotic hyperglycemic nonketotic state		ORT	Oral rehydration therapy
HHS	Hyperosmolar hyperglycemic state		PAC	Pulmonary artery catheter
HRS	Hepatorenal syndrome		PAOP	Pulmonary artery occlusion pressure
IABP	Intra-aortic balloon pump		PAWP	Pulmonary artery wedge pressure
IBD	Inflammatory bowel disease		PCC	Prothrombin complex concentrate
ICF	Intracellular fluid		PCWP	Pulmonary capillary wedge pressure
ICP	Intracranial pressure		PE	Preeclampsia
ICU	Intensive care unit		PEEP	Positive end-expiratory pressure
IDDM	Insulin dependent diabetes mellitus		PICC	Percutaneous inserted central catheter
IHD	Ischemic heart disease		PN	Parenteral nutrition
ILE	Lipid injectable emulsion		PNALD	Parenteral nutrition-associated liver disease
IM	Intramuscular		PPH	Postpartum hemorrhage
ITP	Intrathoracic pressure		PPI	Proton pump inhibitor
IV	Intravenous		PPN	Peripheral parenteral nutrition
IVC	Inferior vena cava		PPV	Pulse pressure variation
JVP	Jugular venous pressure		PRBCs	Packed red blood cells
KCI	Potassium chloride		PTH	Parathyroid hormone
kg	Kilogram		PVI	Plethysmographic variability index
LCT	Long chain triglycerides		RAASi	Renin-angiotensin-aldosterone system inhibitor
LFT	Liver function test		RAS	Reninangiotensin system
LUS	Lung ultrasound		RBC	Red blood cells
LV	Left ventricle		RCA	Regional citrate anticoagulation
LVEDP	Left ventricular end-diastolic pressure		REE	Resting energy expenditure
LVP	Large volume paracentesis		RFT	Renal function test
MAP	Mean arterial pressure		RL	Ringer's lactate
MCT	Medium-chain triglyceride		RQ	Respiratory quotient
mEq/L	Millie equivalents per liter		RRT	Renal replacement therapy
MRI	Magnetic resonance imaging		RTA	Renal tubular acidosis
MS	Molar substitution		SAM	Severe acute malnutrition
MUFA	Monounsaturated fatty acid		SBP	Systolic blood pressure
MW	Molecular weight		SBS	Short bowel syndrome
NG	Nasogastric tube		SIADH	Syndrome of inappropriate antidiuretic hormone secretion
NIV	Noninvasive ventilation			
NO	Nitric oxide		SID	Strong ion difference

SLED	Sustained low-efficiency dialysis	TG	Triglyceride
SLKT	Simultaneous liver-kidney transplantation	TIPS	Transjugular intrahepatic portosystemic shunt
SPS	Sodium polystyrene sulfonate	TPE	Therapeutic plasma exchange
SVC	Superior vena cava	TPN	Total parenteral nutrition
SVV	Stroke volume variation	TRALI	Transfusion-related acute lung injury
SZC	Sodium zirconium cyclosilicate	TTE	Transthoracic echocardiography
TBI	Traumatic brain injury	TTKG	Transtubular potassium gradient
TBSA	Total body surface area	TURP	Trans urethral resection of prostate
TBW	Total body water	UAG	Urinary anion gap
TCA	Tricyclic antidepressant	UC	Ulcerative colitis
TEB	Thoracic electrical bioimpedance	V/Q	Ventilation-perfusion
TEE	Total energy expenditure	VTI	Velocity-time integral
TF	Thermal factor		

Made in United States
Orlando, FL
12 June 2024

47790130R00422